D1265863

DREXEL UNIVERSITY
HEALTH SCIENCES LIBRARIES
HAHNEMANN LIBRARY

Principles and Practice of Geriatric Psychiatry

■ **MARC E. AGRONIN, M.D.**

Director of Mental Health Services
Miami Jewish Home and Hospital for the Aged
Assistant Professor of Psychiatry
Miller School of Medicine at the University of Miami.
Miami, Florida

■ **GABE J. MALETTA, Ph.D., M.D.**

Clinical Professor
Department of Psychiatry
Department of Family Practice/Community Health
University of Minnesota Medical School
Consultant in Geriatric Psychiatry
Mental Health Patient Service Line
VA Medical Center
Minneapolis, Minnesota
Consultant in Geriatric Psychiatry
Department of Medicine
Bethesda Rehabilitation Hospital
St. Paul, Minnesota

LIPPINCOTT WILLIAMS & WILKINS
A **Wolters Kluwer** Company

Philadelphia • Baltimore • New York • London
Buenos Aires • Hong Kong • Sydney • Tokyo

Acquisitions Editor: Charles W. Mitchell
Managing Editor: Lisa Kairis
Production Project Manager: Bridgett Dougherty
Senior Manufacturing Manager: Benjamin Rivera
Associate Director of Marketing: Adam Glazer
Design Coordinator: Holly McLaughlin
Production Services: Techbooks
Printer: Quebecor World

WT
150
P9575
2006

© 2006 by LIPPINCOTT WILLIAMS & WILKINS

530 Walnut Street
Philadelphia, PA 19106 USA
LWW.com

All rights reserved. This book is protected by copyright. No part of this book may be reproduced in any form or by any means, including photocopying, or utilized by any information storage and retrieval system without written permission from the copyright owner, except for brief quotations embodied in critical articles and reviews. Materials appearing in this book prepared by individuals as part of their official duties as U.S. government employees are not covered by the above-mentioned copyright.

Printed in the USA

Library of Congress Cataloging-in-Publication Data
Principles and practice of geriatric psychiatry / [edited by] Marc E.
    Agronin, Gabe J. Maletta.
        p. ; cm.
    Includes bibliographical references and index.
    ISBN 0-7817-4810-0 (alk. paper)
    1. Geriatric psychiatry.   I. Agronin, Marc E.   II. Maletta, Gabe J.
    [DNLM: 1. Geriatric Psychiatry—methods. 2. Mental Disorders—
    diagnosis—Aged.   3. Mental Disorders—therapy—Aged.   4. Psycho-
    therapy—methods—Aged.   WT 150 P9575 2006]
    RC451.4.A5P725 2006
    618.97'689—dc22

                                          2005020861

Care has been taken to confirm the accuracy of the information presented and to describe generally accepted practices. However, the authors, editors, and publisher are not responsible for errors or omissions or for any consequences from application of the information in this book and make no warranty, expressed or implied, with respect to the currency, completeness, or accuracy of the contents of the publication. Application of this information in a particular situation remains the professional responsibility of the practitioner.

The authors, editors, and publisher have exerted every effort to ensure that drug selection and dosage set forth in this text are in accordance with current recommendations and practice at the time of publication. However, in view of ongoing research, changes in government regulations, and the constant flow of information relating to drug therapy and drug reactions, the reader is urged to check the package insert for each drug for any change in indications and dosage and for added warnings and precautions. This is particularly important when the recommended agent is a new or infrequently employed drug.

Some drugs and medical devices presented in this publication have Food and Drug Administration (FDA) clearance for limited use in restricted research settings. It is the responsibility of the health care provider to ascertain the FDA status of each drug or device planned for use in their clinical practice.

To purchase additional copies of this book, call our customer service department at (800) 639 -3030 or fax orders to (301) 824-7390. International customers should call (301) 714-2324.

Visit Lippincott Williams & Wilkins on the Internet: at LWW.com. Lippincott Williams & Wilkins customer service representatives are available from 8:30 am to 6pm, EST.

10 9 8 7 6 5 4 3 2 1

Dr. Marc Agronin:
Dedicated to
My wife Robin
My three sons Jacob, Max, and Sam
And my parents Ronald and Belle Agronin,
for the constant wellspring of love and support

Dr. Gabe Maletta:
For Barbara Zink Maletta
Advisor, Critic, Confidante, Soul mate
Dedicated with love and gratitude

Contents

Contributors

MARC E. AGRONIN, M.D. Director of Mental Health Services, Miami Jewish Home and Hospital for the Aged, Assistant Professor of Psychiatry, Miller School of Medicine at the University of Miami, Miami, Florida

STUART A. ANFANG, M.D. Assistant Professor of Psychiatry, University of Massachusetts Medical School, Western Massachusetts Area Medical Director, Massachusetts Department of Mental Health, Worcester, Massachusetts

FRANCESCA CANNAVO ANTOGNINI, Ph.D. Director, Psychotherapy and Geropsychology Training, Geriatric Service, McLean Hospital Clinical Instructor in Psychiatry, Department of Psychology, Harvard Medical School, Belmont, Massachusetts

PAUL S. APPELBAUM, M.D. A. F. Zeleznik Distinguished Professor and Chairman of Psychiatry, Director, Law and Psychiatry Program, University of Massachusetts Medical School, Worcester, Massachusetts

PATRICIA A. AREÁN, Ph.D. Associate Professor, Department of Psychiatry, University of California, San Fransisco, San Francisco, California

DEBORAH K. ATTIX, Ph.D. Assistant Clinical Professor, Department of Psychiatry, Division of Medical Psychology, Department of Medicine, Division of Neurology, Duke University Medical Center, Durham, North Carolina

PAMELA M. BASEHORE, M.P.H. Assistant Director of Education, New Jersey Institute for Successful Aging, University of Medicine & Dentistry of New Jersey, School of Osteopathic Medicine, Stratford, New Jersey

ASHOK J. BHARUCHA, M.D. Assistant Professor, Department of Psychiatry, University of Pittsburgh School of Medicine, Pittsburgh, Pennsylvania

DAN G. BLAZER, M.D., Ph.D. JP Gibbons Professor, Department of Psychiatry and Behavioral Sciences, Duke University Medical Center, Durham, North Carolina

DONALD L. BLIWISE, Ph.D. Professor of Neurology, Emory University School of Medicine, Director, Program in Sleep, Aging and Chronobiology, Wesley Woods Geriatric Hospital, Atlanta, Georgia

JASON BORENSTEIN, Ph.D. Visiting Assistant Professor, School of Public Policy, Georgia Tech, Editor, Journal of Philosophy, Science, & Law, Atlanta, Georgia

SOO BORSON, M.D. Professor, Department of Psychiatry and Behavioral Sciences, Director, Geriatric and Family Services Clinic and the Alzheimer's Disease Research Center Satellite, University of Washington, Seattle, Washington

LISA L. BOYLE, M.D. Geriatric Psychiatry and Interdisciplinary Geriatrics Fellow, Program in Geriatrics and Neuropsychiatry, Department of Psychiatry, University of Rochester Medical Center, Rochester, New York

ALISTAIR BURNS, M.B.Ch.B., F.R.C.P., F.R.C.Psych, M.D., M.Phil, D.H.M.S.A. Professor, Division of Psychiatry, University of Manchester, Professor of Old Age Psychiatry, Department of Psychiatry, Wythenshawe Hospital, Honorary Consultant Old Age Psychiatrist, Manchester Mental Health and Social Care Trust, Wythenshawe Hospital, Manchester, United Kingdon

ROBERT N. BUTLER, M.D. President and CEO, International Longevity Center, Professor of Geriatrics, Mount Sinai School of Medicine, New York, New York

SALLY CALAHAN Educator, Massasoit Community College, Brockton, Massachusetts, Chair, Patient and Family Services Committee, Alzheimer's Association of Cape Cod and the Islands, Cape Cod, Massachusetts

DANIEL CARLAT, M.D. Editor-in-chief, The Carlat Report on Psychiatric Treatment, Newburyport, Massachusetts

ANITA CHOPRA, M.D., F.A.C.P., A.G.S.F., C.M.D. Deputy Director, New Jersey Institute for Successful Aging, Professor of Medicine, University of Medicine and Dentistry of New Jersey, School of Osteopathic Medicine, Stratford, New Jersey

HELENA C. CHUI, M.D. McCarron Professor and Chair, Department of Neurology, University of Southern California School of Medicine, Los Angeles, California

GENE. D. COHEN, M.D., Ph.D. Director, Center on Aging, Health & Humanities, Professor of Health Care Sciences and Professor of Psychiatry and Behavioral Sciences, George Washington University, Washington, District of Columbia

ELIZABETH COLLUMB, M.D. Clinical Instructor of Psychiatry, University of California, San Diego

YEATES CONWELL, M.D. Center for the Study and Prevention of Suicide, Department of Psychiatry, University of Rochester School of Medicine and Dentistry, Rochester, New York

COLIN A. DEPP, Ph.D. Geriatric Psychiatry Research Center, Department of Psychiatry, University of California, San Diego School of Medicine, La Jolla, California

ISABELLE DESJARDINS, M.D. Assistant Professor of Psychiatry, University of Vermont College of Medicine, Medical Director of Inpatient Psychiatry, Fletcher Allen Health Care, Burlington, Vermont

PAUL R. DUBERSTEIN, Ph.D. Professor, Department of Psychiatry, University of Rochester School of Medicine, Clinical Psychologist, Department of Psychiatry, University of Rochester Medical Center, Rochester, New York

YOHANNES ENDESHAW, M.D., M.P.H., F.A.C.P. Assistant Professor of Medicine, Division of Geriatrics and Gerontology, Emory University School of Medicine, Wesley Woods Geriatric Hospital, Atlanta, Georgia

SHANE A. FISHCO, Pharm.D. Oncology Pharmacist, James A. Haley Veterans Hospital, Tampa, Florida

KEVIN C. FLEMING M.D. General Internal Medicine, Mayo Clinic, Rochester, Minnesota

BRENT FORESTER, M.D. Instructor in Psychiatry, Harvard Medical School, Boston, Massachusetts, Medical Director Special Care Dementia Unit, Director, Mood Disorders Division, Geriatric Psychiatry Research Program, McLean Hospital, Belmont, Massachusetts

DOLORES GALLAGHER-THOMPSON, Ph.D. Professor of Research, Department of Psychiatry and Behavioral Sciences, Stanford University School of Medicine, Stanford, California, Director, Older Adult and Family Center, VA Medical Center, Menlo Park, California

YONAS ENDALE GEDA, M.D. Alzheimer's Disease Research Center, Mayo Clinic College of Medicine, Rochester, Minnesota

KENNETH W. GOODMAN, Ph.D. Director, Bioethics Program, Associate Professor of Medicine and Philosophy, University of Miami, Miami, Florida

SHELLY L. GRAY, Pharm.D., M.S., B.C.P.S. Associate Professor and Director, Geriatric Pharmacy Program, School of Pharmacy, University of Washington, Seattle, Washington

ROBERT M. GREENBERG, M.D. Associate Clinical Professor, Department of Psychiatry, University of Medicine & Dentistry of New Jersey, School of Medicine, Stratford, New Jersey, Medical Director, Geriatric Psychiatry and ECT Services, St. Mary's Hospital, Hoboken, New Jersey

AMBER GUM, Ph.D. Assistant Professor, Department of Aging and Mental Health, Florida Mental Health Institute, University of South Florida, Tampa, Florida

JOSEPH T. HANLON, Pharm.D., M.S., B.C.P.S., F.A.S.C.P., F.A.S.H.P., F.G.S.A., Professor, Department of Medicine, Division of Geriatrics, University of Pittsburgh School of Medicine, Research Scientist, Center for Health Equity Research and Promotion, VA Pittsburgh Healthcare System, Pittsburgh, Pennsylvania

ANSAR M. HAROUN, M.D. Clinical Professor of Psychiatry and Pediatrics, Departments of Psychiatry and Pediatrics, University of California, San Diego, Adjunct Professor of Law, Department of Law, University of San Diego, La Jolla, California, Supervising Psychiatrist, Forensic Psychiatry Clinic, San Diego Superior Court, San Diego County Courthouse, San Diego, California

MARNIN J. HEISEL, Ph.D. Senior Instructor of Psychiatry (Psychology), Department of Psychiatry, University of Rochester School of Medicine and Dentistry, Rochester, New York

MONIKA HELLWIG President, Association of Catholic Colleges & Universities, Washington, District of Columbia

REV. THEODORE M. HESBURGH, C.S.C. President Emeritus, University of Notre Dame, Notre Dame, Indiana

JOHN P. HIRDES, Ph.D. Professor, Department of Health Studies and Gerontology, University of Waterloo, Waterloo, Ontario, Scientific Director, Homewood Research Institute, Homewood Health Centre, Guelph, Ontario, Canada

STACY HORN, D.O. Clinical Assistant Professor, Department of Neurological Sciences, University of Pennsylvania, Philadelphia, Pennsylvania

M. SALEEM ISMAIL, M.D. Assistant Professor of Psychiatry, Department of Psychiatry, University of Rochester, Director, Psychiatric Consultation Service, Monroe Community Hospital, Rochester, New York

MATTHEW P. JANICKI, Ph.D. Research Professor, Department of Disability and Human Development, University of Illinois at Chicago, Chicago, Illinois

LISSY JARVIK, M.D., Ph.D. Professor Emeritus, Department of Psychiatry and Biobehavioral Sciences, University of California, Los Angeles, Distinguished Physician Emeritus, U.S. Department of Veterans Affairs, Los Angeles, California

DILIP V. JESTE, M.D. Professor, Department of Psychiatry, University of California, San Diego, La Jolla, California,

Staff Physician, Department of Psychiatry Service, VA San Diego Healthcare System, San Diego, California

SALMAN KARIM, M.B.B.S. Clinical Lecturer in Old Age Psychiatry, University of Manchester School of Psychiatry and Behavioural Sciences, Wythenshawe Hospital, Wythenshawe, Manchester

JORDAN F. KARP, M.D. John A. Hartford Physician-Investigator Fellow, Center for Excellence in Geriatric Psychiatry, Department of Psychiatry, University of Pittsburgh School of Medicine, Western Psychiatric Institute and Clinic, Pittsburgh, Pennsylvania

CHARLES H. KELLNER, M.D. Professor and Chair, Department of Psychiatry, University of Medicine & Dentistry of New Jersey, School of Medicine, Stratford, New Jersey

KACIE KELLY, M.H.S. Project Coordinator, National Center for PTSD, VA Boston Healthcare System, Boston, Massachussets

ANDREW KERTESZ, M.D., F.R.C.P.C. Professor, Department of Clinical Neurological Sciences, University of Western Ontario, Director, Cognitive Neurology, Department of Clinical Neurological Sciences, St. Joseph's Hospital, London, Ontario, Canada

DAVID KNOPMAN, M.D. Professor and Consultant of Neurology, Department of Neurology, Mayo Clinic, Rochester, Minnesota

ELISABETH KOSS, Ph.D. Assistant Director, Alzheimer's Disease Centers Program, Neuroscience and Neuropsychology of Aging Program, National Institute on Aging, Bethesda, Maryland

MICHAEL KOTLYAR, Pharm.D. Assistant Professor, Department of Experimental and Clinical Pharmacology, University of Minnesota College of Pharmacy, Minneapolis, Minnesota

MELINDA LANTZ, M.D. Associate Professor, Department of Geriatrics, Mount Sinai School of Medicine, Director of Psychiatry, The Jewish Home & Hospital, New York, New York

MARIA I. LAPID, M.D. Assistant Professor of Psychiatry, Department of Psychiatry and Psychology, Mayo Clinic College of Medicine, Geriatric Psychiatrist, Department of Psychiatry and Psychology, Mayo Clinic, Rochester, Minnesota

SEAN A. LAUDERDALE, Ph.D. Assistant Professor, Department of Psychology and Counseling, Pittsburg State University, Pittsburg, Kansas

HELEN LAVRETSKY, M.D., M.S. Associate Professor, Department of Psychiatry and Behavioral Sciences, University of California, Los Angeles, Los Angeles, California

TSAO-WEI LIANG, M.D. Assistant Professor, Department of Neurology, Jefferson Hospital for Neurosciences, Philadelphia, Pennsylvania,

JANET M. LIETO, D.O., C.M.D. Assistant Professor of Family Medicine, New Jersey Institute for Successful Aging, University of Medicine and Dentistry of New Jersey, School of Osteopathic Medicine, Stratford, New Jersey

CATHERINE I. LINDBLAD, Pharm.D. Assistant Clinical Specialist and Assistant Professor, Department of Experimental and Clinical Pharmacology, University of Minnesota College of Pharmacy, Clinical Pharmacist Specialist in Geriatrics, Department of Pharmacy, Minneapolis VA Medical Center, Minneapolis, Minnesota

MARIA D. LLORENTE, M.D. Professor, Department of Psychiatry and Behavioral Sciences, Miller School of Medicine at the University of Miami, Chief of Psychiatry Service, Department of Mental Health and Behavioral Sciences, Miami VA Medical Center, Miami, Florida

GABE J. MALETTA, M.A., Ph.D., M.D., D.F.A.P.A. Clinical Professor, Departments of Psychiatry and Family Practice/Community Health, University of Minnesota School of Medicine, Consultant in Geriatric Psychiatry and Psychopharmacology, VA Medical Center, Minneapolis, Minnesota, Private Practice, Edina, Minnesota

JULIE MALPHURS, Ph.D. Assistant Professor, Miller School of Medicine at the University of Miami, Department of Psychiatry & Behavioral Science, Investigator, Miami VA Medical Center, Mental Health & Behavioral Science Service Miami, Florida

CHITRA MALUR, M.D. Staff Psychiatrist, Department of Psychiatry, The Zucker Hillside Hospital, Glen Oaks, New York

ELLIOTT L. MANCALL, M.D. Professor, Department of Neurology, Jefferson Medical College, Attending Neurologist, Department of Neurology, Thomas Jefferson University Hospital, Philadelphia, Pennsylvania

RICHARD MARGOLIN, M.D. Visiting Professor of Clinical Psychiatry, Director, Division of Consultation-Liaison Psychiatry, Department of Psychiatry, Keck University of Southern California School of Medicine, Los Angeles, California

KIMBERLY M. MATTOX, Pharm.D. Clinical Pharmacy Specialist, Department of Geriatrics, James A. Haley Veterans Hospital, Tampa, Florida

JOCELYN SHEALY MCGEE, M.S.G., Ph.D. Aging Treatment Studies Program, VA Palo Alto Healthcare System, Menlo Park, California

IAN G. MCKEITH, M.D., F.R.C.Psych., F.Med.Sci. Professor of Old Age Psychiatry, Institute for Ageing and Health, University of Newcastle-upon-Tyne, Newcastle General Hospital, United Kingdom

DAVID J. MEAGHER, M.D., M.R.C.Psych., MSc (Neuroscience) Consultant Psychiatrist and Clinical Research Tutor, Department of Adult Psychiatry, Midwestern Regional Hospital, Dooradoyle, Limerick, Ireland

DAVID NAIMARK, M.D. Associate Clinical Professor, Department of Psychiatry, University of California, San Diego, La Jolla, California, Forensic Psychiatrist, Forensic Psychiatry Clinic, San Diego County Courthouse, San Diego, California

SELAMAWIT NEGASH, Ph.D. Postdoctoral Fellow, Alzheimer's Disease Research Center, Mayo Clinic, Rochester, Minnesota

JOHN W. NORTON, M.D. Associate Professor of Psychiatry and Human Behavior, Associate Professor of Neurology, University of Mississippi School of Medicine, Medical Director, Medical Psychiatry Inpatient Unit, University of Mississippi Medical Center, Jackson, Mississippi

WILLIAM B. ORR, Ph.D., M.D. Assistant Professor of Psychiatry, Department of Psychiatry, University of Minnesota School of Medicine, Geriatric Psychiatrist, Psychiatry Service, Minneapolis VA Medical Center, Minneapolis, Minnesota

DAVID W. OSLIN, M.D. Associate Professor, Department of Psychiatry, University of Pennsylvania, Associate Professor, Department of Behavioral Health, Philadelphia VA Medical Center, Philadelphia, Pennsylvania

RONALD C. PETERSEN, Ph.D., M.D. Cora Kanow Professor of Alzheimer's Disease Research, Department of Neurology, Mayo Clinic College of Medicine, Director, Alzheimer's Disease Research Center, Mayo Clinic College of Medicine, Rochester, Minnesota

BRUCE G. POLLOCK, M.D., Ph.D., F.R.C.P.(C) Sandra A. Rotman Chair in Neuropsychiatry and Head, Division of Geriatric Psychiatry, Department of Psychiatry, University of Toronto, The Rotman Research Institute, Baycrest Centre for Geriatric Care and Centre for Addiction and Mental Health, Toronto, Ontario, Canada

ANTON P. PORSTEINSSON, M.D. Associate Professor of Psychiatry, University of Rochester School of Medicine, Rochester, New York

ROBERT B. PORTNEY, M.D. Clinical Instructor, Harvard Medical School, Geriatric Neuropsychiatrist and Supervising Physician, Massachusetts General Hospital/McLean Hospital Training Programs, Boston, Massachusetts

TERRY RABINOWITZ, M.D., F.A.P.A., F.A.P.M. Associate Professor of Psychiatry and of Family Medicine, University of Vermont College of Medicine, Director, Psychiatric Consultation Service and Clinical Director of Telemedicine, Fletcher Allen Health Care, Burlington, Vermont

BARRY ROVNER, M.D. Professor, Departments of Psychiatry and Neurology, Thomas Jefferson University, Jefferson Hospital for Neuroscience, Philadelphia, Pennsylvania

TERESA A. RUMMANS, M.D. Professor of Psychiatry, Department of Psychiatry and Psychology, Mayo Clinic, Rochester, Minnesota

NATALIE SACHS-ERICSSON, Ph.D. Research Associate in Clinical Psychology, Department of Psychology, Florida State University, Tallahassee, Florida

KENNETH SAKAUYE, M.D. Professor of Clinical Psychiatry, Director of Geriatric Psychiatry, Louisiana State University Health Sciences Center School of Medicine, New Orleans, Louisiana

BRITT SANFORD, M.D., M.S. Assistant Professor, Department of Neurology, Assistant Professor, Department of Pathology, Anatomy, and Cell Biology, Jefferson Medical College, Philadelphia, Pennsylvania

STEPHEN M. SCHEINTHAL, D.O., F.A.C.N. Director, Clinical Geriatric Psychiatry, Assistant Professor of Psychiatry, University of Medicine & Dentistry of New Jersey, School of Osteopathic Medicine, Stratford, New Jersey

KATHRYN PEKALA SERVICE, M.S., R.N.C./N.P., C.D.D.N. Postgraduate Student, School of Health, Community, and Education Studies, Northumbria University, Newcastle-upon-Tyne, England, Nurse Practitioner, Franklin-Hampshire Area Office, Massachusetts Department of Mental Retardation, Northampton, Massachusetts

JAVAID I. SHEIKH, M.D., M.B.A. Associate Dean for Veterans Affairs, Professor of Psychiatry and Behavioral Sciences, Stanford University School of Medicine, Chief of Staff, VA Palo Alto Healthcare System, Stanford, California

ALAN SIEGAL, M.D. Associate Clinical Professor of Psychiatry, Yale University, Geriatric and Adult Psychiatry LLC, Hamden, Connecticut

JEANNE JACKSON-SIEGAL, M.D. Assistant Clinical Professor, Department of Psychiatry, Yale University, Medical Director, Alzheimer's Resource Center of CT, Geriatric and Adult Psychiatry LLC, Hamden, Connecticut

LEN SPERRY, M.D., Ph.D. Clinical Professor of Psychiatry and Behavioral Medicine, and past Director of the Center for Aging and Development at the Medical College of Wisconsin, Milwaukee, WI, Professor, Florida Atlantic University, Boca Raton, Florida

ADAM P. SPIRA, Ph.D. Postdoctoral Fellow, Department of Psychiatry, VA Palo Alto Healthcare System, Menlo Park, California

ANDREW STOLL M.D.   Associate Professor, Department of Psychiatry, Harvard Medical School, Director, Psycho-pharmacology Research Laboratory, McLean Hospital, Belmont, Massachusetts

DARREN J. THOMPSON, M.D., A.B.P.N., F.R.C.P.(C)   Clinical Faculty, Department of Geriatric Psychiatry, University of British Columbia, Vancouver, British Columbia, Canada

LARRY W. THOMPSON, Ph.D.   Goldman Family Professor of Psychology, Pacific Graduate School of Psychology, Palo Alto, California

PAULA T. TRZEPACZ, M.D.   Clinical Professor of Psychiatry, University of Mississippi Medical Center, Jackson, Mississippi, Adjunct Professor of Psychiatry, Tufts University School of Medicine, Boston, Massachusetts, Clinical Professor of Psychiatry, Indiana University School of Medicine, Lilly Research Laboratories, Indianapolis, Indiana

JOHN A. TSIOURIS, M.D.   Clinical Assistant Professor, Department of Psychiatry, SUNY- Downstate Medical Center, Brooklyn, New York, Associate Director, Psychological/ Psychiatric Services, George A. Jervis Clinic, New York State Institute for Basic Research, Staten Island, New York

RABBI ABRAHAM J. TWERSKI, M.D.   Founder and Medical Director Emeritus, Gateway Rehabilitation Center, Pittsburgh, Pennsylvania, Associate Professor of Psychiatry, University of Pittsburgh School of Medicine, Pittsburgh, Pennsylvania

LADISLAV VOLICER, M.D., Ph.D.   Courtesy Full Professor, School of Aging Studies, University of South Florida, Tampa, Florida

DEBRA K. WEINER, M.D.   Associate Professor, Department of Medicine, University of Pittsburgh, Director, Older Adult Pain Management Program, UPMC Pain Medicine at Centre Commons, Pittsburgh, Pennsylvania

RUTH K. WESTHEIMER, Ed.D.   Sex Therapist and Educator, Adjunct Professor, New York University, New York City, New York, Lecturer, Yale University, New Haven, Connecticut, Lecturer, Princeton University, Princeton, New Jersey

MARY F. WYMAN, Ph.D.   Staff Psychologist in Geriatrics, Division of Mental Health and Rehabilitation, Zablocki Veterans Affairs Medical Center, Milwaukee, Wisconsin

RICHARD A. ZWEIG, Ph.D.   Assistant Professor of Psychology, Ferkauf Graduate School of Psychology, Yeshiva University, Assistant Professor of Psychiatry, Department of Psychiatry, Albert Einstein College of Medicine, Bronx, New York

Foreword

Just as they struggle to comprehend mental illness, it is important for practitioners in a field such as geriatric psychiatry to understand how health and science policy is made. They need to appreciate the art and, might I say, the science of politics. Psychiatrists must understand that in a democracy one must speak up effectively and be willing to go to all lengths to meet the needs of our patients and our profession. This is especially true when confronted with public prejudice and fear of mental illness, particularly when coupled with ageism or prejudice with respect to age—that older people are not as important as other age groups and are unproductive.

As recently as the 1970s, Alzheimer's disease was considered by many to be a rare neurological condition and "senility" to be inevitable, unpreventable, and untreatable. The word *senile* was still used as a prefix to other conditions such as osteoporosis, also regarded as beyond scientific study, prevention, and treatment. When given a choice, physicians were encouraged to diagnose "psychosis with arteriosclerosis" rather than "senile psychosis," the diagnosis of old age then used, because it was believed that organic brain syndromes in old age were due to "hardening of the arteries." And what of aging research? It was regarded as frivolous, prolix, and futile.

In 1975 there were only twelve grants related to all aspects of brain aging provided by both the National Institutes of Health (NIH) and the National Institute of Mental Health (NIMH). These averaged $60,000 each, for a total of $720,000. It was obviously important to elevate Alzheimer's disease to be a national priority, as we did at the National Institute on Aging (NIA) in 1976. One might ask about other reasons why a marked and rapid increase in interest and evolution of increased research funding in aging occurred in a relatively short time period. Along with the obvious pressure exerted from the realization by some that the huge number of "baby boomers" would eventually age, an important catalyst for this reaction was the work of a number of extremely effective public policy advocates over the years, both in the private sector and government—Congressman Claude Pepper; the American Association for Retired Persons (AARP); the American Association for Geriatric Psychiatry (AAGP); and the Department of Veterans Affairs (VA) come to mind, among many others.

One of these, a great citizen health advocate who believed wholeheartedly in the value and consequence of education and scientific research, Florence Mahoney, helped mobilize changes in Washington D.C. that affect us to this day; she illustrates the importance of personal influences in making health and science policy. An extremely well-connected doyen, Florence successfully "worked" the White House and the halls of Congress in the halcyon days when James Shannon was the iconic director of the NIH. She collaborated with disease advocacy groups, as well as with Senator Lister Hill and Congressman John Fogarty, congressional leaders concerned with health research. Together they established the parameters of the present-day NIH, and eventually, the NIA. During her most productive period, Florence was already an older person, which makes her an appropriate symbol to introduce a book like this one that specifically focuses on and celebrates older people. She died at 103 years of age.

This unique textbook of geriatric psychiatry exemplifies the enormous strides made in aging over the past 30 years. It offers not only clinical science, but also a sense of advocacy and a broad social context; it does an excellent job spotlighting the importance of understanding the immediate relevance to our lives of the field of aging in general, and the relationship of mental health and illness in older persons in particular. The "demographic imperative" of aging has arrived.

The following chapters comprise a massive, comprehensive, wide-ranging, informative, scientifically rigorous, and eminently practical text. It is in the tradition of Florence Mahoney. The broad approach is successful because the authors are not only respected academics but also experienced clinicians. Some of the important and timely topics include forensic issues; palliative and end-of-life care; chronic pain; medications; ethics; spirituality; sexuality; and intellectual disability. In addition, the book addresses the specific, important clinical syndromes of geriatric psychiatry in a lucid and practical fashion. It understands well the impact of social and cultural traditions upon the lives of older people and suggests opportunities and strategies to care for them. Today's practitioner of geriatric psychiatry will want to have this book available in the clinical setting.

What about the future? One can speculate as to where the field of aging, and particularly brain aging, is headed. Should the research and clinical context simply continue to focus on studying the old and oldest-old, important as that approach is? Or, should attention also be paid to other directions, as well; for example, emphasizing additional so-called "critical developmental periods" of brain function, such as is studied in children. These two developmental periods of life—young and old—historically have been described as polar opposites (anabolic vs. catabolic; synthesis vs. breakdown), but they are actually more similar from a physiological view than previously thought. Already, many present-day research studies describe brain aging, not as a time of overall decline in function, but rather, in its own way, an anabolic period of growth and development. One can only imagine the developments yet to come, or the new crop of public-policy advocates who, like their predecessors, will help ensure the funding necessary to meet the resource demands for brain aging clinical practice and research.

Robert N. Butler, M.D.
President and CEO
International Longevity Center, USA

Foreword

The publication of *Principles and Practice of Geriatric Psychiatry* signifies that the field has successfully taken its place among medical subspecialties. Progress has been swift indeed. Seventeen years ago there were just 258 pages covering the "essentials of geriatric psychiatry" (1). Perusal of the current text with its 43 chapters and three appendices (one of them a very useful review of neuroanatomy) substantiates that in less than two decades, geriatric psychiatry has evolved into a discipline with a solid knowledge base, both clinical and scientific. I am delighted that the editors have given me the opportunity to share some recollections on the development of geriatric psychiatry as a subspecialty. As one of those few who actually can remember what it was like before there was geriatric psychiatry in the United States, I will give you my personal perspective of its development. Clearly, it is impossible to recapture all of the important events and condense them to fit into this foreword. Space limitations force me to omit far more that I can include. I have tried to verify and supplement my recall with information from several sources, but I know that my recollections are bound to be incomplete and apologize for the inevitable unintended omissions.

It is hard to imagine today the Zeitgeist of the mid-twentieth century when all debilities of later life, including physical as well as mental disorders, were considered merely the consequences of advancing chronological age, to be dismissed as unavoidable, unalterable, and unworthy of serious attention. In other words, they were part of "normal aging." Thus, Webster's dictionary defined senility (other than senile psychosis) as "old age," "weakness or infirmity due to old age" (2). That was the situation confronting the early researchers and clinicians who studied aging and age-associated mental changes. However, by the 1980s the pendulum had swung so far in the opposite direction that anyone who associated old age with intellectual decline was branded as ageist (3). That change in attitude was not limited to intellectual decline, but applied to mental disorders as well.

I will give only two examples—viz., depression and dementia—the most frequent mental disorders in the elderly. Old people, especially if they had life-threatening illnesses such as cancer or heart disease, were expected to be depressed, despite the fact that anyone who visited a cancer ward could plainly see that, even there, many of the patients were not depressed. Today, we know that coexistence of medical and psychiatric morbidities calls for treatment of both, as discussed in Chapter 25 of this book. Also, there have been dramatic advances in the treatment of depression, particularly in pharmacotherapy. For a long time after effective antidepressant drugs became available, it was believed that elderly patients responded so poorly to such drugs that it was hardly worth trying them, particularly in light of the complications so often resulting from drug-drug and drug-disease interactions. As data began to accumulate on results of antidepressant drug treatment of the elderly, it became clear that the 50% frequency of responders (4) was not so very different from the 60% average responder rate in nongeriatric patients (5).

With regard to psychotherapeutic interventions, data are scarce in general, and even more so for depressed patients over the age of 65. Yet, there is some indication that the response of elderly depressed patients to psychotherapy may not differ significantly from their response to antidepressant drugs (4). More data are needed, but today it is generally agreed that clinical depression is not part of normal aging and requires treatment in the elderly just as it does in other age groups.

Similarly, we no longer accept the once widely prevalent belief that disengagement, with its ensuing isolation, is the appropriate response to growing older (6,7). Starting more than 25 years ago (8), research results have shown that for most older people continued engagement, not disengagement, is associated with successful aging, supporting the advocates of activity theory (9,10). Today, "civic engagement" is becoming a topic of much interest (11). Indeed, an active social network as well as exercise (both mental and physical), nutritional discretion, and pursuit of wide-ranging interests have been associated with successful aging (12,13).

As mentioned earlier, there has also been a profound change in our attitude toward cognitive decline in old age, i.e., age-associated memory impairment (AAMI), mild cognitive impairment (MCI), and especially dementia. No longer are they accepted as the inevitable consequences of advancing chronological age; instead, they are regarded as abnormalities for which treatments are sought. Unfortunately, the search for consistently effective treatment is still ongoing. Since 1995, when the first acetylcholinesterase inhibitor (i.e., tacrine) became available, three more have come into use. They are superior to the original because of better side-effect profiles, but all have modest efficacy only. Many other drugs are in development, and most experts are optimistic that truly effective drugs for the treatment of Alzheimer's disease (AD) will become available in the future. At that point, the distinction between the early changes of AD and those of "normal aging" will assume ever-increasing importance. The current volume devotes five chapters to providing up-to-date information on memory disorders and specific forms of dementia (Chapters 19–23) in addition to depression/anxiety and dementia (Chapter 38), neuropsychological assessment (Chapter 9), and dementia work-up (Chapter 10). Further, Chapter 36 comprehensively reviews intellectual disabilities in adults at or beyond middle age, an area with but limited information in the current literature.

Some of the key information on dementia derives from longitudinal studies, one of the earliest having been concerned with genetic influences on cognitive decline. That prospective study of normal community-residing twins, 60 years of age or older, demonstrated that intellectual decline after age 60 was not inevitable but was associated with disease and predictive of mortality many years later—even for members of monozygotic twin pairs (3). Long-term follow-up is the most direct way to determine how individuals change over time. However, not many researchers want to invest decades of their career in such studies. Thus, the follow-up for most of the 35 studies listed in a recent review (14) was 6 years or less. Fortunately, there exists a number of long-term studies, some dating as far back as the 1940s, to increase our understanding of the mental and physical changes associated with aging. Among the best known are the Framingham Heart Study (15), Honolulu-Asia Aging Study (HAAS) (16), Western Collaborative Group Study (17), NHLBI Twin Study (18), the Study of Dementia in Swedish Twins (19), the UCLA/VA 20-Year Follow-Up Study of AD Families (20), the Baltimore Longitudinal Study of Aging (21), the Nun Study (22), the Duke Veteran Twin Study of AD (23), MIRAGE (24), and BIOCARD (25).

The data from these studies are ready to be mined and will add substantially to our understanding of the very early changes in AD (and other dementias), as well as their differentiation from the nonprogressive (or slowly progressive) mental changes not likely to interfere with daily functioning that are characteristic of "normal aging" (26). There are some, including myself , who believe that, just like wrinkles, osteoporosis and other age-associated changes, even the memory changes that today we consider part of normal aging, may become remediable, if not preventable. "Successful aging" has become of great interest to the marketplace because of the *demographic imperative*. The proportion of the U.S. population over the age of 65 doubled between 1900 and 1950 (4.1%–8.2%) (27), with life expectancy at birth increasing during the same period by nearly 20 years for men (from 46.3 years to 65.6 years) and even more than that for women (from 48.3 years to 71.1 years) (28). Projections for 2000–2050 are that the proportion of the population over the age of 65 will increase more than one and one-half times (from 12.4% to 20.7%), while the total population over the age of 65 will more than double (35.1 million to 86.7 million).(29). Life expectancy during the coming half-century is projected to increase for men from 74.1 years to 81.2 years and even more than that for women (from 79.8 years to 86.7 years) (30). This demographic imperative has been the single most important factor in the rise of gerontology, geriatrics, and geriatric psychiatry.

The Group for the Advancement of Psychiatry (GAP) was among the first to recognize the importance of this trend and published *The Problem of the Aged Patient in the Public Psychiatric Hospital* in 1950 (31). It took more than 10 years before the American Psychiatric Association (APA) established the Committee on Aging (later Council on Aging), largely as a result of the pioneering efforts of Jack Weinberg. He has been memorialized by the APA's annual presentation of the Jack Weinberg Memorial Award. The first journal, the *Journal of Geriatric Psychiatry*, was established in 1967 by a group of Boston psychoanalysts (including Martin Berezin, David Blau, Stanley Cath, and Ralph Kahana), 26 years before the *American Journal of Geriatric Psychiatry* published its first issue. The demographic imperative helped to make available funding for research, education, training, and clinical care in geriatrics and geriatric psychiatry, with the Department of Veterans Affairs (then the Veterans Administration) in the forefront thanks to the pioneering efforts of Paul Haber—the "godfather" of the present-day Geriatric Research, Education and Clinical Centers (GRECC). Others included the National Institutes of Health (NIH), through the Center on Aging, established within the National Institute of Mental Health (NIMH) in 1975 under the outstanding leadership of Gene Cohen, and later Barry Lebowitz. Just 4 years earlier, the second White House Conference on Aging (1971) had provided a big impetus for advancing the study of aging, culminating in the establishment of the National Institute on Aging (NIA) in 1974. Prior to that time, from the mid 1960s, the aging branch of the National Institute of Child Health and Human Development (NICHD), and its first director, James Birren (followed in the late 1960s by Leroy Duncan, along with Gabe Maletta, Don Gibson, and Don Murphy), helped initiate, develop, and expand academic and federal government interest and national funding in aging research, training, and education. NIA supported a broad array of biopsychosocial research in aging. Psychiatrists were involved in all of these activities, and to one of them, Robert Butler, the first Director of NIA, much credit is due for the development of geriatrics as well as geriatric psychiatry in the United States. After leaving NIA, he was appointed the first chair of the first department of geriatrics in the United States (Mount Sinai Hospital, NY). The Alzheimer's Disease and Related Disorders Association (ADRDA), an association of family members (founded in 1980 by Jerome Stone), with its Medical and Scientific Advisory Board (especially

Drs. Robert Katzman and Robert Terry), was a moving force at the time. Not only did ADRDA secure financial support for the study of AD and the care of the afflicted, but it helped transform AD from a rare familial presenile disorder, known only to the specialists, into a disease familiar to the public-at-large. Among ADRDA's many other accomplishments was the formulation of the diagnostic criteria for AD, which are still in use today (32).

Many other organizations were involved in the birth, growth, and development of geriatric psychiatry, prominent among them, for example, the Gerontological Society of America (GSA). It was founded in 1945 "to promote the scientific study of aging, to encourage exchanges among researchers and practitioners from the various disciplines related to gerontology, and to foster the use of gerontological research in forming public policy" (33). The interaction of psychologists, biologists, nurses, sociologists, pharmacologists, and epidemiologists with internists and psychiatrists became both a characteristic and a major strength of early gerontology, geriatrics, and geriatric psychiatry. Psychologists specializing in child development had begun to expand their interests to development extending beyond the attainment of adulthood. In 1945, their influence resulted in the creation of a new Division of Adulthood and Old Age, Division 20 (now called Division of Adult Development and Aging) in the American Psychological Association. They played a pivotal role also in the development of the GSA, as did a variety of other professionals, as mentioned above. The American Geriatrics Society (AGS), too, welcomed psychiatrists and led the way in securing added qualifications for geriatric medicine (1988); geriatric psychiatry followed, with the first added qualifications examination for the sub-specialty of geriatric psychiatry, in 1991.

Over the years, fellowship programs in geriatric psychiatry have been established throughout the United States. Currently there are 60 of them (which can be found at www.acgme.org/adspublic/). The collaborative efforts of diverse disciplines were vital components in the development of these programs. The first major academic program in geriatric psychiatry was established in the mid 1960s at Duke University, thanks to the efforts of Ewald (Bud) Busse and his associates. It endures to this day and can take credit for having members of the original faculty, as well as graduates of the program (e.g., Carl Eisdorfer, Murray Raskind, and Burton Reifler) set up programs of their own. Among other early university training programs were those at Cornell, Harvard, and Stanford and the Universities of Pennsylvania, Texas, Pittsburgh, Rochester, and California–Los Angeles (UCLA). The early training programs initiated throughout the country were essential elements in the development of geriatric psychiatry.

I will conclude by citing just one more ingredient in the conception, birth, and growth of geriatric psychiatry as a sub-specialty—i.e., the people who made it happen. Working together, community clinicians and academics gave unstintingly of their time and generously devoted their own resources and efforts to educate themselves, their colleagues within the profession, other professionals, students, trainees, and the public-at-large. They also worked with local, regional, state, and federal agencies, as well as legislative, executive, and judicial leaders. Moreover, as far as I know, none of them received any financial compensation for either the time or the efforts devoted to these activities. A few names not already mentioned come to mind: George Alexopoulos, Jeff Foster, Charles Gaitz, Gary Gottlieb, George Grossberg, Hugh Hendrie, Ben Liptzin, Eric Pfeiffer, Bill Reichman, Joel Sadavoy, Charles Shamoian , Elliott Stein, and I. As time went by, they were joined by a very able second generation (among them, Steve Bartels, Chris Colenda, Don Hay, Dilip Jeste, Gary Kennedy, Susan Lieff, Ken Sakauye, Alan Siegal, Gary W. Small, and Dave Sultzer). And, most important was the organizational work done initially by Sandy Finkel, founder of the American Association for Geriatric Psychiatry (AAGP) and later founder of the International Psychogeriatric Association (IPA). I apologize to those many others who should be in the above listing but are not, due to my less than perfect memory. Perhaps the best testimony to the success of their efforts is the fact that there are now so many expert geriatric psychiatrists that only 11 of the 101 authors of the current text have contributed to either of the previously published texts (34, 35). The current list of outstanding authors includes 54 geriatric psychiatrists and 47 others drawn from psychology (19), neurology (9), pharmacology (6), philosophy/ethics/religion (5), geriatrics (2), and miscellaneous other backgrounds (6), including a family caregiver. The editors are to be congratulated for having recruited them and for having successfully completed the monumental task resulting in the publication of *Principles and Practice of Geriatric Psychiatry*.

Lissy Jarvik, MD, PhD
Professor Emeritus
Department of Psychiatry and Biobehavioral Sciences
University of California–Los Angeles
and
Distinguished Physician Emeritus
U.S. Department of Veterans Affairs

REFERENCES

1. Lazarus LW, Jarvik LF, Foster JR, Lieff JD, Mershon SR, eds. *Essentials of Geriatric Psychiatry: A Guide for Health Professionals.* New York: Springer; 1988.
2. *Webster's New International Dictionary of the English Language.* 2nd ed. Springfield, MA: G. & C. Merriam; 1936.
3. Jarvik, LF: Aging of the brain—how can we prevent it? (Robert W. Kleemeier Lecture) *Gerontologist.* 1988;28:739–747.
4. Gerson S, Belin TR, Kaufman A, Mintz J, Jarvik L. Pharmacological and psychological treatments for depressed older patients: a meta-analysis and overview of recent findings. *Harv Rev Psychiatry.* 1999;7(1):1–28.
5. NIH Consensus Statement. *Diagnosis and Treatment of Depression in Late Life.* November 4-6, 1991:9(3):1–27.

6. Cumming E, Henry W. *Growing Old: The Process of Disengagement.* New York: Basic Books; 1961.

7. Kastenbaum RJ. *Death, Society, & Human Experience.* St. Louis: Mosby; 1977.

8. Berkman L, Syme S. Social networks host resistance and mortality: a nine-year follow-up of Alameda County residents. *American Journal of Epidemiology.* 1979;109:186–204.

9. Maddox GL. Disengagement theory: a critical evaluation. *Gerontologist.* 1964;4:80–83.

10. Lemon BW, Bengtson VL, Petersen JA.. An exploration of the activity theory of aging: activity types and life expectation among in-movers to a retirement community. *Journal of Gerontology.* 1972;27(4):511–523.

11. Harvard School of Public Health, Center for Health Communication. *Reinventing Aging: Baby Boomers and Civic Engagement.* Boston: Harvard School of Public Health; 2004.

12. Rowe JW, RL Kahn. *Successful Aging.* New York: Pantheon Books; 1998.

13. Small GW. *The Memory Prescription: Dr. Gary Small's 14-Day Plan to Keep Your Brain and Body Young.* Hyperion: New York; 2004.

14. Schaie KW, Hofer SM. Longitudinal studies in aging research. In: JE Birren, KW Schaie, eds. *Handbook of the Psychology of Aging.* 5th ed. San Diego: Academic Press; 2001:53–77.

15. Tan ZS, Seshadri S, Beiser A, et al. Plasma total cholesterol level as a risk factor for Alzheimer disease: the Framingham Study. *Arch Intern Med.* 2003;163(9):1053–1057.

16. Schmidt R, Schmidt H, Curb JD, Masaki K, White LR, Launer LJ. Early inflammation and dementia: a 25-year follow-up of the Honolulu-Asia Aging Study. *Ann Neurol.* 2002;52(2):168–174.

17. Carmelli D, Swan GE, LaRue A, Eslinger PJ. Correlates of change in cognitive function in survivors from the Western Collaborative Group Study. Neuroepidemiology. 1997;16:285–295.183.

18. Caffery JM, Niaura R, Todaro JF, Swan GE, Carmelli D. Depressive symptoms and metabolic risk in adult male twins enrolled in the National Heart, Lung, and Blood Institute twin study. *Psychosom Med.* 2003;65(3):490–497.

19. Gatz M, Fratiglioni L, Johansson B, et al. Complete ascertainment of dementia in the Swedish Twin Registry: the HARMONY study. *Neurobiol Aging.* 2005;26(4):439–447.

20. Jarvik LF, Harrison TR, Holt L, et al. Children of Alzheimer patients: more data needed. *J Gerontol A Biol Sci Med Sci.* 2004;59(10):1076–1077.

21. Kawas CH, Corrada MM, Brookmeyer R, et al. Visual memory predicts Alzheimer's disease more than a decade before diagnosis. Neurology. 2003;60(7):1089–1093.

22. Mortimer JA, Gosche KM, Riley KP, Markesbery WR, Snowdon DA. Delayed recall, hippocampal volume and Alzheimer neuropathology: findings from the Nun Study. *Neurology.* 2004; 62(3):428–432.

23. Plassman BL, Welsh KA, Helms M, Brandt J, Page WF, Breitner JC. Intelligence and education as predictors of cognitive state in late life: a 50-year follow-up. *Neurology.* 1995;45(8):1446–1450.

24. Yip AG, Green RC, Huyck M, Cupples LA, Farrer LA (MIRAGE Study Group). Nonsteroidal anti-inflammatory drug use and Alzheimer's disease risk: the MIRAGE Study. *BMC Geriatrics.* 2005;5(1):2.

25. Greenwood PM, Lambert C, Sunderland T, Parasuraman R. Effects of apolipoprotein E genotype on spatial attention, working memory, and their interaction in healthy, middle-aged adults: results from the National Institute of Mental Health's BIOCARD Study. *Neuropsychology.* 2005;19(2) 199–211.

26. Jarvik LF, Blazer D. Journal of Geriatric Psychiatry and Neurology. In-Press.

27. US Bureau of the Census. *Actual Life Expectancies 1900–1990 from U.S. Bureau of the Census. Current Population Reports, Special Studies, P23-190, 65+ in the United States.* Washington, DC: US Bureau of the Census; 1996.

28. US Bureau of the Census. *Current Population Reports, Special Studies, P23-190, 65+ in the United States.* Washington DC: US Bureau of the Census; 1996.

29. US Bureau of the Census. *U.S. Interim Projections by Age, Sex, Race, and Hispanic Origin.* www.census.gov/ipc/www/usinterimproj/. Accessed March 18, 2004.

30. US Bureau of the Census. *Projected Life Expectancy at Birth by Race and Hispanic Origin (NP-T7-B) 1999 to 2100.* National Projections Program, Population Division, Washington, DC: US Bureau of the Census; 2000.

31. Group for the Advancement of Psychiatry, Committee on Aging. *The Problem of the Aged Patient in the Public Psychiatric Hospital.* New York: Group for the Advancement of Psychiatry; GAP Report 14; 1950

32. McKhann G. Mental and clinical diagnosis of Alzheimer's disease: report of the NINCDS-ADRDA Work Group under the auspices of the Department of Health and Human Services Task Force on Alzheimer's Disease. Neurology. 1984;34(7): 939–944.

33. Gerontological Society of America Web site. *50th anniversary of the Gerontological Society of America* (1995). Available at www.geron.org/history.htm#beginnings. Accessed June 2, 2005.

34. Blazer DG, Steffens DC, Busse E, eds. *The American Psychiatric Publishing Textbook of Geriatric Psychiatry,* 3rd ed. Arlington, VA: American Psychiatric Publishing; 2004.

35. Sadavoy J, Jarvik LF, Grossberg GT, Meyers BS, eds. *Comprehensive Textbook of Geriatric Psychiatry,* 3rd ed. New York: Norton; 2004.

Preface

Like a fine piece of classical music, a book needs a central theme, with variations running throughout. The theme inherent in this book can best be described as the integration of clinical expertise in psychiatry, medicine, and neurology, focused on treating the individual elderly patient, the family, and other caregivers. The variations of the theme encompass the multiple and varied professions essential for the provision of optimal care. Nowhere in the mental health field is the integration of psychiatry and medicine more important than in geriatric psychiatry. It isn't enough in this population to simply treat "emotional" problems. Elderly patients regularly have psychiatric symptoms that are either due to—or exacerbated by—underlying medical problems, which, unless addressed, will continue despite treatment with psychotropic drugs. Conversely, medical problems can be initiated and exacerbated by psychiatric problems. Anxiety is but one of several excellent examples of this phenomenon of co-morbidity. Consideration of this mind–body integration and the importance of treating the entire patient, using a "team" approach, should be most prevalent in the older population.

Although this book provides an up-to-date compendium of information and research findings, it is, at its core, a clinical, patient-based, practical resource written to assist practicing clinicians of geriatric psychiatry in evaluating and managing their patients. By definition, the book includes the scientific principles of geriatric psychiatry, as well as its clinical practice. *Practice* here encompasses evaluation ("*by careful appraisal and study*") and management ("*judicious use of means to accomplish an end*"), both implying ongoing action, which is the best way to assess and treat elderly patients. It is a process rather than a discrete event, and fits well with the geriatric psychiatry principle of continuing, comprehensive, and flexible overall care. *Empiric*—that is, a scientific, reasoned trial and error approach over time—is often a more valid model of care in this population than is the classic *rational* one—that is, problem–solution.

The authors in this book were carefully selected, not only for their ability as fine writers (concise, thorough, understandable) and thought leaders, but also because of their extensive practical knowledge and experience in treating geriatric patients. The knowledge found herein is based on the most recent, evidence-based guidelines for care and relies on field-accepted outcome measures to optimize that care. When relevant to the chapter, useful and interesting research studies also are incorporated. Nearly every chapter provides in-depth, real-world case studies to illustrate approaches to diagnosis and treatment. Section I of the textbook provides a practical context for geriatric psychiatry; it focuses on the patient from a developmental, strengths-based perspective (Chapter 1), the geriatric psychiatrist and how to establish a private practice (Chapter 2), the geriatric practice setting with a focus on long-term care and pharmacologic guidelines (Chapter 3), and the all-important caregiver for geriatric patients (Chapter 4). Dr. Cohen's opening chapter, in particular, challenges the reader with an enlightened perspective on aging that emphasizes the potential for growth and wellness and the clinician's role in promoting its wide-spread appreciation, on a par with the more traditional clinical role of identifying decline and treating pathology.

Section II is wholly comprised of the principles of clinical evaluation and includes eight chapters that focus in depth on psychiatric, medical, neurological, radiographic, neuropsychological, and forensic examinations. Chapter 10 reviews all modalities with respect to the dementia workup, a significant central component to geriatric psychiatry practice. Chapter 11 reviews the relevance of cultural factors to any geriatric examination.

Section III is devoted to explicating general principles and treatment and provides three comprehensive chapters on psychotherapy, pharmacotherapy, and electroconvulsive therapy in older patients. We insisted that this section also contain several key but often neglected topics: spirituality, hospice and palliative care, and ethical issues. We are honored to have in Dr. Len Sperry's chapter on spirituality (Chapter 17) brief commentaries by the President-emeritus of the University of Notre Dame, Reverend Theodore Hesburgh; the noted Catholic theologian, Monika Hellwig; and the prolific and popular author and psychiatrist, Rabbi Abraham J. Twersky, M.D.

Section IV is the anchor of the text, covering all major psychiatric disorders seen in late life, without exception. Major voices in the field of geriatric psychiatry and their junior colleagues have covered: the most prevalent forms of dementia, in separate chapters; all mood, anxiety, and psychotic disorders; delirium; suicide; adjustment disorders and disorders of personality; substance use; somatoform, sleep, and sexual disorders; and intellectual disabilities. The noted sex therapist and radio and television personality Dr. Ruth Westheimer lent her voice to a wide-ranging interview on late-life sexuality that is woven throughout the chapter on sexual disorders. The chapter on intellectual disabilities is the first of its kind in a geriatric psychiatry text, providing a review of clinical care for the aging individual with intellectual and developmental disabilities.

Section V truly makes this a comprehensive text by covering, in separate chapters, many seminally important geriatric psychiatry issues: dementia-related mood and behavioral disturbances, the impact of medications, Parkinson's disease, movement disorders, pain, and apathy. Three practical appendices follow, which provide a comprehensive guide to the dosing and monitoring of psychotropic medications, a neuroanatomy primer to guide clinical practice, and a list of major educational resources available for clinicians, patients, and caregivers.

Regrettably, it seems to be *de rigueur* among some of the cognoscenti of medicine and psychiatry to minimize the usefulness of clinical textbook preparation as not being cost effective, either personally or professionally, primarily because of the long latency inherent between preparation of the information and its publication. The argument reasons that much of the evaluation and treatment approaches described already may be outdated on the day of the books' delivery. Our approach in producing this book was to recognize this argument as potentially valid and attempt to address it by having authors stress, wherever possible, principles and practice of care that have enduring clinical relevance. One unique approach used was to include in many of the syndromic chapters short commentaries that contain useful and timeless messages highlighting particular clinical situations involving geriatric patients and their caregivers—both family and professional.

Our primary goal from the outset in the development of this book was to assist direct-care psychiatric clinicians by providing them with useful, comprehensive, cutting-edge information, along with practical approaches to optimize care, in a variety of practice settings, for their older patients—who comprise an ever-increasing and important segment of our society.

Marc E. Agronin, M.D.
Gabe J. Maletta, Ph.D., M.D.
2005

Acknowledgments

Both editors would like to sincerely thank Charley Mitchell, Executive Editor at Lippincott, Williams & Wilkins for offering us the opportunity to create this text and for his support along the way. We offer our admiration and gratitude to our own editor Lisa Kairis, for her guidance, shepherding, and patience throughout the course of developing this text. We are particularly honored to have two of the founders of the field of geriatrics and geriatric psychiatry in the United States provide forewords: Robert Butler, M.D., and Lissy Jarvik, M.D., Ph.D. Their introductions to this textbook speak to their ongoing ability to inspire our own efforts and those of our colleagues in the ever-growing and important field of geriatric psychiatry.

Dr. Agronin:

It has been of considerable joy to create and co-edit this textbook with my mentor, colleague, and close friend Gabe Maletta. Our work together has taught me over and over again the timelessness and great meaning to be found in both friendship and intellectual pursuit—and where the two meet is a particularly wonderful place to be. I offer my gratitude, as well, to so many friends and colleagues who wrote chapters for this text. Special thanks for their assistance throughout the preparation of this text go to Stephen M. Scheinthal, D.O., Katya Miloslavich, Eli Feldman, and Jacobo Forma. Dr. Ruth Westheimer was exceptionally generous with her time and encouragement in preparing our chapter on sexual disorders. Finally, I would like to acknowledge the training provided by my grandfather Simon Cherkasky, M.D., and uncle Alan Cherkasky, M.D., which laid the foundation for my role as a physician and psychiatrist.

Dr. Maletta:

The original idea for this important book was conceived in the fertile imagination of my friend, Marc Agronin; and it's been a pleasure for me to work with him, as a contributor and as a co-editor. He's made the evolution—from scholarly Fellow to respected colleague—a seamless one. Although this project was extremely long and labor intensive, the knowledge I gained throughout its course was well worth the time and effort spent.

I want to acknowledge the support, patience, humor, and strength of my family during this work, particularly my children—Elizabeth (and her husband Rick, and especially my graceful grandson Richie) and my sons Keith and Matthew, all of whom I cherish (*everywhere they are, there I'll be*). Thank you for everything.

I'm indebted to my mentors (and a special maestra), colleagues, and students—past and present, many of whom I count as friends. I'm also indebted to my patients, their families, and other caregivers. A day doesn't go by without my learning something from these wise ones. It reinforces my original reason for deciding to work with older people in the first place; their wisdom, experience, and creativity should be respected, honored, and celebrated by all of us.

Thanks to the authors of this book for their excellent contributions, which will certainly benefit the health of those a bit ahead of us on this exciting journey.

Geriatric Psychiatry: An Introduction to the Patient, Clinician, Setting, and Caregiver

The Geriatric Patient

Gene D. Cohen

1

This chapter is being written for the clinician with the geriatric patient presented as an older person. It is critical to understand patients as people in order to balance a focus on the patient's problems with attention to the person's potential. Understanding the individual's strengths, capacities, hopes, and desires points to the path toward health promotion and disease prevention with aging.

Accordingly, today's older adults will be examined by how they differ from previous generations of older people. The capacity to change with age has been much misunderstood and maligned. Without an understanding of an older person's capacity for positive change, the clinician is less well prepared to motivate the geriatric patient to adopt new therapeutic and health-promoting strategies. Hence, the latest thinking on human development in the second half of life will be delineated.

Given findings from research on the positive effects on overall health and brain vitality that come from being challenged and engaged in productive endeavors along with social activities, the clinician needs to know how to help geriatric patients reassess and better plan their activities. Toward this goal, the concept of a *social portfolio* is presented, better equipping the clinician to give more informed and specific advice to patients on social and behavioral strategies that can promote health with aging. Within this context, advice for reinvigorating marriages and other significant relationships in later life is offered.

Retirement has become ever more varied, so the clinician is provided a retirement readiness questionnaire that can be shared with patients who are approaching retirement or re-evaluating plans already in place. Finally, the clinician is provided a list to share with patients of 10 ways to challenge one's mind and improve health in aging.

OVERALL HEALTH STATUS OF TODAY'S OLDER ADULTS

In its "Older Americans 2000 Report," the Federal Interagency Forum on Aging-Related Statistics provided the following data on the overall health status of today's older adults (Table 1-1)[1]. Given the enormous interplay between physical health and mental health in later life, it is important to be aware of the potential influence and interaction of coexisting health conditions and treatments in older patients.

In addition, the percentage of older adults with moderate or severe memory impairment ranged from about 4% among people aged 65 to 69, to about 36% among people aged 85 or older, and approximately 30% of all prescription medications are used by people 65 and older.

Disability

It is noteworthy that the proportion of Americans 65 or older with a chronic disability declined from 24% in 1982 to 21% in 1994. Despite the decline in rates, however, the number of older Americans with chronic disabilities increased by about 600,000 from 6.4 million in 1982 to 7 million in 1994 [1]. This is because the overall population of older people was growing fast enough to outweigh the decline in disability rates. However, if disability rates had not declined from 1982 to 1994, then the disabled population would have increased by almost 1.5 million, bringing the total number of older Americans with chronic disabilities close to 7.9 million.

TABLE 1-1
CHRONIC HEALTH CONDITIONS AMONG PEOPLE AGED 70 AND OLDER

Arthritis: 58%
Hypertension: 45%
Heart disease: 21%
Cancer: 19%
Diabetes: 12%
Stroke: 9%

Adapted from Reference 1.

The decline in disability rates occurred for both sexes since 1982, when 27% of older women and 20% of older men had a chronic disability. By 1994, about 25% of older women and 16% of older men had a chronic disability.

Self-Rated Health Status

Asking people to rate their own health as excellent, very good, good, fair, or poor provides a common indicator of health that is easily measured in surveys. It represents physical, emotional, and social aspects of health and well-being. Good-to-excellent self-reported health correlates with a lower risk of mortality.

Seventy-two percent of older Americans reported their health as good, very good, or excellent. Women and men reported comparable levels of health status (1).

Positive health evaluations decline with age. Among non-Hispanic White men aged 65 to 74, 76% reported good-to-excellent health, compared with 67% of non-Hispanic White men 85 or older. A similar decline with age was reported by non-Hispanic Black and Hispanic older men, and by women, with the exception of non-Hispanic Black women.

Among older men and women in every age group, non-Hispanic Black and Hispanic people were less likely to report good health than non-Hispanic White people.

CHANGING OLDER COHORT GROUPS

It has been only recently that we have witnessed the true picture of aging in older people. For so long, life expectancy was short due to the prevalence of death due to disease, war, famine, complications of child birth, poor public health conditions, poor health habits, the absence of modern medical interventions, and the lack of sound preventive and health-promotion strategies. Not only did these factors limit the number of people who reached age 65, but they increased the likelihood of life for many by that age to be accompanied by considerable frailty. Even at the start of the 20th century, life expectancy in the United States was still less than 50 years of age. This historical legacy, along with accruing negative stereotypes about aging, led to great negative expectations about life in one's later years.

By the start of the 21st century, the situation surrounding aging had changed dramatically, undergoing a profound transformation. By the year 2000, compared to 1900, those aged 65 and older had increased more than 10-fold, totaling approximately 35 million—more than the total population of Canada at that time. In effect, by the turn of the 21st century in America, there was a veritable nation of older people within the overall nation, with all the diversity of any country. By 2000, compared to 1900, the number of people aged 75 and older had increased nearly 19-fold, and the number of people 85 and older had increased nearly 38-fold (2).

The educational level of older people by the end of the 20th century further reflected the profound changes in the older cohort group in the population, again illustrating how, for the first time in history, we were witnessing what was indeed possible and increasingly common with aging and advancing years. In 1970, images of aging in America were perhaps at their nadir. Many of the negative myths about aging became pronounced around that time, along with the prevalence of descriptors such as *age gap* and *intergenerational conflict.* It was also at this point in American history when one commonly heard the phrase, "You cannot trust anyone over 30!" But rather than an age gap, what was operating was more fundamentally an *education gap.* The median level of education among those 65 and older in 1970 was 8.7 years (less than a high school education), compared to 12.1 years among those 25 and older. But by 1989, that education gap had largely closed. The median level of education among people 65 and older had risen to 12.1 years (greater than a high school education), compared to 12.7 years among those 25 and older. In hardly a generation, the median educational level of older people had gone from less than a high school education to greater than a high school education. And during that period from 1970 to 1989, sociological studies showed positive, collaborative intergenerational relationships to have soared (3–5).

From the start of the 20th century to the start of the 21st century, life expectancy in America increased by more than 50%. And this was accomplished without modifying the human genome—illustrating the impact on longevity and quality of life of improved public health practices and personal health habits, along with advances in medicine and research on aging. Not only had life expectancy substantially increased, but frailty by age 65 had greatly diminished. By the mid 1970s, a new era in gerontology had begun, characterized by an awareness of the difference between aging *per se* and problems that can accompany aging. By alleviating the problems, the quality of aging was improved. By 2000, a change in thinking about aging was occurring. In addition to growing sophistication in addressing problems associated with aging, for the first time significant scientific and societal interest was mounting about what could be done to promote potential in later life (4). The ramifications of this new orientation for promoting further improvements in the level of health and independent functioning with aging and the quality of later life are profound. The discussion that follows addresses this new focus on potential in the second half of life.

Perspectives on Health and Wellness

In 1948, the World Health Organization officially asserted that health is "a state of complete physical, mental, and social well-being, and not merely the absence of disease and infirmity" (6). This perspective on wellness—with its emphasis on not being merely the absence of disease—is relevant regardless of age. Moreover, a strong case can be made that even without being completely free of physical or mental illness, areas of physical and mental health persist and are subject to enhancement. Certainly this applies to the vast majority of people over 65 who have one or more chronic illnesses (7).

One can have high blood pressure and diabetes, yet still experience a feeling of wellness, especially if the symptoms of these disorders are treated and under control. Similarly, one can manifest areas of mental wellness even in the midst of coping with manifestations of mental disorder or impairment, especially during periods of remission. And even when a person is symptomatic with a mental health problem, mental health and mental illness can coexist, with the individual exhibiting a strong orientation toward mental wellness. For example, one can struggle with anxiety, and yet still experience psychological growth in later life—a powerful orientation toward wellness. Despite suffering from Alzheimer's disease (AD), an overwhelming disorder affecting the mind, one can still have a quest for joyous intervals of time with a loved one, or still have the desire to tap into a partially preserved skill. In the years immediately following his diagnosis of AD, Willem de Kooning continued to tap his preserved skill as an artist, creating paintings sought after by museums for public exhibition.

The clinical significance of the coexistence of health and illness is that while a problem-oriented plan of interventions is indicated for addressing a patient's illness or illnesses, a potential-oriented plan should similarly be developed to tap into a person's healthy aspects, where quality of life and dimensions of wellness can still be promoted. Classic applications of this concept have focused on enhancing the sense of control or sense of coherence, both of healthy individuals and those struggling with illness. Research on sense of control and coherence shows positive outcomes in older people, measured in terms of health promotion and improved coping with disease (8,9,10).

If clinicians and geriatric patients are going to collaborate on potential-oriented intervention plans, both must understand the nature of capacity in later life—the ability of the geriatric patient as a person to promote areas of physical and mental health. Psychological growth in later life is particularly important to understand, for the state of the mind with aging significantly influences the state of the body. But for too long, the capacity for psychological and intellectual growth has been seen as being largely completed by the end of adolescence. To better help the person who is the geriatric patient, one needs a much more in-depth understanding of human development in the second half of life.

HUMAN DEVELOPMENT IN THE SECOND HALF OF LIFE: IMPACT ON HEALTH, MENTAL WELLNESS, AND ACCESSING POTENTIAL WITH AGING

To have a sense of possibility for positive change in one's future is to have a sense of hope along with all that is therapeutic and life enhancing through experiencing that hope. The human body experiences a powerful gravitational pull in the direction of hope. That is why the patient's hopes are the physician's secret weapon. They are the hidden ingredients in any prescription.

Norman Cousins

The very least you can do in your life is to figure out what you hope for. And the most you can do is live inside that hope.

Barbara Kingsolver

But throughout so much of the history of science—from evolutionary biology to human development—little has been offered regarding what is possible in the future associated with aging. Until recently, classical evolutionary biology saw no value to aging *per se*, because it saw no natural selection benefit once one became too old to reproduce, a stage relatively early in the aging process (e.g., typically around age 50 in humans). From a human development perspective, little highly developed theory about psychological development has been offered past early adulthood, there is very little theory about middle age, and almost none about later life.

Theories of Human Development

Human development has largely been viewed as a phenomenon occurring in the first half of life, with its biggest effects in the very early years. Many, in fact, have asserted that our brain potential is for the most part determined in the first 3 years of life; they believe that the neurological hard-wiring for both brain development and behavior is essentially completed by the age of three (5).

In comparison, little attention has been paid to developmental stages in the second half of life—as if by then everything is programmed, locked in motion, and ready to decline. The primary exception to this pattern has been the work of Erik Erikson, whose work in stage theory has been viewed as the most comprehensive. Briefly, Erikson's description of different stages of life is framed in terms of dichotomies, indicating different polar directions that an individual's psychodynamic path may take, depending on whether one resolves or comes to terms with new life issues and conflicts confronted at each developmental stage (11). An outline of Erikson's eight developmental stages is presented in Table 1-2.

What becomes evident is that even in Erikson's thoughtful schema, six of the eight developmental stages are in the first half of life, while five occur by adolescence, and only one addresses later life. In fact, when one reviews his seminal work, *Identity and the Life Cycle*, one finds that in the 50-page

TABLE 1-2
ERIKSON'S EIGHT DEVELOPMENT STAGES

Stage	Psychosocial Issue or Crisis
I. Infancy	Trust vs. mistrust
II. Early childhood	Autonomy vs. shame, doubt
III. Play age	Initiative vs. guilt
IV. School age	Industry vs. inferiority
V. Adolescence	Identity vs. identity diffusion
VI. Young adult	Intimacy vs. isolation
VII. Adulthood	Generativity vs. stagnation
VIII. Mature age	Integrity vs. disgust, despair

Adapted from Reference 11.

theoretical discussion of the eight stages, the final three occupy only three pages, with only one page for the eighth stage, Mature Age.

Newly Described Developmental Potential in the Second Half of Life

While Erikson's developmental overview does not represent the only example where stage theory has been attempted with attention to the second half of life, it has been regarded the best effort or the best elaboration of such thinking. Jung theorized about the developmental significance of the second half of life in terms of its task, but he dealt with it as a single stage. He posed the question, "Could by any chance culture be the meaning and purpose of the second half of life?" Daniel Levinson contributed to stage theory, but the major focus of his work was on middle-to-late middle age, without the same depth of analysis on older age groups. Many other attempts focusing on later life have taken more of a categorizing approach as opposed to advancing developmental understanding, with descriptions of the *third age* or Neugarten's classification of the *young-old* versus the *old-old*.

Hence, developmental considerations of the second half of life have been limited and thin. But today, growing interest in aging has generated new research and fresh insights into human development and potential, and new human potential phases in later life have been described (5,12,13). Research is showing how psychological growth and creative expression can continue independent of age, with age, in fact, associated with new internal (psychodynamic) and external (psychosocial) sources of positive stimuli.

Biological Considerations

The first 3 years of life are no longer seen as the period when hard-wiring or development of the central nervous system is completed. Those who study human development are finding more evidence that learning and psychological development is lifelong, and greatly influenced by the ongoing diversity of human experience. Moreover, findings from biological research reveal that brain plasticity and creative potential continue to unfold through new phases of adult physical and emotional development. One of the most fascinating findings in understanding the ongoing capacity for learning and creative development in the second half of life comes from the discovery that when we challenge the mind, the brain biologically responds in positive ways—both anatomically and physiologically—regardless of age (14,15). And not challenging the brain has negative effects (16,17). How brain cells communicate was a great 19th-century debate between Golgi (a network of connected neurons) and Ramon y Cajal (individual neurons, somehow separated from each other). Ramon y Cajal won the Nobel Prize for being correct, thanks to Sherrington's later descriptions of the synapse. Science has shown that a stimulating environment results in individual neurons sprouting new dendritic branches, in turn affecting neurotransmission.

Moreover, a number of other changes, both neuroanatomical and neurochemical, also result from increased brain challenge. Nerve cell bodies and nuclei increase in size. Glia—supportive cells in the brain that help nourish, support, and protect the neurons—increase in number. Choline acetyltransferase, the enzyme involved in the synthesis of acetylcholine—a neurotransmitter that influences memory—becomes more active. It is interesting to note that acetylcholine is the neurotransmitter found to be at deficit levels in AD. Research shows that all of these changes continue independent of age, illustrating neurobiological underpinnings for maintaining a well-functioning mind with advancing years. Newer findings reveal that between one's early 50s and late 70s, there is actually an increase in the density of the dendritic growth at the ends of individual neurons in different parts of the cerebral cortex (18). Yet more recent research discovered that from one's early 50s to late 70s, the length of individual dendrites increases in different parts of the brain (19). Both of these changes—density and length, further reflect the plasticity or modifiability of the brain as it ages. George M. Martin has referred to these changes with aging as reflecting *sageing*. And the most recent discoveries find that *de novo* neurons actually continue to form in different parts of the brain over time (20). Anyone who claims you cannot teach an old dog new tricks is not up to date on brain research. Old dogs can learn, and older humans can as well.

In fact, the more we think and do, the more we contribute to vibrant cell life in the brain. The latest findings from research on the neuroplasticity point strongly to the remodeling effects that lifelong experiences and constructive challenges have on the brain, especially in modifying synapses. Neuroplastic changes associated with aging not only promote new compensatory and adaptive capacities, but also most likely contribute to new neurogenic influences on the psychological manifestations of the mind. It is theorized that among these new manifestations of the aging psyche are the four human potential phases in the second half of life, which will be described later in this chapter (5,21).

Psychological Considerations

When we talk about developmental growth, we are talking about changes at different points in the life cycle—changes in how we view and experience life in a combined psychological, emotional, and intellectual sense. Just as you cannot teach a child to read before he or she is developmentally ready to read, certain qualities of mind and action in adulthood are developmental in nature and unfold in their own good time.

For instance, *wisdom* cannot be taught. It is a developmental mix of age, knowledge, emotional and practical life experience, and brain function, which allows us to integrate those pieces to achieve insight that we can then apply to a variety of life circumstances. Similarly, with aging it is typically easier to define problems with competing solutions and envision multiple strategies to deal with them— what in Piagetian terms is described as *postformal thought* (22). Postformal reasoning helps integrate the subjective and the objective, feeling and thinking, the heart and the mind, and becomes more facile with enhanced dialectical thinking to deal with conflicting opposites in the second half of life. The quality we refer to as *maturity* is itself developmental, as are other aspects of personality that, as they become more highly developed with age, open up new opportunities for us. At different times in our adult lives we can take advantage of this developmental impetus to energize our creativity and jump-start our efforts to explore new ideas or make desired changes.

Creativity can be defined as bringing something new into existence that is valued, be it a great work of art, innovative volunteerism, or a fabulous new recipe (5,18).

Keep in mind that creativity applies not just to artists, but is apparent in all aspects of life, including the social realm where, over the history of civilization, older adults have assumed the creative role of keepers of the culture, transmitting accumulated knowledge and perspective. Creativity also needs to be looked at not just in terms of *big-C* creativity that can change the course of a society or culture through gifts such as great art, ideas, and inventions, but also *little-c* creativity—everyday creativity—that can change the course of an individual or family through personal innovation. Sometimes, little-c creativity can evolve into to big-C creativity, as with Maria Ann Smith who, during her 60s in the 1860s, was experimenting in Australia with different recipes. One was a hardy French crabapple seedling that bore the late-ripening Granny Smith apple, bearing her name, which because of its outstanding taste and keeping qualities, formed the bulk of Australia's apple exports for many years.

The author's own research has demonstrated the significant influence on mental health—even in the midst of

mental disorder—of accessing what he has referred to as *human-potential phases* in the second half of life. They reflect evolving mental maturity, ongoing human development, and psychological growth as we age, and provide new opportunities for accessing human potential throughout midlife and older adulthood. They occur sequentially, but overlap one another time-wise in their transitions. These phases represent the combination of neurobiological, cognitive, and emotional development with the passage of time, expressed in the positive push from within us toward new perspectives, new impetuses for change, and new forms of creative expression from mid-to-later life. These human potential phases are, in effect, inner orientations toward mental wellness that continue throughout the life cycle, right to the end. Descriptions of these four second-half-of-life developmental phases follow:

1. The Mid-Life Re-evaluation Phase (Mid-to-Late 30s Through the Mid-60s): Characterized by a Developmental Impetus—an Internal Drive for Re-evaluation, Exploration, and Transition

Typically occurring in our 40s and 50s, powerful inner stirrings motivate us toward re-evaluating our lives, often leading to new exploration of inner feelings and outer activities, resulting for many in a transition regarding how we deal with thoughts and emotions and the choices we make. Although mid-life crisis is the phrase we hear so often during this period in the life cycle, most middle-age adults are actually more affected by *quest energy* rather than *crisis anxiety*. They are motivated by a new developmental inner push to re-evaluate their lives and work in order to make them more gratifying. The mid-life re-evaluation phase combines the capacity for insightful reflection with a powerful desire to create meaning in life.

Alex Haley in the mid-life re-evaluation phase. Alex Haley poignantly illustrated this inner push for exploration in his Pulitzer Prize-winning book, *Roots*, published when he was 55 and portraying his well-researched seven-generation family history, stimulated by rich memories related by his maternal grandmother. Reminiscent of the midlife quest of Odysseus, Haley pursued leads from his grandmother's oral history and spent 12 years traveling three continents, tracking his maternal family back to Kunta Kinde, a Mandingo youth kidnapped into slavery from the small village of Juffure in Gambia, West Africa. Haley's quest, and *Roots*, catalyzed a soaring interest in family roots on the part of America as a whole.

Madeline Albright in the mid-life re-evaluation phase. Madeline Albright, at age 45, following a devastating divorce after 23 years of marriage, re-evaluated her life and began a new quest. She started teaching government at Georgetown University and hosting insightful foreign-policy discussions in her Washington home. This led to her emergence as a valuable source of political knowledge and perspective, with a world view that attracted Democratic presidential contenders to seek her advice. Her midlife re-evaluation culminated in 1993 at age 56, when she was chosen UN ambassador, and then again in 1997 at age 60, when she was appointed as the United States' first female Secretary of State.

2. The Liberation Phase (Mid-50s to Mid-70s):
Characterized by a Developmental Impetus—an Internal Drive for Liberation, Experimentation, and Innovation
Typically occurring as we approach our 60s to early 70s, creative endeavors are charged with the added energy of a new degree of personal freedom that comes both psychologically from within us, and externally through retirement. Creative expression in this phase often includes translating a feeling of *If not now, when?* into action. People tend to feel comfortable about themselves by this time in life, knowing that if they make a mistake it will not undo the image others have of them, and more importantly, it will not undo the image they have of themselves. This provides a new context, a new comfort level for experimentation and innovation. And retirement often provides a new feeling of finally having time to try something new. Retirement or partial retirement, for many, is like a patron, providing the external freedom to focus on activities other than making ends meet. Both the influence of new inner psychological liberation and the impact of new outer social freedom synergize to produce a powerful and comfortable feeling of being liberated to experiment and to innovate. New comfort and confidence in trying something different is often accompanied by a desire to do the right thing, and a feeling of *What can they do to me?* if the experimentation proves provocative or elicits resistance in the response of others.

Laura Ingalls Wilder in the liberation phase. It was not until her mid-60s that Laura Ingalls Wilder felt sufficient inner freedom to record and share with the public the many fascinating stories from her private childhood memories; until then, she did not feel ready to write them down. Encouraged by her daughter, Laura Ingalls Wilder, at age 64, began work on her first Little House book, *Little House in the Big Woods.* This was followed by her immensely successful *Little House on the Prairie,* at age 68. *Little Town on the Prairie* was published when she was 74, and *Those Happy Golden Years* when she was 76. Her books draw upon her childhood experiences that reflect the spirit, independence, and values of family life on a Midwest farm in the mid-to-late 19th century. They capture the pioneering quality and spirit that characterized the dominant American culture of the late 1800s.

Jim Jeffords in the liberation phase. On May 24, 2001, Senator Jim Jeffords of Vermont changed parties, from Republican to Independent. He consequently altered the control of the Senate, changing it from a Republican to a Democratic majority. While the predominant discussion to explain his actions focused on political and ideological issues, the fact was that Jeffords, at age 68, was right in the middle of the liberation phase. As Jeffords agonized about

the decision, he explained, "I can see more and more instances when I will disagree with the President on very fundamental issues." In *My Declaration of Independence,* Jeffords explained the issues that led to this dramatic break with the President and the Republican Party. With that liberation-phase quality of a growing inner pressure—an inner push to do the right thing—in his declaration Jeffords wrote, "But in the end I had to be true to what I thought was right, and leave the consequences to sort themselves out in the days ahead." So many of the words he used during this period were charged with liberation-phase associations, such as the title of his book that followed in 2003, *An Independent Man: Adventures of a Public Servant.*

3. The Summing-Up Phase (Late-60s into the 90s):
Characterized by a Developmental Impetus—an Internal Drive for Recapitulation, Resolution, and Contribution
In this phase, typically occurring in one's 70s and older, individuals feel more urgently the desire to find larger meaning in the story of their lives through a process of looking back, summing-up, and giving back. They also begin to experience themselves even more strongly as keepers of the culture, and wish to contribute to others more of whatever wisdom and wealth they may have accrued. Creative expression in this phase often includes a recapitulation and review of one's life through personal story-telling, memoirs, and autobiography. In the process of reviewing what one has experienced, received, and gained, there is often a feeling of wanting to contribute to society—a desire to give back through volunteerism, community activism, and philanthropy. And, in looking back and summing-up, there is also reflection on what remains unresolved or unfinished—unresolved conflicts or issues, and unfinished business or unfulfilled dreams. Passion or commitment in any of these areas can translate into community-focused actions reflecting social creativity.

Martha Graham in the summing-up phase. Martha Graham reigned for more than half a century as the indisputable high priestess of modern dance. She danced until she was 75, and then continued to influence dance through her choreography. Her choreography represented a summing-up process that, on the one hand, offered a way of giving back what she had gained to an even larger audience, while on the other hand, provided an impetus to satisfy not yet fulfilled dreams of further accomplishment. In the process, she contributed enormously to keeping the culture of modern dance alive. Her method of dance training has been widely adopted in classes and colleges around the world. Her dance language was intended to express universal human emotions and experiences beyond displays of graceful movements; both her work and her life demonstrated that the poignancy of these emotions knows no endpoint in the life cycle. These later works included *Mendicants of Evening* (age 79), *Lucifer* (age 81), *The Owl and the Pussycat* (age 84), and

Frescoes (age 86). In the early 1980s, she created neoclassical dances, beginning with *Acts of Light* (age 87). Her last work was *Maple Leaf Rag*, choreographed in 1990 at age 96.

Giuseppe Verdi in the summing-up phase. Critics marvel that Guiseppe Verdi was in his 80th year when he composed his celebrated opera, *Falstaff*. But what motivated Verdi to compose *Falstaff*, rather than a different opera? The dynamics of the summing-up human potential phase offer an explanation. Many older people going through their summing-up phase look back at any unfinished business. Verdi had unfinished business that gnawed at him for more than half a century. When he was 25, Verdi attempted to compose an opera buffa—a comic opera—*Un Giorno di Regno* (King for a Day). It opened in 1840 in the famous theater La Scala, but was received so poorly that it was canceled after that one performance. Verdi had recently lost his wife and a year earlier his infant son; he became overcome with despair, vowing never to compose another opera. The director of La Scala tactfully and sensitively released Verdi from his contract, but when he felt Verdi's emotional trauma was healing, he gently encouraged him to write a new opera. The result was *Nebucco* in 1842, the success of which established Verdi's reputation in Italy. Fifty-five years after *Un Giorno di Regno* flopped, Verdi, at the top of his field and in his summing-up phase, looked back at unfinished business—his failure to compose a successful comic opera. Deciding it was time to set the picture straight and provide the missing chapter, he composed a great comic libretto, *Falstaff*. And to leave no stain unremoved, he arranged to have *Falstaff* open in the same theater where the earlier sad disappointment had occurred, La Scala. *Falstaff*, of course, was greeted at La Scala as a resounding success, one of the finest operas ever written. For Verdi, it was a moment of triumph and resolution.

4. The Encore Phase (Late-70s to the End of the Life Cycle): Characterized by a Developmental Impetus—an Internal Drive for Reflection, Continuation, and Celebration of Self, Family, Community, Culture, and Spirituality

The encore phase generally starts during one's late 70s, becoming more pronounced during one's 80s to the end of life. Plans and actions are shaped by the desire to restate and reaffirm major themes in one's life, but also to explore novel variations on those themes. There may be the desire to make a final statement, or to seize a further opportunity to take care of unfinished business or unresolved conflicts, or to surprise people with something new. One continues to be motivated by life's energy and the audience of others, reflecting upon and affirming life by continuing to live it in a vital way, and celebrating one's place in family, community, and in the spiritual realm. Often at this stage of life, one is also a catalyst for families and communities to celebrate, through reunions and honorific recognition focused on these long-

lifers. Celebratory reunions promote solidarity by bringing families together, while special recognition events model the value of lifelong contribution to one's community. Thus, the vital continuation of the older individual fosters continuity in extended family relationships and community togetherness in celebrating valued older members.

The Delany Sisters in the encore phase. At the age of 104, retired teacher Sarah Delany collaborated with her 102-year-old sister, retired dentist Dr. Bessie Delany, to write *Having Our Say: The Delany Sisters' First 100 Years*. It was a wonderful example of an encore phase celebration of something quite remarkable—a relationship that had most satisfyingly endured for more than a century, one of the longest human relationships ever. The book became a *New York Times* bestseller and a Broadway hit. In 1994, the sisters, at 105 and 103, published a sequel, as they drew further upon the potential for creative expression associated with the encore human potential phase. Two years later Bessie Delany died, and suddenly, for the first time in over a century, Sarah Delany felt alone. Among her creative coping strategies was another encore human potential phase product, writing the book *On My Own* at age 107.

George Abbott in the encore phase. George Abbott (1887– 1995), the American director of theater and film, playwright, actor, and producer, had a career that spanned more than eight decades and 120 productions. These productions ranged from *Love 'em and Leave 'em* (in 1925 at age 38) to *Frankie* (in 1989 at age 101), which was a two-act musical remake of *Frankenstein*. The shows he was involved with accrued an awesome 40 Tony Awards, including five for George Abbott on his own. It was remarkable enough that he wrote *Damn Yankees* when he was 68, but he also decided on an encore by collaborating on a Broadway revival of *Damn Yankees* at age 107.

To know that the natural course of one's inner development in the second half of life can bring one closer at different times to accessing unexpressed capacity, improved coping, or one's creative potential, should increase an individual's incentive to work at seizing the moment while in the midst of one of these human potential phases. These phases can set the stage for creative expression that commences in the second half of life; they can precipitate a change in the direction of one's creative expression; they can provide new energy to promote a continuation of one's ongoing creative work; they can enable one to become creative in response to loss.

These phases do not automatically produce growth or creative expression, but they have the potential to do so. What is most critical is that individuals, significant others, and society know that these phases are there, waiting to be nurtured and tapped, through one's own efforts and/or through the help of others.

Anaïs Nin, a central figure in the new feminism of the 1970s, wrote her seven *Journals* from age 63 to the time of her death at 74, providing a passionate and candid account of her voyage of self-discovery. Among her poignant insights was the realization: "And the day came when the risk to remain tight in a bud was more painful than the risk it took to blossom."

THE SOCIAL PORTFOLIO: PROMOTING HEALTH AND INDEPENDENCE THROUGH SOCIAL ENGAGEMENT AND PRODUCTIVE ACTIVITIES

Among the most common questions raised about aging is, "What can one do to increase the likelihood of a healthy and satisfying later life?" and the related question, "What can one do to promote independence and access potential with aging?" Usually, advice is offered in two domains:

- *Adopting good health habits* that can reduce the risk of physical disease and disability—such as not smoking, following good nutrition practices, maintaining regular exercise, addressing somatic symptoms when they occur, scheduling regular doctor visits, etc.
- *Developing a diversified and balanced financial portfolio* to ensure economic comfort and security in one's later years—a plan that considers both sufficient assets to draw upon in retirement, and special resources that would become available should disability occur.

In contrast, advice of a mental health nature is given short shrift; the succinct old standby "stay active" is commonly delivered, though not elaborated on. The idea of developing a social portfolio has not even been in the shadow of the sense of importance of building a financial portfolio (5,24,25).

Historical Controversy and Confusion about the Relationship of Activity to Aging

Historically, considerable controversy was generated around the concept of *activity* through interpersonal involvement and mental challenge in gerontology (25). This may in part explain why mental health promotion efforts relating to staying active socially were on a slow track, if not derailed, for so long. Controversy was generated by the *disengagement theory*, which maintained that high satisfaction in old age was associated with accepting the inevitability of reduction in social and personal interactions (26). Misinterpretation and misuse of the disengagement theory undermined both personal and societal motivation to actively foster social opportunity and activity for older adults; many rationalized that the goal or norm of aging was to disengage. Proponents of the *activity theory* challenged this thinking, asserting that maintaining activity for most individuals in later life is important for obtaining and sustaining satisfaction, self-esteem, and overall health (27). Findings from longitudinal studies on aging added support to the activity theory. The disengagement versus activity debate highlighted

both the confusion around mental health promotion practices in later life, and the sparse research on such strategies.

Late-20th-Century Findings from Brain and Behavior Research on Aging

In the midst of confusion about the role and impact of activity with aging, new findings from brain and behavior studies emerged, introducing a growing impetus for promoting not only social activity, but mental challenge for older people. This research, as discussed earlier, showed that in response to mental and behavioral challenge, the brain and its neurons responded both neuroanatomically and neurophysiologically to cognitively and environmentally stimulating environments. And, in contrast to the stereotype of brain anatomy and function being on an irreversible course of reduction with age, all of the changes in response to environmental and behavioral challenge continued with aging. The brain was found to maintain plasticity—the ability for positive modifiability—independent of age. In effect, the aging brain was found to respond to mental exercise in much the same way that muscle responds to physical exercise, regardless of age. This dramatic influence of behavior on biology has profound ramifications for the role of stimulating social activities in promoting both mental and physical health with aging. Modern neuroscience supported common sense advice from longstanding folk wisdom to *use it or lose it*, but took it a step further, showing there was no age limit for using it to prevent losing it.

Moving from research examining the influence of social activity on the aging brain to investigations studying its effect on the aging body, a study by Glass et al. is of note (28). In this collaborative project that selected for older "couch potatoes"—human subjects aged 65 and older involved in limited physical exercise—the positive impact of social activity on overall health was remarkable. The investigators reported: "Social and productive activities that involve little or no enhancement of fitness lower the risk of all cause mortality as much as fitness activities do."

The findings from this study suggest that in addition to increased cardiopulmonary fitness, activity may confer survival benefits through psychosocial pathways. Social and productive activities that require less physical exertion may complement exercise programs and constitute alternative intervention for elderly people. Research on social and mental activity for older people is demonstrating not only significant effect on mental health with aging, but also on physical health and survival in later life (Table 1-3)(29,30).

The Social Portfolio

With late 20th-century research bringing us back on track in understanding the role of social and mental stimulation influencing, and indeed promoting, mental health as well

TABLE 1-3

SELECTED BENEFICIAL ACTIVITIES FOR OLDER PEOPLE

Social Activities	Productive Activities	Physical Fitness Activities
▪ Church attendance	▪ Gardening	▪ Active sports or swimming
▪ Visits to cinema, restaurants, sporting events	▪ Preparing meals	▪ Walking
▪ Day or overnight trips	▪ Shopping	▪ Physical exercise
▪ Playing cards, games, bingo	▪ Unpaid community Work	
▪ Participation in social groups	▪ Paid community work	
	▪ Other paid employment	

See reference 28.

as physical health in later life, the question then becomes how to translate research findings effectively into practice. At the same time, the need for additional research addressing the application of mental health and aging advances into new health promotion practices for older adults becomes apparent.

Returning to the question about how to promote a healthier and more satisfying later life, what can be said at present from a mental health and social activities perspective? One approach relates to the eloquent advice that Samuel Johnson, at age 70, wrote in a letter to his friend, Boswell, in 1779:

If you are idle, be not solitary;
if you are solitary, be not idle.

An attempt to adapt Samuel Johnson's sage advice, along with findings from activity theory research and brain stimulation studies, into a practical protocol led to the development of the social portfolio approach. While people in the modern work force are advised to plan for economic security for their future—to strive for a balanced financial portfolio—too little attention is paid to developing a balanced social portfolio based on sound activities, mental challenges, and interpersonal relationships that can be carried into old age.

The diagram of a social portfolio (Figure 1-1) in preparation for later life reflects efforts to plan for the future, balancing individual with group activities, and balancing high mobility/energy endeavors (activities that require significant physical exertion) with low mobility/energy ones (5). Four categories of equal importance are thereby created: group/high mobility, group/low mobility, individual/high mobility, and individual/low mobility. The social portfolio is a way of helping people develop new

strengths and satisfactions while aging, even in the face of loss.

The financial portfolio has three major concepts that influence its growth and development:

▪ Assets to draw upon, with emphasis on diversification;
▪ Insurance back-up, should disability or related loss occur; and
▪ The idea that you start early and build over time, though it is never too late.

The social portfolio is designed with an analogous three major concepts in mind.

1. One's assets are the diversified interests and relationships that one can develop and draw upon.
2. The insurance back-up is addressed by focusing on two dichotomies:
   a. Individual versus group activities, and
   b. High energy/high mobility versus low energy/low mobility activities.

The concept here is that should loss occur in the form of a decline in physical health, not all the interests one has developed should require high energy or high mobility; similarly, if loss of a spouse or friend occurs, in the transition of dealing with such loss one should have interests that he or she can draw upon that do not require the involvement of another.

3. The idea that one starts early and builds is the third concept. Thus, if one has an interest in writing, he or she can start by taking a course in creative writing, and in retirement, when one has more time, write the great American novel.

Tapping Creative Potential in Later Life

	GROUP EFFORTS	INDIVIDUAL EFFORTS
HIGH MOBILITY HIGH ENERGY	*GROUP-HIGH MOBILITY* • Coordinating a new volunteer group in a neglected area • International folk-dance lessons in host countries • Running for an elected office in your local community	*INDIVIDUAL-HIGH MOBILITY* • Creating neighborhood showcase garden • Creating an annotated walking tour of your town • Documentary photographer of family mementos
LOW MOBILITY LOW ENERGY	*GROUP-LOW MOBILITY* • Creating best joke and pot-luck dinner group • Creating family newspaper with children/grandchildren • Hosting *provocative novels* book club at your home	*INDIVIDUAL-LOW MOBILITY* • Creating the *secret recipes* family cookbook • Creating family tree with dynamic commentary • creating *ultimate e-Mail letters to grandchildren*

Figure 1-1 The Social Portfolio: Examples of Group and Individual Efforts. Adapted from Reference 5.

Social Portfolio Planning Strategies

Older people seeking practical social portfolio planning strategies could be encouraged to arrange a round-robin advice-giving dinner with close friends, to get the perspectives of those who know them best as to what might be areas of interest or strength to further develop. The way this works is that everyone in the group takes turns focusing on one individual in the group, with each sharing views about the strengths, talents, and areas that the person in the spotlight might consider for further involvement. For example, someone who takes interesting snapshots might be encouraged to take a course on photography in their middle years, and in retirement go on to become the family's documentary photographer through camera visits with the extended family (*group active*). Someone who likes exotic foods might be encouraged to take up cooking more formally, and in retirement to develop an evolving loose-leaf notebook of the latest-rage recipes (*individual passive*). Someone who likes reading and book reviews might be encouraged to set up a book club on bestsellers (*group passive*). Someone who enjoys both physical activity and architecture might develop a walking tour of interesting buildings in the community for the local chamber of commerce (*individual active*).

In addition to the round-robin social portfolio planning strategy described above, there are some other straightforward planning approaches that can be followed, allowing individuals to invest in their own social portfolios to identify new activities and new relationships. These approaches themselves can contribute to an older person's sense of control in everyday life (5,25).

Conduct an audit. For each social portfolio category, individuals should list the activities, friendships, or other relationships that are already part of their lives. What portion of one's time is spent in solo activity? Group activity? With close friends? Family? Coworkers or new acquaintances? How much of one's activity is low energy or low mobility, and how much of it requires more energy and mobility? If one's list under any particular category is thin or empty, that's the type of activity or relationship he or she needs to build.

Create a reserve of ideas by listing several things one does well. Individuals should expand their options and be bold. One does not have to skydive like the first President Bush did in his 70s. But individuals should be wary of limiting their options based on their past, or on the wishes of family and friends. They should be open to the idea of trying something new—tapping into the dynamics of the liberation phase that developmentally they are likely to be experiencing.

Aim for diversity and balance in the way one invests his or her time and energy among people and activities. Depending on the nature of social interaction that is underrepresented in one's current portfolio, one could develop opportunities for group and solo activities, low-mobility and high-mobility options, and low-energy and high-energy options.

Call local colleges, universities, community colleges, community centers, and other resources, looking for programs one might attend to advance one's learning or experience in an interest area. Individuals might recruit company from among those they believe will make their venture more enjoyable, or simply less daunting. Attending a community college could bring the added dimension of an intergenerational learning environment.

Visit a local bookstore's hobbies and jobs section. This a good way to jog new ideas for a potential new hobby, interesting part-time work, or small business venture in areas that one did not have the time or opportunity to pursue in the past. It could be an opportunity to address unfinished business or unfulfilled dreams.

Consult community-based information and referral programs for older adults. Consulting organizations such as Area Agencies on Aging and Senior Centers is another way of gathering information about local programs targeted toward older people.

Make the commitment to oneself. Whether one chooses to develop a solitary interest, attend a class, travel, or socialize in another way more often or with different people, he or she should follow through with this plan. One should look for ways to get the most out of the experience by investing one's time and attention in the activity and in any new relationships it offers. These are pathways to developing new individual mastery and interpersonal growth.

Be adaptable. One should have a rainy day plan for an unforeseen change in his or her social network of significant others and/or physical health status.

Social Portfolio Marriage/Relationship Enrichment Tracks

Collaborative approaches can be used to strengthen one's relationships and deepen emotional intimacy or connectedness—goals that many individuals hold to build upon the foundation of or to revitalize their marriage or other relationships. The following exercises are designed to expand, through various activities and efforts, the opportunity for personal growth for both partners in a significant relationship (5). These kinds of positive experiences enhance self-esteem and satisfaction with each other and the relationship. To set the stage for this work:

■ Individuals should start with a better understanding of their relationship's beginnings, for example, thinking about the basic internal and external forces at work in

their marriage. People marry for different reasons: love, intimacy, sex, close and enduring companionship, having a soul mate, personal identity and a sense of completion in the marriage partnership, having children and cultivating a family life. What brought the two individuals together? What has kept them together? What more or different aspects do they desire from the relationship?

■ Individuals should identify aspects of their relationship they feel need improvement. Too often, personal dissatisfaction with one's own situation is taken out on the marriage. Partners should sort out the issues that undermine emotional intimacy and connectedness.

■ Individuals should identify opportunities for growth in their relationship and in their individual lives. Appealing new activities nourish the chemistry of a close relationship, enriching the relationship by helping both partners feel good about themselves and each other and, consequently, about the marriage. Appealing new activities not only help maintain and repair a relationship, they influence even more its growth. Fundamentally, they are pathways for discovering new aspects of oneself and of those close to the individual. Interesting new activities with friends and family promote interaction, sharing, and communication, as well as enhanced individual mastery and interpersonal growth.

Track I Activity Plan: Personal Inner Growth

These activities focus on inner growth for an individual and his or her partner, on a personal level and in relation to others, but not involving the two partners together.

■ One could explore new activities separate from one's partner, and new activities just by oneself. For example, one could create a new home-based self-learning program on an engaging topic, which one could build upon over time. One could read and collect books and other materials that support one's interest. Such activities enhance one's sense of control and individual mastery.

■ One could explore new activities separate from one's partner and involving others. This approach reduces the risk of too much pressure being placed on any one relationship. For example, one could take a class with others (not including one's partner), especially one that is exciting and could be built upon, and where there is active interaction with the others. Or one could create a family tree or write a family history, ideally a project that has personal meaning for the individual and enables him or her to better understand oneself and one's roots.

■ One could encourage and support his or her partner's inner growth through activities that are separate from oneself and solitary for one's partner. Similarly, one could encourage and support activities that involve one's partner with others, but not with oneself.

Track II Activity Plan: Shared Activities for Growth as a Couple

These activities focus on efforts in one's relationship together with one's partner, first as a couple alone, and then as a couple in relation to others. These activities promote new exploration, with a sense of novelty and revitalization.

- The couple could together explore new activities that are exciting for both people and offer the opportunity to build on the activity over time—for example, a sport or recreational pastime, music, dancing, travel, theater, or sampling ethnic cuisine.
- The couple could explore new activities that enable both partners, as a couple, to share meaningful time with old friends, or to develop new ones to expand their shared circle of social relationships.
- Each member of the couple should save something special just for each other. Some activities that can be enjoyed as a couple alone may also be fun to share with others, but partners should find ways to develop facets of these activities in ways that are uniquely intimate for each partner.

Conclusion about the Social Portfolio

The social portfolio represents, on the one hand, an attempt to articulate common sense and folk wisdom about fostering overall health in aging through a balanced plan of action, with built-in contingencies, to keep one socially and intellectually stimulated in later life. On the other hand, it offers research-based practical advice for maintaining both mental and physical health with aging, and reminds us of the broader need and opportunity to advance research on health promotion in later life. Ultimately, the social portfolio provides the opportunity to increase individual mastery and to enhance interpersonal growth, while promoting overall health and quality of life as one ages.

The journey of a thousand miles begins with one step.
Lao-Tse

RETIREMENT

A sound social portfolio helps one prepare for the second half of life in general, and for retirement or partial retirement in particular. But, fewer than 10% of retirees have had any formal retirement planning focused on how they will actually spend their retired time (31). The development of at least a preliminary social portfolio increases the likelihood of a more satisfying and fulfilling retirement experience. In addition to working on a social portfolio, the following retirement readiness questionnaire can be useful for individuals contemplating retirement, by helping them

assess if they are indeed ready and reasonably prepared (Table 1-4) (31).

Strategies to Challenge One's Mind and Improve One's Health in Aging and Retirement

The 10 strategies in Table 1-5 represent an attempt to apply scientific findings, showing that when older people are involved socially and challenge themselves with productive and everyday creative activities, both their overall health and sense of well-being improve. These strategies similarly reflect an effort to apply landmark results from neuroscience studies revealing that when we continue to challenge our minds in the second half of life, our brain cells sprout new dendrites and develop new synapses, which improve communication within the brain, regardless of age. These strategies are useful during later life in general, and in retirement in particular. They represent useful advice that practitioners can provide to older patients and to older people as a whole in a health promotion context.

TABLE 1-4
RETIREMENT READINESS QUESTIONNAIRE

Directions for Completing the Retirement Readiness Questionnaire

---

Take some time to think about the following questions and what your answers tell you about your thoughts on retirement. If you have not given much thought to any of these questions, or if you do not have many good answers for them, you are probably not well-prepared for retirement. Using these questions as a guide, how can you improve your preparation?

1. Why are you thinking about retirement now?
2. Do you want to retire?
3. Have you attended a retirement preparation program or seminar focused on financial planning?
4. Have you attended a retirement preparation program or seminar focused on social planning (e.g., community activities and interpersonal endeavors)?
5. How would your finances be if you retired now?
6. Have you developed any outside interests, hobbies, volunteer activities, or areas of new learning?
7. Have you planned new activities where you would interact with people on a regular basis, offering opportunities for new friendships?
8. What do your family and friends say about you retiring?
9. Have you considered whether you want a complete or partial retirement? In other words, have you considered part-time or temporary work, or even a less than full-time small business venture? The emphasis here is on *consideration*.
10. During retirement, will the process of making at least a modest contribution through helping out in various volunteer or other activities be sufficient for you, or do you feel you need to make an immediate major difference in what you do?
11. What is important and fulfilling for you? How do your retirement plans relate to your thinking here?
12. What gives you a sense of meaning and purpose in life? How do your retirement plans relate to your thinking here?

TABLE 1-5
TEN WAYS TO CHALLENGE YOUR MIND AND IMPROVE YOUR HEALTH IN AGING

Here are just 10 of the ways you can reinvent yourself, tap hidden potential, challenge your mind, be productive, and utilize creativity in everyday life throughout the second half of life. These suggestions represent doable components of a social portfolio, offering new opportunities for individual mastery, interpersonal growth, and enhanced health.

1. *Play games and do crossword puzzles that challenge your mind.* Word games in particular provide both social stimulation and mental challenge. Studies show that you can continue to increase your vocabulary at least into your 80s.
2. *Plan a dinner and book or video discussion group for a circle of friends.* Provocative discussion and food for thought in a stimulating and entertaining social activity is as good for the mind as it is for the palate.
3. *Travel to someplace new—locally or away.* Identify a new place you would like to visit and go there, either alone or with a friend or family. It can be as close as a new museum exhibit in town, or as far away as the Orient. Develop a diary on these visits, and be creative in what you write or sketch.
4. *Take an educational course—explore a new area.* Lifelong learning provides for lifelong growth and development. Today's increasing intergenerational mix in continuing education classrooms provides opportunities for interesting new knowledge and relationships. Combine learning and travel through programs like Elderhostel.
5. *Explore the hobby or crafts section at a bookstore for new ideas.* Even if you are not sure what you might be interested in, browsing through the enormous diversity of books on hobbies and crafts may ignite new curiosity, or remind you of a long-standing interest that you never had time to pursue in the past.
6. *Volunteer.* Volunteering is a way of sharing special skills or learning new ones while interacting with people and providing community service, or even just helping neighbors. It can be an avenue to experiment with new approaches and to work with all age groups. Even among those in their early 80s, more than one-fourth still volunteer.
7. *Consider new work or a new career—perhaps part-time.* Part-time and temporary work as well as involvement in small businesses increases with age. And attitudes toward older workers are improving, particularly in our expanding service-oriented society, where the experience and conscientiousness of seasoned workers pays off. Check out books on jobs, visit a career counselor, and venture ahead.
8. *Write letters or email regularly to family members and friends.* Letters have become so scarce these days that receiving one will thrill a friend or loved one. Feel free to be creative and funny in your writing. You will be stimulating your creative side while at the same time entertaining the recipient. E-mail keeps you up with the times and in touch with grandchildren, who typically return e-mails but not letters.
9. *Develop a dream journal.* Dreams and day dreams are among the best illustrations of our inner creativity. Their form and content are the essence of creative expression. Write them down and/or draw them. They may open your eyes to inner thoughts and desires, and help you tap into your creative potential.
10. *Write your memoirs or autobiography, or a family history.* Autobiographies are not just for the famous. Developing a genealogy, family history, or memoirs provides a wonderful, valuable gift to the family. It can also launch you on a new creative journey of personal exploration and discovery, getting you in touch with fascinating historical and inner psychological roots.

Adapted from Reference 5.

In the past few years, I have made a thrilling discovery . . . that until one is over 60, one can never really learn the secret of living. One can then begin to live, not simply with the intense part of oneself, but with one's entire being.

Ellen Glasgow (Pulitzer Prize winner at age 67)

REFERENCES

1. Older Americans 2000. In: Federal Interagency Forum on Aging-Related Statistics. http://www.agingstats.gov/chartbook2000/default.htm. Accessed Dec 10, 2004.
2. US Department of Commerce. *We the American Elderly.* Washington, DC: US Department of Commerce, Economics and Statistics Administration, Bureau of the Census; 1993.
3. Bengtson VL, Cutler NE, Mangen DJ, et al. Generations, cohorts, and relations between age groups. In: Binstock RH, Shanus E, eds. *Handbook of Aging and the Social Sciences.* New York: Van Nostrand Reinhold; 1985:415–449.
4. US Senate Special Committee on Aging. *Aging America: Trends and Projections.* Washington, DC: US Department of Health and Human Services; 1991.
5. Cohen GD. *The Creative Age: Awakening Human Potential in the Second Half of Life.* New York: AVON Books; 2000.
6. World Health Organization website. http://www.who.int/about definition/en. Accessed Dec 10, 2004.
7. Cohen GD. Development and personal growth in middle age and older adulthood. *Dimensions.* 2004;11(1):1.
8. Cohen GD. Mental wellness and aging: human development and personal growth in mid-life and older adulthood. *Generations Today.* In press.
9. Rodin J. Aging and health: effect of the sense of control. *Science.* 1986;233(4770):1271–1276.
10. Lutgendorf SK, Vitaliano PP, Tripp-Reimer T, Harvey JH, Lubaroff DM. Sense of coherence moderates the relationship between life stress and natural killer cell activity in healthy older adults. *Psychol Aging.* 1999;14(4):552–563.
11. Erikson E. *Identity and the Life Cycle.* New York: International Universities Press, Inc.; 1959.
12. Cohen GD. Human potential phases in the second half of life: mental health theory development. *Am J Geriatr Psychiatry.* 1999;7(1):1–7.
13. Cohen GD. Creativity with aging: four phases of potential in the second half of life. *Geriatrics.* 2001;56(4):51–57.
14. Diamond MC, Krech S, Rosenzweig MR. The effects of an enriched environment on the histology of the rat cortex. *J Comp Neurol.* 1964;123:111–120.
15. Diamond MC. An optimistic view of the aging brain. In: Smyer MA, ed. *Mental Health and Aging.* New York: Springer Publishing Co.; 1993:59–63.

16. Krech D, Rosenzweig M, Bennett E. Environmental impoverishment, social isolation and changes in brain chemistry and anatomy. *Physiol Behav.* 1966;1:99–104.

17. Maletta GJ, Timiras PS. Acetylcholinesterase and butyrylcholinesterase activities in optic areas of rats after complete light deprivation from birth. *Exp Neurol.* 1967;19:513–518.

18. Flood DG, Buell SJ, Defiore CH, Horwitz GJ, Coleman PD. Age-related dendritic growth in dentate gyrus of human brain is followed by regression in the "oldest old." *Brain Res.* 1985;345(2): 366–368.

19. Flood DG, Coleman PD. Hippocampal plasticity in normal aging and decreased plasticity in Alzheimer's disease. *Prog Brain Res.* 1990;83:435–443.

20. Gould E, Reeves AJ, Graziano MS, Gross CG. Neurogenesis in the neocortex of adult primates. *Science.* 1999;286(5439): 548–552.

21. Cohen GD. Presentation on human potential phases. International Congress of the International Psychogeriatric Association. Chicago, IL, Aug 22,2003.

22. Sinnott JD. Creativity and postformal thought: why the last stage is the creative stage. In: Adams-Price CE, ed. *Creativity & Successful Aging.* New York: Springer Publishing Co.; 1998:43–72.

23. Cohen GD. Creativity and aging: ramifications for research, practice, and policy. *Geriatrics.* 1998;53(Suppl):S4–S8.

24. Cohen GD. Mental health promotion in later life: the case for the social portfolio. *Am J Geriatr Psychiatry.* 1995;3:277–279.

25. Cohen GD. The social portfolio: the role of activity in mental wellness as people age. In: Ronch JL, Goldfield JA, eds. *Mental Wellness in Aging.* Baltimore: Health Professions Press; 2003: 113–122.

26. Cumming E, Henry EW. *Growing Old: The Process of Disengagement.* New York: Basic Books; 1961.

27. Havighurst RJ, Neugarten BL, Tobin SS. Disengagement, personality, and life satisfaction in the later years. In: Hansen P, ed. *Age with a Future.* Copenhagen: Munksgoard; 1963:419–425.

28. Glass TA, de Leon CM, Marottoli RA, Berkman LF. Population-based study of social and productive activities as predictors of survival among elderly Americans. *BMJ.* 1999;319: 478–483.

29. Avlund K, Damsgaard MT, Holstein BE. Social relations and mortality: an eleven year follow-up study of 70-year-old men and women in Denmark. *Soc Sci Med.* 1998;47(5):635–643.

30. Welin L, Larsson B, Svardsudd K, Tibblin B, Tibblin G. Social network and activities in relation to mortality from cardiovascular disease, cancer and other causes: a 12 year follow up of the study of men born in 1913 and 1923. *J Epidemiol Community Health.* 1992;46(2):127–132.

31. Cohen GD. Retirement: advising older adults who are contemplating this change. *Geriatrics.* 2002;57(8):37–38.

The Geriatric Psychiatrist

2

Alan Siegal   Jeanne Jackson-Siegal

The geriatric psychiatrist is a relatively new subspecialist in the field of psychiatry; in fact, it has only been since the late 1970s that geriatric psychiatry has emerged as a career in its own right. Before that, although they had always treated older patients with mental disorders, psychiatrists did not have the benefit of formalized geriatric training or the support of a professional organization. Much has changed in the few decades since geriatric psychiatry was formally recognized by the American Psychiatric Association (APA). These developments were motivated by the tremendous need for psychiatric skills in long-term care settings, and by the growing number of individuals suffering from Alzheimer's disease (AD) and other dementias. As a result, the opportunities for geriatric psychiatrists have continued to expand. The first section of this chapter will briefly review the history of geriatric psychiatry, its current training requirements, and the range of career opportunities. The remainder of the chapter serves as a practical guide to those interested in setting up a private practice in geriatric psychiatry.

The demographic demands of this country's growing population continue to drive the field of geriatric psychiatry at a rapid pace. For example, in 1997 approximately 12.7% of the US population—or 35 million Americans—were over the age of 65. By 2030 this number is anticipated to increase to 20% of the population (1,2). Currently, there are over 1.6 million individuals in over 16,000 long-term care facilities in the United States, and it is estimated that over 80% of them suffer from mental illness (3). Dementia represents the most common psychiatric diagnosis, followed by depression (3). High rates of mental illness are also seen in older populations across both community and clinical settings (4). On the basis of these statistics, it has been estimated that 5,000 clinically-based geriatric

psychiatrists and 400 to 500 academic geriatric psychiatrists will be needed by 2010 to adequately care for the nation's elderly (1,5). Unfortunately, the current number of board-certified geriatric psychiatrists provides only slightly more than half of this number. These figures, however, illustrate both the great need and the burgeoning opportunities for the geriatric psychiatrist.

A HISTORY OF GERIATRIC PSYCHIATRY

Geriatric psychiatry, initially called Old Age Psychiatry, originated in England. The growth of the field in the United States began in 1978 at the annual APA meeting in Atlanta, GA, when a small group of psychiatrists conceptualized the vision of a national organization. The American Association for Geriatric Psychiatry (AAGP) was subsequently established by a number of leaders and experts in the field, including Sanford Finkel, MD, who became AAGP's first president in 1979. The initial goals of AAGP included:

- The dissemination of information to psychiatrists caring for the elderly
- The expansion of the APA's focus on geriatric training and research
- Policy development for late-life mental health issues
- The encouragement of local societies throughout the United States whose concerns would concentrate on the mental health aspects of aging

Over the past 25 years, the AAGP has grown to over 1,700 members and employs a full-time staff of 13. The AAGP exemplifies a vibrant, growing, and dynamic organization. Through the commitment of the board and dedicated editors, the *American Journal of Geriatric Psychiatry* now ranks as a premier psychiatric journal. In 2003, the mission of the AAGP expanded, as did the professional disciplines of its members. In addition to psychiatrists, membership is now comprised of neurologists, primary care physicians, psychologists, social workers, and nurse clinicians dedicated to the care of the elderly.

TRAINING REQUIREMENTS FOR GERIATRIC PSYCHIATRY

The AAGP successfully lobbied for added qualifications for board certification in geriatric psychiatry, and thus far, nearly 2,600 psychiatrists have obtained this rank. Despite attaining board certification, many of the 2,600 do not practice geriatric psychiatry full-time. Added qualifications in geriatric psychiatry require that a candidate first achieve board certification in adult psychiatry, and complete a 1-year fellowship in geriatric psychiatry (in the fifth postgraduate year) at a site approved by the Accreditation Council for Graduate Medical Education (ACGME). The certification is valid for 10 years before proficiency testing is required for renewal. Twenty years ago, only a handful of first-rate academic settings offered geriatric psychiatry fellowship training programs. The explosion in geriatric psychiatry research and training has resulted in many medical schools now having geriatric medicine, as well as geriatric psychiatry sections providing clinical care, training for medical students and residents, and an expanded number of fellowship training positions.

A complete list of geriatric psychiatry fellowship programs is available from the AAGP website (www.aagponline.org). As of 2005, there are 56 accredited programs offering 137 positions. In 2002, however, only 61% of these positions were filled. ACGME criteria require that geriatric psychiatry fellowship programs offer a mix of experiences including inpatient and outpatient care, consultation and liaison psychiatry, and nursing home care. The 1-year fellowship allows candidates to acquire important clinical knowledge and exposure to research methodology. Some programs also offer a second research year as an option.

During the fellowship year, there are numerous funded opportunities for fellows to become involved in the AAGP and begin to network with colleagues and leaders in the field. These additional fellowships usually provide funding to attend the AAGP annual meeting, and sometimes committee meetings as well. Such contacts can be invaluable in terms of research collaboration, joint writing projects, and both academic and practice opportunities. One unique program for early career psychiatrists, psychologists, and nurse clinicians is the week-long Summer Research Institute, sponsored by the National Institute of Mental Health (NIMH) and the AAGP. This research "boot camp" covers the nuts and bolts of academic research skills, and provides opportunities to network and interact with senior geriatric researchers and staff from NIMH. It has proven to be an incubator for many of the best and brightest researchers in geriatric psychiatry.

PRACTICE OPTIONS FOR GERIATRIC PSYCHIATRISTS

Choices abound as to where one might practice geriatric psychiatry. Regardless of the career path chosen, a fellowship in geriatric psychiatry is extraordinarily valuable. Professional opportunities include:

- Academic psychiatry
- Pharmaceutical industry
- Government-based (state or Veterans Affairs [VA] hospitals, community mental health centers)
- Institutions (community hospitals, long-term care facilities)
- Private practice

Academic Geriatric Psychiatry

For the geriatric psychiatrist wanting to pursue a career in academia, a growing number of university medical schools have geriatric psychiatry programs providing tenure-track, clinical-track, and adjunctive-track positions. In this setting, the geriatric psychiatrist can focus his or her efforts on research, clinical work, teaching, administration, or a combination of all four. Research opportunities abound, and involve both clinical and laboratory projects. Before actually conducting research, however, a great deal of time is spent writing grant proposals, or applying to some of the numerous research fellowships offered by national aging organizations (e.g., the American Geriatrics Society, AAGP). Primary teaching roles are becoming more remunerative, and provide the opportunity to serve as a role model and mentor for medical students, residents, and fellows.

Both academic research and teaching tracks almost always require the geriatric psychiatrist to work at a university inpatient unit, outpatient clinic, or memory disorder center. Individuals from a variety of medical and mental health disciplines train at these sites, so teaching responsibilities are common. Additionally, research projects and clinical drug trials are encouraged, both for the income stream they provide and for the training opportunities. Medical schools and university hospitals have increasingly come to rely on the income stream from clinical care. Much of the information on private practice provided later in this chapter can be applied to any academic position where patient care is delivered and billed.

Pharmaceutical Industry

Many pharmaceutical companies have developed medications used widely to treat late-life psychiatric disorders. The pharmaceutical industry can provide consistent funding for research in areas such as AD, behavioral disorders, late-life depression, and anxiety disorders. There are potential career opportunities in both the research divisions and the marketing and educational areas. Both early career and seasoned psychiatrists are finding their expertise in great demand. Marketing to clinicians about medication use in the elderly has become increasingly important particularly as the older population continues to grow. Medical Associates or Medical Directors with experience in geriatric psychiatry are being added to many sales, marketing, and research teams. These positions call for a great deal of travel, but can be immeasurably rewarding, with the opportunity to help shape the research and marketing approaches used by the industry.

Government-Based Careers

Historically, VA hospitals have been the backbone of academic geriatric psychiatry programs. In fact, many fellows have trained in VA facilities, in part because these settings have become *de facto* geriatric care centers. In 1990, 26% of veterans were older than 65, and this number is expected to rise to nearly 40% by the year 2010 (6). The opportunity to step into a position of leadership (e.g., running a geriatric psychiatry team, ward, or fellowship program) and improve the care of elderly patients has never been greater. Of particular relevance are the federally funded Geriatric Research, Education, and Clinical Centers (GRECCs) around the country, each with a unique focus in geriatrics. The GRECC system generates numerous career opportunities for the geriatric psychiatrist, all with the benefit of providing a multidisciplinary environment.

In addition to the VA system, both state psychiatric facilities and community mental health centers frequently employ geriatric psychiatrists to run both inpatient units and outpatient clinics. These positions have the advantages of full-time salaried employment with benefits and good job security, but without the billing hassles that are part and parcel of private practice or the "publish or perish" pressures of academic positions.

Institutions

Due to the growing emphasis on decreasing hospital length of stay, as well as increased competition for patients among hospital systems, geriatric psychiatry expertise remains in high demand. Geriatric psychiatry staffing is needed for memory disorder clinics, inpatient geriatric psychiatry units, outpatient clinics, and consultative relationships with local nursing homes. Clinicians may work as full-time or part-time employees, or may work on contract

and bill their services separately. In the contractual relationship, it is common for a small stipend to be provided. The stipend allows the psychiatrist to be available for administrative tasks and staff education. The risk with salaried positions is that the clinician must generate sufficient billing to cover his or her salary and benefits. This can result in pressure to see many patients and minimize non-billable activities. In such circumstances, the geriatric psychiatrist must design his or her services so they are not so expensive that the costs cannot be captured in the available billing codes. Do not assume that great clinical care guarantees profit; good clinicians can find themselves in conflict with administrative staff motivated more by the bottom line than by their skills as a psychiatrist. There are numerous ways in which staff clinicians can maximize their revenue, including using competent billing services, conducting clinical drug trials, serving as training sites for other institutions, and contracting services out to smaller institutions in need of a geriatric psychiatrist.

PRIVATE PRACTICE

Achieving a successful private practice in geriatric psychiatry can be done. In order to maximize the potential for a geriatric psychiatrist to pursue his or her chosen and much needed profession, a great deal of information needs to be assimilated. It is our hope that the remainder of this chapter will prove useful and reassuring to those embarking on the private practice track.

Many skills and attributes are required to be successful. These include good clinical skills, willingness to gain knowledge of the Medicare billing and payment system, and motivation to learn a great deal about running a business. Setting up a private practice also requires a good accountant and attorney to help get started on the right foot. The greatest mistake clinicians make is to believe that success in business results solely from taking good care of their patients. This section will describe the numerous elements that can make or break the viability of a practice, and offer practical suggestions for running a successful geriatric psychiatry private practice. For most early career psychiatrists, neither psychiatry residency nor fellowship training taught the necessary information to develop, run, and succeed in private practice. Be prepared for a steep learning curve, as well as some emotional adjustments along the way. To be successful, the geriatric psychiatrist must be clear in his or her motivation, and must be willing to consider the financial aspects of how a successful practice must be run.

The initial process of starting a private practice should begin months before the first patient is anticipated. It is helpful to develop a time-line that begins at least 6 months before the expected opening of the office. Obviously, many of these steps are completed or are considerably easier if the geriatric psychiatrist chooses to join an existing private practice. Five areas will be discussed:

- Private practice as a business
- Office space and structure
- Getting office papers in order
- Hiring a staff
- Establishing a good reputation

Private Practice as a Business

In order to deliver psychiatric care in your chosen way, you must keep the business financially solvent. Maintaining a profit or financial solvency includes taking a careful look at both vendors and customers. A vendor is anyone that must be paid for goods and services in order to do business. Examples of vendors include: accountant, answering service, attorney, billing service, cleaning service, computer technologists, insurance agent, and property owner. In any type of medical private practice there are two types of customers, the patients themselves, and the insurance companies (also called third-party payers). The practice must be organized to provide services in ways that consider the needs of both these customers. For example, the psychiatrist must help the patients define their needs and requests, provide information about what services are offered, and negotiate changes in their expectations when necessary. Psychiatrists may choose to deny some requests or limit the kinds of patients accepted according to their professional or financial judgment. It may also be preferable to use or avoid certain insurance companies due to their fee schedule or reputation for handling billing problems. It is critical to make these financial and practice-related determinations before opening, based on a careful analysis of how each choice will affect expenses and income. Talking with other colleagues in similar private practices, as well as their billing and office managers, can provide valuable information and insights that may aid in making these decisions.

Customer Service

For many clinicians, thinking of the patient as the customer may feel quite foreign. However, the interaction between the psychiatrist and patient is an exchange of service for payment, and many principles of customer relations apply. If the practice as a whole does not adequately address a patient's needs, that patient's business may be lost. Patients choose a psychiatrist based on many factors, including the quality of service, reputation, or relationship with the referring parties. These issues, therefore, become significant elements in any psychiatrist's success in business. Important factors in satisfying patient/customer needs include the following:

Communication: Patients want the ability to contact the psychiatrist or covering psychiatrist quickly and easily (e.g., telephone calls from the patient or family). This requires both a friendly and accurate secretary and/or answering service, and that the psychiatrist returns phone calls promptly. The psychiatrist must be willing to speak to the patient or family about the pertinent symptoms, illnesses, and treatment plan in a clear and understanding manner. Some consideration may be worthwhile regarding specific situations when phone calls are numerous or lengthy. In such a scenario, developing a policy for case management services that can be billed in addition to patient appointments may be helpful. Case management services are not paid for by Medicare. Services that are never paid by Medicare can be billed to the patient if certain requirements are met before the service is delivered. Medicare regulations require that before the patient is billed, the service agreement is written and agreed upon by the patient or responsible party, and that the claim has been submitted and denied by Medicare. If used, presenting this service should be done at evaluation or early in the treatment process, before expectations become untenable. Another option is to set up family meetings to capture appropriate billing while addressing concerns face-to-face.

Compassion: It is important that the patients feel the psychiatrist has a genuine interest and concern for them. This is a particularly vital factor for older individuals. One major influence is the interaction between the patients' experience and the office staff. Examine the experience—from the first phone call, scheduling, leaving messages, and payment—from the patients' points of view.

Confidence: Patients need to feel the psychiatrist understands their problem and has a plan about what can be done. The doctor does not need to define all the answers, but must indicate a grasp of the situation and some ideas for approach. This helps provide structure to what is often a strange and frightening experience. Empathy for the patient's distress is very helpful; for example, explaining to the patient that he or she is not the worst case the doctor has ever seen (a common fantasy). The support staff is very important in subtle but powerful ways to reassure the patient that getting treatment is the right thing to do, and getting better is a reasonable goal.

Cost: Reasonable fees are defined as those that are customary and accepted by Medicare or other insurance companies. Patients need access to helpful staff that can explain billing matters and work with the patients and/or families regarding payments.

Office Space and Structure

If the decision is made to establish an office, remember the real estate adage: "location, location, location." Other specific factors include the type of community, nearby resources, the type of building, office site considerations, space utilization, and acquisition.

Type of community: There should be an adequate number of elderly in the community, including the number of aging adults and retirement areas nearby to which elderly people are moving. Each type of community—whether urban, suburban, or rural—has pros and cons for the elderly in terms of lifestyle, resources, and access to treatment. The psychiatrist must also consider the environment in which he or she wishes to live, work, and raise a family, and the distance and commuting time from home to office.

Nearby resources: The presence of other geriatric psychiatrists must be taken into consideration, since they could be viewed as competition. The number of general psychiatrists not specializing in geriatrics must also be taken into account, but for other reasons. If a new psychiatrist establishes a reputation as a geriatric specialist, this may prompt other psychiatrists in the area to refer patients to them. Ideally, the location chosen will have an adequate numbers of local physicians for patient referrals, including geriatric medicine specialists, neurologists, and primary care physicians with largely geriatric practices. It is vitally important to nurture these referral sources, and to actively develop new ones. Other key resources that are helpful, if nearby, include a clinical laboratory, pharmacies, senior centers, day programs, assisted living facilities, and nursing homes—in particular, those with associated dementia units.

Knowledge of the community and its resources is imperative when working with seniors. Although physical proximity is less crucial, important community resources include a local chapter of the Alzheimer's Association, Visiting Nurse Association (VNA) services, Meals on Wheels, services for hearing and visually impaired individuals (e.g., Lighthouse for the Blind), transportation services, and legal aid societies. In addition to providing support services for patients, they provide volunteer opportunities for patients and clinicians alike, and can ultimately serve as referral sources. Finally, knowledge of local social events, clubs, museums, and libraries is also beneficial when treating older individuals.

Type of building: Traditionally, psychiatric offices were not located in medical office buildings due to the increased costs associated with this type of building. For the geriatric psychiatrist, however, it can be beneficial to have referral sources in close proximity to the office site. Proximity breeds ease of referrals and collegial relationships. If the geriatric psychiatrist's office is down the hall in the Medical Arts Building from neurologists, geriatricians, and primary care physicians with large geriatric practices, it is easier for them and the patients to make use of it. It may also be beneficial to be close to the hospital to do consultations on the medicine and surgery services. While consultations in the hospital are time-consuming, they are a great way for the geriatric psychiatrist to get his or her name out in the physician community. Rents may be more reasonable in buildings owned by community hospitals than in privately owned medical buildings. Because of Stark II and Medicare Fraud and Abuse Regulations, as well as Internal Revenue Service concerns, buildings owned by hospitals and other healthcare delivery systems must rent at fair market rates.

Sharing an office or subletting it—may be an attractive option when first starting out in practice. Locating the office in a senior retirement building or community allows immediate and very easy access for a large group of potential patients.

Office site considerations: The ideal office is handicap accessible; has minimal physical barriers such as stairs, varying levels, or long, narrow, corridors; is on the first floor (or has reliable elevator service); and has plenty of free parking spaces. Simple driving instructions to the office and information about public transportation in the area should be available through handouts, faxes, and a website. Some settings (e.g., larger hospitals) may have a shuttle bus system, and may extend this service to patients if the practice is leasing space from them. Bear in mind that cold or snow will interfere with patients' abilities to get to the office. Some communities have senior transportation services that take people with limited mobility to physicians if reservations are made 24 to 48 hours in advance. Some hospitals may transport patients from the hospital to physicians' offices in adjoined buildings.

Space utilization: Office space may be new and without walls, or might be already built out. Many elderly patients and their families are quite sensitive to the environment, particularly with regard to crowding and noise. A space with a slightly larger than normal waiting room, patient restrooms, and hallways adds greatly to patients' comfort. More space also decreases the likelihood that behaviorally distressed patients will become overwhelmed. Six to 8-foot-wide hallways not only make the office suite appear larger, but also allow for a safer traffic pattern. Consider patient flow when laying out the space, taking into account patients in wheelchairs or movement in both directions simultaneously. Depending on the available options, it may be worthwhile to hire a consultant to help plan the space.

Basic needs include an office for each clinician and the office manager, a waiting area separated from the offices, bathroom(s), and a reception/administrative area. It can be very helpful, and even critical for confidentiality, to have a separate office to talk to patients privately about billing issues. A larger space will be needed for family and group meetings. Each clinical office should be sound-proofed with wall insulation and sound-absorbing ceiling tiles. There must be adequate space in rooms and hallways for wheelchairs or motorized scooters to enter and exit. Bathrooms must be handicap accessible and should have an emergency call button. Having a bathroom off the reception area for patients and a separate facility for staff reduces congestion. Other important space considerations include storage areas for patient records, office machines and supplies, and medication samples, and a kitchen or break room for staff lunches and training.

Acquisition of the office site: An office, condo, or small building can be purchased or leased. Some of the issues to consider are listed in Table 2-1.

TABLE 2-1

FACTORS TO CONSIDER WHEN BUYING OR LEASING OFFICE SPACE

- Cost of space per square foot
- Length of lease and options for renewal
- Cost and availability of routine services (e.g., utilities, cleaning, parking, basic maintenance)
- Renovations (e.g., carpet, repainting, upgrades)
- Hours and days during which the building is open
- Parking
- Type of building security (e.g., locks, alarms, guards)
- Temperature control and building maintenance (e.g., heating and air conditioning, pest control, etc.)
- Signage allowed (outside the building, and in the lobby, halls, and on the office door)
- Amount of other professional office space in the area
- History of property values in the area (sales and leases)

Getting Office Papers in Order

Gone are the days of renting office space, hanging out a shingle, and waiting for patients to arrive. A successful business requires careful advance planning to address both the clinical care and financial aspects of the practice. This section on paperwork is subdivided into three broad categories: information related to insurers/hospitals, papers related to setting up an office, and information regarding office equipment.

Insurers and Hospitals

While there are many benefits in running a psychiatric practice, the complexity and amount of work required can be daunting at times. A common complaint is the frustration experienced due to the complex Medicare reimbursement system and low reimbursement rates. Each Medicare carrier has wide discretion for policy development, and thus the rules for covered services and payment rates vary significantly from region to region. The arbitrary nature and variability in policy makes learning reimbursement rules quite difficult. Many clinicians have complained of the hassle factor when trying to get clarity from their carriers. Although a slow process, organizations like the AAGP, APA, and American Medical Directors Association are working diligently with the Center for Medicare and Medicaid Services to standardize the policies and procedures regarding Medicare reimbursement and documentation requirements.

Medicare: Every clinician in the practice must apply for an individual Medicare provider number. Be sure to do this well in advance, because it may take several months for the number to be received, and it is required for billing. Applications for a Medicare number are available from the Medicare carrier providing reimbursement services for the practice location. Unless the practice will only have a single practitioner, a group Medicare billing provider number will also be needed. The group Medicare billing provider number and the individual Medicare number are needed for billing submissions. The reports of the annual gross income from Medicare to the practice will be associated with the group Medicare billing provider number.

Credentialing—insurance companies: It is worthwhile to talk with potential sources of referral, such as local primary care physicians, to find out which health maintenance organizations they participate in, and where they prefer to admit their patients when hospitalization is needed. Managed care organizations often have their panels closed. If they are taking new providers, most insurance companies (e.g., United Behavioral Health, Anthem Blue Cross, CHAMPUS) require that the geriatric psychiatrist be credentialed with them, and an application must be submitted to each one. Typically, insurance companies require the clinician to have hospital privileges prior to being accepted. Some insurance providers contract only through hospital-based independent practice associations (IPAs). Many practices have privileges at a number of hospitals, and have membership in multiple IPAs or physician hospital organizations.

Credentialing—hospitals: Each hospital must be called in order to obtain a credentialing application and to determine the specific requirements for acceptance. In either case, it normally takes about 3 months to be credentialed by a hospital's medical board. Obtaining hospital credentials typically requires notarized copies of the geriatric psychiatrist's medical school diploma, state medical and Drug Enforcement Agency licenses, certification of malpractice insurance, documentation of residency completion and board certification, a physician statement attesting to health, and several letters of support.

Practice insurance: The various types of insurance required of a private practice are listed in Table 2-2. Note that the relative costs of these insurances vary widely by

TABLE 2-2

TYPES OF INSURANCE NEEDED IN PRIVATE PRACTICE

- *Malpractice insurance* is available from the American Psychiatric Association, local medical societies, or independent insurers.
  - Occurrence policies cover any alleged incident *occurring* during the period of time the policy is, or was, in effect.
  - Claims-made policies cover any alleged incident *claimed* during the period when the policy is in effect. Tail coverage can be purchased to cover future claims filed.
- *Office liability insurance* covers injuries sustained by people while on the office premises.
- *Unemployment compensation insurance* requirements vary from state to state.
- *Workers' Compensation* requirements vary from state to state.
- *Health and disability insurance* is available from many sources, including individual policies from insurance companies and group policies through professional associations, hospitals, and some payroll service providers.

region, and depend on the scope of practice and the size and type of staff.

Office Paperwork and Services

It is critical to be very practical when thinking about all the paper requirements when starting up a practice. The following items require an office address to get started: practice name and logo, announcements, stationery and business cards, prescription pads, and yellow page listings. The style of each of these items will affect costs, and it is more important to select effective and professional items rather than ones with gimmicks or excessive glitz.

The office should have a minimum of three telephone lines; the first should be listed, the second is a rollover, and the third is to be used primarily for outgoing calls. The rollover can also be hooked up to the fax machine. In terms of services, the practice will need telephone and cellular phone service, a fax number, a paging service, an answering service, and a transcription service. As the number of ancillary staff grows, a centralized payroll service is a good idea. This service is relatively inexpensive and convenient, and handles all filings such as state and federal taxes, as well as providing excellent reports for tax purposes. Some also provide extensive and reasonably priced human resource services, as well as reduced rates on insurances and other benefits.

One of the most critical services will be a computer system consultant to set up, manage, and maintain the computer hardware and practice management software. A good computerized practice management system will include modules for scheduling, billing, collections, and accounts receivable. Training is a critical feature, and is required for optimal use of these systems. Even with such a system, outside accounting services are recommended, especially to get advice on their experience with different systems and to determine the report required.

Office Equipment

Office equipment can be leased or purchased. Consider differences in costs, maintenance, the ability and cost to upgrade, and potential tax consequences. Often leasing is relatively economical and saves headaches if the equipment malfunctions. Items commonly leased include fax machines, copiers, and phone systems for more than two lines. Office furniture can be purchased, rented, or leased. All leases are negotiable, and most come with a $1 buyout after 3 to 5 years. In this age of expanding electronic capabilities, most computer leases run for 3 years, after which time much of the currently leased computer hardware is obsolete. If a phone system is leased, make sure that a future expansion of that system is financially possible. Many local and most long-distance phone companies can now tie together phones, computers, cell phones, and beepers. It is worth the time to talk with salespeople from the phone company to see what kind of package they can put together. Lease rates can be below the market average for borrowing money.

Hiring a Staff

Since medical schools and residency training programs do not teach the business side of medical care, these skills must be learned and then taught to the clinicians and office staff. An option is to hire office staff with experience and learn from them. It would be unusual, however, to find staff with exactly the sort of experience and knowledge that fits the anticipated work approach. Some changes on one or both sides will likely have to be made. Depending on the size of the practice and the skill sets of each employee, there will likely be overlap among the job duties.

How to Find Office Staff

At the beginning of office set-up, particularly if initial funds are low, psychiatrists may opt to schedule their own appointments, submit billing, and maintain the books. If the clerical workload is small, this may be appropriate. A spouse, significant other, or other family member may be enlisted to do part or all of the above, depending on that individual's availability, inclinations, and circumstances; but as the clerical workload increases, this option quickly becomes markedly less cost-efficient. Hiring a good employee can occasionally be done quickly, but often the search requires weeks or months. Be prepared to conduct a lot of interviews, if necessary. If a candidate is selected for reasons of expedience but is not truly fit for the position, problems are likely to follow. Sources of possible candidates for administrative staff include:

- Word of mouth: from other doctors, hospitals, or health care facilities. If hiring staff from another practice, inquire about why they left and call their previous employers
- Other businesses
- Secretarial schools
- Temporary agencies or employment agencies
- Newspaper ads

Candidates should fill out an application for the position and come in for an interview. Be aware of things that cannot be asked by law, including age, race, ethnic background, religion, health, marital status, or disability. In each interview, inquire about his or her experience for the job requirements, other work background, skills, past experiences that are directly relevant, reasons for leaving past or current employment, strengths and weaknesses, and what he or she is looking for in terms of salary and benefits. Give information about what the job entails, expectations, and some information about salary range and any benefits. Typically, most practices employ staff-at-will rather than for a guaranteed length of time. Upon hiring, an initial probationary period of up to 3 months is common. During the probationary period, employment can be terminated without a reason. A person terminated during a probationary period is not considered laid off and is not eligible for unemployment insurance. Consequently, state employment compensation taxes for the practice (which vary from state to state) do not increase. Indicate whether there may be a further adjustment of salary or eligibility for benefits following the end of the probationary period.

The various types of employees or consultants that may comprise staffing for a private practice are listed in Table 2-3, along with basic job responsibilities. Note the overlap between job responsibilities. Every practice will use staff members in somewhat different ways depending on the size and scope of the practice.

Employing Clinicians

Clinicians that might work in a private practice include psychiatrists, psychologists, advanced practice registered nurses (APRNs) or nurse practitioners, and social workers. To bill for an employee's clinical services, the Medicare group practice billing number is required. The clinical services of physician extenders can be billed to Medicare under *incident*

TABLE 2-3
PRIVATE PRACTICE STAFF AND CONSULTANTS

Position	Responsibilities
Accountant	• Help set up an office financial management system, including billing, collections, and payroll • Maintain the financial books • Assist in arranging for bank loans • Prepare tax returns
Healthcare law attorney	• Assist with arranging bank loans for office space, equipment, etc. • Help secure malpractice insurance • Develop contracts for employees, hospitals, insurance companies, and nursing home consultant agreements • Risk management • Monitor compliance with state and federal employment laws, as well as Medicare rules and regulations
Office/business manager	• Set up and maintain office management system and software • Coordinate contacts with accountant and attorney • Hire and supervise other staff • Serve along with clerical staff as the "friendly face" of the practice • Assist in patient scheduling • Troubleshoot patient requests and complaints • Promote relations with other doctors and facilities • Insures that all licenses, fees, and reappointment forms for hospital privileges and professional societies are completed and submitted in a timely fashion • Monitor physician's schedule to verify that clinical time, on-call time, and vacations do not conflict • Assist in purchase and maintenance of office equipment • Facilitate staff training and morale
Receptionist/secretarial	• Manage appointment book or software program • Field inquiries on appointment changes, directions to office, transportation • Organize and maintain waiting room • Manage intake forms, medical records, requests for records • Collect fees or copays
Billing and bookkeeping staff	• Receive and record payments from patients, insurers, and other third-party payers • Monitor balances due from patients and/or supplemental and secondary payers • Send out bills, track receipts, and catch and correct errors • Monitor changes in fee schedules from third-party payers • Provide regular tabulations of information on amounts billed, received, etc.

to, provided the physician is in the office suite and available as needed. *Incident to* services are allowed in the office, but not in the nursing home. *Incident to* services are paid at the full physician rate without the 15% reduction in Medicare rate normally applied to psychologists, social workers, or nurse clinicians when working alone.

Staff may be hired for specific clinical work (e.g., psychotherapy), and be paid per hour of service delivered. A second option is to provide billing services and office space for clinicians, and pay the clinician a percentage of the fees collected (e.g., 60/40, 70/30, and so forth). This may be considered fee-splitting by some state medical licensing boards or Medicare intermediary. Seeking local advice regarding these possibilities is advised. If clinicians are paid only for the work performed, there are no costs associated with any down time. A final approach is to rent or lease office space (at fair market value) to clinicians, refer them patients and, when appropriate, serve as the medical backup. In this situation, there are no fixed costs associated with the clinician. Income is earned as a property owner and no additional income is derived when the entire practice is very busy.

Each approach has its own merits and drawbacks. A social worker or clinical nurse specialist who commands a salary of $50,000 to $80,000 per year costs the practice $30 to $45 per hour, including benefits. Optimally, they can generate $80+/hour doing clinical work, which provides for a good profit margin. If, however, the clinician is not seeing a sufficient number of patients, the cost remains unchanged. Usually, employing clinical staff will allow the practice to better meet the needs of the community if there are more referrals than a solo practitioner can respond to in a timely fashion. Additionally, benefits include sharing the responsibilities for clinical duties such as refill requests, telephone calls, and on-call responsibilities.

Determining the salary and benefits package for clinical and administrative employees is crucial before advertising and interviewing prospective employees. While a high salary will draw employees, care must be taken to ensure this cost is sustainable considering the anticipated income and other practice expenses. A salary that is too low will not attract or keep good employees. Rarely can a fledgling practice compete with the financial packages offered by large healthcare centers, so it is important to highlight the advantages of joining a smaller practice. For example, incentives might include factors such as more flexibility, closer working relationships, a more comfortable atmosphere, and more control over the types of patients accepted.

Determine the salary and benefits package being offered in the area. Call the office manager or psychiatrist in offices advertising in the newspaper, trade journals, or online. Attend local medical and psychiatric society meetings and discuss the issue with colleagues. Search the internet for information on the local professional societies for APRNs, social workers, and psychologists. If another practice is actively interviewing, ask that any additional applicants be referred to your practice after their position is filled.

Establishing a Good Reputation

The greatest asset a geriatric psychiatry practice can establish is a reputation for superior treatment and innovative approaches when caring for the elderly. Initially, this will likely require greater availability than would be expected long-term. There are a myriad of ways to become well-known and respected in the community. For example, consider doing emergency consultations in local hospitals or seeing crisis patients after office hours or on weekends. Respond to emergency requests for consultation in nursing homes, even if the practice does not have an established contract with that nursing home. This will allow the nursing home administrator and director of nursing to experience the benefits of psychiatric expertise and training when considering a future contract. Think about doing home visits for important primary-care referral sources. Meet with the staff of Adult Protective Services, or provide educational in-services to their staff at no charge. Speak to community groups about important issues of aging. Write letters to the editor or op-ed pieces for the local newspaper. Draft short, thoughtful pieces that can be run in small local publications to get the practice name in front of many potential referral sources and patients. Volunteering to serve in community service organizations or on their boards is also an important marketing tool. Any of these activities put the practice in the public eye and demonstrate how the practice provides care.

Organizations of particular interest include the Alzheimer's Association, Parkinson's Support Group, American Association for Retired Persons groups, Area Agency on Aging, various home health agencies, and local hospice organizations. Identify other resources that may arrange for speaking engagements, such as the pharmaceutical industry or corporations. Numerous venues could be available, including hospital grand rounds, local newspapers, television and radio, nursing home and pharmacist associations, and state medical and psychiatric societies' annual meetings. While each attempt to establish a reputation of excellence and expertise may yield only small rewards initially, the collective effort over time becomes the foundation of success for years to come.

REFERENCES

1. Halpain MC, Harris MJ, McClure FS, Jeste DV. Training in geriatric mental health: needs and strategies. *Psychiatr Serv.* 1999;50(9):1205–1208.
2. Himes CK. *Elderly Americans.* Washington, DC: Population Reference Bureau; 2001.
3. Rovner BW, German PS, Broadhead J, et al. The prevalence and management of dementia and other psychiatric disorders in nursing homes. *Int Psychogeriatr.* 1990;2:13–24.
4. Gurland BJ. Epidemiology of psychiatric disorders. In: Sadavoy J, Jarvik LF, Grossberg GT, Meyers BS, eds. *Comprehensive Textbook of Geriatric Psychiatry.* 3rd Ed. New York: W.W. Norton and Company; 2004:3–38.
5. Personnel for health needs of the elderly through the year 2020. NIH pub 87-2950. Washington DC: National Institutes of Health, 1987.
6. Proceedings of the Future of Geriatrics in the VA Health Care System. Ann Arbor, MI: VA Medical Center, Geriatric Research, Education, and Clinical Center, June 4–5, 1990.

The Geriatric Setting

3

Stephen M. Scheinthal   *Anita Chopra*   *Janet M. Lieto*
Pamela M. Basehore   *Barry Rovner*

There has been an incredible expansion in the number and types of clinical settings in which geriatric psychiatrists provide care. Although the traditional expectation is that geriatric patients are seen in a clinic or hospital setting, today they may be evaluated and followed across a spectrum of other settings. These include the patients' own homes, assisted living facilities (ALFs), nursing homes, continuing care retirement communities (CCRCs), rehabilitation facilities, day programs, and partial hospitalization programs. For any institutional setting, it is critical for the geriatric psychiatrist to have a basic understanding of the main rules and regulations that will govern psychiatric care. This chapter will devote most of its content to an extensive and important set of rules pertaining to nursing home care, known as OBRA (Omnibus Budget Reconciliation Act of 1987). Understanding OBRA guidelines is integral to successful clinical practice in long-term care (LTC) settings.

ASSISTED LIVING FACILITIES

ALFs are the fastest-growing type of residential facilities for the elderly, with an estimated 11,000 to 30,000 facilities in the country (1) housing up to 1.2 million individuals (2,3). ALFs provide room and board, along with 24-hour staffing to monitor residents' well-being and assist with medication management, activities of daily living (ADLs), and access to medical and nursing care. Some ALFs have dementia units with restrictive access and more intensive nursing assistance for ADLs. Sizes of ALFs range from small homes or buildings with up to a dozen residents, to well-appointed apartment complexes with hundreds of residents and an array of amenities, including dining rooms, meeting halls, beauty parlors, exercise rooms, and pools, to name but a few. Many ALFs cater to specific populations, such as religious or minority groups,

mentally ill individuals, or those with mental retardation (2). In terms of medical and psychiatric care, some facilities have office space for periodic visits by clinicians, but most residents go out for appointments. For the geriatric psychiatrist, ALFs offer important sources of referrals and potential sites for clinics, educational programs, and research projects.

To date there are no clearly established federal rules regulating psychiatric care or the use of psychiatric drugs in ALFs, although some states do regulate these facilities and conduct annual inspections. As an example, ALFs are not required to assess residents with the Minimum Data Set (MDS), which is the standard measure of patient status in LTC facilities. Despite these regulatory differences, the psychiatric problems in ALFs tend to mimic those in LTC, including dementia, behavioral problems, mood disorders, and anxiety disorders. ALFs, however, lack the intensity of nursing care, patient monitoring, and clinical attention found in LTC settings. As a result, psychiatric disorders can cause disproportionate problems in the ALF setting. As the number of ALFs grow, along with the dilemma of providing effective psychiatric management, the imposition of regulations is likely on the horizon.

CONTINUING CARE RETIREMENT COMMUNITIES

CCRCs provide a continuum of care for elderly individuals through a range of living settings on a single campus. For example, there may be an independent living facility, an ALF, and a skilled nursing facility. Some also include subacute or rehabilitation units for individuals transitioning back from hospitalization. Providing care at a CCRC may be very rewarding for a physician, due to the ability to easily follow patients through different levels of care as their needs change. Currently, formal federal guidelines for psychiatric care exist only for the subacute and skilled nursing portions of the CCRC. These guidelines will be described in the sections that follow.

OMNIBUS BUDGET RECONCILIATION ACT OF 1987—AN INTRODUCTION

Regulation of care in the LTC setting was born of necessity. As the numbers of individuals in nursing homes grew through the 1970s and 1980s, more and more psychiatric problems were seen and dealt with. However, psychiatric care in LTC varied widely in its safety and efficacy, and lacked the presence of trained geriatric psychiatrists. The resulting situation often led to overuse of heavily sedating psychotropic medications, without clearly documented indications, dosing guidelines, behavioral tracking, or appropriate follow-up (4–6). Concern in LTC went beyond just psychiatric care, and focused on the impact of polypharmacy and multiple medical illnesses on patient status. Regrettably, with the multiple prescribers, patients were sometimes adversely affected through inappropriate use of medications, again without clear documentation justifying and tracking their use. The legacy of this era still exists, to some extent, in the fears of many LTC residents and their caregivers that psychiatric treatment uses medications to turn agitated individuals into "zombies."

In an attempt to restore some sanity to care, legislators became involved in devising a set of guidelines for medical and psychiatric care in subacute and nursing home settings. The resultant Nursing Home Reform Amendments were attached to OBRA, and consisted of new federal regulations for nursing home care (7). After considerable public comment, debate, and revision, the rules became effective in 1991. OBRA mandated the Health Care Financing Administration (HCFA—now known as the Center for Medicare and Medicaid Services, or CMS, in the Department of Health and Human Services) to develop a set of interpretative guidelines for the implementation and monitoring of the regulatory requirements (8). These guidelines helped standardize the survey process nationally, and improve the monitoring of quality of care in all nursing facilities. When noting a deficiency, surveyors are required to cite a specific OBRA/HCFA regulation and to specify how patient care outcome was compromised by lack of adherence to the regulation. In July of 1995, the federal government released the enforcement regulations, which include civil fines to nursing homes found in noncompliance with OBRA.

The overall impact of OBRA in improving the quality of medical and psychiatric care in nursing homes has been dramatic (9,10). Since the adoption of the regulations, it is estimated that restraint usage has decreased over 50% (11), psychotropic medication usage has dropped by over one third (12–15), behavioral management interventions have increased by almost 30%, hearing aid usage has increased by almost 30%, toileting programs have almost doubled, and family involvement has significantly increased. The following sections will serve as a primer on OBRA, detailing the specific guidelines relevant to both medical and geriatric psychiatry practices in nursing homes in the following areas: physician responsibilities, resident assessment and care planning, drug therapy, use of physical restraints, residents' rights, and quality of care.

Physician Responsibilities

OBRA provides direct guidelines to ensure that a physician supervises the medical care of each LTC resident. Physicians must see the patients every 30 days during the first 3 months of admission to a facility, and then a minimum of every 60 days after that. After the initial visit, at the option of the physician, visits may alternate between the physician and a physician assistant, nurse practitioner, or clinical nurse specialist. Under OBRA, the attending physician is expected to be involved, available and responsive, and to focus on maintaining or improving functional status. The medical director of the facility is responsible for ensuring the attending physicians comply with the regulations and provide quality care. If the attending physician fails to fulfill the requirements, OBRA guidelines give the facility the right to recommend to the resident that he or she seek alternate physician care.

Clinical Recommendations—the Attending Physician Should:

- Authorize admission orders in a timely fashion.
- Provide accurate information regarding medical history, current medical status, diagnosis, medications, and treatments for all new admissions.
- During follow-up visits, review a patient's current condition and the status of any acute episodes of illness since the last visit, identify potential medical problems that may affect functional status, and manage chronic illnesses to maximize function and personal comfort.
- Manage acute illnesses or significant changes in condition promptly and as aggressively as is indicated by the resident's goals, condition, and progress.
- Always consider reversible medical causes, such as medications and infections, when a decline in function is noted.

Resident Assessment and Care Planning

Since 1990, all LTC facilities are required to complete a comprehensive assessment of each resident's needs and functional capacity using a standardized instrument called the Resident Assessment Instrument (RAI) (16,17). The RAI has two major components: the MDS and the Resident Assessment Protocols (RAPs) (18). Data points included in the RAI include demographic information, cognitive status, communication, vision, mood and behavior patterns, psychosocial well-being, physical functioning, disease diagnoses and health conditions, dental and nutritional status, skin conditions, activity pursuits, medications, special treatments and procedures, and discharge potential. Data from the MDS are used not only for clinical assessment, but also for deriving quality indicators and quality measures (used for facility grading and comparisons), and for determining Medicare and Medicaid payments for nursing homes (18).

This comprehensive assessment must be performed within 14 days of admission, and must be repeated yearly and promptly after a significant change occurs in the resident's condition. The MDS is a standardized form containing a core set of screening, clinical, and functional status indicators in 16 sections with over 400 items. It is completed by an assigned coordinator based on input from members of the interdisciplinary team. A revised version known as the MDS 2.0 has been in use since 1996.

Certain answers on the MDS serve as triggers for RAPs. The RAPs help nursing staff to recognize and evaluate certain common clinical problems in nursing home residents that require more in-depth assessment. There are 18 trigger conditions covering the domains of ADLs, mobility, continence, pressure ulcers, sensory and communication impairments, mental status, medication use, mood and behavioral state, nutritional status, and psychological well-being.

Clinical Recommendations—the Attending Physician Should:

- Familiarize him or herself with the MDS and help ensure the accuracy and completeness of information placed in the assessment by an interdisciplinary team.
- Promptly evaluate an individual with a significant change in condition, and document pertinent history and physical findings.
- Review the care plan to ensure it is consistent with the medical assessment and orders.

Use of Physical Restraints

One of the areas of OBRA that has had the greatest impact is the statement that the resident has the right to be free of any physical restraints imposed for purposes of discipline or convenience and not required to treat the resident's medical symptoms. Physical restraints are defined as any manual method or physical device, material or equipment, attached to or adjacent to the resident's body that they cannot easily remove and that restricts freedom of movement or normal access to one's body.

The attending physician's order alone is no longer sufficient justification for a restraint. The comprehensive assessment done by an interdisciplinary team must show the presence of specific medical symptoms requiring use of restraints, and document how the restraints are expected to

help. The care plan should contain a schedule for attempts at progressive reduction of restraint use, where possible. The care plan must address any declines in functioning or overall status resulting from the use of a restraint. OBRA guidelines state that the facility is obligated to demonstrate that less restrictive measures were tried, and the physical or occupational therapist was consulted prior to using restraints. Consent of the resident or family must be documented in cases where restraints are used, and it must be documented that the restraining device actually enables the resident to attain and maintain his or her highest practical physical, mental, and psychosocial function.

Clinical Recommendations—the Attending Physician Should:

- Document or explain medical symptoms that justify the use of restraint.
- Instruct the staff to monitor for potential major side effects; for example, incontinence, pressure sores, contractures.
- At each visit, review the need for continuing the order for restraints and the staff's documentation of the frequency and nature of target symptoms.

Drug Therapy

OBRA regulations state that each resident's pharmacological regimen must be free from unnecessary drugs. Unnecessary drugs are defined as any drug used in excessive dose, for excessive duration, without adequate monitoring, without adequate indications for its use, when adverse consequences indicate the dose should be reduced or discontinued, or in any combinations of the reasons above. OBRA interpretive guidelines for evaluating whether a drug is unnecessary are extremely detailed, and include regulated lists of the following drugs:

- Long-acting benzodiazepines (Table 3-1)
- Short-acting benzodiazepines (Table 3-2)
- Other anxiolytic/sedative drugs (Table 3-2)
- Drugs used for sleep induction (Table 3-3)
- Miscellaneous hypnotic/sedative/anxiolytic drugs (Table 3-4)
- Antipsychotic drugs (Table 3-5)

Although the concepts in Tables 3-1 through 3-11 are important, the geriatric clinician must keep in mind that they are somewhat dated, are not necessarily specific to elderly patients, and may be of limited use in clinical practice given more recent trends in drug selection, common dosing strategies, and diagnostic classification. Please refer to Appendix A for up-to-date and comprehensive information on psychotropic pharmacotherapy specific to the elderly.

One goal of these guidelines is to stimulate appropriate differential diagnosis of behavioral symptoms, so the underlying cause of the symptoms is recognized and

TABLE 3-1
INTERPRETIVE GUIDELINES FOR LONG-ACTING BENZODIAZEPINES

Generic	Brand	Maximum Recommended Daily Dose
Flurazepam	Dalmane	15 mg
Chlordiazepoxide	Librium	20 mg
Clorazepate	Tranxene	15 mg
Diazepam	Valium	5 mg
Clonazepam	Klonopin	1.5 mg
Quazepam	Doral	7.5 mg
Halazepam	Paxipam	40 mg

Use of these long-acting benzodiazepines should not occur in residents unless an attempt with a short-acting drug has failed. After an attempt with a short-acting benzodiazepine has failed, a long-acting benzodiazepine should not be used unless:

- Evidence exists that other possible reasons for the resident's distress have been considered and ruled out.
- Its use has resulted in maintenance or improvement in the resident's functional status.
- Daily use is less than 4 continuous months, unless an attempt at gradual dose reduction is unsuccessful.
- Its use is less than or equal to the daily doses listed, unless higher doses are necessary for the maintenance of improvement in the resident's functional status (as supported by the resident's response and documented in the clinical record).

This guideline does not apply in the following instances:

- When diazepam is used for neuromuscular syndromes.
- When long-acting agents are used to withdraw residents from short-acting agents.
- When clonazepam is used for bipolar disorder, tardive dyskinesia, nocturnal myoclonus, or seizure disorders.

Adapted from Reference 21.

TABLE 3-2
INTERPRETIVE GUIDELINES FOR SHORT-ACTING BENZODIAZEPINES AND OTHER ANXIOLYTIC/SEDATIVE DRUGS

Generic	Brand	Maximum Recommended Daily Dose
Short-Acting Benzodiazepines		
Lorazepam	Ativan	2 mg
Oxazepam	Serax	30 mg
Alprazolam	Xanax	0.75 mg
Estazolam	ProSom	0.5 mg
Other Anxiolytic and Sedative Drugs		
Diphenhydramine	Benadryl	50 mg
Hydroxyzine	Atarax, Vistaril	50 mg
Chloral hydrate	Many brands	750 mg

Use of the listed anxiolytic/sedative drugs should occur only when:

- Evidence exists that other possible reasons for the resident's distress have been considered and ruled out.
- Use results in maintenance or improvements in the resident's functional status.
- Daily use at any dose is less than 4 continuous months, unless an attempt at a gradual dose reduction is unsuccessful.
- Use is for one of the following indications as defined by the DSM-IV:
  - Generalized anxiety disorder.
  - Organic mental syndromes (now called *delirium, dementia, and amnestic and other cognitive disorders* by DSM-IV) with associated agitated behaviors that are quantitatively and objectively documented and that constitute sources of distress or dysfunction to the resident or represent a danger to the resident or others.
  - Panic disorder.
  - Symptomatic anxiety that occurs in residents with another diagnosed psychiatric disorder.
- Use is equal to or less than the listed total daily doses, unless higher doses are necessary for the improvement or maintenance in the resident's response and documented in the clinical record.

For drugs in this category, a gradual dose reduction should be attempted at least twice within 1 year before one can conclude that a gradual dose reduction is clinically contraindicated.

DSM-IV, Diagnostic and Statistical Manual of Mental Disorders, 4th Edition.
Adapted from Reference 21.

treated appropriately. This treatment may include the use of environmental and/or behavioral therapy, as well as pharmacotherapy. Another key goal is to prevent the exclusive use of psychopharmacological drugs when the behavioral symptom is caused by reversible environmental or psychosocial stressors, or treatable medical conditions.

Residents should only be prescribed any of the above drug types when there is documentation of an appropriate diagnosis from an approved list. The guidelines include specific conditions that justify the use of antipsychotic medications (Table 3-6), and indications for which antipsychotic medications cannot be used in the absence of other justifying criteria (Table 3-7). It is also important to monitor for and document the presence or absence of significant side effects, particularly extrapyramidal symptoms and tardive dyskinesia, when using antipsychotics. Gradual dose reductions should be considered (and if

appropriate, attempted) every 4 to 6 months (depending on the agent, with greater frequency for sedative/hypnotics), with documentation to justify continuing use of the agent.

As of July, 1999, HCFA has added a list of drugs and diagnosis/drug combinations that are judged to place a person over the age of 65 at greater risk of adverse drug reactions. These guidelines incorporate what have been termed the *Beers criteria* (19,20). These criteria were developed to predict when the potential for adverse drug reactions is greater than the potential for benefits. Beers criteria are

TABLE 3-3
INTERPRETIVE GUIDELINES FOR DRUGS USED FOR SLEEP INDUCTION

Generic	Brand	Maximum Recommended Daily Dose
Temazepam	Restoril	7.5 mg
Triazolam	Halcion	0.125 mg
Lorazepam	Ativan	1 mg
Oxazepam	Serax	15 mg
Alprazolam	Xanax	0.25 mg
Estazolam	ProSom	0.5 mg
Diphenhydramine	Benadryl	25 mg
Hydroxyzine	Atarax, Vistaril	50 mg
Chloral hydrate	Many brands	500 mg
Zolpidem	Ambien	5 mg

Diminished sleep in the elderly is not necessarily pathologic. Drugs used for sleep induction should only be used if:

- Evidence exists that other possible reasons for insomnia have been ruled out (e.g., depression, pain, noise, light, caffeine).
- The use of a drug to induce sleep results in the maintenance or improvement of the resident's functional status.
- Daily use of the drug is less than 10 continuous days, unless an attempt at gradual dose reduction is unsuccessful.
- The dose of the drug is equal to or less than the listed doses, unless higher doses are necessary for maintenance or improvement in the resident's function, as evidenced by the resident's response and documented in the clinical record.

For drugs in this category, a gradual dose reduction should be attempted at least three times within a 6-month period before one can conclude that a gradual dose reduction is clinically contraindicated.

Adapted from Reference 21.

TABLE 3-4
INTERPRETIVE GUIDELINES FOR MISCELLANEOUS HYPNOTIC/SEDATIVE/ANXIOLYTIC DRUGS

Generic	Brand
Barbiturates	Many brands
Glutethimide	Doriden
Methyprylon	Noludar
Ethchlorvynol	Placidyl
Meprobamate	Equanil, Miltown
Paraldehyde	Many brands

The initiation of the above sedative/hypnotic/anxiolytic drugs should not occur in any dose for any resident. Residents currently receiving these drugs or residents admitted to the facility while using these drugs should receive gradual dose reductions as part of a plan to eliminate or modify the symptoms for which they are prescribed. A gradual dose reduction should be attempted at least twice within 1 year before one can conclude that the gradual dose reduction is clinically contraindicated. Newly admitted residents using these drugs may have a period of adjustment before a gradual dose reduction is attempted. *Caution*: Do not encourage rapid withdrawal of these drugs due to the risk of severe physiologic withdrawal symptoms.

Phenobarbital is exempted from this guideline when used in the treatment of seizure disorder.

Adapted from Reference 21.

divided into several broad categories, based on a high potential for severe or less-severe adverse outcomes for specific drugs and drug-disease combinations (Table 3-8 through to Table 3-11).

It should be noted that alterations in the use of medications based on the Beers criteria may not be appropriate for some residents, especially if they have been on the medications (and tolerated them) for years. Of course, sometimes they have tolerated the medications with undetected problems, such as electrocardiogram changes due to tricyclic antidepressants. Regardless of the reason for their use, changes to potentially problematic medications should not be considered without a period of observation and information gathering. Therefore, medications under Beers criteria may be continued for 7 days after admission, unless there is an immediate threat to health and safety.

In general, an attending physician or geriatric psychiatrist may prescribe any drug, in any dosage, for any legitimate reason, even if this does not fall within OBRA guidelines. Many clinicians misinterpret OBRA guidelines, however, and believe that dose reductions are mandatory, or Beers criteria medications are absolutely prohibited. Sometimes they overreact to suggestions from a reviewing pharmacist reminding them of the length of treatment, or the potential for side effects.

Keep in mind that the term *interpretive guidelines* simply means that the clinician must consider whether a dose reduction or the use of a specific agent is appropriate given the clinical situation, and then document his or her thinking. Such documentation must include the diagnosis, clinical justification for treatment, attempts at nonpharmacological intervention, and side effects. When continuing use beyond 4 to 6 months, or in a higher than recommended dose, the clinician might also cite the unsuccessful results of previous trials at lower doses, or the adverse consequences of previous taper attempts. The intent of OBRA to prompt consideration of dose changes is reasonable, however, given the fact that many of the causes of agitation or psychosis in LTC patients abate within months, leading to symptom reduction with or without the use of psychotropic agents.

Clinical Recommendations—the Attending Physician Should:

- On admission and at each revisit, consider whether each medication is still needed and ensure there is a clear reason or problem accompanying each medication order.

TABLE 3-5
INTERPRETIVE GUIDELINES FOR ANTIPSYCHOTIC DRUGS

Generic	Brand	Maximum Recommended Daily Dose
Chlorpromazine	Thorazine	75 mg
Promazine	Sparine	150 mg
Triflupromazine	Vesprin	20 mg
Thioridazine	Mellaril	75 mg
Mesoridazine	Serentil	25 mg
Acetophenazine	Tindal	20 mg
Perphenazine	Trilafon	8 mg
Fluphenazine	Prolixin, Permitil	4 mg
Trifluoperazine	Stelazine	8 mg
Chlorprothixene	Taractan	75 mg
Thiothixene	Navane	7 mg
Haloperidol	Haldol	4 mg
Molindone	Moban	10 mg
Loxapine	Loxitane	10 mg
Clozapine	Clozaril	50 mg
Prochlorperazine	Compazine	10 mg
Risperidone	Risperdal	2 mg
Olanzapine	Zyprexa	10 mg
Quetiapine	Seroquel	200 mg

The facility ensures that residents who are undergoing antipsychotic drug therapy receive adequate monitoring for significant side effects of such therapy, with emphasis on the following potential side effects:

- Tardive dyskinesia
- Postural hypotension
- Cognitive/behavioral impairment
- Akathisia
- Parkinsonism

Note: The guidelines have not yet been updated with established maximum dosing recommendations for ziprasidone or aripiprazole in nursing home populations.

Adapted from Reference 21.

TABLE 3-6
SPECIFIC CONDITIONS THAT JUSTIFY THE USE OF ANTIPSYCHOTIC DRUGS

Antipsychotic drugs should not be used unless the clinical record documents that the resident has one or more of the following specific conditions:

- Schizophrenia
- Schizoaffective disorder
- Delusional disorder
- Psychotic mood disorder
- Acute psychotic episodes
- Brief reactive psychosis
- Schizophreniform disorder
- Atypical psychosis
- Tourette's disorder
- Huntington's disease

Or: Organic mental syndromes (including delirium and dementia) with associated psychotic and/or agitated behaviors as defined by:

- Specific behaviors as quantitatively (number of episodes) and objectively (e.g., biting, kicking, scratching) documented by the facility which causes the resident to:
  - Present a danger to themselves
  - Present a danger to others (including staff)
  - Interfere with the staff's ability to provide care, *or*
- Continuously crying out, screaming, yelling, or pacing, if these specific behaviors cause an impairment in functional capacity and if they are quantitatively (e.g., periods of time) documented by the facility, *or*
- Psychotic symptoms (e.g., hallucinations, paranoia, delusions) not exhibited as specific behaviors listed above, if these behaviors cause the resident distress or impairment in functional capacity

Or: Short-term (7 days) symptomatic treatment of hiccoughs, nausea, vomiting, or pruritus

Adapted from Reference 21.

- Try to reduce the use of multiple medications for the same problem.
- Taper and discontinue medications when no longer needed.
- Order appropriate clinical and laboratory monitoring of medications with potential risks or complications.
- Review and acknowledge the pharmacist reviewer comments on medications used.
- Be familiar with approved indications/diagnoses for prescribing antipsychotic drugs, along with symptoms that are inadequate indications.
- Gradually reduce the dosage of antipsychotic medications to minimum effective doses.
- Be knowledgeable about inappropriate medication use in the elderly because it relates to a high potential for adverse outcomes.

Residents' Rights

According to OBRA, a resident has the right to exercise his or her rights as a resident of the facility and as a citizen or resident of the United States. Exercising of rights means that residents have autonomy in choice, to the maximum extent possible, about how they wish to live their everyday lives and receive care, subject to the facility's rules, as long as those rules do not violate a regulatory requirement. Several of the specific rights outlined in the regulations that have a direct effect on attending physicians practicing within the nursing facility include:

- The resident has the right to choose a personal attending physician.
- The resident has a right to be able to contact his or her attending physician.
- The resident and/or his or her legal representative has the right to be informed by the facility about the resident's

TABLE 3-7
INTERPRETIVE GUIDELINES FOR ANTIPSYCHOTIC DRUGS

Antipsychotics should not be used if one or more of the following is/are the only indications:

- Wandering
- Poor self-care
- Restlessness
- Impaired memory
- Anxiety
- Depression (without psychotic features)
- Insomnia
- Unsociability
- Indifference to surroundings
- Fidgeting
- Nervousness
- Uncooperativeness
- Unspecified agitation
- Agitated behaviors that do not represent a danger to self or others

As needed (PRN) antipsychotic drug orders should not be used more than five times in any 7-day period without a review of the resident's condition by a physician.

The facility must assure that residents who use antipsychotic drugs receive gradual dose reductions and behavioral interventions, unless clinically contraindicated, in an effort to discontinue these drugs.

In residents with organic mental syndromes (dementia, delirium), "clinically contraindicated" means that a gradual dose reduction has been attempted twice in 1 year, and that attempt resulted in the return of symptoms for which the drug was prescribed to a degree that a cessation in the gradual dose reduction, or a return to previous dose levels, was necessary.

In determining whether an antipsychotic drug is without a specific condition, or that gradual dose reduction and behavioral interventions have not been performed, the facility should be allowed an opportunity to justify why using the drug outside the guidelines is in the best interest of the resident.

Although the facility can refer to a physician's justification as a valid justification for the use of a drug, the facility may not justify the use of a drug, the dose, its duration, and so forth solely on the basis that the doctor ordered it.

Adapted from Reference 21.

TABLE 3-8
LIST OF DRUGS WITH HIGH POTENTIAL FOR SEVERE ADVERSE OUTCOMES

Amitriptyline[a] (Elavil)
Chlorpropamide (Diabinese)
Digoxin, if dose is greater than 0.125 mg/day[b]
Disopyramide (Norpace)
Doxepin (Sinequan)
Gastrointestinal antispasmodics (belladonna alkaloids, clidinium, dicyclomine, hyoscyamine, propantheline)[c]
Meperidine (Demerol), oral if started within past month
Methyldopa (Aldomet), if started within past month
Pentazocine (Talwin)
Ticlopidine[d] (Ticlid)

[a]Amitriptyline may be used for neurogenic pain (e.g., trigeminal neuralgia, peripheral neuropathy) if an evaluation of risk versus benefit of the drug is documented, including consideration of alternative therapies.
[b]Digoxin should be used in a dose of no more than 0.125 mg/day in the elderly, unless an atrial arrhythmia is being treated. High severity is considered if started within the past month.
[c]Use of these medications for short periods (not over 7 days) on an intermittent basis (not more frequently than every 3 months) does not require review by the surveyor.
[d]Review by the surveyor is not necessary in individuals who receive ticlopidine because they have had a previous stroke or have evidence of stroke precursors (transient ischemic attacks), and cannot tolerate aspirin.
Adapted from References 19 and 20.

Clinical Recommendations—the Attending Physician Should:

- Document discussions with residents/families about care and medical conditions, and specifically note that medical and functional status was discussed.
- Avoid examining nursing home residents while they are sitting in public areas of the facility, because this practice is not consistent with maintaining the privacy or dignity of residents.
- Examine residents who may have been subjected to abuse, and document and report the findings.
- Be knowledgeable regarding state laws and assure that resident preferences regarding end-of-life care and treatment are honored.

The Facility Must:

- Facilitate resident selection of a personal physician.
- Inform each resident of the name and best way of contacting his or her attending physician.

Quality of Care

OBRA regulations state that a facility must provide each resident with necessary care and services to attain the highest degree of physical, mental, and psychosocial well-being

total health status (functional status, medical care, nursing care, nutritional status, rehabilitation and restorative potential, activities potential, cognitive status, oral health status, psychosocial status, and sensory and physical impairments) in a language they understand.

- The resident has the right to personal privacy, which includes privacy during medical treatment.
- The resident has the right to be free from verbal, sexual, physical, and mental abuse, corporal punishment, and involuntary seclusion.
- The resident has the right to refuse treatment, and can exercise this right within the context of state laws governing advance directives and surrogate decision-making.

TABLE 3-9

LIST OF DIAGNOSIS-DRUG COMBINATIONS WITH HIGH POTENTIAL FOR SEVERE OUTCOMES

Use of sedative/hypnotics in residents with COPD. Short-acting benzodiazepines are acceptable.

Use of NSAIDs in residents with active or recurrent gastritis, PUD, or GERD. Cox-2 inhibitors (e.g., Celebrex) are not included on the HCFA list of NSAIDs.

Use of metoclopramide in residents with seizures or epilepsy.

Use of aspirin, NSAIDs, dipyridamole, clopidogrel, or ticlopidine in residents taking anticoagulants.

Use of anticholinergic drugs in residents with BPH. Drugs listed include: anticholinergic antihistamines, anticholinergic antidepressants, anti-Parkinson medications, and GI antispasmodics. Antihistamines and GI antispasmodics do not require review by the surveyor if used intermittently (every 3 months) for short periods (7 days).

Use of tricyclic antidepressants in residents with arrhythmias (if started within past month).

Use of aspirin, NSAIDs, dipyridamole, or ticlopidine in residents taking anticoagulants.

BPH, benign prostatic hypertrophy; COPD, chronic obstructive pulmonary disease; GERD, gastroesophageal reflux disease; GI, gastrointestinal; HCFA, Health Care Financing Administration; NSAIDs, nonsteroidal anti-inflammatory drugs; PUD, peptic ulcer disease. Adapted from References 19 and 20.

possible, limited only by the individual's presenting functional status, and potential for improvement or reducing the rate of functional decline. The facility must ensure that the resident obtains optimal improvement or does not deteriorate within the limits of a resident's right to refuse treatment, and within the limits of recognized pathology and the normal aging process. In any case in which there has been a lack of improvement or a decline, the survey team must determine if the occurrence was unavoidable, based on the following information:

- An accurate and complete assessment
- A care plan which is implemented consistently and based on information from the assessment
- An evaluation of the results of treatment, with appropriate revisions to the intervention

As of July, 1999, a series of markers known as Quality Indicators (QIs), derived from the MDS, have been incorporated into the survey process. The QI report provides an overview of potential problem areas in the facility. The Facility Quality Indicator Profile lists 24 QIs in a total of 11 domains (Table 3-12). Some of the QIs have subsections, with residents divided into high risk and low risk. The report shows all the QIs for that facility and compares them to statewide averages for all facilities. In addition, the facility will have a percentile ranking for each indicator to show how it compares with all others in the state. QIs which rank

it above the 90th percentile in comparison to other facilities in the state will be flagged. In addition, three sentinel event QIs will be flagged if there is at least one resident who triggers it. The three triggers are:

- Prevalence of fecal impaction
- Prevalence of dehydration
- Prevalence of pressure ulcers in low-risk residents

The following QIs are related to medication use:

- Prevalence of symptoms of depression without antidepressant therapy
- Prevalence of residents who take nine or more medications
- Prevalence of antipsychotic use, in the absence of psychotic or related conditions
- Prevalence of antianxiety/hypnotic use
- Prevalence of hypnotic use of more than two times in the previous week

Several QIs have now been converted to Quality Measures (QMs), listed on the CMS website, to be used as markers of quality of care that consumers can review and compare amongst facilities. Although QMs as listed on the website give a snapshot of a single facility, they are limited regarding comparisons, since not all facilities are alike. The LTC facilities with more high-acuity patients may compare less favorably simply looking at the numbers, even though this is not an accurate portrayal of actual quality of care. Similarly, the presence of a full-time geriatric psychiatrist at a facility might result in higher-than-average numbers of individuals on psychotropic drugs. These numbers could be higher due to over-prescribing, or could reflect optimal use of these medications given the more intensive psychiatric surveillance. Ultimately, clinical documentation must justify the QI or QM numbers, wherever they lie.

Clinical Recommendations—the Attending Physician Should:

- Document observations of each resident's progress.
- Check that the staff has implemented medical orders consistently and appropriately.
- Address potential risk factors for decline.
- Order appropriate tests, consultations, or evaluations to help decide the potential for improvement and effectiveness of treatments.
- Be familiar with QIs and potential sentinel events.

SUMMARY

While OBRA is not perfect, it has had a remarkable impact on nursing home care, and has led to significant improvements in the quality of patient life. It set a uniform national standard for quality of care in nursing homes, including standards for certifying Medicare and Medicaid. The regulations emphasize not only quality of care, but also quality of life.

TABLE 3-10
LIST OF DRUGS WITH HIGH POTENTIAL FOR LESS SEVERE OUTCOMES

Antihistamines (i.e., with anticholinergic properties)
Cyclandelate (Cyclospasmol)
Diphenhydramine[a] (Benadryl)
Dipyridamole (Persantine)
Ergot mesyloids (e.g., Hydergine)
Indomethacin[b] (Indocin)
Muscle relaxants (e.g., Carisoprodol, Chlorzoxazone, Cyclobenzaprine, Dantrolene, Metaxalone, Methocarbamol, Orphenadrine)[c]
Phenylbutazone (Butazolidin)
Reserpine (Serpasil)
Trimethobenzamide (Tigan)

[a]Review by the surveyor is not necessary if use is for short duration (7 days or less) on an intermittent basis (once every 3 months) for treatment of allergies.
[b]Short-term use (e.g., 1 week) is considered acceptable for treatment of gouty arthritis.
[c]Review by the surveyor is not necessary if use is for short duration (7 days or less) on an intermittent basis (once every 3 months) for symptoms of an acute, self-limiting condition.
Adapted from References 19 and 20.

TABLE 3-11
DIAGNOSIS-DRUG COMBINATIONS WITH HIGH POTENTIAL FOR LESS-SEVERE OUTCOMES

Corticosteroids in residents with diabetes, if started within past month
Potassium supplements or aspirin (greater than 325 mg/day) in residents with active or recurrent gastritis, PUD, or GERD[a]
Antipsychotics in residents with seizures or epilepsy[b]
Narcotic drugs, including propoxyphene, in residents with BPH[c]
Bladder relaxants (flavoxate, oxybutynin, bethanechol) in residents with BPH[c]
Constipation can be worsened by:

- Anticholinergic antihistamines[c]
- Anti-Parkinson medications
- GI antispasmodics[c]
- Anticholinergic antidepressants
- Narcotic drugs, including propoxyphene[c]

Insomnia can be worsened by:

- Decongestants
- Theophylline
- Methylphenidate
- SSRI antidepressants and desipramine
- MAO inhibitors
- Beta agonists

[a]Use of potassium supplements to treat low potassium levels until they return to normal range is permissible in these residents if the prescriber determines that the use of fresh fruits and vegetables or other dietary supplementation is not adequate or possible.
[b]Treatment of acute psychosis for 72 hours or less is permissible.
[c]Review by the surveyor is not necessary if use is for short duration (7 days or less) on an intermittent basis (once every 3 months) for symptoms of an acute, self-limiting condition.
BPH, benign prostate hypertrophy; GERD, gastroesophageal reflux disease; GI, gastrointestinal; MAO, monoamine oxidase; PUD, peptic ulcer disease; SSRI, selective serotonin-reuptake inhibitor.
Adapted from References 19 and 20.

TABLE 3-12
FACILITY QUALITY INDICATORS

Domain/Quality Indicator

Accidents
1. Incidence of new fractures
2. Prevalence of falls

Behavioral/Emotional Patterns
3. Prevalence of behavioral symptoms affecting others
   High risk
   Low risk
4. Prevalence of symptoms of depression
5. Prevalence of symptoms of depression without antidepressant therapy

Clinical Management
6. Use of nine or more different medications

Cognitive Patterns
7. Incidence of cognitive impairment

Elimination/Incontinence
8. Prevalence of bladder or bowel incontinence
   High risk
   Low risk
9. Prevalence of occasional or frequent bladder or bowel incontinence without a toileting plan
10. Prevalence of indwelling catheter
11. Prevalence of fecal impaction*

Infection Control
12. Prevalence of urinary tract infections

Nutrition/Eating
13. Prevalence of weight loss
14. Prevalence of tube feeding
15. Prevalence of dehydration*

Physical Functioning
16. Prevalence of bedfast residents
17. Incidence of decline in late loss ADLs
18. Incidence of decline of ROM

Psychotropic Drug Use
19. Prevalence of antipsychotic use, in the absence of psychotic or related conditions (High risk/Low risk)
20. Prevalence of antianxiety/hypnotic use
21. Prevalence of hypnotic use more than two times in last week

Quality of Life
22. Prevalence of daily physical restraints
23. Prevalence of little or no activity

Skin Care
24. Prevalence of stage 1–4 pressure ulcers* (High risk/Low risk)

ADLs, activities of daily living; ROM, range of motion;*,sentinel events.
Adapted from Reference 22.

OBRA set the standard for a patient's ADLs to be maintained or improved. The regulations laid the groundwork for individual treatment plans for each LTC resident. Residents' rights to remain in a skilled facility were ensured, with excep-tions for behavioral disturbances, nonpayment, or significant changes in their medical condition.

REFERENCES

1. Meyer H. The bottom line on assisted living. *Hosp Health Netw.* 1998;72(14):22–26.
2. Zimmerman S, Sloane PD, Eckert JK, eds. *Assisted Living: Needs, Practices and Policies in Residential Care for the Elderly.* Baltimore: John Hopkins University Press; 2001.
3. Chapin R, Dobbs-Kepper D. Aging in place in assisted living: philosophy versus policy. *Gerontologist.* 2001;41(1):43–50.
4. Sabin TD, Vitung AJ, Mark VH. Are nursing home diagnosis and treatment inadequate? *JAMA.* 1982;248:321–322.
5. Burns BJ, Larson DB, Goldstrom ID, Johnson WE. Mental disorders among nursing home patients: preliminary findings from the national nursing home survey pretest. *Int J Ger Psychiatry.* 1988; 327–335.
6. Avorn J, Dreyer P, Connelly K, Soumerai SB. Use of psychoactive medication and the quality of care in rest homes. *N Eng J Med.* 1989;320:227–232.
7. Public Law No. 100-203, Omnibus Budget Reconciliation Act of 1987, 22 December 1987. *Annu Rev Popul Law.* 1987;14:473–475.
8. Health Care Financing Administration. Medicare and Medicaid: requirements for long-term care facilities, final regulations. *Federal Register.* 1991;56(187):48865–48921.
9. Snowden M, Roy-Byrne P. Mental illness and nursing home reform: OBRA-87 ten years later. Omnibus Budget Reconciliation Act. *Psychiatr Serv.* 1998;49(2):229–233.
10. Colenda CC, Streim J, Greene JA, Meyers N, Beckwith E, Rabins P. The impact of OBRA '87 on psychiatric services in nursing homes. Joint testimony of the American Psychiatric Association and the American Association for Geriatric Psychiatry. *Am J Geriatr Psychiatry.* 1999;7(1):12–17.
11. Siegler EL, Capezuti E, Maislin G, Baumgarten M, Evans L, Strumpf N. Effects of a restraint reduction intervention and OBRA '87 regulations on psychoactive drug use in nursing homes. *J Am Geriatr Soc.* 1997;45(7):791–796.
12. Rovner BW, Edelman BA, Cox MP, Shmuely Y. The impact of antipsychotic drug regulations (OBRA 1987) on psychotropic prescribing practices in nursing homes. *Am J Psychiatry.* 1992;149: 1390–1392.
13. Semla TP, Palla K, Poddig B, Brauner DJ. Effect of the Omnibus Reconciliation Act 1987 on antipsychotic prescribing in nursing home residents. *J Am Geriatr Soc.* 1994;42(6):648–652.
14. Lantz MS, Giambanco V, Buchalter EN. A ten-year review of the effect of OBRA-87 on psychotropic prescribing practices in an academic nursing home. *Psychiatr Serv.* 1996;47(9):951–955.
15. Borson S, Doane K. The impact of OBRA-87 on psychotropic drug prescribing in skilled nursing facilities. *Psychiatr Serv.* 1997;48(10): 1289–1296.
16. Morris JN, Hawes C, Fries BE, et al. Designing the national resident assessment instrument for nursing homes. *Gerontologist.* 1990;30(3):293–307.
17. Health Care Financing Administration. Medicare and Medicaid: resident assessment in long-term care facilities. *Federal Register.* 1992;57(249):61614–61733.
18. Rantz MJ, Zwygart-Stauffacher M, Popejoy LL, et al. The minimum data set: no longer just for clinical assessment. *Ann Long-Term Care.* 1999;7(9):354–360.
19. Beers MH, Ouslander JG, Fingold SF, et al. Inappropriate medication prescribing in skilled nursing facilities. *Ann Int Med.* 1992;117(8):684–689.
20. Beers MH. Explicit criteria for determining potentially inappropriate medication use in the elderly: an update. *Ann Int Med.* 1997;157:1531–1536.
21. Health Care Financing Administration. *Survey Procedures and Interpretive Guidelines for Skilled Nursing Facilities and Intermediate Care Facilities.* Baltimore: US Department of Health and Human Services; 1990.
22. Center for Health Systems Research and Analysis, University of Wisconsin–Madison. *Facility Guide for the Nursing Home Quality Indicators;* 1997.

The Geriatric Caregiver

4

Larry W. Thompson   *Adam P. Spira*   *Colin A. Depp*

Jocelyn Shealy McGee   *Dolores Gallagher-Thompson*

WHO ARE THE FAMILY CAREGIVERS?

Ada is a 69-year-old college-educated, retired teacher who has been caring for her 75-year-old husband, Bill, for the past 6 years. When Bill was in his mid sixties, he began to complain about forgetting names of people and not being able to think of the right words to describe a particular event or object. A year later, Ada noticed that he was forgetting to deposit checks and sometimes acted inappropriately in mixed company. She knew that something was not "right," but delayed asking his doctor about it, thinking that the problem might take care of itself in time. Shortly after Bill's 68th birthday, she received a call from a police officer who informed her that Bill had been stopped in a shopping mall parking lot, because he was acting strangely and had accused several people of stealing his car. When Ada arrived at the shopping mall she discovered that Bill had actually forgotten where he had parked his car, resulting in panic. The police assisted Ada in finding Bill's car, and then released him in her custody with the strong admonition that Bill should be seen by his primary care physician (PCP) as soon as possible.

After a medical examination and laboratory tests were completed, a diagnosis of Alzheimer's disease (AD) was made and Bill's doctor prescribed donepezil in combination with small doses of vitamin E and C. Despite some initial improvement in cognitive symptoms, Bill gradually began to have more memory and behavioral problems, which required that he eventually receive constant supervision by another adult. As his functioning decreased, Ada began to make more frequent appointments with Bill's PCP to see if there were additional options for his care. At these appointments, she served as an informant regard-

ing behavioral changes and called the PCP's attention to new interventions that had been reported in the news. Over time, Ada's level of functioning began to change. She lost weight and became increasingly anxious and dysphoric. Ada complained of sleep problems and openly questioned whether she provided good care for Bill. However, as per her request, the focus of these visits remained on strategies for remedying Bill's condition. In an attempt to deal with Ada's explicit requests to help Bill, the PCP spent little time focusing on Ada's health care needs. Realizing that, given his time constraints, he was not equipped to resolve the needs of this family, he referred them to a local geropsychiatrist.

Although specific details vary from family to family, the clinical picture portrayed in the case of Ada and Bill is being seen with increasing regularity. The need for assistance with activities of daily living (ADLs) due to dementias such as AD increases with age (1), and the continued growth of the elderly population in the United States has led to an unprecedented demand for such assistance. In the year 2000, 4.5 million Americans had AD; by the year 2050 this number will grow to 13.2 million (2). All of these individuals will require some form of care, and the burden of the care will fall heavily on family caregivers. Between 1987 and 1997, the proportion of individuals who required some form of care rose from 7.8% to approximately 23% of the U.S. population (3). Although formal or professional caregivers (e.g., home health aides, visiting nurses, nursing staff within long-term care facilities) provide an important service, approximately 95% of community-dwelling older adults with severe ADL impairments receive care from a family or community member (1), totaling more than five million informal caregivers for older adults with dementia (4).

Definitions of informal/family caregiving vary across studies, but it is generally accepted that this activity includes the rendering of personal care to a family member who can no longer provide adequate self-care in some or all aspects of his or her daily life, such as dressing, bathing, toileting, feeding, and other personal and household management activities (4). Caregiving of persons with dementia typically begins informally within the family and remains as the responsibility of family or close friends until such time that they believe they can no longer provide adequate care. Factors associated with this turn of events include the development of severe cognitive impairment in the care recipient, more time required to provide adequate care than the caregivers can actually allot, low functional status of the care recipient, the development of serious physical health problems in either the caregiver or care recipient, and a poor relationship between caregiver and care recipient (5–7). Thus, often the decisive factors for terminating family caregiving are either a substantial increase in behavior problems (e.g., wandering, incontinence, assaults), which overwhelm the caregiver's management ability, or increased medical and/or psychological problems in either party that make it difficult for the caregiver to be effective in their role. At such points, it generally becomes necessary to implement formal caregiving strategies through institutionalization or through intensive in-home supportive services.

The marked cost differential between formal and informal caregiving attests to the significance of the family caregiver as an essential resource in the health care system. Thus, it behooves us to develop ways to improve the caregiver's quality of life, while at the same time prolonging their effectiveness in this role. However, in many instances there comes a time when families must deal with the enormously difficult issue of when and how to place a loved one in an institutional care setting. When confronted with this issue, caregivers often need increased instrumental and emotional support that many physicians are not equipped to provide, given the time constraints in their practice. At such times, referral to other community agencies with appropriate information and referral resources and skilled counselors to assist the caregiver in working through this transition is recommended.

For the past two decades, the modal family caregiver has continued to be a married woman in her forties (mean age = 46 years) who works full time (4). However, since the 1980s, the proportion of male caregivers has increased. More family caregivers are now living apart from the care recipients than in the past and a greater percentage are employed (3). Ethnic characteristics of caregivers are also beginning to change. Today, non-Hispanic Whites make up 81% of the U.S. population aged 55 and over, but only 66% of the population under age 55 (8). As these younger Americans age,

the older segment of the population and its family caregivers will become much more ethnically diverse. For example, in the year 2000, ethnic minority groups made up 16.5% of the population age 65 and over. This figure is expected to rise to almost 38% by the year 2050 (9).

This increased ethnic diversity is particularly noteworthy, since recent research has shown that significant differences in cultural attitudes and beliefs regarding disability and illness can influence how family members actually perceive dementia, what types of care are provided, who provides the care in the family, and how formal services might be utilized (10). Also, it is likely that members of different ethnic groups experience different levels of psychological distress in response to distinct aspects of caregiving (11). For example, caregivers in some ethnic groups experience little distress when assisting with feeding and toileting, but have considerable difficulty when confronted with embarrassing behavior in social situations (12). Greater familiarization with the needs of ethnically diverse caregivers is an important goal for psychiatrists working with these individuals (13).

POTENTIAL PITFALLS OF CAREGIVING

Caregivers of individuals with dementia face a particularly stressful situation, and are at increased risk for both physical illness and psychiatric morbidity (14). Compared to other caregivers, AD caregivers spend more hours per week actually providing care, provide help with more ADLs, are twice as likely to provide care related to incontinence and feeding, and are more likely to be living with care recipients (15,16). Often, the task of providing care for a dependent older adult causes significant disruptions in sleep, physical health, privacy, leisure, finances, and household management (17). Family caregivers for individuals with dementia are more likely to experience occupational problems, emotional and physical distress, and disturbance in social functioning, than are caregivers of individuals without dementia (16). Further, they tend to have lower self-rated health and altered immune function (18). Spousal caregivers who experience mental or emotional strain related to caregiving have mortality risks that are 63% higher than spouses who provide similar care but do not report significant stress associated with their role (19). Although some positive aspects of caregiving, including role satisfaction and increased self-worth have been reported (20), the fact remains that, compared to non-caregiving control samples, caregivers experience more negative physical health effects, increased rates of psychiatric disorders (11), and a greater preponderance of financial strain (14). Thus, as a group, they are likely to be in need of medical, psychiatric, psychological, and social services as their loved ones' dementia progresses over time. Despite these increased risks, health and psychiatric care for caregivers is often overlooked until they develop a clinical disorder.

Referring back to the example of Ada, there clearly was increased evidence of psychiatric distress. However, her choice was to focus her interactions with the health care system on improving Bill's health, with little concern for her own welfare. She continued to maintain this focus when first meeting with the geropsychiatrist. Understandably, the initial focus of the psychiatrist was to evaluate Bill's condition and then prescribe a treatment regimen. In this task, Ada again became an ally, providing extensive information about Bill's present and past symptoms. Little thought was given to her mental health. However, Bill's intellectual functioning did not improve as she had hoped, and her symptoms of psychological distress began to increase.

At this point in the course of Bill's treatment, the psychiatrist began to focus more on Ada's current status. She asked Ada to take several psychological screening tests which clearly showed that she was experiencing substantial psychological distress. Although Bill was her patient of record, the psychiatrist inquired more directly about Ada's general welfare in subsequent meetings. While Ada was uncomfortable with this, she did accept the logic that she had to take care of her own health in order to be able to care for Bill.

Eventually, she acknowledged that she needed help with her emotional condition, so the psychiatrist started Ada on an antidepressant medication and made a referral to a mental health provider with skills and experience working with distressed family caregivers. Ada began attending a psychotherapy group for family caregivers where she was taught an array of specific skills to improve her mood and increase her use of adaptive coping strategies. After completing this program, she began to use other community-based resources, such as support groups through the local chapter of the Alzheimer's Association. While Ada continued to experience mild symptoms of anxiety and depression, her overall quality of life was greatly improved. Her contact with others in her support group helped her finally to accept the fact that Bill's condition was irreversible, and that her caretaking of Bill was as professional and competent as it could possibly be. She took comfort in the knowledge that she was doing the best job she could, given the circumstances. Along with acceptance of her situation, Ada understood that she needed to take better care of herself. She learned how to be more assertive with family members in getting them to assist with Bill's care on a short-term basis. This enabled her to have time to occasionally engage in other pleasant activities and to manage other family affairs that needed attention. At this point in Bill's illness, Ada appeared to be doing reasonably well. One wonders how her situation might have turned out had the physicians involved with this family not been persistent in their efforts to help her receive care for herself as well as Bill.

Ada's case raises several questions pertaining to the identification and treatment of clinical disorders in caregivers. What strategies can be used to assist in the identification of caregivers who have or are at risk for developing psychiatric disorders? What are some of the risk factors? What resources are available to help prevent the development of clinical disorders? What kinds of interventions are effective in treating caregivers who have psychiatric problems?

While many of these questions remain unanswered, information is available that in several ways can be helpful to geropsychiatrists and, particularly, to PCPs, who initially see the large majority of these patients. First, even though many caring for the elderly may not have the time or resources to integrate comprehensive psychosocial procedures into their practice, it is recommended that at least some assessment and treatment of caregiver concerns be done on a regular basis. Doing so leads to high levels of both physician and consumer satisfaction (21), and often can be accomplished with only a few additional resources. For example, most screening instruments can be administered with a minimum of training on the part of existing allied health professionals (e.g., nurses, social workers), and then referrals can be made, as necessary, to appropriate psychological and social service providers in the community.

It is encouraging that numerous medical and allied health professional organizations have become more sensitive to the need for information pertaining to the care of dementia patients at home, and are developing consumer-friendly publications to this end. For example, the Alzheimer's Society has a free interactive tutorial CD-ROM on diagnosis and care management (available from www.alzheimer's.org.uk) that can be helpful to primary care professionals. Similarly, the International Psychogeriatric Association has recently released an educational packet on the behavioral and psychological symptoms of dementia that includes information on the caregivers' role and the problems they encounter. Information regarding these and other useful publications can be obtained at their website: www.ipa-online.org. Other websites, such as www.caregiving.com, provide practical information on how to cope with the perils of caregiving, and some also implement online support groups.

CAREGIVER ASSESSMENT

Although the caregiver's role in an office visit may most commonly be viewed as "informant," a clinical interview with a caregiver–care recipient dyad should include assessment of the caregiver's functioning and level of distress. As we saw in Ada's situation, the caregiver may suffer an array of symptoms that are not yet at threshold level but may be prodromal to a clinical disorder. Interventions to reduce symptoms and improve overall coping are warranted, since these symptom clusters often reduce caregivers' effectiveness in their roles. Assessment of the caregiver's mental status and psychosocial functioning can guide the clinician in selecting cost-effective treatment.

A useful guideline for a comprehensive assessment is depicted in Figure 4-1, which considers the interplay among a variety of factors, including sociodemographic

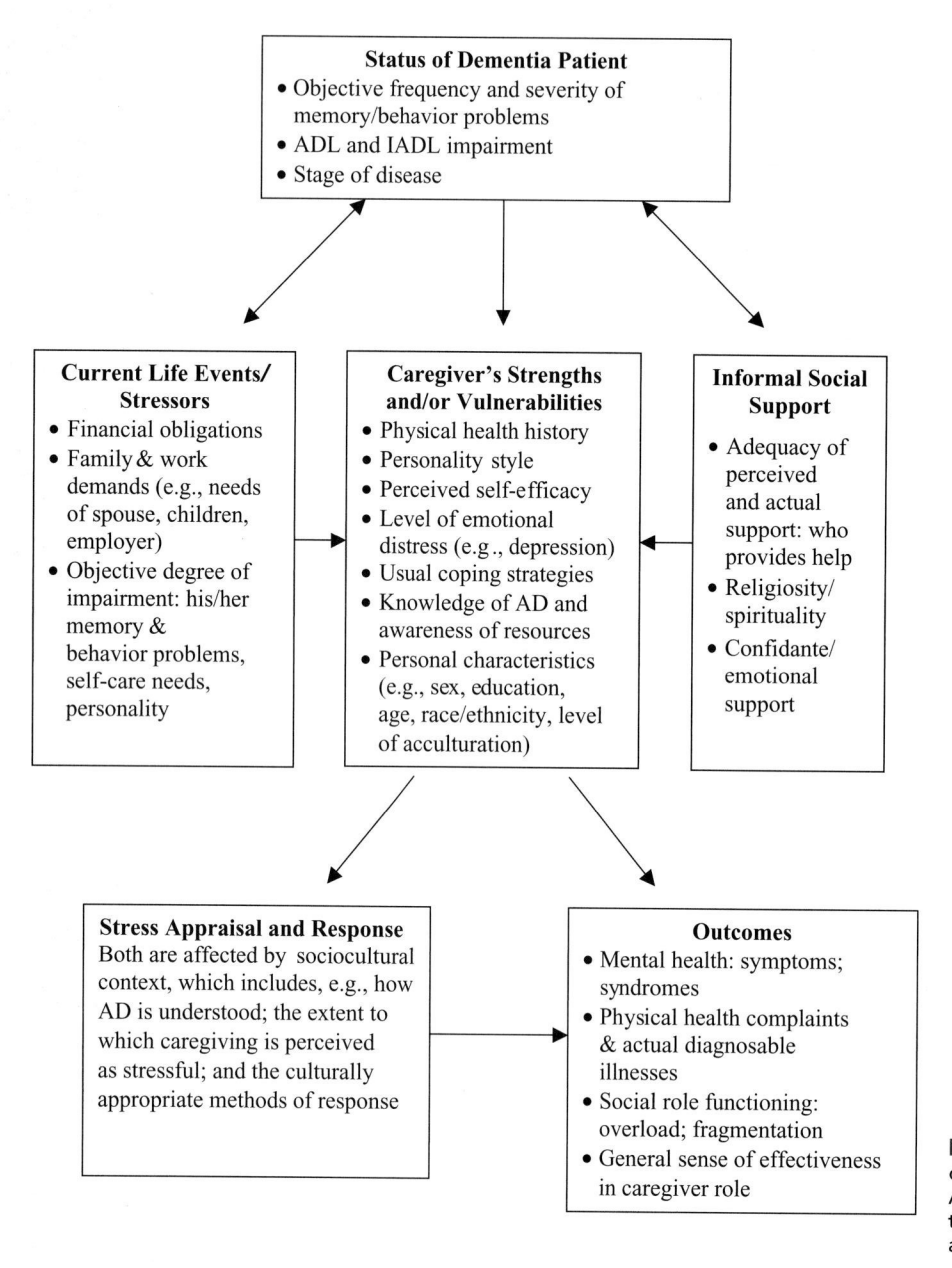

Figure 4-1 Sociocultural context of dementia caregiving.
AD, Alzheimer's disease; ADL, activities of daily living; IADL, instrumental activities of daily living.

information, extent of objective and subjective burden (the actual number of memory and behavior problems and self-care needs that are present in the situation, and how one appraises and reacts to these demands), the variety of coping mechanisms or strategies that the caregiver has at his/her disposal, perceived self-efficacy for handling stressful caregiving situations, and perceived adequacy of the social support network (22,23,24). Since many caregivers are older adults, the practitioner should be familiar with the fundamentals of geriatric assessment (25). Finally, since caregivers are coming from diverse ethnic and cultural groups, appropriate assessment requires knowledge of the caregiver's cultural background and culturally appropriate assessment devices (26,27). The geriatric psychiatrist is in a pivotal position to implement such a biopsychosocial assessment model, thereby identifying caregivers who

are at risk for poor health and/or poor mental health outcomes. While it may not be practical for the psychiatrist to complete a detailed assessment in the office, he/she can coordinate assessment information from referrals in cases where detailed assessment seems warranted.

Identifying the "At Risk" Caregiver

Given the very challenging—and often unrelenting—demands of caregiving, we believe it is unreasonable to expect that caregivers will be completely free of symptoms such as dysphoria, anxiety, anger, frustration, and feelings of grief and loss (28). Many who are captive in this role feel as if they are "going crazy" and need assistance to recognize that their reactions are within reason, considering the circumstances. It is very helpful to validate and normalize caregivers' feelings about their experience, while also not downplaying their significance (29).

Many caregivers may be at risk for the development of more serious problems, but it is not always easy to identify these individuals. The more relevant information there is available, the more effective one can be in identifying such individuals. If, however, it is not possible to obtain detailed information in all of the domains mentioned when screening a caregiver, then a good rule of thumb is to consider at least the ratio of current psychological complaints to available resources. Consider these case examples:

Cynthia, who is a 45-year-old businesswoman, was caring for her moderately demented mother at home. She complained of stress, problems with sleep, and frequent worry and anxiety about the future. Cynthia's husband and her two sisters, however, were quite supportive. They provided regular financial and emotional support (e.g., paid for in-home health care workers while Cynthia was at her job) and helped with personal care on weekends so that Cynthia could get some respite and engage in other activities that she enjoyed. Thus, although she was experiencing psychological distress, the adequacy of her support system was such that she was not likely to experience any further loss of functioning. Nevertheless, caregivers with Cynthia's profile can still benefit from psychoeducational programs to help develop improved skills for coping with stress, and it is useful to suggest that they explore such programs.

Laura, on the other hand, was in a similar situation and frame of mind, with virtually no immediate support network. She is a 55-year-old divorced woman who worked long hours in her position as a sales manager and was also trying to provide care at home for her mother. Laura's adult children and sister did not live nearby and seemed uninterested in her plight. Although she had some in-home help for her mother, Laura was becoming more distracted at work and was unable to perform adequately due to stress. She was in danger of losing her position or being demoted to a job that paid much less. At that point, Laura recognized that she needed help, sought psychiatric care, was started on an antidepressant, and referred for individual therapy to a social worker skilled in working with family caregivers' issues.

As previously noted, medical practitioners are in a prime position to identify caregivers who are at risk for developing more serious stress-related disorders. We recommend evaluating the following factors in several relevant domains:

First: Determine whether the caregiver has access to educational material on dementia. Learning more about the disorder, what to expect from loved ones who have dementia, and tips on how to provide care for them often reduces the stress of caregiving substantially, and little else is needed until later phases of caregiving. Ask if the caregiver has information about memory loss and dementia. Does the caregiver have brochures or pamphlets that review problems one can expect and possible solutions? Does the care recipient have a living will? Have issues such as durable power of attorney or guardianship been resolved? Having information pertaining to such questions in the office can be a real time-saver. Additionally there are many organizations, such as the Alzheimer's Disease Education and Referral Center (ADEAR) clearinghouse sponsored by the National Institute on Aging, as well as the Alzheimer's Association and state or local organizations, particularly local Area Offices on Aging that have this type of information readily available—often in multiple languages. Low-cost or free websites sponsoring online chat rooms and online support groups, such as www.caregiving.com, are becoming more readily available. Resources on the Internet can be particularly helpful late at night when all other agencies are closed. If they have not already done so, encouraging caregivers to utilize resources provided by these agencies may be sufficient help to prevent, or at least delay, the development of a later stress-related disorder.

Second: Determine the relevance of specific safety issues that may arise in caregiving situations. For example, is the patient still driving? Often it is difficult for the impaired individual to give up driving. Men, in particular, are likely to insist that they be allowed to continue to drive, and families are usually extremely grateful for any support they receive from a physician or other allied health professional in effecting this change. Another important question is whether the patient can be safely left alone. One should inquire whether there are features in the home that are potentially dangerous for a patient with severe cognitive impairment and/or poor judgment. Are poisons and harmful medicines locked up securely? Does the care recipient have access to dangerous knives or a gun? Does the care recipient ever smoke in the house when he/she is alone? Does the home have appropriate fire alarms and are fire extinguishers readily available? Also, encourage the caregiver to obtain identification for the care recipient that indicates the medical diagnosis, in the event that he/she might wander too far from the home. Finally, is there evidence of abuse initiated by either the caregiver or care recipient? Many professionals find it difficult to ask about this, but caregivers, though often reluctant to acknowledge the problem at first, typically are relieved when this information is disclosed, and most often they collaborate in active problem solving to prevent any subsequent occurrence. The initial response may be to deny that abuse has occurred, but the seed is sown, which makes it easier to discuss the problem at a later time.

Third: Evaluate whether or not the caregiver has the intellectual ability or the personality structure to carry out the skills required to cope adequately with the demands of their unique situation. Consider this case example:

Bob was a successful midlevel executive in a large corporation who remained oblivious to the severity of his wife's impairment. Sarah was doing things like putting soap powder in the sugar bowl, fixing herself cereal, and then throwing it on the living room floor because of the terrible taste. Even in the face of such behavior, Bob remained convinced that Sarah did not need supervision while she was at home. Much to Bob's dismay, it became necessary to involve Adult Protective Services (APS) to ensure that an appropriate care plan was put into effect. When contacted by staff from APS, Bob delayed arranging a meeting as long as possible. However, he was finally convinced that other arrangements had to be made when Sarah started a fire on top of the kitchen stove to roast hot dogs. Thus, although he was intellectually competent, he was emotionally in denial about the severity of his wife's condition, and this clouded his judgment.

Screening measures can be helpful in making this decision. Determining caregiver skills to deal with the problems can also be facilitated by obtaining specific information about their perception of how effective they are in handling tasks and problems that occur in family caregiving. For example, do they have difficulty completing household chores? Are they able to help with toileting or cleaning up accidents without getting upset? Are preparing meals for and feeding the care recipient a problem? Is the caregiver able to help with bathing, brushing teeth, dressing, etc.? Does the care recipient frequently engage in any behaviors that are disturbing, like socially inappropriate behaviors or repeatedly asking the same question? As with Bob, do they deny possible risks when questioned about them?

A *fourth* area to assess is the degree of instrumental and social support available to caregivers. Their stress can be decreased substantially by availability of adequate transportation, financial assistance, legal and other professional consultation, along with emotional support from family and friends. If these are lacking, then caregivers should be encouraged to obtain such resources through available social service agencies and by linking up with support groups offered free of charge by local and regional chapters of the Alzheimer's Association. They can also check with the local office of the Administration on Aging (AoA) to learn about available resources.

Fifth: it is clear that the caregivers' emotional and physical well-being should be evaluated carefully and repeatedly while a psychiatrist is treating care recipients who have dementia. Caregivers with significant levels of depression, anxiety, guilt, fear, and/or anger function less effectively in their role and typically need treatment themselves. Office screening measures to assist with this continual monitoring are readily available and are noted below.

Specific Areas of Assessment and Possible Measures

The Caregiver Self-Assessment Questionnaire, developed by the American Medical Association (30), is a helpful entry point. This self-report scale has 16 "yes/no" items and two global items designed to assess emotional and physical distress, such as perceived stress or feelings of depression. It was developed for use in physician offices to quickly pinpoint areas of concern. It can be completed by the caregiver while their loved one is in for an office visit. It is available on the AMA website (http://www.ama-assn.org/ama/pub/category/5037.html), along with tips on how best to use it and basic information on how to help caregivers to prevent further decline in their psychological or physical functioning.

Health and Health-related Behaviors. Overall health is a primary concern, and caregivers should be encouraged to have an annual physical evaluation. Often caregivers become so concerned about their care recipient that they neglect and abuse their own health status (e.g., begin overeating, smoking, increasing alcohol use). Thus, the physician should ask about health issues that might make it difficult for caregivers to function. For example, are they getting adequate rest? Inadequate sleep is a common problem for dementia caregivers, and can contribute significantly to caregiver burden (31).

Emotional Functioning. The proportion of mood and anxiety disorders is clearly higher in dementia caregivers than in age-matched individuals who are not caregivers. Some studies have found that one in every two caregivers has a sufficient level of depression or other emotional problem to warrant therapy (32–34). Thus, it is important to assess for these potential psychiatric morbidities. The Center for Epidemiological Studies-Depression Scale (CES-D) (35) and the Geriatric Depression Scale (36,37) are often used as screening measures for symptoms of depression in caregivers. These are brief, self-report measures (in the public domain) that can be administered easily in the waiting room of a busy office practice. Both have acceptable reliability and validity, are available in several languages, and have been used frequently in studies of older adults (38). Other useful measures can be found in the Handbook of Psychiatric Measures (39). It includes a wide array of interview and self-report instruments, references, and a CD-ROM that contains a number of instruments available in the public domain.

Cognitive Functioning. Intact cognitive functioning on the part of the caregiver is essential for adequate role performance. There are several brief cognitive screening tests that can be quickly and easily administered with minimal training. The most popular of these is the Mini-Mental State Examination (MMSE) (40). However, a cautionary note about the MMSE is that it tends to overestimate the presence of severe cognitive deficits in persons with limited education, and underestimate cognitive difficulties in those who are more highly educated. Referral for a more comprehensive neuropsychological evaluation can be useful if the caregiver performs poorly on screening tests.

Perceived Stress/Burden. This construct is particularly important with family caregivers, because the degree to which individuals perceive life events or situations as stressful influences the actual psychological impact on their lives. The Burden Interview (41) is a tool to collect information about caregivers' stress. It asks a series of questions about the extent to which caregivers perceive that their current responsibilities are having a negative impact on their physical, psychosocial, and financial status. It is noteworthy that the perception of burden by the caregiver is often more highly correlated with placement of the care recipient than are more objective measures of the severity of the dementia.

Social Support. In general, persons who have a high degree of social support tend to have decreased physical and psychiatric morbidity, above and beyond standard medical risk factors (42). For example, caregivers with high social support tend to have less impairment in immune system function (43). Several self-report measures exist for this purpose; one that has frequently been successfully used with caregivers is the Yale Social Support Index (44).

Coping. Certain coping styles are associated with better outcomes (e.g., use of active, problem-oriented cognitive and behavioral strategies), whereas other coping styles, such as denial or avoidance strategies, are associated with poorer outcomes (45,46). The Revised Ways of Coping Checklist has been widely used with family caregivers in both clinical and research settings to assess coping style (47). Caregivers who assume a positive problem-solving mode are less likely to be depressed or dysphoric, compared to caregivers who tend to avoid and withdraw from the situation (48).

Religious Coping. Religion and spirituality share a generally positive relationship with ability to cope with stress, although the exact mechanisms are not clear (49,50). Calling on the resources of something greater than oneself (e.g., God, or a higher force), attending religious services, and the use of prayer to help reduce stress are more common in African Americans and Latino caregivers than in Caucasians (51,52). The Religious/Spiritual Coping Scale (53) is one of the most widely used to assess this domain.

In summary, we recognize that it would be difficult and time consuming to incorporate use of all of these measures into a busy psychiatric practice where the identified patient is the demented individual. Referrals for clinical assessment can be helpful, and familiarity with these tools can serve as guidelines for developing individual clinical interviews with caregivers.

INTERVENTIONS FOR CAREGIVERS

Substantial evidence is accumulating that interventions for caregivers are variously effective with African American and Hispanic/Latino caregivers, as well as Caucasians, in reducing symptoms of distress, improving quality of life, increasing adaptive coping strategies, and delaying institutional placement of the care recipient (54–58). This is true despite the fact that providing care to an individual with progressive dementia represents a "moving target," where the specific challenges of caregiving change as the disease progresses. Below are some of the intervention techniques found to be helpful with caregivers.

Psychoeducation and Skill-Building Interventions

Psychoeducational interventions are typically conducted in small groups of eight to 10 participants. They are time-limited and closed-ended, and involve a structured agenda, trained leader, detailed leader and participant manuals, and a primary goal of skill acquisition. The number of sessions and actual skills taught vary, but usually skills are taught to manage disruptive behaviors, to relax in stressful situations, and to increase daily pleasant events (10,48). Content and methods are derived from cognitive-behavioral therapies, and the focus is on skill practice, both in and out of the session. They typically range from four to 12 sessions, which are usually held weekly for 1 to 2 hours in a community location. These programs are quite flexible and can be easily tailored to meet specific needs of specialized subgroups of caregivers such as ethnic and cultural minorities or male caregivers (10).

Support Groups

Support groups are the most common intervention for caregivers. These are most often offered free of charge by relevant agencies in the community (e.g., the Alzheimer's Association), and some may be designed for particular subgroups of caregivers (e.g., "early stage" groups). The goals of these groups are most often to foster emotional expression among caregivers and promote informal exchange of information. They vary widely in their frequency, whether they are peer or professionally led, and whether outside speakers are invited to discuss emerging information in the field. There are very few empirical studies at present that demonstrate the effectiveness of this modality (54). Despite the lack of empirical support, this intervention continues to be popular. Caregivers report that they feel less isolated and find the sharing in the group comforting. Clearly, some strengths of support groups include their minimal burden to the caregiver, their ease of application, the lack of associated costs, and the strong infrastructure of the Alzheimer's Association and other organizations, which are able to promote them effectively.

Respite Care Programs

The goal of respite care is to give the caregiver a break from the multiple burdens associated with providing direct supervision and personal care to their demented relative. Many formats for respite exist, such as adult day programs, in-home respite, and short-term residential placement. Although few empirical studies have been conducted with caregivers, (54) moderate effects have been reported in the reduction of caregiver burden and depression and in the enhancement of well-being. Caregivers often use respite for short periods, particularly at more severe stages of dementia when their personal resources are being over-taxed and outside assistance is needed to keep the elder at home. A clear limitation for many caregivers in obtaining formal respite is the high cost of these services.

Individual and Family Psychotherapy

Individual psychotherapy has been used with caregivers for several decades. Common theoretical frameworks used are cognitive-behavioral and psychodynamic: the former emphasizes skill acquisition, whereas the latter focuses on development of understanding about one's emotional responses to caregiving. Most of the empirically-based studies have emphasized controlling negative thoughts and increasing the frequency of engagement in pleasant events between the caregiver and care-receiver (59,60). Recent evaluations of family therapy (57,61) have also reported significant reductions in depressive symptoms, along with other indicators of improved well-being and more adaptive interaction patterns. A meta-analysis reported that psychotherapy, along with psychoeducational programs, had significant positive effects on all outcome domains that they reviewed, including burden, depression, subjective well-being, knowledge of the disease, and how troublesome the behaviors of the care recipient were (54).

Technological Interventions

In light of the time, transportation, and financial restrictions of many caregivers, technological interventions, such as dedicated telephones connected with computer systems, websites, and home instruction on video, have begun to spring up. These allow caregivers to utilize services and gain information and support in their own home at their convenience. Potential advantages of these interventions are their ability to be very individualized, their *transportability*, and their low cost. There are few empirical studies to support their efficacy at the present time, but utilization rates of available services are encouraging.

Care Management

Care or case management generally refers to the work done by a professional provider who assesses a caregiver's identifiable needs, links him or her to community resources, provides emotional support, and monitors the caregiving dyad over time. These interventions may include some training for caregivers in how to improve caregiving skills

(62), or may be restricted to assessment, referral to agencies, and follow-up. This model is widely available in most communities in the United States, often funded by the state or county or through special national funding available from the AoA (63). Case management services have rarely been systematically evaluated for their impact on caregiver well-being or functioning.

Other Interventions

Other interventions under study deserve mention for their promise to relieve at least some aspects of caregiver distress. These include:

■ Environmental interventions, which focus on improving the home environment and thus reducing objective burden on the caregiver. Most typically, modifications are made that increase home safety and accessibility (e.g., installing grab bars, labeling cabinets). Caregivers in one study of environmental interventions reported less upset with memory problems, less need for assistance from others, and improved affect (58). Interventions of this type require skilled occupational therapists to implement the program, along with monitoring and intervention delivery over long periods of time, since the care-recipient's needs change as the dementia progresses.

■ Multi-component interventions, which include various combinations of education, support, counseling, case management, and respite care. Such programs are reported to have delayed placement of care recipients (64), improved caregiver well-being, and reduced perceived burden (54). The most effective interventions studied provided care over at least a one-year period, which can be quite costly to arrange and maintain, and requires a coordination among various care providers not easily arranged in the community. Thus, it is not clear yet to what extent multi-component programs will really be able to be paid for and implemented in actual community settings.

■ A more cost-effective direction for intervention may be the timely dissemination of relevant information about caregiver stress and coping in the primary care office setting, offered by nurses or other appropriately trained personnel. One study evaluating this procedure reported positive results over a two-year period (65). Information about multiple subjects of concern was flexibly provided as caregivers asked for it. This model may work more efficiently when it is combined with technological intervention strategies (e.g., use of information kiosks in waiting areas) and referral to support groups or psychoeducational programs in the area.

SENSITIVITY TO ETHNIC AND CULTURAL DIVERSITY AMONG FAMILY CAREGIVERS

Caregivers are an extremely heterogeneous group that will continually challenge the clinician to adapt intervention strategies to suit individual needs. There is likely to be significant variability within any given census-designated group, which must be taken into account in treatment planning. For example, the term Hispanic/Latino American is used to encompass individuals whose families or themselves came from Mexico; Puerto Rico; South and Central American countries such as El Salvador and Chile; Cuba; or regions in the United States such as Texas, New Mexico, Florida, New York, and California. Although they share a common language, unique cultural manifestations are readily apparent among these different ethnic groups in customs, beliefs, health care practices, and so on. When setting up a treatment regimen, one must be extremely cautious in generalizing from one ethnic group to another. Understanding the differences among several large ethnic groups will facilitate the individualization of treatment for family caregivers (see also the chapter on Cultural Issues in this textbook).

Chinese Caregivers

Traditional Chinese beliefs emphasize the importance of family structure and support. According to traditional roles, first-born sons provide care for aging parents; but changing times have begun to decrease adherence to such values (66). This has introduced conflicts about who in the family should accept responsibility and the proper way to engage family members in the caregiving process. Spouses, who are the most common family caregivers of Chinese patients in this country, may need—and by tradition expect—help from the first-born son. However, the son may not accept this traditional role, and therefore not spontaneously volunteer help. This poses a dilemma for the caregiver, because to ask for help from children if it is not forthcoming freely would result in a "loss of face." Children, on the other hand, might think that help is not needed if no direct requests are being made by the parent.

Furthermore, mental illness is highly stigmatized within the Chinese American community and dementia is often perceived as a mental illness. To avoid stigma, families try to avoid the dementia label and attempt to characterize cognitive decline as normal aging (67–69). Chinese American healthcare professionals have been known themselves to assist families in the avoidance of this labeling and stigmatization, and even to view this service as part of their professional roles (70). However, avoidance does not eliminate the negative psychological impact of caregiving. Approximately one third of mainland Chinese family caregivers for AD are depressed (71), although most elders would not acknowledge this. They prefer to focus on words such as *stress* or *physical health needs*. Risk factors for depression include being a spousal or daughter-in-law caregiver, a high rate of disruptive behavior problems, and caregivers' use of passive coping strategies. Younger Chinese American are more likely than their elders to seek out support from Western-style agencies, whereas older, more traditional Chinese Americans might wish to obtain Chinese medicine interventions, such as herbal preparations and acupuncture.

Hispanic Caregivers

Hispanic/Latino caregivers are the most rapidly growing group in this country at the present time, yet culturally sensitive services are sorely lacking. Important cultural values that impact the caregiving process include the following: (1) a sense of social obligation or dedication to community; (2) *personalismo*, the value of informal over professional relationships; (3) *familismo*, the importance of the family unit over the individual; and (4) *respeto*, strong respect toward older family members. These values may affect what services are sought for the demented elder, and how the family might respond to intervention attempts.

Hispanic families may attribute dementia symptoms to a temporary *nervous* condition, past transgressions, or the *evil eye* (72). A lack of education regarding the physiological changes underlying dementia may lead family members to attribute negative intentional causes to the irrational behaviors of the demented family member. *Respeto* can result in dismay and confusion on the part of family caregivers, since their value system calls for them to revere, and hence obey, their elders. Yet this is difficult to do when the demands of the care recipient are irrational. As is the case within the Chinese American community, mental illness is highly stigmatizing. Embarrassment about dementia symptoms discourages caregivers from seeking support outside the family (73). In terms of coping, church service attendance and other forms of religious coping are more common among Hispanic caregivers than Caucasian caregivers and are reported to be very helpful in dealing with caregiving demands (74). Often, a mono-lingual Spanish-speaking elder may expect to be cared for at home regardless of the difficulties that presents, whereas the younger daughter or daughter-in-law may wish to alleviate some of the stress by bringing outside help into the home or using daycare or other kinds of respite services. This can be very difficult to negotiate among family members, since seeking help outside the family is tantamount to acknowledging that the primary caregiver cannot handle things anymore *and* that the family is not providing adequate support and help.

African American Caregivers

Within the African American community, the definition of family often includes individuals who are not blood relatives but who share a close relationship with the biological family. These individuals have been described as *fictive kin* (75) and they may participate in caregiving to an extent equivalent to actual family members. Several studies have found that African Americans report less psychological distress than any other ethnic or racial group to which they are compared (76). This has been related to their strong reliance on religion, church networking, and frequent prayer, to help mitigate daily stress (52,76). Health and financial concerns are common for many, along with lack of education about dementia and medications or treatment programs that can help both their relative and themselves. African Americans with more education and socioeconomic resources tend to be more able to recognize dementia as a disease process and to initiate efforts to obtain diagnostic and treatment information (77), although they are still very much under-represented nationally in the dementia care delivery system.

Men as Caregivers

Although the majority of family caregivers are women, the proportion of males who provide care for relatives with dementia is growing (3). Educational support groups have been used successfully with males (78). Unfortunately, there is little empirical research at present to guide us in the development of interventions for this group, yet it seems intuitively obvious that men will have different needs in their caregiving careers, and so will require interventions that address these needs. Clearly, more research is needed so that well-informed treatment recommendations can be made.

OTHER IMPORTANT ISSUES

In addition to the need to tailor interventions to caregivers' diverse backgrounds, other circumstances can present challenges to the clinician. For example, given the increasing availability of genetic testing for the apolipoprotein E-4(APOE-4) allele, family members may desire testing to determine their own risk for AD (e.g., to inform financial, medical, or reproductive decisions). Whether testing is performed or not, just the thought of possibly having AD is enough to cause significant stress among blood-relative caregivers. It is important for the clinician to be aware that significant anxiety and depression will accompany this topic (79). It is helpful to normalize these concerns and also point out that the likelihood of developing AD is relatively low, even though present data suggest a genetic association in some patients.

Another difficult but common circumstance is the transition to institutionalization. The decision to place a loved one in an institution is often a central issue in working with caregivers. Among the most common causes of institutionalization are behavior problems, particularly aggressive behaviors and psychosis, as well as incontinence. Here again, cultural factors influence decision-making. A common challenge for the clinician is disagreement among family members with regard to whether, when, and where to place the patient. The task of the clinician is often to provide objective information regarding the risks and

benefits of community vs. institutional residence, and more complex disagreements between family members may need to be formally dealt with in counseling. Another common problem faced in this situation is the intense guilt one may have over placement. It is helpful for caregivers to realize and accept that they have done the very best job that one can do in this role, but the problems encountered now have finally overcome their abilities to handle the situation, and anyone else in their situation would likely seek placement as well. Finally, neglect and emotional, financial, and/or physical abuse of frail older adults occur all too frequently. Thus, it is incumbent on the clinician that assessment of elderly patients include investigation of any signs of neglect or abuse, and a working knowledge of community agencies, such as Adult Protective Services, is essential for ethical geriatric care.

CONCLUSIONS AND RECOMMENDATIONS

The number of older adults with AD is increasing rapidly (2) and this has resulted in a boom in caregiving (4). Family caregiving is becoming increasingly common (1), and family caregivers, as a group, are becoming increasingly diverse (9). Because significant differences exist among caregivers, assessment and treatment programs must meet the unique needs of these specific caregiver–care-recipient family constellations. Several interventions have empirical support, and new ones are being developed. New research in the past decade has yielded many forms of assessment that can be used to help characterize the caregivers' strengths and weaknesses, before deciding on intervention targets.

Caregivers commonly experience a range of physical and psychological problems. Stressed spousal caregivers are at a 63% greater mortality risk than non-stressed spousal caregivers; dementia caregivers are more likely to report problems with occupation, emotional and physical distress, and social functioning than non-dementia caregivers (16). Therefore, there are significant reasons to think of the caregiver as the *hidden victim* and to proceed to assess and treat that person, along with the demented patient.

Careful psychiatric assessment of caregivers is critical to their effective treatment, and an important role of the psychiatrist is to differentiate between clinical problems and normal responses to the ongoing stresses of caregiving. Domains addressed in Figure 4-1 can serve as a practical guide for this process. Results from this process should guide the choice of intervention from among the many that now have at least some empirical support.

The physician–caregiver relationship cannot be overemphasized. A decade ago the American Medical Association called for the recognition of partnership between and the informal caregiver and the primary care physician

(80) through the development of initiatives that would promote this model in primary practice. A delicate balance is required to maintain the concept of *caregiver as a colleague*, while still remaining sensitive to the fact that the caregiver may also be in need of medical and psychiatric help. Doing so, however, may create the kind of reciprocal relationship where the physician can be both partner and doctor, as needed, when interacting with the caregiver and the care recipient.

REFERENCES

1. Administration on Aging. *Family Caregiver Fact Sheet*. Washington, DC: Author; 1999.
2. Hebert LE, Scherr PA, Bienias JL, Bennett DA, Evans DA. Alzheimer disease in the US population: prevalence estimates using the 2000 census. *Arch Neurol*. 2003;60(8):1119–1122.
3. Wagner D. *Comparative Analysis of Caregiver Data for Caregivers to the Elderly: 1987 and 1997*. Bethesda, MD: National Alliance for Caregiving; 1997.
4. National Alliance for Caregiving & American Association of Retired Persons. *Family Caregiving in the US: Findings from a National Survey*. Bethesda, MD and Washington, DC: Author; 1997.
5. Heyman A, Peterson B, Fillenbaum G, Pieper C. Predictors of time to institutionalization of patients with Alzheimer's disease: the CERAD experience, part XVII. *Neurology*. 1997;48(5):1304–1309.
6. Spruytte N, Van Audenhove Ch, Lammertyn F. Predictors of institutionalization of cognitively impaired elderly cared for by their relatives. *Int J Geriatr Psychiatry*. 2001;16(12),1119–1128.
7. Mausbach BT, Coon DW, Depp C, Rabinowitz R, Wilson-Arias E, Kraemer HC, Thompson LW, Lane G, Gallagher-Thompson D. Ethnicity and time to institutionalization: A comparison of Latino and Caucasian dementia caregivers. *J Am Geriatr Soc*. (in press).
8. Smith D. *The Older Population in the United States: March 2002*. Washington, DC: U.S. Census Bureau Current Population Reports; 2003.
9. U.S. Bureau of the Census. *Population Projections of the United States by Age, Sex, Race, Hispanic Origin, and Nativity: 1999–2100*. Washington, DC: U.S. Government Printing Office; 2000.
10. Gallagher-Thompson D, Haley W, Guy D, Rupert M, Arguelles T, Zeiss L, et al. Tailoring psychological interventions for ethnically diverse dementia caregivers. *Clinical Psychology: Science and Practice*. 2003;10:423–438.
11. Harwood DG, Barker WW, Cantillon M, Loewenstein DA, Ownby R, Duara R. Depressive symptomatology in first-degree family caregivers of Alzheimer disease patients: a cross-ethnic comparison. *Alzheimer Dis Assoc Disord*. 1998;12(4):340–346.
12. Aranda M, Knight B. The influence of ethnicity and culture on caregiver stress and coping process: a sociocultural review and analysis. *Gerontologist*. 1997;37:342–354.
13. Gaw AC. *Culture, Ethnicity, and Mental Illness*. Washington DC: American Psychiatric Press; 1993.
14. Connell CM, Janevic MR, Gallant MP. The costs of caring: impact of dementia on family caregivers. *J Geriatr Psychiatry Neurol*. 2001;14(4):179–87.
15. Alzheimer's Association & National Alliance for Caregiving. *Who Cares? Families Caring for Persons with Alzheimer's Disease*. Washington, DC: Author; 1999.
16. Ory MG, Hoffman RR, Yee JL, Tennstedt S, Schulz R. Prevalence and impact of caregiving: a detailed comparison between dementia and nondementia caregivers. *Gerontologist*. 1999;39(2):177–85.
17. McKinlay JB, Crawford SL, Tennstedt SL. The everyday impacts of providing informal care to dependent elders and their consequences for the care recipients. *J Aging Health*. 1995;7(4):497–528.
18. Schulz R, O'Brien AT, Bookwala J, Fleissner K. Psychiatric and physical morbidity effects of dementia caregiving: prevalence, correlates, and causes. *Gerontologist*. 1995;35(6):771–791.
19. Schulz R, Beach SR. Caregiving as a risk factor for mortality: the Caregiver Health Effects Study. *JAMA*. 1999;282(23):2215–9.
20. Kramer B. Gain in the caregiving experience: where are we? what next? *Gerontologist*. 1997;Apr;37(2):218–32.
21. Lawton MP, Moss M, Kleban MH, Glicksman A, Rovine M. A two-factor model of caregiving appraisal and psychological well-being. *J Gerontol*. 1991;46:P181–P189.
22. Pearlin LI, Mullan JT, Semple SJ, Skaff MM. Caregiving and the stress process: an overview of concepts and their measures. *Gerontologist*. 1990;30:583–594.
23. Schulz R, Gallagher-Thompson D, Haley W, Czaja S. Understanding the interventions process: a theoretical/conceptual framework for intervention approaches to caregiving. In: R Schulz, ed. *Handbook on Dementia Caregiving*. New York: Springer; 2000.
24. Stewart AL, Ware JE, eds. *Measuring Functioning and Well-being*. Durham and London: Duke University Press; 1992.
25. Lichtenberg P. *Handbook of Assessment in Clinical Gerontology*. New York: John Wiley & Sons, Inc; 1999.
26. Skinner J, Teresi J, Holmes D, Stahl S, Stewart A. Measurement in older ethnically diverse populations. *Journal of Mental Health and Aging*. 2001;7:5–200.
27. Chun KM, Organista PB, Marin G, eds. *Acculturation: Advances in Theory, Measurement, and Applied Research*. Washington DC: American Psychological Association; 2003.
28. Gottlieb B, Thompson L., Bourgeois M. Monitoring and evaluating interventions. In: Coon DW, Gallagher-Thompson D, Thompson LW, eds. *Innovative Interventions to Reduce Dementia Caregiver Distress: A Clinical Guide*. New York: Springer; 2003:28–49.
29. Castleman M, Gallagher-Thompson D, Naythons M. *There's Still a Person in There*. New York: Putnam; 1999.
30. American Medical Association. *Caregiver Self-assessment Questionnaire*. 2002. Available at: http://www.ama-assn.org/ama/pub/category/5037.html. Accessed February 3, 2004.
31. McCurry SM, Logsdon RG, Vitiello MV, Teri L. Successful behavioral treatment for reported sleep problems in elderly caregivers of dementia patients: a controlled study. *J Gerontol B Psychol Sci Soc Sci*. 1998 53: P122–P129.
32. Gallagher D, Rose J, Rivera P, Lovett S, Thompson LW. Prevalence of depression in family caregivers. *Gerontologist*. 1989;29:449–456.
33. Schulz R, O'Brien AT, Bookwala J, Fleissner K. Psychiatric and physical morbidity effects of dementia caregiving: prevalence, correlates, and causes. *Gerontologist*. 1995;35:771–791.
34. Schulz RN, Newsom J, Mittelmark J, Burton M, Hirsch L, Jackson C. Health effects of caregiving: the caregiver health effects study: an ancillary study of the Cardiovascular Health Study. *Ann Behav Med*. 1997;19(2):110–116.
35. Radloff L. The CES-D scale: a self-report depression scale for research in the general population. *Applied Psychological Measurement*. 1977:1:385–401.
36. Yesavage JA, Rose J, Lum TL, Huang O, Adey V, Leirer M. Development and validation of a geriatric depression screening scale: a preliminary report. *J Psychiatr Res*. 1982;17(1):37–49.
37. Sheikh JI, Yesavage JA. Geriatric Depression Scale (GDS): recent evidence and development of a shorter version. *Clin Gerontol*. 1986;5:165–73.
38. Mui AC, Burnette D, Chen Mei LM. Cross-cultural assessment of geriatric depression: a review of the CES-D and GDS. In: Skinner JH, Teresi J, eds. *Multicultural Measurement in Older Populations*. New York: Springer; 2002:147–177.
39. American Psychiatric Association. *Handbook of Psychiatric Measures*. Washington, DC: Author; 2000.
40. Folstein MF, Folstein SE, McHugh PR. "Mini-mental state." A practical method for grading the cognitive state of patients for the clinician. *J Psychiatr Res*. 1975;12(3):189–98.
41. Zarit SH, Todd PA, Zarit JM. Subjective burden of husbands and wives as caregivers: a longitudinal study. *Gerontologist*. 1986;26:260–270.
42. Seeman TE, McEwan BS. Impact of social environment characteristics on neuroendocrine regulation. *Psychosom Med* 1996;58(5):459–471.
43. Kiecolt-Glaser JK, Dura JR, Speicher CE, Trask OJ, Glaser R. Spousal caregivers of dementia victims: longitudinal changes in immunity and health. *Psychosom Med*. 1991;53(4):345–362.

44. Seeman T, Berkman LF. Structural characteristics of social networks and their relationship with social support in the elderly: who provides support? *Social Science and Medicine.* 1988;36: 737–749.

45. Sinyor D, Amato P, Kaloupec DG, Becker R, Goldenberger M, Coopersmith H. Post-stroke depression: relationships to functional impairment, coping strategies, and rehabilitation outcome. *Stroke.* 1986;17(6):1102–1107.

46. Schulz RT, Tompkins CA, Rau MT. A longitudinal study of the psychosocial impact of stroke on primary support persons. *Psychol Aging.* 1988;3(2):131–141.

47. Vitaliano P, Russo J, Carr J, Maiuro R, Becker J. The ways of coping checklist: revision and psychometric properties. *Multivariate Behavioral Research.* 1985;20:3–26.

48. Gallagher-Thompson D, Coon DW, Solano N, Ambler C, Rabinowitz Y, Thompson LW. Change in indices of distress among Latino and Anglo female caregivers of elderly relatives with dementia: site-specific results from the REACH National Collaborative Study. *Gerontologist.* 2003;43:580–591.

49. Dein S, Stygall J. Does being religious help or hinder coping with chronic illness: a critical literature review. *Palliat Med.* 1997;11:291–298.

50. Koenig H. Use of religion by patients with severe medical illness. *Mind Body Med.* 1997;2:31–36.

51. Janevic MR, Connell CM. Racial, ethnic, and cultural differences in the dementia caregiving experience: recent findings. *Gerontologist.* 2001;41:334–347.

52. Haley WE, Roth DL, Coleton M, Ford GR, West CAC, Collins RP. Appraisal, coping, and social support as mediators of well-being in Black and White family caregivers of patients with Alzheimer's disease. *J Consult and Clin Psychol* 1996;64: 120–129.

53. Pargament KI, Koenig HG, Perez LM. The many methods of religious coping: development and initial validation of the RCOPE. *J Clin Psychol.* 2000;56(4):519–543.

54. Sorensen S, Pinquart M, Duberstein P. How effective are interventions with caregivers? An updated meta-analysis. *Gerontologist.* 2002;42(3):356–72.

55. Brodaty H, Green A, Koschera A. Meta-analysis of psychosocial interventions for caregivers of people with dementia. *J Am Geriatr Soc.* 2003;51:657–664.

56. Burgio L, Stevens A, Guy D, Roth DL, Haley WE. Impact of two psychosocial interventions on White and African-American family caregivers of individuals with dementia. *Gerontologist.* 2003;43: 568–579.

57. Eisdorfer C, Czaja S, Loewenstein D, Rubert M, Arguelles S, Mitrani V, Szapocznik J. The effect of a family therapy and technology-based intervention on caregiver depression. *Gerontologist.* 2003;43:521–531.

58. Gitlin L, Belle SH, Burgio L, Czaja S, Mahoney D, Gallagher-Thompson D, et al. Effect of multicomponent interventions on caregiver burden and depression: the REACH multisite initiative at 6-month follow-up. *Psychol Aging.* 2003;18:361–374.

59. Gallagher-Thompson D, Steffen AM. Comparative effects of cognitive-behavioral and brief psychodynamic psychotherapies for depressed family caregivers. *J Consult Clin Psychol.* 1994;62(3): 543–9.

60. Teri L, Logsdon R, Uomoto J, McCurry S. Behavioral treatment of depression in dementia patients: a controlled clinical trial. *J Gerontol Psych Sci.* 1997;52B(P159–166).

61. Marriot A, Donaldson C, Tarrier N, Burns A. Effectiveness of a cognitive-behavioral family intervention in reducing the burden of

carers of patients with Alzheimer's disease. *British Journal of Psychiatry.* 2000;176:557–562.

62. Brodaty H, Gresham L, Luscombe G. The Prince Henry Hospital dementia caregivers' training program. *Int J Geriatr Psychiatry.* 1997;9:195–204.

63. Bass D, Clark P, Looman W, McCarthy C, Eckert S. The Cleveland Alzheimer's managed care demonstration: outcomes after 12 months of implementation. *Gerontologist.* 2003;43: 73–85.

64. Mittelman MS, Ferris S, Shulman E, Steinberg G, Levin B. A family intervention to delay nursing home placement of patients with Alzheimer's disease. *JAMA.* 1996;276:1725–1757.

65. Burns R, Nichols L, Martindale-Adams J, Grainey M, Lummus A. Primary care interventions for dementia caregivers: 2-year outcomes from the REACH study. *Gerontologist.* 2003;43:547–555.

66. Braun KL, Browne CV. Perceptions of dementia, caregiving, and help seeking among Asian and Pacific Islander Americans. *Health and Social Work.* 1998;23:262–274.

67. Elliot KS, Di Minno M, Lam D, Tu AM. Working with Chinese families in the context of dementia. In: Yeo G, Gallagher-Thompson, D, editor. *Ethnicity and the Dementias.* Philadelphia: Taylor & Francis; 1996:89–108.

68. Smedley BD, Stith AY, Nelson AR, eds. *Unequal Treatment: Confronting Racial and Ethnic Disparities in Health Care.* 2002, Washington, DC: Institute of Medicine.

69. Guo Z, Levy BR, Hinton, L, Weitzman, PF, Levkoff SE. The power of labels: recruiting dementia-affected Chinese American elders and their caregivers. *Journal of Mental Health and Aging.* 2000;6: 103–112.71.

70. Fuh JL, Wang SJ, Liu HC, Liu CY, Wang HC. Predictors of depression among Chinese family caregivers of Alzheimer's patients. *Alzheimer Dis Assoc Disord.* 1999;13:171–175.

71. Cooney RS, Di J. Primary family caregivers of impaired elderly in Shanghai, China. *Research on Aging.* 1999;21:739–761.

72. Arean PA, Gallagher-Thompson D. Issues and recommendations for the recruitment and retention of older ethnic minority adults into clinical research. *J Consult Clin Psychol.* 1996;64(5): 875–80.

73. John R, McMillian B. Exploring caregiver burden among Mexican Americans: cultural prescriptions, family dilemmas. *Journal of Aging and Ethnicity.* 1998;1:93–111.

74. Mausbach BT, Coon DW, Cardenas V, Thompson LW. Religious coping among Caucasian and Latino dementia caregivers. *Journal of Mental Health and Aging.* 2003;9:97–110.

75. Chatters LM, Taylor RJ, Jayakody R. Fictive kinship relations in Black extended families. *Journal of Comparative Family Studies.* 1994;25:297–312.

76. Knight BG, Silverstein M, McCallum TJ, Fox LS. A sociocultural stress and coping model for mental health outcomes among African American caregivers in southern California. *J Gerontol Psych Sci.* 2000;55B: 142–150.

77. Dilworth-Anderson P, Williams SW, Cooper T. Family caregivers to elderly African Americans: caregiver types and structures. *J Gerontol Psych Sci.* 1999;54:S237–S241.78.

78. McFarland P, Sanders S. Educational support groups for male caregivers of individuals with Alzheimer's disease. *Am J Alzheimer's Dis Other Demen.* 2000;15:367–373.

79. Coon DW, Davies H, McKibben C, Gallagher-Thompson D. The psychological impact of genetic testing for Alzheimer disease. *Genet Test.* 1999;3:121–31.

80. Council on Scientific Affairs. Physicians and family caregivers: a model for partnership. *JAMA.* 1993;269:1282–1284.

Principles of Clinical Evaluation

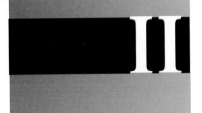

5

The Psychiatric Interview of the Older Patient

Daniel Carlat

Interviewing the older patient really should not be all that different from interviewing the younger patient. All our patients are human beings, regardless of age, and as such we have to evaluate their personal histories as well as their emotional and cognitive states. Nonetheless, the experience of interviewing an older patient *is* different. How? The obvious difference is that the emphasis of the evaluation tends to be on scrutinizing cognition, since the chances of finding impaired cognition are statistically higher in older people. But beyond this, interviewing older patients *feels* different, at least for those of us who might be considered "younger" psychiatrists. The oft-repeated dictate "respect your elders" echoes in our heads during the interview, subtly altering our demeanor. On the other hand, we are not immune to our culture's youth-centered, anti-aging attitude, and we may have to battle with an impulse to disparage an older patient as "out-dated" or "washed up." Ultimately, working with older people brings up transference and countertransference issues in all of us, making it particularly challenging but also immensely rewarding if we rise to that challenge. This chapter is meant to guide you through some of the particular challenges of working with this population.

LOGISTICAL ISSUES

The psychiatric interview actually begins with your patient's first phone call requesting an appointment. Whether you are in solo practice and take these calls yourself, or work in a clinic where support staff does this for you, you can enhance everyone's experience of your first face-to-face meeting by taking care of some preliminaries.

Transportation Issues

If parking is a problem, this is likely to be much more of an issue for the elderly. Likewise, if you have stairs, you had better let your prospective patient know, as this factor alone may convince many elderly to skip to the next psychiatrist on their list.

Informants

Strongly encourage your new patient to bring an informant (a friend or family member). Your interview will be covering terrain such as cognitive impairment and ability to manage basic functions of daily living, and you will want to corroborate your patient's report with an informant's. Obviously, some elderly patients come across so clearly intact over the phone that you will not have to insist on an informant. If an informant is unavailable during the appointment time, plan for them to be available by phone so that you can still have the benefit of this collateral information during the interview. If you are as busy as most psychiatrists, you will want to avoid committing to calling an informant at a time other than the scheduled appointment, but this may sometimes be your only option.

Medical Documentation

Insist on obtaining copies of primary care medical records, either to be brought with the patient during the appointment or to be sent or faxed to you before the appointment. It is also nice to obtain a printout from the patient's pharmacy of all medications prescribed over the past year or so. You will not believe how handy this information will be when you are faced with a patient who is telling you that he takes "a bunch of pills" everyday and cannot specify further!

ESTABLISHING RAPPORT

Establishing rapport is a crucial part of the interview with any patient, because this allows you to obtain the clinical information you need for a diagnosis, and also helps to ensure that your patient will comply with any treatment that you suggest. Your elderly patient may not be as psychologically minded or sophisticated as your younger patients. So do not "go psychiatric" on elderly patients too quickly—this may be confusing or alienating. You may want to start your interview as a pleasant, meandering chat. A handy way to do this is by glancing through the initial registration/encounter form as you begin.

Sample Interview

Psychiatrist (Psych): So, Mrs. Jones, I see you live in Chelsea. How long have you lived there?

Mrs. Jones (Jones): Fifty-seven years. I moved there right after I married my dear husband—may his soul rest in peace.

Psych: I expect the neighborhood has changed over the years?

Jones: It is so different now. It is all the foreigners! I used to know everyone on my block, but they have all either died off or moved away.

Psych: But you have staying power.

Jones: Well, I have it pretty good there. The rent is a lot cheaper than Boston, and my sister still lives in the same building. Plus, I can walk to the grocery story.

Of course, a wealth of psychiatric information has been communicated here in the guise of a "non-psychiatric" exchange. Dementia seems unlikely, given the patient's ability to respond to questions appropriately, her command of dates, and her apparent ability to shop for groceries independently. There are strains of possible depression or unresolved grief, given her immediate reference to her deceased husband. Later in the interview, you will likely pick up on some of these strands, but at this point, your job is to learn more about your patient's life in a nonthreatening way.

In general, maintaining an attitude of respect and dignity will go far for your elderly patients. You communicate such an attitude in innumerable nonverbal ways, such as smiling, showing sustained interest, and making sure that your patient is physically comfortable throughout the interview. You also communicate respect by asking questions that show your interest and appreciation in your patient as a human being who has lived through a lot and has accumulated some wisdom over the years.

Of course, there are times when cautious rapport-building can wait until later, because the issue at hand requires immediate attention:

Sample Interview

The patient appears visibly anxious and distressed, is wringing her hands and rocking her body in the chair.

Psych: How are you, Mrs. Jones?

Jones: Not good, not good. I do not know what to do, I just do not know.

Psych: You look like you are very nervous.

Jones: Oh, I just do not know how I can get through this, doctor!

Psych: Tell me exactly how you have been feeling?

The clinician begins exploring criteria for DSM-IV anxiety and depressive disorders.

ASKING QUESTIONS IN A NON-THREATENING WAY

While techniques for phrasing questions with finesse are not specific to the geriatric interview, they are certainly necessary in this setting and it is worth reviewing these, because clinicians often have never been taught them in explicit terms during the course of training. The problem with any clinical interview (and, in particular, with the psychiatric interview), is that you are getting very personal with your patient, very quickly. And while it is easy for us to take for granted the kinds of questions that we ask, it is rarely as easy for our patients to hear them. The techniques that clinicians tend to use in approaching sensitive topics fall into the following three categories: 1) normalization, 2) symptom expectation, and 3) symptom exaggeration (1).

Normalization

A bread and butter technique of accomplished interviewers, normalization begins with a statement implying that the symptom or behavior under question is normal. Here are two examples:

Q: Sometimes, when people experience the death of a spouse, they begin to wonder whether their own life is worth living anymore—has that been true for you?

Q: It is very common for people to become a little absent-minded as they age—have you noticed that this has been happening to you?

Symptom Expectation

This is similar to normalization, but in this case you offer a statement or question showing that you assume that the patient is doing or feeling something. This is best reserved when your index of suspicion for a behavior is already quite high; otherwise, patients may find it offensive. Consider the following example:

The patient is a 70-year-old man who came in with a chief complaint of anxiety. His son had called to say that he was concerned that his father had been drinking too much, but halfway into the interview, the patient seems to have gone to lengths not to mention drinking. So you use the symptom expectation technique.

Q: Mr. Jones, I assume you have been drinking more than usual to cope with all this stress?

A: I cannot lie to you doc, I've been back to the scotch every night.

Symptom Exaggeration

In order to encourage your patient to admit to an embarrassing behavior or symptom, you suggest a much higher frequency of the behavior than is likely. The patient then feels that if they admit to a lower frequency you might be pleasantly surprised. Here is an example:

Q: How often do you come close to hitting your wife? Two, three times a week? More?

A: Oh no, nothing like that. Maybe once a month at the most, and I have only actually hit her a handful of times ever.

Asking questions in non-threatening ways is often critically important for patients with dementia, who may present with paranoia as a complication of their cognitive impairment. Such patients may perceive you as being one of the "villains" who are trying to commit them or steal things from them. In such cases, it may help to explicitly acknowledge your patient's concerns, using what Leston Havens has called a *counterprojective statement* (2). Here is an example of such a statement used in an interview:

Q: Have you been able to manage your affairs at home on your own?

A: Oh, now you are asking!

Q: I am just wondering—

A: I know what you are wondering, you are wondering how you can get a little piece of my life savings too, just like those kids.

Q: I see. Even though I am a doctor saying that I am trying to help you feel better, you suspect that I am in cahoots with your family, trying to get my hands on your money. Wow, is your family really trying to put one over on you? Tell me what they are up to.

A: OK, but everything stays in this room!

Q: Fine.

MOVING THROUGH THE INTERVIEW RAPIDLY

It is quite common for us to evaluate patients who have difficulty coming to the point, or at least, the point that we feel is most crucial. Often, this is a good thing, especially early in the interview when you are supposed to let your patient talk for a while anyway. Furthermore, many elderly patients have had such fascinating lives that you are captivated by their stories. Nonetheless, you have a job to do, and a limited time in which to do it, so here are some tried-and-true techniques for hurrying patients along—in a friendly way.

Closed-Ended Questions

Once considered anathema in the psychiatric interview, in this age of DSM-IV criteria, closed-ended questions have their place. They are questions that can be answered with only a finite number of responses. Usually, there are only two possible answers: "yes" and "no." In multiple-choice questions, there may be a few more. But long meandering stories and anecdotes are not options when it comes to closed-ended questions. Here are several examples:

Q: Do you typically sleep the whole night through, or not?

Q: Do you get your panic attacks daily, weekly, or monthly?

Q: If I were to ask you if you considered yourself to have a drinking problem, how would you answer: "yes" or "no"?

Gentle Interruptions

Interrupting patients is OK, if done gently. Often, when patients are really excessively talkative, the entire interview becomes a gentle process of educating them about the need to keep answers a little briefer. In order to interrupt gracefully, consider the following techniques: 1) smile, 2) use a gentle but firm tone of voice, 3) personalize the interruption by using their name or asking a question about their concern, 4) express empathy and interest in them as you interrupt. Here is a clinical example:

Q: Mrs. Smith, do you sleep the whole night through, or not?

A: Well, last night, I had eaten cucumbers, and they repeated on me, so around the middle of the night I got up to have big glass of milk, but that did not help much, so then I asked my husband what to do, because he has these terrible problems with—

Q: I am sorry to interrupt, Mrs. Smith, but it is important that I learn the answer to this question, because you have been having such difficulties lately and I really want to help you to feel better. In general, and not specifically last night, are you a good sleeper?

A: Usually, I would say I am, but last week when my daughter was having trouble with that strange boyfriend of hers—I cannot believe the kinds of choices she has made, . . . (!)

As the interview progresses, your interrupting statements may have to become more elaborate:

"Mrs. Smith, I am sorry to interrupt once again, but today we have a lot of material to cover, and it is very important that I get to ask several more questions, so that I can come up with an accurate idea of what has been going on with you, and most importantly, so that I can suggest a treatment that is going to help you. So I may have to interrupt you a few more times during our time together, which I hope will not offend you."

Point Redirection

When listening to a rambling patient, try to interrupt by focusing on one point that you may have heard earlier in the interview, and use that point to logically redirect them back to the relevant topic. Consider this approach:

Q: How have you been?

A: I have to tell you this, because I am worried, you see, because where I used to live, they called me Jimmy even though my real name is James, here they do not do that! And the staff should use Jimmy, even when they care for me. I remember being a teacher and how important the name of each child was—but here, boy, its terrible! The staff just does not understand that—

Q *(Interrupting on the point of how terrible it is)*: "Excuse me, Jimmy, but I must ask you—when you tell me the situation is terrible, does this mean you feel depressed?

INTERVIEWING DIFFICULT PATIENTS

When patients are particularly difficult, none of these techniques is likely to work very well. Two common examples of difficult situations (with suggestions on how to resolve them) include the following:

The Hostile Patient

You realize quickly that the patient is not answering your questions because of an undertone of anger and hostility. The best approach here varies. Making a direct comment about the affect sometimes works:

Q: Mr. Jones, would you mind talking a little more about how you have been sleeping . . .

A: What do you think, traipsing in here without even knocking. You cannot even get a bit of privacy in this place.

Q: I would be very angry about that, like you are. And I would like to offer you my sincerest apology for not having had the decency to knock!

A: It's OK, I know you didn't mean it; you seem like a better sort than the other doctors who work here.

But this can always backfire if your patient feels that your efforts at empathy are too intrusive. If so, simply being quiet while allowing your patient plenty of time for catharsis allows him to feel that he is back in control; the interview may proceed more smoothly thereafter.

The Confused Patient

Confusion is a nonspecific symptom that can reflect underlying dementia, ruminative depression, and overwhelming anxiety, among other states. Frequently, a confused patient will be accompanied by an informant and you will be tempted to direct your questions to this person, rather than the patient, in order to more efficiently attain information. However, this can increase your patient's sense of anxious confusion as he fights a losing battle to try to understand what is being said. In these cases, carve out time explicitly for interaction with the patient. Here is a sample interview:

Patient *(suffering from a ruminative and nearly psychotic depression)*: What is he saying? (referring to the psychiatrist's last question directed toward the patient's husband)

Psych: I was just asking how you have been sleeping.

Patient: Fine, fine, I always sleep fine (contradicting her husband's report).

Psych: Tell me a little about your room—What does it look like? (Bringing up a concrete topic that the patient may be more comfortable with).

Patient: There is a bed, and a night stand.

Psych: Do you have a book on the night stand? (And so on, for a few minutes, after which the interviewer makes the following transition.) I have a few more questions for your husband now, would you mind if I talked to him?

SPECIFIC DATA TO OBTAIN

The second goal in conducting the psychiatric interview, after establishing rapport, is to come up with a psychiatric diagnosis that is consistent with current nomenclature. For this, you need cold, hard data, and plenty of it. This is accomplished partly through unstructured listening (usually during the first 5 minutes of the interview), and partly through diagnostic questioning. Studies of diagnostic masters reveal that they share a common technique (3). After the first few minutes of the interview, accomplished clinicians already have generated four to five hypothetical diagnoses. The rest of the interview is spent methodically ruling in or ruling out each of these.

So which diagnoses are most likely in the elderly? While all of the diagnostic categories can be seen in patients of almost any age, prevalence figures of disorders do shift a bit with advancing age. Some of the most common disorders to be seen in the elderly include depressive disorders, dementia of all types, and anxiety disorders. (4). Other disorders that are certainly seen in late life but with less frequency include bipolar disorder, schizophrenia, alcohol abuse, and personality disorders. You are advised to take these lists with a grain of salt. They might help to orient your thinking toward the most likely diagnostic culprits, but they do not let you off the hook in ruling out some of the less frequently seen disorders.

As you ask your diagnostic questions, be aware that there are several sources of potential data distortion that may be more common in elderly patients. These include:

- Lack of records or excessively old records. Having family informants accompany the patient helps to compensate for this problem.
- Poor memory for needed information. Methods to jog your patient's memory include anchoring questions to memorable events, such as historic events or holidays; tagging questions with specific examples of possible answers, which converts a question into a multiple choice format; and clearly defining technical terms whenever possible.
- Conflicting stories from family, caregivers, and inpatient staff. Obviously, this requires a judgment call on which sources are most reliable, and usually requires quite a bit of sensitivity when confronting your patient with differing accounts of functioning.

THE HISTORY OF PRESENT ILLNESS

While the initial interview is traditionally broken up into separate sections, such as the history of present illness (HPI) and the past psychiatric history (PPH), the actual flesh-and-blood interview rarely proceeds so systematically. The HPI is supposed to be a more recent history of what led the patient to your office, but it usually blends into the PPH. In the elderly in particular, excessively structuring the interview can backfire and threaten your rapport.

Nonetheless, it is certainly important to obtain the history of the patient's chief complaint over the course of the interview, as this will help you to gather all the data you need to piece together a psychiatric diagnosis.

THE PSYCHIATRIC REVIEW OF SYSTEMS (PROS)

The term *psychiatric review of symptoms* is stolen from our non-psychiatric medical colleagues who routinely ask an anatomically guided series of questions in order to make sure not to miss an important symptom (5). The PROS works the same way for psychiatrists. Furthermore, it is a convenient way to structure the entire interview.

Mnemonic buffs out there may choose to use the following to remember all the diagnoses to cover: "*Depressed Patients Seem Anxious, So Claim Psychiatrists.*"

Depressive Disorders (including bipolar disorder)
Personality Disorders
Substance Abuse
Anxiety Disorders
Somatoform Disorders
Cognitive Disorders and Dementia
Psychotic Disorders

While each of these disorders is covered in detail elsewhere in this book, below are some issues of particular relevance to the initial psychiatric interview. As you ask your diagnostic questions, be aware that psychiatric symptoms in late life may be altered or obscured by the aging process and by other comorbid diagnoses, especially dementia. For example, elderly patients with depressive and anxiety disorders may not describe mood states *per se*, but instead may describe their medical problems, financial woes, or that poignant loneliness of old age that comes when most of one's friends and family members have died.

Depressive Disorders

Diagnosing late-life depression can be quite difficult because the neurovegetative symptoms of fatigue, insomnia, and poor appetite may also reflect non-psychiatric illnesses or concurrent medication effects. Your interview then focuses on teasing apart *medical* from *psychiatric* symptoms—no small task. Commonly, elderly patients dwell on somatic symptoms as a metaphor for depressive symptoms, so if you find yourself tiring of hearing your patient ruminate about constipation for the *umpteenth* time, consider yourself lucky: you may have just diagnosed depression, possibly with psychotic features.

Personality Disorders

While borderline pathology may tend to diminish or change with age, we have all had the experience of interviewing an elderly person who seems to come at us swinging for no obvious reason other than to punish us for reminding them of a past abuser. In clinical practice, more common than borderline elderly patients are those with dependent personality disorder who do not answer questions without turning toward their spouse for confirmation. This may affect your treatment, because the patient with long-standing dependent personality disorder may not respond as well to your typical treatments for anxiety or depression.

Substance Abuse

Do not be fooled! Many people drink excessively well into late life, but may have never been asked about it. This seems especially true for alcohol-abusing elderly women. Consider this case example:

> A 64-year-old woman who continued to manage a successful home-based sales business was being treated for bipolar disorder, apparently successfully, with a combination of divalproex sodium and bupropion. Her visits had gradually decreased in frequency to every 4 months, during which she and her psychiatrist would chat affably for 15 to 20 minutes, and she would leave with a prescription and another appointment. One day, the psychiatrist received a phone call from her husband, who requested an urgent visit with himself and the patient. At the visit, the husband reported that the patient's drinking, which had always been a mild to moderate problem, had been increasing. This was the first time the psychiatrist had ever heard of it.

Anxiety Disorders

Usually this is fairly easy to diagnose, as many anxious elderly patients are less adept at hiding their agitation during the interview than their younger counterparts. As the mnemonic above mentions, patients may often come in complaining of "nerves" or anxiety when the true underlying problem is major depression with an anxious component.

Somatoform Disorders

While one might assume that somatoform disorders are more common in the elderly because of the plethora of organic physical symptoms they experience, epidemiologists tell us this is not the case. When somatization *does* occur, it is devilishly difficult to treat, because there is usually some real pathology there as well, making the outcome of treatment something of a moving target. Depression more often masks as somatic preoccupations in the elderly, sometimes bordering on psychosis.

Cognitive Disorders and Dementia

See below, under MMSE.

Psychotic Disorders

Assessing psychosis in an elderly patient with long-standing schizophrenia is easy. The trick is uncovering covert paranoia, ideas of reference, and hallucinations in someone with no known history and who appears pretty much intact. This requires that you have the discipline to ask screening questions about psychosis for most patients. Normalization is a good technique to use here. Consider the following statement:

> Q: Often, when people get really depressed, they start to believe things that may seem strange to others. Has this happened to you?

MEDICAL HISTORY

You may have already gotten much of this in the HPI part of your interview, because unfortunately, much of what is noteworthy in the lives of people as they age is unpleasant medical stuff. It has been drummed into our heads over and over during training not to miss an underlying organic cause of psychiatric symptoms, but complacence inevitably sets in. And, to be fair to those complacent psychiatrists among us, truly reversible organic factors are uncommon. Nonetheless, a review of medications and the medical history should rightly be a part of the initial psychiatric interview of an elderly person. As mentioned already, your job here is infinitely easier if you can get records from the primary care doctor and the pharmacy.

In your medical history, ask specifically about:

- Thyroid disease (hypothyroidism can cause depression, while hyperthyroidism can cause anxiety symptoms)
- Anemia (a potential cause of depression)
- Head injury or seizures (this may explain any cognitive dysfunction)
- Cardiovascular disease (you will need to know this before prescribing certain medications)
- Liver or kidney problems (again, largely because problems with either of these organs will affect medication selection and dosing decisions)
- Metabolic disease (e.g. diabetes)

Current medications, both prescription and over the counter, must be accounted for in the history. Medications that may induce cognitive impairment include: anticholinergics such as benztropine, atropine, and dicyclomine; anticonvulsants such as divalproex sodium; low-potency antipsychotics such as chlorpromazine and thioridazine; lithium; tricyclic antidepressants; and benzodiazepines.

THE MENTAL STATUS EXAM

By *mental status exam*, I am referring primarily to the *cognitive* component of the evaluation. It should go without saying that you will be closely evaluating appearance, mood, affect, speech, thought process and content, and behavior while you are asking questions pertaining to the PROS. The cognitive evaluation is easy or difficult depending on your philosophy. There are psychiatrists who avoid structured memory questions, maintaining that they can evaluate all the cognitive domains adequately in the course of the normal interview. Others swear by the Folstein Mini-Mental State Examination (MMSE) (6) because they were raised on this in residency and have developed a good sense of how to interpret patients' responses.

Research evidence has increasingly pointed toward the view that the MMSE is an inefficient way to test cognition (7). Consider, for example, the famous "serial sevens subtraction test" that is part of the MMSE and is often used as a test of concentration. Studies have found an alarming error rate among high functioning and highly educated people who carry no psychiatric diagnosis. In one study, only 42% of highly educated professionals had errorless performances (8). Another limitation of the MMSE is that, while it has a high sensitivity for picking up cases of dementia, its specificity is low. This means that many patients who are cognitively normal may be misclassified as demented by the MMSE. This is particularly true of patients who never graduated high school. Age- and education-adjusted norms are available for more accurately interpreting MMSE scores (9).

Recently, a very streamlined dementia screen has been validated, called the Mini-Cog (10). This combines two tests: the three-item recall of MMSE fame and the clock drawing task (CDT). Studies comparing the Mini-Cog with the MMSE have shown no real differences in sensitivity or specificity, and the Mini-Cog is much faster to administer and avoids most of the cultural and language problems associated with the MMSE.

The Mini-Cog is administered in two steps. First, you ask your patient if you can test his memory by asking him to repeat and memorize three simple words (the specific words are up to you). Then you give him a paper and pen, and ask him to draw a clock, with the hands pointing to ten minutes after eleven (or pick another time in which there is a hand on each side of the clock). Once the clock is drawn, ask him to repeat your three words.

Here is a practical way of interpreting the results of the Mini-Cog. Use the results of the three-item recall as a screen. Patients who recall all three words are probably not demented, those who can remember none of them are probably demented, while those who remember one or two might be demented. For patients in the middle, their performance on the CDT portion of the Mini-Cog provides crucial information that may or may not convince you to seek neuropsychological testing.

If you are allergic to structured cognitive testing, that is okay, because you have some good research support for a more conversational approach to the cognitive evaluation (11). You can test short-term memory pretty well by establishing over the course of your initial greetings that your patient is oriented to place and date. Recall of current events is another good test of recent memory (memory over the past day or two.) Just ask about some important event from the morning paper. Of course, this is no better than a screening test, because some people never read the paper or they live the lives of hermits, etc. Ultimately, the entire cognitive component of your initial interview is no more than a screening procedure anyway, enabling you to decide on a referral for more detailed testing.

DEALING WITH FAMILIES

Assessing and treating elderly patients often brings you face-to-face with their family members, usually either a spouse and one or more adult children. While this contact is generally quite helpful, it can also bring up some tricky situations, as the following case example illustrates:

A 78-year-old woman was brought in by her son for the evaluation of depression. The psychiatrist identified symptoms of loneliness, anhedonia, hopelessness, and anergia, and prescribed an antidepressant. The next day he received a phone call from a different son, who disagreed with the prescription of an antidepressant, stating that his mother was simply lonely and not "depressed." The psychiatrist responded that it was actually up to the patient to decide whether she wanted to take the medication, since she had no significant cognitive impairment and had not legally given up decision-making authority. The following day, the original son called, irate that his mother had been "taken off" the antidepressant by his brother, and demanding to know why. Ultimately, the psychiatrist held a meeting with the entire family, where it became apparent that there was an active feud between the brothers, with origins that ran deep, largely related to a large inheritance expected upon the mother's death. On the psychiatrist's insistence, a single family member was identified as the contact person for all future clinical conversations.

As is made clear by this case example, contact with family can be a double-edged sword. Still, we need to rely on family informants to help us make our diagnoses, particularly when there is a question of dementia. In fact, studies that have compared results of the mental status exam with family interviews have found that family interviews have greater diagnostic sensitivity (7). When interviewing family members and other informants, I suggest that you follow the format of the Informant Questionnaire on Cognitive Decline in the Elderly (12). To do so, ask the informant, compared with 10 years ago, how good is this person at:

- remembering things that have happened recently?
- remembering where things are usually kept?
- remembering things about family and friends, such as names, occupations, birthdays, or addresses?
- making decisions on everyday matters?
- handling financial matters?
- finding the right word when talking about things?
- knowing how to do everyday things around the house, such as cooking and cleaning?

Although this approach with informants can be helpful, keep in mind that sometimes the caregiver may be nearly as impaired as the patient, whether the impairment is due to dementia, medical problems, or psychiatric disorders. In that case, it is important to insist on speaking with another informant in order to get a reliable picture of your patient's situation. Also be on the lookout for a caregiver who has an ax to grind, either with the medical establishment, you personally as a psychiatrist, or with other family members. Such an attitude may get in the way of good patient care by leading to cancelled or missed visits, the caregiver not giving the patient the proper medication, and so on. If you think this is an issue, you should bring it up as a topic, and you may need to personally ensure that a visiting nurse is involved in the patient's care.

Much research has been published over the last several years documenting the dramatic effect of dementia on caregivers (see Chapter 4). In general, the caregivers of demented patients are at high risk for depression and other psychiatric problems, and interventions targeted toward them are helpful. You should prepare caregivers for the potential frustrations of caring for their loved one and offer psychiatric services to them, either your own or a colleague's. Many nursing homes and professional organizations offer free support groups for caregivers.

CONCLUSION

Interviewing elderly patients requires extra sensitivity, compassion, and skill. Making the diagnosis requires much more of us than simply asking all the right questions; it requires being attuned to underlying conditions and attitudes that may interfere with the reliability of the information we obtain. Treating older patients is immensely fulfilling, but it is also one of the more challenging tasks in psychiatry. As in the rest of medicine, practice helps us aspire to perfection. As the distinguished physician William Osler said, "Start out with the conviction that absolute truth is hard to reach in matters relating to our fellow creatures, healthy or diseased, . . . that errors in judgement must occur in the practice of an art which consists largely in balancing probabilities, and you will draw from your errors the very lessons which may enable you to avoid their repetition" (13).

REFERENCES

1. Carlat DJ. *The Psychiatric Interview*. Philadelphia: Lippincott Williams & Wilkins; 1999.
2. Havens L. *Making Contact*. Cambridge: Harvard University Press; 1986.
3. Kaplan C. Hypothesis testing. In: Lipkin MJ, Putnam SM, Lazare A, eds. *The Medical Interview*. New York: Springer-Verlag; 1995.
4. Blazer DG. Epidemiology of psychiatric disorders in late life. In: Busse EW, Blazer DG, eds. *American Textbook of Geriatric Psychiatry*. 2nd Ed. Washington, DC: American Psychiatric Press; 1996.
5. Carlat DJ. The Psychiatric Review of Symptoms: A Screening Tool for Family Physicians. *Am Fam Physician*. 1998;58:1617–1624.
6. Folstein, MF, Folstein SE, McHugh PR, et al. "Mini-mental state": a practical method for grading the cognitive state of patients for the clinician. *J Psychiatr Res*. 1975;12:189–198.
7. Harwood DMJ, Hope T, Jacoby R, et al. Cognitive impairment in medical inpatients. I: Screening for dementia—is history better than mental state? *Age and Ageing*. 1997;26:31–35.
8. Smith A. The serial sevens subtraction test. *Arch Neurol*. 1967;17:78–80.
9. Crum RM, Anthony JC, Bassett SS, Folstein MF. Population-based norms for the mini-Mental State Examination by age and educational level. *JAMA*. 1993;269:2386–2391.
10. Borson S, Scanlan JM, Chen P, et al. The Mini-Cog as a screen for dementia: validation in a population-based sample. *J Am Geriatr Soc*. 2003;51:1451–1454.
11. Keller MB, Manschreck TC. The mental status examination. II. Higher intellectual functioning. In: Lazare A, ed. *Outpatient Psychiatry: Diagnosis and Treatment*. Baltimore: Williams & Wilkins; 1989.
12. Jorm A, Scott R, Cullen JS, MacKinnon AJ. Performance for the Informant Questionnaire on Cognitive Decline in the Elderly (IQCODE) as a screening test for dementia. *Psychol Med*. 1991;21:785–790.
13. Osler W. *Counsels and Ideals from the Writings of William Oster*. Birmingham, AL: The Classics of Medicine Library; 1985.

Medical Assessment of the Elderly Psychiatric Patient

6

Kevin C. Fleming   *Teresa A. Rummans*   *Gabe J. Maletta*

Medical issues are important considerations in the management of the elderly person with mental illness. Acute illnesses and chronic comorbidities may be confused with psychiatric disease, exacerbate behavioral symptoms, or interfere with therapy. Presentations of these illnesses in older people can vary greatly. This variation is a result of many factors including the person's genetic background, previous medical status, living environment, diet, level of physical activity, and use of alcohol, nicotine, and other drugs. However, any abrupt change in an older person's mental or physical health is a problem, and is due to a disease or external factors and should not be considered a part of normal aging.

Abrupt mental status changes producing psychiatric symptoms such as depression, anxiety, psychosis, or cognitive changes are often the product of one of more organ system problems that are usually not associated with that symptom in younger people. For example, acute cognitive impairment or confusion in the elderly is less likely to be due to a new brain lesion than it would be in a much younger person. Consequently, it is important for older people to have a thorough medical and neurological evaluation when psychiatric problems present acutely.

When psychiatric problems develop in the elderly, close scrutiny of the person's physical and neurological status must be pursued before attributing symptoms to a mental illness alone. Often, the problems are the result of multiple rather than single causes. For example, agitation in a demented individual might not be a direct result of the dementia itself. With further evaluation and examination, one may discover that the person has pain from severe constipation, caused by an anticholinergic medication. Addressing this issue may completely resolve the agitation without the use of psychotropic medication. This example highlights the importance of close attention to details of the patient's history, which may uncover the existence of a medical problem. Likewise, attention to the physical exam may point to subtle physical changes contributing to the problem. Finally, changes in screening laboratory tests may identify underlying organ dysfunction that significantly affects the care of the patient. This chapter focuses on the importance of the history, physical examination, and laboratory assessment of the older person presenting with psychiatric symptoms.

As individuals grow older, maintaining social independence, functional mobility, and cognitive abilities becomes increasingly important. Functional impairments frequently accompany the aging process, and can lead to an inability to meet the demands of daily life. Medical illnesses can lead to a similar decline in physical function. Indeed, functional decline is often the presenting symptom of medical illness in older people, and in some instances may be the only symptom (1). Such impairments may greatly affect quality of life, and will have a significant impact on future care. The older patient frequently has multiple complex illnesses, and loss of function is the net effect of these interacting disease processes. Functional assessment must be part of the evaluation of any geriatric

TABLE 6-1

COMMON MEDICAL ILLNESSES IN THE ELDERLY

Disease	Prevalence
Eye disease (cataracts, glaucoma)	53%
Hypertension	52%
Arthritis	50%
Dementia	42%
Cerebral vascular disease	35%
Coronary artery disease	30%
Peripheral vascular disease	25%
Diabetes mellitus	25%
Ear disease (hearing loss)	24%
Depression/anxiety	23%

Adapted from Reference 20.

patient. Clinicians must recognize that preventive practice is still necessary and can have an important effect on quality of life in later years. Most studies evaluating preventive services use reduction of disease-specific mortality as an outcome, but in the elderly there are more relevant health outcomes to be considered. While prevention and modern disease management can prolong life, death cannot be indefinitely deferred. Recognizing this inescapable finality and the accumulation of illnesses over a lifetime, good health in old age entails the maintenance of optimal function, stability in chronic disease, and adequate support systems (2). Table 6-1 lists the frequency of the most common medical illnesses in the elderly, while Table 6-2 details the leading causes of death among those 65 and older.

Chronic medical conditions frequently result in limitation of activity. According to government figures from 2001, health conditions cause impairment in activities

TABLE 6-2

LEADING CAUSES OF DEATH: 65 YEARS AND OVER

Heart diseases
Malignant neoplasms
Cerebrovascular diseases
Chronic lower respiratory diseases
Influenza and pneumonia
Alzheimer's disease
Diabetes mellitus
Nephritis, nephrosis, and nephrotic syndrome
Accidents
Septicemia

Adapted from Reference 21.

of daily living (ADLs) for 13.1% of those 45 to 54 years old, 20.7% of those aged 55 to 64, and 26% of those 65 to 74 years old. In contrast, the frequency of impaired activity among noninstitutionalized people 75 years and older reaches 44.7%, and nearly 19% of those older than 75 need the help of other people for handling routine needs such as everyday household chores, shopping, managing money, or getting around (3). In addition, symptoms of mental illness are increasingly common in old age, notably occurring in the context of comorbid medical illness. The significant prevalence of depression alone in various medical illnesses is shown in Table 6-3.

THE MEDICAL HISTORY

The medical history retains its central importance in the clinical encounter with the geriatric patient. There are, however, challenges to gathering the medical history that must be anticipated. The patient should be addressed by his or her surname unless directed otherwise. While the interviewer usually assumes the patient is competent, accurate, and reliable, the high frequency of cognitive impairment (especially among those older than 80) warrants caution. Family members can provide corroborating or corrective information about the patient's illness and medical history. Determining patient reliability can be a useful indicator of cognitive status. In addition, assessing the arc of behavioral change in psychiatric disease frequently requires family and

TABLE 6-3

DEPRESSION IN MEDICAL ILLNESS

Disease	Prevalence of Associated Depression
Cushing's syndrome	33–67%
Diabetes mellitus	19–33%
Hypothyroidism	15%
End-stage renal disease	5–8% (18% minor depression)
Coronary heart disease	26%
Parkinson's disease	40–50%
Cerebrovascular accidents	30–50% (major and minor depression)
Alzheimer's disease	15–55%
Colon cancer	13–25%
Gynecologic cancers	12–23%
Lymphoma	8–19%
Oropharyngeal cancer	22–57%
Breast cancer	1.5–46%
Lung cancer	11–44%
Pancreatic cancer	33–50%

Adapted from References 22–25.

caregiver input. However, family involvement should be negotiated with the patient, reflecting a balance between patient safety and autonomy. Except in severe cases, an interview between the clinician and family that appears to exclude the patient while present (such as discussing him or her in the third person) should be avoided.

As with any patient, the preferred interview setting is both quiet and private. Busy hospital wards, nursing home units, or daycare centers are often ill suited for this requirement, with noise and commotion interfering with the assessment. Vision and hearing impairments common to old age may also impede the interview. Patients should be instructed to wear needed eyeglasses, hearing aids, and dentures to the appointment. Clinicians may find that having a pocket amplifier on hand is helpful when interviewing the hearing impaired, especially when ambient noise and distractions are significant. Office ergonomics should be designed with the older adult in mind, with bright lighting, higher chairs (with arms), and a minimum of clutter to reduce barriers and avoid falls. In order to avoid delays and embarrassment, the patient should be advised to use the toilet prior to the interview. The need to urinate or defecate can be urgent in the elderly with incontinence and mobility problems, triggered by medication effects, or affected by concurrent diagnostic studies.

History of Present Illness

In older adults, the number and complexity of patient concerns and comorbidities can be significant. Patients frequently suffer from multiple medical problems in various stages of activity. Consequently, while some patients may have one chief complaint, frequently there are many. In addition, when slower memory retrieval, sensory impairments, or speech disorders are present, more time may be required to extract and record the history. However, given the reality of time constraints, the priority for a particular visit should be negotiated. The history of each medical condition of concern should be obtained, detailing the chronology of symptoms, pertinent tests and procedures, diagnoses reached or entertained, and treatments attempted (with their results available, whether positive, negative, or neutral). The interviewer should remain aware of the atypical presentation of illness common in the elderly. For example, falls, confusion, incontinence, or functional loss can be the initial sign of an underlying illness, and may be the only sign.

The medical assessment of the older patient with new-onset behavioral changes such as confusion, agitation, or psychosis may be broad, although certain historical features can be helpful. For example, in the nursing home patient with agitation or confusion, pertinent narrative details may be lacking due to the absence of consistent caregivers. However, useful clues are often contained in the nursing home chart among the narrative nursing notes. At times, a behavior sheet may detail the frequency of events, timing, environmental cues, and therapeutic attempts. Historical patterns may be recognized, for instance when similar changes were previously associated with an illness such as urinary tract infection or pneumonia. In contrast to psychotic or agitated behaviors, the presence of falls, incontinence, or functional impairment (e.g., the loss of independence in ADLs) may be the only sign of an underlying depression or delirium. Consequently, a psychiatrist should view the new onset of any geriatric syndrome as a flag, warranting further cognitive and behavioral assessment.

While patients are often encouraged to bring all of their medications to each visit for review, this can be quite time consuming for the physician. Allied staff should update the list from patient notes, medical records, and the "bag of pills" for physician review and verification. The list should include prescriptions for daily and as-needed medicines, including over-the-counter medications, vitamin and nutritional supplements, herbal preparations, and other complementary therapies (e.g., skins creams or rubs, culturally based drinks or teas). It is advised to specifically ask the patient what he or she uses for pain, and whether he or she takes any sleeping pills, as patients often inadvertently exclude these agents. Medication allergies should be reviewed, and modified if simple intolerances or nonallergic symptoms are identified, rather than true allergies.

The current and past use of tobacco and alcohol should be ascertained. The type, amount, and duration of tobacco use should be recorded, and the reasons for attempted or successful cessation(s) explored, as these may uncover useful information on symptoms or diseases. The CAGE questionnaire is a simple and reliable screening instrument for possible alcoholism (Table 6-4). One affirmative answer should raise suspicion. Two affirmative answers indicate an alcohol use problem that requires further assessment and intervention (4).

Past Medical History

A complete medical history is essential to the care of the geriatric patient. Obtaining an accurate and comprehensive

TABLE 6-4
THE CAGE INTERVIEW

Cut down	Have you ever felt you that should *cut down* on your drinking?
Annoyed	Have people *annoyed* you by criticizing your drinking?
Guilt	Have you ever felt bad or *guilty* about your drinking?
Eye Opener	Have you ever had a drink first thing in the morning (an *eye opener*) to steady your nerves or get rid of a hangover?

medical history, however, may be difficult in older patients due to complex illnesses, multiple treating physicians, and insufficient or unavailable medical records. While forms completed by the patient and family are useful, accuracy can be improved by requiring patients to bring referral letters, clinic notes from prior practitioners, nursing home records, medication lists, surgical procedures, and hospital discharge summaries. A nurse or midlevel provider can categorize these documents, freeing the physician for the task at hand. Not surprisingly, the history may require multiple visits for completion. Notably, remote or childhood illnesses such as rheumatic heart disease and tuberculosis may remain important into old age. Due to its impact, it is important to inquire about the occurrence of delirium during hospital stays or after surgery, as this event is frequently left unrecorded. This might only be discovered by direct questioning (usually of family that were present), or on close examination of contemporaneous notes.

Family History

While family history may seem less useful once an older patient outlives the average life expectancy, certain aspects remain important. The presence of longevity, neurodegenerative disorders such as dementias and parkinsonism, and mood disorders in the family may provide useful information, even among the very old.

Social History

Psychiatric problems in an older patient, as in a younger one, are often the result of or aggravated by factors other than the individual's physical status. Some factors that should be explored with the older person and his or her family include living environment, family support, daily activities, and advance directives.

Living Environment
Questions that should be addressed to explore the patient's living environment include the following:

- What is the current living environment of the person? For example, is this person living independently or in an assisted-living facility or nursing home?
- If living independently, is he or she capable of continuing this arrangement? Formal assessment utilizing one of the many instruments designed to evaluate ADLs will help answer this question.
- Is this person still driving? If yes, do current physical or cognitive problems exist that can impair his or her driving?
- Is the patient's home environment safe? Is there safe access to the home, within the home, and in the bathroom?
- Is the living environment suitable for his or her disabilities?
- Does the patient have access to transportation to physicians, shopping, day programs, etc.?

Support
Questions that should be addressed to explore the level of support include the following:

- Does the patient have family (especially a spouse or adult children) who can support them if and when they need additional help?
- Does the patient have friends or other social supports that they see on a regular basis?
- Do they have religious or spiritual guidance, or attend a particular house of worship?
- Is the patient involved in any social, civic, or religious groups that provide socialization and support?
- Have they experienced significant losses of family and friends who previously provided support? How have these losses impacted mood and level of functioning?
- Is there a good relationship between the older person and the identified caregiver, or are there concerns about neglect or even abuse occurring?
- If no family or close friends exist, what other resources are available to help the patient maintain their independent living status? Should assisted living or nursing home placement be considered at this time?

Daily Activities
Questions that should be asked to explore daily activities include the following:

- What does the person do with his or her time?
- Is the patient still employed?
- Are they involved in other activities?
- What did the patient enjoy doing in the past?
- Do they still drive?
- Is the patient able to see or hear well enough to enjoy reading, television, radio, etc.

Advance Directives
Questions that should be asked to explore the extent that future medical care has been considered include the following:

- Does the person have an advance health care directive, and if so, is a copy in the medical record?
- If they do not have a health care directive, it must be explored as to whom would be designated as a spokesperson if the person were unable to make informed decisions about his or her own care.

Review of Systems

The review of systems for the older adult is similar to that obtained in younger cohorts, with a few additions. Standard questions regarding the neurologic, cardiovascular, pulmonary, gastrointestinal, genitourinary, endocrine, and musculoskeletal systems are appropriate, even in advanced old age. However, some issues in geriatrics merit special attention.

Neurologic

Memory, falls, orthostatic hypotension, weakness, poor sleep quality, and restless legs are frequent concerns in the elderly. Stroke, dementia, Parkinson's disease, and sleep apnea can result in symptoms of depression. Anxiety and agitation can occur in vertigo, Alzheimer's disease and other dementias, delirium, and Parkinson's disease. Notably, unintentional weight loss in the elderly appears to be an early harbinger of dementia, presenting prior to the onset of cognitive symptoms. Sensory losses such as impairments in vision or hearing may contribute to isolation and depression, provoke fear or anxiety when mobility exceeds ability, or heighten confusion when coupled with delirium or cognitive impairment (5).

Cardiovascular

The prevalence of heart failure increases with age, from 0.8% in the 50- to 59-year age group, to 9.1% in the population 80 years and older. Peripheral vascular arteriosclerosis can result in reduced blood flow to the brain, extremities, kidneys, and intestines. As a result, older patients are more susceptible to cardiac ischemia and stroke, systolic hypertension, and congestive heart failure. Common symptoms attributable to cardiovascular disorders include fatigue, exertional dyspnea, dizziness, and edema. In addition, vascular disease can cause claudication and intestinal angina. Anxiety, agitation, or panic symptoms may arise as a result of angina, arrhythmias, congestive heart failure, myocardial infarction, or vascular collapse. In addition, depression can be present in coronary disease, especially following bypass surgery (6).

Pulmonary

Increased dead-space and related declines in thoracic compliance and elastic lung recoil create a ventilation-perfusion mismatch. As a result, the total work of breathing increases, limiting the maximum breathing capacity at age 70 to just one-half of that present at age 30. Symptoms such as exertional dyspnea and fatigue are a common result (7). Depression, anxiety, agitation, or panic symptoms may occur in the context of asthma, emphysema, chronic obstructive pulmonary disease (COPD), pneumonia, pneumothorax, or pulmonary embolus. The presence of cough or aspiration should be noted when assessing delirium, as these might reveal an underlying asthma, pneumonia, or COPD exacerbation (8).

Gastrointestinal

With aging, the liver declines in mass, cytochrome P-450 enzyme efficiency, and oxidative metabolic capacity. As a result, it contributes to reduced drug metabolism and clearance; therefore, medication side effects need to be reviewed with the patient. Teeth are often lost due to receding gum lines, osteoporosis, and reduced saliva. Dry mouth and dental caries are common, as are dysphagia and aspiration. Esophageal peristalsis and lower esophageal sphincter relaxation become delayed, and colonic transit may be slowed. Constipation is common, and often exacerbated by drugs. Peptic ulcer disease, irritable bowel syndrome, and constipation can result in anxiety, agitation, or panic symptoms. Undernutrition and weight loss are common findings in mental illness, dementia, malignancy, and other disorders. Thus, it is important to inquire whether the patient has lost weight recently. Involuntary weight loss of more than 5% of body weight (or at least 5 pounds) in 1 month, or more than 10% of body weight (or 10 pounds) in 6 months is considered significant.

Genitourinary

The aging kidney is progressively impaired by glomerulosclerosis, cortical atrophy, and a reduction in functioning glomeruli. Combined with diminished total body water and renal blood flow, these changes result in a progressive decline in renal filtration. However, because of diminished skeletal muscle mass in the aged, serum creatinine underestimates true renal function. In addition, bladder changes and mobility problems result in urinary incontinence, affecting one-third of community-dwelling older adults and 50% of older nursing home patients (9). Older individuals are thus more susceptible to dehydration and renal failure from fever, drugs, and disease. At the same time, fluid replacement can easily result in edema or heart failure. Bladder infections, distension, and obstruction also are more common. These disorders can contribute to symptoms of dizziness, anxiety, agitation, or panic. Electrolyte disturbances may cause confusion and malaise. Depression can occur in renal failure or with dialysis, and incontinence may result in self-isolation (10).

Endocrine

Symptoms of agitation, confusion, or anxiety in the elderly may reflect underlying hyperthyroidism, hypothyroidism, hypercalcemia, hypocalcemia, hyperglycemia, or hypoglycemia. Parathyroid, thyroid, and adrenal disorders may result in depression.

Musculoskeletal

In the elderly, musculoskeletal problems such as inflammatory arthritis and degenerative joint disease are common. However, disuse will quickly lead to muscle weakness, atrophy, and deconditioning. Elderly people who are bed or chair-bound may develop edema, contractures, incontinence, pneumonia, pulmonary embolism, orthostatic hypotension, or pressure sores. Joint pain combined with limited mobility can contribute to social withdrawal and depression. Rheumatologic disorders such as systemic lupus may be associated with anxiety (11).

Miscellaneous

Hematologic conditions like anemia can result in dizziness and anxiety. Similarly, the immunologic phenomenon of anaphylaxis can result in prominent anxiety symptoms. Infectious diseases that cause fever may provoke anxiety or even delirium.

FUNCTIONAL ASSESSMENT

In the elderly population, the assessment of independent functional status is advised. The ADLs, generally defined as the capacity to perform the functional tasks necessary to meet the demands of daily life, should be assessed. Basic ADLs include the elemental activities necessary for an individual to care for him or herself within a limited environment (e.g., getting dressed, using the toilet, walking). Higher-level activities, known as *instrumental ADLs*, are those abilities necessary to function in the community (e.g., driving, shopping, paying bills). A specific evaluation of functional status is essential, because impairment cannot be predicted by the number or severity of medical diagnoses in an individual patient. Identifying functional impairments allows the practitioner to attempt to modify those factors that may contribute to any disability, and can affect other treatment decisions (12). For example, impairments in the ability to purchase or cook food, or even to feed oneself, can have enormous nutritional consequences. Impairments in ADLs have also been identified as risk factors for falls and institutionalization. In long-term care settings, functional assessment is performed as part of the admission database, such as the Minimum Data Set used in nursing homes.

THE PHYSICAL EXAMINATION

After completing the medical history, the clinician performs a physical examination of the patient. As with younger patients, first impressions are telling. Observations of grip strength when shaking hands, deformities, skin rash or pallor, muscle tremor, speech character and content, eyeglasses, hearing aids, use of a cane or walker, and mobility can be incorporated into the assessment. Examination of the frail, demented, confused, or bedridden individual presents a special challenge. While the examiner might devise resourceful ways to accommodate these difficulties, compromise is often necessary. Remaining mindful of missed findings, the physician may need to examine the patient in a wheelchair rather than on an exam table or hospital bed.

Vital Signs

The examination should include the patient's height and weight. Comparison with prior weight measurements is helpful for finding unintentional weight loss. A body mass index (calculated as [weight in kg]/[height in meters]^2) of less than 18.5 kg/m^2 is considered underweight (13). Older people have a tendency toward temperature dysregulation, and may have serious infections that do not pro-

duce much temperature rise. Thus, fever is a less reliable marker of infection.

Head and Neck Examination

Temporal wasting, while common in advanced old age, may indicate significant weight loss in some patients. The ears should be checked for cerumen impaction, which can impair hearing. The temporal arteries should be palpated in patients suspected of giant cell arteritis or polymyalgia rheumatica. However, a high index of suspicion for temporal arteritis is needed, because symptoms may be atypical, including new-onset headache, hallucinations, visual loss, dry cough, sore throat, tongue pain, hoarseness, toothache, a choking sensation, claudication, and fever of unknown origin (14). When examining the mouth, it is important to remove dentures so that the mucosa can be inspected, especially in patients with a history of significant tobacco or alcohol use. Dry mouth should be noted. The neck should be palpated for adenopathy. Palpation of the thyroid gland for enlargement, texture, or nodules is advised.

Cardiovascular System

Pulse and blood pressure should be measured at each visit. While individual goals may vary, the recommended blood pressure of 135/85 or less also applies to older adults. Careful detection of pulses, bruits, and capillary refill can assist in identifying atherosclerotic blockages. Orthostatic blood pressures should be measured when the patient complains of dizziness, lightheadedness, or falls. Signs of heart failure such as an elevated jugular venous pulse, S3 gallop, or enlarged apical impulse can be valuable. The murmurs of aortic stenosis, aortic insufficiency, and mitral regurgitation should be recognized due to their impact on this population. Pulses should be palpated in the neck, abdomen, groin, and feet.

Pulmonary System

The presence of kyphosis or scoliosis often reflects underlying osteoporosis. Auscultation of the chest may reveal crackles, wheezes, or the dullness of poor ventilation, indicating underlying pulmonary pathology. Cough, dyspnea, or rapid breathing may suggest infection or heart failure. Tachypnea alone can be a subtle clue to an underlying illness such as pneumonia, hypoxia, acidosis, or a cerebrovascular event.

Abdominal Examination

Surgical scars should be recorded and their origins confirmed. As in younger patients, examination for masses and organomegaly is required. Experience can teach the clinician to discern stool in the colon from worrisome masses. An aortic aneurysm is easier to detect in thinner

TABLE 6-5
RECOMMENDED LABORATORY TESTING FOR GERIATRIC PSYCHIATRY PATIENTS

Anxiety, Psychosis, Altered Mental Status, or Acute Behavioral Changes
Electrolytes plus calcium and magnesium
Glucose
Complete blood count
Renal function (BUN/creatinine)
Liver function tests (ALT/AST, bilirubin, alkaline phosphatase)
Thyroid function tests (T4, TSH)
Erythrocyte sedimentation rate
Urinalysis (consider culture)
Pulse oximetry (and blood gas if signs of hypoxemia)
Electrocardiogram
Chest radiograph
Brain CT or MRI

Mood Disorders (Depression, Mania)
Electrolytes plus calcium and magnesium
Glucose
Complete blood count
Renal function (BUN/creatinine)
Liver function tests (ALT/AST, bilirubin, alkaline phosphatase)
Thyroid function tests (T4, TSH)
AM cortisol
Vitamin B12, folate
Erythrocyte sedimentation rate
Urinalysis (consider culture)

New Onset Psychiatric Disorder or Change in Personality, Mood, Behavior, or Cognition
In selected patients, check all of the labs and tests listed above for altered mental status, plus one or more of the following tests based on clinical suspicion:
- Toxicology screen for blood alcohol level and illicit substances (for altered mental status)
- Medication levels (e.g., lithium, tricyclic antidepressants, anticonvulsants)
- Vitamin D (for diffuse pain)
- Syphilis and HIV serologies (for personality, mood, and cognitive changes)
- Lumbar puncture, including infectious stains and titers (for altered mental status)
- Lyme testing (for mood or cognitive changes due to Lyme disease)
- 24-hour urine cortisol (for mood changes due to Cushing's disease)
- Cortrosyn stimulation testing (for mood changes due to Addison's disease)
- Heavy metal screen
- Antinuclear antibody (to rule out lupus)
- Ceruloplasmin (to rule out Wilson's disease)
- Phosphorus (to rule out parathyroid disease)
- Ammonia (in suspected hepatic encephalopathy)
- Viral titers (depression due to Epstein-Barr virus, Cytomegalovirus, etc.)
- Long-chain fatty acids (to rule out adrenoleukodystrophy)
- Arylsulfatase A (to rule out metachromatic leukodystrophy)
- Porphobilinogen, ALA in 24-hour urine (to rule out acute intermittent porphyria)
- Spirometry (for anxiety in COPD)
- Postvoid residual urine (for agitation due to urinary retention)
- EEG (if altered consciousness of unknown etiology)
- Radiograph of painful sites (for agitation due to pain)
- Colonoscopy (for mood changes associated with colon cancer)
- Neck, chest, and/or abdominal CT or MRI (for depression due to lymphoma or cancers of the pancreas, lung, or ovary)

ALA, amino-levulinic acid; AST, aspartate aminotransferase; ALT, alanine aminotransferase; BUN, blood urea nitrogen; COPD, chronic obstructive pulmonary disease; CT, computed tomography; EEG, electroencephalogram; MRI, magnetic resonance imaging; T4, thyroxine; TSH, thyroid stimulating hormone.
Adapted from References 10, 26, and 27.

TABLE 6-6

LABORATORY STUDIES FOR THE GERIATRIC PSYCHIATRY WORK-UP

Lab Value	Normal Range in the Elderly[a]	Notes	Additional Tests
Hemoglobin	Hgb Male: 13.5–17.5 g/dL Female: 12.0–15.5 g/dL	Anemia is associated with panic symptoms, depression, psychosis.	Anemia: If no cause is apparent, and MCV is low, check iron, TIBC, ferritin, INR, bilirubin, LDH, Coomb's, reticulocytes, sprue antibodies, lead level, peripheral smear, stool occult blood. Hematology consultation.
Hematocrit	HCT Male: 38.8–50.0% Female: 34.9–44.5%	Anemia may be caused by menstruation, GI or other blood loss, hemolysis, B12 or folate deficiency, alcoholism or liver disease, bone marrow failure, hemoglobinopathies.	If no cause is apparent, and MCV is normal or high, check iron, TIBC, ferritin, peripheral smear, stool occult blood, B12, serum and RBC folate, sprue antibodies, AST, ALT. Hematology consultation.

White blood cell count	Males:
	$3.5–10.5 \times 10^9$ cells/L
	Females:
	$3.5–10.5 \times 10^9$ cells/L
		Mild-to-moderate elevated WBC (11–17) can normally be seen with infection, smoking, lithium treatment, glucocorticoids, catecholamines, myocardial infarction, bone marrow disorders, and physical or emotional stress. Anxiety and panic symptoms can occur with infection.
		Leukopenia: Infection, alcoholism, bone marrow disorders, collagen-vascular disorders, liver disease, drug effect.
		Drug-induced neutropenia and agranulocytosis with:
		  Psychoactive drugs: clozapine, phenothiazines, tricyclic and tetracyclic antidepressants, meprobamate.
		  Anticonvulsants: carbamazepine, phenytoin, valproate, ethosuximide.
			Leukocytosis: If no cause is apparent, check peripheral smear, BUN, creatinine, ABG, uric acid, leukocyte alkaline phosphatase. Hematology consultation.
			
			Leukopenia: If no cause is apparent, consider drug effect. Check peripheral smear, B12, folate, ANA, ANCA, SPEP, cold agglutinins. Hematology consultation.

Platelets	$150–450 \times 10^9$ cells/L	Thrombocytopenia: Viral infections (hepatitis, HIV), alcoholism, vitamin B12 and folic acid deficiency. Drug causes: Definite: Thiothixene Probable: Carbamazepine, phenytoin Thrombocytosis: Infections, recent surgery, malignancy, chronic inflammatory conditions (RA), iron-deficiency anemia, cirrhosis, renal failure, myeloproliferative diseases. Rebound thrombocytosis: Alcohol abstinence and resumption of a normal diet.	Thrombocytopenia: If no cause is apparent, check peripheral smear, iron studies, INR, aPTT, Coomb's, bleeding time, platelet antibodies, SPEP, fibrinogen, D-dimer. Hematology consultation. Thrombocytosis: If no cause is apparent, check peripheral smear, iron studies, INR, aPTT, Coomb's, bleeding time, fibrinogen, D-dimer. Hematology consultation.

TABLE 6-6
(continued)

Lab Value	Normal Range in the Elderly[a]	Notes	Additional Tests
Calcium	8.9–10.1 mg/dL	Hypercalcemia: Associated with depression, anxiety, agitation, psychosis. Causes include: Hyperparathyroidism (primary or secondary), lithium, renal failure, malignancy, pheochromocytoma. Hypocalcemia: Associated with depression, irritability, delirium. Causes include: Renal failure, vitamin D deficiency, status post parathyroidectomy. Low calcium and hypoalbuminemia: Serum total calcium concentration falls by 0.8 mg/dL (0.2 mmol/L) for every 1 g/dL (10 g/L) fall in serum albumin concentration.	Hypercalcemia: Check ionized calcium, PTH, 25-hydroxy vitamin D, SPEP, TSH, BUN, creatinine, phosphorous, serum metanephrine, PSA, CXR, mammogram. Endocrine consultation. Hypocalcemia: Check ionized calcium, PTH, 25-hydroxy vitamin D, magnesium, BUN, creatinine, phosphorous. Endocrine consultation.
Potassium	3.6–4.8 mEq/L	If low, consider diuretic or steroid effect. Causes include: Vomiting, nasogastric suction, diarrhea, enema or laxative abuse, diuretics, renal tubular acidosis, Cushing's syndrome, hyperaldosteronism. Hyperkalemia has been associated with anxiety and panic symptoms. If elevated, consider hemolyzed serum, possible drug effect (e.g., ACE inhibitors). Causes include: Renal failure, hemolysis, acidosis, muscle necrosis, adrenal insufficiency, hypoaldosteronism, thrombocytosis, leukocytosis.	Hypokalemia: Check creatinine, BUN, 24-hour urine potassium and cortisol, ABG, bicarbonate, AST, ALT, aldosterone, renin, TSH, urinalysis, ECG. Endocrine or nephrology consultation. Hyperkalemia: First confirm by rechecking potassium level. Check CBC, glucose, serum osmolality, creatine kinase, creatinine, BUN, ABG, bicarbonate, AM cortisol, AST, ALT, aldosterone, renin, urinalysis, ECG. Endocrine or nephrology consultation.
Sodium	135–145 mEq/L	Hyponatremia may result in delirium, anxiety or panic symptoms. Causes: Diuretics, diarrhea, emesis, CHF, SIADH, cirrhosis, nephrotic syndrome, water intoxication, hypothyroidism, hyperglycemia, nephrotic syndrome, adrenal insufficiency. Hypernatremia may be due to: Aldosteronism, Cushing's syndrome, diabetes insipidus, dehydration, diarrhea, diabetes, obstructive uropathy, hypertonic IV fluids.	Hyponatremia: Check urine and serum osmolality, urine sodium, AST, ALT, creatinine, BUN, TSH, glucose, AM cortisol, ABG, urinalysis, 24-hour urine protein. Endocrine or nephrology consultation. Hypernatremia: Check glucose, aldosterone, 24-hour urine cortisol, urinalysis, urine sodium, urine and serum osmolality. Endocrine or nephrology consultation.
Glucose	70–100 mg/dL (fasting)	Sweating, anxiety, palpitations, hunger, and tremor occur as plasma glucose concentrations fall below 55 mg/dL. Impaired cognition is common at or below 50 mg/dL.	If low, check plasma insulin, C-peptide, proinsulin, beta-hydroxybutyrate. Endocrine consultation.

(continued)

TABLE 6-6
(continued)

Lab Value	Normal Range in the Elderly[a]	Notes	Additional Tests
		The earliest symptoms of marked hyperglycemia are polyuria, polydipsia and weight loss. As hyperglycemia worsens, lethargy, obtundation, and coma ensue. Neurologic symptoms occur primarily when the effective plasma osmolality exceeds 320–330 mosmol/kg. Depression is common in diabetes.	If glucose is markedly elevated, check A1c, bicarbonate, phosphate, serum and urine osmolality, ABG, anion gap, sodium, potassium, urinalysis, amylase, lipase, ketones, creatinine, BUN. Endocrine consultation.
Creatinine	Male: 0.9–1.4 mg/dL Female: 0.7–1.2 mg/dL	BUN/plasma creatinine ratio is normal at 10–15:1 in acute tubular necrosis, but may be greater than 20:1 in prerenal disease.	If greater than 2.0, or continuing to increase, check BUN, potassium, urine and plasma sodium, urine and plasma creatinine, urinalysis, urine and plasma osmolality. Check bladder for obstruction by catheter.
BUN	Males: 8–24 mg/dL Females: 6–21 mg/dL Creatinine clearance (male) = $\dfrac{(140 - age\ [yrs]) \times body\ wt\ (kg)}{72 \times serum\ creatinine}$ For women, the calculated value is multiplied by 0.85. Range: 70–135 mL/min/SA	Watch for elevations, especially in response to medication changes. A normal creatinine may underestimate a reduced GFR in the elderly. End-stage renal disease is associated with depression.	Ultrasound kidneys. Nephrology consultation.
AST	12–31 U/L	AST elevated in liver disease, alcohol use, cholestasis, skeletal muscle disease or trauma, hemolysis, CHF, myocardial infarction, malignancy, pancreatitis, renal or pulmonary infarction.	If significantly elevated (more than two or three times normal), check bilirubin, glucose, INR, hemoglobin A1c, alkaline phosphatase, ferritin, iron, amylase, ceruloplasmin, creatine kinase, TSH, AM cortisol, celiac antibodies, hepatitis and HIV serologies, beta-2-microglobulin, ANA, ANCA, smooth-muscle antibody, alpha-fetoprotein, antimitochondrial antibody. CT or ultrasound liver, spleen. Gastroenterology consultation.
ALT	Males: 10–45 U/L Females: 9–29 U/L	ALT often elevated during heparin use. ALT elevated in liver disease, alcohol use, cholestasis, CHF, myocardial infarction, renal infarction, pancreatitis, myopathies. Drugs associated with: ■ Mild elevations in liver enzymes: Alcohol, antidepressants, tacrine. ■ Acute hepatic injury: Ethanol, phenytoin, phenothiazines, valproic acid. ■ Acute cholestatic injury: Chlorpromazine. ■ Acute steatosis: Valproic acid. ■ Chronic liver injury: Ethanol, phenytoin, valproic acid, chlordiazepoxide.	

TABLE 6-6
(continued)

Lab Value	Normal Range in the Elderly[a]	Notes	Additional Tests
		▪ Chronic intrahepatic cholestasis: Amitriptyline, chlorpromazine, haloperidol, imipramine, prochlorperazine, phenytoin, carbamazepine, chlorpromazine, haloperidol, tricyclic antidepressants. ▪ Noncaseating hepatic granulomas: Carbamazepine, diazepam, phenytoin. Phospholipidosis has been described in patients taking amitriptyline, chlorpromazine, and thioridazine.	
Vitamin B12 Methyl malonic acid	B12: 200–650 ng/L MMA: ≤0.40 µmol/L	Vitamin B12 deficiency can cause psychiatric and behavioral symptoms, as well as dementia, without megaloblastic anemia or neurological signs.	If low B12 or MMA, check Schilling test, folate, SPEP, sprue antibodies, 24-hour stool fat. Hematology consultation.
Folate	Folate, serum: ≥3.5 µg/L Folate, erythrocytes Adults: 268–616 ng/mL	Low B12 levels caused by: Inadequate diet or absorption (e.g., pernicious anemia, gastrectomy, small bowel diseases), anticonvulsants, myeloma. High B12 levels caused by: Hepatitis, excessive meat intake, renal failure, myeloproliferative diseases, leukocytosis, oral contraceptives. Increased levels of MMA are an early and sensitive indicator of tissue cobalamin deficiency. Isolated folate deficiency is common in alcoholism. Decreased RBC folate and normal serum folate may occur with pure vitamin B12 deficiency.	If high B12, check AST, ALT, creatinine, BUN, CBC, peripheral smear. Hematology consultation.
TSH	0.3–5.0 mIU/L normal 5.1–7.0 mIU/L borderline hypothyroid <0.3 mIU/L hyperthyroid	Hyperthyroidism and hypothyroidism are associated with anxiety, panic symptoms, psychosis. Decreased TSH: Hyperthyroidism, thyroiditis, Grave's disease. Drugs including exogenous thyroid hormone, steroids, dopaminergic agents. Hypothyroidism is associated with depression. Elevated TSH: Hypothyroidism, Hashimoto's thyroiditis, drug effect (chlorpromazine, haloperidol, dopamine antagonists).	If TSH abnormal, check free thyroxine and antithyroid antibodies, thyroid peroxidase. Endocrine consultation.

(continued)

TABLE 6-6
(continued)

Lab Value	Normal Range in the Elderly[a]	Notes	Additional Tests
ECG	Normal sinus rhythm	Abnormal results: Tachycardia, bradycardia, atrial fibrillation, prolonged pauses or complete heart block. Anxiety and panic symptoms occur with angina, arrhythmias, cardiomyopathies, CHF, myocardial infarction, vascular collapse. Tachycardia and anxiety or panic symptoms occur with asthma, emphysema, COPD, pneumonia, pneumothorax, pulmonary embolus.	If abnormal, according to the clinical setting, check CK-MB, troponin, D-dimer, AST, CBC, BUN, creatinine. Consider evaluation for PE (e.g., CT angiogram). Cardiology or pulmonary consultation.
CXR	Normal	Abnormal results: Heart failure, effusion, malignancy, pneumonia, osteoporosis (may be asymptomatic). Depression occurs in heart failure and malignancy. Anxiety and panic symptoms occur with asthma, emphysema, COPD, pneumonia, pneumothorax, pulmonary embolus.	If abnormal, according to the clinical setting, check ECG, CBC, AST, BUN, creatinine, troponin, D-dimer, ABGs, respiratory rate, bedside spirometry (peak flow), CT angiogram (for PE). Cardiology or pulmonary consultation.

[a]Authors' Notes: This is not an exhaustive list. It is important to note that reference ranges will vary from one laboratory to another. The references presented here come from a large reference laboratory in the Midwest United States. The clinician should be familiar with the ranges from the actual laboratory performing the test.

A "normal" value for a lab test is its mean ± 2 standard deviations in a population of healthy people. Therefore, 5% of abnormal values obtained, even in healthy people, represent simply a statistical concept. Furthermore, if each test in a test battery is independent, the probability that a healthy person will have completely normal results is relatively low.

Reference ranges for lab values are determined by using appropriate population samples obtained under precisely defined conditions. Because cross-sectional studies provide test results from only one point in a person's life, they are not nearly as informative as long-term longitudinal studies of the same individuals.

Variability of organ function is a well-known hallmark of aging. As a result, extrapolating from a normal population to individuals within that population is less valid in the elderly. Determining what are normal lab values in elderly people is further complicated by other factors, including not only physiologic (and anatomic) changes associated with normal aging, but also diseases—both overt and latent, and multiple environmental differences, for example drugs, diet, exercise.

Because of these multiple disparities among even same-aged elderly, it is difficult to choose homogeneous controls to determine normal reference values. These factors confound the determination of valid age-adjusted normal lab values. Thus, the most useful technique to establish presence of disease using lab values is to compare present lab results with previous results obtained, when possible, from that person when disease is not present.

A table of normal reference values may be of limited value when assessing the elderly. In the ongoing assessment process, the strategy of individualized screening lab tests is often considered. However, even in the elderly population, most patients with diseases that can be detected by biochemical profiles present with clinical symptoms and signs of such significance that screening lab tests usually have little value. Consideration of the relative sensitivity of a particular test would be more significant, for example serum cholesterol or blood glucose, which both have a high sensitivity in asymptomatic people.

ABG, arterial blood gas; ACE, angiotensin converting enzyme; ALT, alanine aminotransferase; ANA, antinuclear antibodies; ANCA, antineutrophilic cytoplasmic antibodies; aPTT, activated partial thromboplastin time; AST, aspartate aminotransferase; BUN, blood urea nitrogen; CBC, complete blood count; CHF, congestive heart failure; CK-MB, creatine kinase—muscle-brain fraction; COPD, chronic obstructive pulmonary disease; CT, computed tomography; CXR, chest radiograph; ECG, electrocardiogram; GFR, glomerular filtration rate; GI, gastrointestinal; HCT, hematocrit; Hgb, hemoglobin; INR, international normalized ratio; IV, intravenous; LDH, lactate dehydrogenase; MCV, mean corpuscular volume; MMA, methyl malonic acid; PE, pulmonary embolus; PSA, prostate-specific antigen; PTH, parathyroid hormone; RA, rheumatoid arthritis; RBC, red blood cell; SIADH, syndrome of inappropriate antidiuretic hormone; SPEP, serum protein electrophoresis; TIBC, total iron binding capacity; TSH, thyroid stimulating hormone; WBC, white blood cells.

patients, but can be entirely missed in the obese. In older patients, the absence of rigidity, rebound, or guarding does not reliably exclude a surgical abdomen, making this diagnosis sometimes problematic.

Genitourinary Examination

In women, estrogen loss results in atrophy of the labia and vaginal wall. Inspection of the vulva for abnormalities suggestive of malignancy is important. With advancing age, atrophy of the uterus and ovaries may render these organs nonpalpable. Indeed, the presence of a palpable ovary in an elderly woman should raise the suspicion of malignancy. Breast examination remains important even in late life, since breast cancer increases in incidence through the ninth decade. While much rarer in men, breast cancer occurs with enough frequency to warrant palpation. Although its efficacy in screening for prostate cancer is as yet unclear, the prostate exam should also be performed. When urinary incontinence is present in either sex, a more detailed urologic or gynecologic examination is advised.

Musculoskeletal Examination

Active neck range of motion (ROM) should be tested by having the patient turn the head laterally to its limit. Hands, feet, wrists, elbows, shoulders, knees, and hips should be examined for evidence of arthritis and deformity. Passive and active ROM will detect any pain or limitations in the joints. For example, the shoulders can be tested by having patients reach up with their arms and then clasp their hands together behind their neck. The hip joints can be assessed when the patient attempts to squat and rise. Observation of his or her ability to grasp and pinch (such as when buttoning clothes or tying shoes) can demonstrate sufficient hand function.

Neurological Examination

While the neurologic examination is covered in another chapter of this textbook, certain issues warrant review. Examination should include testing of mental status, vision, and hearing. Falls are a serious problem among older adults, with potentially devastating consequences, including institutionalization and death. One-third of noninstitutionalized older adults fall each year, with costs for the care of related fractures reaching nearly $10 billion annually (15–17). Despite the high degree of concern regarding the implications of falls in the elderly, it remains unproven whether falls can be prevented, or whether reducing the fall rate will reduce fractures (18). Nevertheless, a modified Romberg maneuver (i.e., checking a patient's balance while they stand with eyes closed and arms held out in front of his or her body) and the simple

"get up and go" tests are fast and practical assessments of gait and balance (19).

LABORATORY ASSESSMENT

The utility of routinely performing a set of screening laboratory tests in the asymptomatic patient has been the subject of considerable debate, and the question remains largely unanswered. However, the older adult with mental illness is not, in fact, asymptomatic. As noted, the psychiatric disorders are frequent companions to the myriad of medical illnesses common to old age. In addition, the presence of cognitive impairment, delirium, or dementia may mask or alter the expression of comorbid disease, as can the aging process itself. As a result, and until better evidence clarifies the issue, certain tests may be warranted when assessing the geriatric patient with mental illness. Table 6-5 outlines laboratory and other tests relevant to several major late-life psychiatric conditions. Table 6-6 outlines individual tests in more detail, including comments on interpretation and further workup relevant to geriatric psychiatry practice.

REFERENCES

1. Pinholt EM, Kroenke K, Hanley JF, et al. Functional assessment of the elderly: a comparison of standard instruments with clinical judgement. *Arch Int Med.* 1987;147:484–488.
2. Kennie DC. Health maintenance of the elderly. *Clin Geriat Med.* 1986;2:53–83.
3. US Census Bureau. *Statistical Abstract of the United States: 2003.* 123rd ed. 2003 Library of Congress Card No. 4-18089, Health and Nutrition, Nos. 195–196. Available at: http://www.census.gov/prod/2004pubs/03statab/health.pdf.
4. Lapid, MI, Rummans, TA. Evaluation and management of geriatric depression in primary care [symposium on geriatrics]. *Mayo Clin Proc.* November 2003:1423–1429.
5. Stewart R, Masaki K, Xue QL, et al. A 32-year prospective study of change in body weight and incident dementia: the Honolulu-Asia Aging Study. *Arch Neurol.* 2005;62:55–60.
6. Cheitlin MD, Zipes DP. Cardiovascular disease in the elderly. In: Braunwald E, Zipes DP, Lippy P (eds.). Heart Disease: A Textbook of Cardiovascular Medicine, 6th ed. Philadelphia, PA: W.B. Saunders Company. 2001; 2019–2030.
7. Samuels SC, Neugroschl JA. Delirium. In: Sadock BJ, Sadock VA (eds). Comprehensive Textbook of Psychiatry, 8th ed. Philadelphia, PA: Lippincott Williams & Wilkins. 2005;1054–1068.
8. Tonner PH, Kampen J, Scholz J. Pathophysiological changes in the elderly. *Best Pract Res Clin Anaesthesiol.* 2003;17(2): 163–177.
9. Diokno AC. The epidemiology of urinary incontinence. *J Gerontol Med Sci.* 2001;56A:M3–M4.
10. Beck LH. Changes in renal function with aging. *Clin Geriatr Med.* 1998;14(2):199–209.
11. Harper C, Lyles Y. Physiology and complications of bed rest. *J Am Geriatr Soc.* 1988;36:11.
12. Applegate WB, Blass JP, Williams TF. Instruments for the functional assessment of older patients. *N Engl J Med.* 1990;322(17): 1207–1214.
13. Davison KK, Ford ES, Cogswell ME, Dietz WH. Percentage of body fat and body mass index are associated with mobility limitations in people aged 70 and older (from NHANES III). *J Am Geriatr Soc.* 2002;50:1802–1840.
14. Hellmann DB. Temporal arteritis: a cough, toothache, and tongue infarction. *JAMA.* 2002;287:2996–3000.
15. Aditya BS, Sharma JC, Allen SC, Vassallo M. Predictors of a nursing home placement from a non-acute geriatric hospital. *Clin Rehabil.* 2003;17(1):108–113.

16. Rubenstein LZ, Josephson KR, Robbins AS. Falls in the nursing home. *Ann Int Med.* 1994;121:442–451.

17. Campbell AJ, Borrie MJ. Risk factors for falls in a community-based prospective study of people 70 years and older. *J Gerontol.* 1989;44:M112–M117.

18. Gillespie LD, Gillespie WJ, Robertson MC, et al. Interventions to reduce the incidence of falling in the elderly (Cochrane Review). In: *The Cochrane Library.* Issue 3. Oxford: Update Software; 2001.

19. Mathias S, Nayak U, Isaacs B. Balance in elderly patients: the get up and go test. *Arch Phys Med Rehabil.* 1987;68:305.

20. Branch LG, Coulam RF, Zimmerman YA. The PACE evaluation: initial findings. *Gerontologist.* 1995;35:349–359.

21. Deaths: Preliminary Data for 2002, Table 7. National Vital Statistics Reports, Vol. 52, No. 13, February 11, 2004. Available at: http://www.cdc.gov/nchs/data/nvsr/nvsr52/nvsr52_13.pdf.

22. Sutor B, Rummans TA, Jowsey SG, et al. Major depression in medically ill patients. *Mayo Clin Proc.* 1998;73:329–337.

23. Massie MJ, Popkin MK. Depressive disorders. In: Holland JC, ed. *Psycho-Oncology.* New York: Oxford University Press; 1998: 518–540.

24. Massie MJ. Prevalence of depression in patients with cancer. *J Natl Cancer Inst Monogr.* 2004;32:57–71.

25. Monzani F, Del Guerra P, Caraccio N, et al. Subclinical hypothyroidism: neurobehavioral features and beneficial effect of L-thyroxine treatment. *Clin Investig.* 1993;71(5):367–371.

26. Ciechanowski P, Katon W. Overview of generalized anxiety disorder. *UpToDate Online.* Available at: http://uptodateonline.com /application/topic.asp?file=psychiat/2208&type=A&selectedTitle= 1~51. Accessed on December 2, 2004.

27. Fricchione G. Clinical practice. Generalized anxiety disorder. *N Engl J Med.* 2004;351:675.

NOTES FROM CLINICAL PRACTICE: RECOGNIZING PSYCHIATRIC MANIFESTATIONS OF MEDICAL ILLNESS

Robert B. Portney

Patients suffer behavioral and cognitive changes that are frequently induced or exacerbated by unrecognized and untreated medical disorders. It is essential for geriatric psychiatrists and other clinicians to have an appreciation for the unique frailties of the elderly and these influences on psychiatric functioning. Unless this important connection between medical disturbances and psychiatric symptoms is recognized, the reasons for a thorough medical assessment in psychiatric patients may not be appreciated.

THE AGING PROCESS

Aspects of the aging process contribute to an enhanced vulnerability to alterations in cognition, affect, and behavior. As an example, in a patient aged 30 to 40 years old one would not typically expect a urinary tract infection to induce the kind of marked behavioral changes often seen in elderly patients. With advanced age, however, there is a greater likelihood for the development of psychiatric disturbances due to changes in central nervous system (CNS) functioning. Studies in the elderly suggest that when deficiencies in neurotransmitters exist, diseases or medications that further compromise these levels are likely to induce physical, cognitive, or behavioral difficulties (1–3). For example, the risk of both cognitive decline and delirium increases in older individuals with greater serum anticholinergic activity (1), typically resulting from taking medications with anticholinergic properties (2).

The geriatric clinician should first consider the physical state of the brain before moving towards psychopharmacologic treatment. If factors contributing to cognitive and behavioral change are not identified and treated, the efficacy of psychiatric interventions could be limited. This might help explain why a meta-analysis of studies examining the effects of conventional antipsychotics versus placebo to treat agitation in dementia patients demonstrated only modest efficacy (4). It is quite possible that underlying medical illnesses went untreated in many subjects.

PRERENAL EQUALS PREBRAIN

An adequate flow of blood is necessary for the appropriate functioning of the brain and all other organ systems in the body. Inadequate blood flow compromises organ function; for example, consider the *prerenal* state that exists when kidney function is compromised by the inadequate delivery of blood through the renal arteries, producing a serum blood urea nitrogen to creatinine ratio greater than 20:1. Similarly, the term *prebrain* can be postulated to refer to a condition in which insufficient blood, oxygen, or nutrients reach the brain, enhancing the potential for cognitive and behavioral difficulties, as well as the development of delirium. In theory, many medical conditions could lead to a prebrain state, including anemia, cardiac disease, dehydration, infection, metabolic disturbances, renal or hepatic failure, and endocrine disorders.

CARDIAC DISEASE AND DEPRESSION

Most geriatric clinicians have noticed that patients suffering from cardiac disease experience poorer outcomes when they are also depressed. What appears to logically follow is that treatment of an underlying mood disorder might improve cardiac status. One would obviously not want to ignore depression in a sick cardiac patient if successful treatment might both make them happier and improve overall survival.

From a psychological perspective, encouraging a healthy lifestyle with alterations in diet and exercise might provide a patient with a feeling of control over cardiac or other medical disorders, and possibly result in mood elevation. Cardiac rehabilitation might help restore a sense that life can still be enjoyed, and help the patient feel as though he or she is not just waiting to die. This may be especially important for individuals who were in extreme denial about the risks associated with past behaviors, and who now fear that almost any activity might bring on another heart attack. It is always important for clinicians to be aware that the loss of a sense of control and independence in life can be devastating to one's psyche, and risks making a patient feel worthless and depressed.

PULMONARY DISEASE AND ANXIETY

Many older patients with pulmonary disease have long-standing histories of tobacco abuse. Whether emotional difficulties impart a greater vulnerability to becoming addicted or make quitting more difficult is currently unknown. However, some have observed that the average smoker of today appears to possess greater psychopathology than the typical smoker of 50 years ago. This may relate in part to increased societal pressures against smoking, allowing healthier, less-vulnerable individuals to resist peer pressure to continue smoking. Unfortunately, when attempting to treat patients who remain addicted to cigarettes, our therapeutic options become somewhat limited. This is why patients with advanced pulmonary disease who suffer from depression or anxiety can be amongst the most challenging patients to treat.

When a pulmonary patient complains of heightened anxiety, it is necessary to assess what organic factors might be contributing to current symptoms. The anxiety may be psychological in origin, or may be due to one of several organic factors: a reduction in arterial oxygen tension, an elevation in arterial carbon dioxide (CO_2) levels, or alterations in blood flow to the CNS. Sorting out the causes of anxiety can be complex, especially in those individuals with significant hypoxia. Failure to improve oxygenation can result in increased shortness of breath, anxiety, and confusion. Some individuals become hopeless and even suicidal, viewing daily life as miserable with little hope for improvement.

Physicians typically attempt to treat chronic obstructive pulmonary disease (COPD) patients who are CO_2 retainers with low levels of inhaled oxygen, in the hope of decreasing the sensation of air hunger and anxiety, without compromising respiratory drive. However, as COPD becomes more severe, the relative lack of blood oxygen and excess CO_2 invariably results in an enhanced sensation of dyspnea and an increase in anxiety. In addition to careful titration of oxygen, antidepressants that increase serotonin levels may diminish the anxiety associated with elevated CO_2. Benzodiazepines may also be used to reduce anxiety, but with the small risk of further compromising respiratory status.

RENAL DISEASE AND DEPRESSION

Kidney failure frequently occurs as a manifestation of systemic disease. It is not uncommon for patients with renal pathology to have already suffered hypertension or diabetes for many years before reductions in creatinine clearance or hematocrit levels are noted. A tragic cause of deterioration in renal function is sometimes patient nonadherence with a therapeutic regimen. Complaints of sadness or fatigue are not uncommon in renal patients. However, in older cognitively impaired individuals who are also prerenal, anxiety, confusion, agitation, or even delirium can occur. With advanced disease, patients frequently become anemic due to reductions in erythropoietin synthesis, and suffer increased fatigue, lack of concentration, confusion, and behavioral disturbances. All of these symptoms can diminish the motivation to comply with complex treatment regimens. Sometimes primary treatments aimed at improving the underlying renal failure and/or cardiac output may improve the clinical situation. The addition of an antidepressant or antipsychotic medication may be necessary, but is only variably effective.

HEPATIC DISEASE

Patients suffering from hepatic disease are highly vulnerable to numerous complications capable of inducing cognitive and/or behavioral disturbances. Psychiatric disorders with an enhanced risk of hepatic disease include drug and alcohol abuse, as well as certain mood, psychotic, or personality disorders associated with high-risk behaviors. Depression, eating disorders, and psychosis can also be associated with the development of liver disease due to chronic malnutrition and resultant loss of hepatic function. Unfortunately, despite adequate psychiatric treatment, such patients are frequently left to cope with the devastating effects from past behaviors. The same can be said of older individuals, although they may be less likely to engage in high-risk behaviors that might lead to hepatic disease.

INFECTIOUS DISEASES AND DELIRIUM

Many older individuals become susceptible to symptoms of a delirium during periods of infection. For example, urinary tract infections (UTIs) represent a leading cause of delirium, particularly for elderly female patients in long-term care facilities. One of the reasons these individuals become so vulnerable to recurrent UTIs is because urogenital tissue atrophy following menopause diminishes the physical barrier to bacteria in the urethra. Furthermore, if the patient suffers from cognitive impairment with reduced awareness of the importance of wiping from front to back after defecating or voiding, a greater vulnerability to infection occurs. The risk is further increased when a patient takes medications with anticholinergic properties that relax bladder smooth muscle, resulting in increased postvoid urine residuals. In addition to UTIs, respiratory, abdominal, dental, and skin infections (e.g., from decubiti) can lead to delirium and associated behavioral disturbances. It is unclear why elderly patients are more sensitive to CNS alterations from infectious processes, since they typically did not experience difficulties during similar situations in prior years. Numerous theories suggest that baseline neurotransmitter vulnerabilities—particularly in cholinergic, dopaminergic, and glutaminergic systems—are involved. Chemical mediators of infection and inflammation, such as cytokines and cortisol, may also increase the vulnerability to delirium.

GASTROINTESTINAL DISORDERS AND ANXIETY

Patients suffering gastrointestinal problems have historically been thought to suffer emotional difficulties that trigger somatic complaints. However, many of the illnesses once thought to be closely associated with anxiety or personality disorders have turned out to be the result of infectious or other organic disease states. Despite the lack of a clear association between many diseases of the bowel and proven psychopathology, a few important issues deserve mention.

Patients suffering bowel disease capable of inducing acute symptoms necessitating multiple visits to the bathroom might easily experience nervousness that mimics an anxiety disorder. If an individual does not know when the sudden urge to defecate might arise, precautions must be taken on a chronic basis to prevent fecal incontinence. Such concerns can easily resemble anxiety or phobic difficulties suggestive of a patient with panic disorder, and an almost agoraphobic lifestyle can develop. It may be difficult for the clinician experienced in the treatment of anxiety disorders to differentiate avoidance due to anxiety as opposed to limitations imposed from bowel disease. Some patients might be embarrassed to divulge the role of their bowel habits. It is interesting to note that some agents used to treat irritable bowel symptoms possess antianxiety effects.

AUTOIMMUNE/COLLAGEN VASCULAR DISORDERS

Patients presenting a variety of physical symptoms in the absence of diagnosable pathological processes frequently turn out to suffer from either autoimmune diseases or ill-defined psychiatric disturbances. They may present with symptoms highly suggestive of depression, but at other times appear to suffer from psychosis or even a personality disorder. Many individuals require chronic interventions for painful conditions for which objective evidence of disease may not be found. Unfortunately, this makes caregivers suspicious that patients are exaggerating symptoms, or perhaps using complaints of physical symptoms as a means of gaining access to substances of abuse. In the absence of definitive laboratory abnormalities or other objective evidence of medical pathology, clinicians must try to decide if symptoms suggest malingering or psychopathology. Clinicians are never quite certain as to the true nature of many illnesses, and are frequently left wondering whether they are encouraging inappropriate drug-seeking behaviors in their patients. In response to such issues, it is not uncommon for clinicians to decide to withhold all medications possessing significant addictive potential, in the hope of decreasing the risk for abuse and dependence. What this typically does is increase the desire on the part of the patient to seek other clinicians whom they believe might be more likely to accept their somatic complaints. It is essential that clinicians search for the most effective manner in which to assess and treat complex clinical conditions, while still encouraging patients to be both honest and open. This continues to be true, even when symptoms are not well supported by objective findings and concerns remain about the true nature of the pathology.

MALIGNANCIES AND DEPRESSION

When a patient is informed that he or she is suffering from a malignancy, and then told that no known cure exists, it is an extremely devastating experience. Any attempts to separate the normal psychological response from the physical manifestations of disease may not only be difficult, but probably impossible. When we ask cancer patients how they are feeling, they may not know how best to answer the question. They may think, "How do I feel about having a life-threatening illness?" or perhaps, "How am I feeling at this moment?" It is obviously challenging to differentiate depression due to an endogenous affective disorder from the sadness and emotional suffering associated with malignancy. Physicians must remain positive and not let emotions interfere with the ability to provide care for terminally ill patients. Effective therapeutic interventions should be provided, including treatment of pain, while remaining honest and as encouraging as possible.

ENDOCRINE DISORDERS

Disorders of the endocrine system can induce significant alterations in mood and cognition. Thyroid disorders are probably the most common endocrine causes of psychiatric disturbances, followed by adrenal and parathyroid disease. Psychiatric disturbances, when present, can range from subtle to profound, and can be difficult to distinguish from manifestations of other metabolic abnormalities. However, if the psychiatric symptoms are treated without regard to influences of the untreated endocrine disorder, the chance for remission of either process is poor.

As an example, patients suffering from hypothyroidism can display symptoms of depression, psychosis, or dementia. Patients may complain of weakness or intolerance to cold, become bradycardic, and display symptoms suggestive of congestive heart failure. Some individuals develop electrolyte imbalances that can exacerbate heart failure, making an accurate diagnosis extremely difficult unless one is already considering the endocrine disorder. Older individuals may not initially complain of typical symptoms of hypothyroid disease, but instead develop constipation or confusion. Or they may identify common manifestations only when asked. Patients may be incorrectly diagnosed with depression, since symptoms can mimic those of a mood disorder; however, treatment of the depressive symptoms alone will never resolve the systemic manifestations of disease. Left untreated, dramatic alterations in behavior and cognition may occur and, in rare instances, patients may become psychotic. This is one of the reasons that tests for thyroid function are considered an integral part of the dementia workup. When treating hypothyroidism, the clinician should not expect to see a reversal of depressive symptoms or significant improvement in cognitive dysfunction until at least several weeks after thyroid treatments have been started and the thyroid stimulating hormone begins to approach the normal range.

REFERENCES

1. Flacker JM, Cummings V, Mach JR Jr, et al. The association of serum anticholinergic activity with delirium in elderly medical patients. *Am J Ger Psychiatry.* 1998;6:31–41.
2. Street JS, Clark WS, Gannon KS, et al. Olanzapine treatment of psychotic and behavioral symptoms in patients with Alzheimer disease in nursing care facilities: a double-blind randomized, placebo-controlled trial. *Arch Gen Psychiatry.* 2000;57:971.
3. Samuels SC, Neugroschl JA. Delirium. In: Sadock BJ, Sadock VA, eds. *Comprehensive Textbook of Psychiatry.* 8th ed. Philadelphia, PA: Lippincott Williams & Wilkins; 2005:1054–1068.
4. Schneider LS, Pollock VE, Lyness SA. A meta-analysis of controlled trials of neuroleptic treatment in dementia. *J Am Geriatr Soc.* 1990;38:553–563.

Neurological Assessment of the Elderly Psychiatric Patient

7

Elliott L. Mancall

Competence in aspects of clinical neurology is a *sine qua non* for the successful geriatric psychiatrist, particularly in the domains of the neurological assessment itself and of the more common and often confusing psychiatric manifestations of organic neurological disease. Both will be discussed in this chapter.

NEUROLOGICAL ASSESSMENT

The neurological examination in the elderly patient follows the ordinary pattern of examination in younger individuals. For the most part, in patients with no neurological disease the examination yields normal responses. However, several changes are well recognized on examination in older individuals who have no demonstrable disease of either the central or peripheral nervous system (Table 7-1) (1–3). These changes include impaired ocular convergence and upgaze; reduced or lost Achilles reflexes; impaired vibratory sense, especially in the lower extremities, with some occasional blunting of position sense as well; tremor that is not otherwise explained, particularly involving the head and neck; and, at times, a gait reminiscent of a parkinsonian gait. In assessing such alterations, it is of course essential to not only exclude neurological disease *per se*, but also to consider systemic disorders such as thyroid disease or diabetes mellitus, which themselves might be responsible for one or more of these changes. In general, however, the unimpaired elderly demonstrate no other consistent alterations, and as a result, a specific explanation for observed changes must be sought.

A necessary prelude to the neurological examination itself is a careful and concise neurological history, comprising not only the chief complaint but also a detailed history of the present illness, since in fact the vast majority of neurological diagnoses are based on the history rather than the examination. Unfortunately, some elderly are circumstantial in presenting their history. Symptoms as recounted by a patient often lack precision, and the skilled historian must pursue complaints to establish their neurological significance. For example, a complaint of dizziness may simply refer to light-headedness or a sense of instability, but in some instances reflects true vertigo. Heaviness in the limbs may actually represent a sense of weakness, or may imply sensory loss. The complaint of numbness should be pursued in terms of, for example, the presence of tingling paresthesiae. Loss or blurring of vision may indicate a true reduction of visual acuity, but these terms are often used by patients to describe diplopia or constriction of the visual fields. Complaints such as headache are in isolation imprecise, and a detailed description of the headache including its exact location, qualitative character, severity, accompanying symptoms such as nausea, vomiting, or visual impairment, and factors that alleviate or intensify the headache should all be defined. In the final analysis, although the patient is ordinarily given free rein in recounting his or her history, the examiner must often guide the patient in an attempt to be as exact as possible. Family members may be of substantial help in obtaining a careful and detailed history. Indeed, an elderly patient, particularly one with dementia, may actually be unaware of why he or she is in the consultant's office,

TABLE 7-1

NEUROLOGICAL CHANGES
IN THE NORMAL ELDERLY

Reduced ocular convergence
Impaired conjugate upgaze
Tremor (primarily head and neck)
Muscular atrophy (hands)
Nonspecific gait disorder
Reduced vibratory sense (ankles)
Hypoactive Achilles reflexes

and may categorically deny the existence of neurological problems.

Other aspects of the history are often critical in establishing a correct diagnosis. There is increasing awareness of a genetic background for many neurological diseases, even in the elderly, and a careful family history is essential. For instance, it is very difficult to clinically establish a diagnosis of Huntington's disease (HD) without a positive family history. Also, a diagnosis of migraine in the headache patient becomes more tenable when information of the family constellation is available.

The medical history is pertinent, not only in terms of significant systemic illness such as diabetes or hypertension, but also in search of prior neurologically significant events such as craniocerebral trauma. The social history, although often neglected, is similarly important as the medical community becomes increasingly aware of the effects of occupational and environmental factors in the pathogenesis of neurological disease. Finally, a review of systems may elicit complaints, at least potentially, of neurological importance that have perhaps been overlooked by the patient or family.

The Neurological Examination

An outline of the neurological examination pertinent to the geriatrician is found in Table 7-2. A general physical examination should accompany this neurological assessment.

Mental Status

To the neurologist or geriatrician seeking signs of organic brain disease, parameters in the cognitive sphere that are relatively easily assessed in the clinic or at the bedside are:

- Orientation in time, place, and person.
- Adequacy of the attention span, which may be assessed in the give and take of the history, but may also be determined by a test of digit retention.
- Memory for recent events, evaluated to some extent while taking the history, but more specifically documented by asking the patient to repeat several test items or phrases after 5 to 10 minutes (memory for events of the more remote test are much more difficult to evalu-

ate, and often require the presence of a knowledgeable family member for confirmation).
- Fund of general knowledge.
- Ability to calculate, most commonly tested with the serial sevens test, but at times requiring a more concrete problem solving approach, for example with a shopping list.
- Ability to think in the abstract, determined by the ability to explain proverbs and/or similarities in an abstract rather than concrete manner.
- Judgment in a test situation, for example, reaction to smelling smoke in a theater.

In the individual found to have cognitive impairment, it may be difficult to separate dementia, in terms of an acquired impairment of cognition and memory, from mental retardation; the presence of another historian is clearly important in this respect.

During the course of the examination, the patient's language performance is also assessed on the basis of spontaneous speech, fluency, response to verbal commands, ability to express himself or herself appropriately, ability to repeat, and the ability to name a variety of objects. A detailed testing of language function and of praxis and gnosis is at times warranted.

The Mini-Mental State Examination (MMSE) has been widely utilized in evaluating mentation, but has also been criticized on a number of grounds, including the lack of behavioral measurements (4). It does, however, provide a reasonable quantitative assessment, and may be particularly useful in following a patient with evolving cognitive dysfunction. See Chapter 5 in this textbook for more information

Although clearly not needed on a routine basis, formal neuropsychological testing is at times helpful for distinguishing dementia from a so-called pseudodementia, for separating organic from functional disease in general, for identifying and quantifying behavioral and emotional changes that may not be evident during the routine examination, such as executive dysfunction, and as part of preparation for epilepsy surgery.

Cranial Nerves

I   The *olfactory nerve* is often ignored in a routine examination, but loss of the sense of smell is sometimes encountered in instances of cranial trauma with basal skull fracture, or with subfrontal tumors.

II   Evaluation of the *optic nerve* demands the determination of the visual acuity, confrontation visual fields, color perception, pupillary reflexes to light and accommodation, and funduscopic examination. Because of the remarkable neuroanatomic precision of the visual apparatus from retina to calcarine cortex and beyond, such visual parameters are often of extreme importance clinically in localizing disease. In the older patient, the presence of cataract or other local ocular disease may make evaluation particularly difficult.

TABLE 7-2
THE NEUROLOGICAL EXAMINATION

Mental Status
Level of consciousness
Affect
Orientation
Memory

Immediate
Short term
Long term

Fund of general knowledge
Calculation (serial 7s)
Abstract thinking
Judgment
Insight
Appearance and Behavior

Speech/Language
Fluency
Verbal comprehension
Naming
Repetition
Reading/writing

Cranial Nerves
I   Olfactory: odor discrimination
II   Optic: visual acuity, fields, color vision, fundi, pupillary
          light reactions
III, IV, VI Oculomotor, trochlear, abducens: extraocular
          movements, pupils, lids, diplopia, nystagmus or other
          abnormal movements
V   Trigeminal: sensory, motor
VII   Facial: facial expression, taste over anterior two-thirds
          of tongue
VIII   Auditory: hearing threshold
IX, X   Glossopharyngeal, vagus: palatal movements, gag
          reflex, voice
XI   Spinal accessory: movement of sternomastoid and
          trapezia
XII   Hypoglossal: tongue movements

Motor System
Bulk
Tone
Strength (0–5)
Grading:

0 – no movement
1 – muscle contracts but does not move the joint
2 – can move the joint but not against gravity
3 – can move against gravity but can offer no resistance

4 – can offer some resistance
5 – normal strength
Involuntary movements

Rhythmical: tremor, repose, postural, intentional
Nonrhythmical: chorea, dystonia, myoclonus, tics
Reflexes (0–4)

Upper extremities: biceps, triceps, radial
Lower extremities: knee (patellar) and ankle (Achilles) reflexes
Grading:

0 – none
1 – hypoactive
2 – normal
3 – hyperactive
4 – very hyperactive (with clonus)

Pathological reflexes
Babinski (plantar response)
Jaw jerk
Glabellar
Suck reflex (tactile or visual)
Rooting reflex
Palmomental reflex
Cerebellar testing
Gait and station
Finger to nose
Heel-knee-shin
Rapid alternating movements
Rebound
Dexterity

Sensation
Primary modalities
Light touch
Pinprick
Vibration
Temperature
Proprioception
Integrative (discriminatory, cortical) modalities
Stereognosis
Graphesthesia
Two-point discrimination
Double simultaneous stimulation

Miscellaneous
Carotid auscultation
Vertebral column
Autonomic function

III, IV, VI The *oculomotor, trochlear,* and *abducens nerves* (i.e., nerves concerned with movements of the globes) are assessed in terms of adequacy of ocular mobility, with or without diplopia, and the presence of nystagmus. Ocular motility may normally be somewhat reduced in the elderly, with particular reduction of ocular convergence and perhaps of vertical gaze.

V Evaluation of the motor and sensory components of the *trigeminal nerve* is generally straightforward. The motor contribution from the trigeminal nerve is relatively small, involving primarily the muscles of mas-

tication. The more important functions of this nerve are sensory. Testing follows the three prime radicular zones (ophthalmic, maxillary, and mandibular) of this nerve. Assessment of the corneal reflexes is helpful. As elsewhere in the examination, the patient serves as his or her own control, and one side is always being compared with the other. There is no obvious difference in trigeminal function between older and younger patients.

VII The *facial nerve* is primarily involved with mobility of the facial muscles. In terms of localization of neurological disease, a distinction between upper and lower motor neuron facial weakness is fundamental, the former being characterized by preservation of the frontalis muscle, and the latter by complete paralysis in the entire distribution of the nerve. It may be useful to assess the sense of taste over the anterior two-thirds of the tongue as well, since this may provide evidence of the exact location of the lesion.

VIII The auditory component of the *auditory nerve* can be checked crudely by asking the patient to repeat whispered words or phrases. An accurate assessment of hearing, however, demands formal audiologic testing that is very often of importance in the elderly, and of particular significance in defining the presence and extent of cognitive decline. The vestibular component is judged by a search for nystagmus, and also by a history of vertigo.

IX, X The *glossopharyngeal* and *vagus nerves* are tested by observing movements of the palate and uvula, the presence of a gag reflex, the adequacy of pharyngeal sensation, and the presence of hoarseness, nasality, or other articulatory disturbance.

XI The *spinal accessory nerve* supplies the sternomastoid muscles and the trapezia. These are easily observed and tested and ordinarily pose no problem in evaluation.

XII The *hypoglossal nerve* is investigated by virtue of inspection and protrusion of the tongue, observing changes such as fasciculations or atrophy as well as weakness. In view of the fact that many elderly eat poorly, often without vitamin supplementation, the tongue should be inspected carefully for evidence of nutritional depletion.

Motor System

The examiner should assess muscle tone, bulk, and power, bearing in mind the fundamental symmetry of the nervous system and the need to compare one side of the body with the other as a form of control. Tendon reflexes (muscle stretch reflexes) should be tested in all limbs. Routinely tested are the biceps, triceps, and brachioradialis in the arms, and the patellar and Achilles reflexes in the legs. There is substantial variation in reflex between individuals at all ages. The presence and character of involuntary movements (e.g., tremors, tics, orofacial dyskinesias, myoclonic jerks) must be noted. Tremors are particularly common in older individuals and should be characterized as precisely as possible, distinguishing, for example, a parkinsonian repose tremor from the postural tremor of so-called essential or, in this population, senile tremor.

The patient's station and gait must be observed, and cerebellar function is then tested in the limbs. Cerebellar function is assessed by determination of the patient's ability to perform coordinated and rapidly alternating movements in all limbs, as well as with the finger-to-nose and heel-to-shin maneuvers.

Sensory System

Sensory testing for routine screening purposes should involve pain perception, touch, vibratory sense (using a 128 cycle [Hertz] tuning fork), position sense, stereognosis, and double simultaneous stimulation. Again, one side of the body should be compared with the other. As cited previously, vibratory sense is progressively reduced in the middle aged and elderly as part of normal aging of the nervous system. For the most part, however, other modalities are well preserved.

As required in individual cases, assessment of the vertebral column and autonomic functions may be undertaken following the initial evaluation. It should be emphasized that the ultimate goal of the examination is to arrive at a preliminary determination as to whether organic disease is present, the location of the lesion, and, if possible, a determination of its nature and pathogenesis, with the aim of establishing a logical program of study and therapeutic intervention.

LABORATORY TESTING

Remarkable strides in diagnostic testing have been made in the clinical neurosciences over the past two decades. It is clearly not possible here to cite every laboratory test that may be found useful in the occasional case of neurological disease. The more commonly employed tests will be reviewed, with stress on their indications, complications, and potential impact in terms of patient management. Selection of the most appropriate laboratory test to be pursued in any given patient will depend upon the clinician's conclusions based on the neurological history and examination as outlined above.

Lumbar Puncture

There is no indication for routine lumbar punctures in patients of any age with neurological disease. Technically, performance of a lumbar puncture may be especially difficult in the elderly because of arthritic/spondylitic changes in the lumbosacral spine. Examination of the cerebrospinal fluid (CSF) is most useful in situations of meningeal or intracranial hemorrhage or infection. Great care must be exercised in the performance of lumbar puncture in the face of increased intracranial pressure (as determined, for example, by funduscopic examination), or in patients with posterior fossa mass lesions. Nonetheless, important information can be gleaned from careful assessment of the CSF and, when indicated, a lumbar puncture can and should be performed. In terms of central nervous system (CNS) infection, it should be pointed out that not only classic bacteriologic techniques should be employed, but also a host of others ranging from cryptococcal antigen to Lyme and West Nile titers, including a search for the 14-3-3 protein in presumed cases of Creutzfeldt-Jakob disease (CJD) (although the specificity of the latter has recently been questioned). In general, there is no indication for performance of a lumbar puncture in the face of neurodegenerative diseases, in instances of toxic or metabolic encephalopathy, or routinely in cases of cerebrovascular disease (CVD). A therapeutic lumbar puncture may be carried out in highly selected cases of normal pressure hydrocephalus (NPH), but this should not be done indiscriminately. In fact, it is very difficult if not impossible to predict in advance which elderly patient will actually benefit from such a procedure. It should be pointed out in this context that the diagnosis of NPH may be especially problematic in the elderly, because ventriculomegaly may have a variety of causes, such as cortical atrophy and loss of central tissue with diffuse vascular lesions.

Electroencephalography (EEG)

The EEG is a well-established diagnostic test and requires no detailed discussion here. Although potentially helpful under many circumstances, the EEG achieves its maximal application in instances of seizures, in metabolic encephalopathies, and in rapidly progressive dementing disorders such as CJD (Figure 7-1). EEG monitoring is particularly important in the context of potential surgical intervention for management of uncontrollable seizures. Monitoring is also extremely useful in distinguishing true seizures from so-called pseudoseizures. Intracranial monitoring may be necessary to identify an epileptogenic focus prior to epilepsy surgery. In the elderly with delirium or impaired consciousness, the EEG often demonstrates diffuse slowing. Slowing is also typically encountered in

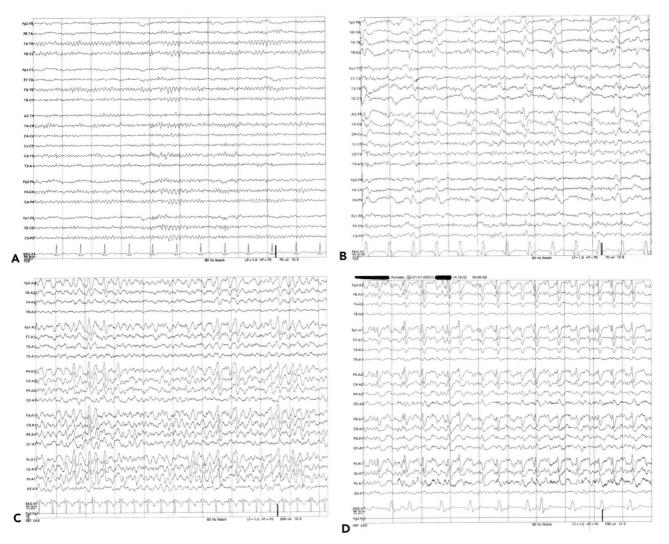

Figure 7-1 Representative EEGs **A.** *Normal EEG* in a slightly drowsy elderly man. **B.** *Periodic lateralized epileptiform discharges* (PLEDs) in a 70-year-old patient with stroke. **C.** *Triphasic waves* in a 60-year-old woman with hepatic encephalopathy. **D** *Triphasic waves* in a 72-year-old man post-anoxia following cardiac arrest.

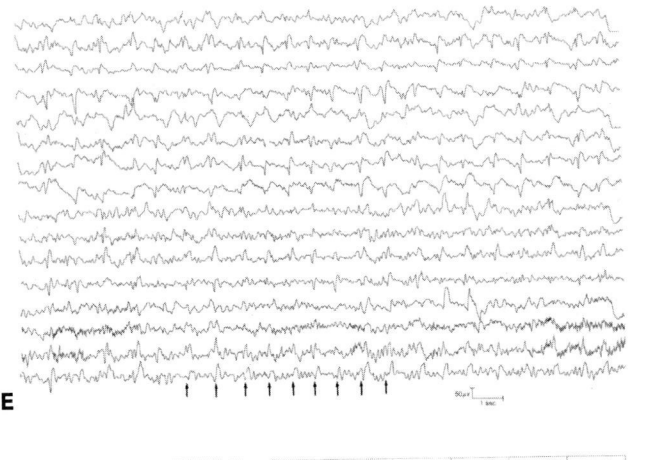

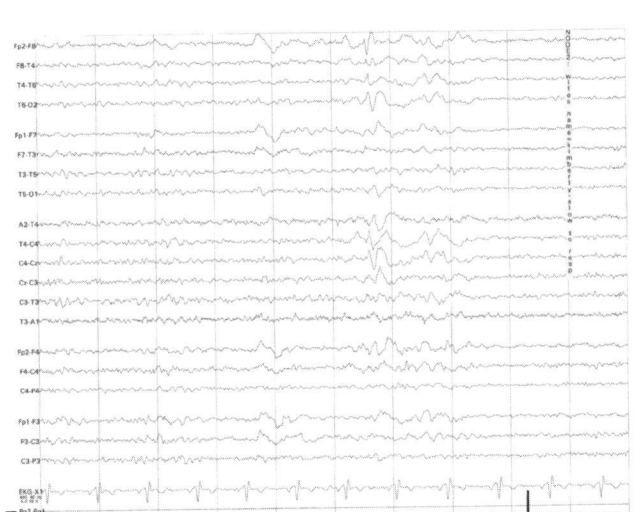

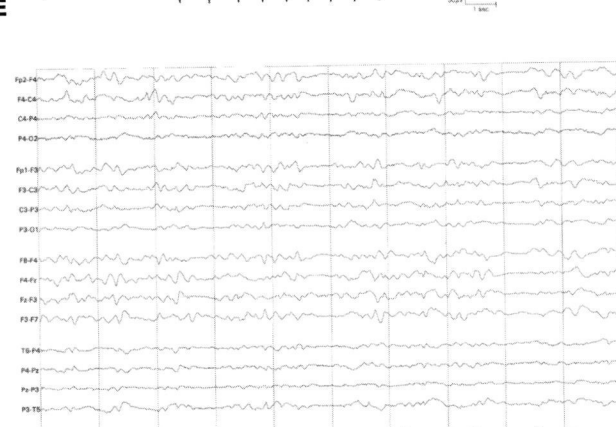

Figure 7-1 *(continued)* **E.** *Periodic complexes* in a 68-year-old man with Creutzfeldt-Jakob disease (CJD). This patient exhibited dementia, cortical blindness, and random myoclonic jerks; This "classical" EEG only appeared late in the course. **F.** *Anterior temporal sharp waves* in a man of 63 with a long history of complex partial seizures with incomplete control. **G.** *Background slowing* in a 55-year-old woman with poly-substance abuse.

patients with a variety of metabolic encephalopathies, many of which are common in the elderly.

Evoked response testing (visual, auditory, and somatosensory) may be very helpful diagnostically, for instance in cases of multiple sclerosis.

Electromyography/Nerve Conduction Testing

Electromyography is useful under many circumstances, but is perhaps most helpful at any age in distinguishing between intrinsic disease of muscle (e.g., myopathy) and denervation due to peripheral neuropathy and anterior horn cell diseases such as amyotrophic lateral sclerosis. The utility of nerve conduction studies is well recognized in a variety of circumstances from youth to old age, ranging from the Guillain-Barré syndrome, to neuropathies characterized by conduction block, to the garden variety carpal tunnel syndrome, and is also helpful in distinguishing between the principle forms of neuropathy (i.e., demyelinating versus axonal). The determination of changes (either decay or increment) in evoked muscle action

potentials in response to repetitive stimulation of a motor nerve is of importance in disorders of the neuromuscular junction, such as myasthenia gravis and the Lambert-Eaton syndrome, which are both of importance in older patients.

Neuroimaging

Computed Tomography (CT)

Computed tomography (CT) is a well-established diagnostic tool that is extremely useful in documenting the presence of intracranial hemorrhage or ventriculomegaly, most dramatically in the setting of an evolving obstructive hydrocephalus, in demonstration of calcification in tumors, in the neuroectodermal dysplasias, and in assessment of the bony structures of the cranial vault and base. Because of artifact generated by the petrous bones, CT is of relatively less value in disease of the posterior fossa. It is of variable benefit in demonstrating ischemic vascular lesions of the brain. CT angiography is useful in evaluating the presence and extent of carotid stenosis or dissection. In geriatric psychiatry, CT is perhaps most widely used to exclude a chronic subdural hematoma that may be responsible for an evolving dementing illness. It is also very useful in distinguishing ventricular enlargement associated with cortical atrophy (as in Alzheimer's disease [AD]) from NPH, the latter characterized by enlarged ventricles but generally with a relatively normal cortical mantle. Some degree of central atrophy is frequently encountered in the apparently normal elderly (age-dependent atrophy).

Magnetic Resonance Imaging

Magnetic resonance imaging (MRI), with or without gadolinium enhancement, is of major importance in assessing a variety of diseases of both the brain and the spine. Its impact may be measured by the fact that the technique has nearly eliminated myelography in the study of patients with spinal disease. Frequently used in diffusion/perfusion and fluid attenuated inversion recovery studies, MRI is extraordinarily helpful in identifying early vascular lesions, with ultimate therapeutic benefits. Diffusion weighted imaging, reflecting reduced water molecule diffusion, is capable of demonstrating an acute cerebral infarction within less than an hour of onset of ischemia, while regional cerebral perfusion differences can be imaged with perfusion studies, which may indicate very early reduced blood flow that progresses to frank infarction in many instances. There may be a region, or zone, of diffusion/perfusion discrepancy as, for example, in the ischemic penumbra, an observation that could have major therapeutic implications in terms of restoration of blood flow.

Magnetic resonance angiography is often helpful in defining degrees of carotid stenosis, complementing *carotid Doppler imaging*, and may be useful in demonstrating at least proximally-placed intracranial aneurysms. *Magnetic resonance venography* is extremely important when considering disorders of the cerebral veins and sinuses. *Magnetic resonance spectroscopy* is at times useful in identifying intercranial tumors and distinguishing such mass lesions from demyelinating processes or infarction. *Functional MRI* is an extraordinarily informative research tool, but at the moment has little clinical application. Its potential future application in geriatrics remains unclear.

Other forms of imaging include *single photon emission computed tomography*, which is useful in patients considered to be likely candidates for AD by demonstrating reduced perfusion in the parietal lobes, but relatively less helpful under other circumstances. *Positron emission tomography* is increasingly available but has been predominantly a research tool in clinical neurology, although with increasing clinical applications recently, (e.g., in terms of differential diagnosis of dementia). *Sonography* (i.e., carotid ultrasound or Doppler) is useful in the setting of presumed carotid disease with stenosis and transient ischemic attacks. At times, in cases of carotid or vertebral artery dissection, transcranial Doppler is applicable, especially in a setting of subarachnoid hemorrhage with vasospasm and resultant cerebral ischemia. A comprehensive review of Neuroimaging can be found in Chapter 8 of this textbook.

Genetic Testing

Genetic testing represents the most rapidly growing segment of clinical neuroscience assessment, with extraordinary advances over the past two decades identifying an increasing number of genetic defects found to underlie a host of neurological and neuromuscular disorders at all ages. Genetic testing may be of paramount importance in establishing a correct diagnosis in, for example, HD, with the characteristic trinucleotide repeat, but has found increasing application in a number of other disorders involving both central and peripheral nervous systems. Unfortunately, at this time identification of specific gene abnormalities such as Parkinson's disease (obviously of importance in older patients) or dystrophin in muscular dystrophy has not yet led to significant therapeutic interventions. Similarly, identification of frontotemporal dementia (e.g., Pick's disease), as among the so-called tauopathies, has not yet proven to be therapeutically of importance. The widely recognized genetic alteration in AD related to apolipoprotein E, a specific risk factor on chromosome 19, has unfortunately no meaningful diagnostic or therapeutic application at this time, and APO4E genotyping cannot be recommended as a routine test.

PSYCHIATRIC MANIFESTATIONS OF NEUROLOGICAL DISEASE

Many neurological disorders exhibit a variety of psychiatric/psychological abnormalities among their clinical manifestations. When the neurological disease is advanced, there is generally no difficulty separating the organic from the psychological components. However, when a neurological disorder is in its early stages of evolution, it may be far more difficult to distinguish the two. In fact, it is in these early stages that significant and at times serious diagnostic errors are made by virtue of failure to recognize, or to realize the underlying potential for, organicity in the patient. Further complicating the issue is the comorbidity of both organic and psychological factors in the same patient, and as a given disease advances, it may become impossible, even with contemporary diagnostic testing, to clearly separate the two. It must be emphasized that rational, therapeutic interventions must be directed towards both organic and psychiatric factors when identified. Patients in the early stages of disease are a major concern to the geriatric psychiatrist and/or geriatrician; therefore, early psychiatric manifestations in these individuals should receive the most attention, stressing the potential implications of these symptoms in the context of the ultimate neurological diagnosis. For additional information on the variety of diseases that follow, see the appropriate chapters in this textbook.

The Dementias

No practicing physician has difficulty recognizing the existence of an advanced dementing illness (sometimes referred to, at least historically, as an organic or chronic mental syndrome). However, although a large majority of all dementing illnesses are necessarily associated with significant psychiatric comorbidity, early cases of dementia not uncommonly vex the clinician. In these cases, failure to appreciate the potential for an evolving organic disease not uncommonly leads to diagnostic errors, and thus significant therapeutic misadventures, for example treating a patient with early AD as an instance of schizophrenia.

Alzheimer's Disease

The classical clinical phenotype of AD needs no emphasis here. The combination of insidiously progressive cognitive deterioration with judgmental and memory failure is so well recognized that it requires no further comment, and the psychological and behavioral components of the disorder, seen as the disease advances, are widely appreciated. AD sometimes manifests itself initially with psychiatric symptoms, and it is these that commonly prompt a family to bring the patient to medical attention, before recognition of significant memory or other clinical manifestations. Thus, in advance of clinically obvious dementing features, early AD patients may exhibit one or more of a variety of psychological/behavioral abnormalities, including depression and other alterations of mood such as anxiety, irritability, apathy, and delusions; and/or behavioral changes such as aggression, apathy, impulsivity, social disinhibition, hypomania, compulsions, and alterations in sexual behavior (5,6). Judgmental errors, for example in a business setting, are common and may be the first abnormality to arouse concern among family members.

As AD evolves, many of these symptoms worsen progressively, while cognitive changes become increasingly apparent. The practicing psychiatrist needs no reminder as to the development of such florid psychological, or perhaps more accurately, neuropsychological alterations as AD inexorably progresses. The patient often becomes increasingly reclusive, withdrawn, and neglectful of personal hygiene, and may wander or direct unwarranted aggression toward caregivers. The niceties of table manners break down, and choking on food or drink may result. Anorexia may lead to significant weight loss. Paranoid or other delusions may be prominent, with the patient accusing family members of theft and/or the spouse of marital infidelity. These delusional expressions often suggest a primary psychiatric disorder (5,6). As the disease evolves, a language disorder commonly appears, most typically anomia, at least in the earlier stages of the disease, with more severe forms of aphasia appearing with the passage of time. Focal neurological findings are otherwise very unusual.

CASE EXAMPLE

A 78-year-old man is brought for further assessment of failing memory. He had initially been seen 1 year before, at which time he exhibited only mild difficulty with memory, achieving an MMSE score of 26. He was considered mildly

---

depressed and somewhat withdrawn from his usual social contacts. A CT of his head at that time was interpreted as normal. Since then he is said to have become confused sometimes and to occasionally become lost in familiar surroundings. He has been verbally abusive to his wife, accusing her of stealing his money and of sexual indiscretions with several neighbors. Now he often loses his train of thought in conversation, has occasional problems with word finding, and tends to repeatedly ask the same questions. There is no history of trauma or of antecedent neurological disease. There is no family history of a similar disorder.

Examination demonstrates a moderately severely demented man (MMSE score 18), who has a short attention span and thus limited cooperation with the examiner. There is a definite anomia, but language function appears otherwise normal. He exhibits visual and tactile sucking, bilateral positive palmomental responses, and bilateral forced grasping. Strength is excellent, and there is no reflex asymmetry. Plantar responses are flexor. There are no myoclonic jerks.

Comment: This patient demonstrates the typical clinical progression of AD. There are no features that suggest meaningful CVD (the possibility of vascular or multi-infarct dementia) and no parkinsonian features, which could support a diagnosis of diffuse Lewy body disease. CT now shows moderate ventriculomegaly with appropriate cerebral convolutional atrophy.

Diffuse Lewy Body Disease (DLBD)

Considered by some to be the most common dementing illness after AD itself, DLBD may similarly present with psychiatric symptoms in advance of, or along with, a progressive dementia, with an admixture of parkinsonian signs. Visual hallucinations are prominent early in the course in over half the cases, and may be the presenting complaint, with more obvious signs of parkinsonism and cognitive failure appearing later. Cummings has emphasized the importance of formed visual hallucinations and delusions and of rapid eye movement sleep behavior disorder in establishing the correct diagnosis in these individuals (5,6). Ferman et al. have described clinical fluctuations involving, for example, daytime drowsiness, staring, and disorganized speech, symptoms which appear specific to DLBD and serve to separate this disorder from AD (7).

It should be noted that features of dementia also appear in many cases of seemingly otherwise uncomplicated idiopathic Parkinson's disease (PD), with estimates of cognitive dysfunction in individuals ranging as high as 40% or more. Unfortunately, there are no consistent or widely accepted clinical features that permit an accurate prediction of the likelihood of developing dementia in these patients, although increasing age, gender (male), and postural and gait disorders are important in this respect. Depression to some degree is common in the great majority of PD patients as well. Neuropsychological alterations may also reflect therapeutic interventions in the PD patient. Patients treated with dopaminergic drugs may develop hallucinations, illusions and delusions, changes in mood, and altered sexual behavior, while anticholinergic medication may induce an acute confusional state or frank psychosis, especially in the elderly. It may be impossible in any given patient to separate the adverse affects of medication from the naturally occurring manifestations of the basic disease process itself. A broad variety of other neuropsychiatric disorders such as sleep disorders may also be encountered in PD (5,6).

CASE EXAMPLE

A 63-year-old man has complaints of depression and memory impairment, with prominent visual and occasional auditory hallucinations. He becomes increasingly demented over time. Examination demonstrates cogwheeling rigidity in the limbs, masking of the facies, and a variable tremor of the hands. Treatment with antiparkinsonian agents provides little meaningful relief. Autopsy demonstrates widespread Lewy bodies throughout the gray matter of the cerebral cortex and the brainstem, establishing a diagnosis of diffuse Lewy body disease.

Comment: This case illustrates the difficulty clinically in distinguishing AD from DLBD and from parkinsonism with dementia. In this instance, definitive diagnosis was achieved only with postmortem examination.

Multi-Infarct (Vascular) Dementia

The appearance of dementia in association with CVD (primarily infarctions involving either the cerebral white matter or deep gray structures), often called vascular dementia (VaD) or multi-infarct dementia (MID), is well recognized and indeed is considered among the most common causes of dementia, particularly in older patients. Since many patients with AD may also develop symptoms of CVD in the later decades of life, it may be extremely difficult in any individual case to separate Alzheimer's degenerative dementia from VaD diagnostically, and both may be of clinical importance in the same patient. These patients are often referred to as comprising a *mixed dementia* population. A history of stroke-like episodes, recognition of significant risk factors for CVD such as hypertension or diabetes, a stuttering clinical course, and the presence of focal neurological signs such as aphasia, hemiparesis, or visual field loss favor a diagnosis of VaD. Note that focal neurological signs are generally lacking in the typical patient with AD. The appearance of executive dysfunction, or of an abulic state, may at times lead to diagnostic confusion. Aharon-Peretz et al. have emphasized the behavioral differences between MID and AD in some patients, with memory impairment being less prominent in the former, while agitation and depression appear more commonly in the latter (8). Nonetheless, the clinician must be alert to the appearance of significant depression in either setting (8).

Binswanger's Disease

Binswanger's disease is best looked upon as a form of MID characterized by multiple and diffuse subcortical ischemic lesions, often associated with pyramidal tract signs, disordered gait, and loss of sphincter control. There are no clinical features unique to this form of vascular encephalopathy.

Fronto Temporal Degeneration

Patients with fronto temporal degeneration (FTD) (of which Pick's disease may be considered a subset) often exhibit prominent neuropsychiatric abnormalities, especially executive dysfunction, impulsivity, behavioral disinhibition with grossly inappropriate behavior, distractibility, and apathy. Cummings (5,6) has called attention to significant neuropsychiatric differences between FTD and AD, which have been elaborated on by Snowden et al. (9) and Hirono et al. (10).

Miscellaneous Dementing Diseases

Creutzfeldt-Jakob Disease (CJD)

CJD is a rapidly evolving dementing illness, generally accompanied by myoclonic jerks, seizures, and a variety of organic neurological signs. Visual abnormalities may appear very early in the *Heidenhain variety*. Patients suffering from this prion disorder exhibit a host of nonspecific neuropsychological abnormalities as the disease evolves over its usual course, as measured in weeks to months.

CASE EXAMPLE

A 74-year-old physician, previously well, develops a primary dementing illness associated with a short attention span, cortical blindness, bilateral pyramidal tract signs, and random myoclonic jerks involving the trunk and limbs. Over a period of several months he becomes increasingly lethargic, eventually lapsing into coma. Early EEG studies demonstrate diffuse slow and sharp waves, but eventually demonstrate a burst suppression pattern considered typical of, but not confined to, CJD. Spinal fluid contains an elevated 14-3-3 protein, and a brain biopsy ultimately demonstrates a spongiform encephalopathy with widespread neuronal loss and a brisk astrocytic proliferation. Therapy with antiviral agents and corticosteroids provides no benefit.

Comment: CJD is characterized by subacutely evolving dementia associated with a variety of neurological signs and myoclonic jerks, and the patient eventually lapses into coma. This man's EEG ultimately demonstrated the typical burst-suppression pattern of CJD, and his spinal fluid contained the elevated 14-3-3 protein considered typical, but not pathognomonic, of CJD. Brain biopsy definitively established the correct diagnosis.

Huntington's Disease

HD is a dementing illness characterized by a combination of involuntary movements, in particular chorea or choreoathetosis, with a progressive dementia. Although often looked upon as a disease of mid-life or of the young, cases occasionally appear in the sixth to seventh decade of life. As is true of most so-called subcortical dementias, here affecting the sub-thalamic nucleus, HD is associated with depression that may be severe and long standing, antedating the more widely recognized features of the disease for many years. There is a remarkably high rate of suicide among HD patients, presumably reflecting the prevalence of depression. By reviewing the available literature, Hayden has estimated that suicide is between seven and 200 times more common in HD than in the normal population (11). There is also a heightened rate of suicide in at-risk offspring. Behavioral abnormalities such as child abuse and alcoholism are often encountered, and serious structural disruption is noted among family members, perhaps especially among at-risk offspring. When the diagnosis of HD is unclear, demonstration of the characteristic elevation of trinucleotide (CAG) repeats on chromosome 4 in genetic DNA testing is critical. DNA analysis has been suggested as a predictive test among those at risk, but this carries serious ethical and psychological weight, and psychological counseling is best undertaken before such testing is performed.

CASE EXAMPLE

A 48-year-old man has a long history of depression and alcohol abuse. His judgment in his business has become increasingly erratic, and he has difficulty maintaining focus on tasks both at home and at work, which his family attributes to his depression. His movements have become clumsy, and he tends to lurch or stagger while walking. His mother is said to have had schizophrenia, with symptoms developing in mid-life, and a maternal uncle is said to have died of parkinsonism.

On examination, the patient demonstrates facial grimacing, an inability to maintain the tongue in a protruded posture, and ineffective saccades. At times twitching movements of the fingers are observed. The gait is lilting in quality, but he does not fall. His memory is poor. He has a short attention span, which initially precluded detailed cognitive testing.

Comment: This is a typical instance of HD developing in mid-life, with features of depression, motor impersistence, and a movement disorder, and with a family history that in retrospect is clearly supportive of the clinical diagnosis. Neuropsychological testing subsequently confirmed the presence of a mild dementia, and DNA analysis demonstrated an increased number of trinucleotide repeats, unequivocally substantiating the clinical diagnosis.

Traumatic Brain Injury

Traumatic brain injury is unfortunately common in the elderly by virtue of the tendency for many seniors to fall, for a variety of reasons. Head injury under such circumstances may result in concussion, itself a self-limited disorder, but often followed by a distressing complex of complaints including headache, difficulty concentrating, memory impairment, insomnia, apathy, sexual dysfunction, and dizziness. In general, these features of *postconcussive syndrome* are benign, tending to disappear over a period of weeks to months, but occasionally they persist indefinitely. Dementia and a variety of behavioral changes may also appear under these circumstances, suggesting diffuse axonal injury in a pathogenetic sense, although it should be emphasized that this tends to follow more serious head injuries.

Of particular importance in the elderly, following trauma, is the development of a chronic subdural hematoma, which usually appears insidiously days to weeks after an injury. There are unfortunately no specific clinical manifestations of subdural hematoma; many patients experience intermittent headache, confusion, a mild and at times evolving dementia, and a mild, often fluctuating, hemiparesis. An accurate diagnosis of subdural hematoma requires appropriate imaging. Surgical evacuation of the clot may result in remarkable clinical improvement in such patients. Significant craniocerebral trauma may also be followed by NPH, a disorder that appears under other circumstances as well, such as prior subarachnoid hemorrhage or meningitis. Patients with NPH often present with dementia, along with gait ataxia (or perhaps more accurately apraxia), pyramidal tract signs in the lower extremities, and bladder difficulties. Diagnosis is often not straightforward in these individuals, and selection of patients appropriate for ventricular shunting is difficult. Some patients improve dramatically after ventricular shunting, but unfortunately this is not always the case.

Miscellaneous Causes of Dementia

Features of dementia also appear under circumstances of metabolic abnormality, most noteworthy in the context of hypoxic encephalopathy following cardiac arrest, anesthetic, or surgical misadventure during the course of coronary artery bypass surgery. Dementia may also develop from severe and chronic hypoglycemia, but this is much less common. Other metabolic abnormalities responsible for the appearance of dementia include chronic lead intoxication, chronic B12 deficiency and, although a matter of some disagreement, chronic alcoholism. Nutritional depletion, particularly related to thiamine, may appear in the chronic alcoholic as well as in other circumstances of chronic malnutrition, and is responsible for the development of such disorders as *Wernicke-Korsakoff syndrome* and *Marchiafava-Bignami disease*. Dementia is also a component of paraneoplastic limbic encephalitis.

A variety of infectious disorders may be responsible for the development of a dementing process at virtually any age. HIV dementia is a well-recognized and common complication of AIDS, although this is relatively less important statistically in elderly individuals. Lyme disease and West Nile are both capable of producing a dementing illness, although dementia as the presenting clinical manifestation of these disorders would be most unusual. In contrast, features of dementia are not uncommon acutely with, or following recovery from, herpes simplex encephalitis. Tertiary syphilis, in the form of *general paresis of the insane*, presents with features of dementia often associated with a striking delusional or confusional state. This is a relatively minor hazard in the elderly today, but certainly one that can be treated effectively if a diagnosis can be established.

The appearance of features of a dementia, with or without other neuropsychiatric abnormalities such as depression or abulia, may be found under many other circumstances including, for example, neoplasm (perhaps especially butterfly gliomas of the corpus callosum), and occasionally with demyelinating illness such as multiple sclerosis (although the latter would be most unusual in the older patient population).

Memory Disorders

It is self evident that memory impairment appears as a clinical characteristic of dementing illnesses in general, usually in the context of diffuse disease of either gray or white matter, as *reviewed above*. Under such circumstances the memory difficulty, commonly described as a loss of recent memory but in fact a reflection of an inability to form or store new memories, is usually accompanied by other neuropsychiatric manifestations such as depression, agitation, or apathy, as already described. As these diseases progress, memory loss becomes more profound, and extends ultimately to memories of the more remote past as well. Confabulation may appear, perhaps as a corrective device (i.e., a conscious filling in of memories in those patients aware, to at least some extent, of the memory impairment).

In addition to such instances of memory loss with global dementia, more specific *amnestic dementias* have been recognized, defined as disorders characterized by significant memory impairment but with relative preservation of other cognitive functions. The best known of these disorders is *Korsakoff's psychosis*, the chronic manifestation of the Wernicke-Korsakoff syndrome, in which the memory deficit is commonly accompanied by apathy and disinterest on the part of the patient. Confabulation may appear but is not a diagnostic *sine qua non*. Residual features of a prior bout of acute Wernicke's encephalopathy, in particular nystagmus or mild gait ataxia, may be noted, and recognition of these signs is of major diagnostic assistance. In terms of memory difficulty, the pertinent lesions in the Wernicke-Korsakoff syndrome appear to be symmetrical lesions, often quite small, comprising subtotal tissue necrosis in the mammillary bodies and/or thalamus. Victor et al. have pointed out that the disease may appear at any age, with the highest incidence in the fifth and sixth decade. In 25% of cases, however, symptoms first develop at age 60 or later (12).

In addition to the classical Wernicke-Korsakoff syndrome, a number of other disorders are also characterized by a more or less isolated amnestic dementia. These include herpes simplex encephalitis, bilateral posterior cerebral artery occlusions with medial temporal/occipital infarctions (particularly important in the elderly with CVD), extensive and perhaps overenthusiastic bilateral temporal lobectomy, tumors of the floor of the hypothalamus or of the third ventricle, surgical resection of the fornix, and traumatic destruction of medial temporal structures. The common thread among all of these disorders is bilateral affection of the primitive hippocampal/limbic circuitry buried deep in the medial aspect of the cerebral hemispheres and comprising the hippocampus, fornix, mammillary bodies, and thalamus. The early appearance of memory defects in AD may be explained by the relatively early development of lesions in the hippocampus, and the amnesia characteristic of complex partial seizures presumably reflects transient suppression of activity in the same structures, especially in the medial temporal lobe.

The syndrome of transient global amnesia (TGA) is characterized by the abrupt onset of mental confusion and bewilderment associated with an inability to process memory traces, and appears particularly prevalent in older individuals. The duration of TGA is ordinarily measured in hours, with a gradual return to normal memory performance, and the patient generally preserves few if any memories of the acute confusional episode. Although the pathogenesis of TGA is not entirely clear, it is generally held that the disorder reflects either transient vascular insufficiency or unrecognized epileptic activity involving medial temporal structures. Patients with *Klein-Levin syndrome*, a curious disorder most commonly involving young males and characterized by episodic hypersomnolence interspersed with bouts of excessive eating with irritability and aggressive behavior when awake, exhibit few if any memories of these episodes. Dysfunction of the temporal lobe or the hypothalamus is implicated in causation of this disorder as well.

Delirium

Delirium, readily recognized by the practicing psychiatrist, is characterized by an acutely developing confusional syndrome associated with hallucinations, delusions, illusions, insomnia, agitation, and autonomic abnormalities. Most commonly encountered in the elderly, the disorder appears on a background of fever, dehydration, azotemia, hypothyroidism (myxedema madness), hypoxia, or hepatic failure, *inter alia*. Withdrawal from alcohol or drugs may precipitate an episode. Myoclonic jerks, asterixis, tremulousness, seizures, and hyperactive reflexes are frequent, but focal neurological signs are unusual. Sloane has described in detail the many neuropsychological manifestations of delirium, including, for example, short attention span, incoherent thought processes, variable mood, memory impairment, poor judgment and absence of insight, and disordered sleep, as well as delusions, illusions, and hallucinations (13). Demented patients may present with a concomitant delirium, which itself intensifies pre-existing behavioral problems in these individuals. The appearance of delirium as a manifestation most commonly of a metabolic encephalopathy makes it mandatory to exclude a variety of underlying toxic and metabolic abnormalities, so as to permit appropriate therapeutic interventions on an individual basis.

Hallucinations and Perceptual Distortions

As described at length previously in this chapter, a number of diffuse disorders of cerebral dysfunction, whether structural (e.g., DLBD) or metabolic (e.g., drug induced), are associated with the appearance of perceptual distortions (illusions and hallucinations). Of additional interest, however, is the appearance of such neuropsychological manifestations as a reflection of more focal neurological disease. In *complex partial seizures* (temporal lobe epilepsy, TLE), hallucinations and illusions are often prominent but only rarely comprise the only clinical manifestations of the underlying seizure disorder. Both auditory and visual hallucinations are well recognized under these circumstances. It has been suggested that crude visual hallucinations such as flashes of light or simple geometric figures reflect posteriorly placed epileptogenic activity in the occipital (calcarine) cortex, and more formed visual hallucinations appear with foci within the medial temporal lobe itself. Auditory hallucinations may similarly vary from crude and unformed experiences (noises, tinnitus) to more readily recognizable phenomena, such as voices. Some patients experience mixed auditory and visual hallucinations.

Hallucinations of smell and/or taste (olfactory and gustatory hallucinations) may also appear in patients with complex partial seizures, particularly in those with antero-medial epileptogenic foci, as in the classic uncinate fits described by first Hughlings Jackson. Illusions (perceptional distortions) are also widely appreciated in the patient with TLE. These illusions comprise the *Alice in Wonderland* or *Lilliputian syndrome*, with either macropsia or micropsia as part of the focal seizure activity. Other episodic neuropsychological abnormalities in these patients include a sense of depersonalization and forced thinking. The occurrence of *déjà vu* and, much less commonly, of its reverse, *jamais vu*, is well recognized in these individuals and is often independent of frank seizure activity. It will be recalled, however, that déjà vu is normally encountered in individuals in their teens or early 20s. It should be emphasized that patients are often reluctant to volunteer such symptoms to the physician for fear of being considered psychotic, and a determined search should be made for these clinical manifestations in all patients in whom a diagnosis of complex partial seizures is considered.

As noted above, lesions in the calcarine cortex, including tumors, may present with predominantly crude visual hallucinatory experiences. Patients with classical migraine also experience visual hallucinations (generally poorly formed and comprising colored balls or other geometric figures, bright flashes of light, or fortification spectra) as part of the aura and preceding the onset of headache by 5 to 20 minutes. Visual distortions, often limited to one hemianopic visual field, and often described as looking through rippled glass or running water, may be described by the migraineur, sometimes associated with transient impairment of visual acuity. Experiences of this sort may occur without a frank headache (migraine sine migraine, retinal or ophthalmic migraine), leading at times to diagnostic confusion. It should be emphasized that in migraine, visual symptoms may be either cortical or retinal in origin. Although it is often thought that migraine is a disease of the young, in fact typical migraine may have its onset in the later decades of life; this is perhaps especially true of ophthalmic migraine.

Hallucinations, generally visual, may also appear in patients with brainstem and posterior thalamic lesions, as in *Lhermitte's peduncular hallucinosis*. Hallucinations are relatively common in patients with narcolepsy, in addition to the more characteristic episodes of uncontrollable sleep, cataplexy, and sleep paralysis. In the narcoleptic, visual or auditory hallucinations tend to occur most commonly as the patient is falling asleep (*hypnagogic hallucinations*), but may also occur as a patient awakens in the morning (*hypnopompic hallucinations*). Hypnagogic hallucinations are not rare among normal individuals; patients may describe, for example, hearing someone call their name as they are falling off to sleep.

Finally, as is well known to the clinical psychiatrist, hallucinations, primarily visual, also occur in association with the use or abuse of a variety of prescribed medications as well as illicit drugs, and are common in individuals withdrawing from drugs such as alcohol or barbiturates, *inter alia*. Unfortunately, the development of hallucinations, for example as a result of the use of antiparkinsonian agents in older patients, often seriously interferes with therapeutic interventions.

Mood Disorders

The occurrence of depression with diseases involving either gray or white matter has been repeatedly noted clinically. Although generally lacking focal significance *per se*, it should be noted that depression often appears in instances of CVD with left hemispheral infarction in the immediate poststroke period. During recovery depression may appear with infarctions in either hemisphere, and later appears more commonly among those with right hemispheral lesions. It is tempting to attribute the depression in those with left hemispheral lesions to awareness of the aphasia which so commonly appears under those circumstances, with resultant loss of the ability to communicate effectively.

In many circumstances of depression associated with neurological disease, it must be admitted that the appearance of mood change may simply represent a reactive depression rather than being an intrinsic part of the disease. Thus, for example, young patients with multiple sclerosis are often depressed, almost certainly as a response to the disability engendered by such a disease. Depression, with or without associated anxiety, is common in patients after serious head injury, perhaps especially among those with prefrontal or orbital frontal lesions.

As noted earlier, severe depression may appear in older individuals with a host of organic neurological diseases, for example in PD or AD.

Patients with seizure disorders of all sorts are often depressed or angry, and at times exhibit overtly paranoid delusions. Such responses perhaps reflect an individual patient's resentment of the many societal restrictions, if not overt discrimination, to which he or she is exposed. Mood changes are particularly prominent in the patient with TLE. Many of these patients are irascible, obsessive, overly sharply focused on immediate goals, and often simply difficult to get on with.

Euphoria (mania, hypomania) appears in many neurological disorders, and certainly in individuals with recognized pre-existing bipolar disease. Lesions in the right cerebral hemisphere appear to be more frequently associated with manic manifestations than those in the left. Frontal and temporal regions, thalamus, and basal ganglia are most commonly implicated in causation of this mood disorder. So-called secondary mania appears with a wide variety of other neurological diseases, including CVD, HD, treated PD, and tumors and trauma, among others (2,3). It was once commonly stated that euphoria/hypomania is characteristic of multiple sclerosis, but this is in fact not the case. Depression is far more common among such patients. Mood disorders may also appear in the Klein Levin syndrome.

Patients with the rarely encountered complete *Klüver-Bucy syndrome*, as a consequence of bilateral temporal lobe disease or ablation, are typically apathetic and indifferent, with reduced emotional responses along with other, more readily recognized behavioral changes such as altered sexual activity, oral tendencies, and memory disorder.

Individuals with bilateral cerebral disease, generally associated with bilateral signs of corticospinal dysfunction, may exhibit what is commonly referred to as pathological laughter and/or pathological crying, or *emotional incontinence* (i.e., emotional expression not clearly related to external stimuli) as part of the syndrome of *pseudobulbar palsy*. This may reflect a variety of organic disorders including CVD, but may appear in the setting of trauma, motor neuron disease, and tumors involving the brain stem. Such emotional outbursts may be very puzzling to caretakers looking after demented patients, especially in long-term care facilities. The affective manifestations of pseudobulbar palsy should not be confused with the appearance of uncontrollable laughter as an automatism in complex partial seizures, so-called *gelastic seizures*. Such laughter may appear briefly before more obvious manifestations of the seizure disorder. It is said that gelastic seizures appear especially with right hemispheral disease involving the anterior cingulate and/or anteromedial temporal regions.

As is widely appreciated, patients with TLE may describe striking emotional experiences as part of the seizure. A sense of fear or dread is common, whereas a sense of well being, frank exhilaration, or exaltation is less common. The appearance of laughter preceding or accompanying TLE in gelastic epilepsy is generally without emotional content, and is at times accompanied by undirected running (cursive epilepsy).

Behavioral Disorders

The occurrence of apathy and/or unusually placid behavior in neurological disease has been previously noted. The appearance of abulia in association with tumors, primarily butterfly gliomas involving the anterior cingulate gyri or the genu of the corpus callosum, or in association with CVD with bilateral infarctions in the territory of the anterior cerebral arteries, is especially noteworthy, particularly in older patients. The development of aggressive behavior in a variety of settings, and appearing at all ages, has also been commented upon. The appearance of random episodic violence, either during the course of a seizure or in the immediate postictal phase, is well-recognized. The issue as to whether more structured, antisocial, violent, aggressive, or frankly criminal behavior can be attributed to interictal abnormalities in seizure patients remains vexing, but appears unlikely. The existence of so-called dyscontrol syndrome in epileptic patients with disease of the temporal lobes remains a matter of dispute. This is said to be characterized by anger or fury developing in response to minor provocation. It is likely that underlying psychiatric disease explains such aggressive behavior in many individuals. Especially in those with head injury, dysfunction of the frontal lobes appears related to violent behavior. Whether affection of the orbital frontal components of the limbic apparatus plays a significant role in this respect remains undetermined. Rage reactions have been described in patients with frontal lobe disease and in association with disorders of the hypothalamus, most commonly tumor. It is clear that episodic aggressive manifestations may reflect either organic or psychiatric disease, or a combination of both. The patient so afflicted must be carefully studied to exclude epilepsy or other intermittent disorders of the nervous system. It must be emphasized that the elderly are not immune to such dramatic behavioral changes under a wide variety of circumstances.

Sexual dysfunction is a common consequence of neurological disease involving the cerebral hemispheres, the spinal cord, and the peripheral nerves. Infarction of the cerebral hemispheres, perhaps particularly but not exclusively involving the temporal lobes, may be responsible for reduced libido or impotence. Contrary to popular and widely accepted belief, impotence may be of major concern in elderly patients, and cannot be ignored in management. Hypersexuality may appear, as seen most dramatically in the human Klüver-Bucy syndrome, but also following temporal lobectomy for seizure control, as postictal behavior in patients with temporal lobe epilepsy, or in demented individuals, some of whom may respond to the use of an estrogen patch. Exhibitionism has been described in those with temporal lobe seizures, and orgasm may appear as part of the aura or as a late ictal phenomenon. Hypothalamic lesions are well-recognized as a cause of impotence, with reduced libido in the male and amenorrhea in the female.

Numerous spinal diseases, ranging from spinal cord trauma to multiple sclerosis and cervical myelopathy, are responsible for sexual dysfunction, in particular impotence and difficulty achieving or maintaining an erection. Among diseases of the peripheral nervous system, autonomic neuropathy as a result of diabetes mellitus is most commonly recognized as a cause for impotence.

Disorders of the Body Scheme

Awareness of the relationship of one part of the body to the other, and of the body to extracorporeal space, comprises the body image, or body scheme, which is an unconscious construct (gestalt) of these relationships based on visual, tactile, and proprioceptive inputs during infancy. Clinical experience indicates that the body scheme is localized in a functional sense primarily in the nondominant (i.e., right) parietal lobe, although there is at least some clinical evidence suggesting bilateral representation. In any case, under certain circumstances acute disorders such as infarction of the parietal lobe can be responsible for clinical manifestations which represent a breakdown of the body scheme. In view of the relationship to vascular lesions, these extraordinary abnormalities are much more frequent in the elderly than in younger individuals. Symptoms of body scheme disorders are usually associated with impairment of proprioception on the left (i.e., contralateral) side of the body, along with varying degrees of mental confusion. Several levels of affection can be identified in terms of severity. The most common, and in a sense most benign, is the syndrome of *left-sided neglect* (inattention, extinction). Patients so afflicted tend to ignore the left side of their body, for example when dressing or shaving, and exhibit sensory inattention with double simultaneous stimulation. The patient may perceive pain or tactile stimuli normally on either side independently, but when both sides of the body are stimulated simultaneously, he or she perceives only the right-sided stimulus, ignoring or neglecting that on the left. A similar deficit appears to involve spatial relationships. Thus, the patient may be capable of perceiving visual stimuli applied in either the right or left visual field, but when both are presented simultaneously he or she will not recognize the stimulus in the left field (attention hemianopsia). When asked to draw something, for example a clock face or a flower, or to copy a design or drawing, the patient typically ignores the left side of space. Similar dysfunction may be found in the auditory sphere. Although such deficits almost always involve the left side of the body or of space, as a consequence of a right hemispheral lesion, on occasion sensory inattention may be found on the right side in a patient with a left hemispheral infarction. It has been suggested that the explanation for the seeming right hemispheral predominance in this respect reflects the development of aphasia in patients with infarction involving the left hemisphere, the language disorder precluding the detailed testing necessary to bring out such deficits.

Somewhat more dramatically, a patient with a left hemiparesis or hemiplegia with a right hemispheral lesion may deny the existence of his or her hemiplegia, a condition called *anosognosia*. While sensory inattention may persist, at least in mild form, for months or years after a stroke, anosognosia in general disappears after several days to weeks. On those few occasions when anosognosia persists, rehabilitation becomes a virtual impossibility since the patient simply is not aware of, or denies the existence of, the incapacitating neurological deficit.

A particularly disturbing form of anosognosia is *Anton's syndrome*, defined as cortical blindness without awareness of such blindness. Usually a consequence of bilateral parieto-occipital lesions, often vascular, this is not infrequently misinterpreted as an hysteric manifestation or as evidence of malingering, at least until appropriate studies demonstrate the organic basis for this remarkable syndrome. Patients are not only unaware of their cortical blindness, but actively deny it, confabulating readily when asked to describe objects around them in the visual sphere.

Still more dramatic is the syndrome of amorphosynthesis, or *hemisomatotopagnosia*, defined as denial of existence of the left side of the body. Immediately following a stroke with left hemiplegia, usually with marked confusion, patients may deny the existence of their own left arm or leg. This deficit is often fleeting, and may disappear within a day or two of onset, but not infrequently leads to considerable perplexity on the part of those attending the patient, who may misinterpret this symptom as hysterical or as evidence of psychosis. Again, since this dramatic symptom appears most commonly with an acute ischemic lesion, it tends to be noted especially in the older individual with cerebrovascular insufficiency.

Movement Disorders

Movement disorders are generally readily recognized as organic in origin, although some may be misinterpreted as psychogenic, for example the tics of Tourette's syndrome, or focal dystonic manifestations such as writers cramp, torticollis, lingual dystonia, and orofacial or hemi-facial spasm (the latter sometimes occurring together in the Meige syndrome). Patients with Tourette's syndrome, particularly young individuals, frequently exhibit an obsessive-compulsive disorder as well. The disorder is variously considered to reflect disease of the orbital frontal cortex, the globus pallidus, or the thalamus. Stereotypic movements appear in psychotic patients and in those who are intellectually disabled or autistic, while repetitive behaviors with self-mutilation are found in some demented individuals and in the Lesch-Nyhan and Rett syndromes, among others.

Neuropsychiatric abnormalities are typically encountered in the classic choreic illnesses, i.e., Sydenham's chorea, and HD. As noted previously, depression is prominent in HD and may antedate the development of the more obvious clinical features of the disease by years. Although perhaps of only theoretical interest to the geriatrician, it is a common observation in Sydenham's (rheumatic) chorea that affected children are irritable, easily distracted with a short attention span, and occasionally have obsessive-compulsive behavior. Sydenham's is widely considered to be an autoimmune disorder. It has recently been suggested that compulsive disorder and Tourette's syndrome are similarly autoimmune disorders, as so-called pediatric autoimmune neuropsychiatric disorders associated with streptococcal infection.

REFERENCES

1. Critchley M. The neurology of old age, II: clinical manifestations in old age. *Lancet.* 1931;2:1221–1230.
2. Jenkyn LR, Reeves AL. Neurological signs in uncomplicated aging (senescence). *Semin Neurol.* 1981;1:21–30.
3. Benassi G, D'Alessandro R, Gallassi R, et al. Neurological examination in subjects over 65 years: an epidemiological survey. *Neuroepidemiology.* 1990;9:27–38.
4. Folstein MF, Folstein SE, McHugh PR. Mini-mental status: a practical method for grading the cognitive status of patients for the clinician. *T Psych Res.* 1975;12:189–198.
5. Cummings JL, Mega MS. *Neuropsychiatry and Behavioral Neuroscience.* New York: Oxford; 2003.
6. Cummings JL. *The Neuropsychiatry of Alzheimer's Disease and Related Dementias.* London: Martin Dunitz; 2003.
7. Ferman TJ, Smith GE, Boeve BF, et al. DLB fluctuations: specific features that reliably differentiate DLB from AD and normal aging. *Neurology.* 2004;62:181–187.
8. Aharon-Peretz J, Kliot D, Tomer R. Behavioral differences between white matter lacunar dementia and Alzheimer's disease: a comparison on the neuropsychiatric inventory. *Dement Geriatr Cogn Disord.* 2000;2:294–298.
9. Snowden JS, Bathgate D, Varma A, et al. Distinct behavioral profiles in frontotemporal dementias and semantic dementia. *J Neurol Neurosurg Psychiatry.* 2001;70:323–332.
10. Hirono N, Mori E, Tanimukai S, et al. Distinctive neurobehavioral features among neurodegenerative dementias. *J Neuropsychiatry Clin Neurosci.* 1999;11:498–503.
11. Hayden MR. *Huntington's Chorea.* New York: Springer-Verlag; 1981.
12. Victor M, Adams RD, Collins GH. *The Wernicke-Korsakoff Syndrome.* Philadelphia: F.A. Davis; 1971.
13. Sloane RB. Organic brain syndrome. In: Birren JE, Sloane RB. *Handbook of Mental Health and Aging.* Englewood Cliffs, NJ: Prentice-Hall; 1980.

Neuroimaging in the Geriatric Patient

Richard Margolin

8

It has been almost 30 years since the potential of neuroimaging to revolutionize psychiatric practice was first heralded. This potential is grounded in neuroimaging's ability to provide detailed anatomical and physiological information about both normal mental function and psychopathology. In the ensuing years, several imaging methods have matured and contributed greatly to our evolving understanding of a number of important neural systems and processes. Imaging data have helped to elucidate the ways that individual brain structures, circuits, and chemical mechanisms work together to enable major elements of mental activity, for example, sensation, perception, and cognition. Other mental and behavioral domains, such as mood and affect, have likewise been probed with imaging, in health as well as in psychiatric and neurological diseases. The effect of aging on neuroanatomy, physiology, and brain chemistry has been an important focus of neuroimaging research, and mental disorders commonly afflicting the elderly, especially the cognitive disorders and depression, have also been targets of substantial research.

In recent years neuroimaging has also taken a prominent—perhaps even an essential—place in the geropsychiatrist's diagnostic toolset, alongside established methods such as interview, physical, neurological, and mental status examination, and laboratory testing. Imaging represents a valuable addition to traditional methods because it adds a completely different kind of information, which is both complementary and in some ways closer to the locus of pathological processes in geropsychiatric disorders. The term *neuroimaging* actually denotes a set of disparate techniques that have in common the production of representations of brain structure or function. The most widely known techniques are computed tomography (CT), magnetic resonance imaging (MRI), positron emission tomography (PET), and single photon emission computed tomography (SPECT). Because of both the importance of the body of knowledge that

neuroimaging has provided about aging and geropsychiatric disorders, and the impact that it has had on practice, in-depth consideration of neuroimaging is a worthy and important activity for students of geropsychiatry.

In that context, the overall goal of this chapter is to review the nature of neuroimaging methods and their application in geropsychiatry. The content includes selected information about methodology, research findings, and clinical applications. The order of considering these topics has been designed to support the overall goal. Presented in sequence are some basic concepts about imaging in general, the fundamentals of the major neuroimaging modalities, results of important research studies on aging and the major geropsychiatric disorders, clinical use of the key techniques, and some emerging methods and directions. For readers seeking more detail, comprehensive reviews of neuroimaging generally (1) and psychiatric aspects in particular (2,3) are recommended. More extensive discussions of specific topics such as the methodology of individual techniques (4,5), research findings in normal aging and specific neurological and psychiatric disorders (6), and clinical applications in psychiatry (7) are also available. One important neurodiagnostic method, electroencephalography, will not be considered here, even though it is sometimes considered a neuroimaging technique; however, an excellent recent review exists (8). Other methods, for example angiography and cranial/carotid ultrasound, will likewise not be discussed because they are somewhat peripheral to geropsychiatry. Again, however, reviews are available (1).

METHODOLOGY

General Concepts

Before considering the imaging methods individually, it will be helpful to address several topics common to them

TABLE 8-1
COMPARISON OF IMAGING TECHNIQUES

Category	CT	MRI	PET	SPECT
Type	Structural	Structural and Functional	Functional	Functional
Resolution (mm)	~1	~1	3–5	8–10
Radiation exposure	Yes	No	Yes	Yes
Approximate cost	$500	$1,000	$2,000	$1,000
Accessibility	Wide	Wide	Fairly wide	Wide
Tolerability	Good	Fair	Fair	Good
Slices per set	~30	~20	~30	~60
Study time (min.)	1–2	~30	10–20	30

CT, computed tomography; MRI, magnetic resonance imaging; PET, positron emission tomography; SPECT, single photon emission computed tomography.

as a group. In addition to the following discussion, these topics are summarized in Table 8-1.

One of the most basic concepts meriting attention is the nature of the information depicted—whether it is structural or functional. Structural imaging techniques identify various features of cerebral anatomy such as the size, location, and shape of brain regions, as well as the presence of pathology such as tumors or infarcts. By contrast, functional imaging techniques reveal elements of cerebral physiology such as blood flow, metabolism, and parameters of neurotransmission. Until relatively recently it was possible to divide the imaging methods into structural and functional categories, with CT and MRI considered structural imaging methods, and PET and SPECT classified as functional imaging tools. However, with the advent of certain MRI methods, the distinction has become blurred.

Another important subject is the spatial character of the data obtained. All the modern techniques are tomographic or volumetric. A tomogram literally means a picture of a slice, and the techniques being considered generally produce sets of multiple parallel, thin, slice-like images of the brain. Newer CT methods, some MRI and PET techniques, and SPECT actually capture volumetric (three-dimensional) slabs of data, in some cases with approximately the same level of detail as is usual in single-slice imaging methods, or even better. Such volumetric data acquisition can also be approximated by image manipulation, as discussed later in this chapter. Whether tomographic or volumetric, data are usually collected in one of several standard orientations, namely, the transverse, sagittal, and coronal planes. The transverse plane is also called the axial or horizontal plane, and the sagittal plane is sometimes called the frontal plane. The transverse plane is the primary orientation for data collection in CT, PET, and SPECT, whereas any of the planes can be used for data acquisition in MRI, and often more than one are used. The planes can be defined by either external or internal landmarks; they are not as exactly perpendicular to each other if external landmarks

are used, because of variability in the definition of key external landmarks. Research has also shown that external landmarks correlate unsatisfactorily with internal landmarks because of individual variation, and thus internal landmarks are increasingly used, especially in MRI and PET. A widely used internal landmark system uses the anterior and posterior commissures and the interhemispheric fissure to create a three-dimensional coordinate system (9). This system has achieved wide use in imaging research because it enables quantitative spatial measurements in individual brains, as well as group comparisons.

A number of brain structures are best visualized and/or their size quantified in one or another of the standard planes. For example, the hippocampus is preferentially imaged in the coronal plane. Clinical image review often incorporates examination of data in all three orientations. The "ideal" tomographic data set might consist of a very large number of very thin slices, with no interslice gaps or even with overlap. However, practical limitations govern the number of slices obtained in a study, for example the increasing quantity of data that must be stored and examined, and, in the case of CT, increasing radiation exposure associated with obtaining more and thinner slices. Still, a trend toward collection of an increasing number of slices of decreasing thickness exists for all the modalities and in both clinical and research applications.

One concept that is critical for proper understanding of the spatial nature of neuroimaging data is resolution. Technically, this term connotes the smallest two structures that can be discriminated within an image. The resolution of scanning methods is important because it limits the structures and features of the brain that can be accurately identified. There are significant differences in resolution between the imaging methods (Table 8-1) and theoretical limits for PET, but as with the number and thickness of slices, a steady increase in resolution has occurred for all the modalities over the years. Also, in-plane resolution and resolution perpendicular to the imaging plane (z-axis resolution) are distinct concepts, and both are important. While in-plane resolution is the more common concept, z-axis resolution also significantly affects images qualitatively and quantitatively.

Another general topic relevant to all the techniques is the way in which data are represented and displayed. Though acquired by very different means, all the modern imaging modalities are inherently digital in nature, which means the imaged space is represented by an array of picture elements called *pixels*. Because slices have finite thickness, the term *voxel* is also used to express the truly three-dimensional nature of data elements. Neuroimaging studies are most commonly displayed in a gray scale. The particular meaning of the scale varies among applications (e.g., tissue density, water content). Color display scales are also used, particularly for PET and SPECT. It is important to note that an individual shade of gray or a particular color only has meaning in relation to the tissue characteristic being imaged. The purpose of such scales is simply to facilitate appreciation of distinctions in such characteristics. For certain physiological imaging methods, though (e.g., PET-based cerebral glucose metabolism imaging), color bands represent truly quantitative ranges of physiological function.

Specialized image processing systems have lately enabled volumetric display of assembled slices (Figure 8-1), including surface representations created from slice data. Such systems also increasingly provide the ability to manipulate the orientation of displayed volumes. This facilitates the appreciation of three-dimensional relationships among brain structures and can dramatically aid the study of normal and pathological anatomy. Contemporary image processing systems also enable the superimposition of one modality's display on another, for example a PET image on an MRI background. This capability assists the identification of the anatomical location of physiologic phenomena. Cutting-edge capabilities also include techniques for automated or semiautomated analysis of brain images, for example the quantification of brain structure size. Such methods are already widely used in neuroimaging research, and are also becoming employed clinically. While clinical interpretation of brain images is still the province of the radiologist, neuroradiologist, or neurologist, steady advances in image analysis methods are leading to useful tools to automate and otherwise enhance the process. This trend is driven at least in part by the vastly increasing size of scan data. Inspecting 30 slices individually may be manageable, but reviewing 100 is not.

Technological progress is also influencing data storage approaches. While photographic film was for many years the ultimate repository of scan data, the ability to store large amounts of digital data in permanently accessible electronic and, more recently, optical media has increased dramatically in recent years. Digital storage approaches have also become progressively less expensive. Thus, their use is becoming the norm, with data now often transferred to film only when necessary.

General topics worth consideration also include radiation exposure, cost, accessibility, and tolerability (Table 8-1). CT, PET, and SPECT involve radiation exposure. While not insignificant, the exposures are comparable to or less than those of other radiologic procedures patients commonly undergo, and given the age of geropsychiatric patients, long-term risks of radiation exposure are perhaps less significant in this population than in younger adults. Cost varies somewhat among the techniques, although in some cases (e.g., CT and MRI) much less so nowadays. Reimbursement by major payors is customary for common clinical indications, except for PET, although that is slowly changing. All the techniques except PET are generally available in acute care hospitals. Tolerability varies somewhat across techniques, with MRI being the most challenging for geropsychiatric patients.

Computed Tomography

Introduced in the 1970s, CT quickly achieved wide use in neuropsychiatry because of the great value of the tomographic images of brain structure it provided. Moreover, these images were obtainable noninvasively and relatively rapidly. In CT images, cortical and subcortical gray matter structures, as well as white matter areas and the cerebrospinal fluid (CSF) space can each be visualized. Furthermore, both normal anatomy and pathological structural changes can be detected. In cranial CT, a patient

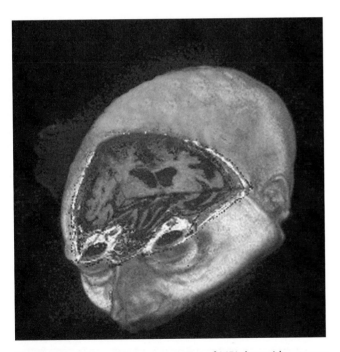

Figure 8-1 Volumetric representation of MRI data with cutaway demonstrating white matter and subcortical structures. Also note marked frontal lobe atrophy (especially prefrontal areas and orbitofrontal cortex) and widening of the Sylvian fissure in this patient with frontotemporal dementia. (courtesy of Tiffany Chow MD, University of Toronto)

lies on the scanner's bed with the head positioned in the center of the gantry (a frame that holds an x-ray source and a detector system). An x-ray beam is passed through the head, and the intervening tissues absorb it in proportion to their relative densities (bone > gray matter > white matter > CSF). The magnitude of the residual beam is measured by a detector system across the head from the x-ray source. As originally implemented, the beam was linear, and a single detector 180 degrees away was used. After the x-ray source and the detector were rotated together around the head, the bed was advanced and the process repeated. Each slice was thus acquired sequentially. Subsequently, a computer converted the absorption patterns into images through a mathematical procedure called reconstruction. This procedure involves the solution of multiple simultaneous equations to determine the unique characteristics of an object that would produce the absorption pattern found.

Progress in CT led to modifications of the data acquisition scheme. One improvement was the replacement of a linear beam with a fan-shaped beam. This allowed the use of a number of adjacent detectors at once, with software improvements permitting the coding of individual rays. Spiral CT was introduced around 1990. In this technique, the patient was moved slowly through the gantry while the beam and detectors operated in a continuous circular motion around the head. Spiral CT produced faster scans and thinner slices, and became the standard for CT in the following decade. More recently, multislice CT has been introduced. In this method, multiple detector banks are arranged in parallel along the gantry; the number of slices obtained simultaneously has increased from two to 16, with 64-slice scanners on the horizon. Spiral/multislice CT technology has dramatically decreased the time required for head CT imaging, which has led to a considerable reduction in the need for stabilization and immobilization of the head. In fact, faster scans and less need for head restraint, together with the large aperture of the CT gantry (about 70 cm), account for CT's relatively high tolerability in geropsychiatry. This is important because of the relative uncooperativeness of some elderly patients, for example those with cognitive impairment.

CT can be performed with or without contrast media, which are substances, usually containing iodine, which absorb radiographs well. In CT brain scanning, the primary purpose of using contrast is to highlight intracranial blood vessels (angiography). A contrast scan is actually two studies, an initial noncontrast study and a subsequent postcontrast (contrast-enhanced) study. Comparison of the two studies can provide important information, such as whether a mass lesion is more or less likely to be malignant. This information relates to the greater vascularity of malignancies. Unfortunately, although some abnormalities are better seen with contrast, a small but significant percentage of people are allergic to iodinated contrast media, and at-risk individuals cannot always be identified in advance. Nonionic (low osmolar) contrast media with low allergy potential have become available for individuals with known allergy, and as a result, contrast reactions have decreased in frequency. Contrast-enhanced scans are not indicated for the majority of geropsychiatric purposes.

In the CT gray-scale display scheme, white represents structures of highest density, and black those of least density. While CT can readily distinguish tissues of significantly different density (e.g., brain, CSF, and bone) (Figure 8-2A), it cannot do so as well for tissues of marginally different density, such as gray and white matter. This limitation, as well as the radiation exposure associated with CT, has been a factor in the increasing displacement of CT by MRI in geropsychiatry, despite CT's acknowledged virtues.

Magnetic Resonance Imaging

Since its introduction to clinical practice in geropsychiatry in the mid-1980s, MRI's growth has been nothing short of phenomenal. From its initial application as simply an improved CT for anatomic imaging, MRI quickly came to be recognized as enabling visualization of a variety of chemical and physiological processes. Furthermore, besides its increasingly routine practice use, it has also become a major research tool for studies aimed at elucidating the pathology of the major geriatric mental disorders. MRI has historically been divided into structural and functional imaging subtypes, though the distinction is imperfect. From this perspective the acronym MRI generally refers to structural MR imaging, whereas functional MR imaging is known as fMRI. In contrast to CT, which measures only tissue density, structural MRI is actually a set of distinct procedures that in the aggregate reveal various facets of the physicochemical composition of brain tissue. MRI actually grew out of an older laboratory technique, magnetic resonance spectroscopy, which yields information about the chemical composition of biological samples. That technique has itself been adapted for imaging and is generally referenced by the acronym MRS. MRI therefore specifically refers to anatomic and tissue water content imaging.

The essence of MRI lies in a particular property of certain atoms, namely, those with an odd number of protons/neutrons. This property, called magnetic resonance, refers to the behavior of the nuclei of such atoms when exposed to externally applied magnetic fields and specific levels of radiofrequency (RF) energy. While all atomic nuclei spin about their axes, under ordinary circumstances there is no net orientation of the spins. However, when nuclei with an odd number of protons/neutrons are placed in an externally applied field, they align in relation to its axis and rotate (precess) around it. If specific levels of RF energy are imparted to these aligned nuclei, the energy is transferred to them, and their orientation can be changed. The most common element in the human body is hydrogen, and its most abundant form happens to have a single proton (an odd number). Thus, hydrogen demonstrates magnetic

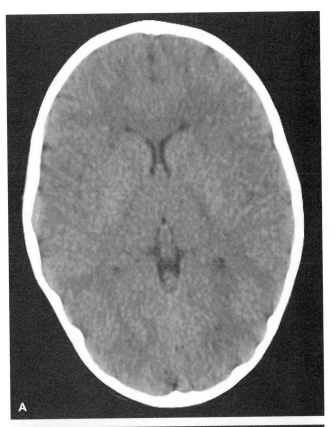

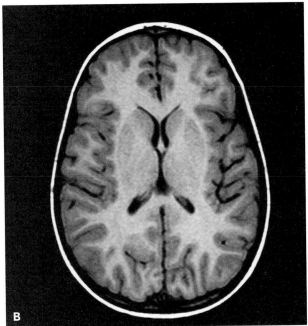

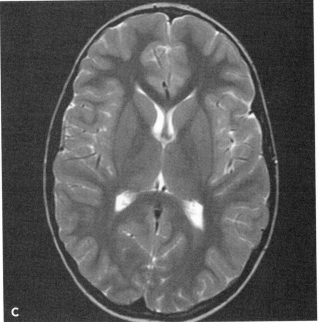

Figure 8-2 Normal brain images in several modalities: a) CT image showing gray and white matter, as well as CSF in sulci and ventricles; b) T1-weighted MRI image showing gray and white matter with excellent contrast; c) T2-weighted MRI image: Note brightness of CSF. (courtesy of Robert Kessler MD/Curtis Wushensky MD, Vanderbilt University Medical Center)

resonance and is the basis of almost all contemporary MRI systems.

A magnetic resonance imager (scanner) is a device that applies a large magnetic field together with one or more pulses of RF energy to an area of an individual's body. The most widely used scanners today, in both research and clinical practice, have a magnetic field strength of 1.5 Tesla, although higher field strength scanners, generally operating at 3 Tesla, are increasingly available. Low field strength scanners also exist, operating at up to 1.0 Tesla. While the quality of the images these devices produce is inferior to regular scanners, these devices do have certain advantages, including a larger scanning environment. This can be beneficial for claustrophobic patients. In the most common scanner design the magnet is cylindrical and housed in a gantry resembling that of CT scanners. The magnetic field is created by an electric current passed through wire coils wrapped closely in a spiral arrangement in the gantry. Because very large currents are necessary to achieve the required magnetic field strength for MRI, the coils are bathed in liquid helium/nitrogen, thus attaining superconductivity. As in CT, an individual undergoing brain MRI lies supine on the scanner's bed with the head positioned in the center of the gantry's aperture. There is no gantry or bed movement during imaging.

In brain MRI, a series of brief, exactly timed RF energy pulses are applied to the head, often in conjunction with nearly simultaneous perturbations of the local magnetic field. These RF energy pulses/magnetic field perturbations are generally referred to as pulse sequences. MRI further involves computerized image reconstruction by mathematical analysis of the pattern of nuclear responses to applied pulse sequences. In order to explain the essential features of MRI, the prototypical pulse sequence for brain imaging, known as the spin echo (SE) sequence, will be used for illustration. While at rest the scanner's magnetic field is steady. During the application of the pulse sequence, a magnetic field gradient is created, with slightly less than the nominal field strength at the base of the imaging volume and slightly more at the top. The purpose of this gradient is to select a specific slice for imaging. The orientation of the gradient is modifiable to achieve the particular slice orientation desired. For example, for a transverse image set, the field gradient orientation is along the long axis of the head.

Very soon (within milliseconds) after application of the gradient, RF energy at a frequency chosen to correspond to the magnetic field strength in the slice being imaged is applied in a perpendicular direction and excites the nuclei, changing their alignment to that of the plane in which the RF energy is applied. Because of a fundamental physical relationship between field strength and RF energy frequency, only nuclei in the slice selected by the field gradient experience this realignment. Besides being flipped into the RF pulse's plane, the rates of spin of the proton nuclei are also synchronized. When the RF pulse ends, the protons desynchronize and ultimately reorient themselves with the scanner's field. A receiver incorporated in the scanner records several important aspects of the temporal response to the RF pulse of nuclei in the volume being scanned. Because desynchronization occurs too quickly for recording of all the information possible for image creation, certain maneuvers are used to extend the signal over time. In one of earliest and most widely used pulse sequences, for example the SE sequence, refocusing gradients are employed just after the RF pulse to generate one or more echoes, each of which can be used for data collection.

Two key MRI parameters reflect distinct tissue responses to the RF-induced magnetic field perturbation and govern the quantitative nature of the response. These parameters are called the T1 and T2 relaxation times. The T1 relaxation time indicates the release of RF-imparted energy back to the surrounding environment and ultimately the realignment of the deflected protons with the orientation of the scanner's magnetic field. The T2 relaxation time, by contrast, reflects the release of energy between adjacent protons. Importantly, images representing either T1 or T2 relaxation times (called *T1-weighted* or *T2-weighted images*, respectively) can be created by varying certain aspects of the pulse sequence. The T1-weighted image is best understood as resembling a noncontrast-enhanced CT in that it reflects primarily anatomy (Figure 8-2B). It reveals spatial relationships among structures in the brain extremely well and also provides good visualization of contrast between gray and white matter. T1-weighted MRI is distinctly superior to CT in this regard. The T2-weighted image, on the other hand, is heavily influenced by tissue water content and does not correspond as closely to anatomic detail. While demonstrating CSF in sulci and ventricles very well (Figure 8-2C), it has proven particularly useful in revealing pathology not evident on T1-weighted images. These two image types are generally considered complementary and are acquired together in an SE sequence.

A large number of pulse sequences besides SE imaging have been developed over the years and are commonly referred to by acronyms. Such sequences have been created for three main reasons: to accelerate data acquisition, to better image tissue water content, and to identify aspects of tissue structure/chemistry other than anatomy and water content. The development of novel pulse sequences has in general been made possible by one interesting physical property inherent in MRI, which is the nonsimultaneity of the nuclear excitation and response processes. While excitation is quite brief (several milliseconds), the response can last up to a few seconds. This phenomenon permits remarkable control over sequence details, for example, varying the angle of inflection of the nuclei, inverting their initial inflection, and other maneuvers that allow highlighting of specific tissue types. The newer anatomical and water content imaging sequences include fast (turbo) spin echo (FSE/TSE), magnetization-prepared rapid gradient-echo (MP-RAGE), spoiled GRASS (gradient refocused acquisition in the steady state) (SPGR), and fluid attenuated inversion recovery (FLAIR). These methods, which are now widely used clinically for examining older adults, have dramatically shortened study times in the past decade. A typical clinical study in geropsychiatry consists of several sets of images, of different types and durations, and in different orientations, for example, a T1-weighted sagittal SE set, an axial T2-weighted FSE set, an axial FLAIR set, and an axial T1-weighted SE set. Each set might require about 3 minutes for data collection, with the whole procedure consuming less than 15 minutes of imaging time. Each set produces about 20 parallel 5-mm-thick images, with 1.5 mm interslice gaps.

Besides anatomic/tissue water content MRI, MRS and fMRI have also developed robustly in recent years. In MRS, signal strength corresponds to the concentration of nuclei of hydrogen, phosphorus, and a few other elements in certain nonwater biomolecules. Among these are a molecular marker of neuronal integrity (n-acetyl aspartate), an indicator of metabolism (creatine/phosphocreatine), measures of phospholipid metabolism, and the concentration of the neurotransmitter γ-aminobutyric acid (10). While a significant amount of MRS research has been conducted in relation to the major psychiatric disorders, little of it to date has focused on the elderly. An in-depth review of MRS is available (10).

Functional MRI is an enormously important research domain with great potential for geropsychiatry. Comprehensive discussions of it (11) and an aging-focused review (12) are available. Briefly, in the main implementation used to date, called the *blood oxygenation level dependent method*, the relationship between neuronal activity and the oxygenation level of hemoglobin (itself indicative of regional cerebral blood flow [rCBF]) is exploited to enable the mapping of local brain blood flow responses to sensory stimulation, motor tasks, or mental activity. In the category of mental activity, this method has been extensively applied to the study of elemental cognitive and affective processes in healthy adults, as well as patients with psychiatric disorders. The fastest anatomical imaging pulse sequence yet developed, echo-planar imaging (EPI), is commonly used in fMRI. In EPI a whole plane is imaged in one acquisition period. As with MRS, though, relatively little fMRI research has yet focused on the elderly.

MRI, like CT, customarily uses a gray-scale image display scheme; however, the term signal intensity is used instead of density, reflecting the heterogeneity of MRI data. In this scheme, white represents areas of highest signal intensity, gray represents intermediate values, and black depicts areas of lowest signal intensity. It is important to realize that a given brain structure can appear very different on images produced by different pulse sequences. For example, in a T1-weighted SE image, gray matter is brighter than white matter and CSF is dark (Figure 8-2B). In a T2-weighted SE or FSE sequence, CSF is bright and gray and white matter are dark (Figure 8-2C). By contrast, in the complementary FLAIR sequence, CSF is dark. However acquired, MRI must be reconstructed from the raw data. Though in a general sense similar to CT's reconstruction process, the mathematics involved in MRI reconstruction are different. It uses Fourier transformation, a process in which the frequency and magnetic phase data acquired during scanning are converted to a spatial representation of the image that was scanned. Explanation of the Fourier transformation process is beyond the scope of this chapter, but detailed discussion is available (13).

Several practical aspects of MRI in geropsychiatry deserve mention. First, MRI's ability to produce images in any plane, not just the transverse plane, without requiring flexion or extension of the head, is an important advantage over CT. Second, MRI has some absolute and relative contraindications, which must be considered before scanning. Absolute contraindications include the presence of a pacemaker or internal ferromagnetic material such as some aneurysm clips. Relative contraindications include known claustrophobia. MRI is somewhat more challenging than CT for several reasons. The scanner aperture is smaller, which sometimes produces a feeling of confinement, the scans take longer, and the procedure is accompanied by rather loud repetitive banging noises, which are disturbing to some people. Although a screening questionnaire is routinely administered prior to scanning in order to identify contraindications, their anticipation by the referring geropsychiatrist and proactive communication with the radiology department is important. Claustrophobia can be minimized by the presence of a friend or family member, and the distress caused by the scanner's loud sounds can be minimized by use of earplugs or headphones. If necessary, sedation is administered, usually with lorazepam or midazolam. Care must be taken when using more potent sedation than oral lorazepam, including respiratory and cardiac monitoring. In the case of extreme anxiety/agitation in the context of clinical necessity, general anesthesia can be administered. This, of course, requires the presence of anesthesiology staff.

Positron Emission Tomography

PET is a functional neuroimaging modality of great promise. As with MRI, it is made possible by a remarkably creative convolution of interesting features of physics and facets of human biology. PET is a nuclear medicine technique that depends on the behavior of positrons introduced into the body. Positrons are subatomic particles with the same mass as electrons but opposite charge. They exist transiently in nature in conjunction with the radioactive decay of certain isotopes of various elements, including carbon, oxygen, nitrogen, and fluorine. Positron-emitting isotopes of these elements (called radioisotopes or radionuclides) can be produced artificially in significant quantity with a medical cyclotron. They can then be chemically attached to a molecule of biological interest in a process known as radiochemistry. Molecules so produced are called radiotracers. In neuropsychiatric PET, a radiotracer is injected intravenously or inhaled while the individual being scanned lies supine with the head centered in the PET scanner's aperture. PET scanners physically resemble CT and MRI devices, with a gantry and a bed. The PET scanner's gantry contains multiple parallel banks of crystals made of materials optimized to detect the radiation produced by positron-electron interactions (called annihilation reactions). Because electrons are ubiquitous in biological tissues, an emitted positron collides with an electron within a short distance (2–3 mm). Since the two particles have opposite charge, they annihilate each other and, in accord with the law of conservation of energy, emit two photons of a particular energy level 180 degrees apart. Within a very narrow time window, these photons strike crystals on opposite sides of the head. PET scanners' crystal banks are connected to high-speed electronic circuits in a way that enables localization of the source of the coincidently deposited energy. This in turn permits images of the distribution of positron concentration (and thus indirectly, of tracer presence) to be reconstructed. A recent and detailed explanation of these concepts by one of the pioneers of PET is available (5).

The potential of PET to provide unique information about pathophysiology in psychiatric disorders has been recognized since its introduction over 25 years ago. The basis for this perspective is twofold. First, as mentioned above, positron-emitting isotopes of some of the key component elements of biologically important molecules exist, specifically, ^{15}O, ^{11}C, and ^{13}N (^{18}F is also a positron-emitter, and while not a natural component of biomolecules, resembles hydrogen sufficiently well physicochemically to substitute for it). Using these radioisotopes and radiochemistry, PET radiotracers can be created for investigation of various normal physiologic processes and their disturbance in relevant psychiatric disorders.

Second, PET can measure these physiologic processes quantitatively. Upon introduction to the body, the fate of a PET radiotracer depends on the way the various cellular systems and organs it encounters "see" it. For example, some tracers are extensively metabolized, whereas others are not. Some are trapped intracellularly in the brain or in the extracellular space, while others remain in the vascular compartment. Although the PET scanner detects only the spatial distribution of total radioactivity and creates corresponding images, mathematical models can be applied to such data. This approach, called tracer kinetic modeling, enables creation of images that precisely reflect physiological processes.

Although PET brain research began in the 1970s, its applications in psychiatry, and certainly in geriatric psychiatry, are still developing. Among the important physiological processes that can be imaged by PET, regional cerebral blood flow (CBF), also called perfusion, regional cerebral metabolic rate for glucose (CMRglu), and regional cerebral metabolic rate for oxygen (CMRO$_2$) have been perhaps the most thoroughly studied so far. Under normal physiologic conditions, CBF and CMRglu are tightly coupled, and CBF is thus a valid surrogate for CMRglu. This is not the case, however, in some neurological disorders involving structural brain damage, and it may not be the case in certain psychiatric disorders either. Extensive research over more than two decades has clarified many fundamental aspects of CBF/CMRglu in adults, for example normal range, regional distribution, and the response of relevant areas to sensory stimulation. Gray matter, for example, has a CMRglu about three to four times that of white matter, and the somatosensory and visual cortices, as well as the basal ganglia, typically have relatively high metabolic rates. More complex aspects of neurophysiology, which are of great interest to psychiatry, have also been probed, for example the activity of association cortices during performance of psychological tasks.

A substantial amount of research on neurotransmission has also been conducted. Tracers have been developed for several systems, including dopamine, serotonin, and acetylcholine synapses. Within these systems, in fact, agents have been created for imaging specific processes such as synthesis, vesicular packaging, release, reuptake, receptor binding/occupancy, and transmitter degradation. Opiate and benzodiazepine receptors have also been studied with imaging methods. Some major tracers (called radioligands in the case of receptor binding agents) and the systems they image are listed in Table 8-2. These methods are of great value because they may help explain important aspects of aging and the pathophysiology of relevant psychiatric disorders. An excellent and thorough discussion of the various methods and issues in physiological imaging, with particular reference to aging, have been described in further detail by Kessler (12). A related area that has increasingly been probed by PET is the neuropharmacology of psychotropic drug action. Radiolabeled psychotropic drugs and analogs of them have been created and administered, with interesting and provocative results.

Like CT and MRI, PET also generates tomographic images, the number of which per scan has increased substantially over the years. The most current PET scanners produce at least 30 parallel slices simultaneously. For some applications this number is sufficient; if additional detail is desired, the acquisition can be repeated after moving (indexing) the patient a fraction of the slice thickness. Scanning duration depends on the injected tracer dose and a number of other factors. For example, a single set of slices can be acquired in as little as 40 seconds with the intravenous (IV) bolus [^{15}O]-H$_2$O CBF method, while imaging may require several hours for some neurotransmission studies. A typical clinical CMRglu study takes 10 to 20 minutes. In some applications (e.g., the IV bolus [^{15}O]-H$_2$O CBF method) scanning begins essentially simultaneously with tracer administration; in other procedures, there is a delay. For example, in CMRglu imaging with the widely used tracer [^{18}F]-fluorodeoxyglucose (FDG), scanning is typically initiated 30 to 40 minutes after tracer administration. From the patient's perspective, PET's tolerability is intermediate between CT and MRI. Most tracers are introduced intravenously, so an IV line is generally required. Another method (sometimes arterial catheterization) is used for blood sampling if quantification of a physiological process is desired.

In addition to many research applications, PET has achieved some significant clinical use in geropsychiatry. Clinical PET is usually performed with only semiquantitative data analysis. An important practical aspect of PET is that, as a nuclear medicine procedure, it does produce radiation exposure. This varies with the tracer and the dose. For

TABLE 8-2

PHYSIOLOGICAL PROCESSES AND TRACERS FOR PET AND SPECT RESEARCH

Process	Tracers
Cerebral blood flow	$[^{15}O]H_2O$; $[^{15}O]CO_2$; $[^{15}O]$-butanol
Cerebral glucose metabolism	$[^{18}F]$-fluorodeoxyglucose
Cerebral oxygen metabolism	$[^{15}O]O_2$
Acetylcholine Synapse	
Vesicular transporter	$[^{18}F]$-fluoroethoxy-benzovesamicol; $(-)$-5-$[^{123}I]$-iodobenzovesamicol
Muscarinic receptor	$[^{123}I]$-QNB; N-$[^{11}C]$-methyl-benztropine; $[^{11}C]$scopolamine; $[^{11}C]$-N-methyl-4-piperidyl benzilate
Nicotinic receptor	$[^{11}C]$-nicotine; 6-$[^{18}F]$-fluoro-A-85380
Acetylcholinesterase	N-$[^{11}C]$-PMP; $[^{11}C]$-MP4A
Dopamine Synapse	
Synthesis	$[^{18}F]$-6-Fluoro-DOPA
Reuptake transporter	$[^{11}C, {}^{127}I]$-altropane; $[^{123}I]$-β-CIT; $[^{123}I]$-FPCIT; $[^{11}C]$-d-threo-methylphenidate
D1 receptor	$[^{11}C]$-NNC-112; $[^{11}C]$-SCH 23390
D_2 receptor	$[^{11}C]$-raclopride; $[^{18}F]$-fallypride; $[^{123}I]$-IBZM; $[^{18}F]$-N-methyl-spiperone
Serotonin Synapse	
Reuptake transporter	$[^{11}C]$-McN 5652; $[^{123}I]$-β-CIT
$5HT_{1A}$	[Carbonyl-^{11}C]-WAY 100635
$5HT_2$	$[^{18}F]$-altanserin; $[^{18}F]$-setoperone; $[^{18}F]$-N-Methyl-spiperone
Vesicular monoamine transporter	$[^{11}C]$-dihydrotetrabenazine
Monoamine oxidase B	L-$[11C]$deprenyl-D_2
Amyloid deposition	$[^{18}F]$-FDDNP; $[^{11}C]$-PIB

PET, positron emission tomography; SPECT, single photon emission computed tomography.

example, an FDG scan typically produces an exposure equivalent to 8 months of natural background radiation.

Single Photon Emission Computed Tomography

SPECT can be considered a hybrid between PET and standard nuclear medicine imaging in that it combines the PET's tomographic nature with the widely distributed gamma camera methodology of clinical nuclear medicine. Currently used SPECT tracers for neuropsychiatric applications generally employ radioisotopes of technetium (^{99m}Tc) or iodine (^{123}I). In contrast to PET, these radioisotopes emit single photons, as indicated in the acronym SPECT. The primary neurophysiologic function imaged by SPECT, which is of relevance to geropsychiatry, is CBF. Three tracers of CBF have been commercially developed for the US market: $[^{123}I]$-iofetamine (Spectamine); $[^{99m}Tc]$-exametazime, also known as HMPAO (Ceretec); and $[^{99m}Tc]$-bicisate, also known as ECD (Neurolite). Only the latter two agents are used today. Both are lipophilic, rapidly taken up by the brain after IV administration, in rough proportion to blood flow, and cleared very slowly—properties that permit imaging with gamma cameras. There are interesting differences between these agents in such areas as the minimum injection/imaging interval,

appropriate dose, compound stability, and the correlation with CBF as obtained by other means. However, the tracers are more similar than different (14).

SPECT radiotracers for some components of the dopamine, serotonin, and acetylcholine synapses have also been developed (Table 8-2). As with PET, both research and clinical applications have been explored in geropsychiatry. A distinct virtue of SPECT is its availability and affordability, properties that result from not requiring a dedicated cyclotron or coincident photon-detecting scanner. SPECT's virtues are accompanied by several drawbacks as compared to PET, however. These include inferior spatial resolution, the lack as yet of truly quantitative models for CBF imaging, and the lack of useful single-photon emitting radionuclides among the common elements of biomolecules. For example, the best current SPECT system resolution is about 8 mm, as opposed to 3 mm for PET. Each of the aforementioned drawbacks has been at least partially overcome, however. Limited spatial resolution, which stems from single photon/gamma camera imaging systems' lack of PET's natural photon beam collimation, has been addressed by steady advances in instrumentation. In lieu of truly quantitative CBF imaging, semiquantitative approaches have been developed and widely adopted. These methods reveal abnormal patterns and their relative magnitude. They are adequate for clinical use and have also been used successfully in research. Lastly, the paucity of SPECT radionuclides for introduction into naturally occurring biomolecules has been approached by creative radiochemistry. Like PET, SPECT also produces tomograms, usually about 60 per study. The procedure is quite tolerable for patients because gamma cameras are not confining. As in the methods previously discussed, an individual lies supine on an open bed. In this case, three cameras rotate in a slow circular motion.

Image Processing and Quantitative Image Analysis

Although the visual inspection of individual slices has historically been the basis of the clinical interpretation of neuroimaging studies, the limitations of that approach for clinical use, and particularly for research applications, have become increasingly apparent. As previously mentioned, both the number of slices produced in studies and their detail has steadily increased for all the modalities. This phenomenon, along with certain technical problems in the interpretation of some kinds of images (e.g., the effect of atrophy on PET CMRglu imaging in dementia), has stimulated dramatic developments in computerized image processing, both to enhance clinical image interpretation and as a foundation for optimal use of imaging data in research applications. Although this area is highly technical and largely beyond the scope of the present chapter, a few tools and applications will be discussed.

Like SPECT, semiquantitative methods have been developed for PET CBF and CMRglu measurements. Although this approach sacrifices methodologic elegance, it is much more practical. For example, instead of multiple samples from arterial or heated venous ("arterialized") blood, partial quantification involves limited blood sampling and the construction of ratios of active areas of metabolism/blood flow to relatively invariant areas (e.g., for dementia evaluation, the cerebellum) or the whole brain average. Based on studies comparing such approaches to the gold standard, these techniques have achieved wide use clinically (and to a lesser extent in research), even though some issues exist.

Image processing and image analysis are related procedures that together enable maximal extraction of data contained in the raw images. Image processing includes several distinct elements, for example, "removal" of non-central nervous system tissue from images, correction for movement and other artifacts, alignment of images of interest with standardized reference images, and, in the case of physiological imaging, calculation of quantitative measures.

Image processing supports the multiple and diverse contexts and goals of image analysis, for example, the comparison of image sets obtained on a given person at different times or with different modalities. Very often an individual's image sets need to be integrated into a class (e.g., patients or controls, elderly or young) or analyzed in the context of an experimental manipulation (e.g., a drug treatment or a cognitive task). Diverse software systems have been developed by numerous research groups to carry out these various tasks. The most advanced systems combine a number of processing steps and even automate the analysis.

A particularly valuable and consequently widely implemented use of image processing is the exploitation of MRI's superior spatial resolution so as to permit the best possible analysis of lower resolution functional images. For this purpose an individual's functional image set (e.g., a PET/FDG CMRglu study) is coordinated with a matching MRI set, for example, a scan acquired relatively contemporaneously on the same individual. This matching process is called *registration*, and the development of software for this purpose (15), together with its subsequent refinement and automation, were important advances. With MRI registration, regional physiologic measures can be obtained with more certainty about the underlying anatomy than would be possible by analyzing the functional images alone.

The MRI set used for matching need not necessarily be obtained from the same individual as the one whose functional images are to be analyzed. Doing so is not always possible; sometimes the number of scans to be analyzed is large, and in the case of group comparisons, statistical reasons dictate use of an "average" anatomical brain template. Thus, considerable efforts have been aimed at creating standardized MRI-based atlases (16). In these endeavors MRI data from a number of normal individuals are pooled to create a representative image set for use as a template for analysis of test images. Whether images are being registered to an individual's own MRI data or to a digital atlas, statistical maneuvers are required to "deform" them appropriately. This process is often called *normalization*.

Once normalized, images can be optimally subjected to analysis. Early methods for analyzing brain images involved identifying relevant brain structures and/or tissue types by hand-drawn regions of interest (ROIs). Many issues with this approach were identified, such as a priori assumptions and operator error and bias (17). It was also labor intensive, which limited applicability in large research studies. Consequently, the manual ROI analysis strategy has gradually given way to semiautomated or fully automated techniques. As a group these methods have been termed computational neuroanatomy (18), and the Talairach and Tournoux (9) stereotaxic coordinate system is generally employed as a common basis for image consideration in them. Several robust systems of this kind have been developed and made available to research groups. In fact, a number of large and even multinational collaborative working groups have been created to validate and refine the methods. One particularly widely used system that incorporates both normalization and automated image analysis is called statistical parametric mapping (SPM) (19). The most advanced automated analytic application of SPM in structural imaging is called voxel-based morphometry (VBM) (20). Hybrid computer/human approaches have also been developed and may have unique value in specific situations.

A particularly important application of image processing in geropsychiatry is the correction of errors introduced by atrophy. This is a particular issue in both structural and functional geropsychiatric imaging because of the well-appreciated extent of brain atrophy in late life. In structural imaging studies of the volume of specific structures or tissue types as a whole (e.g., gray matter volume), the need to relate the absolute size of areas under study to skull size/total brain volume was recognized early on (21). In functional imaging, error is introduced into measurements of physiological processes by the effect of inert tissue (e.g., CSF) or differentially functional tissue (e.g., white matter adjoining gray matter) contained in individual image voxels (22). Because of the relatively low spatial resolution of PET and SPECT (as compared to CT or MRI), such tissue type averaging is more likely to occur in these methods, erroneously reducing the measured level of processes being assessed (e.g., CBF/CMRglu or parameters of neurotransmission). This phenomenon, called the *partial volume effect*, is strongly associated with atrophy and thus profoundly affects geropsychiatric imaging. Consequently, considerable efforts have been devoted to developing and validating methods to correct for it. Sophisticated systems for this purpose, which use an MRI-based anatomical template and the above-referenced automated image registration methods, have recently been created (23).

NEUROIMAGING RESEARCH FINDINGS IN AGING AND THE GERIATRIC MENTAL DISORDERS

Aging

Before considering the body of research findings and clinical applications in the various geropsychiatric disorders, it is worthwhile to briefly review the imaging data that have been accumulated in the study of normal aging. Understanding aging-related changes in cerebral structure and function is important because these changes interact with and confound disease-specific changes. Both structural and functional changes in the brain have been investigated with regard to aging. It should be noted that considerable variability exists in these studies with regard to the age of participants. Many studies investigated aging from young adulthood to late middle age, while relatively few have examined changes within late life.

Structural Changes

From a geropsychiatric imaging perspective, the intracranial space is essentially composed of the brain and CSF.

Other structures such as the meninges and large blood vessels constitute a very small percentage of the intracranial space and are not a major focus for geropsychiatric imaging. The brain is in turn composed of gray and white matter compartments, while the CSF is composed of the sulcal space, which surrounds the cortical gyri, and the ventricles (third, fourth, and lateral). The major age-related structural changes identified to date through neuroimaging include reductions in gray and white matter density, reductions in the size of their compartments (with corresponding increase in measures of sulcal and ventricular volumes), atrophy of specific brain regions, and the development of certain focal abnormalities in the white matter and basal ganglia. Many cross-sectional and a few longitudinal studies have been conducted. Since the early 1990s, CT investigations have been largely supplanted by MRI studies. Brain density reductions and atrophy were associated with aging in early CT studies (24). Age-associated atrophy has also been demonstrated for both the brain as a whole (25) and specific structures in many MRI studies. Interestingly, this process seems to affect gray matter more than white matter, and the frontal lobes more than other cortical regions (26). Subcortically, the hippocampus shows the most significant age-related atrophy, with its prevalence increasing from 15% in healthy 60- to 75-year-olds to 48% in 76- to 90-year-olds (27). Gender differences in age-associated atrophy have also been reported (28), and the rate of atrophy has been asserted to be increased in the elderly by common age-related medical problems such as diabetes mellitus, hypertension, and cardiovascular disease (29).

While cross-sectional studies have produced extensive and intriguing data, longitudinal studies are best for investigating the neurobiological effects of aging, because they are less subject to some of the major drawbacks of cross-sectional studies (e.g., large individual differences and secular effects). In one such study, for example, Jack and associates found annual hippocampal volume loss of about 1.5% in people aged 70 to 89, no correlation of the rate with advancing age, and no effect attributable to either key medical comorbidities (hypertension, diabetes mellitus, or ischemic cardiac disease), gender, or apolipoprotein E genotype (30). In a large long-term study, 4-year follow-up data confirmed both the linearity of gray and white matter volume atrophy rates across the span of old age and the lack of a gender effect, but identified a slower rate in very healthy people (31).

In addition to brain atrophy, age-associated changes have been identified in the white matter. Visible to some extent on CT as zones of low density (and called leukoaraiosis there), these changes are much better appreciated in T2-weighted MRI as areas of increased signal (hyperintensity). MRI white matter hyperintensities (WMH) are often termed periventricular hyperintensities (PVH) or deep (subcortical) white matter hyperintensities (DWMH), respectively, based on their location (Figure 8-3). WMH mainly reflect localized increased tissue water, a condition

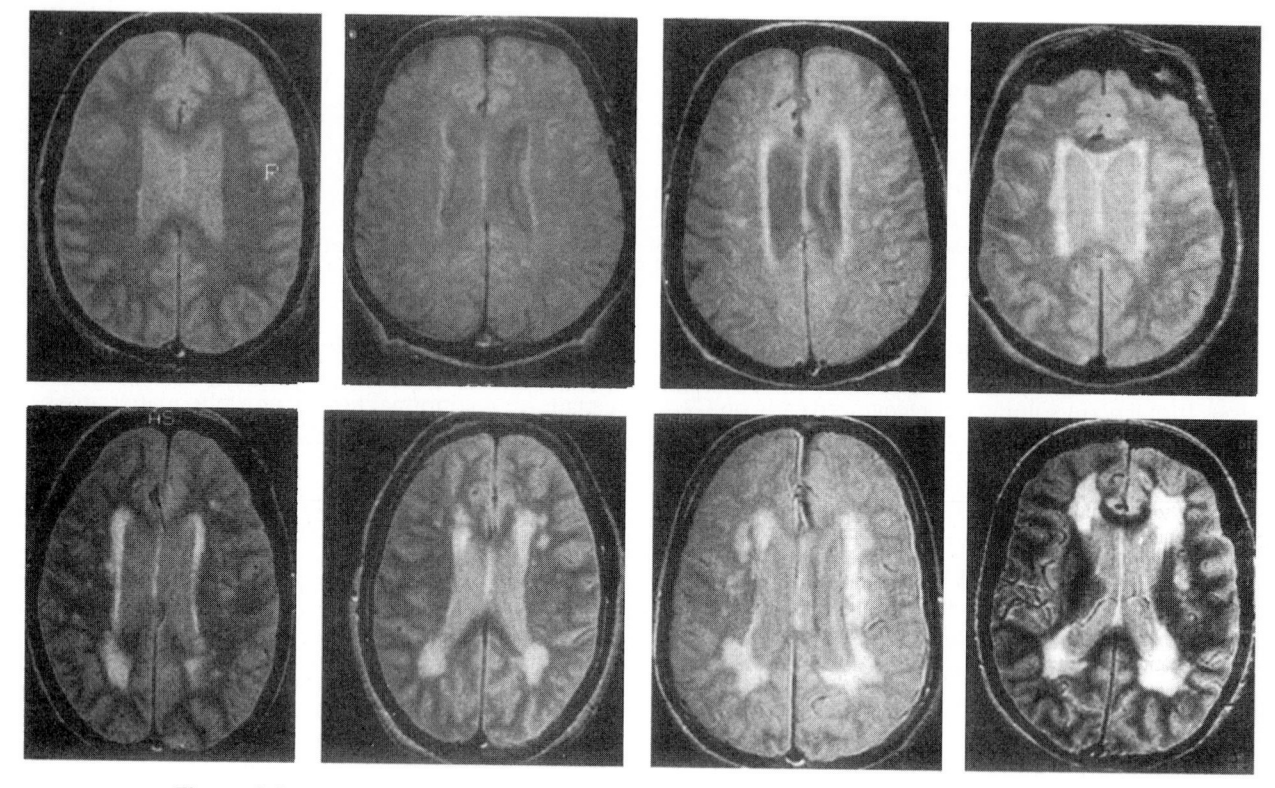

Figure 8-3   T2-weighted MR images showing periventricular and deep white matter abnormalities. Note variation in grades. From Longstreth et al. (36), with permission.

caused by several distinct pathologic derangements of small cerebral arteries, including arteriolosclerosis, tortuosity caused by vessel elongation and dilatation, and enlargement of the perivascular spaces (32,33). Demyelination may also be involved (34), and transependymal CSF migration into adjacent brain tissue may be a factor in PVH (35). A consensus holds WMH to be markers of small-vessel cerebrovascular disease (CVD), and some may actually represent silent (incomplete) infarcts (36).

An increased prevalence of WMH in the elderly was reported from the early days of MRI (37) and has been associated with increasing age in a recent large population-based study (38). However, the strength of this association has been debated over the years, because these abnormalities are at least as strongly correlated with several medical disorders (e.g., hypertension, atherosclerosis, and perhaps diabetes mellitus), which are themselves common in the elderly (32). The number, size, and location of WMH can all be quantified with imaging. Individual differences in the extent of both PVH and DWMH are striking (Figure 8-3); overall, PVH are more common. As with atrophy, longitudinal studies have investigated the progression of these lesions over time. In one such study, for example, very small (punctuate) DWMH seemed stable, but larger DWMH and PVH grew and even became confluent over 5 years (39).

A final age-associated structural change deserving mention is iron deposition. While the basis for this phenomenon is obscure, it has been noted in several basal ganglia structures in the form of foci of decreased signal on T2-weighted MRI (40). Although iron deposition may be normal after age 80 in the putamen, it is likely abnormal at any age in other areas, for example the caudate and thalamus.

Functional Changes

Age-related functional changes have also been well documented in such physiological domains as CBF, CMRglu, and elements of neurotransmission. CBF and CMRglu were among the first aspects of brain function to be examined with PET. Numerous cross-sectional studies conducted over the years examined age-related changes in these processes, with varied findings For example, one study (41) found linear CBF and $CMRO_2$ decrements in various cortical regions, but another (42) found no age association with CMRglu in an examination of many cortical regions in healthy men from 21 to 83 years old. Studies of glucose metabolism somewhat consistently show age-related declines, particularly in the frontal lobes (43), while CBF studies have done so less regularly. Of note, in a recent well designed CBF study, after correction for partial volume effect, no significant reduction in CBF with aging was found in any brain region (44). Moreover, in a SPECT hexamethylpropylene amine oxime CBF study, Mozley et al. found decrements only in young adulthood, with stable flow throughout late middle age (45). A number of factors may explain such discrepant findings, including environmental differences (e.g., the level of sensory stimulation during scanning [eye opening status, ambient noise]), cognitive parameters (e.g., instructions, mental activity), age-related cortical atrophy, aspects of physiology (e.g., alterations in CBF coupling with CMRglu and $CMRO_2$), and differences in scanner resolution.

Evidence of age-related changes in elements of several neurotransmission systems of great importance to cognitive and affective functioning in health and illness has also accumulated (46,47). The acetylcholine synapse, for example, has been studied in detail by Kuhl and associates (48). This group found an approximately 4% decline per decade of the adult life span in presynaptic cholinergic system integrity with the SPECT tracer $[^{123}I]$-IBVM (48), no significant decline in acetylcholinesterase (AChE) function, as assessed with the PET tracer $[^{11}C]$-PMP, and some regional age-associated decrements in muscarinic receptor binding using the nonselective receptor subtype PET tracer $[^{11}C]$-NMPB (49). The dopamine synapse has also been investigated extensively. Rather consistent age-associated declines in tracer binding in several synaptic components have been identified: 7% per decade at the D1 receptor (50), a 1% annual decrement at the D2 receptor (51), and almost 7% at the dopamine transporter (52). The serotonin synapse has been likewise well-dissected. For example, 5HT transporter availability declined approximately 4% per decade (53), $5HT_{1A}$ binding potential was found to be reduced about 10% per decade in most brain regions (54), and $5HT_{2A}$ binding was noted to be almost 60% less in the elderly than in young adults (55).

Cognitive Impairment

Cognitive disorders, particularly Alzheimer's disease (AD), have been among the most extensively studied neuropsychiatric conditions. Both structural and functional investigations have been conducted; initial studies were largely descriptive, but more recent ones have incorporated experimental manipulations such as cognitive tasks and drug administration. In the following discussion, important imaging findings will be reviewed by category of cognitive impairment, namely, AD, dementia due to CVD (also called vascular dementia [VaD]), mixed AD/VaD, dementia due to various other etiologies, and finally mild cognitive impairment (MCI).

Alzheimer's Disease

AD has without question received the greatest amount of neuroimaging research attention of any geropsychiatric condition. Beginning in the 1970s, CT studies revealed global brain atrophy (56) with other findings, for example

density reductions, regional atrophy, and ventriculomegaly (57), and white matter abnormalities (58) being reported soon afterward. In ensuing years, larger sample sizes and better scanners added detail to these findings. For example, Jobst and colleagues (59) found that medial temporal lobe thickness a year before death reliably predicted a postmortem diagnosis of AD. Longitudinal studies identified a more rapid rate of ventriculomegaly (60) and medial temporal atrophy in AD (61), as compared to controls. However, the radiation exposure associated with CT and also MRI's superior resolution eventually led to MRI generally replacing CT for structural investigations.

Since the early 1990s there has been a veritable explosion of MRI-based structural imaging research on AD, as recently reviewed comprehensively by Atiya et al. (62). Briefly, in addition to generally confirming earlier CT-based findings, MRI studies quantified the atrophy of medial temporal lobe structures known to be involved in the pathogenesis of AD, especially the hippocampus (63) and entorhinal cortex (ERC) (64). Reductions ranging from about 20% in mild AD to 40% in more severe patients were reported (62). Relatively recently, atrophy in other structures of interest, specifically the cingulate and superior temporal gyrus, has also been identified. In a large sample, hippocampal volume loss was found to be correlated with clinical severity, as assessed by the Clinical Dementia Rating scale (65). In the past few years, results of several valuable longitudinal MRI studies of structure volume changes in AD have been reported. One such study revealed a rate of hippocampal atrophy of 4% per year, 2.5 times the rate in normal aging (30). Another (66) found the ERC rate to be even higher, and still another (67) calculated whole brain atrophy to be 2% per year.

The white matter abnormalities in established AD initially reported in CT studies have been extensively investigated with MRI. While some early investigations found WMH of all types to occur at an increased frequency in AD (68) and to be correlated with dementia severity, others found only PVH to be increased (69), or no difference (70) and no correlation with severity (71). In several creative studies, Bronge has shown that apolipoprotein E4 homozygosity is associated with more extensive WMH in AD, and that *in vivo* WMH correlate with but underestimate postmortem white matter pathology (72). WMH are also more severe in late-onset AD, but the association of WMH with aging itself makes the independence of this relationship uncertain.

Physiological disturbances in AD have also been intensively investigated since the early 1980s using PET, SPECT, and more recently, other methods. This work has involved studies of blood flow, metabolism, and neurotransmission. Early reports identified widespread coupled $CBF/CMRO_2$ (73) and cortical CMRglu reductions (74). The CMRglu decrements were most prominent in the parietal and temporal lobes (75), were usually present bilaterally (although sometimes asymmetrically), and were correlated with

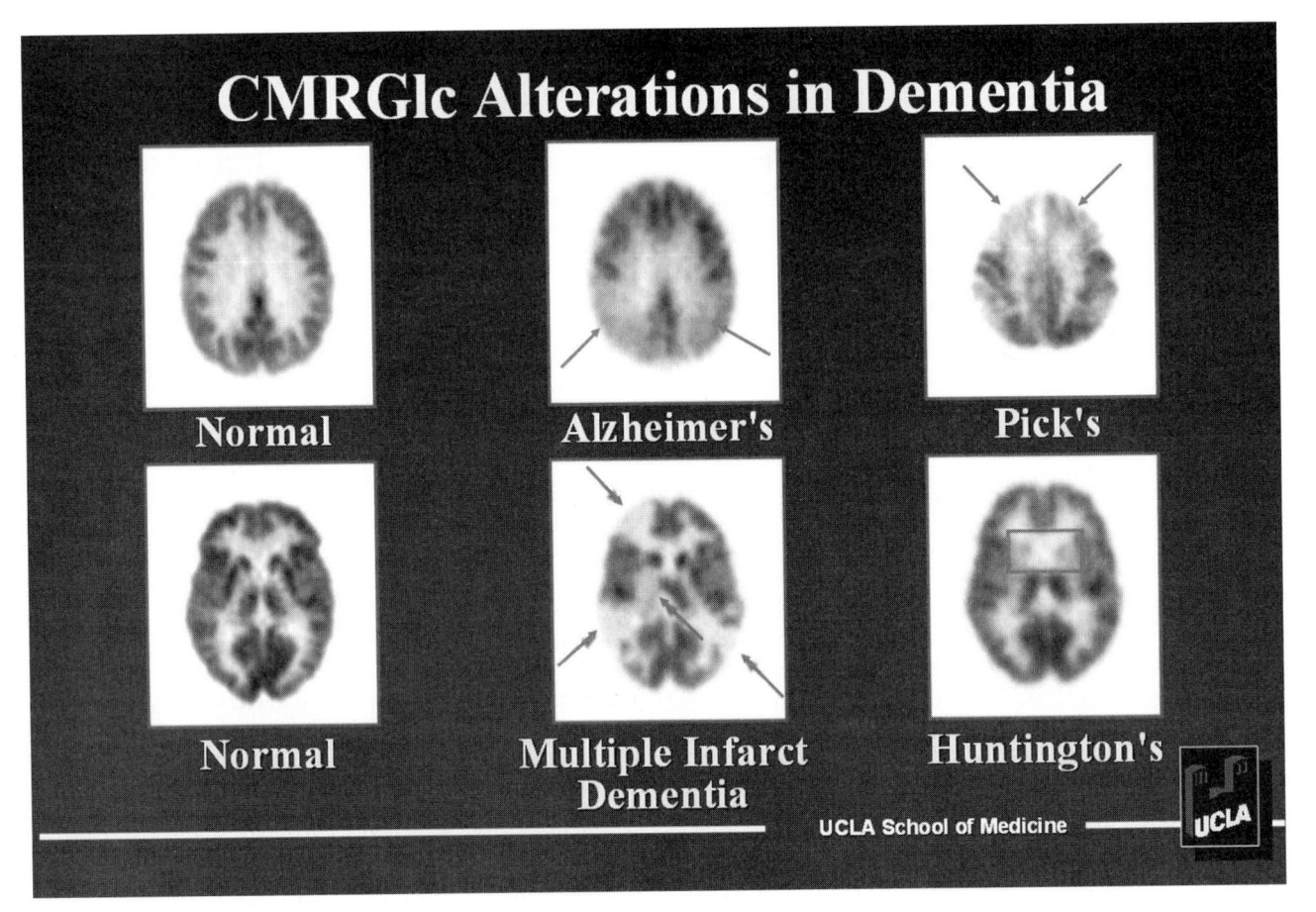

Figure 8-4 Normal transverse PET CMRglu images and images demonstrating some common causes of dementia (courtesy of Gary Small MD, University of California, Los Angeles; From Phelps et al (eds). *Positron Emission Tomography*. Raven Press, New York, 1986.). Note Alzheimer's disease, frontotemporal dementia (Pick's disease) and multi-infarct dementia (vascular dementia) patterns in particular.

clinical severity (76) (Figure 8-4). Later studies found posterior cingulate hypometabolism as well (77). The primary visual and sensorimotor cortices were usually spared until advanced disease. Longitudinal studies revealed that metabolic deficits were present even in mild AD and preceded nonmemory cognitive deficits (78); importantly, their severity predicted the rate of clinical decline (79). SPECT rCBF studies have generally confirmed the major PET-based findings, such as the parietotemporal hypometabolism pattern (80), although direct comparisons have found significant differences in some areas (81). While most early studies were conducted at rest, with reduced sensory stimulation, performance of cognitive activation tasks was found to increase metabolism in various brain regions, including areas hypometabolic at rest (82).

In addition to CMRglu and CBF studies, the neurochemical pathology of AD has also been probed with PET and SPECT. For example, the cholinergic system has been studied presynaptically and postsynaptically. Presynaptically, Kuhl's group demonstrated severity-correlated reduction of terminal integrity in the hippocampus and temporal lobe with [123I]-IBVM, a marker of the vesicular acetylcholine transporter (48). This group also imaged AChE activity using the tracer [11C]-PMP in an elegant and provocative study (83) of 14 moderate AD patients, 11 of whom underwent concomitant IBVM and CMRglu imaging. Approximately 30% reductions compared to controls were found in widespread cortical regions and the hippocampus, which correlated with IBVM-identified terminal reductions but not CMRglu. Other groups are investigating milder patients with similar methods. Studies of muscarinic receptors have used a variety of tracers and reported discrepant findings; nicotinic receptor integrity reductions have also been reported (84). Other neurotransmitter systems have been investigated to a much lesser extent. For example, marked reductions in $5HT_2$ receptor binding of a PET tracer have been reported (85). Such findings may have implications for the understanding of psychotic and/or depressive phenomena in AD.

Vascular Dementia

Dementia due to CVD (VaD) is heterogeneous clinically, neuropathologically, and in its imaging manifestations. After AD, it has perhaps been the type of dementia next most studied with imaging. Both structural and physiological imaging studies have been performed, usually contrasting this condition to AD and normal controls. Optimal understanding of the results of VaD-focused imaging studies requires some preparatory consideration of the condition's diagnostic subtypes and the pathophysiology underlying them. As set forth in an excellent and thoughtful review (86), as well as being discussed elsewhere in this textbook, VaD can be considered as encompassing large and small artery syndromes. The first category denotes dementia that follows one or more large cortical infarcts. VaD subsequent to two or more such infarcts is widely known as multi-infarct dementia (MID). Small artery syndromes include dementia due to one or more infarcts in strategic subcortical locations, as well as the lacunar state and Binswanger's disease. The latter two conditions have been lumped under the rubric subcortical ischemic vascular dementia (SIVD). The reader will encounter several terms for vascular dementia and related conditions in the literature besides VaD, MID, and SIVD, including ischemic vascular disease (IVD), subcortical vascular dementia (SCVD), and vascular cognitive impairment (VCI). Also, the term SIVD is used to denote both dementia and disease (neuropathology) associated with subcortical ischemic vascular pathology. Pathologically, infarcts may be complete or incomplete. Complete infarctions in turn can be caused by hemorrhagic or ischemic brain damage; the latter is more common in VaD. Small complete infarcts (<10 mm in length), generally occurring in the white matter or subcortical gray matter, are called lacunes. Incomplete infarcts are mainly appreciated subcortically, especially in the white matter, where they manifest as the WMH (or leukoaraiosis on CT) discussed above. They can also be found in the cortex.

Several imaging-related aspects of infarcts merit discussion. Cortical infarcts often appear wedge-shaped, bright on T2-weighted MRI, and dark on T1-weighted sequences. Small infarcts can be seen on MRI with more certainty than on CT. Although WMH resemble lacunes on T2-weighted MRI, the two phenomena can be distinguished on T1-weighted imaging, where WMH demonstrate less signal intensity reduction than lacunes. Lastly, differentiating lacunes from other radiographic entities, especially dilated perivascular spaces, can be difficult, but the task has been made easier by the development of unambiguous definitions and operational criteria (87).

The findings of imaging studies of VaD would ideally be considered with regard to the specific types of VaD on which they focused. Unfortunately, this is not entirely possible because some studies, especially early ones, did not always or fully present critical clinical information (e.g., prestroke cognitive status) or commingled VaD subtypes (e.g., cortical infarcts and the lacunar state) in their samples. Nevertheless, a number of findings emerge from the various studies, as cataloged by Erkinjuntti and associates (88). Volume, location (lobe, arterial territory), side, and

number of infarcts have all been related to the development of dementia in at least some CT and MRI studies, as have atrophy and the site and extent of WMH. The rate of whole brain atrophy is similar to that of AD and, like AD, increases with disease severity (67). In poststroke dementia, the relatively low predictive power of individual imaging parameters, as well as the complex interactions among them, was recently highlighted in a large study (89). The ability of even quite small but strategically located infarctions to produce dementia (or related neurobehavioral disturbances) is well recognized (90). Such infarcts are those occurring in the caudate, the paramedian nuclei and left anterior pole of the thalamus, and the genu of the internal capsule (91).

The subcortical ischemic forms of VaD have been studied as well, and in recent years increasing attention has been paid to the lacunar state in particular. Surprisingly, generalized cortical atrophy and atrophy of key medial temporal lobe structures (hippocampus and ERC) (92), rather than the extent of lacunar volume (93), best characterize SIVD. WMH burden also separates such patients from controls (92). The imaging signature of Binswanger's disease remains somewhat murky. Very large areas of decreased periventricular density on CT (and corresponding confluent PVH on MRI) were noted in some early imaging studies of dementia, and clinicopathological correlations supported the idea that these findings were manifestations of Binswanger's disease (94). However, no large-scale studies of this condition have yet been conducted.

A modest number of functional imaging studies of VaD have also been conducted over the years, examining CBF, CMRglu/CMRO$_2$, and their coupling, as well as a physiological process potentially even more proximate to the pathophysiology of VaD, *oxygen extraction fraction* (OEF). (OEF is a measure of the metabolic reserve of tissue; in conditions of marginally inadequate perfusion, relatively more oxygen is extracted than predicted.) The findings of functional VaD studies have been well summarized by Mori et al. (90). Even more than in structural studies, VaD subtypes have been commingled in this work, and several major findings have emerged. First, parietotemporal CBF and CMRglu decrements occur in VaD as well as AD (95), but decrements can also be seen elsewhere. Also, the volume of hypometabolic tissue correlates with clinical severity in this condition as it does in AD (96). In an elegant and potentially quite important study, De Reuck and colleagues reported coupled CBF/CMRO$_2$ reductions in MID and SIVD (lacunar type), but increased OEF only in SIVD when dementia was present (97). This finding suggests that pathologically significant lacunes might be differentiable from asymptomatic ones by this method. Finally, small but intriguing studies by several groups, including Mori and colleagues (90), have identified large ipsilateral areas of cortical hypometabolism, or in some cases bilateral hypometabolic zones, resulting from small thalamic or caudate infarcts.

Dementia can also develop in connection with certain uncommon central nervous system vasculopathies, but these syndromes are not usually considered under the term VaD. The vasculopathies associated with dementia include cerebral amyloid angiopathy, cerebral autosomal dominant angiopathy with subcortical ischemic leukoencephalopathy, and cerebral vasculitides associated with autoimmune disease (temporal arteritis, primary intracranial arteritis, and the antiphospholipid syndrome associated with systemic lupus erythematosus). A few imaging studies have been performed in these conditions, but are beyond the scope of this chapter.

Mixed Dementia

The concept of mixed dementia (MxD) (the combination of AD and VaD) is long established, yet many epidemiologic, neurobiological, and clinical questions remain unsettled. Two of the most basic are whether or not this condition exists as a discrete entity, and if so, how the two pathophysiologic processes interact to produce or magnify dementia. MxD would seem to be an ideal target for neuroimaging research, but in fact very few studies have examined it. This results at least in part from the difficulty of selecting patients who have clear-cut contributions from both etiologies. The findings that have emerged from the available studies are that a significant percentage of AD patients have evidence of CVD beyond WMH (e.g., lacunar infarcts) (98), and that the risk of dementia is tripled in AD patients with typical atrophy and substantial WMH (99), suggesting a clinically significant interaction.

Other Dementing Disorders

The list of other etiologies that can cause dementia or with which it is sometimes associated is very long. Some of these conditions have been studied with imaging to a moderate degree, and others with only a few small studies. The relatively well-studied group includes dementia with Lewy bodies (DLB), Parkinson's disease with dementia (PDD), frontotemporal dementia (FTD), and normal pressure hydrocephalus (NPH), which are discussed in detail elsewhere in this textbook.

Dementia with Lewy Bodies

DLB is a relatively recently identified and still evolving clinicopathologic entity. Despite this, and perhaps because of both its apparently substantial frequency as a cause of dementia and the challenge its diagnosis and management present, DLB has been explored in quite a number of structural and functional studies in recent years. The major findings to date have been thoroughly discussed by Small in an excellent recent review (100). Unfortunately, structural studies have been somewhat disappointing. While investigations of global atrophy (101) and its rate of progression (67), as well as the size of some specific structures, have demonstrated differences between DLB and controls, studies comparing such parameters between DLB and AD have been

conflicting. The hippocampus and medial temporal lobe (102), for example, have been reported to show less atrophy than in AD, while the occipital lobe (103) does not differ. The last study is important because it had been thought that visual hallucinations, one of the most prominent symptoms in DLB, might relate to structural changes in the occipital lobe. Studies of DLB/AD differences in WMH parameters have also been negative (104).

By contrast, functional studies have shown replicable and interesting differences between DLB and AD, as well as between DLB and controls. Albin and colleagues (105) reported occipital lobe glucose hypometabolism (both primary and association cortices), and Imamura et al. (106) found that the posterior cingulate CMRglu reduction known to occur in AD was not present in DLB. SPECT and PET CBF studies have generally mirrored the findings of CMRglu studies. Dopamine neurotransmission studies have also produced interesting results, for example, reduced striatal synthesis (107) and reuptake (108) as compared to AD.

Parkinson's Disease with Dementia

Parkinson's disease (PD) alone and PDD share a number of clinical and neuropathological features with DLB. PDD in its own right has received a modest amount of neuroimaging research interest, mainly using functional methods. While early structural studies did not reveal evidence of atrophy in PDD, some more recent studies have reported significant changes. For example, Camicioli et al. (109) identified hippocampal atrophy in both PD and PDD. Functional studies have examined CBF, CMRglu, and dopamine terminal parameters. CBF studies have reported global and especially parietotemporal (110) reductions in PD with cognitive impairment or dementia, as opposed to PD alone. A study of dopamine synthesis found reductions in the striatum, midbrain, and anterior cingulate (111), and an investigation of AChE activity reported greater reductions in PDD than in AD (112).

Frontotemporal Dementia

FTD, another neurodegenerative dementia, is of increasing interest in geropsychiatry, and it has been the focus of a number of structural and functional neuroimaging studies. FTD is thought to be related to two other less common neurodegenerative dementias, semantic dementia (SD) and primary progressive aphasia (PPA), with some patients manifesting overlapping symptoms. It also includes Pick's disease. Neuroimaging studies of FTD are somewhat challenging to interpret, in part because they have often included patients with symptoms or diagnoses of SD and/or PPA, and subgroups have not always been distinguished. Nevertheless, the following findings have emerged. Corresponding to FTD's frontal lobe-based symptoms, atrophy in this area has generally been found (113) (Figure 8-1), and in some studies is especially prominent on the right. Superior and lateral temporal lobe and hippocampal atrophy (114), along with an increased rate of generalized atrophy, has also been demonstrated. The degree of hippocampal atrophy as well as that found in related medial temporal lobe structures is probably less than in AD. WMH abnormalities have also been reported, with an extent indistinguishable from that seen in AD and VaD (115). Functional studies have generally identified frontal and sometimes temporal or more widespread hypoperfusion/hypometabolism (116).

Normal Pressure Hydrocephalus

Imaging abnormalities in NPH have been appreciated for decades. The hallmark of NPH is ventriculomegaly disproportionate to sulcal enlargement, especially in the frontal and temporal horns of the lateral ventricles. While this finding can be readily seen on CT, other findings can be better identified (or in some cases only identified) on MRI. These include an enlarged cerebral aqueduct, upward bowing of the corpus callosum, and flattening of the cortex against the inner table of the skull. Because the risk of NPH treatment (ventricular shunting) is substantial, a number of studies have investigated structural and functional imaging correlates of this condition's clinical features, as well as treatment response or the lack of it. The primary aim of these studies has been to identify potential markers of shunt-related benefit. Among such markers identifiable in the workup phase are CBF change pre/post high-volume lumbar puncture, and WMH-related parameters. Treatment-related markers include the degree of reduction in ventricular volume after shunting, as well as CBF and CMRglu changes. Hurley et al. have conducted an excellent review of the established uses of MRI (117).

Uncommon Dementias

The less common causes of dementias have had correspondingly limited imaging attention. These conditions include progressive supranuclear palsy, corticobasal degeneration, Huntington's disease, multiple sclerosis, benign and malignant neoplasms, epilepsy, Creutzfeldt-Jakob disease, and viral diseases (e.g., HIV dementia and the viral encephalitides), among others. Although intriguing findings have been reported, either no pathognomonic signs or clinically useful tools have emerged, or the disorders do not primarily affect the elderly. One other condition that does cause dementia in seniors, though, subdural hematoma, will be discussed with regard to diagnosis.

Mild Cognitive Impairment

Great interest has developed in recent years in the clinical and neurobiological aspects of mild cognitive disturbances in the elderly. MCI, the most common form of these disturbances, often progresses to frank AD. Recognition of MCI as a discrete subclinical entity has focused and accelerated research (118), including a substantial number of imaging studies. This work, which has usually compared MCI to normal aging and/or AD, has been comprised of mostly cross-sectional studies, but a few longitudinal investigations have also been performed. The majority of studies have been structural, but CMRglu and CBF studies have also been conducted. The aim of this work has generally been descriptive, but a few studies have addressed some important and unsettled questions about MCI, such as whether imaging parameters can predict conversion to AD, and whether they can explain the neural basis of memory impairment. The body of MCI-related imaging research has been comprehensively reviewed by Wolf et al. (119) and also by Atiya and colleagues (62).

The principal finding of structural studies is reduced hippocampal and ERC size compared to normal controls. Volume losses of 12% in the hippocampus and 21% in the ERC have been reported in one representative study (120). Other structures, including the amygdala, posterior cingulate and precuneus, thalamus and caudate, as well as gray matter volume quantified by VBM (121), have also shown size reductions (119). Both baseline hippocampal atrophy (122) and a relatively greater rate of hippocampal atrophy during longitudinal follow-up (123) have been found to predict conversion to AD, as have ERC (124) and cingulate atrophy (125). The relative prevalence of WMH in MCI is uncertain, but their extent has also been associated with conversion to AD (126). Functional studies have revealed reduced CMRglu/CBF in the temporoparietal cortex, the posterior cingulate (127), and the hippocampus (128). Posterior cingulate flow reduction (129) and left temporal CMRglu reduction (130) have also been reported to predict conversion to AD.

Mood Disorders

The various mood disorders represent another psychopathologic domain that has received enormous neuroimaging research attention. Extensive research, mainly conducted on nonelderly adults, has explored a number of specific disorders, including major depression, dysthymia, bipolar disorder, and the anxiety disorders. Besides description, these studies' results have contributed to the formulation of provocative hypotheses about the mechanisms underlying mood disorders, particularly depression. These hypotheses postulate interlinked anatomical and chemical disturbances in putative neural circuits subserving mood and affect (131). They further assert that focal atrophy of key brain structures, mediated by hypercortisolemia and excitatory amino acid action, either causes depressive symptoms and recurrence/chronicity, or results from episodes of depression. In the elderly, other factors could be operative, for example, hypertension and cardiovascular disease, which are associated with increased WMH. The role of vascular factors in particular has been highlighted as a prominent cause of geriatric depression (GD), under the term *vascular depression* (132,133). The relative role of atrophy and vascular factors, and the importance of specific aspects of vascular lesions, for example their side, location (cortical [and specifically, which lobe] or subcortical [and specifically, gray matter structures or white matter]), and type (completed infarct or WMH), in causing GD is uncertain and debated (134,135).

Geriatrically oriented imaging studies have largely focused on major depression, with some work also being done on depression due to medical disorders, particularly neurological conditions (e.g., poststroke depression and AD). As with the cognitive disorders, both structural and functional studies have been conducted. The previously discussed imaging research defining age-related anatomic and physiologic brain changes (i.e., atrophy, WMH, and neurotransmitter-related changes) has strongly influenced GD research by clarifying the normal substrate from which depression-related changes can be considered deviations. One interesting variable unique to GD research that has had some neuroimaging attention is the distinction between early-onset recurrent depression and late-onset depression. Both types of patients are commonly encountered, and neuroimaging studies have suggested differences between them, which may relate at least in part to cerebrovascular risk factors and disease.

Kumar (136) has discussed and Narayan et al. (137) have reviewed the key findings of structural imaging research in GD. These findings include focal brain atrophy and increased WMH as compared to appropriate controls. In the setting of preservation of global brain volume, atrophy of key structures implicated in the above-referenced mood-subserving neural circuits has often been observed, for example, the frontal lobe (138), right hippocampus (139), and caudate. Some studies have localized frontal atrophy in late-life depression to the orbitofrontal (140) or middle-frontal (141) gyri, and frontal atrophy has also been noted in late-life minor depression (138). Some but not all studies have suggested that hippocampal atrophy may correlate more strongly with recurrence or lifetime extent of depression than age itself (142). At the same time, intriguingly, left hippocampal atrophy in GD has been linked to subsequent development of AD (143), and is a well-recognized clinical phenomenon. Some but not all studies have found WMH to be more common in GD (144), and particularly prominent in the frontal lobes (145). Greater WMH extent in GD has also been correlated with late-onset depression (146), more cognitive impairment (147), poor treatment response (148), impaired activities of daily living (149), and even increased mortality (150). How much of the effect of WMH is due to CVD and/or medical burden remains uncertain.

A number of functional imaging studies of mood disorders have also been performed in adults over the years, again mainly focused on depression (151). Very few of these studies, however, have specifically addressed GD. The research on nonelderly adults has involved correlation of CBF/CMRglu and neurotransmission-related parameters with both the existence of depression and the presence of various clinically important features of depression, for example severity, specific symptoms, and treatment response. While reports have been sometimes discrepant, certain findings have emerged with fair consistency, including resting (mainly left-sided) dorsolateral prefrontal cortex, and anterior cingulate CBF and/or CMRglu reductions (152). Some regional abnormalities have been reported to normalize with successful treatment, while others may be trait markers. Specifically, anterior cingulate hypermetabolism may predict treatment response (153). No definite CBF/CMRglu correlate of disease severity or depression type (unipolar versus bipolar) has as yet been identified, but recent research has demonstrated various CBF/CMRglu changes attendant to treatment with specific contemporary antidepressants and psychotherapy, and fairly consistent frontal lobe CBF reductions following electroconvulsive therapy. Limited but fascinating neurotransmission research has also focused on the serotonin system. This work has specifically examined 5HT transporter (5HTT), $5HT_{1A}$ (154), and $5HT_{2/2A}$ receptor differences in depression. Significantly reduced 5HTT availability (155) but variable postsynaptic receptor binding has been reported. Finally, the response of these systems to antidepressant treatment has been studied.

Against this backdrop, the extremely limited geriatrically focused functional imaging research, most recently reviewed by Nobler et al. (47), has rather consistently identified more extensive CBF/CMRglu reductions than in younger adults, involving not only the frontal lobes (156) and subcortical gray matter structures, but also, at least in late-onset GD, the temporal lobes as well (157,158). One small $5HT_{2A}$ receptor binding study (159) did not reveal differences in the cortex, striatum, or hippocampus/amygdaloid complex in GD as compared to controls.

Psychosis

The final major psychopathologic domain that has received substantial imaging attention is psychosis. As with other disorders, both structural (volume and WMH parameters) and functional (CBF/CMRglu and neurotransmission parameters) studies have been conducted. Here as well, the great majority of studies have been conducted on young and middle-aged adults and, not surprisingly, they have principally targeted schizophrenia. While it is impossible to summarize the findings of this voluminous research here, a few key findings stand out. For example, volume reductions in specific temporal and frontal lobes areas have been repeatedly demonstrated. In the elderly, late-onset schizophrenia (LOS) and paraphrenia diagnoses are important areas for imaging research. Overall, only a few geriatrically oriented studies of psychosis have been performed, mainly focusing on LOS. Characteristics of this condition identified through MRI include ventriculomegaly and larger thalami, as compared to aged early-onset schizophrenics (160). Smaller size of the anterior part of the superior temporal gyrus compared to controls has also been reported (161). Of note, the last finding has been made frequently in younger adult schizophrenics. Finally, LOS has been differentiated from late-life depression and bipolar depression (162).

CLINICAL APPLICATION OF NEUROIMAGING

The preceding discussion has focused on the nature of neuroimaging methods and the resultant body of data acquired about aging and geriatric mental disorders. The goal of the present section is to review the clinical use of imaging modalities in geropsychiatry, as well as research aimed at determining the methods' value in this setting. Arguably the most frequent neurodiagnostic challenge geropsychiatrists encounter is the need to identify the cause of cognitive impairment. Unfortunately, the primary symptom of late-life cognitive dysfunction, short-term memory loss, is nonspecific. It also shows variable severity, sometimes fluctuates, and is often accompanied by confounding symptoms such as depressed mood. Also, no laboratory tests are available with results pathognomonic of the specific cognitive disorders being considered, for example AD. In this context, the potential of neuroimaging to provide valuable objective information about brain structure and/or function has long been recognized. Such information might inform treatment-related decision-making and also guide clinicians in communication with patients and their families about relevant illness parameters (e.g., course and prognosis).

Since AD is the predominant cause of significant late-life cognitive impairment in most developed countries, neuroimaging is commonly used in evaluating patients with AD as the focus (163). Two clinical goals exist: excluding certain alternate etiologies (differential diagnosis), and distinguishing AD from normal aging or MCI. When cognitive impairment is already present at the established dementia level, only the first goal matters; however, in milder cases both goals are pursued simultaneously. Structural and functional methods have been applied to both goals, alone and in combination. The use of structural imaging in dementia diagnosis is a standard radiologic practice activity, endorsed by relevant professional organizations (164) and consequently accepted by most payors. Functional imaging has been relatively less accepted, though it has vocal advocates. In the case of PET, reimbursement has also been limited. For certain differential diagnostic distinctions, quantitative image processing methods have been developed to augment radiologists' visual inspection skills. These tools have been used in both structural and functional modalities.

The main alternate dementing disorders amenable to neuroimaging differentiation from AD are VaD, NPH, neoplasm, subdural hematoma (SDH), FTD, and DLB. These conditions have specific structural or functional imaging signatures, which radiologists identify clinically by image inspection. For example, multiple cortical or subcortical infarcts (CT or MRI), extensive white matter density reductions (CT), hyperintensities (MRI) in the Binswanger's disease pattern, or multiple foci of CBF/CMRglu reduction (Figure 8-4) support the diagnosis of VaD. Using WMH extent alone to diagnose VaD, however, is problematic, and geropsychiatrists should be aware that this linkage is all too common in radiologic reports. Ventriculomegaly disproportionate to sulcal enlargement (CT or MRI) or excessive aqueductal CSF flow on phase-contrast cine-MRI (165) suggests NPH. Subdural blood collection (CT or MRI) defines SDH (Figure 8-5), and marked frontal lobe atrophy (CT or MRI) (Figure 8-1) or CBF/CMRglu reduction (Figure 8-4) favors FTD. Occipital lobe hypometabolism or blood flow decrement indicates DLB (166).

Distinguishing AD from aging/MCI is a very different process. It involves either visual rating or computer-assisted measurement of atrophy or CBF/CMRglu reductions in specific brain areas. In structural imaging, the hippocampus and ERC are the main regions currently used (167), because whole brain and lobar atrophy, as well as ventricular size, has not proven reliable. In functional imaging, mainly parameters of the temporoparietal cortex CBF/CMRglu reduction have been assessed (168). Despite progress in automating volumetric and physiological measurements, neither structural nor functional methods are as yet widely used clinically.

Many studies over the years have been aimed at defining the clinical value of the various imaging modalities, both for separating AD from normal aging/MCI and aiding differential diagnosis. These studies have been increasingly

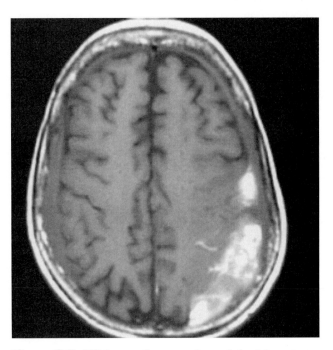

Figure 8-5 MR image demonstrating subdural hematoma. (courtesy of Robert Kessler MD/Curtis Wushensky MD)

influenced by concepts and methods arising from the evolving discipline of evidence-based medicine (EBM). As applied to diagnostic tests such as neuroimaging, EBM research goals are to determine the validity of proposed tests, their importance, and whether they can be applied in specific patient care or screening settings. Among the key elements of validity assessment are whether a proposed diagnostic test was compared to a gold standard, and whether its performance was evaluated in a representative sample of individuals likely to undergo it. Importance is determined quantitatively by traditional measures (e.g., sensitivity and specificity), and newer ones (e.g., positive and negative likelihood ratios, LR+ and LR−, respectively). The value of a proposed test in specific clinical/screening situations is assessed in terms of practical considerations (e.g., availability and cost), through quantitative measures (pretest and posttest probabilities), and with regard to the test's impact level on patient management.

Structural and functional imaging methods have both been subjected to EBM analysis, individually and in the aggregate (169), and their cost-effectiveness in diagnostic use has also been considered. Two types of standards have been used. The gold standard for evaluating imaging, also called ideal evidence, is postmortem neuropathology, but very few correlative imaging/pathological studies have been conducted, largely due to the slow course of AD and the speed of advances in imaging. Consequently, most studies have compared imaging findings to the established clinical diagnostic approaches, NINCDS/ADRDA criteria (170) and DSM-IV. This standard is called strong evidence. The clinical criteria themselves are reported to have sensitivities of 92% and 79% in academic and community-based settings, respectively; corresponding specificity figures are 98% and 84% (171). Thus, a key question is whether imaging adds value (i.e., improves accuracy) to the traditional approach.

CT-based exclusion of NPH, astrocytoma, and SDH was found to be moderately efficient (LR+ 5–10) (172), but these disorders are uncommon. Assessments of atrophy were generally less efficient (LR+ 0–5), but identification of infarcts/VaD was more so. One MRI study, however, reported a robust LR+ (10.24) using severe or asymmetric frontal atrophy to distinguish FTD from AD or VaD (173). MRI-based visual rating and/or volumetry of hippocampus or ERC atrophy to distinguish AD from normal/MCI has shown an LR+ range of 2 to 8 in about 20 studies (174). Perhaps surprisingly, quantitative approaches were not superior to rating methods and were definitely more cumbersome. A substantial number of studies exploring SPECT and PET-based discrimination of AD from normal/MCI have been performed, including a few with pathologic correlation (175). In general, LR+ in the 1 to 4 range was calculated for differential diagnosis and distinction of AD from aging/MCI (the latter being lower). Importantly, the functional methods were not in general superior to either structural imaging or the clinical diagnostic system, and they also did not add predictive value to structural imaging

when combined with it, except perhaps in discriminating DLB from AD.

Other clinical uses of imaging in geropsychiatry include the evaluation of causes of delirium, refractory depression, and new-onset psychosis. Although not a primary diagnostic modality in these settings, imaging can be helpful if answers are not revealed by other means. For example, the data presented above regarding WMH in GD (increased prevalence, frontal lobe predominance, and poor treatment response) suggest a role for structural imaging in this setting.

EMERGING TECHNIQUES AND APPLICATIONS

Magnetic Resonance Imaging

A number of MRI techniques currently under development will likely impact geropsychiatry significantly in coming years. These include diffusion tensor imaging (DTI), diffusion weighted imaging (DWI), perfusion imaging by arterial spin labeling (ASL), magnetization transfer imaging (MTI), and phase contrast cine-MRI, among others.

DTI detects nonrandom water diffusion in tissue, which may indicate white matter pathology (176) in a different way than established T2-weighted pulse sequences. Of interest, one study has identified DTI abnormalities in refractory late-life depression (177). DWI reveals tissue abnormalities associated with very recent infarction and might be of value in evaluating acutely altered mental status.

ASL-based perfusion imaging maps CBF by subtracting T1-weighted images from images representing the delivery of magnetically labeled water to the brain, in conjunction with several mathematical maneuvers (12). It is highly correlated with PET-determined CBF and has advantages over the blood oxygenation level dependent method for fMRI, especially at high field strength (12).

MTI detects differences between free tissue water and macromolecularly bound water. While it has only been applied so far to a very limited degree in geropsychiatry, one study found the free/bound water ratio to be reduced in AD and MCI (178), and another identified MTI abnormalities in geriatric depression (179).

Phase contrast cine-MRI is a specialized sequence for quantifying parameters of CSF flow, which is being explored in the diagnosis of NPH.

The ascendancy of high field strength scanners (generally 3 Tesla or more) represents another significant development in MRI. The chief virtue of these scanners—increased signal-to-noise ratio—enables greater spatial resolution, briefer scanning times, and better image quality with certain newer pulse sequences. The application of fMRI to questions in aging and geriatric mental disorders is particularly exciting. For example, the effects of both aging and dementing disorders on key cognitive operations (e.g., working memory) are being probed (180). Finally, important advances in structural imaging data analysis methods are occurring. Among them is the advent of sophisticated and automated atlas-based morphometric systems, increasingly based on probabilistic approaches to interindividual variation and creatively addressing the effects of aging (181). Of note, such systems are enabling structural imaging parameters to be explored effectively as outcome measures for clinical trials in neuropsychiatric disorders (182).

Positron Emission Tomography/Single Photon Emission Computed Tomography

Advances in functional imaging methodology are also occurring rapidly. These include hybrid PET/CT scanners and ever more powerful imaging agents for components of neuro-transmission. Improved tracers for both elements already under study (e.g., the dopamine and serotonin transporters) and systems previously unable to be assessed (e.g., the glutamate N-methyl-D-aspartate receptor) (183) are under development. Neurotransmission imaging agents, as well as CBF/CMRglu (184), are also being used to improve the drug development process in geropsychiatry (185) by adding biologically-based outcome measures (e.g., neural mechanisms of psychotropic drug action) to the traditional measures of what has been historically a clinically-based system. Finally, of exceptional interest, the design and testing of tracers for amyloid deposition (186,187) and neurofibrillary tangle accumulation (188) is proceeding rapidly (189). Human studies have begun (Figure 8-6), and much progress can be anticipated.

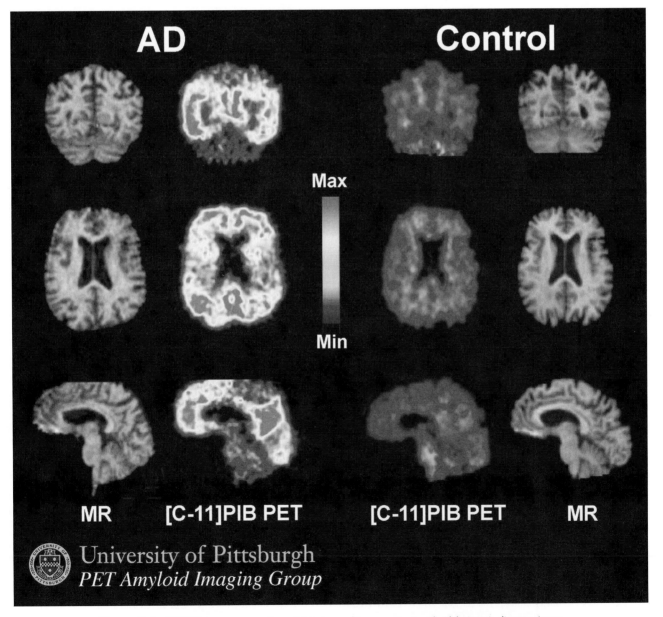

Figure 8-6   PET PIB appearance of amyloid plaque from a patient with Alzheimer's disease. (courtesy of William Klunk MD, PhD and Chester Mathis PhD, University of Pittsburgh School of Medicine)

SUMMARY

In the several decades since the advent of modern neuroimaging, tremendous advances have occurred in methodology, both for structural and functional imaging purposes. Steady improvements in spatial resolution now permit detailed study of small brain regions. Important domains of cerebral physiology such as blood flow and glucose metabolism have been clarified. Aging and geropsychiatric disorders have been a major focus of the application of neuroimaging methods, and a considerable body of knowledge has developed about structure and function in aging and the cognitive disorders. Some data, if less, have been developed about mood disorders (particularly depression), as well as psychosis. The future is increasingly bright for the further application of evolving methods to important questions in geropsychiatry. The impact of methods such as the imaging of amyloid plaques in AD, though presently in their infancy, may prove to be revolutionary in coming decades.

ACKNOWLEDGEMENT

The assistance of Robert Kessler, MD, Roentgen Professor of Radiology, Vanderbilt University Medical Center, in reviewing the accuracy of information about neuroradiologic methods and practices is gratefully acknowledged.

REFERENCES

1. Orrison WW Jr, ed. *Neuroimaging*. Philadelphia: W.B. Saunders Company; 2000.
2. Fu CH, Murray R, Russell T, Senior C, Weinberger DR, eds. *Neuroimaging in Psychiatry*. Philadelphia: Taylor & Francis; 2003.
3. Ng V, Barker GJ, Hendler T, eds. *Psychiatric Neuroimaging*. Burke, VA: IOS Press; 2003.
4. Bushong SC. *Magnetic Resonance Imaging*. 3rd Ed. St. Louis: Mosby; 2003.
5. Phelps ME, ed. *PET—Molecular Imaging and Its Biological Applications*. New York: Springer-Verlag; 2004.
6. Meltzer CC, ed. Neurologic applications of positron emission tomography. In: Drayer BP, series ed. *Neuroimaging Clinics of North America*. 2003;13(4). Philadelphia: W.B. Saunders.
7. Dougherty DD, Rauch SL, Rosenbaum JF, eds. *Essentials of Neuroimaging for Clinical Practice*. Arlington, VA: American Psychiatric Publishing; 2003.
8. Leuchter AF, Holschneider DP. Electroencephalography. In: Sadavoy J, Jarvik LF, Grossberg GT, Meyers BS, eds. *Comprehensive Textbook of Geriatric Psychiatry*. New York: W.W. Norton; 2004:429–446.
9. Talairach J, Tournoux P. *Co-Planar Stereotaxic Atlas of the Human Brain: 3-D Proportional System: An Approach to Cerebral Imaging*. New York: Thieme Medical Publishers; 1988.
10. Brandão LA, Domingues RC. *MR Spectroscopy of the Brain*. Philadelphia: Lippincott Williams & Wilkins; 2003.
11. Huettel SA, Song AW, McCarthy G, eds. *Functional Magnetic Resonance Imaging*. Sunderland, MA: Sinauer Associates; 2004.
12. Kessler RM. Imaging methods for evaluating brain function in man. *Neurobiol Aging*. 2003;24(Suppl 1):S21–S35.
13. Hashemi RH, Bradley WG, Lisanti CJ. *MRI: The Basics*. Philadelphia: Lippincott Williams & Wilkins; 2004.
14. van Dyck CH, Lin CH, Smith EO, et al. Comparison of technetium-99m-HMPAO and technetium-99m-ECD cerebral SPECT images in Alzheimer's disease. *J Nucl Med*. 1996;37(11):1749–1755.
15. Woods RP, Mazziotta JC, Cherry SR. MRI-PET registration with automated algorithm. *J Comput Assist Tomogr*. 1993;17(4):536–546.
16. Toga AW, Thompson PM. New approaches in brain morphometry. *Am J Geriatr Psychiatry*. 2002;10(1):13–23.
17. Fox NC, Schott JM. Imaging cerebral atrophy: normal ageing to Alzheimer's disease. *Lancet*. 2004;363(9406):392–394.
18. Good CD, Ashburner J, Frackowiak RS. Computational neuroanatomy: new perspectives for neuroradiology. *Rev Neurol (Paris)*. 2001;157(8–9 Pt 1):797–806.
19. Friston KJ, Ashburner J, Frith CD, Poline J-B, Heather JD, Frackowiak RSJ. Spatial registration and normalization of images. *Hum Brain Mapp*. 1995;2:165–189.
20. Ashburner J, Friston KJ. Voxel-based morphometry—the methods. *Neuroimage*. 2000;11(6 Pt 1):805–821.
21. Zatz LM, Jernigan TL, Ahumada AJ Jr. Changes on computed cranial tomography with aging: intracranial fluid volume. *AJNR Am J Neuroradiol*. 1982;3(1):1–11.
22. Kessler RM, Ellis JR, Eden M. Analysis of emission tomographic scan data: limitations imposed by resolution and background. *J Comput Assist Tomogr*. 1984;8:514–522.
23. Meltzer CC, Kinahan PE, Greer PJ, et al. Comparative evaluation of MR-based partial-volume correction schemes for PET. *J Nucl Med*. 1999;40(12):2053–2065.
24. Schwartz M, Creasey H, Grady CL, et al. Computed tomographic analysis of brain morphometrics in 30 healthy men, aged 21 to 81 years. *Ann Neurol*. 1985;17(2):146–157.
25. Jernigan TL, Archibald SL, Berhow MT, Sowell ER, Foster DS, Hesselink JR. Cerebral structure on MRI, part I: localization of age-related changes. *Biol Psychiatry*. 1991;29(1):55–67.
26. Coffey CE, Wilkinson WE, Parashos IA, et al. Quantitative cerebral anatomy of the aging human brain: a cross-sectional study using magnetic resonance imaging. *Neurology*. 1992;42(3 Pt 1):527–536.
27. De Leon MJ, George AE, Golomb J, et al. Frequency of hippocampal formation atrophy in normal aging and Alzheimer's disease. *Neurobiol Aging*. 1997;18(1):1–11.
28. Gur RC, Mozley PD, Resnick SM, et al. Gender differences in age effect on brain atrophy measured by magnetic resonance imaging. *Proc Natl Acad Sci USA*. 1991;88(7):2845–2849.
29. Manolio TA, Kronmal RA, Burke GL, et al. Magnetic resonance abnormalities and cardiovascular disease in older adults. The Cardiovascular Health Study. *Stroke*. 1994;25(2):318–327.
30. Jack CR Jr, Petersen RC, Xu Y, et al. Rate of medial temporal lobe atrophy in typical aging and Alzheimer's disease. *Neurology*. 1998;51(4):993–999.
31. Resnick SM, Pham DL, Kraut MA, Zonderman AB, Davatzikos C. Longitudinal magnetic resonance imaging studies of older adults: a shrinking brain. *J Neurosci*. 2003;23(8):3295–3301.
32. Roman GC. Age-associated white matter lesions and dementia: are these lesions causal or casual? *Arch Neurol*. 2004;61(10):1503–1504.
33. Soderlund H, Nyberg L, Adolfsson R, Nilsson LG, Launer LJ. High prevalence of white matter hyperintensities in normal aging: relation to blood pressure and cognition. *Cortex*. 2003;39(4–5):1093–1105.
34. Scheltens P, Barkhof F, Leys D, Wolters EC, Ravid R, Kamphorst W. Histopathologic correlates of white matter changes on MRI in Alzheimer's disease and normal aging. *Neurology*. 1995;45(5):883–888.
35. Fazekas F, Schmidt R, Scheltens P. Pathophysiologic mechanisms in the development of age-related white matter changes of the brain. *Dement Geriatr Cogn Disord*. 1998;9(Suppl 1):2–5.
36. Longstreth WT Jr, Manolio TA, Arnold A, et al. Clinical correlates of white matter findings on cranial magnetic resonance imaging of 3301 elderly people. The Cardiovascular Health Study. *Stroke*. 1996;27(8):1274–1282.
37. Awad IA, Spetzler RF, Hodak JA, Awad CA, Carey R. Incidental subcortical lesions identified on magnetic resonance imaging in the elderly. I. Correlation with age and cerebrovascular risk factors. *Stroke*. 1986;17(6):1084–1089.
38. de Leeuw FE, de Groot JC, Achten E, et al. Prevalence of cerebral white matter lesions in elderly people: a population based magnetic resonance imaging study. The Rotterdam Scan Study. *J Neurol Neurosurg Psychiatry*. 2001;70(1):9–14.

39. Schmidt R, Enzinger C, Ropele S, et al. Progression of cerebral white matter lesions: 6-year results of the Austrian Stroke Prevention Study. *Lancet.* 2003;361(9374):2046–2048.
40. Bartzokis G, Mintz J, Sultzer D, et al. In vivo MR evaluation of age-related increases in brain iron. *AJNR Am J Neuroradiol.* 1994;15(6):1129–1138.
41. Leenders KL, Perani D, Lammertsma AA, et al. Cerebral blood flow, blood volume and oxygen utilization. Normal values and effect of age. *Brain.* 1990;113(Pt 1):27–47.
42. Duara R, Margolin RA, Robertson-Tchabo EA, et al. Cerebral glucose utilization, as measured with positron emission tomography in 21 resting healthy men between the ages of 21 and 83 years. *Brain.* 1983;106(Pt 3):761–775.
43. Moeller JR, Ishikawa T, Dhawan V, et al. The metabolic topography of normal aging. *J Cereb Blood Flow Metab.* 1996;16(3):385–398.
44. Meltzer CC, Cantwell MN, Greer PJ, et al. Does cerebral blood flow decline in healthy aging? A PET study with partial-volume correction. *J Nucl Med.* 2000;41(11):1842–1848.
45. Mozley PD, Sadek AM, Alavi A, et al. Effects of aging on the cerebral distribution of technetium-99m hexamethylpropylene amine oxime in healthy humans. *Eur J Nucl Med.* 1997;24(7):754–761.
46. Meltzer CC, Becker JT, Price JC, Moses-Kolko E. Positron emission tomography imaging of the aging brain. *Neuroimaging Clin N Am.* 2003;13(4):759–767.
47. Nobler MS, Mann JJ, Sackeim HA. Serotonin, cerebral blood flow, and cerebral metabolic rate in geriatric major depression and normal aging. *Brain Res Brain Res Rev.* 1999;30(3):250–263.
48. Kuhl DE, Minoshima S, Fessler JA, et al. In vivo mapping of cholinergic terminals in normal aging, Alzheimer's disease, and Parkinson's disease. *Ann Neurol.* 1996;40(3):399–410.
49. Zubieta JK, Koeppe RA, Frey KA, et al. Assessment of muscarinic receptor concentrations in aging and Alzheimer disease with [11C]NMPB and PET. *Synapse.* 2001;39(4):275–287.
50. Wang Y, Chan GL, Holden JE, et al. Age-dependent decline of dopamine D1 receptors in human brain: a PET study. *Synapse.* 1998;30(1):56–61.
51. Wong DF, Young D, Wilson PD, Meltzer CC, Gjedde A. Quantification of neuroreceptors in the living human brain: III. D2-like dopamine receptors: theory, validation, and changes during normal aging. *J Cereb Blood Flow Metab.* 1997;17(3):316–330.
52. Volkow ND, Ding YS, Fowler JS, et al. Dopamine transporters decrease with age. *J Nucl Med.* 1996;37(4):554–559.
53. van Dyck CH, Malison RT, Seibyl JP, et al. Age-related decline in central serotonin transporter availability with [123I]β-CIT SPECT. *Neurobiol Aging.* 2000;21(4):497–501.
54. Tauscher J, Verhoeff NP, Christensen BK, et al. Serotonin 5-HT$_{1A}$ receptor binding potential declines with age as measured by [11C]WAY-100635 and PET. *Neuropsychopharmacology.* 2001;24(5):522–530.
55. Meltzer CC, Smith G, Price JC, et al. Reduced binding of [18F]altanserin to serotonin type 2A receptors in aging: persistence of effect after partial volume correction. *Brain Res.* 1998;813(1):167–171.
56. Fox JH, Topel JL, Huckman MS. Use of computerized tomography in senile dementia. *J Neurol Neurosurg Psychiatry.* 1975;38(10):948–953.
57. Creasey H, Schwartz M, Frederickson H, Haxby JV, Rapoport SI. Quantitative computed tomography in dementia of the Alzheimer type. *Neurology.* 1986;36(12):1563–1568.
58. Erkinjuntti T, Sulkava R, Palo J, Ketonen L. White matter low attenuation on CT in Alzheimer's disease. *Arch Gerontol Geriatr.* 1989;8(1):95–104.
59. Jobst KA, Smith AD, Szatmari M, et al. Detection in life of confirmed Alzheimer's disease using a simple measurement of medial temporal lobe atrophy by computed tomography. *Lancet.* 1992;340(8829):1179–1183.
60. DeCarli C, Haxby JV, Gillette JA, Teichberg D, Rapoport SI, Schapiro MB. Longitudinal changes in lateral ventricular volume in patients with dementia of the Alzheimer type. *Neurology.* 1992;42(10):2029–2036.
61. Smith AD, Jobst KA. Use of structural imaging to study the progression of Alzheimer's disease. *Br Med Bull.* 1996;52(3):575–586.
62. Atiya M, Hyman BT, Albert MS, Killiany R. Structural magnetic resonance imaging in established and prodromal Alzheimer disease: a review. *Alzheimer Dis Assoc Disord.* 2003;17(3):177–195.
63. Jack CR Jr, Petersen RC, O'Brien PC, Tangalos EG. MR-based hippocampal volumetry in the diagnosis of Alzheimer's disease. *Neurology.* 1992;42(1):183–188.
64. Juottonen K, Laakso MP, Insausti R, et al. Volumes of the entorhinal and perirhinal cortices in Alzheimer's disease. *Neurobiol Aging.* 1998;19(1):15–22.
65. Jack CR Jr, Petersen RC, Xu YC, et al. Medial temporal atrophy on MRI in normal aging and very mild Alzheimer's disease. *Neurology.* 1997;49(3):786–794.
66. Du AT, Schuff N, Zhu XP, et al. Atrophy rates of entorhinal cortex in AD and normal aging. *Neurology.* 2003;60(3):481–486.
67. O'Brien JT, Paling S, Barber R, et al. Progressive brain atrophy on serial MRI in dementia with Lewy bodies, AD, and vascular dementia. *Neurology.* 2001;56(10):1386–1388.
68. Scheltens P, Barkhof F, Valk J, et al. White matter lesions on magnetic resonance imaging in clinically diagnosed Alzheimer's disease. Evidence for heterogeneity. *Brain.* 1992;115(Pt 3):735–748.
69. Fazekas F, Kapeller P, Schmidt R, Offenbacher H, Payer F, Fazekas G. The relation of cerebral magnetic resonance signal hyperintensities to Alzheimer's disease. *J Neurol Sci.* 1996;142(1–2):121–125.
70. Kumar A, Yousem D, Souder E, et al. High-intensity signals in Alzheimer's disease without cerebrovascular risk factors: a magnetic resonance imaging evaluation. *Am J Psychiatry.* 1992;149(2):248–250.
71. Kozachuk WE, DeCarli C, Schapiro MB, Wagner EE, Rapoport SI, Horwitz B. White matter hyperintensities in dementia of Alzheimer's type and in healthy subjects without cerebrovascular risk factors. A magnetic resonance imaging study. *Arch Neurol.* 1990;47(12):1306–1310.
72. Bronge L. Magnetic resonance imaging in dementia. A study of brain white matter changes. *Acta Radiol Suppl.* 2002;(428):1–32.
73. Frackowiak RS, Pozzilli C, Legg NJ, et al. Regional cerebral oxygen supply and utilization in dementia. A clinical and physiological study with oxygen-15 and positron tomography. *Brain.* 1981;104(Pt 4):753–778.
74. Benson DF, Kuhl DE, Hawkins RA, Phelps ME, Cummings JL, Tsai SY. The fluorodeoxyglucose 18F scan in Alzheimer's disease and multi-infarct dementia. *Arch Neurol.* 1983;40(12):711–714.
75. Foster NL, Chase TN, Mansi L, et al. Cortical abnormalities in Alzheimer's disease. *Ann Neurol.* 1984;16(6):649–654.
76. de Leon MJ, Ferris SH, George AE, et al. Positron emission tomographic studies of aging and Alzheimer disease. *AJNR Am J Neuroradiol.* 1983;4(3):568–571.
77. Minoshima S, Foster NL, Kuhl DE. Posterior cingulate cortex in Alzheimer's disease. *Lancet.* 1994;344(8926):895.
78. Grady CL, Haxby JV, Horwitz B, et al. Longitudinal study of the early neuropsychological and cerebral metabolic changes in dementia of the Alzheimer type. *J Clin Exp Neuropsychol.* 1988;10(5):576–596.
79. Jagust WJ, Haan MN, Eberling JL, Wolfe N, Reed BR. Functional imaging predicts cognitive decline in Alzheimer's disease. *J Neuroimaging.* 1996;6(3):156–160.
80. Holman BL, Johnson KA, Gerada B, Carvalho PA, Satlin A. The scintigraphic appearance of Alzheimer's disease: a prospective study using technetium-99m-HMPAO SPECT. *J Nucl Med.* 1992;33(2):181–185.
81. Herholz K, Schopphoff H, Schmidt M, et al. Direct comparison of spatially normalized PET and SPECT scans in Alzheimer's disease. *J Nucl Med.* 2002;43(1):21–26.
82. Duara R, Barker WW, Chang J, Yoshii F, Loewenstein DA, Pascal S. Viability of neocortical function shown in behavioral activation state PET studies in Alzheimer disease. *J Cereb Blood Flow Metab.* 1992;12(6):927–934.
83. Kuhl DE, Koeppe RA, Minoshima S, et al. In vivo mapping of cerebral acetylcholinesterase activity in aging and Alzheimer's disease. *Neurology.* 1999;52(4):691–699.
84. Nordberg A, Hartvig P, Lilja A, et al. Decreased uptake and binding of 11C-nicotine in brain of Alzheimer patients as visualized by

positron emission tomography. *J Neural Transm Park Dis Dement Sect.* 1990;2(3):215–224.

85. Blin J, Baron JC, Dubois B, et al. Loss of brain 5-HT$_2$ receptors in Alzheimer's disease. In vivo assessment with positron emission tomography and [^{18}F]setoperone. *Brain.* 1993;116(Pt 3): 497–510.

86. Chui H. Vascular dementia, a new beginning: shifting focus from clinical phenotype to ischemic brain injury. *Neurol Clin.* 2000;18(4):951–978.

87. Longstreth WT Jr, Bernick C, Manolio TA, Bryan N, Jungreis CA, Price TR. Lacunar infarcts defined by magnetic resonance imaging of 3660 elderly people: the Cardiovascular Health Study. *Arch Neurol.* 1998;55(9):1217–1225.

88. Erkinjuntti T, Bowler JV, DeCarli CS, et al. Imaging of static brain lesions in vascular dementia: implications for clinical trials. *Alzheimer Dis Assoc Disord.* 1999;13(Suppl 3):S81–S90.

89. Pohjasvaara T, Mantyla R, Salonen O, et al. MRI correlates of dementia after first clinical ischemic stroke. *J Neurol Sci.* 2000;181(1–2):111–117.

90. Mori E, Ishii K, Hashimoto M, Imamura T, Hirono N, Kitagaki H. Role of functional brain imaging in the evaluation of vascular dementia. *Alzheimer Dis Assoc Disord.* 1999;13(Suppl 3):S91–S101.

91. Tatemichi TK, Desmond DW, Prohovnik I. Strategic infarcts in vascular dementia. A clinical and brain imaging experience. *Arzneimittelforschung.* 1995;45(3A):371–385.

92. Du AT, Schuff N, Laakso MP, et al. Effects of subcortical ischemic vascular dementia and AD on entorhinal cortex and hippocampus. *Neurology.* 2002;58(11):1635–1641.

93. Fein G, Di Sclafani V, Tanabe J, et al. Hippocampal and cortical atrophy predict dementia in subcortical ischemic vascular disease. *Neurology.* 2000;55(11):1626–1635.

94. Revesz T, Hawkins CP, du Boulay EP, Barnard RO, McDonald WI. Pathological findings correlated with magnetic resonance imaging in subcortical arteriosclerotic encephalopathy (Binswanger's disease). *J Neurol Neurosurg Psychiatry.* 1989;52(12):1337–1344.

95. Mielke R, Herholz K, Grond M, Kessler J, Heiss WD. Severity of vascular dementia is related to volume of metabolically impaired tissue. *Arch Neurol.* 1992;49(9):909–913.

96. Mielke R, Heiss WD. Positron emission tomography for diagnosis of Alzheimer's disease and vascular dementia. *J Neural Transm Suppl.* 1998;53:237–250.

97. De Reuck J, Decoo D, Marchau M, Santens P, Lemahieu I, Strijckmans K. Positron emission tomography in vascular dementia. *J Neurol Sci.* 1998;154(1):55–61.

98. Nagga K, Radberg C, Marcusson J. CT brain findings in clinical dementia investigation—underestimation of mixed dementia. *Dement Geriatr Cogn Disord.* 2004;18(1):59–66.

99. Wu CC, Mungas D, Petkov CI, et al. Brain structure and cognition in a community sample of elderly Latinos. *Neurology.* 2002;59(3):383–391.

100. Small GW. Neuroimaging as a diagnostic tool in dementia with Lewy bodies. *Dement Geriatr Cogn Disord.* 2004;17(Suppl 1):25–31.

101. Hashimoto M, Kitagaki H, Imamura T, et al. Medial temporal and whole-brain atrophy in dementia with Lewy bodies: a volumetric MRI study. *Neurology.* 1998;51(2):357–362.

102. Barber R, McKeith IG, Ballard C, Gholkar A, O'Brien JT. A comparison of medial and lateral temporal lobe atrophy in dementia with Lewy bodies and Alzheimer's disease: magnetic resonance imaging volumetric study. *Dement Geriatr Cogn Disord.* 2001;12 (3):198–205.

103. Middelkoop HA, van der Flier WM, Burton EJ, et al. Dementia with Lewy bodies and AD are not associated with occipital lobe atrophy on MRI. *Neurology.* 2001;57(11):2117–2120.

104. Barber R, Scheltens P, Gholkar A, et al. White matter lesions on magnetic resonance imaging in dementia with Lewy bodies, Alzheimer's disease, vascular dementia, and normal aging. *J Neurol Neurosurg Psychiatry.* 1999;67(1):66–72.

105. Albin RL, Minoshima S, D'Amato CJ, Frey KA, Kuhl DA, Sima AA. Fluoro-deoxyglucose positron emission tomography in diffuse Lewy body disease. *Neurology.* 1996;47(2):462–466.

106. Imamura T, Ishii K, Sasaki M, et al. Regional cerebral glucose metabolism in dementia with Lewy bodies and Alzheimer's disease: a comparative study using positron emission tomography. *Neurosci Lett.* 1997;235(1–2):49–52.

107. Hu XS, Okamura N, Arai H, et al. ^{18}F-fluorodopa PET study of striatal dopamine uptake in the diagnosis of dementia with Lewy bodies. *Neurology.* 2000;55(10):1575–1577.

108. Walker Z, Costa DC, Walker RW, et al. Differentiation of dementia with Lewy bodies from Alzheimer's disease using a dopaminergic presynaptic ligand. *J Neurol Neurosurg Psychiatry.* 2002;73 (2):134–140.

109. Camicioli R, Moore MM, Kinney A, Corbridge E, Glassberg K, Kaye JA. Parkinson's disease is associated with hippocampal atrophy. *Mov Disord.* 2003;18(7):784–790.

110. Antonini A, De Notaris R, Benti R, De Gaspari D, Pezzoli G. Perfusion ECD/SPECT in the characterization of cognitive deficits in Parkinson's disease. *Neurol Sci.* 2001;22(1):45–46.

111. Ito K, Nagano-Saito A, Kato T, et al. Striatal and extrastriatal dysfunction in Parkinson's disease with dementia: a 6-[^{18}F]fluoro-L-dopa PET study. *Brain.* 2002;125(Pt 6):1358–1365.

112. Bohnen NI, Kaufer DI, Ivanco LS, et al. Cortical cholinergic function is more severely affected in parkinsonian dementia than in Alzheimer disease: an in vivo positron emission tomographic study. *Arch Neurol.* 2003;60(12):1745–1748.

113. Frisoni GB, Beltramello A, Geroldi C, Weiss C, Bianchetti A, Trabucchi M. Brain atrophy in frontotemporal dementia. *J Neurol Neurosurg Psychiatry.* 1996;61(2):157–165.

114. Boccardi M, Laakso MP, Bresciani L, et al. The MRI pattern of frontal and temporal brain atrophy in fronto-temporal dementia. *Neurobiol Aging.* 2003;24(1):95–103.

115. Varma AR, Laitt R, Lloyd JJ, et al. Diagnostic value of high signal abnormalities on T2 weighted MRI in the differentiation of Alzheimer's, frontotemporal and vascular dementias. *Acta Neurol Scand.* 2002;105(5):355–364.

116. Ishii K, Sakamoto S, Sasaki M, et al. Cerebral glucose metabolism in patients with frontotemporal dementia. *J Nucl Med.* 1998;39(11):1875–1878.

117. Hurley RA, Bradley WG Jr, Latifi HT, Taber KH. Normal pressure hydrocephalus: significance of MRI in a potentially treatable dementia. *J Neuropsychiatry Clin Neurosci.* 1999;11(3): 297–300.

118. Petersen RC, ed. *Mild Cognitive Impairment: Aging to Alzheimer's Disease.* New York: Oxford University Press; 2003.

119. Wolf H, Jelic V, Gertz HJ, Nordberg A, Julin P, Wahlund LO. A critical discussion of the role of neuroimaging in mild cognitive impairment [erratum appears in *Acta Neurol Scand.* 2003;108(Suppl 1):68]. *Acta Neurol Scand.* 2003;(Suppl 179):52–76.

120. Xu Y, Jack CR Jr, O'Brien PC, et al. Usefulness of MRI measures of entorhinal cortex versus hippocampus in AD. *Neurology.* 2000;54(9):1760–1767.

121. Chetelat G, Desgranges B, De La Sayette V, Viader F, Eustache F, Baron JC. Mapping gray matter loss with voxel-based morphometry in mild cognitive impairment. *Neuroreport.* 2002;13(15): 1939–1943.

122. Jack CR Jr, Petersen RC, Xu YC, et al. Prediction of AD with MRI-based hippocampal volume in mild cognitive impairment. *Neurology.* 1999;52(7):1397–1403.

123. Jack CR Jr, Petersen RC, Xu Y, et al. Rates of hippocampal atrophy correlate with change in clinical status in aging and AD. *Neurology.* 2000;55(4):484–489.

124. Dickerson BC, Goncharova I, Sullivan MP, et al. MRI-derived entorhinal and hippocampal atrophy in incipient and very mild Alzheimer's disease. *Neurobiol Aging.* 2001;22(5):747–754.

125. Killiany RJ, Gomez-Isla T, Moss M, et al. Use of structural magnetic resonance imaging to predict who will get Alzheimer's disease. *Ann Neurol.* 2000;47(4):430–439.

126. Wolf H, Ecke GM, Bettin S, Dietrich J, Gertz HJ. Do white matter changes contribute to the subsequent development of dementia in patients with mild cognitive impairment? A longitudinal study. *Int J Geriatr Psychiatry.* 2000;15(9):803–812.

127. Kogure D, Matsuda H, Ohnishi T, et al. Longitudinal evaluation of early Alzheimer's disease using brain perfusion SPECT. *J Nucl Med.* 2000;41(7):1155–1162.

128. De Santi S, de Leon MJ, Rusinek H, et al. Hippocampal formation glucose metabolism and volume losses in MCI and AD. *Neurobiol Aging.* 2001;22(4):529–539.

129. Huang C, Wahlund LO, Svensson L, Winblad B, Julin P. Cingulate cortex hypoperfusion predicts Alzheimer's disease in mild cognitive impairment. *BMC Neurol.* 2002;2(1):9.

130. Arnaiz E, Jelic V, Almkvist O, et al. Impaired cerebral glucose metabolism and cognitive functioning predict deterioration in mild cognitive impairment. *Neuroreport.* 2001;12(4):851–855.

131. Sheline YI. Neuroimaging studies of mood disorder effects on the brain. *Biol Psychiatry.* 2003;54(3):338–352.

132. Krishnan KR, Hays JC, Blazer DG. MRI-defined vascular depression. *Am J Psychiatry.* 1997;154(4):497–501.

133. Alexopoulos GS, Meyers BS, Young RC, Campbell S, Silbersweig D, Charlson M. 'Vascular depression' hypothesis. *Arch Gen Psychiatry.* 1997;54(10):915–922.

134. Krishnan KR, Taylor WD, McQuoid DR, et al. Clinical characteristics of magnetic resonance imaging-defined subcortical ischemic depression. *Biol Psychiatry.* 2004;55(4):390–397.

135. Kumar A, Mintz J, Bilker W, Gottlieb G. Autonomous neurobiological pathways to late-life major depressive disorder: clinical and pathophysiological implications. *Neuropsychopharmacology.* 2002;26(2):229–236.

136. Kumar A. Neuroimaging in late-life mental disorders. In: Sadavoy J, Jarvik LF, Grossberg GT, Meyers BS, eds. *Comprehensive Textbook of Geriatric Psychiatry.* 3rd Ed. New York: W.W. Norton; 2004:391–428.

137. Narayan M, Bremner JD, Kumar A. Neuroanatomic substrates of late-life mental disorders. *J Geriatr Psychiatry Neurol.* 1999;12(3):95–106.

138. Kumar A, Jin Z, Bilker W, Udupa J, Gottlieb G. Late-onset minor and major depression: early evidence for common neuroanatomical substrates detected by using MRI. *Proc Natl Acad Sci USA.* 1998;95(13):7654–7658.

139. Steffens DC, Byrum CE, McQuoid DR, et al. Hippocampal volume in geriatric depression. *Biol Psychiatry.* 2000;48(4):301–309.

140. Lai T, Payne ME, Byrum CE, Steffens DC, Krishnan KR. Reduction of orbital frontal cortex volume in geriatric depression. *Biol Psychiatry.* 2000;48(10):971–975.

141. Bell-McGinty S, Butters MA, Meltzer CC, Greer PJ, Reynolds CF III, Becker JT. Brain morphometric abnormalities in geriatric depression: long-term neurobiological effects of illness duration. *Am J Psychiatry.* 2002;159(8):1424–1427.

142. Sheline YI, Sanghavi M, Mintun MA, Gado MH. Depression duration but not age predicts hippocampal volume loss in medically healthy women with recurrent major depression. *J Neurosci.* 1999;19(12):5034–5043.

143. Steffens DC, Payne ME, Greenberg DL, et al. Hippocampal volume and incident dementia in geriatric depression. *Am J Geriatr Psychiatry.* 2002;10(1):62–71.

144. Greenwald BS, Kramer-Ginsberg E, Krishnan RR, Ashtari M, Aupperle PM, Patel M. MRI signal hyperintensities in geriatric depression. *Am J Psychiatry.* 1996;153(9):1212–1215.

145. Taylor WD, MacFall JR, Steffens DC, Payne ME, Provenzale JM, Krishnan KR. Localization of age-associated white matter hyperintensities in late-life depression. *Prog Neuropsychopharmacol Biol Psychiatry.* 2003;27(3):539–544.

146. Salloway S, Malloy P, Kohn R, et al. MRI and neuropsychological differences in early- and late-life-onset geriatric depression. *Neurology.* 1996;46(6):1567–1574.

147. Jenkins M, Malloy P, Salloway S, et al. Memory processes in depressed geriatric patients with and without subcortical hyperintensities on MRI. *J Neuroimaging.* 1998;8(1):20–26.

148. Taylor WD, Steffens DC, MacFall JR, et al. White matter hyperintensity progression and late-life depression outcomes. *Arch Gen Psychiatry.* 2003;60(11):1090–1096.

149. Steffens DC, Bosworth HB, Provenzale JM, MacFall JR. Subcortical white matter lesions and functional impairment in geriatric depression. *Depress Anxiety.* 2002;15(1):23–28.

150. Levy RM, Steffens DC, McQuoid DR, Provenzale JM, MacFall JR, Krishnan KR. MRI lesion severity and mortality in geriatric depression. *Am J Geriatr Psychiatry.* 2003;11(6):678–682.

151. Videbech P. PET measurements of brain glucose metabolism and blood flow in major depressive disorder: a critical review. *Acta Psychiatr Scand.* 2000;101(1):11–20.

152. Bench CJ, Friston KJ, Brown RG, Scott LC, Frackowiak RS, Dolan RJ. The anatomy of melancholia—focal abnormalities of cerebral blood flow in major depression. *Psychol Med.* 1992;22(3):607–615.

153. Mayberg HS, Brannan SK, Mahurin RK, et al. Cingulate function in depression: a potential predictor of treatment response. *Neuroreport.* 1997;8(4):1057–1061.

154. Drevets WC, Frank E, Price JC, Kupfer DJ, Greer PJ, Mathis C. Serotonin type-1A receptor imaging in depression. *Nucl Med Biol.* 2000;27(5):499–507.

155. Malison RT, Price LH, Berman R, et al. Reduced brain serotonin transporter availability in major depression as measured by [123I]-2 beta-carbomethoxy-3 beta-(4-iodophenyl) tropane and single photon emission computed tomography. *Biol Psychiatry.* 1998;44(11):1090–1098.

156. Kumar A, Newberg A, Alavi A, Berlin J, Smith R, Reivich M. Regional cerebral glucose metabolism in late-life depression and Alzheimer disease: a preliminary positron emission tomography study. *Proc Natl Acad Sci USA.* 1993;90(15):7019–7023.

157. Lesser IM, Mena I, Boone KB, Miller BL, Mehringer CM, Wohl M. Reduction of cerebral blood flow in older depressed patients. *Arch Gen Psychiatry.* 1994;51(9):677–686.

158. Ebmeier KP, Prentice N, Ryman A, et al. Temporal lobe abnormalities in dementia and depression: a study using high resolution single photon emission tomography and magnetic resonance imaging. *J Neurol Neurosurg Psychiatry.* 1997;63(5):597–604.

159. Meltzer CC, Price JC, Mathis CA, et al. PET imaging of serotonin type 2A receptors in late-life neuropsychiatric disorders. *Am J Psychiatry.* 1999;156(12):1871–1878.

160. Corey-Bloom J, Jernigan T, Archibald S, Harris MJ, Jeste DV. Quantitative magnetic resonance imaging of the brain in late-life schizophrenia. *Am J Psychiatry.* 1995;152(3):447–449.

161. Barta PE, Powers RE, Aylward EH, et al. Quantitative MRI volume changes in late-onset schizophrenia and Alzheimer's disease compared to normal controls. *Psychiatry Res.* 1997;68(2–3):65–75.

162. Rabins PV, Aylward E, Holroyd S, Pearlson G. MRI findings differentiate between late-onset schizophrenia and late-life mood disorder. *Int J Geriatr Psychiatry.* 2000;15(10):954–960.

163. Jagust WJ. Neuroimaging in dementia. *Neurol Clin.* 2000;18(4):885–902.

164. Knopman DS, DeKosky ST, Cummings JL, et al. Practice parameter: diagnosis of dementia (an evidence-based review). Report of the Quality Standards Subcommittee of the American Academy of Neurology. *Neurology.* 2001;56(9):1143–1153.

165. Luetmer PH, Huston J, Friedman JA, et al. Measurement of cerebrospinal fluid flow at the cerebral aqueduct by use of phase-contrast magnetic resonance imaging: technique validation and utility in diagnosing idiopathic normal pressure hydrocephalus. *Neurosurgery.* 2002;50(3):534–543; discussion 543–544.

166. Minoshima S, Foster NL, Sima AA, Frey KA, Albin RL, Kuhl DE. Alzheimer's disease versus dementia with Lewy bodies: cerebral metabolic distinction with autopsy confirmation. *Ann Neurol.* 2001;50(3):358–365.

167. Wahlund LO, Julin P, Johansson SE, Scheltens P. Visual rating and volumetry of the medial temporal lobe on magnetic resonance imaging in dementia: a comparative study. *J Neurol Neurosurg Psychiatry.* 2000;69(5):630–635.

168. Minoshima S, Frey KA, Koeppe RA, Foster NL, Kuhl DE. A diagnostic approach in Alzheimer's disease using three-dimensional stereotactic surface projections of fluorine-18-FDG PET. *J Nucl Med.* 1995;36(7):1238–1248.

169. Kantarci K, Jack CR Jr. Neuroimaging in Alzheimer disease: an evidence-based review. *Neuroimaging Clin N Am.* 2003;13(2):197–209.

170. McKhann G, Drachman D, Folstein M, Katzman R, Price D, Stadlan EM. Clinical diagnosis of Alzheimer's disease: report of the NINCDS-ADRDA work group under the auspices of Department of Health and Human Services task force on Alzheimer's disease. *Neurology.* 1984;34:939–944.

171. Massoud F, Devi G, Stern Y, et al. A clinicopathological comparison of community-based and clinic-based cohorts of patients with dementia. *Arch Neurol.* 1999;56(11):1368–1373.

172. Díaz-Guzman J, Millán JM, Muñoz DG, Bermejo F. Utility of CT scanning in diagnosing dementia. In: Qizilbash N, Schneider LS, Helena C, et al., eds. *Evidence Based Dementia.* Oxford, UK: Blackwell Publishers; 2002:138–154.

173. Varma AR, Adams W, Lloyd JJ, et al. Diagnostic patterns of regional atrophy on MRI and regional cerebral blood flow change on SPECT in young onset patients with Alzheimer's disease, frontotemporal dementia and vascular dementia. *Acta Neurol Scand.* 2002;105(4):261–269.

174. Bosscher L, Scheltens P. MRI of the medial temporal lobe for the diagnosis of Alzheimer's disease. In: Qizilbash N, Schneider LS, Helena C, et al., eds. *Evidence Based Dementia.* Oxford, UK: Blackwell Publishers; 2002:154–162.

175. Jagust W, Chui H, Lee A-Y. Functional imaging in dementia. In: Qizilbash N, Schneider LS, Helena C, et al., eds. *Evidence Based Dementia.* Oxford, UK: Blackwell Publishers; 2002:162–170.

176. Jones DK, Lythgoe D, Horsfield MA, Simmons A, Williams SC, Markus HS. Characterization of white matter damage in ischemic leukoaraiosis with diffusion tensor MRI. *Stroke.* 1999;30(2):393–397.

177. Alexopoulos GS, Kiosses DN, Choi SJ, Murphy CF, Lim KO. Frontal white matter microstructure and treatment response of late-life depression: a preliminary study. *Am J Psychiatry.* 2002;159(11):1929–1932.

178. van der Flier WM, van den Heuvel DM, Weverling-Rijnsburger AW, et al. Magnetization transfer imaging in normal aging, mild cognitive impairment, and Alzheimer's disease. *Ann Neurol.* 2002;52(1):62–67.

179. Wyckoff N, Kumar A, Gupta RC, Alger J, Hwang S, Thomas MA. Magnetization transfer imaging and magnetic resonance spectroscopy of normal-appearing white matter in late-life major depression. *J Magn Reson Imaging.* 2003;18(5):537–543.

180. Sperling RA, Bates JF, Chua EF, et al. fMRI studies of associative encoding in young and elderly controls and mild Alzheimer's disease. *J Neurol Neurosurg Psychiatry.* 2003;74(1):44–50.

181. Ashburner J, Csernansky JG, Davatzikos C, Fox NC, Frisoni GB, Thompson PM. Computer-assisted imaging to assess brain struc-ture in healthy and diseased brains. *Lancet Neurol.* 2003;2(2): 79–88.

182. Jack CR Jr, Slomkowski M, Gracon S, et al. MRI as a biomarker of disease progression in a therapeutic trial of milameline for AD. *Neurology.* 2003;60(2):253–260.

183. Waterhouse RN. Imaging the PCP site of the NMDA ion channel. *Nucl Med Biol.* 2003;30(8):869–878.

184. Tune L, Tiseo PJ, Ieni J, et al. Donepezil HCl (E2020) maintains functional brain activity in patients with Alzheimer disease: results of a 24-week, double-blind, placebo-controlled study. *Am J Geriatr Psychiatry.* 2003;11(2):169–177.

185. Matthews B, Siemers ER, Mozley PD. Imaging-based measures of disease progression in clinical trials of disease-modifying drugs for Alzheimer disease. *Am J Geriatr Psychiatry.* 2003;11(2):146–159.

186. Shoghi-Jadid K, Small GW, Agdeppa ED, et al. Localization of neurofibrillary tangles and beta-amyloid plaques in the brains of living patients with Alzheimer disease. *Am J Geriatr Psychiatry.* 2002;10(1):24–35.

187. Mathis CA, Wang Y, Holt DP, Huang GF, Debnath ML, Klunk WE. Synthesis and evaluation of 11C-labeled 6-substituted 2-arylben-zothiazoles as amyloid imaging agents. *J Med Chem.* 2003;46 (13):2740–2754.

188. Small GW, Agdeppa ED, Kepe V, Satyamurthy N, Huang SC, Barrio JR. In vivo brain imaging of tangle burden in humans. *J Mol Neurosci.* 2002;19(3):323–327.

189. Klunk WE, Engler H, Nordberg A, et al. Imaging the pathology of Alzheimer's disease: amyloid-imaging with positron emission tomography. *Neuroimaging Clin N Am.* 2003;13(4):781–789.

Neuropsychological Assessment

9

Elisabeth Koss   Deborah K. Attix

As treatments become available both for early-stage and advanced-stage dementia, the need for proper neuropsychological evaluation is growing in urgency. In the case of suspected early dementia, the primary goal is to identify cognitive performance that is below what would be anticipated for the individual and represents a change from previous performance. For both early and advanced dementias, a secondary goal is to delineate the specific degree and type of deficits that are present, and then to relate the pattern of "abnormal" changes to a specific disease process. Until biomarkers provide this information, neuropsychological evaluations will remain the tool of choice to assist in the diagnosis of dementia and the prognosis of disease progression.

The objective of this chapter is to educate the practitioner about the contribution offered by neuropsychology in the diagnosis and management of dementia. The chapter will delineate when and why to order neuropsychological testing or intervention, clarify what to expect from a neuropsychological report or treatment, highlight aspects of neuropsychological practice of interest to the practitioner, such as the principles underlying test selection for dementia assessment, and highlight the neuropsychological and neurobehavioral presentations of common dementias.

WHAT ARE NEUROPSYCHOLOGICAL EVALUATIONS?

Neuropsychological evaluations vary considerably as a function of their intended purpose and patient factors. These include the referral question driving the evaluation; patient characteristics, such as overall level of cognitive dysfunction and noncognitive physical constraints; and demographic features that would influence test selection.

Individual tests are selected depending on the overall and specific goals of the evaluation. For example, evaluations involving differential diagnosis require a comprehensive approach with assessment across neurocognitive domains, because it is the constellation of findings—rather than any single score—that is diagnostically informative. The referral question may dictate a more comprehensive assessment of one domain, such as when a detailed language assessment is required if diagnostic considerations include progressive aphasia.

If questions involve a patient's ability to manage his or her financial affairs, performance and rating scales of functional capacity are enhanced with cognitive measures delineating arithmetic skills, reasoning, and judgment. The utility of these measures is further increased when based in part on empirical data that support the relevant application. For example, it is well known that progressive cognitive impairment is related to loss of independence in activities of daily living (1), and that specific neuropsychological deficits will affect specific functions, such as driving or the ability to manage a checkbook (2). In contrast, a longitudinal evaluation focusing upon staging, after the diagnosis has already been established, may allow for the administration of an abbreviated but specifically designed screening battery.

In addition to the purpose of the evaluation, patient characteristics will influence construction of the test battery. Patients with moderate and severe degrees of cognitive dysfunction often have difficulty tolerating extensive test batteries, and abbreviated approaches may yield decisive data to many referral questions. Sensory and motor constraints can also confound test results, necessitating particular attention in the elderly population. Amplification devices can assist in situations of clinically significant auditory acuity deficits, and larger stimuli are available for some tests to address visual deficits. Efforts to conserve time and energy should also be made with geriatric patients to avoid fatigue affecting test performance across the examination (3).

Finally, assessment of an agitated or uncooperative patient is of little use since testing reliability will be severely compromised, and is of questionable practice given issues of consent and assent. Older patients may not be cooperative due to limited previous exposure or comfort with mental health services, which may be related to education or ethnic/cultural background. Their perception may be that the evaluation will show them to be incompetent and will be used to place them in nursing homes. It is essential that patients understand the purpose of evaluation and be reassured about the use of the test data. The authors of this chapter, as standard practice, always openly discuss with the patients the purpose of testing, what it entails, and the possible outcomes. Indeed, ethical practice requires consent or assent to evaluation as appropriate. At best, frank disclosure relieves unnecessary (though understandable) anxiety; and at worst, persistent uncooperative behavior will provide useful clinical information about family dynamics, degree of understanding, or mental outlook.

SHOULD NEUROPSYCHOLOGICAL EVALUATIONS OR BEDSIDE EXAMINATIONS BE USED?

Neuropsychological evaluations and bedside examinations of mental and behavioral status share the same general objectives, may ascertain the same information, but serve different purposes. Bedside examinations are exploratory and are used as important screening tools. They provide the clinician with a quick estimate of current mental status. Such exams tend to be shorter, individualized, and reflect the clinician's unique style. An excellent source for bedside mental status examination can be found in Strub and Black (4). Neuropsychological evaluations, by contrast, strive to be standardized, quantitative, reliable, comprehensive, and utilize existing norms for comparative purposes. These features allow findings to be comparable across different time points, different settings, and different groups. On the flip side, neuropsychological evaluations tend to be time consuming, may be stressful, and are often perceived as superfluous.

WHEN SHOULD NEUROPSYCHOLOGICAL EVALUATIONS BE USED?

In many cases, when the diagnosis is relatively straightforward or for everyday patient management, the clinician will not need a full neuropsychological evaluation. The value of a full evaluation is apparent when there is a need to:

- Resolve clinical uncertainty regarding a difficult diagnosis
- Provide medicolegal documentation
- Address specific questions regarding strength or weakness of cognition or functional competence to assist in patient management for choice of treatment or decision regarding placement
- Document changes (progression or decline) over time to track the course of disease and to evaluate the efficacy of interventions

WHEN NOT TO SEND A PATIENT FOR TESTING

- When a patient's current condition will prevent obtaining reliable information, unless it is the fleeting condition itself that is of interest (e.g,. Is delirium present? Is the current treatment successful in abating specific symptoms?)
- Before a patient's temporary condition, which is unrelated to the referral question, is stabilized (e.g., infectious events, physical problems, personal losses).

Although it may be useful to evaluate how much temporary agitation affects performance or how sensory deprivation (e.g., partial blindness, auditory problems, etc.) may distort the patient's understanding of his or her surroundings, the rule of thumb is to strive to optimize a patient's level of functioning before testing, rather than impose undue burden. However, it should be noted that reliable assessments can be obtained with appropriate modifications to accommodate sensory or motor disabilities.

WHICH INSTRUMENTS OR TEST BATTERIES SHOULD BE GIVEN BY A PSYCHIATRIST OR NEUROLOGIST?

This question is akin to asking whether physicians should do their own electroencephalograms, electromyograms, or magnetic resonance imaging. The answer would be the same in all cases and affirmative only if the clinician is properly trained in giving the tests, interpreting the results, and if he or she can spare the time to provide the service. Even though neuropsychological tests appear deceptively simple, significant education, training, and experience is needed for both giving and interpreting them in a meaningful way. Also, be forewarned that **most tests, including the MMSE, are protected by copyright.** Thus, rather than highlighting which instrument the practitioner should use, it is our advice that in complex cases, the neuropsychological service be contacted to confirm or refute the working clinical hypothesis, and to properly evaluate performance.

SHOULD SPECIFIC TESTS OR BATTERIES BE ORDERED?

By ordering specific tests, the clinician does not take full advantage of the clinical neuropsychologist's expertise. This may well result in an imbalanced evaluation, and, at the least, decrease the potential value of the referral. Rather, it is more efficient to frame the referral in terms of concrete questions, either in cognitive or functional terms, depending on the intended use of the report. For example, based on the list above, useful questions might be framed in terms of legal competency, ability to live independently, or cognitive strengths and weaknesses in comparison to peers or previous performance. Vague referral questions such as "assess mental status," will tend to generate nonspecific and less useful answers.

As outlined above, neuropsychologists will consider many factors, relating to both the referral question and patient characteristics, when developing a test battery that is both comprehensive and suited to the needs of the particular case. They will consider what abilities and functions require assessment and in what way, and will consider patient characteristics that are relevant to test selection. They will also consider psychometric features of various instruments (e.g., known reliability or validity coefficients) that can also influence their utility. Finally, neuropsychologists will consider the strengths and limitations of available norms.

HOW TO EVALUATE A NEUROPSYCHOLOGIST'S QUALIFICATIONS

At a minimum, a clinical neuropsychologist residing in the United States must be licensed at the state level to practice clinical psychology. In addition, clinical neuropsychology is a specialty recognized by the American Psychological Association, with a well-delineated model of training (5). Training includes a strong background in functional neuroanatomy, cognitive psychology, clinical psychology and both predoctoral and postdoctoral supervised "hands on" clinical training. Further—although not required to practice neuropsychology, but sought after by a growing minority of practicing neuropsychologists—board certification indicates that these criteria have been met and is excellent evidence of competence in clinical neuropsychology (5).

WHAT TO EXPECT FROM A NEUROPSYCHOLOGICAL REPORT

Reports vary qualitatively, but generally share some relatively standard features. Typically, reports include information about the referring agent and reason for requesting the evaluation; a description of current and past medical and psychiatric history; a description of the clinical presentation of the patient (from interviews, history, and behavioral observations); and a listing of the tests that were administered (6,7). In all cases, tests results should be described so they can be understood by the person asking for the referral. Some practitioners use an actuarial (or quantitative) approach to examine their patients. Although seductive, this approach often relies on a technician to give the tests, and except for an introduction or closing interview, the database is entirely numeric, often computer-processed. At the other extreme, some reports are composed solely of richly detailed observations. Most neuropsychologists will not mention raw scores because they are meaningless by themselves; that is, they do not allow for comparison of performance to those of peers. Standard scores and percentile ranks are usually the scores of choice in reports. Some neuropsychologists do not even include numeric normative information at all because of concerns about misinterpretations that can arise from presenting such numbers without details about the source of such converted scores. For instance, a memory score of 115 using one norm group is not the same as a language score of 115, if the same norm group was not used. These groups control differently for age, education, gender, ethnicity/culture, and regional variations, and thus are not necessarily comparable.

The median length of a clinical neuropsychological report is six pages, with considerable variations in range (from 1 to 30 or more pages) (6,7). Longer reports do not necessarily add clarity or clinical utility. Rather, quality is defined by how well the report answers the referral question and/or offers new insights.

TYPES OF NEUROPSYCHOLOGICAL EVALUATIONS

Screening Versus Evaluation

The objective of a screening test is to detect a problem and determine whether or not a function is abnormal. Such screening instruments are called "dirty" or "noisy" because of their shotgun approach, which optimizes sensitivity at the expense of specificity. By contrast, the goal of a comprehensive evaluation is to describe function, determine the nature and extent of deficits, provide information relevant to everyday functioning, and assist in differential diagnosis. It is important to recognize the value and limits of both approaches and not confuse them. For example, the Mini-Mental State Examination (MMSE) (8) is a widely accepted and frequently utilized screening test that provides a global estimate of cognitive impairment. The MMSE is sensitive to a vast array of conditions (with several serious limitations, as discussed below), but is extremely nonspecific about the nature of underlying deficits, and is highly susceptible to false positive and negative classifications.

Batteries Versus Individual Tests

Heuristically, the domains of interest to neuropsychology usually include the following: general intellect, executive functions, orientation and attention, memory, expressive and receptive language, visuospatial functions, motor skills, mood and personality, and functional status (9). These domains are evaluated in relative independence of one another to fully appreciate the patient's strengths and deficits. However, the brain is not composed of neatly compartmentalized boxes that are independent of each other. Progress in the neurosciences continually underscores the complexity of the brain and the need to consider functional neuroanatomical systems rather than isolated structures or individual pathways. For example, a poor memory score may result from a host of conditions, such as poor hearing or sight, depression, attentional disorders, language difficulties, and/or lack of interest. It is by evaluating all of the domains that a precise understanding is reached of how they interact, and how the sum of a person's current strengths and weaknesses affects functional abilities.

Using the battery approach involves evaluation of preset cognitive domains and has the advantage of providing a fully standardized evaluation. However, test batteries, even when developed explicitly for older and cognitively impaired individuals, tend to be lengthy, tiring, and nonspecific. Most clinical neuropsychological evaluations typically utilize portions of batteries (e.g., the Halstead-Reitan battery) (10), along with additional tests chosen to enhance the comprehensive nature of the evaluation.

Also, one should keep in mind that with progression of dementia, patients' abilities become increasingly more difficult to assess: comprehension and attention span start to fluctuate, cognitive abilities decline in sometimes unpredictable patterns, and eventually patients become untestable with standardized methods. The clinician will have to increasingly rely on clinical observation and informant report to address the referral question. In such cases, the preferred standardized approach will have to be complemented by a qualitative evaluation. It is of little to no interest to report zero scores without a clinical description about how the patient approached the task and his or her failure. Did the person happily gloss over mistakes? Or, by expressing the need to suddenly have to leave the appointment to "go get the children at school," did the patient suggest some level of awareness of their deficits? The term "untestable" is of course a misnomer that reflects our conceptual limitations. Typically, this refers to the inability of a patient with a mini-mental score in the single digits to reliably perform cognitive tasks. Instead, there is an increasing recognition of the practical importance of focusing such evaluations on functional capacity, such as the ability to dress and toilet oneself, understand requests, or cooperate in group settings. These evaluations target management rather than diagnosis, which is appropriate to this stage of illness.

EVALUATION BY DOMAIN

Below is a brief review of constructs typically evaluated in a comprehensive neuropsychological evaluation. As noted previously, specific tests will be selected based on numerous factors, including patient demographics and presentation, the referral question, and instrument-related factors (such as the quality of normative standards). Therefore, no single "best" test can be recommended for any cognitive domain, because it would vary according to these moderating variables. As a matter of fact, administration of a single, individual test may provide a limited and possibly warped view of the patient's strengths and weaknesses if the moderating effects of chronological age, education, gender, socioeconomic status, ethnic background and individual circumstances (such as sensory status, motivation, perceived purpose of the evaluation, etc.) are not taken into consideration. The best practice is to administer several related tests in each domain. These tests will have some shared variance and should yield consistent results, thereby increasing confidence in the findings. However, they will also diverge in important ways that help clarify what systems may or may not be affected.

Table 9-1 presents an example of a comprehensive neuropsychological test battery. Outlined are the domains evaluated and subskills within these areas. Table 9-2 outlines a detailed list of tests that are commonly used, but this, too, is not exhaustive.

Global Mental Status

Screening batteries often are used for identification of cognitive compromise, staging through a general estimate of cognitive dysfunction, or to determine suitability for more extensive testing. However, because of their brevity, there are limits to their sensitivity and specificity. Because of these limitations, screening batteries are rarely used in isolation and are more often retained to characterize clinical and research samples, and to provide some data when more reliable, extensive testing is not feasible.

There are various mental status screening tests available on the market. For all intents and purposes they are equivalent and most will work well in the hands of an experienced clinician. The two best known and most commonly used today are the *MMSE* (8) and the *Blessed Dementia Scale* (11). The MMSE is the most widely known and used screening test of cognitive decline in the United States, and perhaps even the world. Its huge popularity comes from its ease and speed of administration and its astute estimation of global intellectual functioning. The many drawbacks of the MMSE, however, include biases to demographic factors like age, education, ethnicity, lifetime principal occupation, and lateralization of injury/illness. Also, the MMSE is insensitive to upper and lower limits of the cognitive continuum, as well as to some forms of dementia (such as frontotemporal dementia [FTD]) (12,13).

TABLE 9-1

COMPONENTS OF A NEUROPSYCHOLOGICAL EVALUATION FOR DEMENTIA BY COGNITIVE DOMAIN[a]

General Mental Status
General Intellect
  Estimates of premorbid functions
  Estimates of verbal intellect
  Estimates of nonverbal intellect

Executive Functions
  Mental and motor sequencing
  Cognitive flexibility
  Verbal and design fluency
  Verbal abstract reasoning
  Nonverbal abstract reasoning
  Concept formation
  Problem solving
  Judgment

Orientation
Memory
  Attention and concentration
  Verbal learning and recall
  Nonverbal learning and recall
  Free recall skills
  Recognition/cued recall skills

Language
  Spontaneous speech, reading, writing
  Confrontation naming
  Lexical fluency
  Semantic fluency

Visuospatial
  Perception and judgment
  Organization and integration
  Visual-constructions

Sensory-Motor
  Vision-hearing-olfaction-somatosensory
  Fine motor speed
  Dexterity/coordination

Mood and Personality
  Depression
  Psychopathology
  Emotional distress

Functional Status
  Activities of daily living
  Instrumental activities of daily living

[a]Not all components will be assessed in these cognitive domains.

The Blessed Dementia Scale consists of two scales: an activities of daily living (ADL) subscale registering functional behaviors reported by an informant, and a mental status section. The latter has been further narrowed into a brief mental status screening test: the *Blessed Information-Memory-Concentration Test (BIMC)* (14). The widely used BIMC is more sensitive to attentional compromises than the MMSE, and as such may be the instrument of choice to evaluate delirium or early frontal lobe compromise. In contrast to the MMSE and most tests, points are given for failure and a high score is an indicator of dementia.

When in-person, face-to-face screenings are not practical (such as for frequent follow-up documentation on patients already seen in the clinic), brief telephone screenings can be used.

Other screening assessment batteries are commonly used to evaluate global dementia, and have become popular in clinical research trials. Examples of these are the *Mattis Dementia Rating Scale* (15) or the *Alzheimer Disease Assessment Scale* (16), both too lengthy to be practical in a clinical setting.

The *Consortium to Establish a Registry for Alzheimer's Disease Battery (CERAD)* (17) was developed specifically to evaluate cognitive domains affected by Alzheimer's disease (AD). It is composed of short or shortened subtests borrowed from various well-known tests to assess verbal memory (e.g., the ability to learn, recall, and recognize a list of 10 nouns), language (e.g., the ability to name 15 line-drawn objects), and visuospatial construction skills (e.g., the ability to copy geometric shapes). The CERAD battery is well standardized and is sensitive to cognitive features of mild to moderate dementia (18). The evaluation takes an average of 45 minutes.

The *Neurobehavioral Cognitive Status Examination (NCSE, or Cognistat)* (19) is a screening instrument that provides a profile of cognitive performance in the five major cognitive domains: language, visuospatial functioning, memory, arithmetic, and verbal reasoning. However, relatively little normative data have been collected, and scores seem to be sensitive to depression as well as education (20).

Although it is not strictly speaking a neuropsychological instrument, the *Clinical Dementia Rating Scale (CDR)* (21,22) deserves special recognition for its ability to assess the degree of impairment in several domains, and to synthesize dementia severity into a single score. Thus, it allows comparing degrees of dementia across patient to patient and across institutions. This semi-structured interview, which is conducted with both the patient and the caregiver, provides practical estimates of global impairment in six categories of cognitive function related to everyday activities: memory, orientation, judgment and problem solving, community affairs, home and hobbies, and personal care. Although somewhat lengthy to administer, the CDR can be integrated easily into the clinical evaluation and provides valuable information for patient management.

Assessment of Severe Dementia

Several tests have been developed in recent years to evaluate cognition and behavior in severe dementia. The most common instrument is the *Severe Impairment Battery* (23) that is in essence a scaled-down MMSE. The battery is divided into subtests assessing attention, orientation, language, memory, visuospatial abilities, constructive abilities, and social interaction. It takes about 20 minutes on average to administer.

The *Hierarchic Dementia Scale* (24), popular in Canada, includes 20 subtests covering the whole range of cognitive

TABLE 9-2
NEUROPSYCHOLOGICAL INSTRUMENTS

Screening
Short Portable Mental Status Questionnaire (SPMSQ)
Mini-Mental State Examination (MMSE)
Modified Mini-Mental Status Examination (3MSE)
Cognitive Abilities Screening Instrument (CASI)
Blessed Information-Memory-Concentration Test (BIMC)
Neurobehavioral Cognitive Status Examination (NCSE or Cognistat)
Dementia Rating Scale-2 (DRS-2)
MiniCog
MicroCog: Assessment of Cognitive Functioning
Repeatable Battery for the Assessment of Neuropsychological Status (RBANS)
Geriatric Mental State Examination (GMS)
Telephone Interview for Cognitive Status (TICS)

Intellect
National Adult Reading Test (NART)
Wechsler Adult Intelligence Scale-Revised (WAIS-R)
Wechsler Adult Intelligence Scale-Third Edition (WAIS-III)
Wechsler Abbreviated Scale of Intelligence (WASI)
Kaufman Brief Intelligence Test (K-BIT)
Raven's Coloured Progressive Matrices (RCPM)

Executive Functions
Delis-Kaplan Executive Function Test (D-KEFS)
Wisconsin Card Sorting Test (WCST)
Modified Wisconsin Card Sorting Test (MCST)
Booklet Category Test (BCT)
Short Category Test (SCT)
Trail Making Test (TMT)
Stroop Color-Word Interference Test
Ruff Figural Fluency Test (RFFT)
WAIS-III Similarities subtest
Symbol Digit Modalities Test (SDMT)
Gorham Proverb Interpretation Test

Learning and Memory
Verbal learning and memory
Warrington Recognition Memory Test—Words (RMW)
Wechsler Memory Scale—Revised (WMSR)/ Wechsler Memory Scale-III (WMS-III)
California Verbal Learning Test (CVLT)
List Learning and Memory—CERAD
Rey-Auditory Verbal Learning Test (RAVLT)
Selective Reminding Test (SRT)
Free and Cued Selective Reminding Test (FCSR)
Fuld Object Memory Evaluation (FOME)
Hopkins Verbal Learning Test (HVLT)
Rivermead Behavioral Memory Test (RBMT)
Nonverbal learning and memory
Warrington Recognition Memory Test—Faces (RMF)
Rey-Osterrieth Complex Figure Test (ROCFT)
Brief Test of Visual Memory (BVMT)

Visual Reproduction subscale of Wechsler Memory Scale—Revised
Benton Visual Retention Test (BVRT)
Benton Visual Retention Test, Multiple Choice (BVRT—MC)

Language
Multilingual Aphasia Exam (MAE)
Reitan Indiana Aphasia Screening Test
Controlled Oral Word Association—FAS (COWAT)
Boston Diagnostic Aphasia Examination (BDAE)
Western Aphasia Battery (WAB)
Boston Naming Test

Visuospatial
WAIS-R Performance subtests
Clock-drawing test
Figure-copying test
Hooper Visual Organization Test (VOT)
Judgment of Line Orientation Test (JLOT)
Rey-Osterrieth Complex Figure

Sensory-Motor
Finger Oscillation Test (FOT)
Grooved Pegboard Test
Hand dynamometer
Reitan-Klove Sensory-Perceptual Examination

Mood-Personality-Behavior
Geriatric Depression Scale (GDS)
Beck Depression Inventory (BDI)
The Hamilton Rating Scale for Depression (HRS-D)
The Minnesota Multiphasic Personality Inventory-2 (MMPI-2)
The Personality Assessment Inventory (PAI)
Cohen-Mansfield Agitation Inventory (CMAI)
The Revised Memory and Behavior Problem Checklist (RMBPC)
The Neuropsychiatric Inventory (NPI)/NPI-Q
The Cornell Scale for Depression in Dementia
The Behavioral Scale in Alzheimer's Disease Rating Scale (BEHAVE-AD)

Tests that Combine Cognitive Domains
Consortium to Establish a Registry for Alzheimer's Disease battery (CERAD)
Cambridge Examination for Mental Disorders of the Elderly (CAMDEX)
Dementia Rating Scale (DRS-2)

Questionnaires/Scales that Screen for and/or Stage and Severity of Dementia
Clinical Dementia Rating Scale (CDR)
Global Deterioration Scale (GDS)
Hasegawa Dementia Scale
Informant Questionnaire on Cognitive Decline (IQCODE)
The Katz Index of Activities of Daily Living (Katz ADL)
The Instrumental Activities of Daily Living Scale (IADL)
The Functional Assessment Staging (FAST) scale

and motor functions. Each subtest is hierarchically organized from the most-difficult to the easiest items, leading to an extensive cognitive profile. The battery is reliable and takes about 45 minutes to administer. Although the individualized profile allows longitudinal follow-up of each patient, many researchers and clinicians question the theory behind an organized-hierarchical deterioration.

The *Test for Severe Impairment Battery* (25) has not become widely popular, although it provides fast (10 minutes), reliable and valid estimates of cognitive functions for patients with severe impairment.

Does it make sense to have severely impaired patients evaluated? Here in particular, the referral question should be clearly defined if useful information is to be expected.

In severe dementia, it is less important to evaluate cognitive skills than to consider functional abilities, since patients at that stage are rarely called upon to make independent decisions. Also, differential diagnosis at a late stage is difficult to obtain and probably of little practical value. This does not mean that it is useless to evaluate severely impaired patients. Decisions regarding patient management or response to a particular treatment, for example, can be considerably enlightened by use of pre-post evaluations.

Intellect and Premorbid Function

It is important to note that estimates of premorbid functioning are essential in neuropsychological evaluation to minimize underestimates or overestimates of change based on current performance. The ideal way to determine the presence and extent of change in cognitive functioning would be to know at what level the person used to function. Since it is rarely feasible to have exact knowledge of past intellectual abilities, estimates of premorbid cognition functions are made on the basis of regression formulas incorporating educational level and professional achievement, and by relying on tests relatively insensitive to intellectual deterioration. The most common tests used for this purpose are reading words of decreasing frequency, that require semantic knowledge associated with formal education, such as the *National Adult Reading Test-Revised* (26) and the *Wide Range Achievement Test* 3rd Edition (27). For more information about other estimates, the reader should refer to Axelrod et al. (28).

Even though the concepts of intellectual quotient (IQ) and "intelligence" are archaic and of limited value, test batteries like the Wechsler scales (e.g., *Wechsler Adult Intelligence Scale-III*, [WAIS-III]) (29) remain popular instruments for assessing general intellectual skills in adults. Their value lies in their extensive norms that allow for meaningful performance comparisons across different age groups and in the fact that they are comprised of numerous subtests that individually and collectively provide information on specific neuropsychological functions (e.g., arithmetic skills, mental sequencing, verbal and nonverbal abstract reasoning). Acquisition of a full WAIS can be useful in evaluations of high-functioning individuals. Also, in addition to scores on specific subtests, the WAIS-III provides indices of verbal intellect, nonverbal intellect, working memory, and processing speed. However, the WAIS scales have serious drawbacks for testing average older persons: in addition to being lengthy, they do not evaluate all areas of cognitive functioning of interest to dementia. In particular, the WAIS scales are devoid of true memory tests. Still, individual subtests of the full WAIS-III battery can be useful but should be supplemented with tests in other cognitive domains.

Orientation, Attention, Concentration, and Executive Functions

Assessment of orientation for time, place, and person is usually covered in the bedside mental status examination and most memory test batteries. Tests of specific aspects of orientation are indicated when lapses are noted on an informal mental status examination. However, caution must be exercised as poor performance on time orientation has been demonstrated with nondemented individuals with less than 8 years of schooling.

A formal evaluation of orientation may include time estimation, discrimination of recency, body orientation, finger localization, laterality discrimination, topographical localization, route finding, etc. These specialized tests would only be included in an evaluation if there were indications of specific brain damage or to evaluate lateralization of dysfunction (9).

Attention is a complex set of skills that span awareness, reaction to novel stimuli, maintenance of thought processes, and capacity to allocate, sustain, and divide one's attention to several aspects of the environment occurring at the same time. Problems in these areas manifest as high distractibility, or, conversely, difficulty in switching attention to changes in the environment. Such problems, prominent in frontal lobes disease, occur early in FTDs, and later in AD when the illness becomes more global. Tests of simple attention include: *repeating digits forward and backward, reciting the alphabet or months of the year backward, or counting backward.* Lezak (9) correctly warns against combining the forward and the backward scores, as they are differentially sensitive to aging, brain disease and dementia. Spatial nonverbal versions of span involving finger tapping also exist.

Slowed processing speed may underlie attentional deficits. This can be measured with reaction time tests. Simple reaction time requiring response to a stimulus are very sensitive to early dementia, but can be slowed in other conditions, such as brain injury or depression. Complex reaction times, while challenging to older people, may be the tool of choice to evaluate frontal compromise.

Other measures related to attention involve vigilance, such as *letter or digit cancellation tests, or repeating sentences of increasing length.* Selective attention as measured by *visual search tasks* is also of interest, as are tasks requiring tracking, sequencing, and response inhibition. Some tests have simpler components followed by more complex tasks, allowing a direct comparison of performance under increasing complexity. For instance, the *Trail Making Test* first requires patients to connect in ascending order numbers scattered on a page (30). The task is then made more difficult by introducing an alternating element, wherein the patient must alternate between numbers and letters, requiring increasing attention, working memory, and cognitive flexibility. A word of caution: in general, tests of attention are sensitive to brain damage, but often are not specific, and must be interpreted with this known limitation.

Executive functions represent a class of higher-order cognitive functions, such as the ability to plan, perform abstract reasoning, monitor the quality of one's performance, inhibit wrong or inappropriate responses, appreciate the order or sequence of events, and extract information from one's own repertory of response. Executive functions are characterized by flexibility of thinking, independence of decision-making, and ability to adapt to environmental demands. Since such skills are heavily dependent on the anterior structures and systems of the brain, it is not surprising that executive functions are prominently affected early in frontal-lobe dementias, and later in AD.

Evaluation of executive functions skills is challenging and not easily done in a laboratory-type setting. Indeed, testing in a laboratory setting is inherently highly structured, and thus is not conducive to independent decision-making—the very aspect that such tests are supposed to evaluate. Also, tests of executive functions tend to perform best when they are novel and make heavy demands on planning, organization, and control. Commonly used tests include the *Stroop Test* (31), which requires inhibition and mental control over a response; the *Wisconsin Card Sorting Test* (32), while an excellent source of information regarding problem solving and response to feedback, is lengthy and can be frustrating for some patients; the *Delis-Kaplan Executive Function Test* (33), which provides a good general clinical evaluation of most executive functions; and tasks requiring abstract reasoning and judgment (some subtests of the WAIS-III, for example).

Memory

Memory impairment is the earliest and most salient deficit in AD. It is such an inherent part of the disease that the Diagnostic and Statistical Manual of Mental Disorders (DSM-IV-TR) (34) makes it the first condition for a diagnosis of AD. Deficits in verbal memory may precede overt symptoms by many years. However, the clinician should keep in mind that memory deficits may result from various causes, not the least being depression, systemic diseases, infections, or toxic reactions. Further, normal age-related changes affect many, though not all, aspects of learning and memory (35), and therefore must be carefully differentiated from pathological changes.

There are many theories of memory. For the clinician, however, the most useful distinctions are based on acquisition, storage, and retrieval of information. The latter can be further divided into free recall and recognition (i.e., the ability to independently produce the correct information from memory stores, versus the recognition of the correct response from a limited choice panel provided to the patient). Further, it is useful to assess both verbal and nonverbal learning and memory, and to explore how performance varies across tasks with different amounts of struc-

ture inherent to them. Because of the many facets of memory, many memory subtests or tasks are typically administered in a comprehensive evaluation. Usually, this includes a supraspan list-learning task which involves multiple learning trials of unrelated words, one or more free-recall trials of the information to assess retention (over brief and/or long, 30-minute delays), and a recognition trial where the stimuli occur within the context of foils. Assessment also typically includes immediate and delayed recall of logical narrative passages, and complex geometric figures. In addition, assessment of higher functioning individuals who can tolerate more extensive testing may include immediate and delayed recall of faces, drawn scenes, or pairs of words. The dissociations that occur between these types of tasks can have diagnostic utility. For instance, performance of a patient with impaired free recall and retrieval skills is consistent with AD or other mesial-temporal lobe dysfunction, because storage, and thus subsequent recall and recognition, rely on the integrity of the hippocampus. In contrast, performance of a patient with impaired free recall, but accurate retrieval with cues on recognition tasks would be more consistent with striatal dysfunction.

Language

The major distinctions of language include syntax, grammar, verbal fluency, semantic meaning of words, prosody, articulation, and writing. These in turn can be divided into language comprehension (receptive language) and production (expressive language). One will see some disruption in the coherent expression of ideas and flow of knowledge in all types of dementia, as a result of the disruption of basic memory structures and the ability to maintain a train of thought. As with memory, language assessment is multifaceted and divergences can be diagnostic. For instance, lexical verbal fluency is prominently affected in dementias involving more anterior structures and systems, whereas in more posterior dementias, language comprehension may be more affected. Evaluation should assess the following: spontaneous speech, repetition, speech comprehension, semantic and lexical fluency, confrontation naming, as well as reading and writing (9).

Visuospatial Skills

Visuospatial abilities typically tap posterior structures and systems. Assessment involves judgment of angular relationships, copy of simple and complex geometric figures, and constructions using three-dimensional blocks. Visual integration of drawings of fragmented objects might be evaluated. Praxis and facial recognition could also be assessed. In older people, care should be taken to anticipate the contribution of poor vision or age-associated motor difficulties to visuospatial performance.

The extremely popular **clock drawing test** (36) is considered to have both spatial and executive function components. This test is sensitive to various cognitive deficits but is not specific. Some clinicians attempt to tease out the spatial component by asking the patient to also copy a clock after producing one. The amount and type of instructions given lead to different performances and, thus, need to be highly standardized. Many neuropsychologists request the hands to be drawn at "10 after 11" to enhance sensitivity to executive dysfunction. Minor changes in instructions, such as, "draw the hands to show 11:10," may obscure subtle executive dysfunctions, as might the request to draw the hands at other apparently less confusing times.

Other well-known clinical tests of visuospatial abilities include building a design with blocks based on increasingly difficult patterns (*Block design* subtest from the WAIS scales), or *drawing abstract figures (Rosen figures,* as in the CERAD battery) (17), or drawing figurative objects in perspective, such as *a cube or a house* (with elements of perspective) either from copy or (as a more complex task) from memory.

Sensory and Motor Abilities

It goes without saying that a person coming for evaluation should be checked for well-corrected hearing and vision to obtain a valid examination. An example of a test battery designed to accomodate sensory limitations is the CERAD, which uses enlarged print and oral responses to minimize sensory confounding.

Not uncommonly, patients complain of visual difficulties such as finding something among an array of objects, recognizing well-known relatives, or navigating stairs. Such complaints, often considered to be secondary to cognitive decline, may in fact reflect specific visual difficulties such as decreased contrast sensitivity or defective depth perception. Such problems may also affect reading and spatial orientation. However, when related to neurological rather than sensory deficits, they may reflect a posterior variant of AD, or Lewy body dementia, and other clinical features should be evaluated. Such complaints need to be taken seriously and evaluated with a specialized ophthalmologic examination (37). Because of the early entorhinal involvement, olfactory deficits are not uncommon in AD. They are not commonly picked up by, nor should they be considered as, the major diagnostic tool because of cognitive confounding in measurement.

Motor abilities are usually measured in terms of fine motor speed, fine motor coordination and dexterity, and motor strength. Unilateral decreases beyond expected dominance-related discrepancies raises the suspicion of focal or vascular lesions. Frank motor difficulties are uncommon in the early stages of AD, and are thus suggestive of either Parkinsonian features (particularly when slowing is noted) or vascular involvement. Problems with praxis, in contrast, are more indicative of posterior cortical involvement.

Evaluation of Psychopathology

Psychiatric symptoms are frequently seen in the mid-course of AD, may occur earlier in other dementias, and are an integral part of the complex dementia symptomatology. By mid-course it is estimated that close to 50% of patients will have shown psychotic manifestations (38). Because of the nature of the disease, self-rating instruments are of dubious value even in early stage dementia. Most evaluations are based on clinical observations or caregiver ratings. It is important to include psychiatric functions as an integral part of the neuropsychological evaluation to determine the possible influence of disordered mood on cognition and quality of life.

By far, depression is the most common presenting symptom (or, the most commonly observed clinical sign). Depression can result in cognitive impairments similar to those of AD, a condition historically referred to as *pseudodementia*, or as the *dementia of depression*. More often, depression co-occurs within the setting of AD and other dementias, with over half of patients in some series meeting criteria for dysthymia or major depression (39). Significant depression can sometimes be a harbinger or preclinical sign of AD, predating the more ominous cognitive process (40).

Visual hallucinations and delusions may also occur. By contrast, auditory hallucinations are less common in dementias of old age. The current view is that hallucinations and delusions may express different pathologies in AD and have different prognostic values. Delusions seem to be more resistant to treatment but hallucinations represent a worse prognosis for cognitive decline (41).

Rating scales are often tipped toward evaluating depression, such as the *Cornell Scale for Depression in Dementia* (42) and the *Geriatric Depression Scale* (43). The *Behavioral Scale in Alzheimer's Disease Rating Scale* (44) evaluates and follows behavioral disorders in AD. The scale focuses on psychiatric items, such as paranoid ideas and delusions, hallucinations, disruption of activities, aggressiveness, disorders of diurnal rhythms, affective disorders, anxieties, and phobias. Of particular use in long-term care, the *Cohen-Mansfield Agitation Inventory* (45) provides both frequency and intensity of commonly occurring agitated behaviors without making assumptions about the underlying psychopathology. The *Revised Memory and Behavior Problem Checklist* (46), completed by the caregiver, also provides practical estimates of disruptive behaviors for geriatric outpatient clinics.

The *Neuropsychiatric Inventory* (NPI) (47) is rapidly gaining prominence for evaluating the presence and nature of psychopathological disorders in patients with AD as well as other dementias. This informant-based scale assesses behavioral disturbances in 12 common areas: delusions, hallucinations, agitation, depression, anxiety, euphoria, apathy, disinhibition, irritability, aberrant motor behavior, night-time behaviors, and eating disorders. The

NPI is brief (between 10 and 20 min), easy to administer, and provides four scores in each domain: frequency, severity, total, and caregiver's distress. Relatively minor variations have been introduced to adapt this scale to other settings such as long-term care.

Classical personality tests (e.g., *Minnesota Multiphasic Personality Inventory* and Rorschach Ink Blot Test) are not informative in older cognitively challenged folks and are rarely used—if at all. Those tests require more than an eighth-grade reading ability, are lengthy, tend to use difficult language (e.g., double negatives), require unimpaired vision to be valid, and have scant and inadequate age norms. Further, they were not constructed to address the psychopathology observed in age-related dementias.

Functional Status

Activities of daily living (ADL) scales are useful to evaluate loss of autonomy, especially in severe dementia. The most commonly used scales are the *Katz ADL Index* (48), the Lawton *Instrumental Activities of Daily Living* (IADL) scale (49) and the Reisberg *Functional Assessment Staging (FAST)* scale (50).

The ADL Index evaluates six basic activities of daily living and is designed to be used in institutional settings. The IADL evaluates patients' ability to perform basic and instrumental activities of everyday life and is more relevant for outpatients. Part A evaluates current instrumental activities, and Part B evaluates basic daily activities. This scale is extensively used in the assessment of ADL and IADL in dementia, and is only useful in early and moderate dementia before independent functions bottom out. The FAST is a 16-item scale divided into a seven-point staging system from mild to severe dementia that identifies excess disability. Although widely used, particularly in long-term care, the stages do not always follow the unevenness of clinical decline and do not necessarily mirror functional loss across all dementias.

CLINICAL PATTERNS OF MILD COGNITIVE IMPAIRMENT AND DEMENTIAS

A brief summary of the clinical presentations of common dementias is provided to best provide insight about the cognitive profile to expect for dementia subtypes. More extensive and illuminating clinical descriptions will be found in the relevant chapters of this book. Three notes of caution: first, since AD is the most common, best known, and most studied of the dementing illnesses (51), it tends to be over-diagnosed. Given its visibility, it is not surprising that the term is often used as a shorthand for all dementias. Although convenient, this tendency is misleading and tends to obscure recognition of cognitive differences across subtypes. Second, very early and late dementia

stages are both hard to diagnose; the former because deficits may not yet be apparent, either because of relative later emergence or still successful compensatory mechanisms; the latter because of generalized decline. Third, there is overlap in pathology across the different dementing illnesses, and thus similarities of clinical presentation are to be expected, further muddying the waters. Differential diagnosis is not easy, and particularly in early cases requires extensive clinical information to make educated inferences. Thus, errors in early clinical diagnoses may be common, especially for non-AD dementias (52).

Mild Cognitive Impairment

Many older individuals complain of memory loss. When mild enough, they may be dismissed by the practitioner as normal, or associated with depressive mood. In recent years, however, such subjective complaints have come to be associated with a greater risk of developing AD and are now the subject of intense interest for their potential prognostic value. Globally, such complaints are referred to as mild cognitive impairment (MCI) and clinically defined as impairment in one or more cognitive domains, typically memory, or an overall mild decline across cognitive abilities greater than expected for an individual's age or education, but not interfering with social and occupation functioning (53). Other terms describing the interface from normal age-related changes to possible early dementia are *age-associated memory impairment*, *age-associated cognitive decline*, and *cognitive impairment no dementia*.

MCI is of particular concern to the clinician as it carries such a high risk of conversion to AD. The most common and best-studied form is the amnestic type, although other types of MCI (such as vascular, depressed, parkinsonian, and others) are becoming increasingly recognized and may represent the prodromal stage of other dementing illnesses. Unfortunately, the preclinical stages of dementias other than AD are not well understood at this time.

Clinically, it should be noted that a purely amnestic syndrome is relatively uncommon in the community (54), because declines in multiple cognitive functions often occur in conjunction with memory complaints. MCI individuals with neuropsychiatric symptoms, such as depression, apathy, and irritability, may be at even higher risk of developing dementia than those with a pure amnestic syndrome.

Neuropsychological Profile

Despite the current lack of understanding of good predictors of dementia, an individual with believable memory complaints representing a change from earlier performance should be treated with concern and given a thorough evaluation of all cognitive domains, functional ability, and mood. MCI is perhaps the single most important condition for which a comprehensive neuropsychological evaluation is warranted. Even if the evaluation is equivocal (as it will most likely be given the minimal deficits experienced by MCI patients), this will serve as a baseline against which to calibrate future potential changes. Collateral information concerning the complaints should be sought. Memory impairment of at least 1.5 standard deviations below age-adjusted and education-adjusted means is highly suggestive of MCI.

CASE EXAMPLE: MILD COGNITIVE IMPAIRMENT

The patient was a 72-year-old, right-handed, married White male with 12 years of formal education. He had been experiencing a memory problem for approximately 18 months, with a noticeable worsening in the most recent 6 months. Around this time, the patient lost his best friend. His wife accompanied him to his evaluation, and reported that he had poor memory and difficulty with activities requiring concentration and reasoning, such as playing bridge or finance management. The patient was aware of his memory difficulties and brought these to the attention of his local physician, who attributed the symptoms to aging and depression from his recent loss. He referred the patient for psychiatric evaluation and treatment.

The psychiatrist recognized the possibility of a previously undetected neurodegenerative condition, given the reported course of illness and the patient's strong family history of Alzheimer's disease (AD) (e.g., mother and maternal uncle). There was no known or suspected medical history thought to be contributing to or accounting for the memory loss.

At the request of the referring psychiatrist, a comprehensive neuropsychological evaluation was completed. The referral question requested clarification of likely diagnosis, given the presence of depression. The evaluation included assessment of general intellect, attention, executive functions, learning and memory, language, visuospatial abilities, fine motor skills, and mood.

Results indicated a relatively circumscribed, profound memory deficit characterized by rapid forgetting even after short delays, reflecting inadequate consolidation of new information. Mild executive inefficiencies on timed tasks of sequencing and cognitive flexibility were also noted, but in the context of well-preserved abstract reasoning and concept-formation skills. General intellect, language, and visuospatial abilities were all well within normal limits. Not surprisingly, interview and testing suggested a mild-moderate depression.

This profile was consistent with what is typically observed in mild cognitive impairment (MCI) or prodromal AD before a frank dementia is apparent. The profile was not consistent with the typical presentation of cognitive deficits related to depression, which most often are characterized by retrieval (versus storage) memory deficits and executive compromises. While the patient's depression indeed likely exacerbated his cognitive processing difficulties, it did not account for them. Instead, the constellation of findings reflected the behavioral correlates of an illness primarily affecting medial temporal structures.

The diagnosis of MCI was made with follow-up evaluation to be scheduled in 12 months to track the course,

particularly considering the anticipated recovery from depression. A diagnosis of possible AD was considered premature since all the diagnostic features were not present. By definition, "possible AD" rather than "probable AD" should be considered here because of the presence of depression. Because the patient retained insight, clinical intervention was pursued to assist him in adjusting to his memory loss (through compensatory strategies) and the recent loss of his friend.

Alzheimer's Disease

The first and foremost deficit that heralds AD is significant memory impairment, commonly reported by family, friends, and sometimes the patient as well. These memory difficulties are not trivial and are characterized by impoverished new learning and excessive rapid forgetting of recently learned information. By contrast, recognition of previously learned information, well rehearsed knowledge, and memory for past events are all well preserved in the early stages of the disease. In addition, the progressive and insidious nature of the deficits is a cardinal feature of AD. To differentiate AD from other amnesic syndromes, the DSM-IV-TR criteria require that at least one other cognitive domain shows obvious decline. With the disease progressing, other deficits will become manifest, such as problems with word finding, abstract reasoning, attention, and visuospatial difficulties. These and other intellectual deficits may present at different times and will not necessarily progress in unison. However, at moderate stages, cognitive losses will be widespread and serious enough to be evident to a casual observer. Behavioral and psychological problems such as irritability, screaming, depression, hallucinations, and delusions will occur in about 50% of AD patients by mid-course of the disease. It is likely that such difficulties represent a combination of increasingly disturbed brain connectivity, emotional responses to the dissolution of the patient's intellectual capacities, and increased difficulty dealing with the complexity of his or her environment.

Neuropsychological Profile

A typical neuropsychological profile of mild AD would include: disproportionate memory difficulties for newly or recently learned material and mild problems in at least two other domains (such as language, perception, executive function, praxis, or personality). In moderate AD, memory capacities further worsen and are close to bottoming out, despite fairly well-preserved remote memories. Confusion becomes manifest to casual observers and language is obviously impaired. Most, if not all, cognitive domains show clear deficits with varying and unpredictable degrees of severity. The patient may or may not be aware of his or her deficits, and may start to show behavioral problems.

Dementia with Lewy Bodies

Dementia with Lewy Bodies (DLB) accounts for 20% to 30% of dementia cases (55). In contrast to the relatively predictable and progressive deterioration observed in AD, cognitive impairments, and attention and alertness in particular, can fluctuate significantly in DLB. Core manifestations of DLB include spontaneous motor/extrapyramidal features (similar to those seen in Parkinson' disease); prominent visuospatial deficits; recurrent visual hallucinations; and gait disturbances (56). Other features indicative of DLB are recurrent falls and syncope, transient losses of consciousness, intense hallucinations, delusions, depression, and rapid eye movement sleep disorders. One should keep in mind, however, that most DLB cases exhibit some pathologic features of AD, and that the distinction between AD and DLB can be difficult and somewhat arbitrary. As a rule, cognitive abilities dependent on the frontal lobes or on motor organization are more impaired in DLB patients than in patients with AD. Still, it is not easy to clinically distinguish with adequate reliability between DLB and AD (57). How might features specific to DLB then translate into performance on neuropsychological tests?

Neuropsychological Profile

First, in the early phases, a DLB patient's most serious problem or major complaint will *not* be memory. Second, a core neuropsychological feature is fluctuating cognition with pronounced variation in attention and alertness. Early in the course of the disease, DLB patients may experience periods of somnolence and/or confusion, interspersed with normal performance, even in the space of a few minutes. Any attention lapse on tests evaluating sustained performance and requiring vigilance (such as the trails making test, reaction times, letter or design cancellations, digits forward and backward, verbal fluency, mental computation) should be considered as indicative of DLB, especially if other supportive diagnostic features are present. Third, DLB patients may show disproportionate deficits on tests requiring problem solving and visuospatial ability (such as copying figures, block design, picture arrangement from the WAIS-R or WAIS-III, visual counting tasks, form discrimination, etc.), or even verbal tests requiring visual integrity (such as the Boston Naming Test).

Vascular Dementia

Vascular pathology is increasingly recognized as a major factor affecting cognition. There is an increased risk of AD in persons with a history of stroke. By definition, a dementia is considered to be of vascular origin if clinical history can document a vascular accident temporally related to the onset of dementia with abrupt onset, and the patient scores positively on at least four items from the Hachinski ischemic scale (58). Although there is overlap between the cognitive impairments of AD and vascular dementias, vascular dementia tends to present with more focal and asymmetrical cognitive impairments. Also, vascular dementia can have both cortical and subcortical manifestations, including motor slowing, the occurrence of behavioral problems early in the course of the disease, and depression.

Neuropsychological Profile

It is particularly important to evaluate all aspects of cognitive domains to determine the pattern of impairment. Cognitive deficits will vary depending on the location and size of vascular lesions and the associated pathways. Again, in contrast to AD, patients with vascular dementia may not necessarily present with prominent memory deficits early in the disease process. Patients with vascular dementia will tend to show a patchwork profile of impaired and well-preserved skills. This pattern is highly unusual in any other form of dementia where there is usually some deficit in all functions, albeit with great variability in severity. Retrieval memory deficits are common and executive inefficiencies are observed, usually in terms of cognitive inflexibility and slowed ability to do sequencing tasks. Asymmetric fine motor speed is likely to be present, as are motor coordination and dexterity deficits.

Frontotemporal dementias

The clinical diagnosis of early frontotemporal dementia (FTD) can be challenging even to experienced clinicians. Neuropsychological testing may not be sufficiently sensitive or specific to be used as a diagnostic marker. One reason is that many FTD patients present with prominent and early social and personality changes that are not picked up by classical neuropsychological tests. Behavioral features suggestive of FTD will come up during history-taking and clinical observation.

The disease typically occurs in the mid-fifties, tends to be asymmetric with the left-side disorders showing language disturbances, and the right-side exhibiting more psychiatric disturbances. The whole syndrome is more common in males and tends to run in families. People with FTD show early loss of insight, lose the ability to empathize with others, and become impulsive. They may behave inappropriately, making tactless comments, or being rude. Also, they may lose inhibitions and social control (for example, exhibiting sexual behavior in public, becoming aggressive, being easily distracted, or developing routines, such as compulsive rituals). Also, patients may show changes in eating habits, overeating or craving sweet foods (59).

Different behavioral subtypes have been described that are related to anatomical involvement. The *disinhibited type* is marked by a breakdown in social and interpersonal behaviors, and corresponds to orbitofrontal degeneration. An *apathetic type* is characterized by inertia, and involves primarily the dorsolateral and medial-frontal cortex. The *stereotypic type* is marked by mental rigidity, perseveration, compulsive behavior, and ritualistic behavior, and corresponds to degeneration of the striatum, as well as the frontal and temporal cortex (60). In a rare variant of FTD referred to as *semantic dementia,* patients experience progressive semantic aphasia and word blindness.

Because of the inappropriate behaviors associated with FTD, patients are often referred to the psychiatrist. Depression, ritualistic behaviors, and anxiety are not uncommon, even before the dementia become evident.

Neuropsychological Profile

Cognitive deficits are subtle but present. FTD can be distinguished from early AD primarily by the presence of one or more of the following: marked behavioral disinhibition, minimal insight, carelessness, apathy, self-neglect and executive dysfunction, with only mild memory disturbances, primarily on recognition. Any test evaluating reasoning, planning, organizational skills, or independent behavior will show major deficits. However, executive dysfunctions cannot always be demonstrated reliably in a laboratory setting and their severity tends be underappreciated by using standard testing and structured conditions.

Typically, memory is mostly intact during the initial stages of FTD, although specific deficits might become noticeable. Recall may be mildly impaired, mainly because of inattention and apparent lack of motivation. Characteristically, recognition of recently learned items will fare a bit worse than the ability to recall them, presumably because all items appear equally familiar. This feature is extremely rare in AD patients even at relatively advanced stages of dementia, in whom even though memory trace may vanish after 30 seconds, recall can be helped with cuing and presenting with multiple choices. Further, FTD patients tend to be either unaware of mistakes they make, or cheerfully gloss over them. They also may show perseverative behaviors or concreteness of thought beyond what would be expected based on their cognitive and functional capacities. Finally, the most characteristic, though elusive, cognitive deficit in FTD pertains to impairment in executive function tasks. This set of higher-order functions include organizational skills, abstract reasoning, divided attention, capacity to access fund of knowledge, ability to apply knowledge and to apply instructions, and in general the ability to successfully live independently and structure one's own environment. Tasks that require self-motivation, organization, abstract thinking and attention will be particularly affected, even in early and mild FTD cases. This will translate into particularly poor performance on tests of verbal fluency, trail making test Part B, recognition memory, and the Wisconsin Card Sorting Test. By contrast, learning skills, visuospatial abilities, and comprehension will be relatively well preserved (61)

FTD patients may also show language difficulties associated with either the frontal or temporal lobes (62). Patients with primarily frontal lobe deficits will show difficulties finding the right words, lack of spontaneous conversation, and an overall reduction in speech. Patients with more posterior deficits will tend to be fluent but use many words with little content. We had a patient who when asked, "if a hammer is good for pounding nails," looked at her fingers rather puzzled and mused, "Yes—but why would anybody want to do that!" In contrast, nonverbal reasoning skills remain largely intact until the moderate disease stage.

For the clinician, clinical observation, an almost perfect score on the MMSE, paired with concrete responses on bedside evaluation of abstract thinking, disorganization on clock drawing, and inability to maintain attention or monitor the quality of one's behavior should raise the suspicion of frontal damage.

CASE EXAMPLE: FRONTOTEMPORAL DEMENTIA

The patient was a 53-year-old, right-handed, married, White male with 14 years of formal education. He came to the attention of a local psychiatrist when his family grew concerned about changes in his behavior. According to his wife and daughter, over the past 12 months the patient had experienced changes primarily involving personality, although the patient himself denied any changes in his cognition, affect, personality, or functional skills. His family reported that he was now outgoing and jovial, whereas previously he tended to be a conservative and reserved man. In contrast, he reported that he was simply enjoying his recent early retirement. His family further reported that aspects of the patient's new social style seemed somewhat inappropriate or inconsistent with the mood or content of a discussion. Finally, they reported that the patient had been drinking excessively, and questioned whether or not his changed personality was related to his alcohol consumption. When queried about his cognition, his family did not report any marked, notable changes in processing skills. Nonetheless, the psychiatrist recognized the possibility of a previously undetected neurological condition, given the reported symptoms and age. There was no known or suspected medical history thought to be contributing to or accounting for the reported changes.

A comprehensive neuropsychological evaluation was completed, which included the assessment of general intellect, attention, executive functions, learning and memory, language, visuospatial abilities, fine motor skills, and mood. The referral question asked for a clarification of cognitive and affective status. Results indicated cognitive deficits exceeding the changes that are typically associated with normal aging. Specifically, the patient demonstrated disproportionate compromises in executive abilities, along with a milder retrieval memory deficit. The patient's sequencing, cognitive flexibility, abstract reasoning skills, concept formation, and problem solving abilities fell well below expectation. The patient also had some difficulty on a supraspan list-learning task, although his retrieval performance improved with cuing. General intellect, language, and visuospatial abilities were generally within normal limits. No depression was detected, although interview and testing data suggested that the patient was anosognosic. Further, behavioral observations during testing suggested a disinhibited style with poor self-monitoring or appreciation for social context.

The neuropsychological profile of disproportionate executive compromises and a mild retrieval memory deficit, coupled with the reported behavioral changes and the behavioral presentation of the patient, was consistent with what is typically observed in frontotemporal dementia (FTD). While it was understandable that the patient's family was concerned that the patient's alcohol use might be related to the findings, the constellation of findings and relatively brief time course did not support alcohol abuse as the primarily etiology. Rather, FTD was more likely the cause.

Re-evaluation was recommended in 1 year to objectively determine progression versus stability over time, which would further clarify diagnosis. Complete cessation of alcohol use, given the likely exacerbation of cognitive and behavioral compromises, was strongly encouraged. Finally, given what the executive processing deficits revealed, a formal driving evaluation was recommended.

Dementia of Depression

This syndrome is also known as pseudodementia, a term that encompassed various psychiatric disorders with dementia-type symptoms that persisted if not treated, such as depression, and also in some patients with schizophrenia or hysterical disorders (63). Patients with dementia of depression show typical signs of dementia, e.g., apathy, memory problems, confusion, and inability to care for themselves. Closer examination will reveal that in sharp contrast with patients with AD or other dementias, patients suffering from dementia of depression can precisely date the onset of their impairment and are acutely aware that their memory is insufficient. Other signs and symptoms of depression are also usually present.

The difficulty is that in many cases dementia and depression may coexist (64). Aspects of the clinical presentation of both an early dementing process and depression most likely that contribute to misdiagnosis are: depressed mood or agitation; a history of psychiatric disturbance; psychomotor retardation; impaired immediate memory and learning abilities; defective attention, concentration, and tracking; impaired orientation; an overall poor quality of performance; loss of interest in one's surroundings and, often, in self-care (65).

Neuropsychological Profile

The neuropsychological profile of patients with dementia of depression is marked by long response latency; slow, non-spontaneous and monotonous speech; frequent "I don't know" responses; incomplete responses; and impaired attention with particular difficulty to complete tasks requiring mental effort (9). Such patients will show poor word-list generation, and inability (or unwillingness) to do calculations of tasks requiring sustained attention. Memory is impaired, but mainly for retrieving information that involves mental effort. Probing shows that new information can be learned and be well retained over long periods of time. Thus, performance tends to be uneven, with simple and attention-demanding tasks being poorly attended to, and even complex tasks being successfully done as long as little effort is required. Further, lack of motivation, anxiety, and dysphoria color the whole evaluation, which are variable in persons with AD and related disorders.

INTERVENTIONS: MAXIMIZING COPING AND COMPENSATION IN DEMENTIA

Consumers of psychiatric, neurological, and neuropsychological services challenge us when after examination and diagnosis they ask, "How do I fix the problem?" Many of our geriatric dementia patients suffer from illnesses that preclude the application of traditional rehabilitation approaches, but nonetheless they and their families search for a means to treat their illness, with the overarching goals of slowing the disease process, compensation of deficits, and enhanced quality of life. Fortunately the landscape of geriatric neuropsychological care services is evolving and treatment can now go beyond pharmacological agents.

Until recently, dementia patients were not considered in the neuropsychological therapeutic arena because of the prevailing idea that all behavioral problems were secondary to cognitive decline, that dementia patients could not learn and retain new information, and that their lack of insight precluded benefit from intervention. These biases against intervention with dementia patients are slowly dissolving with the emergence of new drugs slowing the disease, better understanding of the pathophysiology of dementia, and evidence that AD patients can learn and retain new information. For example, recent findings of relative sparing of the basal ganglia and primary cortex areas are evidence that motor memory, procedural knowledge, and implicit memory may be preserved in AD (66–69).

Like evaluation, interventions vary considerably given the patient's characteristics and needs. The intervention will vary also based on the targeted goal, which can be influenced by the patient, caregiver(s), environment, or a combination of these elements. Finally, it is important to distinguish between two broad intervention categories: those designed to improve or prevent behavioral problems, and those aimed at slowing or remediating cognitive and functional decline. Although these distinctions can become blurred as one type of intervention affects the other category, it is useful to consider them separately.

Improvement or Prevention of Behavioral Problems

By first attempting to address the underlying reason for agitated behavior rather than considering it as a primary symptom to be treated, and next by modifying the environment or caregiver behavior, it can be possible to reduce the severity of symptoms (70). These interventions target the *excess disability*, or greater-than-warranted functional incapacity (71) that results from treatable factors. Specifically, the prevalence of depression in elders with dementia underscores the need for attention to this domain. Close to half of patients demonstrate minor or major forms of depression (39,72). Even among patients without marked affective disorders, reports of less efficient processing during periods of emotional distress highlight a potentially powerful target to improve functioning.

Interventions Aimed at Decreasing Behavioral Problems

Anecdotal evidence abounds about many therapeutic interventions, although few have been validated with sufficient certainty at this point. Examples include orientation therapy, pet therapy, tactile stimulation, aromatherapy, validation therapy, successful prevention of wandering by camouflaging doorway and elevator buttons, and treating depression and a disordered sleep cycle with bright light therapy. Even while waiting for more definite evidence on the utility of these treatments, and even if the mechanisms of action may rely in part on self-fulfilling prophecy or the placebo effect, the practice of encouraging the caregiver to focus on concrete problem-solving and being proactive has numerous and obvious advantages. Emotional well-being of the caregiver goes a long way in improving patient behavioral problems (73). A recent study indicated that the combined use of physical exercise and behavioral antidepressive techniques improved physical and emotional well-being of both caregivers and patients (74). The caregiver coached the patient, with the added benefit of providing exercise for the dyad as well as the opportunity for positive interactions.

Classic therapeutic techniques could be effective in mild patients. Also, support groups for newly diagnosed AD patients have been useful to decrease the sense of isolation and facilitate grief work (75,76). Behavioral modification techniques have been evaluated more rigorously, and a few have been shown to be as modestly effective as some psychotropics to treat agitation, even in moderately impaired patients (77).

Further, physical modification of the environment should be pursued vigorously as a way to compensate for the patient's noted weaknesses, because this will significantly decrease discomfort and related anxiety. Examples of successful environmental modifications are increase in lighting, use of nightlights in bathrooms, prominent placement of visual cues to decrease disorientation, removal of glass tables and other poorly visible obstacles, removal of doors (if necessary), removal of loose carpets, marking stairs, and use of high-contrast flatware and food (78).

Change in communication strategies also can effectively decrease anxiety and agitation. Strategies aimed at compensating for dementia-related deficits in comprehension include the use of short, simple sentences, slower speech, concrete language, close-ended questions, and modeling a request (79,80).

With their understanding of the neuroanatomical correlates of behavior, their insight into the patient's cognitive strengths and weaknesses, and their knowledge of various behavioral and therapeutic approaches, neuropsychologists can play a significant role in the treatment team and help identify the most feasible goals to target (81,82).

Slowing, Remediation, or Compensation for Cognitive and Functional Decline

Because the multiple potential effects of emotional distress on the individual and his or her functioning can aggregate in a manner that undermines treatment progress, affective dysfunction warrants particular attention in the remediation of cognitive and functional decline. Any intervention efforts targeting cognitive variables may well be unsuccessful if attempted in the context of emotional distress. It is useful to differentiate emotional and personality changes that are a result of neurological changes from those that may have existed premorbidly, because treatment of these vary (83). Targeting depression before memory compensation minimizes inefficiency introduced by the emotional distress and increases the patient's resources that will be applied during any cognitive-based intervention.

Let us be clear from the outset: it is not the underlying neuropathology that is targeted for modification; the goal here is not to cure the disease. Rather, the aim is to use compensatory strategies and residual abilities to optimize coping and adjustment (81,84,85). On the one hand, training can lead to subjective *perceptions* of memory gains by patients and caregivers (86), potentially impacting both memory and emotional well-being. On the other hand, it may be possible, by using combination therapies, to show gains in *actual* memory performance. The key question in evaluating the effectiveness of such therapies may soon switch from the demonstration of an improvement, to the determination of the duration of such retention.

Pioneering studies are beginning to delineate what approaches (such as spaced retrieval or multiple-technique programs) will be effective individually or in combination. For instance, spaced retrieval, a technique combining repetitions at increasingly longer intervals, can be used to successfully teach AD patients to use a calendar, perform a prospective memory task, and improve recall of everyday objects (87–89). Errorless learning and associative techniques also have improved learning or retention duration of face-name pairs among AD patients (90).

Two recent studies have demonstrated that people who have early-stage AD can still be taught to recall important information and to better perform daily tasks. David Loewenstein and colleagues found that mildly impaired AD patients who participated in 3 to 4 months of cognitive rehabilitation, more than doubled their ability to recall faces and names, and showed a marked improvement in their ability to provide proper change for a purchase (91). The participants also could respond to and process information more rapidly, and were better oriented to time and place, compared to a similar group of AD patients who did not receive this targeted intervention. Moreover, these improvements were still evident 3 months after the cognitive training ended.

The Loewenstein report follows a recent study by Lustig and Buckner at Washington University in St. Louis, which found that older people with early-stage AD retained functioning levels of implicit memory similar to young adults and older adults who did not have AD (92). Implicit memory is relatively unconscious and automatic: information from the past pops into mind without a deliberate effort to remember. This unconscious, implicit memory is important for common skills and activities, such as speaking a language, or riding a bicycle. In many cases, people implicitly remember how to perform these activities, without being able to deliberately remember when or where they learned them.

These findings show it is possible to pinpoint what memory capabilities are preserved in early AD through systematic study. As Camp and colleagues have outlined: "it is possible to design effective, pragmatically useful memory interventions" for geriatric patients with memory disorders (88, p. 193). Maximal treatment benefits will be obtained with the development and implementation of a carefully considered treatment plan, wherein intervention *targets* and *strategies* are identified. Many variables will be considered in this process, including the neuropsychological presentation (including diagnosis, strengths and weaknesses, level of severity), degree of insight or anosognosia, patient and family goals, motivation, and affective status (92). These variables will assist the clinician in ruling in or out specific intervention approaches, and will also suggest technique modifications (e.g., simplifying or eliminating more complex steps, altering the timing of the introduction of strategy sections). For instance, patients demonstrating a circumscribed memory deficit may be capable of learning and applying effortful processing strategies based on association (e.g., mnemonics), whereas memory-disordered patients with additional executive deficits may benefit from techniques relying less on judgment and organization, such as spaced retrieval.

We can now answer the question, "How do I fix the problem?" with more optimism than we historically have,

given the promising lines of emerging evidence. Indeed, it is important that psychiatrists, neurologists, and neuropsychologists alike stay abreast of the empirical progress within these areas. Specifically, it is essential that practitioners should stay informed about modified training and psychotherapeutic approaches to enhance memory compensation and coping for early-stage patients, a time when these approaches will likely have the most utility. Equally important, practitioners should know what types of behavioral modification, environmental strategies, and other therapies are available to assist persons with more advanced dementias. By staying aware of the progress of these approaches in becoming empirically validated, practitioners can inform their patients about treatment alternatives for symptom management. Finally, we should encourage and support evidence-based lines of research to further our understanding of how to best impact these dimensions of quality of life.

In conclusion, this chapter focused on the concepts underlying neuropsychological evaluations for dementia that, hopefully, will remain useful for years to come. With the exponential explosion of technology, communication, and knowledge, however, information tends to becomes obsolete at a speed outpacing book publication. The clinician might wish to check the websites provided in appendix C of this book for up-to-date information on clinical aging research, new testing instruments, and current therapeutic interventions. These links can also be used as high-quality, time-saving devices when given to caregivers as educational tools.

This site maintained by the Alzheimer Association is invaluable for both patients with dementia and their caregivers. It provides the latest news on research, treatments, and links to extensive support for families.

REFERENCES

1. Moritz DJ, Kasl SV, Berkman LF. Cognitive functioning and the incidence of limitations in activities of daily living in an elderly community sample. *Am J Epidemiol.* 1995;141:41–49.
2. Marson DC, Sawrie SM, Snyder S, et al. Assessing financial capacity in patients with Alzheimer Disease: a conceptual model and prototype instrument. *Arch Neurol.* 2000;57(6):877–884.
3. Koss E, Barry M. Testing techniques in persons suspected of dementia. *Am J Alz Dis Other Demen.* 1994;3:22–27.
4. Strub RL, Black FW. *The Mental Status Examination in Neurology.* 4th Ed. Philadelphia: FA Davis; 2000.
5. Hannay HJ, Bieliauskas L, Crosson BA, Hammeke TA, Hamsher KdeS, Koffler S. Proceedings of the Houston conference on specialty education and training in clinical neuropsychology. *Arch Clin Neuropsychol.* 1998;13(Special Issue):157–250.
6. Donders J. A survey of report writing by neuropsychologists, I: general characteristics and content. *Clin Neuropsychol.* 2001;15(2):137–149.
7. Donders, J. A survey of report writing by neuropsychologists, II: test data, report format, and document length. *Clin Neuropsychol.* 2001;15(2):150–161.
8. Folstein M, Folstein S, McHugh PR. Mini-Mental State: a practical method for grading the cognitive state of patients for the clinician. *J Psychiatr Res.* 1975;12:189–198.

9. Lezak MD. *Neuropsychological Assessment.* 3rd Ed. New York: Oxford University Press; 1995.

10. Reitan RM, Wolfson D. *The Halstead-Reitan Neuropsychological Battery: Theory and Clinical Interpretation.* 2nd Ed. Tucson: Neuropsychology Press; 1993.

11. Blessed G, Tomlinson BE, Roth M. The association between quantitative measures of dementia and of senile change in the cerebral grey matter of elderly subjects. *Br J Psychiatry.* 1968; 114: 797–811.

12. Launer LJ, Dinkgreve MA, Jonker C, Hooijer C, Lindeboom J. Are age and education independent correlates of the Mini-Mental State Exam performance of community-dwelling elderly? *J Gerontol.* 1993;48(6):271–277.

13. Naugle RI, Kawczak K. Limitations of the Mini-Mental State Examination. *Cleve Clin J Med.* 1989;56(3):277–281.

14. Katzman R, Brown T, Fuld P, Peck A, Schechter R, Schimmel H. Validation of a short orientation-memory-concentration test of cognitive impairment. *Am J Psychiatry.* 1983; 140(6):734–739.

15. Mattis S. *Dementia Rating Scale.* Odessa, FL: Psychological Assessment Resources; 1988.

16. Mohs RC, Knopman D, Petersen RC, et al. Development of cognitive instruments for use in clinical trials of antidementia drugs: additions to the Alzheimer's Disease Assessment Scale that broaden its scope. *Alzheimer Dis Assoc Disord.* 1997;11(Suppl. 2):S13–S21.

17. Morris JC, Mohs RC, Rogers H, Fillenbaum G, Heyman A. Consortium to establish a registry for Alzheimer's disease (CERAD) clinical and neuropsychological assessment of Alzheimer's disease. *Psychopharmacol Bull.* 1988;24(4):641–652.

18. Welsh K, Butters N, Hughes J, Mohs R, Heyman A. Detection of abnormal memory decline in mild cases of Alzheimer's disease using CERAD neuropsychological measures. *Arch Neurol.* 1991;48:278–281.

19. Kiernan RJ, Mueller J, Langston JW. *Cognistat (Neurobehavioral Cognitive Status Examination).* Lutz, FL: Psychological Assessment Resources, Inc; 1990.

20. Macaulay C, Battista M, Lebby PC, Mueller J. Geriatric performance on the Neurobehavioral Cognitive Status Examination (Cognistat). What Is Normal? *Arch Clin Neuropsychol.* 2003; 18:463–471.

21. Morris JC. The Clinical Dementia Rating (CDR): current version and scoring rules. *Neurology.* 1993;43:2412–2414.

22. Morris JC, Ernesto C, Schafer K, et al. Clinical Dementia Rating training and reliability in multicenter studies: the Alzheimer's Disease Cooperative Study experience. *Neurology.* 1997;48: 1508–1510.

23. Saxton J, McGonigle-Gibsons KL, Swihart AA. Description and validation of a new neuropsychological test battery. *J Consult Clin Psychol.* 1990;2:298–303.

24. Cole MG, Dastoor DP. A new hierarchic approach to the measurement of dementia. *Psychosomatics.* 1987;28:298–304.

25. Albert M, Cohen C. The Test for Severe Impairment: an instrument for the assessment of patients with severe cognitive dysfunction. *J Am Geriatr Soc.* 1992;40(5):449–453.

26. Blair JR, Spreen O. Predicting premorbid IQ: a revision of the National Adult Reading Test. *The Clinical Neuropsychologist.* 1989;3:129–136.

27. Jastak S, Wilkinson GS. *Wide Range Achievement Test-Revised.* Wilmington: Jastak Assessment Systems; 1984.

28. Axelrod BN, Vanderploeg RD, Schinka JA. Comparing methods for estimating premorbid intellectual functioning. *Arch Clin Neuropsychol.* 1999;14(4):341–346.

29. Wechsler D. *Wechsler Adult Intelligence Scale.* 3rd Ed. San Antonio: Psychological Corporation; 1997.

30. Armitage SG. An analysis of certain psychological tests used for the evaluation of brain injury. *Psychol Monographs.* 1946;60 (Whole No. 277).

31. Trenerry MR, Crosson B, DeBoe J, Leber WR. *The Stroop Neuropsychological Screening Test.* Odessa, FL: Psychological Assessment Resources; 1989.

32. Heaton RK. *Wisconsin Card Sorting Test Manual.* Odessa, FL: Psychological Assessment Resources; 1981.

33. Delis DC. *Delis-Kaplan Executive Function Test.* San Antonio: Psychological Corporation; 2001.

34. American Psychiatric Association: *Diagnostic and Statistical Manual of Mental Disorders.* 4th, Text Revision Ed. Washington, DC: American Psychiatric Association; 2000.

35. Koss E, Haxby J, DeCarli C, et al. Patterns of performance preservation and loss in healthy aging. *Dev Neuropsychol.* 1991;7: 99–113.

36. Goodglass H, Kaplan E. *Assessment of Aphasia and Related Disorders.* 2nd Ed. Philadelphia: Lea & Fibiger; 1983.

37. Cronin-Golomb A, Rizzo JF, Corkin S, Growdon JH. Visual function in Alzheimer's disease and normal aging. *Ann NY Acad Sci.* 1991;640:28–35.

38. Paulsen JS, Salmon DP, Thal LJ, et al. Incidence of and risk factors for hallucinations and delusions in patients with probable AD. *Neurology.* 2000;54(10):1965–1971.

39. Migliorelli R, Tesón A, Sabe L, Petracchi M, Leiguarda R, Starkstein SE. Prevalence and correlates of dysthymia and major depression among patients with Alzheimer's disease. *Am J Psychiatry.* 1995; 152:37–44.

40. Steffens DC, Plassman BL, Helms MJ, Welsh-Bohmer KA, Saunders AM, Breitner JC. A twin study of late-onset depression and apolipoprotein E 4 as risk factors for Alzheimer's disease. *Biol Psychiatry.* 1997;41:851–856.

41. Wilson RS, Gilley DW, Bennett DA, Beckett LA, Evans D.A. Hallucinations, delusions, and cognitive decline in Alzheimer's disease. *J Neurol Neurosurg Psychiatry.* 2000;69(2):172–177.

42. Alexopoulos GS, Abrams RC, Young RC, Shamoian CA. Cornell Scale for Depression in Dementia. *Biol Psychiatry.* 1988;23:271–284.

43. Yesavage JA, Brink TL, Rose TL, et al. Development and validation of a geriatric depression scale. *Psychiatr Res.* 1983;17:31–49.

44. Reisberg B, Borenstein J, Franssen E, et al. BEHAVE-AD: a clinical rating scale for the assessment of pharmacologically remediable behavioral symptomatology in Alzheimer's disease. In: Altman HJ (ed). *Alzheimer's Disease: Problems, Prospects, and Perspectives.* New York: Plenum; 1987;1–16

45. Cohen-Mansfield J, Billig N. Agitated behaviors in the elderly. I. A conceptual review. *J Am Geriatr Soc.* 1986;34(10):711–721.

46. Teri L, Truax P, Logsdon R, Uomoto J, Zarit S, Vitaliano PP. Assessment of behavioral problems in dementia: the revised memory and behavior problems checklist. *Psychol Aging.* 1992; 7(4):622–631.

47. Cummings JL, Mega M, Gray K, Rosenberg-Thompson S, Carusi DA, Gornbein J. The Neuropsychiatric Inventory: comprehensive assessment of psychopathology in dementia. *Neurology.* 1994; 44(12):2308–2314.

48. Katz S, Akpom CA. 12. Index of ADL. *Med Care.* 1976;14(5 Suppl): 116–118.

49. Lawton MP, Brody EM. Assessment of older people: self-maintaining and instrumental activities of daily living. *Gerontologist.* 1969; 9(3):179–186.

50. Reisberg B. Functional Assessment Staging (FAST). *Psychopharmacol Bull.* 1988;24(4):653–655.

51. Knopman DS, Boeve BF, Petersen RC. Essentials of the proper diagnoses of mild cognitive impairment, dementia, and major subtypes of dementia. *Mayo Clin Proc.* 2003;78(10):1290–1308.

52. Lopez OL, Litvan I, Catt KE, et al. Accuracy of four clinical diagnostic criteria for the diagnosis of neurodegenerative dementias. *Neurology.* 1999;53(6):1292–1299.

53. Petersen RC, Doody R, Kurz A, et al. Current concepts in mild cognitive impairment. *Arch Neurol.* 2001;58(12):1985–1992.

54. Wilson RS, Beckett LA, Bennett DA, Albert MS, Evans DA. Change in cognitive function in older persons from a community population: relation to age and Alzheimer disease. *Arch Neurol.* 1999;56(10):1274–1279.

55. McKeith IG. Dementia with Lewy Bodies. *Br J Psychiatry.* 2002; 180:144–147.

56. McKeith IG. Advances in the diagnosis and treatment of dementia with Lewy Bodies. Introduction. *Dement Geriatr Cogn Disord.* 2004;17 (Suppl 1):1–2.

57. Knopman DS. An overview of common non-Alzheimer dementias. *Clin Geriatr Med.* 2001;17(2):281–301.

58. Chui HC, Mack W, Jackson JE, et al. Clinical criteria for the diagnosis of vascular dementia: a multicenter study of comparability and inter-rater reliability. *Arch Neurol.* 2000; 57(2):191–196.

59. Miller BL, Diehl J, Freedman M, Kertesz A, Mendez M, Rascovsky K. International approaches to frontotemporal dementia diagnosis: from social cognition to neuropsychology. *Ann Neurol.* 2003;54(Suppl 5):S7–S10.

60. Cummings JL. *The Neuropsychiatry of Alzheimer's Disease and Related Dementias*. London: Martin Dunitz Ltd; 2003.

61. Grossman M. Frontotemporal dementia: a review. *J Int Neuropsychol Soc*. 2002;8(4):566–583.

62. Mesulam MM. Primary progressive aphasia. *Ann Neurol*. 2001;49(4):425–432.

63. Dobie DJ. Depression, dementia, and pseudodementia. *Semin Clin Neuropsychiatry*. 2002;7(3):170–186.

64. Lyketsos CG, Lee HB. Diagnosis and treatment of depression in Alzheimer's disease. a practical update for the clinician. *Dement Geriatr Cogn Disord*. 2004;17(1–2):55–64.

65. Fischer P. The spectrum of depressive pseudo-dementia. *J Neural Transm*. 1996;103(Suppl) 47:193–203.

66. Haxby J, Grady CL, Koss E, et al. Longitudinal studies of cerebral metabolic asymmetries and neuropsychological patterns in early dementia of the Alzheimer's type. *Arch Neurol*. 1990;47: 753–760.

67. Backman L, Andersson JL, Nyberg L, et al. Brain regions associated with episodic memory retrieval in normal aging and Alzheimer's disease. *Neurology*. 1999;52:861–870.

68. Backman L. Utilizing compensatory task conditions for episodic memory in Alzheimer's disease. *Acta Neurol Scand Suppl*. 1996;165:109–113.

69. Dick MB, Nielson KA, Beth RE, et al. Acquisition and long-term retention of a motor skill in Alzheimer's disease. *Brain Cogn*. 2003;29:294–306.

70. Teri L, Logsdon RG, McCurry SM. Nonpharmacologic treatment of behavioral disturbance in dementia. *Med Clin North Am*. 2002;86(3):641–656, viii. Review.

71. Brody E, Kleban M, Lawton MP, Silverman H. Excess disabilities of mentally impaired aged: impact of individualized treatment. *Gerontologist*. 1971;11(2):124–133.

72. Ballard C, Bannister C, Solis M, Oyebode F, Wilcock G. The prevalence, associations and symptoms of depression amongst dementia sufferers. *J Affect Disord*. 1996;36:135–144.

73. Mittelman MS, Roth DL, Haley WE, Zarit SH. Effects of a caregiver intervention on negative caregiver appraisals of behavior problems in patients with Alzheimer's disease: results of a randomized trial. *J Gerontol B Psychol Sci Soc Sci*. 2004;59(1): 27–34.

74. Teri L, Gibbons LE, McCurry SM, et al. Exercise plus behavioral management in patients with Alzheimer disease: a randomized controlled trial. *JAMA*. 2003 Oct 15;290(15):2015–2022.

75. Davies H, Robinson D, Bevill L. Supportive group experience for patients with early-stage Alzheimer's disease. *J Am Geriatr Soc*. 1995;43:1068–1069.

76. LaBarge E, Trtanj F. A support group for people in the early stages of dementia of the Alzheimer type. *J Appl Gerontol*. 1995;14: 289–301.

77. Teri L, Logsdon RG, Peskind E, et al. Treatment of agitation in AD: a randomized, placebo-controlled clinical trial. *Neurology*. 2000 Nov 14;55(9):1271–1278.

78. Koss E, Gilmore GC. Environmental interventions and functional abilities of AD patients. In: Vellas B, Fitten J, Frisoni G, ed. *Research and Practice in Alzheimer's Disease*. New York: Springer Publishing Company; 1998.

79. Ripich DN, Wykle ML. *Alzheimer's Disease Communication Training Manual; the FOCUSED Program for Caregivers*. San Antonio: Psychological Corporation; 1996.

80. Small JA, Gutman G. Recommended and reported use of communication strategies in Alzheimer caregiving. *Alzheimer Dis Assoc Disord*. 2002;16(4):270–278.

81. Sohlberg M, Mateer C. *Introduction to cognitive rehabilitation*. New York: The Guilford Press; 1989.

82. Pramuka M, McCue M. Assessment to rehabilitation: communicating across the gulf. In: Vanderploeg RD, ed. *Clinician's Guide to Neuropsychological Assessment*. Mahwah, NJ: Lawrence Erlbaum Associates, Publishers; 2000:337–355.

83. Crossen B. Application of neuropsychological assessment results. In: Vanderploeg RD, ed. *Clinician's Guide to Neuropsychological Assessment*. Mahwah, NJ: Lawrence Erlbaum Associates, Publishers; 2000:195–244.

84. Koltai DC, Branch LG. Considerations of intervention alternatives to optimize independent functioning in the elderly. *J Clin Geropsychol*. 1998;4:333–349.

85. Koltai DC, Branch LG. Cognitive and affective interventions to maximize abilities and adjustment in dementia. *Ann Psychiatry: Basic Clin Neurosci*. 1999;7:241–255.

86. Koltai DC, Welsh-Bohmer K. Influence of anosognosia on treatment outcome among dementia patients. *Neuropsychol Rehab*. 2001;11:455–475.

87. McKitrick LA, Camp CJ, Black FW. Prospective memory intervention in Alzheimer's disease. *J Gerontol*. 1992;47:P337–P343.

88. Camp C, Foss J, O'Hanlon A, Stevens A. Memory interventions for persons with dementia. *Applied Cognitive Psychology*. 1996;10: 193–210.

89. Cherry K, Simmons S, Camp C. Spaced retrieval enhances memory in older adults with probable Alzheimer's disease. *J Clin Geropsychol*. 1999;5:159–175.

90. Clare L, Wilson BA, Carter G, Roth I, Hodges JR. Relearning face-name associations in early Alzheimer's disease. *Neuropsychology*. 2002;16(4):538–547.

91. Loewenstein DA, Acevedo A, Czaja SJ, Duara R. Cognitive rehabilitation of mildly impaired Alzheimer disease patients on cholinesterase inhibitors. *Am J Geriatr Psychiatry*. 2004; 12(4): 395–402.

92. Lustig C, Buckner RL. Preserved neural correlates of priming in old age and dementia. *Neuron*. 2004 Jun 10;42(5):865–875

The Dementia Workup

10

Lisa L. Boyle   *M. Saleem Ismail*   *Anton P. Porsteinsson*

As the longevity of humans has increased during the past century, age-related illnesses, including dementia, have become a major focus for the health care community. Approximately 4.5 million U.S. individuals have Alzheimer's disease (AD), the most common type of dementia. These numbers are projected to increase at least threefold by the year 2050 (1,2). Dementia, a chronic brain illness, affects virtually every aspect of a person's life and erodes an individual's identity and personality while causing significant caregiver and family distress and psychologic burden. The economic burden on individuals, families, and society is huge (2).

Despite advances during the last decade to improve our awareness of and broaden our understanding into the origins and expression of dementia, the early recognition of dementia is often missed. Under-recognition causes significant delay in establishing the diagnosis and implementing necessary interventions (3–6). History, physical examination, and mental status examination (MSE) are essential for reaching an early and accurate diagnosis so that a timely intervention can be instituted. It is anticipated that, with the rise in the geriatric population, practitioners will continue to face the seemingly daunting task of pursuing a dementia workup with less time allotted per office visit. Therefore, an essential skill for those who treat older adults is the ability to complete a thorough assessment in an efficient manner.

This chapter will provide a practical framework and a step-wise approach to the dementia workup. Essential components of the workup and their importance in guiding differential diagnoses are discussed. This approach will provide the foundation for further reading and understanding of the specific diseases that are discussed in greater detail in subsequent chapters.

DEMENTIA

Dementia is a brain disease and not a normal age-related change. A diagnosis of dementia requires demonstration of impairment in memory as well as one other aspect of cognition such as language, orientation, praxis, or executive functions. The impairment should be severe enough to cause deficits in social and occupational functioning and represents a change from a previously attained level. Substance abuse, medication-related, psychiatric, and medical causes should be excluded.

Practically speaking, dementia is not just a cognitive disorder. Despite the heterogeneity of the effects of dementia within and across individuals, it is possible to categorize these changes using four overlapping and somewhat arbitrary conceptual domains: cognition, daily functioning, behavior, and neurological changes. These domains must be assessed when the patient is being evaluated for suspected dementia, and reassessed over time to monitor progression. Finally, these domains must be assessed periodically during the course of therapy to determine whether it has "worked."

Since there is no antemortem confirmatory test, various diagnostic criteria have been developed. These criteria help in clinically differentiating dementia subtypes. Use of these criteria helps to achieve maximum antemortem diagnostic accuracy (7–11). The National Institute of Neurological, Communicative Disorders and Stroke-Alzheimer Disease and Related Dementia Association (NINCDS-ADRDA) criteria are commonly used to diagnose *possible* and *probable* AD. Other commonly used criteria for diagnosing dementias include: Diagnostic and Statistical Manual of the American Psychiatric Association, Fourth Edition, Text Revision (DSM-IV-TR); the National Institute of

Neurological Disorders Stroke-Association Internationale pour la Recherche et l'Enseignement en Neurosciences (NINDS-AIREN) criteria for vascular dementia (VaD); Consortium for Dementia with Lewy Bodies (DLB); and Consensus for diagnostic criteria for Frontotemporal Dementia (FTD). Practice guidelines have also been adopted to assist clinicians in establishing the diagnosis of dementia (12–14).

Cognitive deficits are usually evident early on and include impairments in memory, attention, language in all of its aspects (speaking, understanding speech, reading, and writing), orientation to space and time, visuospatial function, praxis, and executive function (the ability to respond to information in the environment and execute a logical plan). There is loss of complex (or instrumental) and then ultimately more basic functional abilities. There is also about a 90% lifetime risk of experiencing significant psychopathological features at some point in the dementia illness (15). Finally, neurological abnormalities are relatively common in certain types of dementia.

A limitation of the criteria used in the DSM-IV-TR is the emphasis on memory impairment to establish the diagnosis (8). Whereas this finding is typical for AD, other types of dementia, like FTD, may present with impairment in other cognitive domains, while memory is relatively preserved early in the course of the illness. Therefore, it is essential that a work-up includes evaluation of other aspects of cognition as well as assessment of daily functions and behaviors.

In the absence of diagnostic biologic markers or pathognomonic tests, the role of the history and examination in establishing the dementia diagnosis in the majority of cases remains unchallenged. Although pathologic confirmation of diagnosis typically can be established at autopsy, a thorough clinical assessment can accurately identify various causes of dementia in up to 90% of patients antemortem (14). AD (at approximately 60%) remains the most common cause of dementia, followed by VaD (approximately 20%), and DLB (approximately 20%) (10,14,16). VaD and DLB may also present with AD as a mixed dementia (10,17,18). FTD may represent approximately 15% of neurodegenerative dementias (19), while reversible dementias may account for <1% (20).

EARLY AND ACCURATE DIAGNOSIS

Barriers to Early Diagnosis

Despite the recognition that dementia is one of the biggest public health challenges of this century, the early recognition of dementia is often missed (3–6). Several patient, family, and system-related factors contribute to delayed recognition. Some of the barriers to embarking on the dementia work-up and establishing a diagnosis include: patient and/or family denial of symptoms; hesitation on the clinician's part of making the diagnosis because of lack of recognition of early symptoms; uncertainty due to absence of confirmatory diagnostic tests; and a large differential diagnosis with limited time allotted for office visits.

Overcoming these barriers is the first challenge in most clinical practices. Such barriers can be overcome by having a higher index of suspicion for at-risk individuals, by approaching patients in a nonconfrontational style, involving the family or caregiver, and by using directed clinical measures that allow efficient use of trained clinical staff. Provider and economic factors can be eased to a large extent by incorporating questions related to memory impairment at intake or in routine clinical assessments, using self-administered or caregiver-administered assessment scales, scheduling separate visits for cognitive work-up, and regularly using trained nursing staff in order to efficiently screen and obtain necessary information for review prior to the office visit. Physician extenders can provide valuable support to busy practices by coordinating and supervising care of dementia patients.

Benefits of Early Diagnosis and Intervention

While there is no cure at present for this illness, dementia is treatable. Although current treatments are symptomatic, disease-modifying drugs for dementia are in development. Our improved understanding into the origins and expression of dementia has led to efforts to modify the course of disease and lessen the burden on those who are caught in its downward spiral. Early diagnosis can lead to early intervention and thus benefit the patient and their caregivers by:

- Providing a clinical explanation for presenting complaint(s)
- Providing education about dementia to improve the patient's and family's understanding
- Providing time for the patient and family to discuss and plan for the future (advance directives, financial matters, placement) while the patient continues to have capacity
- Providing anticipatory guidance for emerging symptoms
- Providing referrals to support groups and community resources for the patient and family
- Providing options for nonpharmacologic and pharmacologic treatments for behavioral and medical comorbidities.

The ultimate goal of early and accurate diagnosis is to improve quality of life during the patient's remaining years and to reduce caregiver and family burden. Providing the necessary support can help optimize the patient's and family's ability to cope with a life-altering and usually progressive illness. An early diagnosis will help mobilize all supports and community resources to maximize the benefits for patients and their families.

SCREENING FOR DEMENTIA

Given older patients often have a higher share of medical illness and polypharmacy with higher odds of developing cognitive deficits (either delirium or dementia), routine assessment of cognition before a problem arises is clinically valuable. For example, determining cognitive function in geriatric patients anticipating surgical or high-risk procedures can help provide a baseline measure in the event of a postoperative delirium.

Suspecting Dementia

Whether practitioners should incorporate cognitive screening into their general medical practice is a hotly debated topic. In practice, geriatricians and other physicians who commonly treat older patients often perform cognitive screening to establish baseline measures of cognition. However at present, routine screening is not recommended by the U.S. Preventive Services Task Force, as there is insufficient evidence for or against such a recommendation (21). Some argue that the Mini-Mental State Examination (MMSE), a screening tool commonly used, may be of limited utility if applied to a general medical practice as a routine screen because of decreased positive-predictive value in a population with a low base-rate of dementia (21,22).

Typically, clinical suspicion arises when family reports concerns; during direct observation of the patient during routine office visits; or occasionally by the patient's self-report. Any concerns about the patient's cognition or capacity elicited during interactions in the office should be investigated further. Generally the worried family members raise alarm as the affected individual usually has limited insight and may not report any concerns. Informant concerns about patient's memory loss typically are reliable and predictive of dementia (23).

Some Warning Signs

Potential triggers signaling a need for further assessment include:

- forgetting appointments
- not taking medications correctly
- unusual grooming or behaviors
- confusion, forgetfulness, or repetition during the interview
- inability to follow instructions
- lost in parking lot or office building

Age and Other Risk Factors

If general routine screening is not practical, it makes sense to conduct a thorough assessment in those with suspected cognitive impairment and those at higher risk (21). For instance, age is an identified risk factor for cognitive impairment (3,24,25). The incidence of dementia increases with age by doubling every 5 years after the age of 65 (24). The prevalence of dementia increases with age, affecting approximately 3% to 11% of patients over 65 years old and 25% to 47% over 86 years old (25). Therefore, the patient's age can help guide when to screen for cognitive impairment in an asymptomatic patient. Some physicians screen patients over 65 years old who present to the office for the first time and annually thereafter.

Any patient who presents with unexplained change in mental status, including new-onset depression, anxiety, behavioral or personality changes deserves further investigation. Psychiatric symptoms can be early manifestations of many types of dementia. In FTD, the first and early difficulties are subtle changes in personality, affect, or behavior; memory is spared until later in the disease. Pursuing further evaluation of new or evolving neurologic complaints is necessary, as some dementias (e.g., dementia secondary to brain tumor, stroke, or DLB) may present with neurological signs and symptoms. Other patients who should be followed closely include those with extensive vascular disease (i.e., those at risk for cerebrovascular disease), other neurologic illness (such as Parkinson's disease or Huntington's disease) or family history of dementia (especially if early onset <65 years old). A high index of suspicion for dementia in patients who are high utilizers of health services may be appropriate, as demented patients present more frequently to the office for other medical concerns. Table 10-1 serves as a guide to identify patients who are at increased risk.

THE ROLE OF AN INFORMANT

In the clinical assessment of dementia, the role of the informant or caregiver is critical and not secondary. Because of the nature of dementia, the reliability of the history obtained from the patient alone is often in question. Patients, who may have impaired insight, cover up their disability or unintentionally confabulate. It is not uncommon to spend an entire visit with a patient and develop a

TABLE 10-1
DEMENTIA RISK FACTORS

Advanced age
Positive family history (especially early onset)
Alcohol or drug abuse
History of depression
Mental retardation (Down's syndrome)
History of head injury
Cerebrovascular risk factors
History of delirium
Exposure to heavy metals
Neurologic diseases (Huntington's disease, Parkinson's disease, progressive supranuclear palsy, cortical basal degeneration)
HIV infection

sense that everything is fine, only later to receive a frantic call during a crisis from a family member revealing sufficient problems. Therefore, obtaining collateral information from a reliable informant is crucial. Typically, a spouse or child is available. The reliable informant can provide information that the patient is unable to, such as describing cognitive and functional difficulties, characterizing the earliest changes, and determining if there are specific concerns about the patient's safety. The clinician should be aware of the potential barrier to making an early diagnosis when a cognitively impaired spouse serves as the informant. "I also forget," is an all too common statement made by a protective spouse.

APPROACHING THE PATIENT WITH SUSPECTED DEMENTIA

When pursuing a dementia work-up, it helps to determine how the patient was referred. Is the patient self-referred or brought by a worried family member? Has a concern previously been identified by another physician? Along the same line of thought, it helps to determine the extent of the patient's insight into his or her problems. Patients with insight into their illness can provide some direction during the evaluation, while those with impaired insight often have difficulty communicating any problems or concerns. One way to gather information to determine insight is to establish from the patient his or her understanding of why he or she came to the appointment.

Generally, the patient should be assessed alone first. Subsequently, obtain a careful history from accompanying spouse, family member, or close friend. Ideally, the informant should be reliable and someone who knows the patient very well. The informant interview should be done with the patient out of the room to allow concerns to be shared freely, without censor. Afterward, evaluate the patient and the informant together as a model for collaboration but also to observe the dynamics of the relationship. Keep in mind that loved-ones may be hesitant to report the extent of the problems due to denial or incorrectly attributing difficulties to normal aging (4). However, in general, informant reports of memory problems are necessary to establish the dementia diagnosis and predict eventual dementia in patients with early changes (23).

When the patient has some insight, it can be embarrassing and frustrating for the patient who is struggling to answer questions and undergo cognitive testing. Establish rapport and treat the patient with consideration. Provide an environment where the patient can give her best performance by minimizing distractions and interruptions, as patients with dementia may have difficulties attending. At times, extra patience and time are needed in order to allow the patient to answer questions, secondary to slowed cognitive processes and psychomotor retardation. Empathizing and providing support can lessen the embarrassment and

overall level of distress. Adapting to an individual's level of performance is crucial since many patients who struggle with the assessment can become irritated or belligerent. Incorporating questions that can be applied to daily conversations, social interactions, or practical everyday tasks, while de-emphasizing giving the patient a "test," can decrease resistance. Reassurance and attempts to normalize problems such as, "sometimes people who have similar problems tell me that they also have problems with. . . ." can be effective with the patient but also with informants.

SCREENING MEASURES

Various screening tools are available for use in clinical practice. The most valuable screening tools are those which are simple, brief and reliable in detecting impairments. No single tool is ideal for all situations. The MMSE, despite limitations, is a cognitive screening tool commonly used in clinical practice (26,27). In general, it is brief (typically takes less than 5–10 minutes) and easy to administer at bedside. The MMSE assesses orientation, attention, calculation, registration, short-term memory, language and visuospatial construction. The usual cutoff score of <24 out of a total 30 points yields good sensitivity (63–87%) and specificity (96%) as a dementia screen (27,28). In addition to characterizing if cognitive deficits are present, it can also be used to track progression of illness and to determine effectiveness of therapeutic interventions. At the typical cut-off scores, the MMSE loses sensitivity for mild cognitive deficits (27). The MMSE does not test long-term memory and executive function. Additionally, it does not help to determine etiology of illness.

One must also take into consideration the patients' age and educational level when interpreting the score (22,27–30). Published population-based norms based on age and educational attainment assist with interpretation of MMSE in clinical practice (29). Indeed, for patients who are well-educated and high-functioning, even small decrements on the MMSE may be cause for concern. Conversely, for patients without formal education, scores below the usual cutoff may not necessarily indicate a dementing process, especially if the history and exam do not support a change in cognition or functional abilities. It is important to place the value of the data obtained from the MMSE into perspective and pursue more in-depth evaluation. Again, the emphasis is on a change from a prior level of functioning.

Because of the limitations of the MMSE, additional cognitive screening measures to augment the MMSE are used in clinical practice. The verbal fluency (or category retrieval) test is a measure of language function, verbal fluency and executive function. The patient is given 1 minute and asked to generate a word-list by category. The clinician monitors whether the patient uses a strategy to complete the tasks. Also, observing for perseveration or other errors can provide useful information. One reported cutoff is fifteen items in 1 minute with a sensitivity of 87% and specificity of 96% (31); however, like the MMSE, it is likely influenced by educational attainment (32). If the patient appears to falter, prompting is allowed by encouraging the patient to think of any additional items. Usual items include generating a list of animals, but this can be substituted with other lists like grocery or household items.

A variation of the category fluency test is the letter fluency test. Like the category fluency assessment, the patient is asked to generate a word list in 1 minute. However, in the letter fluency test, the patient is asked to think of as many words starting with a particular letter (i.e., F-, A-, S-). The patient is asked to exclude proper names or use of the same root word repeatedly. Again, observing for strategies, perseveration, errors, and level of effort is important in interpreting the scores. A disparity in performance between category and letter retrieval can provide clues to the origin of brain dysfunction with patients with VaD typically having more difficulty with phonemic fluency (31).

Another cognitive screening test that is easily and quickly administered is the Clock Drawing Test (CDT). This is best done by asking the patient to draw a face of a clock spontaneously, as opposed to providing a predrawn figure to copy. The patient is usually asked to place the hands at "10 after 11." The CDT assesses multiple cognitive domains, including executive function, language, construction, and visuospatial abilities. Subtle cognitive changes that can be missed with the MMSE can be detected with this test without requiring extensive amounts of time. Various versions of this task and scoring methods exist (33–36).

As with the MMSE, interpretation of results for fluency tests and the CDT requires clinical judgment and consideration of the patient's age, educational background, as well as any other impairments (such as aphasia, visual, or motor impairments). Additionally, cultural factors may influence performance. Careful consideration of whether a patient struggles to perform the testing or requires considerable effort in order to answer questions correctly can provide additional valuable clinical information. Some patients with early stages of disease, such as Mild Cognitive Impairment (MCI), ultimately may be able to answer questions correctly but may require considerable effort in order to do so. One should keep in mind that the process can be as informative as the end result.

The Mini-Cog assessment instrument combines an uncued three-item recall test with a CDT. The patient is asked to remember three unrelated words and then to repeat the words. CDT is performed next and serves as the recall distractor. The patient is then asked to repeat the three previously presented words (37). Alternative cognitive screening measures (Blessed Information-Memory-Concentration Test, Blessed Orientation-Memory-Concentration Test, Short Test of Mental Status, Seven Minute Cognitive Screen) have also been developed (38,39). Given the

usual limitations of the MMSE and other screening measures to detect executive function impairments, the EXIT interview can be used to detect frontal lobe impairment and executive dysfunction. It has been identified as a good predictor of disability when using a cutoff of 15 or greater out of a 50-point scale. It is a 25-item test that can be completed in approximately 10 minutes, and does not depend on age or educational attainment (40).

THE DEMENTIA WORK-UP

History

The fact that dementia is a clinical diagnosis helps keep the focus on importance of history and clinical exam. When working-up dementia, the clinician needs to hone in on the following vital elements: cognitive impairment, functional decline, behavioral changes, and neurologic disturbance. Again, clinical concern is raised when there is significant decline from baseline. An outline of the necessary features of the history in the dementia work-up is provided in Table 10-2.

TABLE 10-2
COMPONENTS OF THE HISTORY IN THE DEMENTIA WORK-UP

Obtain history from patient and informant separately
Presenting symptoms
- Cognitive changes
- Daily functions
- Behavior
- Neurologic signs and symptoms

Characteristics
- Onset/duration
- Progression
- Severity of symptoms
- Associated symptoms
- Triggers/stressors/precipitating factors

Psychiatric history
- Mood or psychotic disorders
- Delirium
- Substance abuse

Medical history
- Head injury
- Systemic and neurological illnesses
- Exposures to toxins, metals

Medication and substance use history
- See Table 10-10

Family history
- Cognitive/psychiatric/neurological disorders (age at onset)

Social history
- Educational and occupational attainment
- Premorbid personality and level of functioning
- Social supports and resources (caregivers, family)
- Safety issues (home environment, driving, financial)

Cognition

Commonly, patients will present with memory complaints. This can range from forgetting appointments, repetitious speech, or misplacing things. It is essential that the clinician pursues these subjective complaints with careful questions in order to characterize disturbances commonly found in dementia. Please refer to Table 10-3 for a list of questions to help focus the interview. An efficient and successful evaluation requires that questions be adapted to the presenting complaint and redirected to elicit response from a reliable informant.

It is helpful to ask the informant to think back to identify any early or subtle changes in the patient that previously may have been dismissed as insignificant. Again, significant delay from symptom onset to diagnosis, unfortunately, is not uncommon in clinical practice (3–6). Additional questions about changes in the patient's routine and activities can also help determine types of cognitive impairment. Questions that involve the patient's ability to participate in tasks that are complex or require planning (such as playing card games or meal preparation) can identify problems associated with executive functions. Also ask about any events that may raise concerns about the patient's judgment or safety.

Daily Function

To diagnose dementia a key feature required is impairment in daily functioning. A careful assessment of complex and basic daily functions is necessary to distinguish between early dementia and MCI. Patients with MCI have impaired cognitive function, but it is not associated with impairment in social or daily functioning. These patients warrant close follow-up as the amnestic form of MCI, in particular, is considered a risk factor for AD. Approximately 6% to 25% of patients with MCI convert to AD per year, compared with 0.2% to 3.9% in the normal population (13).

It is often helpful to start with the patient's premorbid or baseline functional level. This includes education, employment history, social activities, hobbies, and typical daily routine. Then determine whether there has been any change and assess the patient's and family's understanding of the reason for such changes. The Instrumental Activities of Daily Living (IADLs) are complex tasks that require a higher level of functional independence while Activities of Daily Living (ADLs) are basic daily functions which are relatively preserved in early stages of dementia. Evaluation can be streamlined by asking the patient and family to complete an IADL and ADL assessment questionnaires prior to the office visit. A list of common IADLs and ADLs as shown in Table 10-4 can be used to record the extent of such impairment. The value of assessing daily functions goes beyond helping to establish a dementia diagnosis. The ability of an individual to live safely and independently in the community is typically determined on the basis of ability to perform daily functions. When patients

have more difficulty attending to their own ADLs (especially bathing and toileting), it becomes harder for families to continue to provide the necessary care to keep them at home.

Behavior

Neuropsychiatric symptoms are commonly found in the course of dementing illness. Therefore, one should also determine whether the patient has had any history suggestive

---

TABLE 10-3
QUESTIONS TO ELICIT TYPES OF MEMORY DIFFICULTIES

Have you noticed:
- Being more forgetful?
- Losing your train of thought?
- Problems trying to find the right word or remembering words to use?
- Problems remembering when and how to take medications?
- Problems remembering appointments?
- Losing things around the house only to have them turn up later?
- Remembering the names of family members or close friends?
- Difficulty following conversations?
- Problems forgetting conversations?
- Difficulties using things around the house such as the coffee maker, vacuum, or telephone?
- Forgetting to turn things off such as the lights or stove?
- Getting lost around the house, in the neighborhood, or while driving?
- Keeping track of time?
- Others expressing a concern about your memory?
- Others expressing concern about you repeatedly asking the same question, only to forget the answer?

TABLE 10-4
QUESTIONS TO HELP GUIDE TYPE OF FUNCTIONAL DECLINE

For the following functions, assess if patient is completely independent, needs assistance secondary to cognitive limitations, needs assistance secondary to physical limitations, or is completely dependent.

Activities of Daily Living (ADLs)	Instrumental Activities of Daily Living (IADLs)
Bathing	Driving
Eating	Using Public transportation
Dressing	Managing Medications
Toileting	Managing Finances
Grooming	Doing Laundry
Transferring	Cooking
Walking	Cleaning
	Attending to Hobbies
	Shopping
	Using Appliances
	Using the Telephone

of personality changes or behavioral disturbances. Social withdrawal, apathy, and disinhibition can be either early or late changes associated with dementia. Assessment of behavioral changes is a critical component of a dementia work-up, as up to 90% of patients eventually develop neuropsychiatric complications as the disease progresses (15,41,42).

Behavioral manifestations are fairly common presenting complaints. It is a good idea to screen for depression when older adults present with cognitive symptoms or *vice versa*. Also, survey associated symptoms such as anxiety, anhedonia, anergia, sleep and appetite disturbances. Any concerns in these areas should trigger a more extensive evaluation. A way to make the screening more efficient includes providing a self-report tool, such as the Geriatric Depression Scale (GDS), to be completed beforehand (43). A short-form of the GDS is also useful to screen for major depression in older primary-care patients (44). Also, two quick screening questions for use in the primary care setting include whether the patient has experienced in the past month: (1) mood that is down, depressed, or hopeless, and (2) anhedonia. Positive responses to these two questions are highly sensitive as a major depression screen (45,46).

Any past psychiatric history should be considered in the evaluation. Although a previous psychiatric history does not automatically rule in or rule out a cognitive disorder, it does pose a diagnostic challenge in some cases. In such cases importance of detailed history taking cannot be over emphasized. In some cases, a referral to a neuropsychologist or psychiatrist may be required.

Depression-associated cognitive impairments in attention, memory, and processing have been well described, and historically have been referred to as constituting a *pseudodementia*. Depression is considered a risk factor for dementia and recent studies have raised concerns about how reversible some of the cognitive changes are despite adequate treatment and remission of the depressive episode (47). Generally, if a clinically significant depression is present, it is best to treat the depression and then reassess for persistence of cognitive deficits once the depression is adequately treated.

The presence of psychotic symptoms (hallucination or delusions) can be very distressing and debilitating for patients and families. Significant neuropsychiatric comorbidity can influence need for placement and significantly strain caregiver and family relationships.

Neurologic Signs and Symptoms

Associated neurologic symptoms can provide clues about the etiology, help focus the subsequent neurologic exam (focusing on gait disturbance, focal neurologic and extrapyramidal signs), and determine the need for ancillary studies. Any positive findings can provide clues regarding dementia etiology. A patient and his or her family's ability to provide care at home often can be limited by comorbid neurologic disability (e.g., gait disturbance, falls,

incontinence); therefore, identifying treatment needs and providing anticipatory guidance for potential future comorbidities can significantly influence successful management of illness.

Putting the History Together

After a list of cognitive, behavioral, functional, and neurologic difficulties has been identified, characterizing the duration of these symptoms is important in order to determine progression. Did all of the problems start at once? Were there any precipitating factors (such as loss of a spouse, major medical setback, new medication)? How rapidly has the patient been declining? Which symptoms appeared first? How have the patient and family been able to adjust? Differentiating between sudden or insidious onset, presence or absence of progression, slow or rapid decline, and predominance of cognitive or behavioral symptoms can help in reaching a diagnosis. A thorough assessment of past medical history, substance abuse history, present medication use, positive family history for early-onset dementia (onset of dementia before the age of 65 years old), or family history of neurologic or psychiatric disease are essential components of a comprehensive dementia evaluation. The goal is to rule out other potential causes for memory disturbance and to avoid the need for an exhaustive clinical workup. Refer to Table 10-5 for common causes of reversible dementia.

Physical Exam

A general physical and neurologic exam can also be completed in a short amount of time. Generally, the goal is to determine if there are any findings to suggest an underlying, reversible, medical etiology for the dementia. A focused neurological exam is a must with emphasis on motor abnormalities (e.g., ataxia, focal findings suggestive

---

TABLE 10-5
POTENTIAL REVERSIBLE CAUSES OF DEMENTIA

Central nervous system: brain tumor, normal pressure hydrocephalus, subdural hematoma
Endocrine disorders: hypothyroid or hyperthyroid disease, hyperparathyroidism
Infectious diseases: neurosyphilis, encephalitis, meningitis
Inflammatory disorders: vasculitis, systemic lupus erythematosus
Systemic illness: hepatic encephalopathy, renal failure
Nutritional deficiencies: vitamin B12 deficiency, thiamine deficiency (Wernicke's encephalopathy)
Psychiatric: depression
Toxins: heavy metal toxicity, alcohol withdrawal or intoxication
Other: Wilson's disease, multiple sclerosis

Source: References 20 and 48.

of stroke, extrapyramidal symptoms [EPS]). Visual field deficits may suggest tumor, or abnormal eye movements may point to other neurologic disease, like impaired upgaze in progressive supranuclear palsy (PSP). An Argyll-Robertson pupil may represent findings consistent with neurosyphilis. Abnormal sensory exam with impaired proprioception could be suggestive of a vitamin-B12 deficiency or significant neuropathy from systemic illness or alcohol abuse.

Reflexes and coordination also should be assessed. Helpful screening tests for Parkinson's disease (PD) include observing range of motion of upper and lower extremities with the reach test, and rising from a chair without use of arms. Special attention should be paid to rigidity and parkinsonian signs which suggest possible DLB, as well as spasticity and asymmetric weakness which raise concern for stroke. Gait is an important part of the dementia work-up as gait disturbances can point towards an underlying potentially reversible cause of dementia; for example, a triad of ataxia, amnesia, and incontinence suggest normal pressure hydrocephalus (NPH); ataxia, confabulation, and ophthalmoplegia constitute Wernicke's encephalopathy. An additional physical exam may suggest systemic disease that could contribute to the cognitive deficits or simply be a comorbid illness often seen in older patients (e.g., hypothyroidism, atrial fibrillation, anemia).

Mental Status Exam

After a careful history is obtained, proceed with a mental status exam (MSE). Abnormalities on MSE often can alert clinicians to an underlying cognitive disorder. During assessment pay careful attention to appearance, whether a patient appears well-groomed, disheveled, or malodorous, suggesting impaired ADLs. Observe the degree of cooperation and social interaction. Does the patient present with an unusual speech pattern or dysarthria? Whether speech is fluent or nonfluent, or pressured or impoverished can be valuable clues to establish diagnosis and determine etiology. Does the patient have unusual movements with slowed or heightened psychomotor activity, stereotypies, or tremors? Note the patient's description of mood and whether his or her affect is mood-congruent. Does the patient appear depressed, flat, labile, or agitated? Thought process involves whether the patient can stay on task in a logical or goal-directed manner, or whether he or she becomes tangential, circumstantial, or completely disorganized. Patients with dementia notably have abnormal thought content, with impoverished thoughts and concrete thinking. Additionally, carefully evaluate for the presence of suicidal ideation or homicidal ideation. Depending on the etiology, psychotic features can be prominent early in the course of illness (e.g., DLB) or become more problematic as the illness progresses (as in AD).

TABLE 10-6

PSYCHOMETRICS: COGNITIVE DOMAINS WITH SAMPLE TESTS

Attention—auditory "A" test, spell "world" backwards, count backwards from 100 by intervals of 7 (serial 7s), state months of year or days of week backwards

Baseline IQ—general measure of patient's vocabulary, educational and occupational achievements

Memory

  Long-term—ask about early childhood, details from past life events

  Short-term/working—repeat digit span both forward and backwards, recall 3 objects, note if there is any improvement with practice

Language

  Receptive—comprehension of speech, can patient follow commands?

  Expressive—patient's speech, quality of expressions

  Written—ask patient to write sentence

  Reading—ask patient to read, does patient comprehend?

  Repetition—repeat phrase

Visuospatial—copying objects such as three-dimensional designs, non-representational hand gestures if not able to write

Executive function—Clock Drawing Test, verbal fluency, EXIT interview

  Abstraction—proverbs, similes, test reasoning

  Switching sets—Luria motor tasks, trail-making tests

  Apraxia—demonstrate how to comb hair, use a key, etc.

  Calculation—can patient make change

Psychomotor—finger tapping, fine finger movements, Luria motor tasks

---

Psychometrics

Additional psychometric assessment can be done by targeting any problematic areas that were detected with the screening measures or history. Table 10-6 refers to the different cognitive domains and suggests corresponding tests. Incorporating some memory testing into the interview by asking the patient questions about her past history, usual routine, or hobbies can provide valuable information in a non-threatening manner. One place to start could be asking the patient about her past childhood, information about growing up, where she went to school, when she was married, and the number and names of children. Additionally, one could ask about the current daily routine. Paying attention to how the patient is able to respond to these questions, can impart important clues (e.g., content, organization, how active, how much assistance she requires). If someone has a work or hobby history, asking details about this or how she did something specific can elicit whether the patient can pull together the information and communicate it in a well-thought out fashion. Asking about current events, things one might have read in the newspaper or seen on the news recently, and asking about the specifics of favorite television shows are other ways to assess memory functions.

Further testing of language includes repetition, naming, pointing to named objects in the room, reading, and writing. Assessment for apraxia includes asking the patient to demonstrate how she would do something (e.g., salute, light a cigarette, hammer a nail). Assessment for visuospatial deficits includes having the patient draw different objects, but one could utilize other tests such as mimicking non-representational hand positions. Executive functions can be assessed by asking about similarities (orange and apple, car and train) proverb interpretation ("people in glass houses should not throw stones"), problem-solving, ability to switch sets (trail-making tests; Luria motor sequencing with alternating hand movements) as well as CDT, verbal fluency tests, and EXIT interview (40).

Laboratory Tests and Other Studies

After a complete history and physical exam is performed, obtaining certain labs to rule out reversible causes of cognitive dysfunction is important. Truly reversible causes of dementia are increasingly rare, with approximately 9% of cases being potentially reversible, while <1% truly resolve with intervention (48). Please refer to Table 10-7 for a list of common labs to consider. The patient's history and presentation help tailor what labs and studies to request, as this list is not all-inclusive.

TABLE 10-7
LABORATORY TESTS IN THE DEMENTIA WORK-UP

Standard Labs	Assess For
Chemistries	Electrolyte disturbance, diabetes
Renal function	Renal failure
Liver function	Liver failure—hepatic encephalopathy
Complete blood count	Infection, anemia
Vitamin B12	B12 deficiency
Thyroid studies	Hypothyroidism or hyperthyroidism

Additional labs/studies if history or physical exam warrants

Syphilis tests (e.g., VDRL/RPR)	Neurosyphilis
Urinalysis	Urinary tract infection
Erythrocyte sedimentation rate	Autoimmune disorder
Toxicology screen	Drug use
Heavy metal screen	Heavy metal toxicity
HIV	HIV-associated dementia
Chest x-ray	Lung disease with chronic hypoxia or tumor
Electroencephalogram	Seizure disorder or delirium
Electrocardiogram	Cardiac disease
Lumbar puncture	Infection, neoplasm, Creutzfeld-Jakob disease

Generally, the basic screening labs include checking a complete blood count (CBC), blood chemistries, renal function, liver function, thyroid panel, and vitamin B12 (12). If during evaluation other risk factors or concerns arise, the clinician should obtain additional lab work-up. Syphilis antibody, human immunodeficiency virus (HIV), erythrocyte sedimentation rate, and plasma electrophoresis are some examples. Electrocardiogram is not routinely required. Similarly, lumbar puncture (LP) and electroencephalography (EEG) are seldom needed, but may be helpful when there is diagnostic uncertainty or an atypical presentation. Although the presence of apolipoprotein E-4 (APOE-4) is considered a potential risk factor for AD, genotype testing for the APOE-4 allele is not recommended for routine use in the dementia work-up (49).

Neuroimaging

There has been some controversy regarding whether imaging is an essential component of the dementia work-up (50,51). Generally, a computed tomography (CT) or magnetic resonance imaging (MRI) of the brain is recommended by the American Academy of Neurology during the initial work-up of dementia (12). Brain imaging with either a CT or an MRI may help to diagnose structural abnormalities in up to 5% of cases not detectable by history and physical exam alone (50). In practice, brain imaging is commonly obtained to rule out the possibility of underlying structural central nervous system (CNS) pathology such as subdural hematoma, brain tumor, or vascular etiology. A CT of the brain can rule out any gross CNS pathology such as masses or large strokes, but an MRI of the brain is generally able to provide better structural detail, especially if there is underlying vascular pathology. Although there is some controversy regarding interpreting the changes commonly seen with aging, an MRI can be very useful in determining the extent of vascular changes reflected by white matter hyperintensities and small vessel ischemic changes. A category of mixed dementia involving both AD and cerebrovascular disease is increasingly being recognized based upon clinical presentation of AD in patients with multiple vascular risk factors (e.g., hypertension, hyperlipidemia, atrial fibrillation) and neuroimaging findings of extensive vascular disease. Although an MRI is also helpful in cases when NPH is suspected, cisternography is a more appropriate study in these uncommon cases.

Previously, single photon emission computed tomography (SPECT) and positron emission tomography (PET) imaging were not practical for use in the general office setting and were reserved for research protocols. However, PET imaging will soon become more easily available for use in practice. Recently the Center for Medicare and Medicaid Services (CMS) approved PET imaging as a tool to add to the assessment in cases that are ambiguous despite adequate clinical work-up. PET imaging can assist in establishing a diagnosis or help characterize the etiology

TABLE 10-8
NEUROIMAGING IN DEMENTIA: WHAT TO ASSESS FOR?

CT	▪ Hematomas ▪ Fractures ▪ Calcified lesions ▪ Those who cannot have MRI
MRI	▪ Hippocampal atrophy ▪ Small vessel ischemia ▪ White matter and brain stem changes
With Contrast	▪ Tumors ▪ Multiple Sclerosis
Diffusion weighted imaging	▪ Acute versus chronic ischemia
PET	▪ Helpful in differential diagnosis ▪ Hypometabolism in parietal and temporal lobes in AD ▪ Hypometabolism in frontal, anterior and medial temporal cortices in FTD ▪ Patchy deficits in VaD ▪ In DLB, similar to AD, but also involvement of occipital lobes and cerebellum ▪ Normal in depression

AD, Alzheimer's disease; CT, computerized tomography; DLB, dementia with Lewy bodies; FTD, frontotemporal dementia; MRI, magnetic resonance imaging; PET, positron emission tomography; VaD, vascular dementia.

in patients with an atypical presentation. PET imaging is very sensitive and specific for distinguishing amongst different types of dementia, such as AD, often picking up early changes prior to clinical evidence of cognitive impairment (12). Other new technologies such as amyloid imaging are now being used in research; however, the utility in daily clinical practice remains to be seen. Table 10-8 describes features of different imaging modalities available in clinical practice. For more information, refer to the comprehensive chapter on neuroimaging in this textbook.

Additional Work-up
Typically, after completion of an initial evaluation and the basic workup, a dementia diagnosis and likely etiology can be established. However, additional studies may be required when the history or examination suggests an atypical presentation (e.g., the history does not fit the clinical findings), or if there are concerns about comorbid conditions. Some specific reasons to pursue additional workup include: rapid progression of illness, early onset (<65 years old) of symptoms, abnormalities on physical or neurological exam, gait disturbance, incontinence, prominent behavioral or personality changes, prominent psychiatric symptoms (e.g., depression, psychosis, suicidal or homicidal ideation), or recent trauma or falls. If the diagnosis remains uncertain despite adequate clinical workup, or if there is inconsistency between subjective reports and objective assessments, additional sophisticated neuropsychometric assessment may be needed, and/or further evaluation or referral to a specialist is appropriate.

When to Refer to a Specialist

Geriatrician
Geriatricians specialize in maintaining functional status in older patients. Consultation with a geriatrician can assist in establishing a diagnosis and treatment plan tailored to the management of frail, medically complicated patients. A consultation should also be considered if there is concern about polypharmacy, delirium, or other medical issues. Common issues for consultants to review include: management of risk factors, medical comorbidities, geriatric syndromes (e.g., incontinence, falls, pain), optimizing functional status, and simplifying medication regimens.

Psychiatrist
If a patient has an established psychiatric disorder that can result in cognitive, behavioral, and functional impairment, a referral to a psychiatrist is warranted. The goal is to optimize treatment for the underlying psychiatric disorder, in order to determine the persistence of cognitive impairment. Additionally, psychiatric medications can, at times, cause cognitive slowing and confusion, and consultation with a psychiatrist to assess for alternatives is helpful. Psychiatrists can also assist in the management of behavioral changes associated with dementia. If there is concern about active substance use, referral to substance abuse treatment is necessary in order to clarify the diagnosis and to optimize treatment outcomes.

Neurologist
If a history or exam reveal neurological findings (like EPS, gait disturbance, asymmetric reflexes/strength/tone) that raise questions about comorbidities or uncommon etiologies, it is a good idea to refer for further neurologic assessment. The neurologist can then determine whether to pursue additional diagnostic tests, like an LP, EEG, etc.

Neuropsychologist
Although a thorough office-based assessment is generally sufficient to reach a diagnosis of dementia, more extensive neuropsychological testing is sometimes warranted in clinically challenging patients. Neuropsychologists tailor their examination based upon an individual's symptoms, educational background, motivation, and personality strengths. Common reasons to request an extensive neuropsychological assessment include: an atypical presentation, to obtain a cognitive baseline at the start of treatment, and periodically to follow progression or treatment response. There are instances where findings on clinic-based cognitive testing do not match reported impairments in cognition and function. Sometimes there are inconsistencies in reports by different family members; and occasionally there is concern

about a patient's level of anxiety or depression. In such cases a formal neuropsychological consultation could help corroborate or refute a clinical impression. Such testing is also helpful when symptoms are very mild and in cases where one needs to differentiate between age-associated changes and early dementia. In addition, it can be helpful if there is concern regarding the patient's ability to remain unsupervised in activities.

DIFFERENTIAL DIAGNOSIS

A proposed algorithm for the dementia differential diagnosis and workup is found in Figure 10-1.

Depression

The role of depression in patients with cognitive complaints is a common clinical challenge. Cognitive symptoms are common in depressed individuals and can complicate the

diagnosis of dementia. Once depression is identified, the focus is to treat depression and reassess for persistent cognitive disturbance. Patients who are depressed generally complain of memory problems, whereas dementia patients lack the insight to complain. Depressed patients often give up on tasks with little effort, whereas demented patients often expend a lot of effort, but have trouble completing tasks (see Table 10-9). Recent literature support that although a majority of memory complaints resolve after treatment for depression, certain difficulties, often relating to executive dysfunction, can actually persist after the depression has remitted (47). Once a patient has been identified with late-life depression, this warrants careful follow-up, given depression itself is an independent risk factor for later development of dementia.

Delirium

Patients with multiple medical issues or on complex medication regimens are at risk for development of delirium.

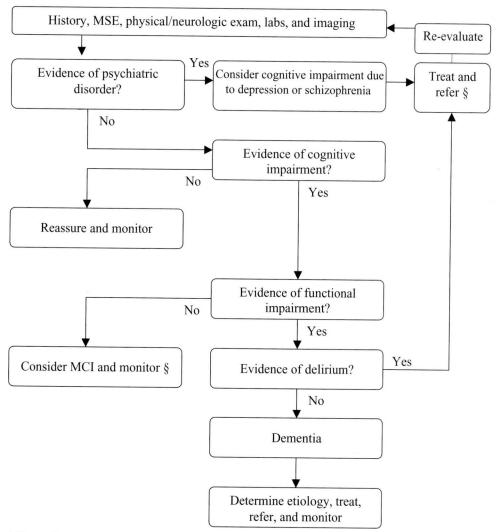

§ Also consider referral for neuropsychological testing

Figure 10-1 An algorithm for the dementia workup.

TABLE 10-9
DIFFERENTIAL DIAGNOSIS: DEPRESSION, DELIRIUM, AND DEMENTIA

	Depression	Delirium	Dementia
Onset	▪ Acute/subacute	▪ Acute/subacute	▪ Acute/subacute (VaD, CJD) ▪ Insidious (AD)
Cognition	▪ Subjective > objective findings ▪ Poor effort	▪ Altered consciousness ▪ Inattention ▪ Fluctuating mental status	▪ Cognitive deficits in multiple domains ▪ Poor insight
Behavior	▪ Evidence of psychiatric disorder ▪ Neurovegetative symptoms (e.g., changes in sleep, apetite, and energy) ▪ Suicidal Ideation ▪ +/− Psychosis	▪ Hypoactive or hyperactive ▪ Dysphoria	▪ Disturbances early on (FTD, DLB) ▪ Depression early with preserved insight (AD) ▪ Neuropsychiatric symptoms common (e.g., apathy, sleep disturbances)
Functional Decline	▪ +/− ▪ Can be out of proportion with objective cognitive findings	▪ Present	▪ Present ▪ Usually difficulties with IADLs before ADLs
Neurologic Exam	▪ +/− psychomotor retardation or agitation	▪ +/− depending on etiology	▪ Evidence of stroke (VaD) ▪ EPS (DLB) ▪ Normal (early AD)
Neuroimaging	▪ Usually normal ▪ +/− white matter hyperintensities on MRI in late-onset depression ▪ Evidence of stroke in vascular depression	▪ +/− depending on etiology	▪ Evidence of stroke on CT/MRI (VaD) ▪ Hippocampal atrophy (AD) or anterior frontal/temporal atrophy (FTD) on MRI ▪ Specific patterns of hypometabolism on PET imaging
Labs/Studies	▪ Rule out medical causes ▪ TSH, CBC, Chem panel	▪ Clues to etiology ▪ TSH, CBC, Chem panel, Calcium, UA, Tox screen ▪ Consider EEG, CXR, LP, other studies as clinically indicated	▪ Rule out reversible causes ▪ Clues to etiology ▪ TSH, CBC, Chem panel, Calcium, B12 ▪ Consider EEG, LP, heavy metal screen, other studies as clinically indicated
Comments	▪ Review Past Psychiatric History	▪ Review medications for offending agents	▪ Informant history essential

ADLs, activities of daily living; AD, Alzheimer's disease; B12, Vitamin B12; CBC, complete blood count; CJD, Creutzfeld-Jakob disease; CT, computerized tomography; CXR, chest x-ray; DLB, dementia with Lewy bodies; EEG, electroencephalogram; EPS, extrapyramidal symptoms; FTD, frontotemporal dementia; IADLs, instrumental activities of daily living; LP, lumbar puncture; MRI, magnetic resonance imaging; PET, positron emission tomography; Tox, toxicology; TSH, thyroid stimulating hormone; UA, urinalysis; VaD, vascular dementia.

Dementia and delirium sometimes go together. Delirium is a risk factor for dementia and *vice versa*. It is not uncommon to see delirium as the first manifestation of underlying dementia and prolonged delirium can mimic dementia. It is recommended that anyone with a delirium diagnosis needs careful follow-up after the delirium itself has resolved. Key characteristics of delirium that distinguish it from dementia include: typically abrupt change in attention, alteration in consciousness, fluctuating mental status, underlying exacerbation in medical condition (e.g., infection, new medication, etc.) (Table 10-9). The Confusion Assessment Method (CAM) is one way to screen for delirium in a high-risk population, such as one finds in a hospital or geriatric outpatient clinic.

Use of the CAM involves confirming that the patient's symptoms are acute and fluctuating, with features of inattention, and with either disorganization or altered consciousness (52). If one suspects delirium, it is important to pursue further investigation into the potential etiology (often multiple ones) and remove or treat offending factors. Delirium should always be considered a medical emergency.

Polypharmacy

Certain medications can impair patients' ability to think efficiently. As patients age, the ability to metabolize certain medications becomes less efficient. Some typical offending agents include sedatives-hypnotics, opiates, psychotropics, anticholinergic agents, and over-the-counter preparations (e.g., diphenhydramine). In frail, older adults, addition of a new, seemingly benign medication can precipitate delirium. Because side effects from medications can be additive, careful assessment of the patient's medication list is important in order to work on streamlining medications and tapering any medications that are non-essential. Table 10-10 provides a representative sample of medications that can potentially cause cognitive changes in older adults.

Common Dementia Etiologies

A table comparing and contrasting features of normal aging and MCI and the most common etiologies for dementia can be used as a guide during the work-up (Table 10-11). More detailed information for the specific diseases is discussed in subsequent chapters. Other potential etiologies of dementia syndromes are: AIDS dementia, Creutzfeld–Jakob disease, Huntington's disease, PD, and other neurologic diseases. There is also a dementia syndrome associated with schizophrenia.

MANAGEMENT

Once a dementia diagnosis has been established, the next step in management is to discuss the ramifications with the patient and family. At times, family members may express hesitance about disclosing the dementia diagnosis to loved ones over fear about how the patient will accept or cope with it. However, patients usually prefer that the diagnosis be discussed with them (56). During the initial evaluation, one can determine the patient's and family's concerns about what the dementia diagnosis signifies and how they anticipate it will affect them. Any misconceptions can be corrected during this time. One can also determine the patient's preference regarding who should accompany him or her during the diagnosis discussion and who will be involved in ongoing management and support during the course of treatment.

The clinician can then also establish a plan for ongoing management, surveillance and close follow-up. It helps to establish a partnership amongst the patient, caregiver, and physician. Helpful referrals to community resources and local or national support groups early during the course of illness can augment office-based education and help alleviate patient and caregiver distress. It is important to provide the patient and family with a sense of support, and alleviate any fears of abandonment or hopelessness. Education about the need to discuss future planning and patient preferences regarding financial and medical decision-making can be introduced at this time and during follow-up visits. One should also establish the importance of regular follow-up visits to evaluate patient and caregiver coping, and to survey for potential medical or psychiatric comorbidities. Nonpharmacologic interventions, such as

TABLE 10-10
SELECTED MEDICATIONS THAT CAN CAUSE COGNITIVE DISTURBANCE IN OLDER ADULTS

Sedatives/Hypnotics
 Benzodiazepines[a]
  lorazepam, clonazepam, alprazolam, oxazepam, temazepam, diazepam, chlordiazepoxide, clorazepate
 Over-the-counter agents
  diphenhydramine[a]
 Alternative agents
  chloral hydrate, hydroxyzine[a], zolpidem, zaleplon
Antidepressants
 Tricyclic agents (TCAs)[a]
  amitriptyline, clomipramine, desipramine, doxepin, imipramine, nortriptyline, protriptyline
 Monoamine Oxidase Inhibitors (MAOIs)[a]
  phenelzine, tranylcypromine
Antipsychotics
 Atypical agents
  clozapine[a]
 Conventional agents
  thioridazine[a], chlorpromazine[a], loxapine, perphenazine
Mood Stabilizers or Anticonvulsants
  lithium, valproic acid, carbamazepine, lamotrigine, tiagabine, topiramate, gabapentin, phenytoin, phenobarbital, levetiracetam
Anti-Parkinsonian Agents
  bromocriptine, benztropine, trihexyphenidyl, carbidopa-levodopa, amantadine, selegiline, entacapone, pergolide, ropinirole, pramipexole, tolcapone, apomorphine
Analgesics/Narcotics
 Non-steroidal anti-inflammatory agents
 COX-2 Inhibitors
 Opiates (meperidine, morphine)
Anti-Emetic agents
  promethazine, prochlorperazine, metoclopramide, ondansetron, dronabinol, trimethobenzamide, droperidol
Antihistamines
 Non-selective
  diphenhydramine, hydroxyzine
 Histamine H$_2$-blockers
  cimetidine[a], ranitidine[a]
Antibiotics
  ciprofloxacin, vancomycin
Antispasmotic agents
  tolterodine, oxybutynin, Donnatal, dicyclomine
Muscle Relaxants
  cyclobenzaprine, baclofen, carisoprodol, orphenadrine, metaxalone
Cardiovascular Agents
 Beta-blockers
  propranolol, metoprolol
 Diuretics
  furosemide[a]
 Anti-arrhythmics
  amiodarone, digoxin[a]
Pulmonary agents
  albuterol, theophylline[a]
Miscellaneous agents
  Steroids[a]

[a]Many of these medications have anticholinergic side effects. Effects can be additive.
Source: References 53–55.

physical exercise, maintaining activities that promote mental stimulation, and social plans can help motivate the patient and caregiver to remain proactive during the course of disease.

TABLE 10.11

DIFFERENTIAL DIAGNOSIS: NORMAL AGING, MILD COGNITIVE IMPAIRMENT, ALZHEIMER'S DISEASE, VASCULAR DEMENTIA, DEMENTIA WITH LEWY BODIES, AND FRONTOTEMPORAL DEMENTIA

	Normal Aging	MCI	AD	VaD	DLB	FTD
Cognitive Change	• Mild decline only in: Word-finding Concentration Multi-tasking Processing speed	• Subjective and objective • Decline in one cognitive domain	• Short-term memory (early) • Language • Visuospatial • Praxis • Executive function	• Executive function • Language • Depends on stroke location	• Fluctuating mental status • Similar to cognitive profile for AD	• Executive function and language > memory (early) • Cognitive changes relatively later in disease progression
Behavioral Changes	• Normal	• +/− Depression • Irritability • Apathy	• Common • Depression, anxiety (early) • Agitation, apathy, psychosis (with disease progression)	• Common • Depression • Apathy	• Well-formed VH or illusions • REM sleep behavior disorder	• Early personality changes • Socially disinhibited • Apathy • Psychiatric presentation
Functional Decline	• Absent	• Absent	• IADLs lost before ADLs • Intact social skills (early)	• Common • Problems planning, completing tasks • Depends on stroke location	• Present	• Present • Usually caregiver more distressed than patient
Neurologic Exam	• Normal	• Normal	• Normal (early) • +/− Paratonias, myoclonus, EPS, frontal-release signs, gait disturbance (later)	• Signs of stroke • Focal exam • Abnormal reflexes, motor, sensory, gait	• EPS • Gait disturbance • Falls	• +/− Gait • +/− Motor abnormalities (can be associated with motor neuron disease)
Neuroimaging	• +/− Mild atrophy (CT) • +/− White matter changes (MRI)	• +/− Mild atrophy (CT) • +/− White matter changes (MRI)	• +/− Mild atrophy (CT) • +/− White matter changes (MRI) • Parietal/temporal hypometabolism (PET)	• Evidence of stroke (CT, MRI) • Scattered deficits (PET)	• +/− Mild atrophy (CT) • +/− White matter changes (MRI) • Similar to AD +/− occipital and cerebellum (PET)	• Frontal/anterior temporal atrophy (CT, MRI) • Same anatomical pattern (PET) • Normal
Labs/Studies	• Normal • +/− Abnormalities associated with comorbidities	• Normal • +/− Abnormalities associated with comorbidities	• Normal • +/−Abnormalities associated with comorbidities	• Evidence of diseases associated with CVA risk factors	• Normal • +/− Abnormalities associated with comorbidities	• +/− Abnormalities associated with comorbidities • Usually younger age of onset
Comments		• Increased risk of AD • Annual conversion to AD: 15% per year	• Usually insidious • Anticipate MMSE decline 2–3 points per year	• Often sudden • Step-wise or static • Stroke risk factors	• Neuroleptic sensitivity	

ADLs, activities of daily living; AD, Alzheimer's disease; CT, computerized tomography; CVA, cerebrovascular accident; DLB, dementia with Lewy bodies; EPS, extrapyramidal symptoms; FTD, frontotemporal dementia; IADLs, instrumental activities of daily living; MMSE, Mini-Mental State Examination; MRI, magnetic resonance imaging; PET, positron emission tomography; REM, rapid eye movement; VaD, vascular dementia; VH, visual hallucinations.

A discussion of appropriate pharmacologic interventions with the necessary disclosure of indications, potential adverse effects, and any available alternatives to treatment will help the patient and family decide their individualized treatment plan. It is necessary to discuss how one should measure a medication's success and expectations for treatment to prevent avoidable disappointments and misunderstandings which may compromise compliance with recommendations. Presently, acetylcholinesterase inhibitors (tacrine, donepezil, rivastigmine, galantamine) are approved by the U.S. Food and Drug Administration for treatment of mild to moderate AD. Acetylcholinesterase inhibitors may also be helpful in other types of dementias, like VaD and DLB. Memantine, an NMDA-receptor antagonist, is approved for moderate-to-severe AD. Newer agents are in development.

REFERENCES

1. Brookmeyer R, Gray S, Kawas C. Projections of Alzheimer's disease in the United States and the public health impact of delaying disease onset. *Am J Public Health.* 1998;88:1337–1342.
2. Sloane PD, Zimmerman S, Scuhindran C, et al. The public health impact of Alzheimer's disease, 200–2050: potential implication of treatment advances. *Annual Review Public Health.* 2002;23: 213–231.
3. Callahan CM, Hendrie HC, Tierney WM. Documentation and evaluation of cognitive impairment in elderly primary care patients. *Ann Intern Med.* 1995;122:422–429.
4. Knopman D, Donohue JA, Gutterman EM. Patterns of care in the early stages of Alzheimer's disease: Impediments to timely diagnosis. *J Am Geriatr Soc.* 2000;48:300–304.
5. Sternberg SA, Wolfson, C, Baumgarten M. Undetected dementia in community-dwelling older people: the Canadian study of health and aging. *J Am Geriatr Soc.* 2000; 48:1430–1434.
6. Webster RG, Abbot RD, Petrovitch H, et al. Frequency and characteristics of silent dementia among elderly Japanese-American men: the Honolulu-Asia aging study. *JAMA.* 1997;277: 800–805.
7. McKhann G, Drachman D, Folstein M, et al. Clinical diagnosis of Alzheimer's disease: report of the NINCDS-ADRDA work group under the auspices of department of health and human services task force on Alzheimer's disease. *Neurology.* 1984;34:939–944.
8. American Psychiatric Association. *Diagnostic and Statistical Manual of Mental Disorders*, 4th Ed, Text Revision (DSM-IV TR). Washington (DC): American Psychiatric Association, 2000.
9. Roman GC, Tatemichi TK, Erkinjuntti T, et al. Vascular dementia: diagnostic criteria for research studies. Report of the NINDS-AIREN international workshop. *Neurology.* 1993;43:250–260.
10. McKeith IG, Glasako D, Kosaka K, et al. Consensus guidelines for the clinical and pathologic diagnosis of dementia with Lewy bodies (DLB): Report of the consortium on DLB international workshop. *Neurology.* 1996;47:1113–1124.
11. Neary D, Snowden JS, Gustafson L, et al. Frontotemporal lobar degeneration: a consensus on clinical diagnostic criteria. *Neurology.* 1998;51:1546–1554.
12. Knopman DS, DeKosky ST, Cummings JL, et al. Practice parameter: diagnosis of dementia (an evidence-based review). Report of the quality standards subcommittee of the American Academy of Neurology. *Neurology.* 2001;56:1143–1153.
13. Petersen RC, Stevens JC, Ganguli M, et al. Practice parameter: early detection of dementia: mild cognitive impairment (an evidence-based review). Report of the quality standards subcommittee of the American Academy of Neurology. *Neurology.* 2001;56:1133–1142.
14. Small GW, Rabins PV, Barry PP, et al. Diagnosis and treatment of Alzheimer disease and related disorders: consensus statement of the American Association for Geriatric Psychiatry, the Alzheimer's Association and the American Geriatrics Society. *JAMA.* 1997; 278:1363–1371.
15. Tariot PN, Mack JL, Patterson MB, et al. Behavioral pathology committee of the consortium to establish a registry for Alzheimer's disease. The behavior rating scale for dementia of the consortium to establish a registry for Alzheimer's disease. *Am J Psychiatry.* 1995;152:1349–1357.
16. Roman GC. Vascular dementia: Distinguishing characteristics, treatment, and prevention. *J Am Geriatr Soc.* 2003;51:S296–304.
17. Knopman DS, Parisi JE, Boeve BF, et al. Vascular dementia in a population-based autopsy study. *Arch Neurol.* 2003;60:569–575.
18. Zekry D, Hauw JJ, Gold G. Mixed dementia: epidemiology, diagnosis and treatment. *J Am Geriatr Soc.* 2002; 50:1431–1438.
19. Rosen HJ, Hartikainen KM, Jagust W, et al. Utility of clinical criteria in differentiating frontotemporal lobar degeneration (FTLD) from AD. *Neurology.* 2002;58:1608–1615.
20. Weytingh MD, Bossuyt PM, van Crevel H. Reversible dementia: more than 10% or less than 1%? A quantitative review. *J Neurol.* 1995;242:466–471.
21. U.S. Preventive Services Task Force. Screening for dementia: recommendation and rationale. *Ann Intern Med.* 2003;138: 925–926.
22. Tangalos EG, Smith GE, Ivnik RJ, et al. The Mini-Mental State Examination in general medical practice: clinical utility and acceptance. *Mayo Clin Proc.* 1996;71:829–837.
23. Carr DB, Gray S, Baty J, et al. The value of informant versus individual's complaints of memory impairment in early dementia. *Neurology.* 2000;55:1724–1726.
24. Bachman DL, Wolf PA, Linn RT, et al. Incidence of dementia and probable Alzheimer's disease in a general population: the Framingham study. *Neurology.* 1993;43:515–519.
25. Boustani M, Peterson B, Hanson L, et al. Screening for dementia in primary care: a summary of the evidence for the U.S. preventive services task force. *Ann Intern Med.* 2003;138: 927–937.
26. Folstein MF, Folstein SE, McHugh PR. "Mini-mental state." A practical method for grading the cognitive state of patients for the clinician. *J Psychiatr Res.* 1975;12:189–198.
27. Tombaugh TN, McIntyre NJ. The Mini-Mental State Examination: a comprehensive review. *J Am Geriatr Soc.* 1992;40:922–935.
28. Kukull WA, Larson EB, Teri L, et al. The Mini-Mental State Examination score and the clinical diagnosis of dementia. *J Clin Epidemiol.* 1994;47:1061–1067.
29. Crum RM, Anthony JC, Bassett SS, Folstein MF. Population-based norms for the Mini-Mental State Examination by age and educational level. *JAMA.* 1993;269:2386–2691.
30. Uhlmann RF, Larson EB. Effect of education on the Mini-Mental State Examination as a screening test for dementia. *Division of Gerontology and Geriatric Medicine.* 1991;39:876–880.
31. Canning SJ, Leach L, Stuss D, et al. Diagnostic utility of abbreviated fluency measures in Alzheimer disease and vascular dementia. *Neurology.* 2004;62:556–562.
32. Cummings JL. The one-minute mental status examination. *Neurology.* 2004;62:534–535.
33. Mendez MF, Ala T, Underwood KL. Development of scoring criteria for the clock drawing task in Alzheimer's disease. *J Am Geriatr Soc.* 1992;40:1095–1099.
34. Royall DR, Cordes JA, Polk M. CLOX: An executive clock drawing task. *J Neurol Neurosurg Psychiatry.* 1998;64:588–1094.
35. Royall DR, Mulroy AR, Chiodo LK, et al. Clock drawing is sensitive to executive control: a comparison of six methods. *J Gerontol.* 1999;54B:P328–P333.
36. Tuokko H, Hadjistavropoulos T, Miller JA, et al. The clock test: a sensitive measure to differentiate normal elderly from those with Alzheimer disease. *J Am Geriatr Soc.* 1992;40:579–584.
37. Borson S, Scanlan JM, Chen P, et al. The Mini-Cog as a screen for dementia: validation in a population-based sample. *J Am Geriatr Soc.* 2003;51:1451–1454.
38. Costa PT Jr, Williams TF, Somerfield M, et al. Early identification of Alzheimer's disease and related dementias. *Clinical Practice Guideline, Quick Reference Guide for Clinicians, No. 19.* Rockville, MD: U.S. Department of Health and Human Services, Public Health Service, Agency for Health Care Policy and Research. AHCPR Publication No. 97-0703. November 1996.
39. Meulen EF, Schmand B, van Campen JP, et al. The seven minute screen: a neurocognitive screening test highly sensitive to various types of dementia. *J Neurol, Neurosurg Psychiatry.* 2004;75: 700–705.
40. Royall DR, Mahurin RK, Gray KF. Bedside assessment of executive cognitive impairment: the executive interview. *J Am Geriatr Soc.* 1992;40:1221–1226.
41. Lyketsos CG, Lopez O, Jones B, et al. Prevalence of neuropsychiatric symptoms in dementia and mild cognitive impairment. Results from the cardiovascular health study. *JAMA.* 2002;288: 1475–1483.
42. Mega MS, Cummings JL, Fiorello T, et al. The spectrum of behavioral changes in Alzheimer's disease. *Neurology.* 1996;46:130–135.
43. Yesavage JA, Brink TL. Development and validation of a geriatric depression screening scale: a preliminary report. *J Psychiatr Res.* 1983;17:37–49.
44. Lyness JM, Noel TK, Cox C, et al. Screening for depression in elderly primary care patients: a comparison of the center for epidemiologic studies-depression scale and the geriatric depression scale. *Arch Intern Med.* 1997;157:449–454.

45. Brody DS, Hahn SR, Spitzer RL, et al. Identifying patients with depression in the primary care setting: a more efficient method. *Arch of Intern Med.* 1998;158:2469–2475.

46. Whooley MA, Avins AL, Miranda J, et al. Case-finding instruments for depression. *J Gen Intern Med.* 1997;12:439–445.

47. Alexopoulos GS, Meyers BS, Young RC, et al. The course of geriatric depression with "reversible dementia": a controlled study. *Am J Psychiatry.* 1993;150:1693–1699.

48. Clarfield AM. The decreasing prevalence of reversible dementias. *Arch Intern Med.* 2003;163:2219–2229.

49. American College of Medical Genetics, American Society of Human Genetics Working Group on ApoE and Alzheimer Disease. Statement on use of apolipoprotein E testing for Alzheimer disease. *JAMA.* 1995;274:1627–1629.

50. Chui H, Zhang Q. Evaluation of dementia: a systematic study of the usefulness of the American Academy of Neurology's practice parameters. *Neurology.* 1997;49:925–935.

51. Gifford DR, Holloway RG, Vickrey BG. Systematic review of clinical prediction rules for neuroimaging in the evaluation of dementia. *Arch Intern Med.* 2000;160:2855–2862.

52. Inouye SK, van Dyck CH, Alessi CA, et al. Clarifying confusion: the confusion assessment method. A new method for detection of delirium. *Ann Intern Med.* 1990;113:941–948.

53. Tune L, Carr S, Hoag E, et al. Anticholinergic effects of drugs commonly prescribed for the elderly: potential means for assessing risk of delirium. *Am J Psychiatry.* 1992;149:1393–1394.

54. Tune LE. Anticholinergic effects of medication in elderly patients. *J Clin Psychiatry.* 2001;62:11–14.

55. Alagiakrishnan K, Wiens CA. An approach to drug induced delirium in the elderly. *Postgrad Med J.* 2004;80:388–393.

56. Samuels SC. Sharing the diagnosis of Alzheimer's disease: methods and expectations. Breaking news to patients requires patience and sensitivity to their needs. *Geriatrics.* 2004;59:38–42.

Cultural Issues in Late Life

11

Kenneth Sakauye

Cultural issues affect many aspects of our daily life, but the degree of ethnic influence on individuals varies widely. It is important for all clinicians to be able to apply a cultural formulation and to be aware of cultural differences, especially when there is a difference between the doctor and patient in the language spoken, race, immigrant status, or marginalization (i.e., social isolation due to low socioeconomic status or prejudicial exclusions so they maintain unique belief systems). One important guide is the Outline for Cultural Formulation in the Diagnostic and Statistical Manual of Mental Disorders, Fourth Edition, Text Revision (DSM-IV-TR). It can help the clinician to supplement the multi-axial assessment, address difficulties that may be encountered in applying the diagnostic criteria in a multicultural environment, and suggest effects on the relationship between the individual and the clinician (1).

Although there are an increasing number of publications on cultural diversity, most remain at the level of case reports and do not deal directly with elderly. The difficulty in doing systematic research in this area is the variability introduced by varying degrees of assimilation and acculturation within every group. There is no single stereotype that fits the majority of African American, Asian, or Hispanic populations, and even less commonality when considering subgroups such as Argentineans versus Nicaraguans, Japanese versus Chinese, or Nigerian versus U.S. African Americans. Racial and ethnic identity can be difficult to define. What does being Asian mean to someone who only speaks English, has never visited their country of origin, honors no unique customs, is married to a White, and has few Asian friends? Studying cultural differences is even harder due to resistance by some minority groups from participating in research. Minority individuals may have developed a cultural paranoia about research after a lifetime of perceived prejudice or victimization.

These issues have led to the current approach of addressing broad principles for working with other cultures, and encourage the clinician to research the individual cultures and backgrounds of groups with whom they work (2–6). However, there is still little information unique to geriatric elderly in the growing body of literature on cultural psychiatry.

The role of ethnicity in health care has many facets. Culture is thought to be the root of our thinking and habits, coping, and treatment efforts; but it is a fluid concept. Some anthropological terms that define what happens to cultural identity in the course of a lifespan are *enculturation* (the process by which an individual acquires a culture), *acculturation* (the process of acquiring a new cultural system), *assimilation* (the process of voluntarily being incorporated into the dominant culture), *cultural uprooting* (restrictions placed on exercising the prior culture), and *cultural diffusion* (bi-directional influences on merging cultural systems). Cultural change and cultural conflict that may occur throughout a lifespan makes it difficult to stereotype ethnic individuals. One does not have a homogeneous cultural group that can be reliably compared and contrasted to others.

This chapter will provide an overview of the major issues that culture affects in psychiatric care: language, different values and beliefs about illness, ethnocentric bias (racial stereotyping), bi-directional effects from prejudice, the culture of poverty that leads to health care disparities, and biological differences. Table 11-1 shows the role of ethnicity in healthcare.

WORKING DEFINITIONS

Race, culture, and *ethnicity* are similar terms but are not synonymous. Race does not imply a cultural or social context. A racial group is comprised of several ethnic groups that generally intermarry and alter the gene pool.

TABLE 11-1
ROLE OF ETHNICITY IN HEALTH CARE

Variable	Clinical Relevance
Language	Often a barrier to treatment
	Implies different cultural values and beliefs
Values and beliefs	Credibility of treatment recommendations
	Disease presentation and communication
	Reason for seeking treatment
	Family issues, social networks, habits
Ethnocentric bias (racial stereotyping)	Misdiagnosis
	Undertreatment
	Treatment errors
	Racial pseudoscience
Prejudice (bi-directional)	Distrust
	Overt hostility or mistreatment
	Problems establishing a treatment alliance
Culture of poverty	Barriers to access to care
	Non-compliance and poor health knowledge
	Higher risk for illness and mental illness
Biological differences	Risk and prevalence of illness
	Pharmacokinetic and pharmacodynamic differences

Culture describes attitudes of a population that are learned or non-biologically determined and which are passed down from generation to generation. Roughly, this represents behavior patterns or beliefs that define a group.

Ethnicity is based on identification with one's place of origin or religion. It incorporates cultural features, such as shared customs and beliefs, but also involves shared language, self-identification, self-concepts, dietary habits, style of dress, and, often, relation to skin color.

These definitions become important as one thinks through the generalizability of findings. It is obvious that genetic and biological differences reflect race, but psychosocial interventions, program needs, and appeal of different approaches may only be applicable to specific ethnic groups. Culture is the underlying core beliefs that we strive to understand and tap, since it much more closely represents the self.

WHAT IS A CULTURAL FORMULATION?

A cultural formulation considers five major issues: cultural identity of the individual; cultural explanations of the individual's illness; cultural factors related to the psychosocial environment and levels of functioning; cultural elements of the relationship between the individual and clinician; and overall cultural assessment for diagnosis and care (1).

Cultural competence involves cultural sensitivity (awareness and empathy for emotions, values, and belief systems of people from other cultures), knowledge of the particular culture, and competence in interaction and treatment. Most professionals must be reminded to ask about ethnic origin,

other family than just those with histories of mental illness, family dynamics, and alternate beliefs of causality. Because of misinterpretation of cultural influences, minority patients are often said to be in denial, to somatize, to have personality disorders, or to lack psychological mindedness.

It is important to sharpen cultural sensitivity through an increase in cultural knowledge about the group one is working with. Reading books and other literature is thought to be the best way to obtain such cultural information, and consulting or talking with local experts on cultural issues is advisable. It is also important to adjust one's interactions to establish a proper and helpful professional relationship with the minority patient. The indicators of a poor relationship include premature termination, noncompliance with treatment, inadequate histories, and failure to establish a therapeutic alliance. Examples of cultural formulations can be found in the Group for the Advancement of Psychiatry (GAP) Report 145 (7).

CASE EXAMPLE:

Mrs. T was an 88-year-old Japanese widow who had been living in the United States since she was in her 20s when she came for an arranged marriage. She had never learned English. She was referred for a psychiatric consult for possible depression and suicidal risk when staff thought her insistence to leave the hospital prematurely on the first anniversary of her son's death was to commit suicide. Staff believed suicide risk was higher in Japanese because they knew about *Seppuku*, or Japanese ritual suicide. However, Mrs. T showed no depressive symptoms and had no intention of suicide. Her intent was just to keep her Buddhist cultural custom of organizing a first-anniversary memorial service for the deceased family member. Suicide rates are no higher among Japanese than the general population. Furthermore, Mrs. T was not a male of a royal class (who might have committed Seppuku a century before).

This case demonstrates the problems that can occur when there is cultural sensitivity, but without cultural competence, and when language barriers are present. Misdiagnosis is common.

WHAT DOES THE LAST CENSUS SHOW?

The U.S. Office of Management and Budget lists seven groupings for data on race and ethnicity: American Indian or Alaska Native, Asian, Black or African American, Hispanic or Latino, Native Hawaiian and other Pacific Islander, White, and other (mixed races with no self-identification with any of the above divisions) (8). The minority populations, especially Hispanic and Asian groups, have been

TABLE 11-2

CHANGE IN U.S. MINORITY POPULATION, 1990–2000

U.S. Census	1990, in millions	2000, in millions	Change
All races	248.7	281.4	+11.6%
White	199.7	211.5	+5.6%
Minority (difference)	49.0	67.0	+29.5%
Minority % of population	19.7%	24.8%	+5.1%

Source: Reference 17.

growing rapidly in comparison to White populations. For all age groups, 12% of the U.S. population (about 35 million individuals) is Hispanic. African Americans comprise a similar 12% of the U.S. population. Of this group, 6% is foreign born, mostly from the Caribbean. Since 1983, more than 100,000 refugees have come to the United States from African nations (4). About 4.1 million people, 1.5% of the U.S. population, are American Indian and Alaska Natives (Indians, Eskimos, and Aleuts). By 2020, it is estimated that 20 million people—about 6% of the U.S. population—will be Asian, with 35% of Asian households being linguistically isolated. This is summarized in Table 11-2.

The demographics show that Asian and Hispanic elderly are largely immigrant and do not speak English as their primary language. Table 11-3 provides an overview of immigrant status of major ethnic groups in the United States. Many elderly immigrants are joining their children, who immigrated first, and are thrown into a socially isolating experience in the suburbs and faced with culture shock. For some from war-torn areas or with refugee status, post-traumatic stress disorder (PTSD) and stress effects are common. Health risks, such as parasitic diseases or toxic exposures, are seen in many refugee populations. For long-term residents or American-born elderly, a history of segregation and racism often play a dominant role in their attitudes, personality, and worldview.

Knowledge of immigration laws and the history of segregation for various minority groups is necessary to understand the statistical differences. For example, because of the Asian Exclusion Law, which was in effect from 1917 to 1943, and other laws that barred naturalization of people from Asia, the only American-born elderly Asians today are those born to pre-1917 immigrants. Only Japanese have high proportions of American-born elderly, because they came pre-1917 as family units.

Refugee status, environmental exposures from low-paying dangerous jobs for many minority elders, and poor education (i.e., low socioeconomic status) have created traumatic experiences, health risks, and nutritional deficiencies that must be considered in a cultural formulation. Although many of these problems may be related to low socioeconomic status or the so-called "culture of poverty," it becomes an ethnic issue when patterns are widespread for particular ethnic groups.

ETHNICITY AND MENTAL HEALTH CARE

Often, minority elderly seem difficult to engage because of cultural differences. When searching for a handle to engage

TABLE 11-3

MINORITY ELDERLY DEMOGRAPHIC PROFILE, 2000[a]

Group	All ages, in millions (% of U.S. Population)	Elderly (>60), in Millions (% of Group)	Foreign-Born Elderly (65+)	% American-Born Elderly (65+)	
All groups	281.2 (100%)	39.4 (14.0%)			
African American	34.7 (12.3%)	3.9 (10.9%)	6% (mainly Caribbean)	94%	
Hispanic American	35.3 (12.6%)	2.5 (7.0%)	65.7%	Not available	
Asian American	10.2 (3.6%)	1.1 (11.2%)	57.4%	Japanese	62.8%[a]
				Chinese	24.1%[a]
				Korean	19.9%[a]
				Filipino	3.7%[a]
				Vietnamese	0%[a]
				Asian Indians	19.3%[a]
Native Hawaiian and other Pacific Islander	0.4 (0.14%)	0.03 (7.8%)	Not applicable	100%	
American Indian and Alaska Native	0.3 (0.9%)	0.2 (8.3%)	Not applicable	100%	

Sources: References 17–19.
[a]Breakdown by nationality is based on the 1990 U.S. Census. Similar reports are not yet available for 2000 census data.

a minority patient, a useful technique is to anticipate common issues from the vantage point of a patient's time from immigration, degree of assimilation, and perceived importance of culture (such as affiliating only with one's own race). Common themes based on immigration status and degree of assimilation are depicted in Figure 11-1.

Core themes are usually different for immigrants than for American-born elderly. New immigrants, especially poorly educated non-English–speaking elderly, face culture shock, language barriers, social isolation, and may have experienced traumatic situations that lead to a spectrum of anxiety and depressive disorders not always recognized. Culture-bound syndromes may be most prevalent in this group. Established residents (defined as residing in the United States for 20 years or more) often show lower psychiatric morbidity than even the dominant Caucasian population, possibly due to a "survivor effect," based on the old Midtown Manhattan study (9). It is not clear if this differentiation continues to hold with new generations of immigrants. American-born minority elderly may differ based on assimilation and degree of conflict over ethnic identity. Poorly assimilated minority individuals who most clearly exhibit cultural isolation from the mainstream may also show problems with language barriers, social issues, more chronic illness and early mortality, fear of the majority group, and impact of prejudice.

Studies have not yet been conducted about efficacy of various psychotherapeutic approaches for different cultural groups, so there are many questions unanswered. For example, what are the most culturally congruent forms of psychotherapy for people from different cultures? Is a psychodynamic approach, or even a cognitive-behavioral approach, meaningful for a culture that endorses a fatalistic view of life, stoicism, or family affiliation above individual autonomy? Instead of questioning suitability of an approach, the patient is often blamed for non-compliance or being resistant to care. Instead, what is needed is a change in the mindset of the clinician and increased evidence-based information from clinical studies.

A large body of literature on minority populations deals with the disparities in access to or utilization of care. For example, racial minorities tend to avoid nursing home care. This may be due to family preference, cost, fear that only substandard facilities will be open to the minority community, or a dearth of offerings specific to their culture (e.g., cultural foods, culturally sensitive activities, and minority residents to affiliate with).

The percentage of minority elderly using public psychiatric clinics is also far below population estimates, assuming rates of mental illness at least equal to other age cohorts. The diagnoses of minority individuals who use

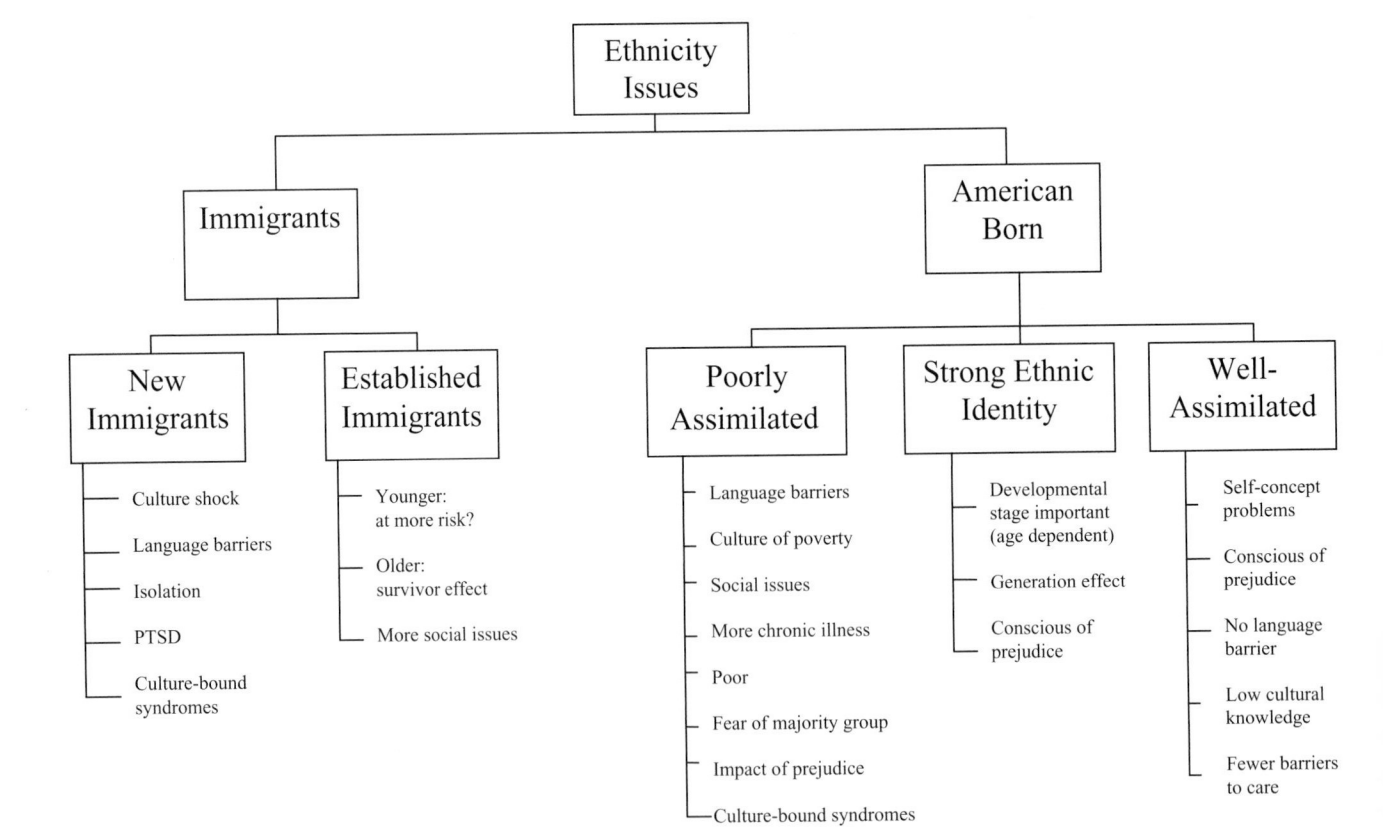

Figure 11-1 Impact of Ethnicity on Mental Health Care. PTSD, post-traumatic stress disorder. (Taken from Reference 20.)

inpatient facilities are often more severe and they come to treatment for different reasons. For example, fewer Black patients are admitted for affective disorders than Whites; more Hispanic patients with psychotic disorders are admitted than Whites with psychotic disorders as the proportion of admissions; and a relatively lower percentage of substance-related admissions occur for Blacks and Hispanics than for Whites (10). These trends may simply reflect different thresholds for when to seek treatment, but also include diagnostic distortions due to different presentations, cultural bias, and stereotyping (11). These factors contribute to the apparent overdiagnosis of schizophrenia and underdiagnosis of affective disorders. Awareness of these problems should make the culturally sensitive psychiatrist more cautious about diagnosis when faced with atypical presentations of disease.

ARE THERE CULTURAL DIFFERENCES IN THE PREVALENCE OF PSYCHIATRIC ILLNESS?

Although some new studies of small, opportunity samples exist, the last large-scale epidemiologic study of rates of mental illness was the Epidemiologic Catchment Area (ECA) program in the 1980s, which used the Diagnostic Interview Schedule. Minority oversampling was conducted in two areas to capture rural cases, African Americans, and Hispanics. An analysis of the ECA data was conducted for the American Psychiatric Association Task Force Report on Minority Elderly (12), which is reproduced in Table 11-4.

Generally, the ECA data showed lower rates of all psychopathology diagnoses for ethnic minority elders as compared to younger patients (under age 55). It was interesting that the rates of somatization disorder and psychotic disorders were not higher than the Caucasian comparison group. Phobias, however, seemed higher in the minority groups.

A major issue in diagnoses lies in the idioms used to describe feelings and distress. A parallel issue is the ethnocentric bias of clinicians that stereotypes the minority patient and distorts the diagnostic process. For example, some depression scales have used phrasing like "Do you feel sad and blue?" instead of "Do you feel depressed." Many people did not understand the idioms used to signify depression. For example, in African American and Asian cultures, color is not the idiom for depression; it is often geography (e.g., "I feel down in the valley."). It is not uncommon for translators to use a whole sentence or paragraph to try to communicate the concept of depression. Yet the World Health Organization has not advised any culture-specific diagnostic tools, because the symptoms defining different major diagnostic syndromes are really not different, only the terminology and interpretation of why the symptoms exist. When in doubt, it is useful to use standardized scales for diagnosis and to use validated translations of scales to monitor progress, even when translators are available. Translated scales exist for many ethnic groups and languages, including the Geriatric Depression Scale, the SCL-90 (Derogatis Symptom Checklist), and even the Minnesota Multiphasic Personality Inventory (MMPI).

TABLE 11.4

ECA 6-MONTH PREVALENCE RATES (%) OF PSYCHIATRIC DIAGNOSES BY AGE AND RACE[a,b,c]

Disorder	White 18–54	White 55 and over	African American 18–54	African American 55 and over	Hispanic 18–54	Hispanic 55 and over
Bipolar[d]	1.1%	—	1.3%	—	—	—
Major depression	4.4%	1.5%	3.7%	1.6%	4.2%	—
Dysthymia	3.7%	2.5%	2.8%	1.8%	4.0%	—
Alcohol abuse	7.5%	2.1%	6.3%	3.3%	8.8%	—
Schizophrenia/ schizophreniform illness	1.1%	0%	1.8%	0%	—	0%
Obsessive-compulsive	2.1%	0.9%	1.6%	1.9%	—	0%
Phobia	8.9%	6.7%	15%	13.9%	8.1%	9.1%
Somatization	0%	0%	0%	0%	0%	0%
Panic	1.2%	—	1.2%	—	—	—
Antisocial personality	1.6%	—	1.2%	—	—	0%
Cognitive impairment	0.3%	2.3%	1.4%	9.2%	—	—
Any DIS[e]/DSM-III diagnosis	23.6%	14.0%	27.3%	24.7%	23.1%	18.5%

[a]Source: Reference 12. ECA, Epidemic Catchment Area.
[b]Inadequate numbers of Asian and Native American individuals were available for analysis.
[c]A dash indicates fewer than 20 unweighted positive cases.
[d]Lifetime diagnosis.
[e]DIS, Diagnostic Interview Schedule; DSM III, Diagnostic and Statistical Manual of Mental Disorders, 3rd Edition.

CASE EXAMPLE:

Mrs. A is a 75-year-old Honduran woman who speaks minimal English despite residing in the United States for over 20 years. She frequently stops eating, necessitating hospitalization for dehydration, and is entering her lifetime limit for Medicare coverage. She was relocated to a nursing home 2 years ago due to restrictive lung disease, but it has no bilingual staff or residents. She stays in bed most of the day and is often seen with the sheet pulled over her head. She refuses to speak in or respond to English, except to select individuals. She says she is not depressed, only weak and sick. Lab parameters show marginally low hemoglobin and albumin. Thyroid function is normal. Despite her denial of depression, her sisters and nursing home staff feel she is depressed. She was referred for consultation for depression only recently. She scored in the major depression range on a Spanish translation of the Geriatric Depression Scale.

This case highlights the difficulty of diagnosis due to cultural factors such as language barriers and belief systems about illness. However, diagnostic criteria for major psychiatric diagnosis are not felt to be significantly different among races.

WHERE DOES BIOLOGY COME INTO PLAY?

There is a growing body of research on the psychobiology of ethnicity. There are important racial differences in isomorphic variations of hepatic enzymes and metabolism of many medications. The cytochrome 2D6 and 3A4 families have been the most studied, with research finding that there are racial differences in subpopulations of slow and rapid hepatic metabolizers of drugs. The frequency of these differences has not been sufficient to create separate dosing recommendations, but occurs frequently enough to alert one to possible problems. Another area is lithium transport mechanisms, which may be altered in many African Americans, necessitating lower lithium doses in affected individuals. (13).

In general, one should use the medication precautions recommended for all elderly; namely, sequential trials of single psychotropic medications rather than polypharmacy, beginning with low doses (one-half usual starting doses), titrating slowly (usually at five half-life intervals to avoid accumulation effects), continuing to advance to an effective dose or tolerance, and not exceeding maximum recommended doses.

Differential rates of and susceptibility to illness occur, but have not yet been clearly linked to racially determined genetic factors.

WHAT IS THE BEST APPROACH?

Several consensus panel reports are now available that help summarize the disparate literature and opinions about minority mental health care. Elderly are usually not specifically mentioned, but cultural issues are frequently most important to elderly because of the largely immigrant status for all minority groups (except African Americans), life-long health disparities and co-morbidities, and exposure to racial prejudice and cultural isolation. Assimilation is least likely to have occurred in the elderly, and cultural themes are most apparent. The following are five major reports that can provide additional detail:

- Curriculum Resource Guide for Cultural Competence, American Association of Geriatric Psychiatry (APA) (3)
- Outline for Cultural Formulation and Glossary of Culture-Bound Syndromes (1)
- Mental Health: Culture, Race, and Ethnicity—A Supplement to Mental Health: A Report of the Surgeon General (14)
- American Psychological Association Guidelines for Providers of Psychological Services to Ethnic, Linguistic, and Culturally Diverse Populations (15)
- Core Curriculum in Ethnogeriatrics, Second Edition (6)

The general approaches are summarized in Table 11-5, covering preparation to work with a person from another culture, what to consider when conducting the interview, and some of the conceptual issues that may influence one's work with a minority elder.

THE EXAMPLE OF DEMENTIA CARE

CASE EXAMPLE:

Mrs. D is an 82-year-old African American woman, from a rural town, who never married. She was brought into treatment by a niece, who is a mental health professional, for evaluation of dementia. The patient did not graduate from grammar school, lived alone and was reportedly doing well until only 1 month before the request, when she began to refuse help from a large family network. Her Mini-Mental State Examination (MMSE) score was 2 out of 30. Functionally, the patient needed standby assistance to dress and bathe, her family had to prepare her meals (though she could feed herself), and she was intermittently incontinent of urine. She had no spontaneous speech, but was able to answer questions with stereotypic answers ("That's fine, dear.") and repeat phrases. She could provide no relevant history and showed minimal insight. An MRI showed marked cortical atrophy with no areas of infarction. The patient was overweight but not obese, and only had a history of mild arthritis. Labs were unremarkable. She was on no medications. Collateral information revealed no history of dementia in the family, but most relatives had died before age 60 from accidents or illness.

This case demonstrates many issues of dementia care in minority populations. The traditional cognitive screening measures like the MMSE are not highly sensitive in assessing

TABLE 11-5
THEMES TO ADDRESS

Prerequisites:
- Sharpen cultural sensitivity (learn from your patients)
- Acquire cultural knowledge (read books and other literature, use consultants)
- Enhance cultural empathy
- Adjust culturally relevant relations and interactions (e.g., encourage negotiating or disagreeing with the therapist as a conscious theme for hierarchical cultures)
- Consider therapist-patient match (e.g., when is same race needed?)

Style of interview:
- Active and direct style is usually best initially
- Allow family to sit in if the patient desires (family-oriented cultures usually demand this)
- Know the social taboos for a culture and proceed cautiously
- Make cultural modifications in questions (e.g., fund-of-knowledge questions should be modified, interpreters may be needed)

Conceptual issues:
- Patient's view of his illness (different classification system for symptoms)
- The phenomenology may be difficult to elicit with language barriers
- The approach to gathering information may be off-putting
- Which issues are common to all people (emic) and which are culture-specific (etic)?
- Equivalency of meaning of words or questions
- Culture-bound syndromes
- Need for special programs or alternative therapies

Adapted from Reference 5.

poorly educated minority individuals. There was little correspondence between cognitive test measures and function. The actual need for an evaluation was for a behavioral disturbance, not cognitive decline. In fact, her cognitive decline was thought to be normal for her age. An extended support network, often including non-family members is common for many minority populations, especially in rural settings with strong community ties. The decision-maker in minority families is frequently the professional in the family, although caregiving is provided by other members. In this case, as is common in many similar situations, dementia services, or even help from primary care physicians, was not utilized until very late, and no services were known in the area. Care was restricted to medication trials and support from the existing support network, heeding the family desire to avoid institutionalization.

The question of increased risk for Alzheimer's dementia (AD) among African Americans has been raised from studies that show increased rates of AD in the United States. Whether this represents genetic factors or environmental influences remains unclear. Cross-cultural studies have often shown *lower* rates of AD in people of color (non-Europeans), even when corrected for survival effects.

One speculation is that diet and obesity in the United States contributes to a situation of increased oxidative stress and cellular damage. No specific differences in genetic predisposition have been discovered up to this point (16).

BENEFITS OF CULTURAL COMPETENCE

Cultural competence in dealing with elderly minority individuals is especially important because of the likelihood of immigrant status for non-African Americans, or a long history of segregation and prejudicial exclusion for elderly African Americans. These situations lead to cultural isolation and poor assimilation.

For the geriatric clinician, in particular, it is necessary to become sensitive to cultural themes by acquiring knowledge about the groups one works with, and to try to maintain empathy for cultural differences. Cultural sensitivity and empathy can enhance compliance and treatment outcomes.

Use of translated diagnostic scales is helpful in treating bilingual or non-English speaking patients, because they reduce subjectivity of the causal attribution for symptoms. At some point, though, one must address the underlying causes of the symptoms. A culturally competent assessment must consider family and community issues, as well as culture-bound syndromes, which are locality-specific patterns of aberrant behavior and troubling experience. The latter may be similar to a DSM-IV-TR diagnosis, but are generally perceived by the patient to have a non-psychological cause. For example, *ataque de nervios* is an idiom of distress among Latinos from the Caribbean and other Hispanic groups that includes uncontrollable seizure-like episodes and a sense of being out of control. It is like panic disorder but lacks the hallmark symptoms of apprehension and acute fear. "Falling-out," where a person claims an inability to move or see but is aware of everything around them, is common among Blacks and Caribbean islanders. This is like a conversion or dissociative disorder but lacks a clear underlying conflictual issue (1,2).

Efficacy of treatment approaches has received less attention than diagnosis. More research is needed on matching psychotherapeutic approaches to different cultural styles, as well as improving culturally sensitive scales for dementia assessment and other psychopathology.

Fortunately, there is growing attention to cultural competence. Federal mandates address cultural competence in areas as far reaching as disaster relief to mental health system reform, and it has already been incorporated into the federal grant process. Requirements for cultural competence in psychiatry training has also been propagated by the Accreditation Council for Graduate Medical Education.

REFERENCES

1. American Psychiatric Association. Appendix I: Outline for cultural formulation and glossary of culture-bound syndromes. In: *American Psychiatric Association, Diagnostic and Statistical Manual of Mental Disorders, Fourth Edition, Text Revision (TR)*. Washington, DC: American Psychiatric Press, Inc; 2000.

2. Mezzich JE, Kleinman A, Fabrega H, Parron DL, eds. *Culture and Psychiatric Diagnosis: A DSM-IV Perspective*. Washington, DC: American Psychiatric Press, Inc; 1996.

3. American Psychiatric Association Committee on Minority Elderly: Curriculum Resource Guide for Cultural Competence (web-based publication). Washington, DC: American Psychiatric Association, 1997.

4. Developing cultural competence in disaster mental health programs: guiding principles and recommendations. U.S. Department of Health and Human Services. pub. no. SMA 3828. Rockville, MD: Center for Mental Health Services, Substance Abuse and Mental Health Services Administration, 2003.

5. Tseng WS. *Cultural Competence in Clinical Psychiatry*. Boston: Academic Press; 2003.

6. American Geriatrics Society Ethnogeriatrics Committee. *Doorway Thoughts: Cross-Cultural Health Care for Older Adults*. vol 1. Boston: Jones and Bartlett Publishers; 2004.

7. Cultural Assessment in Clinical Psychiatry formulated by the Committee on Cultural Psychiatry, Group for the Advancement of Psychiatry. Washington, DC: American Psychiatric Publishing, Inc., 2002.

8. Revisions to the standards for the classification of federal data on race and ethnicity. Washington, DC: U.S. Office of Management and Budget, 1997. Available at: http://www.whitehouse.gov/omb/fedreg/ombdir15.html. Accessed June 7, 2005.

9. Srole L, Langner TS, Michael ST, Opler MK, Rennie TC. *Mental Health in the Metropolis: The Midtown Manhattan Study*. New York: McGraw Hill; 1962.

10. Adebimpe VR. A second opinion on the use of White norms in psychiatric diagnosis of Black patients. *Psychiatric Annals*. 2004;34(7):543–551.

11. Faison, W, Armstrong D. Cultural aspects of psychosis in the elderly. *J Geriatr Psychiatry Neurol*. 2003;16(4): 225–231.

12. Thompson JW. National databases on minority elders. In: *Ethnic Minority Elderly: A Task Force Report of the American Psychiatric Association*. Washington, DC: American Psychiatric Association; 1993;13–19.

13. Lin, KM, Smith, MW, Ortiz V. Culture and psychopharmacology. In: *The Psychiatric Clinics of North America: Cultural Psychiatry: International Perspectives*. Philadelphia: W.B. Saunders Co., 2001;24(3):523–538.

14. Mental health: culture, race, and ethnicity—a supplement to mental health: a report of the Surgeon General. Rockville, MD: U.S. Department of Health and Human Services, Substance Abuse and Mental Health Services Administration, Center for Mental Health Services, 2001.

15. APA guidelines for providers of psychological services to ethnic, linguistic, and culturally diverse populations. Washington, DC: American Psychological Association; 1990.

16. Jarvik L, Mintzer J. Expert panel summary: genetics, response, and cognitive enhancers: implications for Alzheimer's disease (GRACE). Presented at a conference convened by the American Psychiatric Association, the National Institute of Mental Health, the Alzheimer's Association and the American Association for Geriatric Psychiatry at the National Institutes of Health, Bethesda, MD, 2000.

17. U.S. Census Bureau Census 2000 summary file 1 (SF-1) 100-percent data: universe: total population. Washington, DC: U.S. Census Bureau; 2000.

18. He W. *U.S. Census Bureau, Current Population Reports, Series P23-211, the Older Foreign Born-Population in the United States: 2000*. Washington, DC: U.S. Government Printing Office; 2002.

19. Gibson CJ, Lennon E. Historical census statistics on the foreign-born population of the United States 1850–1990. Population division working paper no. 29. Washington, DC: Population Division, U.S. Bureau of the Census; 1999.

20. Sakauye, KM. Ethnocultural aspects. In: Sadavoy J, Boorson S, Grossberg G, eds. *Comprehensive Textbook of Geriatric Psychiatry*. New York: W.W. Norton; 2003.

Forensic Evaluation of the Older Patient

12

Stuart A. Anfang   *Paul S. Appelbaum*

INTRODUCTION/GENERAL ISSUES

> **CASE EXAMPLE:**
>
> You have been treating Mr. B, a 76-year-old, wealthy retired businessman, for depression associated with mild Alzheimer's dementia. He has recently made a number of significant decisions regarding his financial assets and has announced his pending third marriage to his 44-year-old girlfriend and former secretary. You have just received a subpoena for medical records from a lawyer representing Mr. B's children. The new fiancée has left you a voice message about "certifying that he's of sound mind" to sign a new will. She asks if you could give him the letter when Mr. B comes to his next medication appointment, since it should be "covered by Medicare." Later that day, you discover that your patient has been hospitalized with a possible delirium and wants to sign out against medical advice.

Words like *forensic* and *court ordered* often bring a chill of anxiety and trepidation to the clinical psychiatrist, who may anticipate getting involved in a world of unfamiliar terminology, responsibility, and expectations. Psychiatrists often fear being embroiled in time-consuming proceedings—with all the attendant costs—coupled with concerns about the confidentiality of patient information and preserving a carefully nurtured treatment alliance. Treating clinicians may try to avoid or deflect requests for forensic evaluations and reports for the court—and in some cases this may be appropriate. Particularly for the geriatric psychiatrist, however, whose clinical work frequently intersects with legal issues such as competence, it is sometimes impossible (and clinically inappropriate) to deflect these requests (1).

This chapter aims to provide a practical introduction to some relevant legal issues in geriatric psychiatry focusing on those issues most likely to arise in geriatric practice (2). Forensic issues that are of particular importance in geriatric work tend to revolve around issues of decisional competence. Hence, we offer a basic primer on some of the most common competence questions, including how to assess capacities and when to defer to other examiners. We also consider risk assessment issues specific to geriatric psychiatry. First, however, we provide an introduction to forensic psychiatry and the courts (3).

FORENSIC PSYCHIATRY

Broadly defined, forensic psychiatry involves the interface between clinical psychiatry and the legal system—essentially the application of relevant scientific and clinical knowledge to help the legal fact finder (judge or jury) answer the specific legal question (4). It is an important task that makes a valuable contribution to the social demands of justice and fairness. Psychiatric/legal issues—e.g., who is *competent*, who is *insane*—are not straightforward or easily understood by the layperson. Particularly for geriatric patients, where the intersection of medical and psychiatric issues are especially complex, the psychiatrist is in a critical position to help explicate and clarify the issues—ideally in a jargon-free manner, accurate but not overly technical—so that justice may be served.

The introduction of psychiatric information and opinion into the court setting can take many forms. There are occasions when the court will actually request or order an examination of an individual to address a specific question. A common example would be an evaluation for competence to stand trial, where the court would typically order a specific forensic facility or examiner to complete an examination within a specified period of time, often with the cost paid by the court or the state (5). More common for a treating psychiatrist is the request for a medical report or testimony to be introduced into the legal setting, typically at the request of the patient, her family, and/or her attorney. This raises the question of who should do a forensic evaluation: an independent examiner or the treating clinician? There is considerable literature on this question discussing issues such as dual agency, objectivity, interference with the treatment alliance, and differing ethical obligations (i.e., the clinical duties of beneficence and nonmaleficence ["do no harm"] vs. the forensic duties grounded in truth seeking, respect, and fairness) (6–8).

As a general rule, an independent examiner is preferable to provide the legal fact finder with a neutral and objective analysis of the clinical data without compromising the clinician's treatment alliance and inevitable advocacy for his patient. This is particularly true for cases in which the "stakes are high," such as criminally related issues. However, there are times and circumstances when such an independent examiner is not available or would seem unnecessary (or even inadequate) for the question at hand. The treating psychiatrist may be in the best position to comment on questions such as capacity to make treatment decisions or need for guardianship. Particularly for geriatric patients, it is relevant to ask what sort of expertise is necessary to answer the legal question: geriatric or forensic expertise? Ideally, the examiner would be experienced and well-versed in both areas to best address the question. In practice, such optimal expertise may not be easily available, and the treating geriatric psychiatrist who is educated in the basic legal issues can often be the most appropriate expert available (9).

The Legal World

As the clinician enters into the legal world, she needs to recognize it is a realm guided by an entirely different language and paradigm (10). Whereas psychiatrists are accustomed to a scientific language and terminology designed for clinicians, the court is used to a more descriptive language defined by statute or case law. It is an important challenge to translate clinical information into jargon-free-but-accurate descriptions that can be understood easily by the court. Similarly, clinical standards and opinion are rarely absolutes—we often deal with relative odds, likelihoods, and statistical prognoses. Legal standards come in a different language: "beyond a reasonable doubt" (sometimes defined as >95% likelihood, usually restricted to criminal cases), "clear and convincing evidence" (sometimes defined as >75% likelihood), or "preponderance of the evidence . . . more likely than not . . . to a reasonable degree of medical certainty" (sometimes defined as >50% likelihood).

The evaluating psychiatrist needs to understand the specific legal question he is being asked to answer. That would include the relevant standard, definitions, and the burden and standard of proof (i.e., which side has the responsibility of proving the case, and by what degree of certainty). It is essential to know the basics about the relevant statutory law (enacted by the legislature) and case law (precedents based on prior cases, often from higher-level appellate courts) in that jurisdiction. Most civil issues involving competence are derived from relevant state (as opposed to federal) law, although frequently federal law provides a floor standard below which the state law cannot descend (e.g., right to refuse treatment, right to terminate care, etc.) Usually, the attorney involved in the case and asking for an opinion (the retaining attorney) can provide ample education and guidance on these legal issues. However, sometimes the attorney might himself be inexperienced with the specific nuances of the particular forensic psychiatric issues at hand. In those instances, consultation with an appropriate expert (perhaps an elder care attorney or a forensic psychiatrist with geropsychiatry experience) can be very helpful.

It is important to recognize that, while clinical work is often built around a supportive paradigm of treatment alliance, the legal system is designed on an adversarial paradigm, where each side strongly advocates for winning one's position by presenting the facts in the most favorable light to one's side (11). In this process, the zealous opposing attorney may malign the psychiatrist's motives and opinions. Non-lawyers are often amazed to see opposing attorneys, after an afternoon of bitter infighting before the jury, go out for a drink as old friends. A clinician whose reputation is nastily impugned under cross-examination may find that the opposing attorney offers "no hard feelings" after the judge's verdict. To assuage the potential damage of these assaults to their ego and self-esteem, psychiatrists new to the legal process must recognize that this is merely "the way of doing business" in the adversarial legal system.

The psychiatrist working with an attorney must be vigilant about staying true to her role and not overly identifying with the advocacy/adversarial role of the retaining attorney. There may be pressure or temptation to alter or "buff" the expert opinion to bolster the client's case. The psychiatrist best serves the integrity of both herself and her profession by scrupulously sticking to the facts and scientific data in the service of truth and scientific accuracy (to the extent possible), rather than slanting or distorting her opinion for the sake of winning.

In the Courtroom

It is important to emphasize that many legal questions never get to an open courtroom and are resolved earlier in a process of negotiation and settlement between the opposing sides. In that regard, many expert opinions are presented in written form only, and never reach the point of actual verbal testimony. In general, the psychiatrist can be in the courtroom as a fact witness or an expert witness. The treating psychiatrist may be called as a fact witness, testifying to what has occurred in the treatment of the patient. Typically, he is asked to offer only that information, and not offer an expert opinion on the legal issues before the court (e.g., whether the patient is competent to make treatment decisions, or requires a guardianship over financial affairs). Thus, the fact witness may describe his diagnosis and treatment of a patient with Alzheimer's disease and give relevant clinical observations, but is not admitted to offer final opinions regarding the specific legal questions. The expert witness has been accepted by the court and both sides as someone with specialized technical knowledge needed by the legal fact finder to come to a decision. The expert witness is thus allowed to offer opinions specific to the legal question (e.g., the patient lacks appropriate decision-making capacity and meets typical criteria for a finding of incompetence), although the ultimate decision is left to the legal fact finder (judge or jury). The expert draws on multiple data for his opinion, including his direct examination (if appropriate), his knowledge and experience, scientific and medical standards, and relevant collateral information from other sources.

In some cases, the distinction between fact and expert witness may be blurred, as is the qualification process. To be qualified as an expert can be a simple or elaborate process—ranging from a simple admission of one's CV and qualifications into the record, orally or in writing, to a grueling detailed examination and challenging cross-examination by the other side (*voir dire*). The attorney who has retained the psychiatrist to testify can advise her whether she will be presented as an expert witness and the likely qualification process. Giving sworn testimony in open court under the scrutiny of judge and jury can be an intimidating experience; rigorous cross-examination can be frustrating and frightening. The psychiatric witness should resist the temptation to argue back or lose professional composure, leaving the arguments to the attorneys. Preparing for direct and cross-examination in the courtroom is a subject unto itself and beyond the scope of this chapter. The reader is referred to several excellent references for further guidance (12,13).

Release of Medical Records

There are many ways that a patient's medical information can enter the legal arena. The simplest is when the patient signs an appropriate form that allows treaters to release the records and/or speak to an attorney. Psychiatrist and patient should be very clear about the specific information that will be released (e.g., psychotherapy notes, listing of dates/times of sessions, etc.). Confidentiality is the right of the patient to privacy of his medical information, not to be divulged to third parties without consent. State law establishes rights of confidentiality and privilege, often with specific additional rights around psychotherapy notes, substance abuse treatment history, and HIV status, for example. However, the recent federal Health Insurance Portability and Accountability Act (HIPAA) regulations on health information privacy establish a floor of protections in every state, including extra safeguards for psychotherapy notes and specifications for how releases of information must be framed (14). Every psychiatrist should be familiar with these rules, as augmented by state law. *Privilege* is confidentiality applied to testimony in the legal setting, and thus it is the patient's right to waive it. Usually, only the patient can invoke or waive privilege, unless the court waives the privilege for a well-established legal exception. Professionals such as psychiatrists are sometimes allowed to invoke the privilege in the patient's absence. If asked to testify without the patient's explicit consent, the psychiatrist should consult with his own attorney about the specific situation before offering testimony.

If the (presumably competent) patient signs an appropriate release, the psychiatrist does not have the right to withhold medical information, although she can certainly educate the patient prior to the release about the advantages and disadvantages of releasing certain information. Subpoenas can be forbidding and frightening documents, delivered by a sheriff or certified carrier. However, these are merely a mechanism by which a lawyer asks for information, often without a patient's specific consent. The subpoena does not necessarily compel the psychiatrist to release the records, but it does compel her to respond—not merely to ignore the request! The appropriate response to a subpoena for a patient's records is to first notify the patient and/or his attorney, and then notify one's own attorney or risk management advisor for guidance. Depending on their input, it may be appropriate for the psychiatrist to respond to the request for information, or procedures may be initiated to block or quash the subpoena pending further court action. Psychiatrists should not simply release the records in response to a subpoena without attempting to communicate with the patient and/or his attorney.

Court orders are another mechanism by which patient information can be requested, and typically one must comply with such an order unless it is challenged legally. Again, the psychiatrist should attempt to alert the patient and/or his attorney as appropriate, but ignoring a court order puts one at risk of being found in contempt of court and risking penalties (fines and/or incarceration). Finally, the geriatric psychiatrist might be asked to release records of incompetent or deceased patients. If the incompetent patient has a legally authorized representative (LAR, such as a guardian or durable power of attorney, as will be described in more detail later), that person takes on the authority of waiving privilege and confidentiality. For the deceased patient, that authority often rests with the executor of the estate. In situations where a LAR is not available, the court might authorize an appropriate agent (such as a guardian *ad litem* or special executor) to act on the patient's behalf.

Payment Issues

Being asked to participate in legal proceedings can be a time-consuming process in terms of record review, preparation of lengthy reports, discussion with attorneys, and time spent in the actual courtroom. These activities are typically not reimbursed under health insurance or other third-party payments. Prior to any further involvement, it is important to negotiate with the patient and/or the attorney details of hourly rates, retainers, and likely ultimate costs. This can be an awkward discussion for the treating psychiatrist, trying to preserve the alliance with a patient who does not understand why legal evaluations are usually not covered by health insurance. However, it is best to address these issues clearly and early in the process so to avoid any hard feelings later that could impact one's objectivity or comfort working on the case. It is unethical and inappropriate for forensic or treating psychiatrists to accept contingency fees or a "piece of the action" based on potential financial settlement or award (15).

COMPETENCE/CAPACITY

CASE EXAMPLE:

Mrs. A has moderate-stage dementia and was recently admitted to a specialty Alzheimer's "reminiscence unit" within an assisted living facility. On admission, the staff told her that she was required to sign a health care proxy naming her daughter as her agent. Later that month, Mrs. A became agitated and paranoid in the context of a urinary tract infection. With the daughter's consent, the facility wanted to medicate Mrs. A with antipsychotic medication and arrange for voluntary psychiatric hospitalization—both of which Mrs. A adamantly refused.

Competence is a legal concept that refers to the ability to understand, appreciate, and manipulate relevant information in a rational manner as part of an informed decision-making process. From a clinical perspective, this is typically operationalized as decision-making capacity or ability. Although capacity and competence are often used interchangeably, it is important for the clinician to recognize that she is evaluating capacity; only a judge can adjudicate incompetence. Legally, all individuals are presumed to be competent until adjudicated otherwise; however, in some situations (e.g., making medical treatment decisions), procedures allow for surrogate decision making without formal judicial intervention (such as health care proxies or advanced directives, as discussed below).

The legal system may consider two forms of competence: general and specific. General competence is the ability to handle all of one's personal affairs in a reasonable manner, and might be questioned, for example, when advanced dementia renders an elderly patient unable to tend to basic daily needs and decisions. Specific competence usually refers to the specific task in question (e.g., competence to make treatment decisions, to execute a will, or to stand

trial). From the perspective of the clinical examiner, capacity is typically evaluated as task-specific. Distinctions can be made between decisional and non-decisional (or functional) capacities. An example of the former would be capacity to execute a will or health care proxy; an example of the latter would be capacity to drive or to live independently. For that reason, it is critical to clarify the relevant capacities to be evaluated. These include capacity to stand trial, testamentary capacity (ability to execute a will), capacity to make treatment decisions, capacity to consent to research or experimental treatment, capacity to execute a health care proxy or power of attorney, capacity to manage one's financial affairs, capacity to make end-of-life decisions, capacity to drive, and capacity to live independently. We will first review a general framework for capacity assessment, and then go into detail on specific capacity questions that commonly may be encountered by a geriatric psychiatrist.

INFORMED CONSENT

The importance of competence and capacity in treatment decisions derives from the centrality of informed consent. Over the past 50 years, the doctrine of informed consent has become a central pillar of the ethical practice of medicine (16). Although physicians, especially surgeons, were long required to obtain consent before proceeding with invasive treatments, it was common for doctors to provide only a basic explanation of the nature and purpose of treatment to get the patient's agreement (simple consent), with little evaluation or expectation that the patient was truly providing (or able to provide) a fully informed consent. In the 1950s, courts and clinicians began to examine this issue in more depth. With the increased recognition of the importance of patient autonomy and the variety of available treatment options, it was necessary to consider both the patient's need for information and his ability to reach a fully informed decision.

Informed consent is generally separated into three equally important components: information disclosure, voluntariness, and competence (or capacity). Patients need to be provided with the relevant information for a medical decision; the majority of states require disclosure of the information that a reasonable person would find material to the choice at hand. Accepting a consent based on insufficient disclosure of information can constitute malpractice.

Voluntariness requires that the patient give her consent freely, without undue pressure or coercion. Particularly for hospitalized or institutionalized patients, evaluators must be sensitive to potential subtle coercion inherent in such a dependent situation. All individuals, not only psychiatric patients, are subject to transference reactions towards caretakers leading them to be easily influenced or, contrarily, stubborn. The courts prohibit coercion that is clearly illegitimate or that constitutes undue influence. For example, promising an inpatient extra privileges in exchange for consent to try an experimental drug would be considered coercive influence. The clinician or family member can certainly strongly recommend that the patient consent to the proposed treatment, outlining the potential risks and benefits; however, the psychiatrist should always be sensitive to the dynamics of the treatment relationship and strive to make the patient's voluntary choice an enfranchising and therapeutic experience.

Competence or decisional capacity is considered in detail below.

Exceptions

In the clinical setting, the courts have identified several exceptional circumstances where the usual requirements of informed consent do not apply. In medical emergencies, when stopping to obtain informed consent from the patient or substitute decision maker would involve a delay that may threaten life or well-being, clinicians may treat with what is assumed to be *implied consent* (i.e., based on the assumption that any rational patient facing a similar emergent situation would agree to recommended treatment). In psychiatry, such emergencies are usually limited to violent, self-destructive, or delirious patients who require immediate intervention to prevent physical harm to themselves or others. Historically, physicians have argued that, in some situations, full disclosure would actually be emotionally harmful and countertherapeutic for the patient; the common example was disclosure of terminal cancer or advancing dementia. However, attitudes have clearly shifted over time with the advent of improved treatment and increased sensitivity to patients' rights. Arguing for the Hippocratic notion of "first do no harm" (*primum non nocere*), these clinicians have persuaded the courts to allow *therapeutic privilege* as a second exception to informed consent. In psychiatry, this is rarely invoked. If diagnostic or treatment information might damage an emotionally fragile patient, generally the information either can be withheld until the patient is stable enough to consider the data, or the clinician can seek a determination of incompetence and a substituted judgment if appropriate. Another related exception to the usual rules for informed consent is the patient's own waiver: a clinician is not required either to force information on an unwilling patient ("I don't want to know, Doc, just do the surgery.") or to insist that she make the choice ("You do what you think is best."). A patient who *waives disclosure or consent* must clearly understand that she has the right to the information being waived and ultimately the right to decide. For a psychiatric patient in particular, the clinician must consider why the patient is choosing not to know or decide and the meaning of the denial or surrender of decisional rights. Once clarified, the competent waiver of informed consent should be documented clearly in the medical record.

The final exception to informed consent is the *incompetent* patient. Once a court has formally adjudicated a patient incompetent, he cannot give a valid informed consent, which now must be obtained from a substitute decision maker designated by the court. Specific competence to make medical decisions is often determined outside the courtroom. In the hospital, psychiatrists are often asked to make clinical assessments of incompetence; while not legally authoritative, these determinations effectively remove decision-making power from the patient in a specific context. A substitute decision maker, often a family member or designated health care proxy, is allowed to consent for the patient. This non-judicial process balances the need to make urgent decisions without the expensive and cumbersome delay of a judicial proceeding, with the potential for abuse by colluding physicians and families. Hospitals and families continue to rely on these informal medical determinations of decision-making capacity, and it has become a standard practice endorsed by leading legal, ethical, and medical groups (17). The courts often make exceptions for "extraordinary" treatments, including a variety of interventions that require judicial approval for substituted consent even if a general guardianship has been granted. The exceptions vary by state, but typically include procedures such as forced sterilization, psychosurgery, electroconvulsive therapy (ECT), and antipsychotic medication. Psychiatrists must be aware of the regulations in their particular jurisdiction and may need to seek a more formal, often judicial, determination prior to initiating such treatment for a presumably incompetent patient.

Once a court has adjudicated incompetence, the court must be the party to restore legal competence; once the court has become involved, the psychiatrist cannot restore competence, even if a patient clearly has regained capacity. Sometimes a court finding of incompetence is valid only for a specified hospital admission or for a fixed period before automatic expiration or review. If the patient later regains decision-making capacity while still adjudicated incompetent, the psychiatrist should alert the patient's attorney or the court of the patient's improvement and prepare the necessary data for judicial review. These situations are seen more commonly with younger psychiatric patients, whose competence may be restored after appropriate treatment for psychosis or mania. For the patient with advancing dementia, restoration of capacity is unlikely and incompetence is usually permanent. However, for the geriatric patient with an acute delirium, lack of capacity may be temporary and transient, and a time-limited guardianship or adjudication of incompetence may be most appropriate.

CAPACITY ASSESSMENT

Decisional capacity is generally recognized as having four distinct components: *understanding* the information; *appreciating* its relevance for the person's particular situation; rationally *manipulating* (*reasoning* with) the relevant information to reach a decision; and *expressing* a consistent choice (18). Patients may have impairments in all areas, or may be stronger in some aspects than in others. How much capacity is enough? The psychiatrist must probe the patient's decision-making process to assess the degree of competence, factoring in the relative risk/benefit ratio in the setting of treatment consent or refusal. The degree of competence necessary to make an informed decision depends on the nature and context of the decision. The choice to accept an experimental high-risk–low-benefit treatment would require a fairly high level of competence, as would refusal of a low-risk–high-benefit treatment such as antibiotics for a common pneumonia. Particularly for psychiatric patients, issues of appreciation and reasoning are often critical, as will be discussed further below. Finally, when assessing capacity, it is important to consider the underlying etiology of the impaired decision-making capacity, which may help determine whether the incapacity is fluid (as in the case of delirium, drug intoxication, or an acute psychotic mania) or fixed (as in the case of dementia or significant mental retardation).

Conducting the Capacity Assessment

The evaluator must first clarify the specific function or task and decision-making context being assessed. Prior to beginning an assessment, the patient should be told of the purpose of the evaluation, including the limits of confidentiality of the evaluation (i.e., that the evaluator's conclusions may be presented verbally or in writing to outside parties as part of a procedure to determine competence). The patient has the right to refuse to participate in the evaluation, but should be informed that this refusal may be factored into the overall assessment of decision-making capacity, as the evaluator uses collateral information (information from records or family members, diagnostic tests, other clinical observations) to provide data relevant to the capacity assessment.

When interviewing the patient, the evaluator needs to ask specific questions geared to the four elements of capacity. For *understanding*, the psychiatrist must first make sure that the patient has had access to the relevant information, such as the risks, benefits, and alternatives of the proposed medical treatment, or her financial information when preparing a will. If the patient has not yet received adequate information, understanding cannot be adequately determined. The psychiatrist herself must have a clear understanding of the relevant issues in order to ask the appropriate questions. If assessing capacity to consent to colon surgery and a permanent colostomy, the psychiatrist may first need to speak with the surgeon to understand the potential risks, benefits, and alternatives the patient is expected to comprehend. If assessing capacity to stand trial, the evaluator may need to speak to the attorney to understand the charges, potential consequences, and likely judicial process to be faced by the arraigned client.

The clinician needs to explore the aspects of *reasoning* and *appreciation*, which are often closely linked but distinct issues. For psychiatric patients, these are areas that often impair decision-making capacity. Generally, the evaluator wants to follow the patient through his reasoning process as he makes his decision. A patient who has memorized the Physicians Desk Reference (PDR) warnings on antipsychotic medication may still have impaired reasoning if his refusal is based on the delusional belief that his doctor is a CIA agent and the government is intent on silencing his true knowledge about the Kennedy assassination. The patient with psychotic depression who refuses ECT because of concerns about electrocution and brain liquidation may be less competent to consent than the patient who is primarily concerned about the side effects of transient confusion and memory loss. For appreciation, the key issue is often insight: does the patient appreciate that he has a psychiatric illness, or that she is actually charged with a serious felony. The manic patient who refuses treatment because, after all, he really is Napoleon, Emperor of Europe, clearly lacks insight into his illness and need for appropriate treatment. The mentally retarded woman who does not recognize that setting fire to her group home was a crime lacks appreciation of the legal consequences she faces. Often, reasoning and appreciation can be the most challenging aspects to discern fully, and require detailed and probing questioning to examine adequately the rationale and insight underlying the patient's decision.

Expression of choice is often fairly straightforward: what does the patient want, and can she clearly express the decision? Particularly in geriatric patients, however, consistency of choice expression becomes a critical issue, especially for patients with variable cognitive impairment. For the sundowning patient with mild dementia, a clear consent given to the surgeon in the morning might be very different at night when the anesthesiologist comes around. In these situations, it can be useful to anticipate external factors that may impact on transient incapacity, and guide the consent process accordingly (e.g., make sure informed consent discussions occur during the daytime, when the patient is cognitively most intact).

Standardized Assessment Tools

The heart of a capacity evaluation is typically a detailed clinical interview exploring the four aspects outlined above. In addition, researchers have developed a number of specialized and standardized assessment instruments that can help structure formal evaluation of specific capacities (19). The field of forensic assessment instruments is most advanced in the area of criminal and other court-related evaluations. There are well-established instruments to assess issues such as capacity for criminal adjudication, capacity to stand trial for mentally retarded defendants, capacity to comprehend Miranda rights, capacity for criminal responsibility, and capacity for fit parenting. With regard to competence to consent to medical treatment, developments in this field ultimately crystallized during the 1990s in the work of the MacArthur Foundation Research Network on Mental Health and the Law (20). The group developed the MacArthur Competence Assessment Tool for Treatment (MacCAT-T) (21) and a related tool for clinical research (MacCAT-CR) (22), which are structured interviews designed to be clinically useful (taking approximately 20 to 25 minutes to administer) and tailored to the patient's specific context and proposed decision. There is no total competence score, since one could get very "good" scores in understanding and reasoning, for example, but be considered incompetent due to total lack of appreciation that one has schizophrenia. MacCAT-T ratings appear to correlate with overall clinical judgments about competence to consent to treatment, at least in initial studies. In addition, the instrument provides a useful, structured format to guide clinicians through the process of informing the patient about the illness and treatment while simultaneously assessing decision-making capacity. Tools such as these are likely most useful as one part of an overall assessment of capacity to make treatment decisions, especially for the most ambiguous or legally scrutinized cases (23).

For geriatric patients, there are several well-established cognitive screening instruments, beginning with the Mini-Mental State Examination (MMSE) and other dementia rating instruments described elsewhere in this text. It is important to recognize that these instruments do not assess decision-making capacity, *per se*, and should not be relied upon exclusively as part of the capacity assessment. Although the demented patient with a MMSE of 16 may reasonably be expected to have some impairment of decision-making capacity, a more focused assessment will be necessary to assess performance regarding the specific decision-making task at hand (e.g., does the patient still have the capacity to designate an appropriate health care proxy) (24). For patients with Alzheimer's disease, studies have suggested the usefulness of appropriate neuropsychological screening as well as clear exploration of the specific legal standards for competency (25,26). Finally, there are non-decisional capacities that can be evaluated with the assistance of formal functional assessments (e.g., computer simulation for driving skills, occupational and/or physical therapy assessment for independent living and ADL skills) (27).

Increasingly, researchers and clinicians alike have pointed to the key role of aspects of executive functions in decisional capacity, including planning and implementing one's decisions (28). Especially for elderly patients with dementia, executive dysfunction becomes a critical component often overlooked in initial assessments of cognitive impairment and decision-making capacity (29). Tools to assess executive function are well-described elsewhere in this text, ranging from formal, detailed neuropsychological evaluations to briefer, bedside tests (such as clock drawing, Luria hand sequence,

trail making, and category fluency) (30). Again, these tests do not constitute specific assessments of decision-making capacity, but provide data about executive dysfunction relevant to questions of competence.

Documenting the Assessment

After completing the assessment, it is critical that it be well-documented, usually in a formal written report. The vast majority of judicial determinations of competence do not require actual courtroom testimony, so the written report becomes the key medical resource to guide the court's determination. The report should detail in a clear and organized fashion the evaluation of the patient (questions asked, instruments used, responses given) and additional collateral data reviewed (other interviews, test results, relevant records). The basis for the conclusions regarding capacity should be clearly substantiated. For certain situations, it may be useful to record the patient interview by video or audiotape, particularly if this is a high-profile case likely to get greater judicial scrutiny or to evoke expert disagreement (e.g., contested testamentary capacity with a significant estate at issue).

SPECIFIC CAPACITIES

Capacity to Make Treatment Decisions

Over the past 50 years, numerous state and federal court decisions have shaped the analysis by which the law—and clinicians—must assess the right to accept or refuse medical treatment. Landmark cases have outlined how much information must be disclosed for informed consent (*Natanson* (31), *Canterbury* (32)); established that the patient must be competent and uncoerced in making the treatment decision (*Kaimowitz* (33)); clarified that adult patients are competent until proven incompetent, even if they have mental illness and are involuntarily committed (*Rennie* (34), *Rogers* (35)); and identified circumstances where the state can override or allow an appropriate alternate decision maker to substitute for the incompetent patient (*President and Directors of Georgetown* (36), *Saikewicz* (37), *Rogers, Cruzan* (38)). Guided by these decisions and others, state legislatures have enacted statutes clearly outlining the patient's right to accept and reject treatment and the circumstances by which that right can be withdrawn—typically requiring a finding of incompetence.

We have already discussed the basic principles behind informed consent and the general assessment of the four aspects of decision-making capacity. Standardized and structured assessment tools can help supplement the clinical interview described above (39). The evaluator must be value-neutral and avoid projecting her own personal risk/benefit assessment, and should try to gather the most objective information possible from a variety of sources.

Collateral information from others, such as treating physicians and family members, can be essential to clarify the medical risks and benefits as well as quality-of-life considerations for the specific patient.

The evaluator should consider the etiology of impaired capacity, whether it is likely fixed or transient, and whether the incapacity might remit with appropriate treatment. For geriatric patients, the evaluator might consider a broad range of potential factors, including delirium, depression, dementia, delusions/psychosis, cultural perceptions, education, socioeconomic pressures, family dynamics, and psychological denial. Once the etiology is identified, appropriate treatment or other interventions may be indicated. Depending on the etiology and the urgency of the situation, the clinician may decide to delay the consent process until capacity is restored, or may need to seek a substitute decision maker.

Although treating clinicians are usually most concerned about patients who refuse recommended treatment, the geriatric psychiatrist must particularly recognize that some elderly patients are incompetent acceptors, who may agree with recommended treatment despite significantly impaired decision-making capacity. Especially for treatments that entail greater risk, the treating clinician might seek a formal assessment of incapacity and a substitute decision maker and/or judicial intervention if appropriate.

Depending on the jurisdiction, some special treatment decisions (such as ECT, antipsychotic medication, sterilization, termination of pregnancy, psychosurgery) will often require different legal standards and procedures for the incompetent patient. For the psychiatric patient who refuses or is incompetent to accept voluntary inpatient hospitalization, the state will have clear standards for civil commitment, typically based on potential dangerousness. However, even once involuntarily committed, many jurisdictions may still require a separate assessment and procedure to determine competence to reject recommended antipsychotic medications. Both the independent evaluator and the treating psychiatrist must be aware of the legal rules and regulations of their specific jurisdiction.

Testamentary Capacity

Testamentary capacity is the capacity to make a will (i.e., a "last testament"). With some variation by jurisdiction, most states define this as the capacity to (1) understand that the testator is executing (or expressing) a will at the time, (2) understand the nature and extent of his property and assets, and (3) appreciate his natural heirs, namely his relationship to living descendants, spouse, and other relatives whose interests might normally be impacted by the will (40). A testator is presumed to be competent until adjudicated otherwise. Since this question would typically be raised after his death, it is often very challenging to have sufficient data to make a clear retrospective analysis of decision-making capacity. In general, the level of capacity

needed for a competent will is relatively low, and historically there has been a tendency to accept the possibility of lucid intervals even for individuals with some degree of mental impairment.

Since testamentary incapacity may be difficult to prove, many will challenges also raise concerns about *undue influence*—essentially that the will was executed under unfair pressure. Definitions will vary by jurisdiction, usually in case law, but this is often a vaguely defined legal concept that is difficult to operationalize clinically. The courts frequently look at whether the weaker testator was taken advantage of, or had his will substituted by the stronger dominant party. Relevant issues would include whether the named recipient is the natural heir; whether the bequest or the will language was unnatural; whether there was an opportunity for the beneficiary (or a third party) to unduly manipulate or control the execution of the will; and whether the testator was mentally weak, impaired, or susceptible to manipulation or deception (41). Geriatric psychiatrists will be asked to assess these issues of susceptibility due to mental illness or impairment, but it is still necessary for the contesting side to demonstrate that someone exerted improper influence that altered the intention of the donor. Even if there are clear coercive factors, influence is not undue if it did not change the natural disposition of the donor—if the same bequest or gift likely would have been made in any event, despite the influence.

The classic case would be a divorced or widowed wealthy older man with mild dementia who has become involved with a much younger caretaking woman, whom he may ultimately marry or with whom he may otherwise become romantically involved. Depending on the dynamics with other family members who may be opposed to this relationship, this may become a contentious and litigated situation before and after the testator's death, with concerns about potential victimization and abuse. Of course, geriatric patients, even with cognitive impairments, may still make decisions about relationships that are worthy of respect, and such romances may indeed be authentic. These are particularly complicated scenarios for the psychiatrist who is asked to evaluate for undue influence, especially after the testator's death, based on possibly incomplete or biased information.

Because of the difficulties inherent in post-mortem retrospective analysis, some attorneys may seek to have their client's testamentary capacity prospectively assessed and documented at the time of will execution. Typically such cases involve larger estates or potentially challengeable bequests; when requested, it is often by a competent testator or her designated beneficiaries. These evaluations may be audiotaped or videotaped to assure the most complete documentary record likely to survive any later challenge. The evaluating psychiatrist should follow the general approach to decision-making capacity outlined earlier. Detailing the testator's understanding of the nature of her property and assets will require some collateral confirmation from lawyers, accountants, or bankers. Appreciation and reasoning aspects of the bequest must also be explored, e.g., is this a natural heir, and if not, why is the bequest being made (and why is the alternative bequest to a natural heir *not* being granted)? The psychiatrist should confirm that the expression of the will reflects a clear and consistent choice by the testator, with the knowledge that some jurisdictions will recognize the possibility of lucid intervals even in cognitively compromised individuals.

Capacity to Manage One's Financial Affairs/Enter into a Contract

Issues similar to the testamentary capacity questions often arise with regard to a patient's ability to manage his financial affairs, including making large monetary gifts or entering into a contract. One key difference is that these transactions are usually questioned when the patient is still alive, allowing for direct examination. The evaluating psychiatrist must look to the patient's understanding of his financial situation and appreciation of the nature of the potential gift, contract, or other transaction (42). Issues of voluntariness (coercion, undue influence) must also be considered. States will vary in their definition of incapacity to make contracts or gifts, but may generally link this to the requirements for a guardianship of property (called *conservatorship* in some jurisdictions). If an individual is unable to understand his financial situation, appreciate the impact of potential choices, and make reasonable financial decisions with regard to contracts, gifts, and/or payments, these will be grounds for the court appointment of a guardian of property or conservatorship (43). As the psychiatrist assesses the patient's financial understanding and reasoning, it will again be critical to have collateral data from relevant parties, such as family, lawyers, bankers, or accountants. The issue of financial decisional incapacity obviously involves more than a person merely making a bad stock purchase or having a risky business deal go awry; the degree of misunderstanding, impaired judgment and faulty reasoning will be important to consider, particularly in the context of the individual's past (and presumably *competent*) financial affairs.

Elder care attorneys often advise their older clients (and their families) about other mechanisms to manage financial decision-making rather than going through the formal (and sometimes expensive) process of establishing a legal guardian or conservator. These mechanisms might range from having two signatories on a joint checking account, to establishing a durable power of attorney to cover financial and property issues. A power of attorney is standard in every jurisdiction, and allows one person to delegate decision-making authority to another person to act on the first person's behalf in financial or other business/contractual matters. A durable power of attorney is a legal instrument that continues after the delegator is no

longer competent. Obviously, when first executing the durable power of attorney, the individual must have the capacity to appoint a surrogate, but that decision often requires a lower level of capacity than more complicated financial/business decisions. For example, an individual with early dementia may not comprehend all the complex ramifications of selling a particularly valuable piece of property; however, she may fully understand and rationally appreciate the consequences of a decision to designate her trusted daughter or longtime attorney to act on her behalf. The durable power of attorney is becoming an increasingly popular and useful legal instrument, often executed at the same time as a will, to help protect and manage an elderly individual's financial situation when she become less capable, without resorting to the full legal process of adjudicated incompetence.

Capacity to Participate in Court and Other Legal Proceedings

There are distinct competence issues specific to courtroom and other legal proceedings, such as competence to testify as a witness and competence to stand trial (including the capacity to defend oneself [i.e., act as one's own attorney], to plead, and to waive Miranda rights). These are typically specialized exams best done by forensically experienced examiners most familiar with expectations of the court, standards of the jurisdiction, and issues requiring specific assessment.

The standards and procedures for conducting these evaluations are complex, and to describe them in detail is beyond the scope of this discussion. Briefly, competence to stand trial is typically assessed according to the standard described by the US Supreme Court in *Dusky v. United States* (1960): the defendant must have sufficient present ability to consult with his lawyer with a reasonable degree of rational understanding, and have a rational as well as factual understanding of the proceedings against him (44). Competence to plead guilty and competence to defend oneself are considered by that same standard. Capacity to be a witness (testimonial capacity) typically requires the ability to appreciate distinctions between truth and falsehood, and the ability to understand questions, contain oneself appropriately in a courtroom setting, and sustain examination and cross-examination. This testimonial capacity question arises commonly for young child witnesses, as well as for elderly individuals with cognitive or neuropsychiatric impairment.

Capacity to Participate in Research

The same issues relevant to decision-making capacity for medical treatment apply to participation in medical research. Voluntariness, competence, and adequate information are necessary for informed consent. The subject must recognize that this is research, not standard treatment, with its inherent risks, benefits, and alternatives (including the alternative of conventional treatment). Additional issues arise in research studies, including the confidentiality of the data and potential compensation to research subjects. Drawing from the development of the MacCAT-T, Appelbaum and Grisso developed the MacCAT-CR for clinical research (22). It provides a structured interview to assess decision-making abilities relevant to research participation, using each study's specific protocol and informed consent disclosure to structure the MacCAT-CR interview, which takes about 20 to 25 minutes. As is the case with the MacCAT-T, there are no cut off scores or overall competence scores, since the capacity assessment will vary by the individual context, including the specific research study being considered. Other groups have developed instruments to assess specific capacity components, such as appreciation (45,46).

Recently, there has been greater appreciation of the need for appropriate substitute consent for decisionally impaired individuals who may benefit from research participation, including those with dementia or other psychiatric conditions, such as schizophrenia (47) or major depression, with impairment of insight/judgment (48,49). Mechanisms for obtaining substituted informed consent can vary depending on the jurisdiction and nature of the study, ranging from formal judicial involvement (appointment of a guardian or guardian *ad litem*) to non-judicial procedures (accepting consent from a designated proxy or family member in the absence of a relevant advance directive) (50). In 1998, the National Bioethics Advisory Commission issued guideline recommendations on research subjects with impaired decision-making capacity, including risk classification and the role of LARs in protocols with greater-than-minimal risk (51). There has been considerable debate about these guidelines within the professional and scientific community; a clear consensus has yet to be reached about the optimal way to allow research with these subjects (52).

End-of-Life Care/Advance Directives

By legel precedent, the courts have recognized a competent individual's right to refuse treatment, including life-sustaining treatment. While discussion of do-not-resuscitate (DNR) orders and refusing certain procedures (e.g., intubation, feeding tube placement) has become routine today, such openness has increased dramatically over the past 25 years. This capacity assessment is the same as for any other medical treatment decision (53). The law also now recognizes advance directives, by which an individual can legally assure that her desires regarding medical care are followed even after she becomes incompetent. As of 1991, the federal Patient Self Determination Act requires that hospitals, nursing homes, and other health care institutions provide patients with information about these directives (54).

There are two general types of advance directives: *instructional directives* (such as a living will) and *proxy directives* (such as a health care proxy or durable power of attorney for medical decisions). The living will specifies what kind of care the individual wants or does not want, if he later becomes unable to participate competently in medical decision-making. The content can range from general to very specific, and standardized formats are available from a number of organizations, usually including a section where the individual can add his particular preferences. The individual must be competent when he executes the living will, which would not be invoked unless the person loses decision-making capacity. The assessment of capacity to execute the living will would generally follow that of making other treatment decisions, with the caveat that since the decisions will likely be more theoretical at the time of signing the living will, issues of appreciation and reasoning may be more abstract and based on the individual's historical and philosophical perspective.

A proxy directive allows the person to designate another individual as a health care proxy, to act on her behalf when she becomes incompetent to make treatment decisions (55). The proxy directive can have more flexibility than a living will, which cannot anticipate every potential medical decision. The two mechanisms can be combined, directing the proxy to follow the living will where it is explicit, but giving the proxy authority to act according to the appropriate standard in circumstances not addressed in the will. In general, the proxy or surrogate is expected to act, as much as possible, according to the expressed wishes and values of the impaired person. When those values and wishes were not expressed, the proxy may, depending on the law in a given jurisdiction, decide based on what the person would likely have chosen (*substituted judgment standard*), based on what other patients in a similar situation and context would reasonably have decided (*reasonable person standard*), or based on an objective balancing of the overall risks and benefits (*best interests standard*) (56).

As noted earlier, to designate a health care proxy can require a lower level of decision-making capacity than the ability to make a complex medical decision (57). A woman with mild-to-moderate dementia might not be able to understand and appreciate the choice to place a feeding tube but can competently designate her husband of 50 years to be her health care proxy. The individual must understand the purposes of the proxy directive and when it will be invoked, and appreciate the implications of appointing another person to function in this way.

Once competently executed, the advance directive does not take effect until the individual is determined to have lost decision-making capacity. This typically does not involve a formal legal adjudication of incompetence; a medical determination of impaired decision-making capacity *activates* the proxy directive. However, the statutes authorizing advance directives, whether proxy directives or living wills, allow the directive to be revoked or changed by the individual at any time—provided she is competent to do so. Of course, incompetence can only be formally adjudicated by the court. Thus, if a person actively opposes the decision made by her designated health care proxy, treatment cannot take place until a judicial determination of the patient's competence occurs (58). What constitutes active opposition is often a judgment call. If the delirious patient pulls out an IV, does it mean she is actively rejecting the proxy's authorization of antibiotic treatment? Almost certainly not. In contrast, if the moderately demented man actively resists hemodialysis, saying, "No more, I do not want to live like this," this may be more likely to constitute competent opposition to the proxy's decision. In situations where the active opposition to the decision of the health care proxy seems clear and deliberate, the treating physician may need to seek a formal judicial determination of incompetence to validate the health care proxy or provide for another substitute decision maker such as a guardian. In those situations, it may be helpful to consult with the hospital attorney or other lawyer familiar with the procedures for urgent judicial determination of incompetence to make medical treatment decisions.

Finally, many jurisdictions have different procedures for substitute decision-making for ECT, antipsychotic medication, or psychiatric hospitalization. Some states have clarified (either in case law or by statute) whether a properly designated health care proxy is authorized to make such decisions without resorting to the usual full legal process. There has also been increased discussion about psychiatric advance directives (59). For example, a stabilized patient with schizophrenia might sign a living will that anticipates future occasions when she may decompensate and become actively psychotic, directing her psychiatrist to administer neuroleptic medication as appropriate. Again, if the decompensated patient were then to oppose the medication actively, it might be necessary to seek formal judicial determination of competence and validation of the advance directive. Psychiatrists should be familiar with the law in their particular jurisdiction regarding the authority of health care proxies to make psychiatric treatment decisions, as well as the use of psychiatric advance directives (60).

Functional (Non-Decisional) Capacities

There are a group of capacities that involve more than just decision-making, but include functional abilities as well. The capacity to drive safely is a good example, incorporating issues of cognitive decision making along with functional capabilities (vision, reaction time, hearing, etc.) As the elderly population increases and older individuals are maintaining their independence longer, there is increased discussion about when is it appropriate to limit or remove the license to drive. On one hand, driving has become a

commonly assumed "right" (although it is actually a *privilege* of license) in our society. To revoke the driver's license of an older patient often severely restricts his autonomy, independence, self-reliance, and even self-esteem. At the same time, the physician recognizes an obligation to protect society—and the patient himself—from potential serious damage and injury due to his impairment as a driver.

With headlines documenting serious motor vehicle accidents due to older drivers, state legislatures are increasingly grappling with ways to address this challenge. Some legislators have proposed that elder drivers be required to take road tests upon license renewal after a certain age, although this may be an expensive and unwieldy mechanism. Other proposals have looked to physicians to certify the driving safety of their older patients beyond a certain age. Some states require physicians to report to the motor vehicle department concerns about patients with significant cognitive impairment, much in the same way as they may be asked to report patients with an active seizure disorder or other illness impairing the ability to drive. Physicians must be aware of their specific obligations in the jurisdiction where they practice. The challenge becomes to balance the physician's legal and ethical obligations, both to the patient and to the larger society. The potential consequences of allowing an impaired patient to drive are matched by the potential disruption of the doctor-patient alliance if the angry patient mistrusts, fires, or even sues the well-intentioned physician.

Direct methods to assess driving ability are imperfect and not typically within the direct province of the geriatric psychiatrist (61). In addition to cognitive impairment from dementia, other non-psychiatric factors are often relevant, such as visual and hearing impairment, sedation due to medications, delayed response time, and other general medical conditions. Relevant information from other physicians, family members, and other collateral contacts can help inform the assessment of driving capacity. Cognitive assessment, including more detailed neuropsychological testing, can also give valuable information about reaction time, visuospatial abilities, and attentional skills, which allows indirect extrapolation to driving skills. Obviously, the mere diagnosis of early-stage dementia does not preclude the ability to drive safely. However, recognition of disease progression and likely time course can help the doctor, as well as the patient and family, begin to predict and prepare for a future time when the elder is unable to drive. A number of professional organizations, including the American Academy of Neurology and the American Psychiatric Association, have offered clinical guidelines for management of the mild-dementia patient, including when to refer for a more specialized driving assessment (62–64).

Rehabilitation and other facilities are increasingly offering driving simulation programs, where an elder is asked to respond to driving cues, including road signs, hazards, weather conditions, and other potential driving hazards. Although this is still a step removed from an actual road test, it is likely a safer, more practical and less costly screening mechanism to predict dangerous driving behavior. Solid empirical data about the validity and predictive value of these simulators have not yet been widely published. However, the concerned physician might refer an elder patient to one of these programs to get another opinion about driving capacity. The results may reassure that driving capacity is still intact, or may help substantiate the recommendation that the license be relinquished or revoked.

Similarly, the geriatric psychiatrist may be asked to address whether the older patient can live independently, handling activities of daily living (ADLs) ranging from basic dressing and toileting to more complicated tasks such as household management, shopping, cooking, laundry, and taking public transportation. Again, these are areas that the evaluating psychiatrist may not easily assess upon interview in the office setting. Collateral information from family members, friends, or other caretakers will be very helpful. Formal evaluations can be done as part of OT or PT assessments, such as completing cooking tasks in a model kitchen or having an actual in-home assessment. Finally, there are a range of standardized evaluation tools that can be used to assess independent ADL skills based on interview (of patient and/or collateral informant) and direct observation (65). These typically require trained examiners skilled in geriatric assessment, usually nurses, occupational therapists, or other geriatric clinicians. Thus, the role of the geriatric psychiatrist is often to bring together all these data points—cognitive assessment, functional assessments, collateral observations, diagnostic evaluations, clinical history—to offer a comprehensive recommendation about functional capacity, both currently and prospectively.

RISK ASSESSMENT ISSUES

Lastly, we briefly explore risk assessment in two common clinical contexts: elder abuse and the duty to warn/protect third parties (*Tarasoff duty*). These are not formal forensic or competence evaluations, per se, but are common clinical situations that require an assessment by the geriatric psychiatrist due to a legal mandate or duty.

Elder Abuse

As a matter of public policy, every state has specified situations where disclosure of information preempts considerations of confidentiality. Such *mandatory reporter obligations* imposed on physicians range from sexually transmitted diseases and gunshot wounds to abuse of children, the disabled, and the elderly. Cognitively impaired elders may be at higher risk for abuse, especially from frustrated relatives and caregivers (66). All clinicians should be aware of the reporting obligations in their jurisdiction in regard to

detail, responsibility, and practitioners covered. Typically, the legislation provides specific information regarding the reportable circumstances, the information to be released, and the mechanism for notification. The obligation to report generally covers information gathered in the professional context. If the vacationing psychiatrist witnesses elder abuse outside of any professional relationship, most jurisdictions would not mandate a report; however, the physician may feel a moral obligation to contact an authority. Of course, if there is no patient-physician relationship, there is also no expectation of confidentiality, and so the vacationing psychiatrist is free to act as would any concerned citizen.

The statutes typically provide civil immunity to the physician who fulfills her obligation in good faith. Failure to comply with a reporting mandate may subject the clinician to civil penalties. If harm occurs that would have been avoided had the physician reported the situation earlier, civil liability is possible for allegedly negligent practice. If the physician believes that the situation is potentially reportable, it is usually best to notify the appropriate authorities. Sometimes one can call the protective agency anonymously to discuss the situation and determine whether reporting is required. It is not expected that the physician herself will investigate the situation, but she must make a good faith judgment about reporting based on her knowledge and clinical experience. Allegations are then screened by the relevant state agency based on the available information. The clinician may be contacted at a later date for further data. Clinicians should document in the treatment record that a mandated report has been made, and should seek legal consultation for clarification in complicated cases.

Duty to Protect Third Parties

In the well-known 1976 case of *Tarasoff v. Regents of the University of California*, the California Supreme Court established a new precedent, imposing on clinicians a "duty to protect" third parties from harm by dangerous patients, even those who had never been hospitalized (67). That court decided that when clinicians know or should know that their patients represent a danger to others, they have a duty to take whatever steps are reasonably necessary to protect those identifiable third parties. Since 1976, this duty has become a focus of court and legislative activity across the United States. Despite objections from clinicians (regarding the limited ability to predict future dangerousness accurately, the risk of unnecessary breach of confidentiality, and the possibility of excessive protective hospitalization), most states have now adopted some version of the duty to protect by case law or by statute (68).

Although some court decisions suggested that clinicians would have a duty to protect potential victims who are not specifically identified or threatened, the duty is usually limited to situations in which a patient makes an overt threat against a clearly identifiable victim. The statutes defining the duty to protect vary by state, but usually specify one or more possible options for discharging the duty, including warning the victim, notifying the police, and/or hospitalizing the patient voluntarily or involuntarily. If the psychiatrist discharges the duty in good faith and with reasonable clinical judgment, the statutes typically hold the doctor immune from liability for breach of confidentiality and for negligence. It is essential for all clinicians to be familiar with the specific duty to protect in their jurisdiction as defined by statute or case law (69).

Clinical approaches to manage a duty-to-protect situation are covered extensively in the literature (70). Common recommendations are to conduct a thorough clinical assessment of the threat, involve the patient in the decision whenever possible, clearly document reasoning, obtain consultation with a colleague if necessary, and do what is clinically appropriate for the particular situation. When clinically appropriate, either voluntary or involuntary hospitalization can provide a less public means of safely managing a dangerous patient without breaching confidentiality. For some patients, particularly those who pose a chronic threat to others, management outside the inpatient setting may be necessary. Whenever possible, the patient should be engaged in the problem as part of the therapeutic alliance, allowing for an exploration of violent impulses and an acceptance of responsibility for controlling her actions. Some clinicians have advocated for including potential victims who are relatives or acquaintances of the patient in a joint meeting; this may allow for the expression of anger and hostility in a more productive, less dangerous way. For patients who are managed outside the inpatient setting, psychiatrists must monitor closely for any acute change in clinical status that may increase the risk of danger. All of the principles described above apply to general clinical practice with psychiatric patients of all ages; for geriatric patients, sensitivity to the underlying diagnostic etiology (e.g., dementia with psychosis) helps guide appropriate interventions and longer-term management.

CONCLUSION

Practical issues of competence assessment may be more common for a geriatric psychiatrist than for any other general mental health clinician. Thus, it is essential for the geriatric psychiatrist to have a solid, fundamental understanding of both the legal principles underlying competence and the clinical assessment of capacity specific to the activity in question. There may be cases in which the geriatric psychiatrist who feels comfortable and knowledgeable about assessing the patient's capacity is the best evaluator, despite the risk of impact on their therapeutic alliance. In other circumstances, referral to a specialized forensic examiner (ideally, experienced with geriatric

patients) may be indicated. A cardinal principle of risk management also applies to capacity assessment: take appropriate care of the patient and act as a clinician, not as a lawyer. Psychiatrists should respect the patient's clinical needs as well as legal rights, and follow good practice of thorough evaluation, appropriate documentation, and possible consultation to be successful in promoting and protecting the patient's interests, as well as their own.

REFERENCES

1. Kapp MB, Bigot A. *Geriatrics and the Law*. New York: Springer Publishing; 1985.
2. Rosner R, Schwartz HI, eds. *Geriatric Psychiatry and the Law*. New York: Plenum Press; 1987.
3. Anfang SA, Hilliard JT. Legal issues in acute care psychiatry. In: Sederer LI, Rothschild AJ, eds. *Acute Care Psychiatry*. Philadelphia: Williams and Wilkins; 1997;431–456.
4. Gutheil TG, Appelbaum PS. *Clinical Handbook of Psychiatry and the Law*. 3rd Ed. Philadelphia: Lippincott Williams and Wilkins; 2000.
5. Melton G, Petrila J, Poythress N, Slobogin G. *Psychological Evaluations for the Courts: A Handbook for Mental Health Professionals and Lawyers*. 2d Ed. New York: Guilford; 1997.
6. Strasburger LH, Gutheil TG, Brodsky A. On wearing two hats: role conflict in serving as both psychotherapist and expert witness. *Am J Psychiatry*. 1997;154:448–456.
7. Gutheil TG, Hilliard JT. The treating psychiatrist thrust into the role of expert witness. *Psychiatr Serv*. 2001;52:1526–1527.
8. Appelbaum PS. A theory of ethics for forensic psychiatry. *J Am Acad Psychiatry Law*. 1997;25:233–247.
9. Kapp MB. Legal standards for the medical diagnosis and treatment of dementia. *J Legal Medicine*. 2002;23:359–402.
10. Simon RI. *Clinical Psychiatry and the Law*. 2d Ed. Washington DC: American Psychiatric Press; 1992.
11. Gutheil TG. *The Psychiatrist in Court: A Survival Guide*. Washington DC: American Psychiatric Press; 1998.
12. Gutheil TG. *The Psychiatrist as Expert Witness*. Washington DC: American Psychiatric Press; 1998.
13. Brodsky SL. *Testifying in Court*. Washington DC: American Psychological Association; 1991.
14. Health Insurance Portability and Accountability Act of 1996. PL 104–191 (45 CFR 160).
15. American Academy of Psychiatry and the Law. Ethical guidelines for the practice of forensic psychiatry. Bloomfield, CT: AAPL; 1995.
16. Faden R, Beauchamp T. *A History and Theory of Informed Consent*. New York: Oxford University Press; 1986.
17. President's Commission for the Study of Ethical Problems in Medicine and Biomedical and Behavioral Research. *Making Health Care Decisions*. Washington DC: US Government Printing Office; 1982.
18. Appelbaum PS, Grisso T. Assessing patients' capacities to consent to treatment. *N Engl J Med*. 1988;319:1635–38.
19. Grisso T. *Evaluating Competencies: Forensic Assessments and Instruments*. 2d Ed. New York: Plenum Publishing; 2003.
20. Grisso T, Appelbaum PS. *Assessing Competence to Consent to Treatment: A Guide for Physicians and Other Health Professionals*. New York: Oxford University Press; 1998.
21. Grisso T, Appelbaum PS. *MacArthur Competence Assessment Tool for Treatment (MacCAT-T)*. Sarasota FL: Professional Resource Press; 1998.
22. Appelbaum PS, Grisso T. *MacArthur Competence Assessment Tool for Clinical Research (MacCAT-CR)*. Sarasota FL: Professional Resource Press; 2001.
23. Marson DC, Schmitt FA, Ingram KK, Harrell LE. Determining the competency of Alzheimer's patients to consent to treatment and research. *Alzh Dis Assoc Disord*. 1994;8:5–18.
24. Marson DC, McInturff B, Hawkins L, Bartolucci A, Harrell LE. Consistency of physician judgments of capacity to consent in mild Alzheimer's disease. *J Am Geriatr Soc*. 1997;45:453–57.

25. Marson DC, Cody HA, Ingram KK, Harrell LE. Neuropsychologic predictors of competency in Alzheimer's disease using a rational reasons legal standard. *Arch Neurol.* 1995;52:955–959.

26. Marson DC, Earnst KS, Jamil F, Bartolucci A, Harrell LE. Consistency of physicians' legal standard and personal judgments of competency in patients with Alzheimer's disease. *J Am Geriatr Soc.* 2000;48:911–18.

27. Applegate WB, Blass JP, Williams TF. Instruments for the functional assessment of older patients. *N Engl J Med.* 1990;322:1207–14.

28. McCullough LB, Molinari V, Workman RH. Implications of impaired executive control functions for patient autonomy and surrogate decision making. *J Clin Ethics.* 2001;12:397–405.

29. Kennedy GJ, Scalmatia A. The importance of executive deficits. *Geriatrics.* 2002;57:40–42.

30. Royall DR, Mahurin RK, Gray K. Bedside assessment of executive impairment: The executive interview (EXIT). *J Am Geriatr Soc.* 1992;40:1221–1226.

31. *Natanson v. Kline,* 350 P. 2d 1093 (1960).

32. Canterbury v. Spence, 462 F. 2d 772 (1972).

33. Kaimowitz v. DMH, Civ. No. 73-19434–AW (Cir. Ct. Wayne County, 7/10/73).

34. Rennie v. Klein, 720 F. 2d 266 (1983).

35. Rogers v. Commissioner of Mental Health, 390 Mass. 489 (1983).

36. App. of President and Directors of Georgetown, 331 F. 2d 1000 (1964).

37. Super. of Belchertown v. Saikewicz, 373 Mass. 728 (1977).

38. Cruzan v. Director, Missouri Department of Health, 497 US 261 (1990).

39. Kim SY, Karlawish JH, Caine ED. Current state of research on decision-making competence on cognitively impaired elderly persons. *Am J Geriatr Psychiatry.* 2002;10:151–165.

40. Spar JE, Garb AS. Assessing competency to make a will. *Am J Psychiatry.* 1992;149:169–174.

41. Spar JE, Hankin M, Stodden A. Assessing mental capacity and susceptibility to undue influence. *Behav Sci Law.* 1995;13:391–403.

42. Marson DC. Loss of financial capacity in dementia: conceptual and empirical approaches. *Aging Neuropsych Cognition.* 2001;8:164–181.

43. Moye J. Guardianship and conservatorship. In: Grisso T. *Evaluating Competencies.* New York: Plenum Publishing; 2003;309–389.

44. Dusky v. United States, 362 US 402 (1960).

45. Saks ER, Dunn JB, Marshall BJ, Nayak GV, Golshan S, Jeste DV. The California scale of appreciation. *Am J Geriatr Psychiatry.* 2002;10:166–174.

46. Kim SY, Cox C, Caine ED. Impaired decision-making ability in subjects with Alzheimer's disease and willingness to participate in research. *Am J Psychiatry.* 2002;159:797–802.

47. Carpenter WT, Gold JM, Lahti AC, et al. Decisional capacity for informed consent in schizophrenia research. *Arch Gen Psychiatry.* 2000;57:533–38.

48. AGS Ethics Committee. American Geriatrics Society: informed consent for research on human subjects with dementia. *J Am Geriatr Soc.* 1998;46:1308–10.

49. Kim S, Caine E, Currier G, Leibovici A, Ryan J. Assessing the competence of persons with Alzheimer's disease in providing informed consent for participation in research. *Am J Psychiatry.* 2001;158:712–717.

50. Dukoff R, Sunderland T. Durable power of attorney and informed consent with Alzheimer's disease patients. *Am J Psychiatry.* 1997;154:1070–75.

51. National Bioethics Advisory Commission. *Research Involving Persons with Mental Disorder that may Affect Decisionmaking Capacity,* vol. 1. Report and recommendations of the National Bioethics Advisory Commission. Rockville, MD: National Bioethics Advisory Commission; 1999.

52. Carpenter WT. The challenge to psychiatry as society's agent for mental illness treatment and research. *Am J Psychiatry.* 1999;156:1307–10.

53. Grossberg G. Advance directives, competency evaluation and surrogate management in elderly patients. *Am J Geriatr Psychiatry.* 1998;6: S79–S84.

54. Omnibus Budget Reconciliation Act of 1990, PL No. 101–508.

55. Allen RS, Shuster JL. The role of proxies in treatment decisions: evaluating functional capacity to consent to end-of-life treatments within a family context. *Behav Sci Law.* 2002;20:235–252.

56. Perry SJ. Legal implications for failure to comply with advanced directives. *Behav Sci Law.* 2002;20:253–269.

57. Mezey M, Teresi J, Ramsey G, Mitty E, Bobrowitz T. Decision-making capacity to execute a health care proxy. *J Am Geriatr Soc.* 2000;48:179–187.

58. Terry PB, Vettese M, Song J, et al. End of life decision making: when patients and surrogates disagree. *J Clin Ethics.* 1999;10:286–293.

59. Srebnik DS, La Fond JQ. Advance directives for mental health treatment. *Psychiatr Serv.* 1999;50:919–25.

60. Geller J. The use of advance directives by persons with serious mental illness for psychiatric treatment. *Psychiatr Q.* 2000;71:1–13.

61. Dobbs BM, Carr DB, Morris JC. Evaluation and management of the driver with dementia. *Neurology.* 2002;8:61–70.

62. Johansson K, Lundberg C. The 1994 International Consensus Conference on dementia in driving: a brief report. *Alzh Dis Assoc Disorder.* 1997;11(suppl 1):62–69.

63. Dubinsky RM, Stein AC, Lyons K. Practice parameter: risk of driving and Alzheimer's disease. *Neurology.* 2000;54:2205–2211.

64. American Psychiatric Association. Practice guideline for the treatment of patients with Alzheimer's disease and other dementias of later life. *Am J Psychiatry.* 1997;154(suppl):12.

65. Moye J. Guardianship and conservatorship. In: Grisso T. *Evaluating Competencies.* New York: Plenum Publishing; 2003;309–389.

66. Coyne AC, Reichman WE, Berbig LJ. The relationship between dementia and elder abuse. *Am J Psychiatry.* 1993;150:643–646.

67. Tarasoff v. Regents of the University of California, 551 P. 2d 334 (1976).

68. Anfang SA, Appelbaum PS. Twenty years after Tarasoff: reviewing the duty to protect. *Harvard Rev Psychiatry.* 1996;4:67–76.

69. Beck JC, ed. *Confidentiality Versus the Duty to Protect: Foreseeable Harm in the Practice of Psychiatry.* Washington DC: American Psychiatric Press; 1990.

70. Monahan J. Limiting therapist exposure to Tarasoff liability: guidelines for risk containment. *Am Psychol.* 1993;48:242–250.

General Principles of Psychiatric Treatment

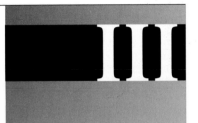

Psychotherapy with Older Adults

Mary F. Wyman   *Amber Gum*   *Patricia A. Areán*

Psychotherapy with older adults is a relatively new field in terms of research and the innovation of effective therapeutic approaches, but one that has been the topic of discussion since the beginnings of psychotherapeutic practice as we know it today. Freud himself, at the age of 49, stated that "... near or above the fifties the elasticity of the mental processes, on which the treatment depends, is as a rule lacking—old people are no longer educable...." (1). Changes in stereotypes associated with aging and the emergence of research evidence regarding successful geriatric psychotherapy outcomes have provided an alternative perspective. We know that psychotherapy is effective with older adults (2), and that many older adults even prefer psychotherapy (3). In a recent study of 1,800 elderly primary care patients being treated for depression, 51% preferred therapy, while only 38% preferred antidepressant medication, when given a choice (4).

Patient preference for treatment may be quite important. Research suggests that engagement in mental health treatment is better when patients, including older adult patients, are allowed to choose type of treatment (5,6). It remains unclear whether matching treatment to patient preferences improves treatment outcome directly, although better attendance points to increased likelihood of better outcomes. Thus, in keeping with current best-practice guidelines for mental health care that recommend honoring patient preferences for treatment (7), a first task for the geriatric clinician is education of the patient about available treatment options and a thorough assessment of his or her preferences. This will be covered again in the section below on socialization to therapy.

The primary aim of this chapter is to provide an overview of psychotherapy with elderly clients. It includes general issues to consider, psychotherapy adaptations that can be made to meet the needs of older clients, and descriptions of specific therapeutic modalities. In addition to our own clinical experience, we rely upon empirical evidence whenever available to inform our discussion and recommendations.

It is important that clinicians be aware of the research process and empirical evidence for their practices. In many clinical settings, there is a growing insistence on the use of empirically supported treatments, and many third-party payers prefer or require the use of evidence-based therapy approaches. An American Psychological Association task force has developed guidelines for evaluating the evidence base for various forms of psychotherapy (8). To be deemed *empirically supported*, randomized clinical trials must demonstrate that the type of therapy in question is: a) superior to placebo or no treatment condition in treating target symptoms; b) comparable to or superior to another gold standard or evidence-based treatment in at least three large trials (by at least two separate investigators); and c) sample sizes in the comparative studies are substantial enough to detect a moderate effect size. Several therapy approaches for older adults already meet these criteria, and several other approaches appear promising but do not yet have the research base to meet these rigorous standards. In this chapter, we will briefly review relevant empirical research as applicable, although the focus will be on the practice of therapy with older adults.

We also focus primarily on psychotherapy for depressive and anxiety symptoms, as they are the most common psychiatric issues for older adults and have received the most research attention (9). While a complete review across the entire range of disorders is not within the scope of the current chapter, the application of psychotherapy, to other psychiatric disorders in later life also appears promising, according to preliminary research (10).

GENERAL ISSUES IN THERAPY WITH OLDER ADULTS

Topics in Therapy

We argue that, in general, psychotherapy with older adults is more similar than different compared to working with younger or middle-aged adults. However, differences related to cohort, biological aging, and life stressors more common in old age can be highly relevant to the psychotherapy treatment. Cohort-specific experiences and coping strategies may differ. Normal age-related changes in physical and mental functioning, while minor, can impact therapy (see below for a discussion of contextual adaptations of therapy relevant to these changes). Older adults often cope with poorer health and a subsequent decline in functioning. The death of a loved one, downsizing of lifestyle and/or possessions, and changes in living arrangements are common. There may be isolation from family and friends due to a move to a retirement community or a child's home, or due to decreased mobility because of disability or illness. In some cultures (especially in Western civilizations), the reduction in community status that comes with old age can bring on a sense of uselessness or uncertainty (11). These challenges and stressors can serve as triggers for new-onset disorders or can exacerbate existing psychopathology. These events and circumstances also may be the primary issues that an elderly client brings to therapy. In discussing specific therapeutic approaches we provide examples that further illustrate the range of problems dealt with by older clients.

Barriers to Therapy

Older adults may also present with substantial barriers to entering or continuing in therapy. Barriers may include practical issues (e.g., financial constraints, transportation) or health-related problems (e.g., hearing or visual impairment, cognitive decline, or mobility). Barriers may be related to perceived stigma surrounding mental illness ("people who go into therapy are crazy or weak"), misperceptions of the therapeutic process ("I will be brainwashed and made to tell all my secrets"), or self-accepted negative stereotypes of aging ("I am too old to change my ways") (11). Some elderly clients will have concerns about the gap in age between themselves and a therapist who may be considerably younger. As therapists, we have experienced several older adults make statements such as, "You are young and healthy; what can you possibly know about getting old and sick?" Such a belief can serve to maintain hopeless feelings and interfere with the development of a therapeutic relationship. Below, we discuss the importance of socialization to therapy in order to address some of these barriers.

Transference, Countertransference, and Boundaries

We use transference and countertransference here in the most general sense, referring to feelings and thoughts that the client has about the therapist (transference) and that the therapist has about the client (countertransference). These feelings and thoughts are based not only on the reality of the current relationship or interaction, but also on previous experiences, stereotypes, and one's own concerns or anxieties. Of primary interest here, of course, are transferential and countertransferential feelings based on age, which can emerge even in the context of very brief, goal-directed therapies (12). Because most of us grow up with some ideas about older adults, and because our society is rife with stereotypes about aging, these are important topics to touch upon briefly. For more information, we refer the reader to two excellent resources, by Knight (12) and Newton and Jacobowitz (13).

An older client's transference toward a therapist can take as many forms as that of a younger client. Indeed, some have noted that because of more years of experience in the older adult, he or she can have feelings about the therapeutic relationship that stem from experiences in any life stage, including the family of origin, nuclear and extended family, and other relationships (12). A therapist must be aware of this range of possibilities, and of the fact that a client can see the therapist as a parent, a spouse, a child or grandchild, an expert, or in an erotic manner. This last type of transference in particular may be overlooked by a therapist, given the ideas in our society about sexuality in old age.

For a therapist, countertransference will likely arise in work with older adult clients. As Knight noted, for many therapists, a lack of professional training with older adults leaves them especially vulnerable to their own countertransferential feelings (12). Often, these feelings stem from the therapist's experiences with parents or grandparents, his or her positive or negative stereotypes about older people, and his or her own fears regarding infirmity and aging. For example, one younger clinician observed that she had difficulty interrupting or confronting her elderly clients while conducting therapy. She connected this to being taught as a child to be extremely respectful to her grandparents and other elderly people. Once she had identified the source of her behavior, she could more accurately assess the therapeutic situations that required her to be more assertive with her clients.

Relevant to both transference and countertransference are the decisions made by therapist regarding boundaries in the therapeutic relationship. For good reasons, many therapists were trained regarding the problems associated with accepting gifts or physical contact from clients, and taught to maintain strict limits in their practices around these issues. However, among the current cohort of older adults, it may be relatively common to offer a small gift or a hug to the therapist and to become insulted if this is not handled appropriately. This may be especially true for older adults from certain cultures. For example, one clinician provided in-home therapy to an elderly Filipino couple, who insisted on serving tea and a snack during each session. The therapist did her research and learned that this behavior was typical of this culture and cohort; despite her initial discomfort with the ritual, she assessed the impact on the therapeutic work to be minimal and decided to allow the tea to continue. The therapy proved quite productive. The main lesson here is to perform a truly comprehensive assessment when conceptualizing the elderly patient and making decisions about boundaries, taking into account personal, cohort-based, and cultural factors.

The following questions may be useful in evaluating transference, countertransference, and boundaries within the therapeutic relationship when working with an elderly patient. Several of these were inspired by the *contextual, cohort-based, maturity, specific-challenge* (CCMSC) model of case conceptualization developed by Knight for use with older adults (12).

Questions to Consider About the Patient

- What cohort does this patient come from? How might that affect how she sees therapy and her interactions with me? How does it affect her coping strategies?
- What is this person's cultural background?
- What is this patient's specific family history, independent of age or cohort?
- What does aging mean to this person?
- What is this person's current social world, and how does it fit with his current needs?

Questions Therapists Can Ask Themselves

- What does *aging* and *old age* mean to me? What are my stereotypes about older people?
- How comfortable am I with my own aging and loss of function, and that of my loved ones?
- What is my cohort and how does that affect my behavior and perspective?
- What did I learn as a child about older people and how to interact with them?
- How I do want to be seen by this older person?

ADAPTING PSYCHOTHERAPY FOR OLDER ADULTS

Despite the overall similarities between working with older and younger adults, experienced geriatric providers agree that some adaptations may be needed to make the treatment maximally effective. These adaptations include taking time to socialize older adults to the process of psychotherapy, adjusting the pace of the psychotherapy to account for age-related changes in information processing, and allowing flexibility in the delivery of psychotherapy to overcome medical and physical barriers to care (14–19). At the same time, older adults bring unique strengths to therapy that therapists can capitalize on, including experience, wisdom, and problem-solving skills. We discuss each of these points in the following sections.

Socialization to Psychotherapy

As noted above, assessing patient preferences for type of treatment is an important step in initiating treatment of psychiatric problems (7). For many older adults, psychotherapy is the preferred mode of treatment when provided with a choice (3). Some older adults still have misconceptions about what psychotherapy involves, however, and are reluctant to engage in mental health treatment (20). Thus, for any type of psychotherapy to be successful, initial sessions should include patient education about the pace, format, and purpose of psychotherapy.

Several studies have looked at the impact of pretreatment socialization on participation in psychotherapy, and have found that such socialization increases patients' attendance and engagement in psychotherapy, regardless of therapeutic approach (21,22). Several studies conducted specifically in elderly populations have reported positive results of pretherapy training. In one comparative study with this population (20), patients who received training demonstrated improved knowledge about psychotherapy and a greater problem-oriented focus in treatment; however, there were no group differences in dropouts, attendance, or outcome. A recent study found that older minorities, who tend to be most underrepresented in psychotherapy use, were more likely to remain in therapy if they received a brief, face-to-face introduction about the process and content of psychotherapy than if no such introduction was provided (23). In fact, when queried about factors contributing to access to and participation in psychotherapy, those patients indicated that the pretreatment socialization was instrumental in motivating them to begin and stay in treatment. Thus, pretreatment socialization can be a very powerful tool for engaging older adults in psychotherapy.

Content of Socialization

Socialization typically begins by addressing common concerns and beliefs older patients have about psychotherapy. In-person socialization will generally begin with a question about the patient's previous experience with psychotherapy. In other words, what does she or he know or expect about psychotherapy in general and the particular therapy that will be provided? Additionally, the pretreatment educator will ask about any stigma concerns the patient may have, such as how to address questions by

TABLE 13-1

ADAPTATIONS FOR PSYCHOTHERAPY WITH OLDER ADULTS

Modification	Sample Methods	Rationale	Effect/Benefit	References
Socialization to therapy (education about pace and course of treatment) Assessment of expectations Address patient-therapist age differences, if necessary	Before start of treatment or in first sessions Group or individual sessions Audiovisual and/or written material plus face-to-face education	Address misconceptions and stigma about therapy Reduce reluctance to initiate or remain in treatment	Increases older adults' attendance and engagement in treatment More likely to initiate and remain in therapy	Latour & Cappeliez, 1994 (20)
Slower pace of treatment, present material over multiple meetings, present using multifaceted methods	"Say-it, show-it, do-it" method to teach new skills Link material to patient's past experiences and knowledge	Adjust for age-related changes in information processing	Ensure adequate learning of concepts and skills	Gallagher-Thompson & Thompson, 1996 (17)
Addition of case management	Assessment of psychosocial and medical needs Link to community services to meet existing needs Advocacy for patient when negotiating benefits	Particularly for low-income patients, this method helps to address crises that interfere with progress in therapy	Ensure patient ability to benefit from therapy	Areán, 1993 (65)
Altering the therapeutic frame	Sessions may occur every other week Sessions may be shorter or delivered over the telephone Sessions may occur in non mental health setting, such as primary care medicine	Accommodate medical illness, fatigue, and psychosocial demands	Ensures patient engagement in treatment Reduce instrumental barriers to treatment	Areán, 1993 (65); Gallagher-Thompson & Thompson, 1996 (17)
Adapting therapy to accommodate disabilities	Sessions in larger rooms Therapy materials on tape or in large print Use of amplifiers	Improve access to therapy for elders with disabilities	Ensures patient engagement in treatment	No citation
More extensive coordination with other care providers	Team approach to providing care Coordination with medical providers to address patient health limitations	Improve treatment plan and coordination Reduce instrumental barriers	Increases use of therapy Facilitates better case formulation	No citation
Use older patient's strengths	Remind patient of existing or previous coping skills	Facilitate learning and processing of new material	Increases effectiveness of therapy, especially for learning-based therapies	Knight & Satre, 1999 (94)
Transference, countertransference, boundary issues	Consider that client's transference may come from any life stage and may take many forms Assess own stereotypes about aging May accept small gifts	Client has number of relationships that may affect transference Therapists generally have preconceived views of aging	Improves rapport Minimizes errors in case conceptualization	Knight, 2004 (12); Newton & Jacobowitz, 1999 (13)

family or friends about mental health appointments, whether receiving mental health treatment may affect judgments of competency in the future, and so forth. Misconceptions or erroneous beliefs are then addressed in the meeting. Next, the educator discusses the process of

therapy, including the type of therapy to be used, frequency and length of sessions, location of therapy, whether or not family members will be involved, and roles of the therapist and patient. Finally, patients are encouraged to ask questions about the process so that any

TABLE 13-2

OVERVIEW OF THERAPEUTIC APPROACHES FOR OLDER ADULTS

Orientation	Focus	Time Frame	Evidence	Strengths	Limitations
CBT	Behavioral and thinking patterns Problem-solving Skills training	Typically brief (i.e., 12–20 sessions) Flexible	Empirically supported for depression (i.e., multiple large RCTs) (34) Smaller studies suggest effective for anxiety (35)	Brief Can address variety of diagnoses/functioning levels Structure helps keep on-task Homework to solidify learning Treatment manuals facilitate therapist training	Learning new skills more difficult for cognitively impaired May dislike structure, homework
IPT	Interpersonal themes: grief, role transitions, conflict, skills deficits	Brief (i.e., 12–20 sessions) Maintenance sessions common (e.g., biweekly or monthly for 12 months)	Empirically supported for depression (i.e., multiple large RCTs) (34)	Can be brief Treatment manuals facilitate therapist training Addresses range of relevant interpersonal and role issues	Less focused on non-interpersonal issues that may be relevant May be longer than other approaches
Psychodynamic	Losses Therapeutic relationship Themes across past and present	Variable Can be brief	Promising (34) Brief dynamic therapy (BDT) comparable to CBT in two studies (58,59)	Useful for grieving losses and reconceptualizing past issues	May be longer than other approaches May need to limit focus on early experiences
RT/Life review	Review of past behavior and events Resolution of past mistakes, regrets	Variable Can be brief	Promising (34) Multiple smaller studies demonstrate helpfulness reducing distress	Specifically designed for older adults Useful for resolving past issues Remote memories intact until very severe cognitive impairment Group format common	Less focused on current issues that may be relevant
PST	Current problems Apply structured problem solving process	Brief: 6–12 sessions	Promising (34) In one study, more effective than RT (65) Part of effective treatment package in two primary care studies (4,95)	Can be used in primary care setting Structure helps keep on-task Homework to solidify learning Treatment manuals facilitate therapist training	Learning new skills more difficult for cognitively impaired May dislike structure, homework Less focused on past issues that may be relevant

Modality	Focus	Time Frame	Evidence	Strengths	Limitations
Group	Variable (e.g., depression, anxiety, health issues, grief)	Variable	Small number of studies and clinical reports support utility (11,74–76)	Cost-effective Normalizing problems Receive support, advice from peers Help peers	Difficult to organize Some elders dislike groups
Couple and family	Relationship issues with partner or other family member(s) Healthcare decision-making Caregiving	Variable	Small number of studies and clinical reports support utility (78,80)	Focus on larger social system Relevant for many elders Helpful for caregiving issues	Difficult to get family members together Challenge of which member(s) is the "patient"

(continued)

TABLE 13-2
(continued)

Special Populations	Focus	Time Frame/ Modality	Evidence	Strengths	Limitations
Individuals with dementia	Coping skills Reduce distress Behavioral disturbance Life review Memory training	Variable/Individual and group	Small number of studies and clinical reports support utility (82)	Make use of preserved cognitive/memory functions Can intervene with patient, environment, caregiver, or staff Can use variety of orientations and modalities	Different therapy approaches may be most effective only in certain stages of impairment
Long-term care setting	Variable, e.g.: Adjustment to new setting Coping skills Reduce distress Behavioral disturbance	Variable/Individual and group	Several small studies and clinical reports support utility (89)	Effective if flexible about location, schedule, disability Proximity to staff for systemic, environmental intervention Can use variety of orientations and modalities	Working within complex system Privacy, scheduling, communication with staff and family can pose challenges

CBT, cognitive-behavioral therapy; IPT, interpersonal therapy; PST, problem solving therapy; RCT, randomly controlled trials; RT, reminiscence therapy.

misunderstandings or concerns can be immediately addressed.

As stated previously, older adults may have concerns about working with a younger therapist. In this case, the therapist's best approach is often to be proactive. Therapists can assuage many of these concerns by attending and responding to patients' comments about age differences, raising the issue themselves during the socialization period, and acknowledging that the difference in experience may indeed limit understanding. A clarification of the collaborative process of therapy is also important; for example, the therapist can explain that the patient is the expert on his or her own life and has important experience to draw from in therapy, and that the patient can teach the therapist what is necessary to design the most appropriate intervention.

Methods of Socialization

Adequate research is lacking on the various methods of socialization and pretherapy training; these recommendations draw from our own experience and that of other geriatric clinicians. The most common format for socialization involves face-to-face discussions between the patient and therapist. Pretherapy training can take place at an initial intake session, a separate presentation after intake but before treatment commences, or in the first therapy session. In addition, the information can be presented as a one-on-one meeting or an informational group presentation. Each method has advantages and disadvantages. Group presentations tend to be more cost effective, as more people can be reached in a session, and questions

raised by some members can be informative to others. Individual meetings, however, allow the socialization to be tailored to each individual's specific concerns and questions, and can be scheduled at the patient's convenience.

In some cases, these face-to-face meetings are accompanied by an educational video or brochure the patient can take home. These materials typically contain the same information that is conveyed in face-to-face meetings. Explicitly addressing stigma issues and providing FAQs (frequently asked questions) are useful to address common concerns older adults may have about psychotherapy. Such materials have the advantage of portability: patients can take them home for review and share the information with family members. Because of research on how older adults process information, most geriatric specialists believe that written information should be brief (no more than four columns of information), succinct, and written at or below a ninth-grade reading level. Video presentation also should be brief (i.e., 30 minutes or less) and should include older adult models discussing their experience with psychotherapy. For many older adults, providing both written materials and verbal presentation of information (face-to-face or videotape) will provide the most effective way of thoroughly communicating information.

Accounting for Changes in Information Processing

Although research shows that older people maintain a significant degree of mental flexibility and can learn new tasks, older adults do learn somewhat differently than younger persons. As detailed in an excellent review by Knight and Satre (24), there are a number of cognitive changes associated with aging that should be attended to when providing psychotherapy to an older patient. The most relevant changes to psychotherapy are those associated with cognitive slowing, decreased fluid intelligence, and working memory. Taken together, these changes indicate that psychotherapy—which relies on the ability to draw inferences, process new material, and recall information—often must be delivered at a slower pace, over multiple meetings, and in a multifaceted way.

Cognitive Slowing

The speed to which we react to stimuli, and hence process information, slows considerably as we age (25). Although slowed reaction time does not necessarily interfere with the ability to process new and/or abstract material, new information should be presented more slowly and over a longer period of time to counteract the effects of cognitive slowing.

Psychotherapies adapted for older populations tend to be slightly longer than the originally developed techniques, and are structured so that new material raised in treatment is reviewed a number of times and presented through a number of modalities. For instance, Gallagher-Thompson and Thompson (17) suggest a "say-it, show-it, do-it" strategy to help older adults to learn new skills. In learning-based therapies (e.g., cognitive–behavioral therapy), this process involves first giving older patients a rationale for a new skill and elucidating the relevance to their problems. Next, the therapist demonstrates the new skill with a generic example, and finally engages the patient in the skill using a patient example. In following this process, the therapist can check to make sure that the older patient understands the application of the new skill and can successfully practice the skill between sessions. In process-oriented or insight-oriented therapies, the therapist can use a similar technique with older patients. The process-oriented therapist can engage in periodic summary of the discussion, connecting the psychotherapeutic process to what the patient has said and to the patient's problems. At the end of the session, the therapist should provide an overall summary of the discussion and of new insights achieved.

Decreased Fluid Intelligence

While the overall reasoning ability of older adults is not impaired because of their vast store of previous learning (crystallized intelligence), the rate at which they can process new information and make inferences (fluid intelligence) is slowed (26). Although the details of memory functioning among older adults are quite complex, there is consensus that working memory, an aspect of memory functioning that is responsible for processing information prior to long-term memory formation, becomes less efficient with age (26). Again, providing repeated exposure to new information is important, to help ensure adequate

learning. Another useful technique, which makes use of intact crystallized intelligence to improve information processing in psychotherapy, is to rely on patients' vast stores of previous experiences. *Life review*, a technique commonly found in reminiscence therapies (see below), is an excellent tool for linking new material to older patients' past experiences. This technique is best illustrated in the following case example.

CASE EXAMPLE: MODIFYING THERAPY BY UTILIZING THE OLDER PATIENT'S PAST EXPERIENCES

Mr. J. was a disabled, 80-year-old man referred to problem-solving therapy (PST, a learning-based therapy; see below) for major depression. During the course of therapy, Mr. J. learned the steps involved in PST through the "say-it, show-it, do-it" method but he was still struggling with understanding the process of PST, and was not applying the model between sessions. More out of frustration than therapeutic gain, the therapist decided to spend a session letting Mr. J. talk about his problems in a free-form fashion. As Mr. J. spoke about his depression, he began discussing the job he had before he became disabled and how good it made him feel to be the "go to" person for the roadblocks faced by his company when rolling out a new product. As the therapist listened to Mr. J. talk about how he managed to solve problems in one particularly complex situation, the therapist noticed similarities between Mr. J.'s problem-solving process at work and the PST model. She then asked, "Is that how you usually solved problems at work? Did you typically follow those steps?" Mr. J. discussed a few more examples of how he solved problems at work, and as he spoke, the therapist tracked the terms he used for his problem-solving steps and used the PST worksheets to record the process Mr. J. took to solve these problems. After a few instances of life review, the therapist then showed Mr. J. what she had done and drew a parallel between his work style and PST. Mr. J. thought for a moment, began nodding his head, and then, as if a light bulb had gone off, he said, "Has this been what you have been trying to get me to do? Well, why didn't you say so?!" By using the patient's life review material, the therapist was able to successfully teach PST skills to Mr. J. and subsequently help him overcome his depression.

Although this example describes using life review in a relatively unstructured manner, therapists may conduct more targeted life review around specific issues. For example, it can be helpful to talk about previous times when the patient faced similar issues and how they managed to resolve or cope with those issues earlier in their life. Ideally, such a review can remind patients of coping skills they already have. Even if patients did not cope effectively with those issues in the past, however, life review discussions can still serve as a valuable learning tool in the therapy.

Contextual Adaptations

For some older adults, a number of practical and health-related barriers may exist, requiring certain contextual modifications to the therapy. The most common therapy adaptations to address contextual issues include: (a) the addition of case management to overcome instrumental barriers to engage in psychotherapy; (b) relaxing the therapeutic frame to accommodate fatigue, illness, and psychosocial demands; and (c) adapting psychotherapy elements to address common physical disabilities and coordinate with other care providers.

Addition of Case Management

For some older patients, instrumental barriers to regular psychotherapy access will need to be addressed before engagement in treatment can commence. Often, there are considerable financial, time, and access problems that will interfere with older patients' use of psychotherapy. For instance, elderly patients may have difficulty with transportation. Many older adults do not drive and often have several regular appointments to attend. Asking family or friends to assist in driving them to yet another appointment (in this case, the psychotherapy hour) is often seen as burdensome, and older patients may be extremely reluctant to make additional demands on their support networks. Further, older patients may have increased difficulty overcoming such barriers, because the systems available to address these problems can be very complicated and difficult to negotiate.

Traditionally, many psychotherapists have believed that patients will resolve these barriers themselves if they are truly motivated for therapy. We believe that the assumption that the patient should solve all problems on his or her own, with minimal assistance by the therapist, is often counterproductive when working with older patients. Many older adults have true and significant instrumental barriers to accessing care that interfere with their ability to engage in psychotherapeutic treatment. Resolutions of issues regarding transportation, conflicts with caregiving obligations, financial constraints, and medical illness may require the assistance of the therapist. In our experience, it is not uncommon for therapists to begin treatment by focusing on case management issues first so that the older patient can attend to and engage in therapy. Although these case management interventions are usually not included as part of a treatment manual, they are crucial to the adequate delivery of care to older patients. In sum, we feel strongly that therapists should not shy away from helping the older patient resolve these common barriers to obtaining psychotherapeutic treatment. In fact, the very process of assisting the patient with these issues will likely increase engagement in the therapeutic process.

The Therapeutic Frame

Gallagher-Thompson and Thompson (17) have found that the traditional therapeutic frame can be a barrier to the delivery of psychotherapy in older populations. The typical expectations that clients come in weekly for appointments, that treatment be delivered during a 50-minute time span, and that it occur in specialty mental health settings may be hard for many older patients to meet. The therapeutic frame must remain flexible with regard to treatment location, session length, and access (15). Because many older adults are coping with caregiving crises, temporary disability due to short-term illnesses or the exacerbation of chronic illnesses, or ongoing medical illnesses that require a number of appointments, being able to participate in regular psychotherapy can be a difficult goal to attain. To account for these factors, therapeutic approaches that allow for flexibility in treatment have been developed for late-life psychotherapy. These include modifying psychotherapy for non-mental health settings, briefer sessions, and using the telephone and/or written materials.

A number of psychotherapies have been adapted for delivery in non-mental health settings. The purpose of adapting psychotherapy to these settings is to allow greater patient access to services by embedding the treatment into the settings where most older persons are likely to come, such as primary care medicine or adult day health centers. In this case, the therapy needs to be modified for the culture of the specific non-mental health setting. In primary care, for example, therapy is often delivered in briefer, more frequent sessions, with flexibility around rescheduling appointments due to illness or crises. Brief treatments are sometimes provided by non-mental health professionals who have received appropriate training (3,14). For example, in the ongoing PROSPECT study (27), interpersonal therapy (IPT) was modified to fit the busy schedules of a primary care practice. Sessions were shorter (reduced from 50 minutes to 30 minutes) and often delivered by a nurse who was supervised by an IPT expert. At times, the treatment was delivered over the phone or at the patient's home, depending on the patient's mobility issues and individual needs.

Telephone-based therapy, home-based therapy, and self-administered therapy using written materials (bibliotherapy) comprises another set of modifications that addresses therapeutic frame issues and has been shown to be successful in use with older adults. The leading researcher in this area of late-life psychotherapy is Scogin (28). One example of his efforts in this area is a modified cognitive-behavioral therapy (CBT) for depression for rural elderly who tend to have difficulty attending regular meetings because of transportation and distance issues (29). In this adaptation, patients meet initially with a therapist who educates and socializes the patient to CBT. Reading materials and behavioral forms are provided. Patients then use the manual on their own and consult periodically with the therapist by phone or through occasional face-to-face meetings. Scogin and his colleagues have found good results in reducing depressive symptoms in older adults using this method.

Accounting for Physical Disabilities

Disabilities common in frail elderly (e.g., impairments in vision, hearing, or mobility) also can impede the progress of therapy, when no adaptations are undertaken. Ideally, the therapist assesses disabilities and attempts to facilitate the patient's receipt of needed medical and social services (e.g., medical treatment, getting new glasses or dentures). The therapeutic process also may benefit from close, ongoing collaboration with other health care professionals, particularly in working with frail elderly with multiple medical problems and medications.

For patients with reading impairments (due to vision loss or illiteracy), audiotaping sessions for at-home review can be used to reinforce session information (30–32). For some patients, treatment forms should be modified with larger print and with larger writing spaces to accommodate changes in fine motor skill (e.g., due to arthritis or stroke).

For patients with hearing loss, hearing problems cannot always be corrected via hearing aids, or patients may refuse to use such devices. When working with these patients, the therapist must be keenly aware of the degree of impairment. In some cases, sitting closer to older patients and near the ear that is less affected by hearing loss can greatly help with communication. Speaking slowly, and in low tones (particularly important for female therapists) also can help the older patient hear the material. If these methods prove ineffective, microphones connected to headphones the patient wears can be used to amplify therapists' voices. Relying on written communication is another option that has been used successfully in some cases.

Finally, chronic or acute physical impairments may interfere with patients' ability to attend and sit through sessions. Therapy sessions may need to be briefer due to fatigue or pain. Therapists also need to assess for and attempt to correct any environmental barriers for these patients, such as lack of transportation, lack of wheelchair accessibility, loose rugs, or poor lighting.

In summary, psychotherapy for older adults typically means more sessions to process information. It also means that new information, whether it is in the form of learning skills or exploration of experience, may need to be reviewed with the older adult to ensure comprehension and assimilation of information. Because of illness and other competing demands on time and energy, the therapeutic frame must be flexible, but not to the detriment of the patient. Finally, adaptations to address physical impairments may be important to consider.

Strengths of Older Adults

In spite of the challenges that may arise in psychotherapy, older adulthood also can be a time of growth, and older adults often retain strengths that therapists can use to maximize therapeutic benefit of the work together. For example, although some cognitive functions may be less efficient, research suggests that compared to younger adults, older adults "have a larger repertoire of experience from which to operate, use more effective strategies, and better integrate emotional information" (33, p. 243). These findings suggest that it can be beneficial for therapists, together with their older patients, to explore the strengths they have developed over their lifetime and ways to use those strengths to approach current issues. Even "mistakes" or regrets can be used to determine different courses of action for the future. Elders in distress are likely to overlook or minimize their assets and past accomplishments, and the therapist may need to be very proactive in assessing and identifying patient strengths during the session. For example, one elderly woman described herself as not accomplishing much in life, then went on to talk about raising three children on her own after her husband's early death. She minimized her role in raising her children, although further discussion revealed that she had worked very hard and frequently expressed love and support to her children. Such discussions can serve to build elders' sense of self-worth and encourage them in dealing with current issues.

Another potential strength of older adults is the presence of more complex emotionality (i.e., multiple emotions in response to an event or issue) to explore and integrate in therapy (12). This ability can be extremely beneficial in psychotherapy and perhaps especially in working on the complex and multifaceted issues common to old age.

SPECIFIC THERAPY APPROACHES

The above adaptations to psychotherapy apply to any psychotherapeutic approach. In the current section, we review specific approaches and modalities to psychotherapy and discuss relevant research and adaptations for older adults. The focus is on CBT and interpersonal therapy (IPT), as they are the primary empirically supported treatments for use with older adults. Other emerging therapeutic approaches that appear promising are then reviewed.

Cognitive–Behavioral Therapies

A significant amount of research demonstrates that CBT is effective for many older adults with depression and anxiety (34,35). The quantity and quality of these studies is sufficient to meet criteria for empirically supported treatments (8). CBT actually comprises a number of specific types of therapy, all of which are founded on learning theory, which assumes that behavior and thinking patterns are learned through processes of reinforcement and punishment. CBT therapeutic approaches focus on changing cognitions and behaviors, which are assumed to result in changes in moods.

The majority of the research with older adults has been conducted using the form of CBT pioneered by Aaron Beck

(36,37). This type of therapy involves behavioral techniques such as scheduling pleasant activities, relaxation strategies, behavioral experiments, and exposure to anxiety-provoking stimuli. Cognitive techniques involve learning to identify and challenge unhelpful thoughts that lead to distressing emotions. More recently, mindfulness techniques have been incorporated into CBT to teach individuals ways to be more aware of their thoughts and feelings, and to accept thoughts and feelings in a nonjudgmental manner without ruminating (38,39). Research indicates that older adults are accepting of all of these types of strategies (40–42).

Treatment Rationale and Therapeutic Relationship

For any type of psychotherapy, it is important that the patient believe in the treatment. In CBT, as with other types of therapy, therapy generally begins by gathering information about the patient's symptoms, problems, and goals, and then discussing the case formulation and treatment rationale with the patient. It is important to explain that: (a) behaviors, thoughts, physical symptoms, and feelings all are interrelated (using examples, preferably from the patient's own experience); and (b) because it is difficult to directly change feelings and physical symptoms, this type of therapy focuses on changing behaviors and thoughts, which should lead to changes in feelings. In order to foster a collaborative therapeutic relationship, the therapist actively involves the patient in this discussion (i.e., seeking the patient's agreement, their conceptualization of their symptoms, and their observations about the links of their experiences to CBT), as opposed to lecturing to the patient about CBT. This may be particularly important for elderly patients, who likely will be working with a younger therapist; a collaborative relationship communicates a sense of respect to the patient and acknowledges the value of their knowledge and experiences. In addition to providing an overall treatment rationale, it is important that patients understand the rationale for each specific strategy being applied, so that they will fully participate in learning and applying the strategy.

Structure of Therapy

CBT relies on a structured, although somewhat flexible, agenda for each therapy session, including review of homework from the previous week, discussion and application of new techniques, homework planning for the upcoming week, and session summary. This structure helps therapist and patient stay focused on the patient's primary goals and target problems, and may be particularly beneficial for older adults who have cognitive impairment and may have difficulty paying attention or staying focused on more relevant topics.

Behavioral Techniques

CBT utilizes a variety of behavioral techniques to directly target behavior change, which also is assumed to lead to changes in thinking and feelings. These strategies are applicable with both younger and older adults and should always be tailored to the individual's specific goals, symptoms, and skills. *Activity scheduling* is an important behavioral strategy; this includes scheduling and engaging in pleasant activities as well as daily activities that may be dropped (e.g., housework, going to work). Patients write down daily schedules and record their completion of activities; this process makes plans concrete and provides clear evidence for success when a patient accomplishes a task. Some depressed patients may claim no activities are enjoyable, in which case they should plan activities they previously enjoyed. Further, by rating level of enjoyment or rating mood before and after an activity, some patients realize they actually enjoyed activities. For example, a vegetative, suicidal elderly inpatient lay in bed all day and claimed no activities were enjoyable. When asked about previous activities, he reported enjoying opera music. He agreed to participate in a *behavioral experiment*, whereby he rated his mood (1 to 10), then listened to opera, and then rated his mood again. He was surprised to find that his mood had indeed improved slightly (from 3 to 5). A *pleasant event schedule* designed specifically for older adults can be useful, such as the one detailed by Lichtenberg (43), which includes events in which even frail elders can engage in a variety of settings. Planning pleasant activities is very important for disabled older adults, who often are lonely and have few pleasant activities. Behavioral experiments can be an effective method for challenging unhelpful thoughts, as in the above example. The use of *graded task assignments* is a similar strategy to activity scheduling, whereby patients concretely plan important tasks that seem overwhelming in incremental, manageable steps. *Social skills training* involves training, practice, and role play of a variety of social skills, such as assertiveness and conflict resolution.

A variety of *relaxation exercises* also may be helpful, particularly for anxious patients; these include progressive muscle relaxation, imagery relaxation, and breathing exercises. Also, for anxious patients, providing *graded exposure* to anxiety-provoking stimuli is important to treatment success (44). This technique involves establishing a hierarchy of feared stimuli, and gradually exposing the patient to these stimuli; this may be done after first teaching relaxation techniques to help manage the anxiety initially experienced in the situation. With older patients, it is important to account for any impairments or disabilities when establishing the hierarchy, ensuring that the person will be able to engage in the planned exposure behaviors.

Cognitive Techniques

Although behavioral techniques likely change some thinking, additional techniques directly target thinking patterns, with the goals of identifying and changing unhelpful thinking patterns. The first step involves learning to identify unhelpful thoughts. This can be very difficult as many thinking patterns are automatic; patients are often only aware that they feel "bad," and additional probing by the therapist is necessary to help them identify what they were thinking to trigger the feeling. Patients learn to use their negative feelings as a red flag, and to identify their unhelpful thoughts. Often, negative feelings result from certain cognitive errors, such as *overgeneralization* ("I always say the wrong thing"), *black-and-white thinking* ("I am a total failure"), or *discounting the positive* ("That was easy, but I could not do anything hard"). Burns provides an accessible and useful discussion of these and other *cognitive distortions* (45). For older adult patients, CBT clinicians report that cognitive distortions tend to be clustered in the areas of unrealistic expectations of themselves and old age, exaggerated meaning given to daily events (e.g., medical experiences), and the necessity for a changing value system (e.g., the value of "work is most important" is not useful for retired individuals, who need to find other sources of personal value and worth) (11). Older adults may have held such beliefs firmly for many years, and may require significant practice and repetition of cognitive techniques.

Once identified, maladaptive thoughts can be challenged through a number of cognitive techniques, including: *examining the evidence* for and against the thought; the *so-what* technique (identifying worst-case scenarios, which often are not as disastrous as feared); and identifying and correcting specific types of cognitive errors.

Some negative thoughts are not irrational and may be less amenable to these strategies. This may be particularly true for older adults with chronic illness, pain, or disability, or those grieving irrevocable losses. Behavioral and cognitive techniques still can be useful in these situations. Consider the example of an elderly woman whose husband was a patient on an inpatient hospice unit. She felt extreme sadness about his impending death, and the most appropriate intervention here was to validate and empathize with her grief. It also was helpful to discuss behavioral techniques she could use to care for herself and better tolerate the distress, and to discuss some of her thoughts about his illness and dying. For example, she had extreme guilt about admitting him to an inpatient hospice, saying to herself that she "should" have been able to care for him at home. By examining the evidence for this thought and considering it from a more objective perspective (e.g., "What would you say to a friend in this situation?"), she was able to see that she had in fact done all that she possibly could. After completing some therapy, she was better able to be present with her partner, focus on their remaining time together, and cope more effectively with the situation.

Mindfulness techniques may be particularly helpful in these types of painful, unchangeable situations in order to help patients tolerate negative feelings and accept difficult situations (38,39). For example, mindfulness meditation has been found to be very helpful with chronic pain patients (46). Mindfulness exercises are based on Eastern meditation practices, with the goal of turning one's attention to current experience. Attending to current experience is often done from a nonjudgmental, observational stand-

point, in which feelings and thoughts are observed but not focused on. To communicate this idea to a patient, analogies often are helpful; for example, a patient might practice observing thoughts float by like clouds or like boxes on a conveyor belt. Mindfulness techniques may include breathing exercises or focusing with full awareness on any one of a variety of simple activities (e.g., washing dishes, eating a meal, without doing any other activity). The result of these activities is that patients often are able to stop ruminating about the past or future, prevent negative thoughts and feelings from spiraling out of control, and tolerate being in pain or distress. Research suggests that older adults are willing to engage in these types of strategies and find them helpful (42).

Importance of Homework

CBT relies heavily on the use of out-of-session assignments to solidify learning and to practice the application of new skills. Research with older adults demonstrates that patients who complete homework assignments are more likely to improve than those who do not (47). Coon and Gallagher-Thompson (48) reviewed strategies to encourage homework compliance in older adults. Patients must understand the rationale for homework: the goal of therapy is to affect change in the person's everyday life, and this change is founded on the patient applying CBT skills in everyday life. Learning these skills takes a lot of practice, given that the targeted patterns of behavior and thinking were learned a long time ago, are well-ingrained, and are sometimes automatic. It is important for the therapist to view homework as a priority, consistently develop homework assignments at the end of each session, and review them at the beginning of each session. Assignments should be developed collaboratively and relate to the themes and goals discussed in that session. In addition, homework should be realistic in order to make achievement more likely. If homework is not completed, direct conversations about potential obstacles and problem solving strategies are very important.

Adapting CBT for Older Adults

Most of the general modifications discussed previously apply to CBT. Some older adults may require additional sessions to solidify learning. In-session and homework assignments often involve reading and writing; therefore, older adults' visual acuity and writing abilities need to be considered. Documents should be created in large fonts, and alternative strategies (e.g., verbal repetition, audiotaping, etc.) may need to be developed for individuals with very poor vision or blindness, or who have difficulty writing (due to arthritis, stroke, etc.). For elders using computers, offering computerized templates may be helpful. For example, one elderly patient found it easier to type than write, and she could easily adjust the font to her visual needs. An example of CBT with a depressed elderly woman is provided below.

CASE EXAMPLE: COGNITIVE–BEHAVIORAL
THERAPY WITH OLDER ADULTS

Mrs. T. was a 70-year-old, widowed African American woman who sought treatment for depression. Although she was in reasonably good health, she reported sleeping most of the day, and was most troubled by the fact that she had completely disengaged from her usual activities. Mrs. T. had been very active in the church, particularly with a foster grandparent program. She indicated that she stopped attending those meetings because of a new member whom she did not like, even though she had met the new member on only one occasion. While she wanted to reengage in the program, she reported not having enough energy to participate in the events. Further, her three adult children lived with her, and she felt they were beginning to control her life. The only solution she could think of was to move away from her home and find an apartment somewhere, but she feared that her children would follow her to her new home and she would find herself in the same unpleasant situation again. Mrs. T. felt trapped by her situation.

Among the many goals Mrs. T. had for therapy was reengagement in the foster grandparent program. Treatment focused first on this issue, as it allowed her to work on a problem that was not as emotionally charged as were her relationship conflicts with her children. Treatment initially focused on behavior change, in the form of graded task assignments. Together with her therapist, Mrs. T. created a series of small steps that she could take to reengage in the program. She began by getting minutes from the meetings to review so she could stay involved without leaving her home. Next, she volunteered to do certain tasks from home, such as calling to remind members about the meeting, updating committee lists, and organizing potlucks through a telephone tree. Because she was still receiving newsletters from the program, these initial steps were relatively easy for her to implement. Her activity level was increased fairly rapidly through engagement in the activities she could do from home with minimal interpersonal involvement. The final steps involved her attending program meetings in person.

Along with implementing her plans for action, Mrs. T. worked on her negative expectations about reengaging with the foster grandparent program. She identified a tendency towards an all-or-nothing thinking pattern in her fear that the organization would not allow her to gradually reinvolve herself in the program. This belief initially prevented her from calling the program and proposing that she help out from home. In addition, Mrs. T. was unsure how to discuss her wishes for this limited involvement with the other program members, as she was concerned about potential suspicions about her health or mental health. With her therapist, Mrs. T. worked on changing her negative thinking by examining the evidence for her belief (for example, thinking about times when other members have participated from home). She also role-played how she might present her plan to the program, which included some *so-what* discussions about

all possible outcomes. In practicing these conversations with the therapist, Mrs. T. found that her emotional connection with the program and her own motivation to reengage was increasing.

Because of this behavioral activation and cognitive restructuring work, she was able to experience success in meeting her goal of becoming reinvolved in the program and improve her mood. As a result, she was in a better position to effectively set limits on her children's demands on her time. By week 6 of therapy, Mrs. T's Hamilton Depression Rating Scale score had dropped from 24 to 6. At week 12, Mrs. T. was actively solving family problems in therapy and was reconnected to many of the activities she had been avoiding when she initially began treatment.

For older adults with cognitive impairment, Coon and Gallagher-Thompson (48) suggest several methods for adapting CBT. These include simplifying concepts and homework, developing a combined calendar and therapy notebook, including only essential material in the notebook, finding a consistent place at home for the notebook, and audiotaping sessions for later review and better learning consolidation. Shorter, more frequent sessions also may be beneficial. For some patients, memory problems will contribute to homework noncompliance. In these cases, techniques such as writing assignments in the same notebook each week, finding one specific time of day to do homework, prearranged reminder calls from the therapist (or from a friend or family member), and simplifying homework assignments may be helpful. For an additional discussion of more general issues in conducting psychotherapy with individuals with dementia, please refer to that section later in the chapter.

Interpersonal Therapy

Interpersonal therapy (IPT) is a second type of therapy that is considered empirically supported for older adults with depression (34). Several studies with older adults have shown IPT to be as effective as nortriptyline in reducing depression, and associated with less dropout than antidepressant treatment (49,50). IPT has also been shown to be effective in combination with nortriptyline in the treatment of initial and subsequent episodes of major depression, and in maintaining remission of symptoms (51–53).

IPT is an approach to treating depression that was developed based on observations of the importance of social relationships to depression (54). Many of the principles of IPT arose from the fundamental assumptions of interpersonal psychiatry, espoused most famously by Harry Stack Sullivan (55). IPT does not make assumptions about the cause of the depression; rather, its central tenet is that depression occurs in a social context, regardless of the specific contribution of genetic, biological, or psychosocial factors (54). IPT is a time-limited (usually 12 to 20 weekly, 1-hour sessions), manualized treatment that focuses on symptom relief and improvement of interpersonal coping strategies. The therapy occurs in three sequential stages: identifying relationship issues, addressing these issues, and termination phase.

Initial Phase: Identify Interpersonal Issues

In the initial phase, the diagnosis of depression is established and psychoeducation is provided regarding the nature of depression, medications (if appropriate), and the connection between depression and psychosocial factors. In this initial phase, the patient is socialized to therapy and rapport is built. The patient is allowed the "sick role" and allowed to feel the full weight of his or her depression. Together, the patient and therapist review current and past relationships in a type of inventory. This review should include all aspects of a patient's social network, including family, friends, coworkers, neighbors, and important professionals (e.g., religious leaders). During this information gathering, the therapist should pay particular attention to patterns of interpersonal interactions that emerge, which may be associated with depression (56).

IPT theory holds that most interpersonal problems relevant for depressed persons fall into one of four categories: a) *grief* (related to loss of an important relationship); b) *interpersonal role disputes* (related to differences in role expectations in important dyadic relationships); c) *role transitions* (e.g., change in job status or change in one's role in the family); and d) *interpersonal deficit* (significant challenges in interacting with others and social isolation; deficits are targeted for improvement but likely will not completely resolve with this short-term therapy). The developers of IPT chose to focus on these areas of treatment not as an attempt to explain the etiology of all depressions, or as a comprehensive formulation, but to provide the therapist with a structure for setting realistic goals and defining treatment strategies for the short-term therapy (54). In this initial phase of IPT, one or two areas of focus are discussed and mutually agreed upon by the therapist and patient. For patients with problems in all of these domains, the main precipitant(s) for the current episode of depression may be most appropriate as a treatment focus.

Middle Phase: Addressing Interpersonal Issues

In the middle phase, therapy is focused on these problem areas, with the emphasis on current interpersonal problems and related feelings and wishes. Treatment techniques in IPT include psychodynamically oriented strategies such as exploration, clarification of affect, and role play, as well as CBT-type elements such as communication analysis, connecting events and mood, and teaching options for behavior and thoughts. In contrast to traditional psychoanalytic therapy, past experiences, while recognized, are not the focus of treatment. Transference and countertransference also are attended to but are not a primary focus of therapy. Similarly, unlike a typical cognitive-behavioral approach, negative thoughts and unpleasant events are emphasized only in the context of the role they play in interpersonal relationships.

Termination Phase: Review

Finally, the termination phase of treatment helps the patient review and consolidate the material and skills he or she has learned in therapy. For example, the patient's progress in therapy and in attaining symptom reduction is emphasized, new skills in handling interpersonal disputes are reviewed, and personal goals of the patient are discussed and problem-solved (for example, how to again engage in pleasurable activities after the loss of a spouse). Unlike traditional psychodynamic therapy, the therapeutic relationship itself is not necessarily explored in depth during termination.

IPT with Older Adults

In general, IPT seems to require little adaptation for work with the elderly (56,57). In terms of structure, IPT has inherent appeal for many older adults: it is short-term, goal-focused, and integrates a psychoeducational component that can help with socialization to therapy (56). The four problem areas covered in the therapy are relevant for persons across the lifespan and have high relevance for a number of problems that are commonly experienced in late life. These include significant changes in social roles, especially those within the family or the work situation (e.g., empty-nest syndrome, retirement, having to rely on family members for caregiving); the death of a spouse and/or friends; and conflict or lack of perceived support in relationships, perhaps most acutely intergenerational relationships. For some elderly, the social roles of most importance may be different than those in younger adults because of cohort differences. For example, the loss of the role of mother and homemaker may be more important for an elderly woman than for a younger adult. In addition, because older adults already have experienced many relationships in their lives, current relationships with the family of origin may not take such prominence in the therapy as they would for younger adults. Finally, with a patient who has already lived much of his or her life, there may be substantial differences in the quality of current versus past relationships and support networks. A thorough understanding of these differences, if any, should be obtained in the initial relationship inventory (56).

Clinicians experienced in using IPT with the elderly have reported that role transition and interpersonal role dispute are by far the most common primary issues dealt with in therapy (56,57). Common types of role transitions implicated in depression include aging issues (for example, patients coping with a loss of an old identity), retirement (patients working on structuring their time and finding meaning in activities), and changes in health that involve adjusting to functional limitations. Aging and health issues are encountered primarily in the context of role transition, and less often in the other categories of interpersonal issues. This suggests that when health and illness are related to depression, they usually are primary issues, over-riding other areas of concern. Miller and Silberman (56), in their work with older adults, found that when interpersonal role disputes were the focus, relationships with spouses were by far the most common source of conflict, followed by relationships with children. A case example is provided to illustrate IPT with an elderly grieving widow.

CASE EXAMPLE: INTERPERSONAL THERAPY WITH OLDER ADULTS

Mrs. A. was a 75-year-old widow referred by her daughter for a psychological evaluation. Mrs. A.'s daughter became concerned when her once very active mother began missing appointments with doctors, friends, and family, claiming that she had forgotten about these commitments. At the time of the evaluation, Mrs. A. had already undergone a thorough neurological and neuropsychological evaluation, with normal findings. She did, however, report significant symptoms of depression, with apparent onset immediately after the death of her husband 1 year prior to the evaluation. She reported that the initially constant tearfulness had subsided over time, but she had begun withdrawing from many social activities. As Mrs. A. discussed her occasional forgetfulness, it emerged that this was largely due to her failure to write the appointments down in her calendar, something she had relied on to organize her day for years. She also admitted that sometimes she used "forgetfulness" as an excuse to not attend an appointment. Mrs. A. connected her depressive symptoms to her husband's death, wondering aloud if her lack of energy was due to a physical ailment or if it was a normal part of grief. Further, she stated that the death of her husband had reminded her of her schizophrenic son's suicide 10 years prior; at that time, her husband had not allowed her to grieve that loss or even talk about it within the family.

Mrs. A. was referred for IPT, which focused on unresolved grief. During the initial phase of the 16-week treatment, socialization to therapy and psychoeducation regarding depression was provided and a relationship inventory was completed, with a special focus on her relationships with her husband and son. Mrs. A. discussed the parallels and contrasts between how she was grieving her husband's death and how she had grieved her son's death. Mrs. A. also talked about how in her culture, one was expected to suppress emotions; to some extent, her husband's refusal to talk about her son's death fit well with her own background. Over the middle phase of treatment, Mrs. A. became more able to openly discuss and tolerate her many conflicting feelings regarding her husband and how he handled his death, and regarding her son's way of handling life. She also began to reengage in social activities and to be more assertive about choosing to socialize or not. By the end of treatment, Mrs. A. was no longer experiencing problems with forgetfulness, and her Hamilton Depression Rating Scale score had dropped from 21 to 3. The termination phase of acute treatment focused on consolidating coping skills to continue to resolve her grief. In addition, Mrs. A. attended relapse prevention therapy over the year following treatment. These monthly sessions served primarily to check in on her mood, which remained stable over the year.

Other Promising Psychotherapies for Older Adults

Whereas CBT and IPT are the two psychotherapies considered to have the most extensive evidence base for treatment of depression and anxiety in older patients, there are other psychotherapies that hold considerable promise for becoming evidence-based practices. The most prominent of these emerging therapies include brief dynamic therapy, reminiscence therapy, and problem-solving therapy. We provide a brief discussion of each approach here that includes theory, research, and application.

Brief Dynamic Therapy

Brief dynamic therapy (BDT) has emerged as a promising intervention for depression in older adults in two comparative studies with CBT or behavioral therapy, matching those approaches in effectiveness as a treatment for depression and caregiver distress in older adults (58,59). Both treatments show improvement in depression symptoms over time. Although BDT has some evidence in support of its efficacy, additional studies are needed to warrant an official designation as an evidence-based practice.

In the research literature, there are several versions of BDT, all emphasizing different aspect of psychodynamic theory and with various practice parameters. Numerous manuals have been published, such as those by Luborsky (60), Strupp and Binder (61), and Book (62). The model used most frequently in the geriatric literature (used by Thompson et al., 59), is based on Horowitz' grief model of depression (63). In this model, depression is viewed as a function of unresolved grief that is re-emerging as a function of recent losses. In order to overcome depression, the patient must first understand the current loss and grief in the context of previous losses. This is done through a process of exploration, discussion, and attempts on the part of the therapist to link past grief to current loss. This therapy consists of 12 weekly, 1-hour sessions. During the session, the therapist and patient discuss depression, losses associated with their low mood, and any previous losses that seem related to the current loss. The therapist helps draw parallels between the past and present through interpretation and exploration of transference in the therapeutic relationship. The treatment is considered successful when the patient's depressive symptoms remit and the patient demonstrates an adequate understanding of the relationship between unresolved grief and current functioning.

Reminiscence Therapy

Reminiscence therapy (RT) was one of the first psychotherapies to be developed explicitly for older adults. Many published reports have examined RT, although most of these studies relied on less rigorous standards of diagnosis (i.e., these studies primarily used age and cutoff scores on questionnaires, as opposed to standard psychiatric diagnostic interviews), or had other methodological flaws that limit their generalizability (64). Therefore, although the research on RT suggests successful resolution of distress, its usefulness in treating DSM-IV-TR Axis I disorders remains unconfirmed. Of the studies that have used diagnostic criteria for major depression to define the sample of older adults, results have been positive, but inadequate to thoroughly evaluate this treatment. One study compared problem solving therapy (PST) to RT using a 12-session, group-based format (65). The results showed that while PST had better treatment outcomes than RT, patients who received RT also improved substantially and did better than a control group of patients on a wait list. Another study with a smaller sample size found similar results in comparing a skills-based group treatment to RT, in that both approaches produced significant improvements in mood and disability (66). Taken together, the research to date suggests that RT has the potential for being an evidence-based treatment for older adults; one or two additional, larger trials with positive results would serve to solidify this status.

Reminiscence therapy was originally based on Erikson's stage theory of personality development (67). In brief, this theory holds that as we age, we are presented with various conflicts that need to be resolved in order for us to continue to function in an adjusted way. Similar to many psychodynamic personality theorists, Erikson posited fixed stages of development that must be resolved in order to successfully negotiate the subsequent conflicts. Unlike many psychodynamic theories, Eriksonian theory holds that people will encounter each stage of conflict, whether or not they have successfully resolved a previous conflict. If a previous conflict has not been resolved, the chances of successfully negotiating subsequent conflicts are reduced. Thus, the model of therapy derived from this theory dictates that some therapeutic work focus on the first conflict that was not resolved successfully, while also moving towards resolution of the current conflict. Reminiscence techniques have been incorporated into various therapeutic frameworks. For example, Viney describes a life review process in which a main goal of reminiscence is for the patient to experience an empowered view of self and affirm self-identity (68). Watt and Cappeliez report on using reminiscence techniques embedded in a cognitive-behavioral framework (69).

The principal psychotherapeutic techniques in RT are life review and reminiscence. The conflict in older age, according to Erikson, is *integrity versus despair,* whereby older persons attempt to process and come to terms with events throughout their lives (67). Older adults deal with this conflict in two basic ways: by accepting past negative and positive events and moving onto new experiences before death (integration), or by continuing to dwell on the past to the exclusion of enjoying the present (despair). Erikson theorized that all older adults engage in a process of reminiscence, whereby the content of their thoughts and discussions focuses on salient times in their lives. For the therapist, these reminiscences during therapy can be indicators of whether the past is being integrated or despaired. They also can indicate at which stage the older person encountered their first unsuccessful resolution, and thus what remedial therapeutic work may be necessary for successful therapy outcome.

In the RT research literature, the delivery of therapy varies from study to study. In many studies, the therapy is delivered over a 12-week period and primarily in a group format. Each week, a different theme is discussed, usually centered on previous stages of development. The discussion is called life review, and patients are encouraged to talk about salient events in each developmental stage in an attempt to come to a positive resolution of that stage. This technique was developed originally by Butler (70). In some treatments, patients are encouraged to bring in photographs, clothing, music and other materials that represent the era in which the developmental stage occurred for them (65). The purpose of these props is to stimulate memories about the conflict and to bring to the present events that occurred in the past. Regardless of how discussion and life review are generated during the course of therapy, these discussions are always raised in an attempt to create better integration of past successes and failures so that the older patient can focus on the here-and-now and reach a point where they feel their lives have been useful and meaningful in some way.

Problem-Solving Therapy

PST also shows great potential as an evidence-based practice for treating depression in older adults. Two versions of PST have been studied: the original PST and PST-PC, adapted for primary care settings. PST has been studied in two trials with older adults with major depression. In one study, PST resulted in more significant improvements in depressive symptoms than RT or a wait-list control (65). In a smaller trial, PST resulted in fewer depressive symptoms and better psychosocial functioning than supportive therapy (71). PST-PC also has been studied in two studies with older adults. In the first trial, use of the antidepressant paroxetine resulted in greater improvement than PST-PC, although PST-PC was somewhat effective; these results appeared to be heavily dependent on site-specific characteristics (72). The second study, labeled IMPACT (4), used PST-PC as one intervention choice in a collaborative care model; however, there was no randomized comparison of PST-PC to another intervention. Overall, preliminary results regarding the effectiveness of PST with older adults are highly promising, but not definitive.

PST is based in social learning theory and posits that depression is due largely to a combination of underdeveloped problem solving skills and feelings of helplessness in taking care of day-to-day problems. Nezu, Nezu, and Perri argue that all therapies implicitly teach patients to solve problems; thus, the most direct approach to overcoming depression is to teach these skills explicitly (73). The main goal of the therapy is to teach patients problem solving skills, using the problems they currently face as opportunities to learn and practice these skills. The therapist is both a teacher and collaborator in the problem solving process.

The therapist teaches the patient six steps that systematically address a psychosocial problem. These steps are 1) problem orientation, 2) problem definition, 3) brainstorming, 4) decision making, 5) planning, 6) solution implementation, and 7) solution verification. In *problem orientation*, patients are taught that there usually is a solution for every problem; however, the goals have to be realistic in order to determine a feasible solution. Patients are taught that when they are feeling depressed, they should attempt to identify thoughts that may be influencing their mood. Much like the cognitive restructuring phase in CBT, the purpose of this skill is to reorient patients to think about their problems as solvable, rather than avoid thinking of solutions. With older adults, many problems may be seen as unsolvable (e.g., the spouse of a grieving widow cannot be brought back, terminal cancer cannot be cured). As with any other type of therapy, it is important to empathize and validate the patient's grief over such losses. In PST, however, the therapist then attempts to orient the patient to recognize that there are aspects of the problem they can solve (e.g., identifying ways to honor the spouse's memory, developing a plan for how one wants to die).

The next skill, *problem definition*, involves teaching the patient to define the problem in concrete and operational terms. Patients are taught to break down larger, ill-defined problems ("I never have enough money") to smaller, specific goals ("I want to pay off my credit card bill by next January"). The focus of intractable problems, such as chronic and untreatable illnesses, is shifted from unachievable wishes ("If only I did not have diabetes") to controllable goals ("I have to make sure I take my blood sugar levels twice a day"). After a problem is defined, patients learn to *brainstorm* at least five to 10 solutions for the problem. Vital to this step is the withholding of any evaluations or decisions about the solution. Often, depressed patients will discard solutions before considering them, simply because they firmly believe that "nothing will work." After solutions are generated, the patient

can engage in *decision making*. The patient learns to think of all the pros and cons of each potential solution, considering issues such as whether or not the solution would meet short-term and long-term goals, whether it would create a burden for the patient or for someone else, and if it is at all feasible. Finally, after comparing the solutions to one another, the patient selects a solution and creates an *implementation* plan. The patient then implements the plan, and with the therapist discusses the success or failure of the solution (*solution verification*).

In the original form of PST, the skills are taught sequentially over five to six sessions. Once each skill is learned well, the therapist and patient work together to use the skills to solve current problems. Typically, patients meet weekly for 50 minutes over a 12-week period of time. In PST-PC, all of the skills are taught in a 1-hour session. After the initial education session, patients meet with the therapist every other week for six to eight 30-minute sessions, in which they apply all of the steps to a problem in each session.

GROUP THERAPY WITH OLDER ADULTS

Although much of the discussion thus far has been regarding individual psychotherapy with older adults, a group therapeutic modality also offers significant benefits to this population. There are numerous reports in the literature regarding group work in the elderly, including the successful use of dynamic and other insight-oriented therapies in group settings (74,75), although most evidence collected to date is related to behavioral and cognitive-behavioral approaches (76).

Group treatment offers several advantages over individual therapy for the elderly patient (77–79). For example, group therapy is usually less costly, a factor which is important to many patients, but can be especially relevant for older adults on a fixed income. In a group there is opportunity to receive positive reinforcement from peers and to practice social skills with other group members. Further, groups usually provide a good deal of enjoyable interaction, which can increase a participant's commitment to treatment, encourage attendance, and increase social confidence (11). Group settings also provide an opportunity to express altruistic needs; there is an opportunity to make contributions to others and to experience being useful. For elderly with little prior experience with mental health treatment, the normalizing function of sharing problems with others and discovering the universality of problems—for example, that forgetfulness is common—can be very important. Finally, it can be helpful for some elderly patients to have a treatment experience with same-age peers, especially when the therapists may be much younger.

The group norms that develop with elderly clients can be somewhat different than those that would emerge among younger adults (11). These norms can be useful in the therapy (for example, strong norms of altruism and commitment to session attendance), but can also be counterproductive (for example, beliefs that one should not air dirty laundry in public; not express emotions; or not disagree with or comment on other members' sharing). Group leaders may choose to proactively address these ideas at the start of therapy and may need to continue to address them as they arise.

Using a structured, psychoeducational approach to group treatment has many advantages. This approach can have inherent appeal to elders for the same reasons discussed above in the individual therapy sections (e.g., structure, review of material, etc). A learning-based group therapy can be desirable for older adults, as it resembles an educational approach; it offers a familiar setting that is like a classroom and the group leader often uses educational tools to structure sessions, such as a blackboard and homework. The emphasis on learning and take-home materials or assignments helps older adults retain the material.

Many of the general adaptations for psychotherapeutic work with older adults enumerated above, in reference to individual therapy, apply equally well to a group therapy setting. In addition, especially for structured approaches such as behavioral and cognitive behavioral approaches, some authors have made further recommendations. Yost and colleagues (11), speaking from extensive experience using behavioral group therapy approaches with depressed older adults, provide the following suggestions for a treatment model:

1. Include several short segments per session (not more than 30 minutes per segment), each with a clear beginning and end, and each accompanied by clear verbal and visual cues related to the material.
2. Include items and methods to cue members' attention and memories. For example, an agenda discussed and posted at the start of each session (which can be modified) provides structure and a way of tracking the therapy session.
3. Give advance warning of tasks during the session (for example, verbal sharing or written work) to allow members to prepare and organize thoughts.
4. Provide ways to assist members in retaining concepts and to practice between sessions (for example, written information sheets or manuals, written homework assignments).
5. Ask questions of members during the session; this is helpful in synthesizing and analyzing information, drawing attention to key issues, providing an organizing focus for sessions, and controlling the pace of the meeting.

COUPLE AND FAMILY THERAPY

Interventions that involve partners and other family members are very important for older adults, as they may spend more time than younger adults with family members, due to retirement or caregiving needs. With retirement, older couples may begin spending significantly more time together, which can raise important therapeutic issues. For example, an older couple in marital therapy had observed increased conflict after the husband's retirement; an important contributor to this conflict was his doing household activities in ways that were not satisfying to his wife (e.g., he did not clean up well in the kitchen due to poor visual acuity). Alternatively, at some times she wanted his help, but he became reticent to help because he expected her to criticize his work. By discussing their perspectives with each other, they were better able to empathize with each other and gradually develop effective ways of working together on tasks. Caregiving for a disabled elderly family member is often distressing to both the patient and caregiver, which may lead to interpersonal conflict. Disability and illness also can lead to serious conflict among various family members about who is responsible for caring for the patient and living arrangements for the patient.

Despite its relevance and importance, very little empirical research has been conducted on couple and family therapy with older adults (78). Experienced clinicians contend that couple and family therapy are helpful with older adults, however, and have made recommendations on working with older couples or families (80). Many considerations are the same as in any other type of couple or family therapy, including considering who the client is, clarifying the therapist's role and allegiance, and remaining neutral and supportive of all family members. Special considerations with older adults include recognition that the older adult family system has longstanding patterns of interactions, and considering cohort-based influences on conflicts (e.g., changes across successive cohorts in expectations about keeping older relatives at home versus the acceptability of placement in long-term care facilities), as well as maturational influences (e.g., older family members may have more wisdom and more stable emotional reactions than younger family members by virtue of age and experience). It is important to understand members' historical role in the family and power relationships. Also, it is important to involve as many family members as possible, and not exclude an older patient due to cognitive impairment or frailty (80).

Psychotherapy interventions have been found effective with caregivers, with some suggestion that dynamic approaches may be more beneficial early in the caregiving process and CBT more helpful for longtime caregivers (58). For patients with moderate-to-severe dementia and depression, caregivers can successfully learn and implement behavioral methods for problem solving around the patient's problematic behavior and increasing the patient's pleasant activities. This intervention results in better emotional functioning for both caregiver and patient (81).

PSYCHOTHERAPY WITH INDIVIDUALS WITH DEMENTIA

Working psychotherapeutically with cognitively impaired older adults is an under-researched area, perhaps due to commonly held, yet unexamined notions of the inefficacy of psychotherapy with these individuals. In particular, impairments in memory and language can seem incompatible with the psychotherapeutic process. However, we are gaining understanding of the existence of various memory systems that remain intact even in advanced dementia, and clinical research data is emerging that indicates promise for various interventions. Interventions with theoretical and some empirical support include supportive therapy, life review therapy, psychodynamic approaches, and memory training (82). In general, goals are to improve coping and reduce distress and symptomatology by maintaining ego functioning and improving perspective (e.g., using psychodynamic or cognitive-behavioral approaches), promoting ego integrity (life review), optimizing daily functioning (memory training, behavioral modification), or improving social interactions (e.g., reality orientation). Many of these therapies have been used in both individual and group formats. The type of approach indicated will vary depending on the extent of the patient's dementia and on the specific goals for each case.

Clinical reports indicate good results with psychodynamic therapy, likely most useful with individuals with mild to moderate impairment, rather than in the later stages of decline (83). Recommendations include keeping interventions concrete, restating interventions several times during a session and across sessions, and keeping abstract interpretations to a minimum. For more structured approaches such as CBT, recommendations include simplifying psychoeducational components, audiotaping sessions, and reducing the amount of information in a client's therapy notebook (48). Life review or reminiscence therapy with a goal of achieving ego integrity may be most appropriate for persons with mild dementia. For those with more severe impairment, reminiscence techniques may be useful to structure social interactions (82). Supportive group and individual therapy have frequently been used to help demented patients cope with impairment and loss and to relieve stress, and in the case of support groups, to promote social interaction and interpersonal connection among members (84).

For persons with moderately-severe-to-severe impairment, reality orientation, behavioral modification, and memory training approaches may be the most useful types of psychotherapy to optimize functioning and reduce distress in the individual and in caregivers (82). Reality orientation aims at reducing confusion through providing orienting information (day, name, and place) and increasing stimulation and interaction with the environment for the patient. Behavioral modifications are focused on decreasing problem behaviors, such as wandering or aggression, and increasing desirable behaviors, such as appropriate hygiene or toileting (85). Finally, memory training aims to improve objective-memory performance through the use of specific techniques such as mnemonics or a memory notebook; to improve functioning through use of environmental cues, such as the use of signs, colors, or pictures to help orientation; and to increase communication and problem solving skills (82).

Intervening with family caregivers and with staff are other approaches that may be useful in improving care and quality of life for persons with dementia. For example, caregivers can be trained to use problem solving to deal with more severely impaired patients' problematic behaviors and to increase patients' engagement in pleasant activities (81), and nursing assistants can be trained to increase verbal interactions and use behavioral management techniques with impaired patients (86,87).

PSYCHOTHERAPY IN THE LONG-TERM CARE SETTING

According to usual estimates, the prevalence of mental disorders among older adults residing in a nursing home can be 50% or more, yet only a very small percentage receives mental health services (88). Thus, providing therapeutic services in long-term care is an area of great need, although very little research has been conducted to guide professionals working in this setting. Working psychotherapeutically with older adults who are residents of an institution such as a nursing home has many challenges, but also many rewards. In general, the same principles of psychotherapeutic intervention that have already been laid out apply in this setting. Below, we briefly review the major additional issues to consider, and provide resources for the reader.

Although the system surrounding a patient is always an important part of the assessment and ongoing therapy, in the long-term care setting it can be particularly complex. The nursing home itself is part of a vast economic and legislative system of care, and each facility is a system and a culture unto itself, comprising staff, family members, and residents. Where the therapist fits into this system (e.g., as a staff member, as a consultant under contract, or as a privately paid therapist following a certain resident), and how the patient is viewed within the system, may impact therapy and therapeutic effectiveness. Not infrequently, effective psychotherapy will involve interventions aimed at other components of the larger system, not just at the patient herself. At the very least, contact with staff and family will almost always be an important adjunct to therapy with the patient.

Secondly, there are practical aspects to the setting that will impact the mode of therapy and how therapy is delivered. Some residents referred for services will have mobility problems that necessitate therapy at the bedside. Private space is at a premium in most facilities, and individual therapy may need to be conducted in a resident's shared room or in a community space. In these settings, interruptions by staff or other residents can be relatively common and must be handled carefully, to protect the patient's privacy without intruding on the other patient's rights or staff member's duties. It can be beneficial to discuss these issues with staff, who can prepare patients for therapy (e.g., help get the patient into a wheelchair, dressed, etc.), suggest times of day when patients are more alert, and suggest strategies to maximize privacy. Staff are more likely to help therapists when they understand the therapist's role in care, goals, and general schedule. Occasionally, family visits, medical appointments, or health crises will conflict with scheduled therapy time. In coping with all of these issues, flexibility is an important characteristic of the long-term care therapist.

Finally, it is important not to fall prey to assumptions regarding limitations on therapy in this setting. Developing rapport and an intensive relationship with the client is important, even though the setting and its inherent challenges can discourage taking the time to do this. Here as in more traditional treatment settings, the therapeutic relationship serves as an important foundation for effective therapy. When considering length and frequency of sessions, each case should be assessed individually. Despite the fact that some older adults will benefit from shorter, frequent therapy sessions due to cognitive or physical frailties, many will do well with 50-minute (or longer) sessions on a weekly basis, with excellent engagement and even feeling energized afterwards (89). Similarly, the goals of therapy should not be limited simply because of the setting; full remission of depression or anxiety symptoms, dynamic-exploratory work toward personal growth, and treatment of longstanding personality traits (90) are perfectly reasonable aims for treatment, taking into account the specifics of the patient situation. As others have noted: meaningful, deep psychotherapy aimed at effecting substantial positive change can be conducted in the long-term care setting (89).

SUMMARY AND CONCLUSIONS

Contrary to long-held stereotypes, psychotherapy with older adults is a feasible and effective approach to treating psychopathology, using a variety of modalities and therapeutic approaches. For several types of psychotherapy, including cognitive-behavioral and interpersonal approaches, a wealth of empirical evidence already exists to support their use with the elderly population. Other emerging therapies have produced promising results thus far and likely will prove to be important best-practice treatments in the future. Depending on each client's needs, specific modifications of standard psychotherapeutic procedures may reduce barriers to client participation and facilitate the effectiveness of the treatment.

We have only summarized some of the central issues in practicing psychotherapy with older adults. Others have written excellent, more detailed descriptions of this work. For interested clinicians, we recommend several books for further reading: a) Knight (12), which reviews aging-related changes and issues and provides a contextual framework for conceptualizing and intervening with older adults and their families; b) Zarit and Knight (91), which includes chapters on a variety of therapeutic approaches (e.g., CBT, IPT, psychoanalytic) and modalities (e.g., individual, family) with older adults; and c) Duffy (92). In addition, Lichtenberg's (43) and Molinari's (93) volumes are very useful for working with older adults and staff in medical and long-term care settings.

In addition to benefiting older clients, psychotherapy with older adults can be extremely rewarding for therapists. Working with older adults allows us to learn about different times and to learn vicariously about a wide array of human experiences and challenges, and often can prepare us for our own aging. We feel strongly that it is a pleasure and an honor to work therapeutically with older adults, and for the reader, we hope for many of these meaningful experiences.

ACKNOWLEDGEMENTS

The authors wish to acknowledge training grant support from NIMH (T32 MH18261) and HRSA (D01 HP 00015-02).

REFERENCES

1. Freud S. *On Psychotherapy*, vol 1. London: Hogarth Press; 1924.
2. Gatz M, Fiske A, Fox LS, Kasl-Godley JE, McCallum TJ, Wetherell JL. Empirically validated psychological treatments for older adults. *Journal of Mental Health and Aging*. 1998;4:9–46.
3. Areán PA, Hegel MT, Reynolds CF. Treating depression in older medical patients with psychotherapy. *J Clin Geropsychol*. 2001; 7(2):93–104.
4. Unützer J, Katon W, Callahan CM, et al. Collaborative care management of late-life depression in the primary care setting: a randomized controlled trial. *JAMA*. 2002;288(22):2836–2845.
5. Bedi N, Chilvers C, Churchill R, et al. Assessing effectiveness of treatment of depression in primary care: partially randomised preference trial. *Br J Psychiatry*. 2000;177:312–318.
6. Rokke PD, Tomhave JA, Jocic Z. The role of client choice and target selection in self-management therapy for depression in older adults. *Psychol Aging*. 1999;14(1):155–169.
7. Schulberg HC, Katon W, Simon GE, Rush AJ. Treating major depression in primary care practice: an update of the Agency for Health Care Policy and Research Practice Guidelines. *Arch Gen Psychiatry*. 1998;55:1121–1127.
8. Chambless DL, Hollon SD. Defining empirically supported therapies. *J Consult Clin Psychol*. 1998;66(1):7–18.
9. American Psychological Association. What practitioners should know about working with older adults. *Professional Psychology: Research & Practice*. 1998;29(5):413–427.
10. Gum A, Areán PA. Recent advances in psychotherapy for older adults with psychiatric disorders. *Curr Psychiatry Rep*. 2004;6: 32–38.
11. Yost EB, Beutler LE, Corbishley MA, Allender JR. *Group Cognitive Therapy: A Treatment Approach for Depressed Older Adults*. New York: Pergamon Press; 1986.
12. Knight BG. *Psychotherapy with Older Adults*. 3rd Ed. Thousand Oaks, CA: Sage; 2004.
13. Newton NA, Jacobowitz J. Transferential and countertransferential processes in therapy with older adults. In: Duffy M, ed. *Handbook of Counseling and Psychotherapy with Older Adults*. New York: John Wiley & Sons; 1999.

14. Coon DW, Higgins AB, Solano N, et al. Behavioral and cognitive interventions for late life depression: special issues in the treatment of older adults. *J Clin Geropsychol.* In press.

15. Coon DW, Rider K, Gallagher-Thompson D, Thompson L. Cognitive-behavioral therapy for the treatment of late-life distress. In: Duffy M, ed. *Handbook of Counseling and Psychotherapy with Older Adults.* New York: John Wiley & Sons, Inc; 1999;487–510.

16. Gallagher-Thompson D, Coon DW, Rivera P, Powers D, Zeiss AM. Family caregiving: stress, coping, and intervention. In: Hersen M, Van Hasselt VB, eds. *Handbook of Clinical Geropsychology.* New York: Plenum Press; 1998;469–493.

17. Gallagher-Thompson D, Thompson LW. Applying cognitive-behavioral therapy to the psychological problems of later life. In: Zarit SH, Knight BG, eds. *A Guide to Psychotherapy and Aging: Effective Clinical Interventions in a Life-Stage Context.* Washington, DC: American Psychological Association; 1996;61–82.

18. Thompson L, Gallagher-Thompson D. Psychotherapeutic interventions with older adults in outpatient and extended care settings. In: Rubenstein RL, Lawton MP, eds. *Depression in Long-Term and Residential Care.* New York: Springer; 1997;169–184.

19. Thompson LW, Powers DV, Coon DW, Takagi K, McKibbin C, Gallagher-Thompson D. Older Adults. In: White JR, Freeman AS, eds. *Cognitive-Behavioral Group Therapy: for Specific Problems and Populations.* Washington, DC: American Psychological Association; 2000;235–261.

20. Latour D, Cappeliez P. Pretherapy training for group cognitive therapy with depressed older adults. *Canadian Journal on Aging.* 1994;13(2):221–235.

21. Larsen DL, Nguyen TD, Green RS, Attkisson CC. Enhancing the utilization of outpatient mental health services. *Community Ment Health J.* 1983;19:305–320.

22. France DG, Dugo JM. Pretherapy orientation as preparation for open psychotherapy groups. *Psychotherapy: Theory, Research, Practice, Training.* 1985;22(2):256–261.

23. Alvidrez J, Areán PA, Stewart AL. Psychoeducation to increase psychotherapy entry for older African Americans: a pilot study. Submitted for publication.

24. Knight BG, Satre DD. Cognitive behavioral psychotherapy with older adults. *Clinical Psychology: Science and Practice.* 1999;6:188–203.

25. Salthouse TA. Speed of behavior and its implications for cognition. In: Birren JE, Schaie KW, eds. *Handbook of the Psychology of Aging.* 2nd Ed. New York: Van Nostrand Reinhold; 1985;400–426.

26. Salthouse TA. *Theoretical Perspectives on Cognitive Aging.* Hillsdale, NJ: Erlbaum; 1991.

27. Schulberg HC, Bryce C, Chism K, et al. Managing late-life depression in primary care practice: a case study of the health specialist's role. *Int J Geriatr Psychiatry.* 2001;16:577–584.

28. Scogin F. Bibliotherapy: a nontraditional intervention for depression. In: Hartman-Stein P, ed. *Innovative Behavioral Healthcare for Older Adults: A Guidebook for Changing Times.* San Francisco: Jossey-Bass; 1998;129–144.

29. Kaufman AV, Scogin FR, Malone-Beach EE, Baumhover LA, McKendree-Smith N. Home-delivered mental health services for aged rural home health care recipients. *J Appl Gerontol.* 2000; 19(4):460–475.

30. Grant RW, Casey DA. Adapting cognitive behavioral therapy for the frail elderly. *Int Psychogeriatr.* 1995;7(4):561–571.

31. Haley W. The medical context of psychotherapy with the elderly. In: Zarit SH, Knight BG, eds. *A Guide to Psychotherapy and Aging: Effective Clinical Interventions in a Life-Stage Context.* Washington, DC: American Psychological Association; 1996;221–240.

32. Rybarczyk B, Gallagher-Thompson D, Rodman J, Zeiss A, et al. Applying cognitive-behavioral psychotherapy to the chronically ill elderly: treatment issues and case illustration. *Int Psychogeriatr.* 1992;4(1):127–140.

33. Blanchard-Fields F, Chen Y. Adaptive cognition and aging. *Am Behav Sci.* 1996;39(3):231–248.

34. Areán PA, Cook BL. Psychotherapy and combined psychotherapy/pharmacotherapy for late life depression. *Biol Psychiatry.* 2002;52:293–303.

35. Nordhus IH, Pallesen S. Psychological treatment of late-life anxiety: an empirical review. *J Consult Clin Psychol.* 2003;71:643–651.

36. Beck AT, Rush AJ, Shaw BF, Emery G. *Cognitive Therapy of Depression.* New York: Guilford; 1979.

37. Beck JS. *Cognitive Therapy: Basics and Beyond.* New York: Guilford; 1995.

38. Linehan MM. *Cognitive Behavioral Treatment for Borderline Personality Disorder.* New York: Guilford Press; 1993.

39. Segal ZV, Williams JMG, Teasdale JD. *Mindfulness-Based Cognitive Therapy for Depression: A New Approach to Preventing Relapse.* New York: Guilford; 2002.

40. Thompson LW, Coon DW, Gallagher-Thompson D, Sommer BR, Koin D. Comparison of desipramine and cognitive/behavioral therapy in the treatment of elderly outpatients with mild-to-moderate depression. *Am J Geriatr Psychiatry.* 2001;9(3):225–240.

41. Wetherell JL, Gatz M, Craske MG. Treatment of generalized anxiety disorder in older adults. *J Consult Clin Psychol.* 2003;71:31–40.

42. Lynch TR, Morse JQ, Mendelson T, Robins CJ. Dialectical behavior therapy for depressed older adults: a randomized pilot study. *Am J Geriatr Psychiatry.* 2003;11(1):33–45.

43. Lichtenberg PA. *Mental Health Practice in Geriatric Health Care Settings.* Binghamton, NY: The Haworth Press, Inc. 1998.

44. Barlow DH, Craske MG, Cerny JA, Klosko JS. Behavioral treatment of panic disorder. *Behavior Therapy.* 1989;20:261–282.

45. Burns DD. *The Feeling Good Handbook.* Revised Ed. New York: Plume/Penguin Books; 1999.

46. Kabat-Zinn J, Lipworth L, Burney R. The clinical use of mindfulness meditation for the self-regulation of chronic pain. *J Behav Med.* 1985;8:163–190.

47. Coon DW, Thompson LW. The relationship between homework compliance and treatment outcomes among older adult outpatients with mild-to-moderate depression. *Am J Geriatr Psychiatry.* 2003;11(1):53–61.

48. Coon DW, Gallagher-Thompson D. Encouraging homework completion among older adults in therapy. *J Clin Psychol.* 2002;58(5): 549–563.

49. Sloane RB, Staples FR, Schneider LS. Interpersonal therapy versus nortriptyline for depression in the elderly. In: Burrows G, Norman TR, Dennerstein L, eds. *Clinical and Pharmacological Studies in Psychiatric Disorders.* London: John Libbey; 1985;344–346.

50. Schneider LS, Sloane RB, Staples FR, Bender M. Pretreatment orthostatic hypotension as a predictor of response to nortriptyline in geriatric depression. *J Clin Psychopharmacol.* 1986;6:172–176.

51. Reynolds CF, Frank E, Perel JM, et al. Combined pharmacotherapy and psychotherapy in the acute and continuation treatment of elderly patients with recurrent major depression: a preliminary report. *Am J Psychiatry.* 1992;149:1687–1682.

52. Reynolds CF, Frank E, Perel JM, et al. Treatment of consecutive episodes of major depression in the elderly. *Am J Psychiatry.* 1994;151:1740–1743.

53. Reynolds ICF, Frank E, Perel JM, et al. Nortriptyline and interpersonal psychotherapy as maintenance therapies for recurrent major depression: a randomized controlled trial in patients older than 59 years. *JAMA.* 1999;281(1):39–45.

54. Klerman GL, Weissman MM, Rounsaville BJ, Chevron E. *Interpersonal Psychotherapy of Depression.* New York: Basic Books; 1984.

55. Sullivan HS. *The Interpersonal Theory of Psychiatry.* New York: Norton; 1953.

56. Miller MD, Silberman RL. Using interpersonal psychotherapy with depressed elders. In: Zarit SH, Knight BG, eds. *A Guide to Psychotherapy and Aging: Effective Clinical Interventions in a Life-Stage Context.* Washington, DC: American Psychological Association; 1996;83–99.

57. Hinrichsen G. Interpersonal psychotherapy for depressed older adults. *J Geriatr Psychiatry.* 1997;30:239–257.

58. Gallagher-Thompson D, Steffen A. Comparative effects of cognitive-behavioral and brief psychodynamic psychotherapies for depressed family caregivers. *J Consult Clin Psychol.* 1994;62:543–549.

59. Thompson LW, Gallagher D, Breckenridge JS. Comparative effectiveness of psychotherapies for depressed elders. *J Consult Clin Psychol.* 1987;55:385–390.

60. Luborsky L. *Principles of Psychoanalytic Psychotherapy: A Manual for Supportive Expressive Treatment.* New York: Basic Books; 1984.

61. Strupp HH, Binder J. *Psychotherapy in a New Key: A Guide to Time-Limited Dynamic Psychotherapy.* New York: Basic Books; 1984.

62. Book HE. *How to Practice Brief Psychodynamic Psychotherapy: The Core Conflictual Relationship Theme Method.* Washington, DC: American Psychological Association; 1998.

63. Horowitz M, Kaltreider N. Brief therapy of the stress response syndrome. *Psychiatr Clin North Am.* 1979;2:365–377.

64. Hsieh H-F, Wang J-J. Effect of reminiscence therapy on depression in older adults: a systematic review. *Int J Nurs Stud.* 2003;40:335–345.

65. Areán PA, Perri MG, Nezu AM, Schein RL, Christoper F, Joseph TX. Comparative effectiveness of social problem-solving therapy and reminiscence therapy as treatments for depression in older adults. *J Consult Clin Psychol.* 1993;61(6):1003–1010.

66. Klausner EJ, Clarkin JF, Spielman L, Pupo C, Abrams R, Alexopoulos GS. Late-life depression and functional disability: the role of goal-focused group psychotherapy. *Int J Geriatr Psychiatry.* 1998;13(10):707–716.

67. Erikson EH. *The Life Cycle Completed: A Review.* New York: Norton Publishing Co; 1982.

68. Viney L. Reminiscence in psychotherapy with the elderly: telling and retelling their stories. In: Haight B, Webster JD, eds. *The Art and Science of Reminiscing: Theory, Research, Methods, and Applications.* Washington, DC: Taylor & Francis; 1995;243–264.

69. Watt LM, Cappeliez P. Reminiscence interventions for the treatment of depression in older adults. In: Haight B, Webster JD, eds. *The Art and Science of Reminiscing: Theory, Research, Methods, and Applications.* Washington, DC: Taylor & Francis; 1995;221–232.

70. Butler RN. Life review: an interpretation of reminiscence in the aged. *Psychiatry.* 1963;26:65–76.

71. Alexopoulos GS, Raue P, Areán P. Problem-solving therapy versus supportive therapy in geriatric major depression with executive dysfunction. *Am J Geriatr Psychiatry.* 2003;11(1):46–52.

72. Williams JW. Treatment of mild depression in elderly patients. *JAMA.* 2000;284(23):2993–2994.

73. Nezu AM, Nezu CM, Perri MG. *Problem-Solving Therapy for Depression.* New York: Wiley-Interscience; 1988.

74. Leszcz M. Integrated group psychotherapy for the treatment of depression in the elderly. *Group.* 1997;21(2):89–113.

75. Saiger GM. Group psychotherapy with older adults. *Psychiatry.* 2001;64(2):132–145.

76. Gallagher-Thompson DE, Thompson LW. Treatment of major depressive disorder in older adult outpatients with brief psychotherapies. *Psychotherapy: Theory, Research, and Practice.* 1982;19:482–490.

77. Finkel SI. Group psychotherapy in later life. In: Myers WA, ed. *New Techniques in the Psychotherapy of Older Patients.* Washington, DC; 1991;223–244.

78. Karel MJ, Hinrichsen G. Treatment of depression in late life: psychotherapeutic interventions. *Clin Psychol Rev.* 2000;20(6):707–729.

79. Tross S, Blum JE. A review of group therapy with the older adult: practice and research. In: MacLennan BW, Saul S, Weiner MB, eds. *Group Psychotherapies for the Elderly.* Madison, CT: International Universities Press; 1988;3–32.

80. Knight BG, McCallum TJ. Psychotherapy with older adult families: the contextual, cohort-based maturity/specific challenge model. In: Nordhus IH, VandenBos GR, Berg S, Fromholt P, eds. *Clinical Geropsychology.* Washington, DC: American Psychological Association; 1998;313–328.

81. Teri L, Logsdon RG, Uomoto J, McCurry SM. Behavioral treatment of depression in dementia patients: a controlled clinical trial. *J Gerontol B Psychol Sci Soc Sci.* 1997;52B(4):P159–P166.

82. Kasl-Godley J, Gatz M. Psychosocial intervention for individuals with dementia: an integration of theory, therapy, and a clinical understanding of dementia. *Clin Psychol Rev Special Issue: Assessment and Treatment of Older Adults.* 2000;20(6): 755–782.

83. Solomon K, Szwabo P. Psychotherapy for patients with dementia. In: Morley JE, Coe RM, Strong R, Grossberg GT, eds. *Memory Function and Aging-Related Disorders.* New York: Springer Publishing Co; 1992;295–319.

84. Reichlin RE. Integrated group approaches with the early stage Alzheimer's patient and family. In: Duffy M, ed. *Handbook of Counseling and Psychotherapy with Older Adults.* New York: John Wiley & Sons; 1999;166–181.

85. Fisher JE, Harsin CW, Hayden JE. Behavior interventions for patients with dementia. In: Molinari V, ed. *Professional Psychology in Long Term Care.* New York: Hatherleigh Press; 2000;179–200.

86. Schonfeld L, Cairl R, Cohen D, Neal KK, Watson MA, Westerhof C. The Florida Care College: a training program for long-term-care staff working with memory-impaired residents. *Journal of Mental Health & Aging.* 1999;5(2):187–199.

87. Bourgeois MS, Dijkstra K, Burgio LD, Allen RS. Communication skills training for nursing aides of residents with dementia: the impact of measuring performance. *Clin Gerontol.* 2003;27(1–2): 119–138.

88. Ponce-Burgos H, Kunik ME. Conducting a medical and psychiatric assessment. In: Molinari V, ed. *Professional Psychology in Long Term Care.* New York: Hatherleigh Press; 2000.

89. Duffy M. Individual therapy in long term care. In: Molinari V, ed. *Professional Psychology in Long Term Care: A Comprehensive Guide.* New York: Hatherleigh Press; 2000;73–89.

90. Rosowsky E, Smyer MA. Personality disorders and the difficult nursing home resident. In: Rosowsky E, Abrams RC, Zweig RA, eds. *Personality Disorders in Older Adults: Emerging Issues in Diagnosis and Treatment.* Mahwah, New Jersey: Lawrence Erlbaum and Associates; 1999;257–274.

91. Zarit SH, Knight BG, eds. *A Guide to Psychotherapy and Aging: Effective Clinical Interventions in a Life-Stage Context.* Washington, DC: American Psychological Association; 1996.

92. Duffy M, ed. *Handbook of Counseling and Psychotherapy with Older Adults.* New York: John Wiley & Sons; 1999.

93. Molinari V, ed. *Professional Psychology in Long Term Care: A Comprehensive Guide.* New York: Hatherleigh Press; 2000.

94. Knight BG, Nordhus IH, Satre DD. Psychotherapy with older adults. In: Stricker G, Widiger TA, eds. *Handbook of Psychology: Clinical Psychology,* vol. 8. New York: John Wiley and Sons, Inc; 2003;453–468.

95. Williams JW Jr, Barrett J, Oxman T, et al. Treatment of dysthymia and minor depression in primary care: a randomized controlled trial in older adults. *JAMA.* 2000;284(12):1519–1526.

Pharmacotherapy in the Elderly

14

Gabe J. Maletta

RATIONAL APPROACH TO OPTIMUM PHARMACOLOGICAL TREATMENT

Treatment of elderly patients with medication (commonly referred to as drugs) is a complex undertaking. Patients in late-life, particularly when frail, are significantly more sensitive to drug effects, including adverse events, than their younger counterparts. A major cause for this increased sensitivity is the pharmacokinetic and pharmacodynamic changes that occur normally as one ages, often exacerbated by a variety of illnesses, e.g., hepatic, gastrointestinal (GI), cardiovascular (CV), renal, endocrine, diabetes, and other metabolic diseases (1,2).

Many factors affect drug use and are obstacles to optimum care. This includes interactions—particularly with other drugs; poor adherence (formerly called compliance), often due to decreased cognitive function; complicated drug regimens; poor instruction, education and follow-up by clinicians; decreased motivation; and co-morbid diseases.

Drug use is further complicated by the vast number of elderly that rely on them for treatment of multiple chronic diseases and associated acute illnesses (80% of people over 65 have at least one chronic disease, compared to 40% under 65). At least one prescription drug is used by 75 to 90% of today's elderly. The number of drugs used increases with aging and women take more drugs than men at all ages. Twenty years ago, when 10% of the U.S. population was over age 65, they used about 25% of all prescription drugs (3). Today, about 13% are over 65 and use 35 to 39% of all prescription drugs, with the over-85 sub-group ("frail elderly"—the fastest growing and most at-risk) using the most drugs (4). An elderly person may take eight to 14 drugs daily, not including those over-the-counter (OTC)

(5). The specific number, type, and access are based on the living situation: community, hospital, or long-term-care (LTC)—which includes assisted living facilities (ALFs), nursing homes (NHs), and dementia units. By 2030, "baby boomers" (those born in 1946 to 1964) will swell the 65+ group to over 20% (about 70 million) and the number of drugs used will be enormous.

In 1980, more than 50% of the federal health-care dollar was spent on the elderly, with a major portion for drugs (3). Medicare—the health insurance program for seniors—will add a prescription drug benefit in 2006, at a huge cost over the next 30 years (6).

Overall, more than 75% of residents in many LTC facilities receive four or more drugs daily, most commonly: central nervous system (CNS) drugs; CV drugs; GI drugs; analgesics; and vitamins (7–11). For example, a small percentage (5%) over age 65 live in NHs, where the average daily number of routinely scheduled drugs per patient is six, and one-third take seven to 10. NH residents using nine or more daily prescription drugs increased from 18% in 1987 to 27% in 2000 (7,12,13).

About 75% of NH residents receive psychotropic drugs (or, more clinically accurate, *psychotherapeutic* drugs). In 1987, an amendment to a federal budget bill—the Omnibus Budget Reconciliation Act (OBRA)—defined strict indicators in NHs for prescribing and dosing psychotropics, particularly the antipsychotics, plus close monitoring and attempts at weaning (14). This was done due to cost and the perception that the drugs were often used as *chemical restraints*; over time, it has resulted in more appropriate use of some psychotropics in this population (6,15).

Other reasons for the disproportionate share of drugs used by elderly are subtle, such as the prescribing habits of clinicians (often primary care physicians and nurse practitioners, who see the bulk of elderly patients); psychosocial issues (e.g., living alone—sometimes with mild-to-moderate cognitive impairment); or the newest (i.e., direct-to-consumer drug advertising now rampant on television, radio, and in print).

Prescribers may have limited drug expertise specific to the elderly. Also, there is a dearth of this information in the clinical literature despite an explosion of knowledge, making it difficult for a clinician to choose the optimum drug in a class, or even the best class to treat a particular older patient. Clinical trials of new drugs seldom include the elderly, especially the over-85 group (5); and inferences about treatment are still derived with evidence from studies done in younger groups. Empirically derived data is growing, but is still minimal compared to young and middle-aged patients.

Age alone is an unreliable criterion on which solely to base drug treatment. The elderly exhibit a unique physiology, i.e., a disparity in functional capability of organs within an individual, as well as in the same organ system compared among multiple elderly. Often, there is greater functional variation among individual same-aged elderly than there are differences between young and old cohorts. Given this diversity and lack of specific drug data, an important concept is *biotitration*. Biotitration is individualizing drug choice, dose, route, and time of administration, and length of treatment for *each* elderly patient, rather than using a general concept that subsumes all elderly. Further, the multiple chronic and acute diseases that randomly occur in same-aged elderly make biotitration even more necessary (16).

Because of these complexities, drug use in the elderly certainly requires "special care" (17). Many psychotropic drugs have been introduced in the past 10 years, so the need to insure continuing safe and effective treatment is essential. When used appropriately, drugs can result in improved functioning and overall quality of life for older patients and their caregivers, be they family or professional (4).

The chapter will emphasize psychotropics in the elderly and will cover basic physiologic principles of pharmacotherapy. Discussion of practical issues will help achieve ongoing benefit, while minimizing problems of management in these complex patients—one person at a time. Underconsidered drug issues particularly relevant to the elderly will be discussed, including the use of psychotherapy, psychosocial and environmental approaches, and dealing with treatment resistance.

The chapter will not discuss specific treatment modalities for each psychiatric disorder. It will not cover a variety of important anatomic and physiologic concepts related to pharmacotherapy (e.g., specifics of CNS neurotransmitter functioning); novel neuromessengers, (e.g., nitric oxide); signal transduction at the sensory receptor; membrane receptor physiology; and second messenger biochemistry and function. Although integral to the clinical responses of all patients, these topics are not practical here, and little is known regarding changes with aging.

General Principles

Use all nonpharmacologic treatment approaches first may seem incongruous in a chapter about pharmacotherapy, but a key issue is whether drug use for a specific presentation is the correct decision.

Nondrug treatment may be the most appropriate approach for the presenting problem (see Table 14-1 for strategies with dementia patients). There are a limited number of psychiatric presentations—singly, or in combination—that are potentially amenable to effective drug treatment, despite the wide variety of behavioral and psychological signs and symptoms seen, particularly in elderly demented patients (see Table 14-2).

TABLE 14-1
SELECTED NON-MEDICATION STRATEGIES FOR TREATMENT OF BPSD

1. Sensory	Music; video or audio-tapes; massage; light touch; familiar smells; tastes
2. Physical and Environmental	A calm safe, structured environment; increase in "personal space"; minimize disruptive, inciting or aggravating stimuli (includes television and human); special-care units with increased structure, appropriate activities, and adequate staffing; optimize lighting and other physical components.
3. Behavioral	Psychotherapy, including *ongoing* supportive (individualized to specific patient); reinforcing alternative behaviors; positive reinforcement; behavioral modeling; validating emotions (empathy); re-direction (verbal/physical); substitution (words, objects); rescue strategy (another staff); re-approach; re-focus attention; reassurance; use of common sense.
4. Communication	Attempt to understand what the behavior is communicating; maximize positive individual psychosocial factors; caregiver awareness of his/her verbal/nonverbal interpersonal communication skills (nonthreatening approach and voice, eye contact, facial expression, touch).
5. Family and Staff Support and Education	Regular family care-conferences and meetings; ongoing support classes and in-services (all staff); written materials and handouts; referral to local support groups; referral to geriatrics experts.

BPSD, behavioral and psychological signs/symptoms of dementia.

TABLE 14-2

SELECTED SIGNS AND SYMPTOMS[a] USUALLY AMENABLE TO APPROPRIATE PSYCHOTROPIC MEDICATION TREATMENT

1. **Psychotic**
   - Disorganized thoughts/speech
   - Delusions causing psychic distress
   - Paranoia
   - Hallucinations causing psychic distress
   - Bizarre, repetitive, or pressured activity
2. **Depressive**
   - Sadness, helplessness
   - Vegetative signs
   - Withdrawal
   - Anger, anxiety
   - Apathy, guilt
   - Dyshedonia, anhedonia
   - Hopelessness, despair
   - Psychosis with or without delusions
3. **Anxiety**
   - Verbal/physical restlessness, unfocused fear, irritability, pressure
   - Nervousness, worry, anger, fidgety
   - Depressive signs
   - Physical signs (nausea, diarrhea; dyspnea, pain, phobia)
4. **Agitation**—episodic
   - Wandering that is pressured or otherwise distressful (initiation or exacerbation)
   - Increased disorientation (especially late afternoon)
5. **Aggression/Assaultive**—episodic or chronic
   - General inappropriate anger often associated with activities/cares (often catastrophic)
   - Focused anger at caregivers, other residents, family, or self
6. **Insomnia**
   - Physical or verbal (i.e., night-time wandering or frequently calling for caregivers)
   - Interrupted sleep, early awakening, excessive daytime naps
   - Morning headaches or fatigue

[a]These behavioral and psychological signs and symptoms are often co-morbid in individual elderly patients.

Every drug has a value, i.e., a ratio of potential clinical benefit (effectiveness in alleviating symptoms) to risk (including safety, tolerability, side effects [SE], interactions, and financial cost). This is described by the equation:

$$\text{Value} = \frac{\text{Benefit}}{\text{Risk}}$$

This classic cost-benefit analysis strategy, ideally evidenced-based, can assist in decisions regarding drug treatment. If the value of a drug is highly positive or negative, there is no debate about use. A problem arises when the value in a particular elderly patient approaches *one*; at that moot point, judgment based on clinical experience becomes relevant, keeping in mind that individual patient response is significantly dependent on multiple, age-related physiological and pathological changes. The ultimate decision about drug use also should consider other factors (i.e., assessment of the patient's degree of emotional distress and functional disabil-ity) and weighing the potential hazards of not treating relative to the probable success of treatment. If drug treatment is chosen, an ongoing monitoring system is an essential component of effective management. Additional guidelines have been compiled that may facilitate drug use, particularly in geriatric patients (see Table 14-3).

Specific Principles

Changes in Physiologic Systems with Aging

With a drug, a relationship exists between its concentration at an effector organ and its beneficial or adverse effects. This relationship is called clinical therapeutics, which connects to basic drug research via the bridge of clinical pharmacology. In the elderly, this bridge can assist the practicing clinician by demonstrating the diversity of drug responses and better defining pertinent concentration and response relationships. This quantitative method helps optimize the individualization of drug treatment by focusing on the physiologic changes known to occur with aging (4,16).

A gradual and progressive decline in performance occurs, even taking into account the diversity and the presence of multiple chronic diseases (18). Fundamental aging can occur at the cellular and subcellular level and physiological changes perhaps represent a molecular disorder, compromising the internal milieu and leading to loss of cell function (19). Also, old cells in general are more vulnerable to pathology than are young cells for as yet unclear reasons (L. Hayflick, personal communication, 2005). There are implications for such changes to impact, either directly or indirectly, on the essential kinetic and dynamic parameters involved with drug use, due to their relative impact on the organ systems involved.

Important changes occur in transporting an appropriate concentration of drug to its site of action (CNS cell membranes in the case of psychotropics), as well as in the ability of membrane receptors to respond appropriately. Detailing these pharmacokinetic and pharmacodynamic changes will help clarify the unique clinical responses of elderly patients.

Pharmacokinetics and Pharmacodynamics

Pharmacokinetics (movement of drugs) is "what your body does to a drug"; pharmacodynamics (changes due to drugs) is "what a drug does to your body." Defined more physiologically, pharmacokinetics is achieving an effective *concentration* of an administered drug with its *specific* pharmacologic *activity* at its site of action (biophase). Pharmacodynamics is the *affinity* of a drug for its particular end-organ *receptor* at the biophase, and the receptors ability to *respond* appropriately, based on number (density) and sensitivity (affinity), at a given point in time. There is a direct relationship between receptor effect and drug concentration; thus, kinetics and dynamics are integrally related.

TABLE 14-3

GUIDELINES FOR TREATING GERIATRIC PATIENTS WITH MEDICATIONS

1. Evaluate patient's present medical/environmental conditions.
2. Establish a therapeutic goal with/for the patient. Clarify specific target signs/symptoms to be alleviated. If possible, ascertain specific cause(s).
3. Review previous treatments and responses.
4. Take a *comprehensive* drug history (prescription, OTC, nutritional supplements, herbals, social, shared, street) for concomitant use (usual in elderly) that may contraindicate new drug choice. Ask about previous adverse SE. Ask about use of alcohol, tobacco, caffeine, and special diets. Ask about other prescribers (communicate with them if possible).
5. Use all nonpharmacologic treatment strategies first. Discontinuing a drug is often better than starting a new one, especially where no diagnosis is clear.
6. Tailor drug class selection and treatment regimen to the specific target signs and symptoms and the specific patient (e.g., a patient with delusional anxiety secondary to dementia who also has Parkinson Disease).
7. Identify physiologic ambience and specific medical conditions of a particular patient that may contraindicate a specific drug choice (drug-system or drug-disease interactions). Be sure to *ask* about allergies (or sensitivities).
8. Select drug based on SE profile (anticholinergic, somnolence, hypotensive and EPS are most common); or select based on previous efficacy in a particular patient. Do not use unless the potential benefit is significantly greater than the potential risk (SE; price).
9. Be familiar with pharmacologic activity, major SE, and toxicity profile of each drug used—prior to using it. Consider possible interactions with drugs already being taken.
10. Consider individual patient pharmacokinetics, pharmacodynamics, and overall decrease in homeostasis with aging when weighing dose versus potential for SE (biotitration).
11. Initiate treatment with low dose and await time to reach steady-state T_{ss} levels before changing dose. Only titrate on basis of drug tolerability and response. Insure that dose is high enough and length of treatment adequate enough to be effective, while continuously monitoring for SE. Achieve MED necessary to obtain desired clinical effect.
12. Use least number of drugs possible. Use one drug to treat more than one sign when possible (e.g., depression and anxiety). Careful polypharmacy is appropriate if clinically justified by complementary actions (and well documented). Remain alert to potential for untoward reactions. Discontinue drugs no longer needed or nonefficacious. Avoid using one drug to treat SE of another. Avoid combination drugs or using multiple drugs from same class.
13. Simplify dosing regimen to enhance adherence (compliance). Once a day is optimum if $T_{1/2}$ and SE allow. Use follow-up (phone calls) to encourage adherence, especially early in the treatment of outpatients.
14. Educate patient, family, and staff about each drug, the therapeutic goal, its planned regimen, potential major SE and/or interactions, and its cost. Provide written instructions when possible.
15. Monitor therapeutic efficacy of drug over time and before prescribing a new one. Add or change one drug at a time, which helps clarify the source of improvement, nonefficacy, or SE. Make use of plasma levels (where readily available), when considering adherence or absorption problems.
16. Consider liquid, rapid-PO-dissolving, or even long-acting IM therapy in patients who do not respond well to standard PO administration (adherence, resistance, dysphagia, or absorption issues). Be alert to potential for enhanced SE (e.g., postural hypotension with some drugs), if IM route is used.
17. Gradually decrease dose of effective drugs over time with goal of eventually discontinuing drug if behavior and safety allow. Observe patient and restart drug only if necessary.
18. PRN psychotropics may be useful on a time-limited or temporary basis, primarily for determining need for a scheduled dosage, e.g., for pain, anxiety. (Monitor frequency of all PRN drugs used by trusted staff and quantify changes in target signs). Comprehensively explain on order sheet (or computerized order entry) the reason for prescribing PRN. Discontinue PRN drugs not being used.
19. Do not withhold drugs simply on basis of patient's advanced age when they may improve quality of life or level of distress.
20. Understand that medications do not always work. Be familiar with usual percentage of effectiveness for particular drugs, if available, and communicate to *all* those involved.
21. Document *all* medication activities. Write a brief progress note *before* writing drug order (not simply noting "dictation to follow").

EPS, extrapyramidal symptoms; IM, intramuscular; MED, minimum effective dose; OTC, over-the-counter; PO, oral; PRN, as required; SE, side effects; $T_{1/2}$, half-life; T_{ss}, steady-state.

Pharmacokinetics

There are four pharmacokinetic variables: absorption, distribution, metabolism, and excretion. Understanding changes due to aging and their clinical implications and relevance is necessary to insure effective drug treatment (20,21) (see Figure 14-1 and Table 14-4).

Absorption. In normal elderly, a range of oral absorptive ability occurs—including no absorption. There is little evidence of diminished nutrient absorption compared to younger individuals. Indeed, most elderly exhibiting low concentrations of vitamins and minerals do so because of poor preparation of food and reduced intake, or interactions with foods or drugs. Individual variability aside, oral absorption of drugs is minimally affected by aging, primarily because most are absorbed into circulation via passive diffusion.

Changes with aging occur in GI physiology that could, in theory, slow absorption (2,22). There is a mild decrease in saliva production. A decrease or absence of gastric acid

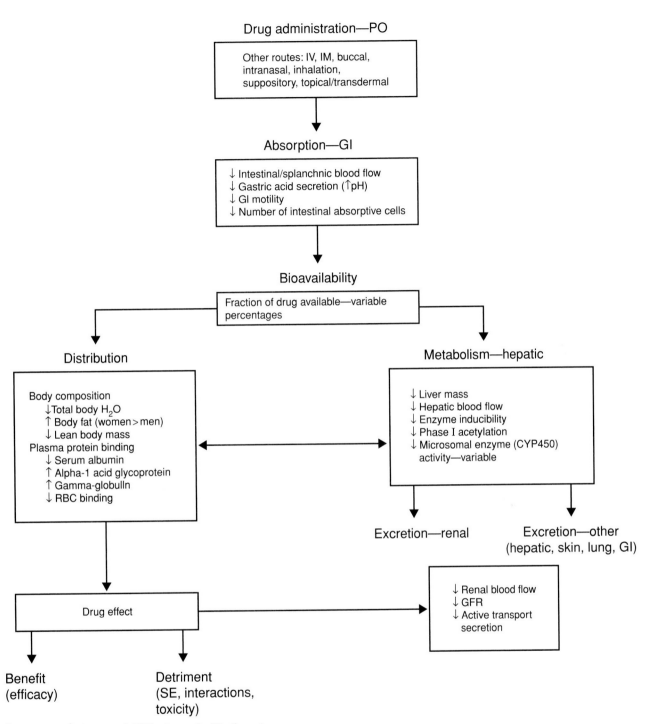

Figure 14-1 Pharmacokinetic aspects of normal physiological changes in the elderly.

production occurs, with a corresponding pH increase in the gut lumen and at villi absorption sites. Also, when acid-suppressive drugs are used in the elderly, they may exacerbate the slow disintegration and dissolution of tablets in GI fluids and the absorption of drugs that are weak acids in solution. With advanced age there is a substantial decrease in esophageal motility and decreased esophagogastric junction tone, a delay in gastric emptying, a slowed transit time in the small and large bowel due to mildly decreased motility, a substantial decrease in intestinal blood flow, and a loss of gastric and intestinal absorptive surface area secondary to villous atrophy. However, an enormous reserve absorptive capacity of small intestine mucosa exists in humans, which may minimize the

TABLE 14-4

CLINICAL RELEVANCE AND IMPLICATIONS OF PHARMACOKINETIC CHANGES IN ELDERLY

1. Absorption
- Unchanged passive diffusion—no change in bioavailability for most drugs
- Decreased dissolution and absorption rate for some drugs
- Drug-food or drug-drug interactions may alter absorption
- Decreased active transport and decreased bioavailability for some drugs
- Decreased first-pass effect and increased bioavailability for some drugs
- Delayed onset of effect

2. Distribution
- Water-soluble drugs have decreased VD and increased plasma concentration
- Lipid-soluble drugs have increased VD. There is delayed onset with subsequent accumulation
- Increased $T_{1/2}$
- Increased free (active) fraction of highly bound acidic drugs[a]
- Decreased free fraction of highly bound basic drugs[a]

3. Metabolism
- Decreased hepatic metabolism and clearance[b]
- Increased $T_{1/2}$ for some oxidatively metabolized drugs and those with high hepatic extraction ratios
- Lower doses may be therapeutic

4. Excretion
- Decreased renal clearance (parent drug and active metabolites)
- Increased $T_{1/2}$ of drugs eliminated via kidneys
- Serum creatinine not a reliable measure of kidney function. Use calculation for CrCl

[a]May have minimal or no clinical effect.
[b]Much influenced by environmental factors.
CrCl, creatinine clearance; $T_{1/2}$, half-life; VD, volume of distribution.

clinical significance of these changes. There is also a decrease in some pancreatic enzyme activity with aging, particularly trypsin.

Of more clinical relevance, for those drugs absorbed by facilitated diffusion or active transport across gut lipoprotein cell membranes, bioavailability (the percent of a drug that enters the systemic circulation after extravascular administration, and the rate at which the entry occurs) may be decreased in the elderly because of changes in pH and in calcium transport. The decrease in *first-pass* hepatic (or intestinal wall) drug extraction that occurs with aging can increase bioavailability for oral doses of some drugs (e.g., morphine, meperidine, and propranolol) (22).

Cross-sectionally, a large variation in serum levels can occur in a same-aged cohort after a single ingestion of the same dose of a drug (e.g., typical antipsychotics and tricyclic antidepressants [TCAs]) (23), which may affect response. This is because bioavailability is crucial to obtain a therapeutic effect. In aged patients, these data are lacking. However, disparity among absorption rates could produce accumulation or even unintentional overdosing in some elderly, due to dosing frequency, e.g., when patients or clinicians perceive that a drug is ineffective.

A practical tip: if no response occurs in a patient—either in symptoms or SE—even after considerable dose increases over time, a serum level may provide data on which to base

the next step in drug adjustment. Despite the limited value of serum levels in determining efficacy for all but a few psychotropics (lithium, valproic acid, carbamazepine, nortriptyline, and desipramine), levels can be of benefit in determining a cause for poor response. If a level is undetectable—or minimal—despite a high oral dose, absorption may be compromised. Insure first that lack of adherence is not an issue before instituting any changes. Consistency of blood-draw timing (at peak or trough levels) will help insure reliability of levels. Although costs vary, levels are available for many psychotropics (24), and are most useful in patients with poor nutritional status, multiple chronic diseases, or on multiple drugs (where competitive receptor-binding displacement or drug interactions may affect response).

Perhaps one in 20 elders has a drug absorption problem significant enough to interfere with treatment. If available, switching to a liquid, a rapidly dissolving oral pill, or even an injectable dosage form, may be beneficial for selected patients. Recently introduced drugs that are rapidly dissolved in buccal mucosa (such as Zyprexa Zydis, Risperdal M-tab, Fazaclo, Remeron Sol-tab, Niravam Rapi-tab, temazepam, and clonazepam wafer) provide little data in elderly. Neither do the *Intensols*, which refers to a few concentrated benzodiazepine liquids developed for use with patients on feeding tubes (they have not been widely used).

The effect of aging changes that occur on absorption from other sites—skin, skeletal muscle and rectum—is not well researched (such as with transdermal fentanyl) (6).

Besides absorption and age, additional factors may affect plasma concentration of some drugs, including: genetics, gender, concomitant medical conditions, smoking, nutrition, enzyme induction or inhibition, and clearance or metabolic inhibitors.

Distribution. Relative distribution of drugs may be altered with aging, due to normal changes in body composition, CV and cerebral blood flow, and drug-binding plasma proteins.

Body Composition
A relative decrease in lean body mass and a corresponding increase in body fat occur with aging (2,25). As a proportion of total body weight, which generally increases, the fat component increases from 15 to 45% (more so in women) from age 25 to age 75, except in the hands, face, and forearms. Lean mass decreases by 19% in men and 12% in women over the same period. Also, total body water decreases 15 to 25%—to about 50%—from age 20 to age 80; and extracellular volume decreases by 40% from age 20 to 65, with a mild increase after age 70 (3,26).

These alterations are important regarding drug activity and clinical effect because they change the *volume of distribution* for some drugs. Thus, the onset and duration of activity of a particular drug can be significantly impacted, depending on whether it is fat-soluble or water-soluble.

The *volume of distribution* of water-soluble (hydrophilic) drugs (e.g., lithium and morphine) is decreased, and is increased for fat-soluble (lipophilic) drugs, including most psychotropics. Increased distribution contributes to prolonging drug half-life, and changes in *volume of distribution* can directly affect loading doses of some drugs (e.g., digoxin, which should be reduced in elderly, especially in the presence of renal dysfunction) (6).

Cardiovascular and Cerebral Blood Flow
Cardiac output decreases linearly about 1% per year starting around age 30, decreasing about 30% by age 65, due to roughly equal changes in heart rate and stroke volume. Coronary vessel flow rates decrease about 0.5% per year after age 25. Organ-specific perfusion also decreases with normal aging, due to decreased blood flow, increased peripheral resistance, and decreased substance clearance. Little is known about in vivo changes in the integrity of the blood-brain barrier. These alterations in the body's primary delivery system result in a delay of drug arrival at its biophase, as well as a delayed removal, and may play a role in the observed activity of a drug, irrespective of prescribed dosage (3).

For psychotropics, the obvious place to observe effects of CV changes is the cerebral circulation, although it is unclear whether changes in cerebral blood flow have clinical relevance. There is a relatively mild but gradual decrease in rate of blood flow in the brain with aging, when comparing 27-year-olds with 68-year-olds (16). The significance is unknown, particularly in terms of oxygen uptake, because in decreased cerebral blood flow due to ischemia, a corresponding increase occurs in the arteriovenous oxygen difference. This indicates that more oxygen is extracted per unit of blood, compensating for the decreased flow.

Drug-Binding Plasma Proteins
Changes in protein-binding are important when a drug is started, the dosage changed (when it displaces other protein-bound drugs), or when plasma protein concentration changes. Plasma albumin concentration does not normally change with aging. However, frailty, malnutrition, cytokine excess, and some diseases—both chronic and acute—may result in a substantial albumin decrease.

Most psychotropics are highly bound to albumin (90% or more for typical neuroleptics). Decreases in albumin can lead to a reduced binding of acidic drugs (e.g., warfarin, phenytoin, and naproxen), which increases *free drug concentration*—that is, the active fraction that crosses membranes into cells—thereby enhancing its pharmacologic effect.

Because the free-fraction of a drug is usually smaller than the bound fraction, normal mechanisms of metabolism and excretion ultimately eliminate the free drug. An increase in the free-drug fraction does not cause an increase in its steady-state plasma concentration (which depends on dose rate and clearance, as well as the drug's saturation kinetics). This suggests a compensatory mechanism for enhancing clearance rate (27). If drug clearance is slowed (as with aging or disease), a relative increase in the free fraction of some drugs may cause a corresponding increase in the intensity of its clinical action and potential for toxicity (e.g., phenytoin, warfarin, and digoxin).

The concentration of alpha-1-acid glycoprotein (α-1-AG), an acute-phase reactant protein that carries basic drugs, is unchanged or rises with aging (28). Increases in plasma α-1-AG (which occurs due to chronic inflammatory disease, heart attack, burns or cancer) leads to an increase in protein binding—and therefore a decrease in free fraction—of basic drugs (e.g., propranolol and TCAs). Because these changes are not large, their clinical relevance is uncertain. The significance of increased gamma globulin and decreased red-blood-cell-binding capacity seen with aging is unknown.

Because of the large number of drugs taken concomitantly by the elderly, a variable displacement of drug binding may occur due to competition for the relatively limited number of membrane receptor sites. Changes in binding may be clinically insignificant and do not imply an altered pharmacologic effect, providing there is no compromise in excretion pathways (27), although plasma drug level measurement becomes more difficult to interpret because most measure total drug concentration (bound plus free). If in doubt, obtaining a free drug level is recommended.

TABLE 14-5

SELECTED INDUCERS[a] AND INHIBITORS[b] OF P450 ISOENZYME ACTIVITY THAT MAY AFFECT PSYCHOTROPICS[c]

CYP1A2[d]	CYP2C 19	CYP2D6	CYP3A4[d]
Inducers	**Inducers**	**Inducers[e]**	**Inducers**
Carbamazepine	Carbamazepine	None known	Carbamazepine
Char-broiled beef	Phenobarbitol		Glucocorticoids
Cruciferous			
vegetables	Phenytoin		Phenobarbitol
Phenobarbitol			Phenytoin
Phenytoin			St. John's Wort
Smoking			
Inhibitors	**Inhibitors**	**Inhibitors**	**Inhibitors**
? Fluoxetine	Fluoxetine	Bupropion	Erythromycin
Fluvoxamine	Fluvoxamine	Celecoxib	Fluoxetine
Paroxetine	Sertraline	Fluoxetine	? Fluvoxamine
? Sertraline	Valproic acid	Paroxetine	Grapefruit juice
		? Sertraline	Haloperidol
		Valproic acid	Ketoconazole
			Nefazodone
			Nifedipine
			? Paroxetine
			? Sertraline

[a]Inducers increase the capacity of rate of activity of the enzyme to metabolize the substrate and potentially decrease therapeutic effect by changing the blood level.
[b]Inhibitors decrease the capacity or prevent the enzyme from metabolizing the substrate, and potentially increase the risk for therapeutic failure or toxicity.
[c]Some interactions presently have in-vivo or in-vitro documentation, while others are theoretical, as this field rapidly evolves.
[d]Most inducible
[e]2D6 (and 2C) activity are genetically determined and not inducible (7–10% of Caucasians have relatively limited 2D6 activity and are considered "poor metabolizers").
? = questionable clinical significance.

Metabolism. Although several body sites (such as GI and kidneys) contain metabolic enzymes, the liver is the primary site of action. Most data in the elderly involve changes in liver function, which, of all organs, is least affected by aging. A gradual decrease in both liver mass and blood flow occurs beginning in one's mid 30s (29). By age 65, blood flow may be 45% less than at age 25, mostly due to the significant decrease in cardiac output (2,16). Its effect on specific drug metabolism is unpredictable (e.g., blood flow changes may reduce clearance of TCAs and other high hepatic-extraction psychotropics).

Although there is no overall age-dependent decrease in cell function, changes do occur in hepatic enzyme activity integral to optimum metabolism or detoxification of both endogenous and exogenous substrates. Drug metabolism occurs via two major pathways: Phase I and/or Phase II. Phase I are primarily oxidation reactions (reduction and hydrolysis are other, less-studied pathways). Oxidation reactions involve dealkylation, hydroxylation, oxidation, deamination, desulphuration, and sulfoxide formation. Most of the reactions are mediated by multiple cytochrome monooxygenase (microsomal) enzymes—the P450 (CYP)

system. The CYP enzymes are composed of 12 or more enzymes of varying clinical interest and importance, and are found primarily in the liver, as well as in smaller quantities in the GI tract, kidney, and lung. These enzymes are affected differentially by age and genetics. Some are clinically relevant because their activity can be induced or inhibited by multiple factors, including a variety of drugs—both prescribed and OTC—and thus can affect metabolism of other drugs (6,30) (see Table 14-5). These interactions are most clinically relevant in drugs with a narrow therapeutic margin (31). Other factors (such as alcohol, smoking, race, gender, frailty, and certain foods) have varying amounts of influence over hepatic metabolism of drugs.

Many psychotropics (e.g., most neuroleptics—both typical and atypical; some cholinesterase inhibitors [ChEI]; most TCAs; benzodiazepines; selective serotonin reuptake inhibitors; valproate; tegretol; and β-blockers) are metabolized by CYP enzymes. Those isoenzymes relatively most involved are: IA2, 2D6, and 3A4 (see Table 14-6). Some psychotropics are metabolized via multiple CYP enzymes, with one usually most prominent, e.g., aripiprazole via

TABLE 14-6

SELECTED PSYCHOTROPIC SUBSTRATES[a] BY P450 ISOENZYME ACTIVITY[b]

CYP1A2	CYP2D6	CYP3A4
Caffeine	Aripiprazole	Alprazolam
Clozapine	Codeine	Buspirone
Olanzapine	Desipramine	Carbamazepine
	Haloperidol	Clonazepam
	Paroxetine	Codeine
	Risperidone	Diazepam
	Thioridazine	Fluoxetine
	Venlafaxine	Nefazodone
		Quetiapine
		Some TCAs
		Trazodone
		Triazolam
		Ziprasidone

[a]Medications primarily metabolized by the isoenzyme.
[b]Most information is obtained from in-vitro metabolic studies in human liver microsomes.
TCAs, tricyclic antidepressants.

2D6(3A4); ziprasodone via 3A4(1A2); olanzapine via 1A2(2D6); clozapine via 1A2(3A4); donepezil and galantamine via 2D6(3A4).

Some theorize the age-related decrease seen in Phase-I metabolism may be more related to the diminished number of hepatocytes than to a specific decrease in enzymatic activity (32). Overall, the decreased metabolism contributes to an increased half-life of some drugs, such as some benzodiazepines, TCAs, L-dopa, propranolol, and morphine (6).

Phase-II metabolism—a separate pathway, not necessarily a continuation of Phase I—involves a group of conjugative or synthetic enzymatic reactions, where an alteration of the drug molecule enhances its water solubility and polarity, thus making the drug available for renal excretion. The major reactions involved are via glucuronide and sulfate conjugation, acetylation, or with an amino acid. Importantly, Phase-II reactions are generally unchanged with aging (except for glucuronidation, which is sensitive to caloric and protein restriction and thus may not always be unchanged) (33). Therefore, use of drugs metabolized by Phase-II pathways generally is recommended for elderly.

In hepatic disease, use of psychotropics is complex. Drugs metabolized by the liver can be highly or poorly extracted from blood, the rate primarily depending on dissociation from protein binding—whether the metabolism is Phase I or II. Highly extracted drugs (e.g., short-acting barbiturates) are dependent on blood flow as well as hepatocyte function and have reduced clearance in all hepatic disease. However, poorly extracted drugs are generally not problematic despite reduced hepatic blood flow if the

remaining hepatocytes are still functioning relatively well (such as in cirrhosis). Metabolism of different poorly extracted drugs varies with acute or chronic hepatitis, and with which pathways are involved. For example, benzodiazepines can generally be used in cirrhosis, but not in hepatitis. However, lorazepam, oxazepam, and temazepam—metabolized via Phase-II glucuronidation—are generally safe even in chronic hepatitis. Diazepam, clonazepam, chlordiazepoxide, and others metabolized via Phase-I pathways should not be used in acute hepatitis (34).

Excretion (Elimination; Clearance). Drugs are excreted from the body primarily by kidneys (and also by liver, lungs, skin, and breast). A gradual decline occurs in renal mass with aging, reaching 45% by age 80, due to a decreased number and size of nephrons. A gradually accelerating decline occurs in renal blood flow, glomerular filtration rate, and active renal tubular secretion. Creatinine clearance (CrCl) (effectively the same as glomerular filtration rate and therefore a valid measure of renal function), may decrease 30% to 40% between ages 35 and 80 (35), primarily due to decreased cardiac output and overall narrowing of renal vessels. A healthy 20-year-old filters 180 liters of plasma per day compared to 120 liters by a 70-year-old.

Exemplifying their disparity, about 33% of healthy elders have no decrease in CrCl over time and presumably no loss of kidney function. Further, when glomerular filtration rate does decrease, it may not do so at the same rate of decline as the active transport mechanism involved in renal tubular secretion (36). Same-aged gender differences occur in clearance of some drugs, with women generally tending toward increased plasma levels compared to men, although olanzapine clearance can be 30% greater in women, thereby decreasing the plasma level at the same dose. It is unknown whether this difference occurs in elderly patients. Age may be a factor with quetiapine clearance, which may be 40% less in aged than young patients.

Although CrCl is a useful measure to evaluate renal function, it has been impractical particularly in some LTC settings because it historically involved collection of a valid 24-hour urine sample. CrCl now can be calculated from an abbreviated, timed urine collection and use of a computer program that extrapolates to 24 hours.

Measuring serum creatinine (sCr) alone to evaluate renal function in normal elderly is imprecise because, although skeletal muscle—from which creatinine is derived—decreases with aging, sCr does not usually decrease (35,37). Because the glomerular filtration rate decrease seen in two-thirds of elderly balances the decreased creatinine production, sCr levels generally remain unchanged. This is clinically important due to the potential for overdose of drugs (e.g., digoxin preparations and some antibiotics) excreted primarily by kidneys that require adjustment to compensate for decreased renal function. The Cockroft-Gault equation can be used to grossly calculate CrCl (38):

$$\text{CrCl (men)} \atop \text{(ml/min)} = \frac{(140\text{-age in years}) \times (\text{body weight in kg})}{72 \times \text{sCr (mg/dL)}}$$

(multiply result by 0.85 for women)

Renal function changes with aging are most important because they can result in a reduction in clearance of many drugs and, importantly, their active metabolites. Thus, the potential exists for adverse clinical consequences for drugs with a narrow margin between therapeutic and toxic levels (e.g., lithium) (2,6).

Pharmacodynamics

Compared to the changes in kinetics with aging, there are much less reproducible data available for changes in pharmacodynamics, which is the study of cell-membrane receptor structure and function. Pharmacodynamics is the integral relationship between clinical effect (onset and duration of action, potency and efficacy) and drug concentration.

There are multiple molecular receptors on neural membranes that are activated via structurally specific portions of various CNS neurotransmitters or drugs. When activated, these receptors alter membrane ionic permeability, causing neural excitation or inhibition. Age-related physiological changes—as well as those caused by disease—may alter receptor function. Sensitivity may decrease, increase, or remain unchanged. This can cause complex alterations at multiple levels (including the molecular), eventually manifested at the person level, and affect the body's ability to maintain homeostasis (39).

Receptor changes can produce less predictable or altered drug responses, even at the usual low doses suggested for the elderly. In theory, this could have benefits (e.g., prolonged pain relief with morphine at lower-than-expected doses), or it may be detrimental (e.g., less pain relief with morphine; altered sensitivity to the effects of β-blockers (40); somnolence; and postural instability with some psychotropics). Other factors, such as drug interactions and disease, confound the situation and may further alter the expected response.

Altered Receptor Sensitivity. Drug-receptor binding is characterized by specificity, saturability, and reversibility. Changes in drug response may be due to receptor sensitivity, number or structural change, a combination of factors, or may occur at the postreceptor (second messenger) level (16). In the elderly, clinically significant pharmacodynamic changes vary. Such variations include lithium efficacy at lower serum levels; an increased sensitivity to benzodiazepines, traditional neuroleptics, dopamine agonists, and opioids; a decreased sensitivity at β-adrenergic receptors (with both agonists and blockers); and in α-2 adrenergic responses (2,39,40). Elderly often have an increased sensitivity to the development of SE, such as anticholinergic (antiChE) SE via altered acetylcholine (ACh) receptor function, and extrapyramidal symptoms (EPS) via dopamine receptors in nigrostriatum. Paradoxical reactions also may occur (e.g., significant anxiety with small doses of benzodiazepines) and may not be related to pharmacodynamics.

The complexities at the neuroreceptor and postreceptor levels, and the variable end-organ capacity to respond remain to be elucidated. At present, poor reliability exists for predicting sensitivity problems in specific elderly, which highlights the need to always individualize drug dosages.

Homeostasis. Homeostasis, described in 1859 by the great physiologist, Claude Bernard (41), is the body's ability to maintain internal physiologic uniformity by adapting with appropriate speed and vigor to marked environmental changes, whether external or internal (42). This beneficial response to daily life challenges is also called allostasis (43). Mediation of this adaptation—an integral part of which is receptor activity—occurs primarily via fast-response neural systems (CNS and autonomic), and slower-response endocrine and immunologic systems; as well as occuring via many chemical mediators, e.g., glucocorticoids, catecholamines, and cytokines. These complex mechanisms are involved when the body adjusts to, or tries to counteract, the effects of a particular drug. However, physiologic mediators that are adaptive in the short-term may actually become damaging over time, perhaps at the membrane receptor level.

Decreased function with aging and disease (including chronic inflammation), gradually alters the effectiveness of the mechanisms responsible for maintaining homeostasis, particularly the *rate* of return to normal after a stress (44). Alterations can lead to multiple problems in various systems, including baroreceptor and chemoreceptor responses; autonomic nervous system dysfunction; circulatory control; impaired thermoregulation; smooth muscle response; immunosenescence; reduced cerebral cortical functional reserve during stress and cognitive dysfunction; impaired postural and gait stability; glucose intolerance; and perhaps even mood disorders (6,18,45). Response to drugs also can be negatively affected by adaptive dysfunction and lead to multiple SE (e.g., orthostasis and falls due to CV effects, CNS and peripheral antiChE changes, and hypothermia), all of which occur at lower doses and serum levels than in younger patients.

Half-Life and Steady State

Half-Life ($T_{1/2}$)

Due to reduced blood flow to liver and kidneys, changes in volume of distribution (VD), and alterations in liver metabolism and renal clearance, a drug's half-life ($T_{1/2}$) is often markedly increased in an elderly patient. $T_{1/2}$ is integral to drug concentration in the blood, and is a dependent parameter, based on an inverse relationship between the VD and renal clearance (Cl), i.e.,

$$T_{1/2} = \frac{VD}{Cl} \times 0.693 \text{ (constant)}$$

This relationship helps clarify the increased $T_{1/2}$ seen in elderly patients, irrespective of dosage. Because Cl is a key factor in determining rate of drug removal from the body, it is relevant to consider it when choosing initial dose, subsequent doses, and dosing schedules, especially because specific age difference in a drug's $T_{1/2}$ is rarely known, even in the healthy elderly (see Appendix A).

Clinically, in the elderly, it is difficult to quantify an optimum drug treatment plan. Therefore, a practical approach in order to minimize adverse SE is to assume a prolonged $T_{1/2}$ for all drugs in individual elderly, and initially to utilize lower doses—taking special caution in those with cardiac, hepatic, or renal disease.

Steady State

The complex interaction of the various physiologic systems previously described can be appreciated by the following equation for steady-state pharmacokinetics (46).

$$\overline{C}_{ss} = \frac{1.44 \times AD \times T_{1/2}}{VD \times di}$$

Where:

$\overline{C}_{ss}$ = average steady-state plasma concentration of the drug

AD = absorbed dose

$T_{1/2}$ = elimination half-life

VD = volume of distribution

di = dosage interval

1.44 = constant

C_{ss} is the point reached where the amount of drug entering the body equals the amount leaving (a dynamic equilibrium, or *flux*), within the periodicity of the peak–trough plasma levels, which is based on the *di*.

The numerator reveals that the concentration at steady state is directly proportional to the dose of the absorbed and bioavailable drug and also its $T_{1/2}$. The more drug absorbed, the greater its plasma concentration. Assuming a constant $T_{1/2}$, the denominator reveals that the average C_{ss} is inversely proportional to the VD and the di. The more frequently a drug is given (therefore a lower di), the higher the plasma concentration. Only two components of this equation—AD and di—are controllable by the patient or clinician (3).

Practically, changes in kinetics with aging or disease affect C_{ss} and influence psychotropic drug actions, e.g., if a decrease in clearance occurs, and the AD is constant and the time interval equally spaced, then the C_{ss} will increase, unless the dosage is decreased. If pharmacologic effects are related to its concentration, a clearance change can influence and alter drug action.

Knowing the time it takes for a particular drug to approximate steady-state (T_{ss}) gives the clinician data regarding the optimum time interval between dose changes (either titrating or tapering). About five times a

drug's $T_{1/2}$ approaches T_{ss}, assuming a constant dose and interval. A reasonable clinical approach is to wait until at least twice the T_{ss} has elapsed before making any change in dose. This tactic takes patience, as well as frequent observation of the patient for signs of effectiveness or SE.

Dose

Although age alone does not always indicate the need for dosage modification, there is good evidence that most elderly should be treated with reduced drug doses, both initially (usually one-half of the adult dose) and during incremental titration. This also holds for incremental decreases during a drug taper as part of a discontinuation strategy. The time interval between dosage changes should also be extended. Ideally, dosing should be biotitrated and continued to an effect.

Initially, taking individualized comprehensive drug histories is paramount because most elderly are already on multiple drugs, which can affect optimum dosage and effectiveness of a target drug. History should include not only information about past and present prescription drugs from all providers that the patient is seeing, but also OTC drugs. (OTC drugs are really *off-the-shelf*, rather than over-the-counter, as most of them are purchased in large multi-purpose stores, without pharmacy consultation, and now include postpatent prescription and some generic drugs, usually at lower doses). Those over age 65 use half of all OTC agents. Chronic OTC use may include drugs for: pain, GI symptoms, cough, colds, eyes, sleep, and vitamins. Common are shared drugs (with a relative or friend) for similar conditions (usually pain, GI, or sleep problems); and social drugs. Often overlooked are minerals and other *nutriceuticals*, herbals (phytomedicines), and special diets. All have potential for causing additive, synergistic, and frequently prolonged SE.

Over time, patients may amass drug sensitivities or allergies—real or questionable. Because this information may not be volunteered and can affect proper dose or use of drugs, patients or their caregivers should be questioned for specifics (47).

Multiple dosing factors must be considered for achieving individualized effectiveness, whether initially or during titration (see Table 14-7). In all cases, achieving the minimum effective dose is the goal.

Use of drugs with very long $T_{1/2}$ or with long-acting metabolites should be minimized (e.g., some benzodiazepines, some TCAs, older SSRIs, and typical antipsychotics). Although such drugs could, in theory, be dosed using long intervals, control of symptoms in this manner is difficult to achieve, and SE tend to be prolonged.

Most drugs exhibit *first-order* kinetics regarding dose; that is, a linear relationship exists between dose and plasma level. Some exhibit *zero-order* (saturation) kinetics; i.e., the linear relationship holds to a point, then a small dose increase causes a significant increase in plasma level (a *saturation curve*). Clinicians should be aware of this, due

TABLE 14-7

TABLE 14-7

CONSIDERATIONS FOR ACHIEVING EFFECTIVE DOSAGE IN ELDERLY PATIENTS

- Age
- Gender and race
- General appearance
- Body size and composition
- Mobility and activity
- Diet and habits (smoking, alcohol)
- Physiologic status (particularly CV, hepatic, renal)
- Presence of acute and chronic physical disease(s)
- Concomitant nonpsychotherapeutic medication use
- Concomitant psychotherapeutic medication use

CV, cardiovascular.

to the potential for unexpected and rapid onset or exacerbation of dose-dependent SE.

Underdosing is as problematic in the elderly as overmedicating. Clinicians should guard against the policy of starting a drug at the lowest possible dose and then not titrating to an effect, leaving the dose at the original, low level. Although the motto of geriatric psychiatry dosing has been "start low and go slow" (attributed to Leo Hollister, a geriatrician at Stanford who coined it in the 1960s), it is incomplete and can cause undertreatment because it views all elderly patients monistically. The statement is made more relevant by adding ". . . but insure an adequate dose, titration, and duration of treatment." This approach would minimize the partial (or no) treatment response seen on inadequate doses. Undertreatment is often seen in depressed and anxious patients, as well as those with chronic pain, particularly demented patients residing in LTC facilities—and not always in the dementia units. Undertreatment with ChEIs also occurs in patients with cognitive impairment, with a woefully small number receiving adequate doses of cognitive enhancing drugs, if any at all. Recent introduction of an n-methyl α-aspartate (NMDA) receptor antagonist adds another treatment option for demented patients. Geriatricians should provide ongoing education for staff and families about all these dosing issues.

Route and Time of Administration

Most drugs are given orally. In the elderly, this is not always the optimum route and may not even be possible for multiple reasons (including nonadherence, dysphagia, and resistance). In these situations, use of alternate dosage forms and routes of administration (such as a liquid version when available), may be useful. Rapidly dissolving oral wafers also can be effective, although older mucous membrane and skin can alter absorption rates and have variable local effects on metabolism. Intramuscular (IM) injection is another route, but chronic administration is not optimum, particularly for frail patients. IM antipsy-

chotics (ziprasidone; olanzapine) are available, as is a long-acting IM (risperidone) (48); however, the utility of present depot preparations remains to be seen in those elderly with dementia, due to dosing issues.

Most once-a-day drugs usually are given in the morning or at bedtime. Recent interest exists in administering some drugs based on the fluctuating daily circadian plasma levels of endogenous glucocorticoids and catecholamines, perhaps optimizing the effect. For example, some pain medications, blood thinners, and antihypertensives might be given at bedtime rather than in the morning to theoretically maximize response. Little data presently support this interesting theory; the field of chronobiology awaits more rigorous study.

Duration of Treatment and Discontinuation

The length of treatment and when (or if) to discontinue a drug in an elderly patient depends on the specific disorder being treated. Two examples are relevant. First, when treatment of major depression is successful, it should be continued for longer periods than with younger patients (49). Although there is contrary evidence, patients show optimum benefit when antidepressants are continued for the long-term (50–52), even indefinitely for some (49).

Second, when neuroleptic (antipsychotic) treatment is effective, it should be tapered and discontinued after a few months, the patient observed for continued need, and the drug restarted only if target signs and symptoms reappear. This is an Omnibus Budget Reconciliation Act (OBRA) guideline and is recommended whether the elderly patient has a primary psychotic disorder, or the psychosis is secondary to dementia. Not only was a 42% placebo response to antipsychotic treatment found in the elderly (53), but also the discontinuation of typical antipsychotics was associated with symptom relapse in only 50% (54). Chronic antipsychotic use runs the risk of causing a tardive (late-onset) dyskinesia (TD) in this very vulnerable population. Discontinuation should not be repeated more than once in a patient who relapses, and comprehensive documentation is essential.

ASSOCIATED PHARMACOTHERAPEUTIC CONSIDERATIONS

Various parameters must be considered to insure optimum drug treatment in the elderly, including safety and efficacy; adherence; common sense approaches; use of social drugs; adverse drug reactions and interactions; SE; and toxicity prevention.

Safety and Efficacy

In clinical therapeutics, two questions are of seminal importance: is the drug safe i.e., what are the risks, and is it effective? These are the components of a drug's value.

One approach to efficacy involves cataloguing the target symptoms and signs to be addressed and then choosing the most appropriate drug. Occasionally, drugs are chosen specifically to take advantage of their SE, e.g., "sedation" (in the elderly, often it is somnolence). Though occasionally effective, this is not an optimum strategy because the effects desired cannot be quantitatively regulated or localized; therefore, adverse responses can occur, such as dizziness, gait instability, and falls, particularly in frail elderly and often at night.

Off-label uses (not Food and Drug Administration approved) of some psychotropics occur, based on substantial clinical evidence of safety and effectiveness. If the treatment is supported by the literature and makes sense scientifically, it can be a useful approach. Well-designed studies should be consulted to assist with current best-drug choices. Pharmaceutical companies utilize information obtained in this manner to guide them in requesting drug approval for additional clinical indications. Examples include atypical antipsychotics and mood stabilizers—alone or in combination—to treat psychosis and assaultive behaviors in demented patients. Also, there is now a role for the atypicals, alone or as augmentors, to treat some mood and anxiety disorders. ChEIs are used to treat agitated behaviors in some demented patients—particularly those with Alzheimer's or Lewy body dementia—where inattention is a prominent sign. As always, comprehensive documentation is essential.

Adherence (Compliance)

Adherence is the correct implementation of a prescribed drug regimen, based on a patient's behavior (55). It has been quantified as missing less than 20% to 25% of prescribed doses, while nonadherence is missing more than 65% to 80% of doses (24). Patients may vary from taking drugs as prescribed, to partial adherence, or complete nonadherence (4). Partial adherence is common in those requiring chronic treatment and is a serious, underappreciated problem (48).

Although age and gender are not directly correlated to the lack of adherence rate, it is common in the elderly for many reasons, such as misunderstanding of prescribing instructions; problems with vision and hearing; confusion and cognitive impairment; or simply lack of interest. In LTC settings, where drugs are administered by staff, nonadherence is less of an issue. However, 95% of people over 65 live independently or in assisted living facilities (ALFs) and self-administer drugs, often without supervision. Problems result from such situations, particularly considering a patient's access not only to prescription drugs—often from multiple doctors—but also to the multiple other sources of drugs.

Drug errors occur often and are directly related to the daily dose frequency. The most common error is omission, either deliberately (self-discontinuation, usually due to SE and without notifying the prescriber), or by accident. Other common errors, alone or combined are: taking the wrong dose, or at the wrong time, or at the wrong frequency.

Additional causes exist for nonadherence. These include failure to receive the drug on a timely basis (many elderly, including military veterans, receive their drugs through the mail), and inability to pay for all drugs prescribed. In these cases a choice is made or the recommended dose is decreased to extend its use.

Adherence improves when younger patients are switched to depot agents. In elderly, follow-up clinician phone calls, particularly soon after a drug is started (or changed), and ongoing involvement with the family significantly increase adherence.

Common-Sense Approaches

Various practical issues are associated with optimizing drug-taking in the elderly. An essential action at the first clinical meeting is the well-known inventory of *all* drugs currently taken. Patients (or families) should be instructed to keep an updated drug record (name, dose, frequency), and monitoring should continue at regular intervals, especially if a relatively rapid onset or change in symptoms occurs.

Before prescribing a drug, ask yourself if the patient really needs it; i.e., will it benefit quality or length of life? If a drug is indicated, explain why it is being prescribed, when, and how it should be taken, with a *reasonable* description of possible SE. Link drug-taking to ingrained daily activities, such as, "take right after brushing your teeth." Ask if the prescription is affordable (most drug companies have programs to help qualified persons). Have these discussions with a family member present, or even have written material for the patient to take home.

Prescriptions should be written legibly and include the purpose for the drug. Similar-looking and confusing abbreviations should be avoided (e.g., hs, qd, qod, ug), and decimal expressions clarified (e.g., put a zero before a decimal, and no zero after a decimal). Also, insure that the suffix is added when using an extended-release preparation (e.g., venlafaxine XR, or bupropion XL), due to differing kinetics. Dose equivalencies among different drugs taken should be clearly explained. Finally, clinician and pharmacist both should insure directions are clear and comprehensive, and the number of refills prominent.

The use of child-proof containers, especially for those living alone, may be a problem. Some elders do not have caregivers to regularly set-up drugs, and because of poor hand or finger strength, chronic pain, or decreased hand/eye coordination, these drug containers may pose an embarrassing barrier. Empathic questioning of patients (and caregivers) about this issue is time well-spent. Proper use of weekly pill-organizers should be discussed with the responsible family member (e.g., reminding that extended-release preparations are generally not meant to be split or crushed).

Decreased visual acuity and color discrimination (leading to decreased depth perception) are normal concomitants of aging. Thus, labels on drug containers should be designed with the elderly in mind and made easier to read. In some pharmacies, print is small, in part due to the increase in information on labels. This maximizes the opportunity for errors—because many elderly keep similar-looking containers all grouped in one place (*the chemical-dresser syndrome*).

Handing the patient an office card with the prescriber's phone number and giving permission to phone between appointments is a small but effective strategy. Occasional follow-up about card location should be done. Patients seldom call, but knowing they can is important to them (and to families and other caregivers).

Following federal guidelines, many LTC facilities (including some ALFs) require informed consent forms for use of psychotropics. Forms usually list drug name, why it is being given, potential SE, and is signed by the patient or proxy. Unfortunately, psychotropics are often loosely defined and the SE listed are not standardized; thus, the main benefit of the form is to highlight psychotropic drug use—important for patients, families, staff, and particularly the prescriber.

Social Drugs

Unmonitored, *social drug* use concomitant with prescribed drugs contributes to the potential for increased SE in elderly. Prescription drugs are calibrated carefully in terms of dose, frequency, mode of administration, optimum time given, and potential risk. Nevertheless, patients may also be ingesting multiple cups of coffee every day, (which may reflect SE, illness, or just habit). Besides coffee or the many soft drinks containing caffeine, chronic and acute alcohol use, smoking (particularly in military veterans), use of tea, chocolate and cocoa (usually candy bars), and illegal drugs, should be listed and monitored.

When treating a population of elderly with chronic medical illnesses, strict monitoring of all drugs is routine. This important tactic happens less often with psychotropics; but as the number of psychotropics increases, a more rigorous social drug history is essential to optimize treatment outcome.

Adverse Drug Reactions and Interactions

A major reason for the increase in Americans over 65 between 1900 and 2000 (3 million versus 34 million), is the effective treatment of chronic diseases. Thus, older people are taking more drugs than ever before. This is both beneficial and detrimental, because the potential for adverse drug reactions (ADR) and interactions increases. The number of ADR is directly proportional to the number of drugs taken. The aged are twice as likely to experience ADR than younger patients. There is a doubling of ADR

TABLE 14-8

ADVERSE DRUG REACTIONS (ADR)

Definition

An unintentional, unexpected, undesired, or excessive patient response (side effect or toxicity) resulting from a drug given at the recommended dose that:

- Complicates the diagnosis
- Requires modifying the dose or discontinuing the drug
- Requires changing the drug treatment
- Necessitates supportive treatment
- Necessitates admission to or prolonging the stay in a healthcare facility
- Results in temporary or permanent harm or disability, or in death

Major Risk Factors

- History of ADR
- Elderly
- Female
- Race (variable)
- Increased number of daily medications
- Increased or inappropriate dosage
- Hospitalization

over age 65; and almost 35% of those 80 and over have had ADR (3) (see Table 14-8).

Elderly account for up to 50% of all ADR and the consequences are significant (56,57):

- Those over age 60 account for about 50% of ADR deaths.
- An estimated 106,000 hospital patients died from an ADR in 1994, making it the fourth to sixth leading cause of death.
- ADR in hospitalized patients increases length of stay between 1.7 and 2.2 days, and increases cost by $2,000 to $2,600 per event.
- 15% to 30% of hospital admissions in patients over 60 may be linked to ADR or toxicity.
- Drug-related problems cost $177 billion in ambulatory care patients, and $4 billion in those in nursing homes (NHs).

Prescriber negligence is responsible for about 30% of ADR; most errors—both commission and omission—are preventable, and drug interactions avoidable. Common problems are misdiagnoses or untreated indication; incorrect, unnecessary or improper use; inappropriate doses; or dangerous combinations (58,59). Redundant, or nonjustifiable selection and concomitant use of drugs is common (*inappropriate polypharmacy*, contrasted with appropriate, carefully used *co-pharmacy*), as is drug use without a clear indication (e.g., treatment for behaviors in demented patients), without first trying nonpharmacologic approaches (see Tables 14-1 and 14-2).

In a study of 1,100 NH patients, the prevalence of potentially inappropriate drug combinations defined by explicit criteria was 40% (60). In another, almost 20% of

NH residents received at least one of 20 drugs considered by experts to be potentially inappropriate (57). Geriatric psychiatrists, especially consultants in NHs and ALFs, should be alert to these practices and available to help optimize care.

Various drug interactions can occur: drug–drug; drug–system (body); drug–disease; and drug–food. Drug–laboratory interactions, causing invalid and unreliable results, can also occur. Incidence of interactions may occur with 2% to 15% of all prescriptions; and although clinically significant interactions causing adverse health outcomes are relatively low, elderly are at high risk. The drug-interaction literature is extremely comprehensive; thus, only basic components will be reviewed (61–64).

Drug–Drug Interactions

These interactions are defined as the effect an administration of one drug has on the action of another (64), and can be organized into kinetic and dynamic categories.

Kinetic Interactions

These occur when absorption, distribution, metabolism, or excretion are affected, either directly or indirectly. There can be *direct interaction* of one drug with another, such that the action of one is detrimentally affected. This *competitive interaction* occurs especially when a number of drugs are taken simultaneously. An example is the interaction between some neuroleptics and multivalent cations (e.g., antacids, causing a decreased absorption of neuroleptic). Others occur during excretion, that is, renal clearance of one drug is inhibited by another. These interactions can involve competitive inhibition of active tubular secretion of anionic or cationic drugs (such as TCAs or benzodiazepines interacting with cimetidine). Effects on lithium excretion vary (e.g., decreased plasma level with hydrochlorothiazide, or increased with non-steroidal anti-inflammatory drugs (NSAIDs)).

An *indirect interaction* is when one drug acts on a physiologic mechanism, altering the effective action of another drug. One example of this would be TCAs and carbamazepine, where a decreased TCA plasma level can occur due to metabolic enzyme activity induction by carbamazepine. Alternatively, increased antidepressant levels may occur due to metabolic enzyme inhibition by other psychotropics.

Because psychotropic combinations are often used to optimize effectiveness for patients who are anxious, depressed, psychotic, or assaultive, the interaction potential increases in these situations. Therefore all combination therapy should be used with caution.

Multiple theoretical metabolic interactions exist with combination therapy. One involves concurrent use of drugs exhibiting Phase-I metabolism with other drugs using the same enzyme system (e.g., risperidone and ChEIs [donepezil and galantamine], all metabolized by CYP2D6). Competition for enzyme receptor binding sites could alter the plasma levels of either drug. Inhibition or induction of some CYP enzymes can occur (for instance, use of a neuroleptic metabolized by a CYP isoenzyme, and an antidepressant that inhibits that isoenzyme's activity, causing an increased neuroleptic level) (see Table 14-5). The magnitude of hepatic enzyme activity inhibitors is similar between young and elderly, while studies of inducers differ—some suggesting a decreased response in elderly to enzyme induction (6,31). Other factors may affect kinetic interactions (e.g., cigarette smoking may induce CYP1A2 activity, causing increased clearance and decreased plasma levels of some drugs).

Interactions involving distribution changes with aging are related to altered plasma protein binding, with one drug displacing another from receptor sites. These are seldom clinically significant with psychotropics.

Dynamic Interactions

These interactions may translate clinically into additive, synergistic, or antagonistic drug reactions. Receptor activation changes may occur when a drug's effect is unexpected or altered, (e.g., NSAIDs and thiazide diuretics). It may involve giving two or more drugs together that exhibit similar pharmacologic effects, which act synergistically (e.g., potassium supplements, potassium-sparing diuretics, and angiotension-converting enzyme (ACE) inhibitors). These interactions often produce detrimental SE.

Among the most common—and problematic—of these synergies are the CNS and peripheral antiChE SE of many drugs used in the elderly—nonpsychotropic and psychotropic alike (5). These include some antipsychotics, antiparkinsons, and antidepressants. A classic SE example is CNS toxicity as seen in anticholinergic delirium (*atropine psychosis*)—a delirium particularly detrimental to frail elderly. Patients being treated with combinations of these drugs, which separately may not cause symptoms, may exhibit impaired attention and disordered thinking. Disorientation, hallucinations, and fluctuating level of consciousness may also be seen. This occurs particularly in patients with Alzheimer's or Lewy body dementia, where a marked loss of CNS acetylcholine already exists; the changes seen may be misdiagnosed as a worsening of the dementia. Treatment may involve ChEIs, which replaced the earlier, short-lived use of physostigmine, a short $T_{1/2}$ drug, which can cause excessive parasympathetic stimulation (*cholinergic crisis*).

Another example is the increased response to combinations of drugs with selected antiadrenergic activity. This synergy can cause heart rate change, postural hypotension (posing a significant danger of falls and fractures), other CV SE, and gait instability. These SE occur more often when multiple CNS depressants are concurrently administered (3,6,58). Daytime somnolence, dizziness, and even diminished level of consciousness secondary to antihistaminic drug synergy are also causes for concern (62).

Drug–System Interactions

This is a variant of drug-drug dynamic interactions, when the mechanism of action of a drug causes a detrimental effect on the overall diminished *physiologic reserve* seen due to normal aging. It involves a direct action on a function already compromised, perhaps leading to a serious consequence. Multiple examples exist, such as a drug with strong, antiChE SE given to a patient already experiencing post-voiding urinary retention because of benign prostatic hypertrophy, causing an increased retention. This discomfort often is displayed in demented elderly as agitation, resistiveness, or even assault. Another example is a patient with existing postural hypotension due to decreased baroreceptor fidelity given a drug that causes symptom exacerbation (16). Finally, perhaps due to a decreased *cerebral reserve*, some elderly respond with marked somnolence to the sedative properties of various psychotropics, especially when combined with drugs with similar SE (3).

Drug–Disease Interactions

A strong potential for drug-disease interactions exists in elderly, where multiple drug use affects—and can be affected by—existing comorbid disease states. Common chronic diseases include cardiac-conduction abnormalities; COPD and asthma; renal insufficiency; diabetes mellitus; hypertension; hypotension; sinusitis; peptic ulcer; hypokalemia; hyponatremia; joint diseases, and dementias.

A variety of psychotropic—as well as other drugs—can cause clinically significant drug-disease interactions. A partial list of nonpsychotropics includes blood thinners, β-blockers and agonists, calcium-channel blockers, antihistaminic sleep aids, antiparkinsons, NSAIDs, corticosteroids, oral hypoglycemics, antiChE drugs used for urinary tract problems, narcotic analgesics, and multiple antihypertensives (5,6).

Drug–Diet/Food Interactions

An important, unique relationship exists in the elderly between drugs and diet. At best, dietary habits may be erratic in terms of frequency, quantity, and quality for a variety of reasons, including finances. At worst, the diet may be a nutritional disaster. Because diet can impinge directly on kinetics, activity, and SE, clinicians should be sensitive to this important aspect of therapy.

Various foods, nutrients, and herbals can alter drug absorption (e.g., warfarin, digoxin, and antibiotics), and therefore effectiveness via direct physical interaction. It also occurs with some psychotropics (e.g., increased ziprasidone absorption when taken with food). Some foods can alter an intended pharmacologic response. For example, foods containing vitamin K (such as broccoli, cabbage, asparagus, and Brussels sprouts) and warfarin; grapefruit juice and CYP3A4 activity; tyramine-containing foods and monoamine oxidase inhibitors (MAOIs). Also, drugs may affect appetite or even the taste of food (some antibiotics, antihypertensives,

ACE inhibitors, lithium), or cause difficulty in chewing or swallowing due to xerostomia. These problems are of particular importance in demented patients, who may be unable to describe or even express them.

In summary, ongoing education about the various drug interactions and their treatment is essential for direct-line staff in LTC settings, as well as for families. Additional useful strategies for prescribers include:

- electronic drug prescribing; use of a pharmacy with updated interactions software;
- association with a Doctor of Pharmacy knowledgeable in elderly patient issue; and
- regularly reviewing the need for chronic use of drugs.

Side Effects and Toxicity Prevention

It is axiomatic that an increased susceptibility to drug SE exists in the elderly, even at *elderly* doses. Up to $1/3$ of patients develop SE. When multiple drugs are taken, or are taken in greater than recommended doses, or patients are relatively more sensitive to the drug effect, the problem is compounded. SE can be relatively benign, while others more severe.

Side Effects

Although introduced previously, the significance of psychotropic drug SE requires additional discussion. They can be variously grouped, e.g., the most common; or those seen in short-term versus long-term treatment. The most common SE are: CNS; autonomic nervous system (ANS) (particularly the peripheral antiChE effects of parasympathetic blockade); hypotensive and other CV effects of α-adrenergic inhibition; extrapyramidal side effects (EPS) due to brain area-specific dopamine (D_2) receptor blockade; neuroendocrine and other effects of histamine receptor blockade (i.e., weight gain, somnolence and hypotension); hypothermia; and occasionally hyperthermia).

AntiChE SE are caused by blockade of muscarinic-ACh receptors and perhaps involve CNS nicotinic-ACh receptors. CNS SE with the most potential for dysfunction in elderly include altered level of consciousness; insomnia; agitation; memory loss; and delirium (often with associated psychosis or assaultive signs/symptoms). Peripheral antiChE SE include decreased salivary flow; sinus tachycardia; cardiac conduction disturbance; constipation and even bowel atony; urinary retention due to dystonic bladder with potential for overflow incontinence (particularly in men); blurred vision and loss of accommodation; exacerbation of narrow-angle glaucoma; impotence (more important in elderly than generally acknowledged); dry skin with an increased potential for skin breakdown; and temperature dysregulation due to decreased sweating.

A potentially hazardous SE of ANS blockade is orthostatic (postural) hypotension, caused by α-adrenergic receptor blockade. Like most ANS SE, it usually appears gradually, is often transient, and directly proportional to dose. Hypotension can be dangerous due to reflex tachycardia, as well as light-headedness and dizziness leading to unsteady gait, falls, and injury. This cascade of problems also can occur with psychotropics that block histamine-H_1 receptors, causing significant somnolence and gait disturbance.

Cardiac conduction problems, including prolonged corrected QT (QT_c) interval, can occur with some psychotropics, such as typical and atypical antipsychotics, TCAs, and lithium. Excess prolongation can cause dangerous arrhythmias, particularly in synergy with other causes (e.g., elderly women, hypokalemia, hypothyroidism, hypocalcemia, hypomagnesemia, bradycardia, and mitral valve prolapse).

EPS are seen in 25% or more of elderly patients treated with typical antipsychotics and increases with ongoing use, due to specific and chronic D_2 receptor antagonism, particularly in the nigrostriatum. These SE are usually dose-dependent. Sometimes, separation of drug-induced EPS from movements caused by normal aging or neurologic diseases is difficult, but must be considered before discontinuing a clinically beneficial drug. Atypical antipsychotics exhibit significantly less EPS and are the first choice for use in the elderly.

EPS seen in the short-term can be separated into dystonias, akathisias, and parkinsonian reactions—including tremor, rigidity, and akinesia. Receptor and/or various neurotransmitter changes are associated with particular EPS. Being aware of these changes—although oversimplified (e.g., serotonin is not taken into account)—may be clinically useful when considering drug treatment approaches.

Dystonia, akathisia, and parkinsonism are all associated with decreased dopamine (DA) brain levels, with a corresponding relative increase in ACh and norepinephrine in parkinsonism; an increase in only ACh in dystonia; and an increase in only norepinephrine in akathisia.

Masking drug-induced parkinsonian and dystonic EPS with antiChE drugs (trihexyphenidyl or benztropine), or a neuroleptic (e.g., olanzapine) is sometimes done rather than changing the offending dose or drug, i.e., using the SE of one drug to treat the SE of another. It is unclear what may be the long-term ramifications of this masking, which is not recommended in elderly.

Dyskinesia, including TD, is a significant problem in elderly patients who are treated long-term with some drugs, particularly the earlier antipsychotics (*typicals*). The etiology is a neurotransmitter imbalance, but unlike EPS, is thought due to an increased number or sensitivity of DA receptors, without a corresponding relative increase in ACh receptor number or sensitivity. AntiChE drugs in this situation may actually exacerbate the symptoms. More than 20% of elderly develop TD within a year of treatment and up to two-thirds within three years (65), which was a major impetus for development of the atypicals. They cause much less TD—about 1/10th the amount of typicals (66). Atypicals bind to and affect both dopamine (primarily D_2, but also D_1—quetiapine, and D_4—olanzapine), and serotonin (primarily

5HT_2a, but also 5HT_2c—quetiapine) receptors, with 65% to 80% range of D_2-binding needed to provide efficacy for psychosis. There is a greater affinity for the 5HT_2a compared with D_2, i.e., the receptor binding ratio is about 10:1 and varies among the atypicals. This receptor antagonism balance of atypicals optimizes treatment both of positive and negative symptoms; and cognitive deficits of schizophrenia (67), minimizes EPS, and also has mood-stabilizing effects. Greater than 80% D_2-binding causes a loss of the 5HT_2a protection, with a corresponding increase in EPS (68).

TD usually appears months or years after beginning treatment, with stereotypical ongoing movements of tongue, mouth, jaw, or trunk. Movements can be temporarily suppressed by the patient and cease during sleep. In some elderly, especially those with progressive dementias, TD may develop in the absence of drug treatment, perhaps due to gradual degeneration of some basal ganglia nuclei/pathways. Effective treatment of TD is currently lacking. Recently, a branched-chain amino acid treatment (Tarvil—designated as a food, therefore not FDA-regulated) has been described in men, some elderly (69). The concept is based on a postulated association between TD and impaired phenylalanine kinetics, and warrants further investigation. Other late-onset disorders, e.g., tardive dystonia, tardive akathisia, and tardive myoclonus, occur in elderly and are all difficult to treat.

Various instruments are available in the public domain to evaluate movement disorders chronically, including: AIMS (Abnormal Involuntary Movement Scale); BARS (Barnes Akathisia Rating Scale); SAS (Simpson-Angus Scale) and ESRS (Extrapyramidal Symptom Rating Scale). Also, movement disorders clinics are useful adjuncts to drug treatment.

Miscellaneous psychotropic SE that may be problematic in elderly include: depressive and manic symptoms; anxiety; fatigue; apathy; insomnia; increased liver-enzyme activity (ALT/AST); and GI upset. Prolactin increase is seen with atypicals, caused by blockade of DA receptors that maintain normal inhibitory regulation between the hypothalamus and anterior pituitary. It has not been shown to be of clinical significance in elderly. Conflicting studies link atypical antipsychotics with cerebrovascular adverse events (70); hyperglycemia and diabetes have also been reported (71). Rare SE include seizures, neuroleptic malignant syndrome, and agranulocytosis. Comprehensive lists and treatments of SE for psychotropics are available elsewhere (58,62,72).

Toxicity Prevention

Drug toxicity (or "overdose") may be due to a deliberate action, an altered pharmacological response, or iatrogeny. Preventable reasons include:

■ Lack of knowledge of the patients' total drug ingestion habits, including the sundry over-the-counter and social drugs, herbals and nutriceuticals. Information also is lacking about the continued use of outdated, previously hoarded drugs, exchange of drugs among friends (particularly those in ALFs), and unhealthy dietary habits.

■ Limited awareness of the uniqueness of individual elders regarding their drug response, particularly psychotropics used in cognitively impaired elderly. Nonspecific use of standard elderly doses is common.

■ Absence of a care coordinator. Long-term treatment of multiple medical problems commonly occurs with multiple drugs, often from multiple prescribers.

TREATMENT, MANAGEMENT, AND MONITORING

General Comments

When considering the practical aspects of treating, managing, and monitoring elderly who need pharmacotherapy for their psychiatric illnesses, common sense should prevail. Based on the overall uniqueness of this pop-

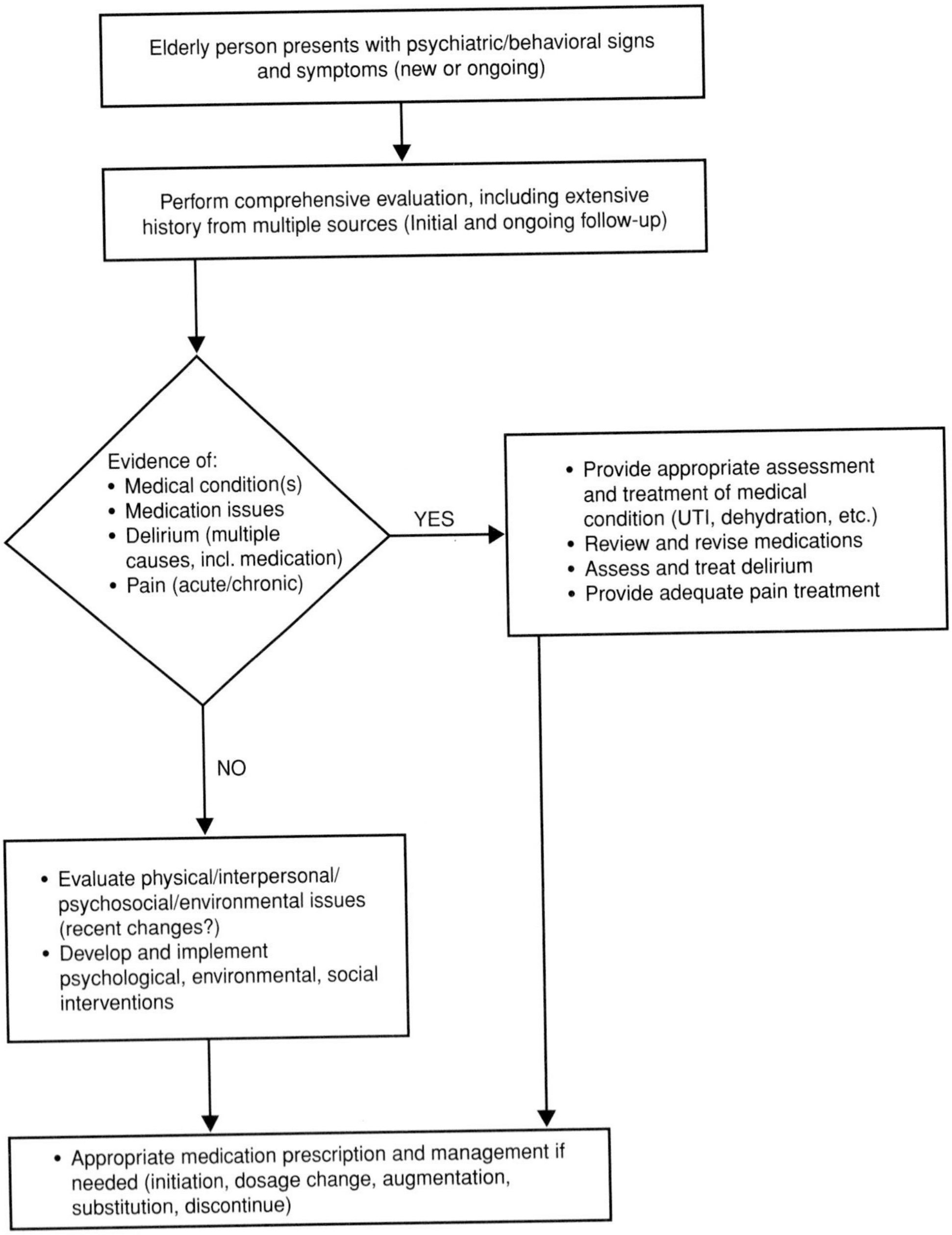

UTI, urinary tract infection.

Figure 14-2   Algorithm for ongoing assessment (evaluation) and treatment (management).

ulation and the disparity among individuals, use of psychotropics—or any drugs—needs to be carefully considered. Certainly, knowing a particular drug's kinetic profile—as well as its potential SE and interactions—will aid in selection, starting dose and frequency, and adjustment(s) necessary to achieve an optimum treatment response. Evolving, best-practice, evidence-based, clinical guidelines are a helpful adjunct, both for optimizing treatment and cost-containment (24).

Clinical Specifics

Comprehensive patient assessment should always preface a drug treatment plan and an algorithmic approach can help standardize care (see Figure 14-2). Present medical and environmental conditions should be evaluated first. Baseline data are necessary (and often not available in the chart), for cardiac, renal, hepatic and hematologic status. Screening for balance, gait, abnormal movements, and pre-existing orthostatic hypotension, as well as obtaining a complete drug list—including PRNs and how often used— are essential. A therapeutic goal should be established clarifying target signs and symptoms to be alleviated and, if possible, specific causes, before a drug is begun. Individualizing starting dose and frequency of titration is necessary. Direct and ongoing assessments of benefit or detriment are important, especially in patients with advanced dementia, before dose changes are made. Often, changes are based on collateral information, which can be misleading because family or staff perceptions of a patient may be more associated with their own mood or need than with an objective evaluation (73).

It should be explained to staff and families that psychotropic drug treatment is mostly *empiric* (trial and error), rather than *rational* (single problem leads to discrete, reliable solution); and that the drugs are unpredictably effective about 50% to 60% of the time (as are most drugs). This observation relates to the unique genetic make-up of individual patients and has led to the emerging field of pharmacogenomics. Research into the pharmacogenetics of psychotropics suggests that specific genes may influence phenotypes associated with drug administration (74). In the future, specific genetic polymorphisms may identify persons predisposed to respond to a specific drug. Indeed, genetic testing prior to drug treatment is now being applied clinically at the Mayo Clinic to identify slow and fast metabolizers of antidepressants, based on CYP2D6 enzymatic activity. This testing predicts potential for SE, assures optimum drug choice and dose, and improves compliance. The future is already here.

Clinicians faced with nonresponding patients should develop an evidence-based protocol to insure that best treatment approaches are utilized. One example of a chronological approach follows:

- Adequate titration with original drug, with appropriate time allowed between changes and for overall length of treatment
- Addition to original drug of an appropriate augmenting agent(s)
- Combination of a drug in a different category
- Switching to a different drug (and beginning protocol again)
- Switching to a somatic treatment, e.g., electro convulsive therapy, if appropriate

This approach requires a prolonged treatment period, which is often possible because many elderly treated by geropsychiatrists reside in LTC settings. Patience in this endeavor is required, particularly by family and staff.

Use of an algorithm facilitates ongoing evaluation of treatment as to continued need and the monitoring of effectiveness (see Figure 14-3). Additional aspects include developing strategies for an inadequate response, for managing relapse, for adjusting dose in stable patients, and for managing complicating problems (25).

TYPES OF DRUGS USED

Novel psychotropics (or alterations of existing drugs regarding dosages, delivery mode, and combinations) are appearing with increasing frequency.

They can be categorized based on their mechanism of action or treatment potential:

- Anxiolytics
- Antidepressants
- Neuroleptics (antipsychotics, thymoleptics)
- Mood stabilizers (including antiepileptic drugs)
- Cognitive enhancers
- Psychostimulants
- Hypnotics
- Miscellaneous (β-blockers, others)

Individual chapters in this book discuss use of their relevant drugs. Additional comprehensive information is also available in Appendix A, and general information on pharmacotherapeutics can be found in several excellent references (4,62,63,75–81).

THE DRUG DEVELOPMENT AND APPROVAL PROCESS

The drug development and approval process is the responsibility of the FDA and is complex, protracted, and expensive. It is important for prescribers to appreciate the general history. It usually takes 10 to 15 years for a drug to proceed from a pharmaceutical research and development laboratory to a patient, at a cost of well over $800 million dollars (82,83). Appendix A contains a flowchart of the process.

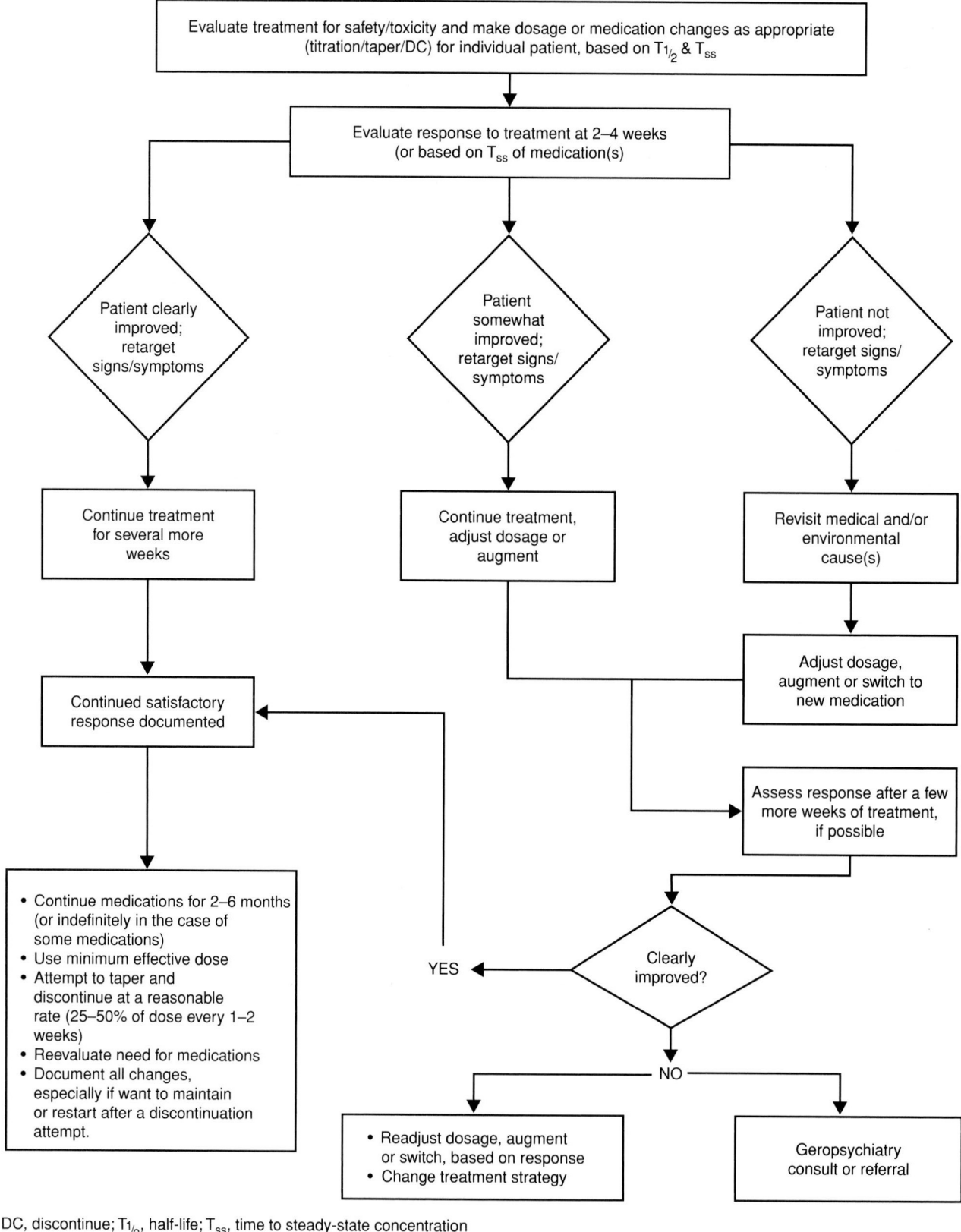

DC, discontinue; $T_{1/2}$, half-life; T_{ss}, time to steady-state concentration

Figure 14-3 Algorithm for ongoing monitoring of medication treatment and management response.

REFERENCES

1. Maletta G, Mattox K, Dysken M. Update 2000: guidelines for prescribing psychoactive drugs. *Geriatrics.* 2000;55(3):65–79.
2. Sakauye K, Maletta G. Pharmacokinetic and pharmacodynamic considerations in psychotropic medication use in the elderly: an overview. *Psychiatric Annals.* 1991;21(1):58–63.
3. Maletta G. Use of antipsychotic medications in the elderly. In: Eisdorfer C, ed. *Annual Review of Gerontology and Geriatrics.* New York: Springer; 1984;4:175–220.
4. Mulsant BH, Pollack BG. Psychopharmacology. In: Blazer DF, Steffans DC, Busse EW, eds. *The American Psychiatric Publishing Textbook of Geriatric Psychiatry.* 3rd Ed. Washington, DC: American Psychiatric Publishing; 2004:387–411.
5. Tune LE. Anticholinergic effects of medication in elderly patients. *J Clin Psychiatry.* 2001;62(21):11–14.
6. Guay D, Artz MB, Hanlon JT, Schmader KE. The pharmacology of aging. In: Talis R, Fillit H, eds. *Brocklehurst's Textbook of Geriatric Medicine.* 6th Ed. London: Churchill Livingstone; 2003:155–161.
7. Hughes CM, Lapane KL, Mar V, et al. The impact of legislation on psychotropic drug use in nursing homes: a cross-national perspective. *J Am Geriatr Soc.* 2000;48(8):931–937.
8. Giron M, Claesson C, Thorslurd M, et al. Drug use patterns in a very elderly population. *Clin Drug Invest.* 1999;17:389–398.
9. Millar WJ. Multiple medication use among seniors. *Health Rep.* 1998, Spring;9(4):11–17.
10. Rathmore SS, Mehta SS, Boyco WL, Schulman KA. Prescription medication use in older Americans. *Fam Med.* 1998;30(10): 733–739.
11. Stoehr GP, Ganguli M, Seaberg, EC, et al. Over-the-counter medication use in an older rural community: the MoVIES Project. *J Am Geriatr Soc.* 1997;45(2):158–165.
12. Tobias D, Sey H. General and psychotherapeutic medication use in 328 nursing facilities. *Consult Pharm.* 2001;16:54–64.
13. Furniss L, Craig SK, Burns A. Medication use in nursing homes for elderly people. *Int J Geriatr Psychiatry.* 1998;13(7):433–439.
14. Stoudemire A, Smith DA. OBRA regulations and the use of psychotropic drugs in long-term care facilities: impact and implications for geropsychiatric care. *Gen Hosp Psychiatry.* 1996;18(2): 77–94.
15. Beardsley RS, Larson DB, Burns BJ, et al. Prescribing of psychotropics in elderly nursing home patients. *J Am Geriatr Soc.* 1989;37(4):327–330.
16. Maletta G. Use of psychotropic drugs in the older patient, with particular emphasis on the antipsychotics. In: Maletta G, Pirozzolo F, eds. *The Aging Nervous System.* New York: Praeger; 1980.
17. DeVane CL, Pollock BG. Pharmacokinetic considerations of antidepressant use in the elderly. *J Clin Psychiatry.* 1999;60(Suppl 20):38–44.
18. Timiras PS, ed. *Physiological Basis of Aging and Geriatrics,* 3rd Ed. Boca Raton, FL: CRC Press; 2003.
19. Hayflick L. How and why we age. *Exp Gerontol.* 1998;33(7–8): 639–653.
20. Chapron DJ. Drug disposition and response in the elderly. In: Delafuente J, Stewart R, eds. *Therapeutics in The Elderly,* 3rd Ed. Cincinnati: Harvey Whitney; 2000:257–288.
21. Hammerlein A, Derendorf H, Lowenthal D. Pharmacokinetic and pharmacodynamic changes in the elderly: clinical implications. *Clin Pharmacokinet.* 1998;35:49–64.
22. Iber FL, Murphy PA, Conner ES. Age-related changes in the GI system: effects on drug therapy. *Drugs Aging.* 1994;5:34–48.
23. Davis J, Garver D. Psychobiology of affective disorders. In: *Current Concepts.* Kalamazoo, MI: Upjohn; 1978:23–45.
24. Kane J, Leucht S, Carpenter D, et al. Optimizing pharmacological treatment of psychotic disorders. *J Clin Psychiatry.* 2003;64(Suppl 12):5–19.
25. Forbes GB, Reina JC. Adult lean body mass declines with age: some longitudinal observations. *Metabolism.* 1970;19:653–663.
26. Fryer J. Studies of body composition in men aged 60 and over. In: Shock N, ed. *Biological Aspects of Aging.* New York: Columbia University Press; 1962:59–78.
27. Greenblatt D, Divall M, Abernathy D, et al. Physiologic changes in old age: relation to altered drug disposition. *J Am Geriatr Soc.* 1982;30(11):9–12.

28. Grandison MK, Boudenet FD. Age-related changes in protein binding of drugs: implications for therapy. *Clin Pharmacokinetics.* 2000;38:271–290.
29. Woodhouse K, Wynne H. Age-related changes in hepatic function. *Drugs Aging.* 1992;2:243–255.
30. Dresser G, Bailey D, Carruthers S. Grapefruit juice-felodipine interaction in the elderly. *Clin Pharmacol Ther.* 2000;68:8–34.
31. Michalets E. Update: clinically significant cytochrome P-450 drug interactions. *Pharmacotherapy.* 1998;18:84–112.
32. Sotaniemi E, Arrants A, Pelkonen O, et al. Age and cytochrome P450-linked drug metabolism in humans. *Clin Pharmacol Therap.* 1997;61:331–339.
33. Korrapati M, Sorkin J, Andres R, et al. Acetylator phenotype in relation to age and gender in the Baltimore Longitudinal Study of Aging. *J Clin Pharmacol.* 1997;37(2):83–91.
34. Williams RI. Drug administration in hepatic disease. *N Eng J Med.* 1983;309(26):1616–1622.
35. Rowe, J, Andres R, Tobin J, et al. Effect of age on creatinine clearance in man. *J Gerontol.* 1976;31:155–163.
36. Ujhelyi M, Bottarff M, Schur M, et al. Aging effects on the organic base transporter and stereoselective renal clearance. *Clin Pharmacol Ther.* 1997;62:117–128.
37. Malmrose L, Gray S, Piefer C, et al. Measured vs. estimated creatinine clearance in a high-functioning elderly sample. *J Am Geriatr Soc.* 1993;41:715–721.
38. Cockroft DW, Gault MH. Prediction of creatinine clearance from serum creatinine. *Nephron.* 1976;16:31–41.
39. Feely J, Coakley D. Altered pharmacodynamics in the elderly. *Clin Ger Med.* 1990;6:269–283.
40. Vestal R, Wood A, Shand D. Reduced β-adrenoceptor sensitivity in the elderly. *Clin Pharmacol Ther.* 1979;26:181–186.
41. Bernard C. *Lecons Sur les Propriete's Physiologiques et les Alterations Pathologiques des Liquides de l'Organisime.* Paris: Bailliere; 1859.
42. Cannon W. The sympathetic division of the autonomic system in relation to homeostasis. *Arch Neurol Psychiatr.* 1929;22:282–294.
43. Sterling P, Eyer J. Allostasis: a new paradigm to explain arousal pathology. In: Fisher S, Reason J, eds. *Handbook of Life Stress, Cognition and Health.* New York: John Wiley; 1988:629–649.
44. Cannon W. Aging of homeostatic mechanisms. In: Cowdry E, ed. *Problems of Aging.* Baltimore: Williams & Wilkins; 1942.
45. McEwen B. Mood disorders and allostatic load. *Biol Psychiatry.* 2003;54:200–207.
46. Solomon K. Haloperidol and the geriatric patient: practical considerations. In: Ayd F, ed. *Haloperidol Update.* Baltimore: Ayd Medical; 1980.
47. Dharmarajan T, Ugalino J. Understanding the pharmacology of aging. In: Dharmarajan T, ed. *Geriatric Medicine Board Review Manual.* Wayne, PA: Turner White Communications; 2001;1(4):1–12.
48. Kane J, Eerdekins, M, Lindenmager JP, et al. Long-acting risperidone: efficacy and safety of the first long-acting atypical antipsychotic. *Am J Psychiatry.* 2003;160:1125–1132.
49. Alexopoulos G, Katz I, Reynolds C, et al. Introduction: Pharmacotherapy of depressive disorders in older patients. *Postgrad Med Special Report.* 2001;5(Oct):1.
50. Delrahim K, Maddux R, Rapaport M. Long-term antidepressant treatment. *Psychopharmacol Bull.* 2002;36(4):26–38.
51. Walters G, Reynolds C, Mulsant B, Pollack B. Continuation and maintenance pharmacotherapy in geriatric depression: an open-trial comparison of paroxetine and nortriptyline in patients older than 70 years. *J Clin Psychiatry.* 1999;60(20):21–25.
52. Wilson K, Mattram P, Ashworth L, Abou-Saleh M. Older community residents with depression: long-term treatment with sertraline. *Brit J Psychiatry.* 2003;182:492–497.
53. Schneider L, Pollack V, Lyness S. A meta-analysis of controlled trials of neuroleptic treatment in dementia. *J Am Geriatr Soc.* 1990;38:553–563.
54. Horowitz G, Tariot P, Mead K, Cox C. Discontinuation of antipsychotics in nursing home patients with dementia. *J Am Geriatr Psychiatry.* 1995;3:290–299.
55. Cramer J, Rosenfeck R, Compliance with medication regimens for mental and physical disorders. *Psychiatr Serv.* 1998;49: 196–201.
56. Hanlon J, Schmader K, Kornkowski M, et al. Adverse drug events in high-risk older outpatients. *J Am Geriatr Soc.* 1997;45:945–948.

57. Beers M, Ouslander J, Fingold S, et al. Inappropriate medication prescribing in skilled nursing facilities. *Ann Intern Med.* 1992;117:684–689.

58. Beers M. Explicit criteria for determining potentially inappropriate medication by the elderly. *Arch Intern Med.* 1997;157: 1531–1536.

59. Fick D, Cooper J, Wade W. et al. Updating the Beers criteria for potentially inappropriate medication use in older adults: results of a US consensus panel of experts. *Arch Intern Med.* 2003;163 (22):2716–2724.

60. Prescription drug use in nursing homes: report 3A. Washington, DC: Office of Inspector General, Department of Health and Human Services, 1997.

61. Pollack BG. Adverse reactions of antidepressants in elderly patients. *J Clin Psychiatry.* 1999;60 (20):4–8,1999.

62. Salzman C, ed. *Clinical Psychopharmacology.* 2nd Ed. Baltimore: Lippincott, Williams & Wilkins; 2002.

63. Pollack B, Mulsant B. Psychopharmacology. In: Crane J, Ford J, eds. *Drugs and the Older Person.* London: Imperial College Press; 2000:275–303.

64. Seymour R, Routledge P. Important drug-drug interactions in the elderly. *Drugs Aging.* 1998;12:485–494.

65. Jeste D, Caligiuri M, Paulsen J, et al. Risk of tardive dyskinesia in older patients: a prospective longitudinal study of 266 outpatients. *Arch Gen Psychiatry.* 1995;52:756–765.

66. Jeste D, Okamoto A, Napolitano, J, et al. Low incidence of persistent tardive dyskinesia in elderly patients with dementia treated with risperidone. *Am J Psychiatry.* 2000;157:1150–1155.

67. Ichikawa J, Meltzer H. Relationship between dopaminergic and serotonergic neuronal activity in frontal cortex and the action of typical and atypical antipsychotic agents. *Eur Arch Psychiatry Clin Neurosci.* 1999;249(4):90–98.

68. Kapur S, Zipursky R, Remington G. Clinical and theoretical implications of 5-HT$_2$ and D$_2$ receptor occupancy of clozapine, risperidone and olanzapine in schizophrenia. *Am J Psychiatry.* 1999;156: 286–293.

69. Richardson M, Bevans M, Read, L, et al. Efficacy of the branched-chain amino acids in the treatment of tardive dyskinesia in men. *Am J Psychiatry.* 2003;160:1117–1124.

70. Herrmann N, Mamdani M, Lanctot K. Atypical antipsychotics and risk of cerebrovascular accidents. *Am J Psychiatry.* 2004;161: 1113–1115.

71. Goldstein L, Henderson D. Atypical antipsychotic agents and diabetes mellitus. *Primary Psychiatry.* 2000;7:65–68.

72. Kennedy A, Satyam J, Venogradov S. Atypical antipsychotics for schizophrenia: their collective role and comparative profiles. *Formulary.* 2001;36:500–517.

73. Light E, Lebowitz B, eds *Alzheimer's Disease Treatment and Family Stress: Directions for Research.* Rockville MD: National Institute of Mental Health, US Department of Health and Human Services, Public Health Service; 1989.

74. Malhotra A, Murphy G, Kennedy J. Pharmacogenetics of psychotropic drug response. *Am J Psychiatry.* 2004;161:780–796.

75. Schatzberg A, Nemeroff C, eds. *Textbook of Psychopharmacology.* Washington, DC: American Psychiatric Publishing; 2003.

76. *PDR Drug Guide for Mental Health Professionals.* Montvale, NJ: Thompson PDR; 2003.

77. Schatzberg A, Cole J, DeBattista C, eds. *Manual of Clinical Psychopharmacology,* 4th Ed. Washington, DC: American Psychiatric Publishing; 2002.

78. Pollack B. Psychotropic drugs and the aging patient. *Geriatrics.* 1998;53(1):S-20–24.

79. Hardman J, Limbird L, Goodman A, eds. *Goodman & Gilman's the Pharmacological Basis of Therapeutics,* 10th Ed. New York: McGraw-Hill; 2001.

80. Jacobson S, Pies R, Greenblatt D, eds. *Handbook of Geriatric Psychopharmacology.* Washington, DC: American Psychiatric Publishing; 2002.

81. Parker B, Cusack B. Pharmacology and appropriate prescribing. In: Reuben D, Yoshikawa T, Besdine R, eds. *Geriatric Review Syllabus: A Core Curriculum in Geriatric Medicine,* 3rd Ed. Dubuque IA: Kendall/Hunt; 1996;33:10–11.

82. Kelly J. The drug development and approval process. In: *New Medicines in Development for Mental Illnesses.* Washington, DC: PhRMA;2003:35.

83. Roses A, Pangelos M. Drug development and Alzheimer disease. *Am J Geriatr Psychiatry.* 2003;11(2):123–130.

Electroconvulsive Therapy in the Geriatric Patient

15

Robert M. Greenberg   *Charles H. Kellner*

Since its introduction in 1938, electroconvulsive therapy (ECT) has remained an important treatment for selected serious neuropsychiatric illnesses, and continues to be one of the most effective treatments in psychiatry. ECT has evolved into a technically sophisticated procedure with a proven track record of safety and efficacy. For this chapter we have reviewed the ECT literature, with a special focus on studies and clinical issues most relevant to elderly patients. Key areas of ECT practice are discussed, and supplemented by relevant research findings and consensus of expert opinion when applicable. Areas of controversy and gaps in our knowledge are pointed out.

Although precise data on the overall use of ECT in the United States are unavailable, practice survey data suggest that approximately 100,000 patients per year receive the treatment. There is a trend towards ECT use in the elderly, as well as a shift towards outpatient ECT.

DIAGNOSTIC INDICATIONS

The clinical literature establishing the efficacy of ECT in specific disorders is among the most robust for any medical treatment and has been extensively reviewed elsewhere (1–5). This literature consists of randomized controlled trials comparing real and sham ECT in the treatment of depression (6–11). However, the nature of ECT makes double-blind controlled studies difficult; furthermore, the overwhelming evidence of ECT's efficacy and conse-

quences of untreated severe mental illness makes comparisons of ECT with sham treatment or other inactive controls unethical today. Other studies have compared ECT with pharmacotherapy (3) and transcranial magnetic stimulation (12), and also ECT trials with differing techniques. The indications for ECT have also been supported by numerous case series, case reports, and surveys of expert opinion.

ECT is used most commonly in the treatment of major depressive disorders, typically in patients who have failed to respond to or tolerate one or more courses of antidepressant medications.

Other principal diagnostic indications for ECT have been reviewed elsewhere (1,3). They include bipolar disorder in depressed, manic, or mixed states; schizophrenia, particularly with recent onset or acute exacerbation of positive symptoms or catatonic subtype; schizoaffective disorders; schizophreniform disorder; and psychotic disorder not otherwise specified, particularly when the clinical features are similar to those of the other major diagnostic indications.

The efficacy of ECT for other diagnoses is less well established and should be considered only after standard treatment alternatives have been tried. However, the presence of such disorders should not preclude the use of ECT for treatment of concurrent major diagnostic indications (e.g., major depression with concurrent obsessive-compulsive disorder).

ECT may be useful in the management of severe affective and psychotic disorders secondary to medical conditions, including catatonic state (13–15). Prior to consideration of ECT, attention should be given to identifying underlying medical causes of the disorder and optimizing their management.

The effects of ECT may benefit certain medical and neurological disorders, including Parkinson's disease, neuroleptic-malignant syndrome, and intractable seizure disorder. ECT has also been reported to benefit deliria of various etiologies; however, these reports are based on uncontrolled case studies, and the use of ECT in the treatment of delirium is largely of historical interest. The use of ECT in other medical and neurological disorders has been reviewed elsewhere (1,3,16–24).

EFFICACY AND PREDICTORS OF RESPONSE IN MAJOR DEPRESSION

The early open trials of ECT generally reported response rates in the 80% to 90% range (103). Among patients who receive ECT as a first-line treatment or who have received inadequate pharmacotherapy prior to ECT, response rates continue to be reported in the 80% to 90% range (25–28). However, patients who have shown relative medication resistance—defined by failure to respond to one or more adequate antidepressant medication trials—may have lower response rates to ECT, falling in the range of 50% to 60% (26,29,30). This finding applies primarily to patients treated with tricyclic antidepressants. In the elderly, one study found that patients who failed to respond to sequential trials of nortriptyline and phenelzine also had low response rates to ECT (31).

Most studies that relate medication resistance to lower ECT responsiveness were conducted prior to currently available classes of medications. Results from a secondary analysis suggest having failed a pharmacotherapy trial may be less relevant to patients treated with selective serotonin-reuptake inhibitors (26), but systemic data on relationships between having failed different classes of medications and responsiveness to ECT are lacking.

Most studies have shown that treatment with ECT leads to higher response rates and superior outcomes when compared to treatment with antidepressant medications (32–35). One naturalistic study focusing on elderly patients with psychotic depression found significantly greater response rates to ECT than to a 6-week trial of nortriptyline plus perphenazine, even when pharmacotherapy nonresponders were given 2 additional weeks of lithium augmentation (27). No studies have compared the efficacy of ECT with newer medications such as venlafaxine, mirtazapine, or bupropion. However, no trial has ever reported any antidepressant medication to be more effective than ECT.

The response to ECT is usually faster than with antidepressant medication. In major depression and mania, substantial clinical improvement usually occurs within several treatments (36,37). In addition, the time to maximal response or remission is typically shorter than with medication (38–40).

Because of the greater certainty and speed of clinical response with ECT, its use should be considered early-on or as a first-line treatment whenever rapid and definitive clinical response is urgent. Examples include patients who are severely agitated, psychotic, actively suicidal, or whose medical status is becoming seriously compromised as a result of severe depression (e.g., significant weight loss due to inanition).

Attempts have been made over the years to determine whether particular subtypes of depression or clinical features predict response to ECT (41). Studies limited to patients with major depression suggest that unipolar versus bipolar subtype, or the presence of melancholia, have little predictive value of response (5,42). There are limited data suggesting that the presence of psychomotor retardation may be a positive predictor of ECT response (43–45). Catatonia, or catatonic symptoms, tend to be positive predictors of ECT response (15,46–52). Patients with major depression and a comorbid personality disorder may have a reduced likelihood of response to ECT (53,54).

Studies that have segregated patients with major depression into psychotic and nonpsychotic subtypes have generally found higher response rates in the psychotic group (45,55–58). This may in part be related to psychotic depression representing a more homogeneous subset of depressed patients. It may also reflect the clinical observation that many patients with psychotic depression referred for ECT have not received combinations of antidepressants and antipsychotic medication in sufficient dosages or duration to represent an adequate trial (59), either due to poor tolerance of such combinations, or illness severity resulting in early consideration of ECT. Thus, they may be less likely to be medication resistant at the time of ECT referral.

Illness chronicity may also be a negative predictor of response, with several studies reporting that patients with a long duration of an index episode of depression had lower response rates to ECT (26,42,60,61).

Many, though not all, studies have found better outcomes with ECT in older compared with younger depressed patients (42,62–65). This is in contrast to the pharmacotherapy literature which does not show any consistent association between age and treatment response (66,67). The positive association between patient age and ECT outcome may be related in part to clinical factors associated with depression in the elderly that influence ECT referral in this population. Elderly patients tend to have higher rates of medication intolerance, medical complications, and psychotic depression, resulting in earlier referral to ECT, with resulting shorter duration of index episode and lower rates of documented medication resistance at the time of ECT. Also, shorter illness duration and lack of medication resistance may correlate with good ECT outcome. Although not well substantiated, the elderly may also have lower rates of comorbid Axis II pathology, and this may also contribute to a higher ECT response rate (42). These findings may explain why the elderly constitute a particularly high proportion of patients who receive ECT (68–72).

Unless effectively treated, depression in the elderly may become a severe, frequently relapsing, or chronic disorder with high associated morbidity and mortality. A number of studies have found that the use of ECT is one of the most important variables associated with a positive outcome in late-life depression (73–76), although further investigation is needed to clarify the impact of ECT on short-term versus long-term outcomes.

A number of investigators have reported that a subgroup of patients with late-life depression have concurrent cerebrovascular disease that appears to be associated with decreased antidepressant responsiveness (77–84). The literature on the impact of cerebrovascular disease and ECT response is more mixed. Some authors have reported excellent responses to ECT in elderly depressed patients with significant leukoencephalopathy, despite poor prior medication response (85). Other reports suggest that a subgroup of these patients continue to have a poor outcome even after ECT (82), including one naturalistic study suggesting that severity of subcortical gray matter hyperintensities correlated with less improvement with ECT (86). To some degree, this variability in reported outcomes appears to reflect differences in study design and patient selection, including severity and location of vascular lesions, degree of medication resistance, and nature of cognitive and functional disability. In general, depression in patients with magnetic resonance imaging findings of confluent white matter lesions, multiple lesions in the basal ganglia and pontine reticular formation, and lesions in frontal subcortical areas lateral to the anterior cingulate with associated executive cognitive deficits, have been linked to poor treatment response (77,82,84). However, the specific predictive value of these findings on ECT response remains unclear.

Depression following stroke has also attracted much interest, and this literature has recently been reviewed by Robinson (87). Prevalence rates for major depression following stroke of 19% to 23% have been reported, likely influenced by lesion location. Effective treatment of poststroke depression can significantly influence cognitive and functional recovery. Clinical reports suggest that ECT can be safe and effective in treating poststroke depression, though this literature is largely limited to retrospective case reports. Currier and associates published retrospective data on 20 geriatric patients with poststroke depression who were treated with ECT (most with unilateral electrode placement) (88). A marked or moderate response was reported in 95% of patients. No patients showed any exacerbation of neurological deficits. However, two patients developed severe interictal delirium, and seven of the 20 patients (37%) relapsed within a mean of 4 months following ECT, despite continuation pharmacotherapy.

PRE–ELECTROCONVULSIVE THERAPY EVALUATION

Each facility should identify a minimal set of procedures for all patients receiving ECT. A psychiatric history and examination should be performed, including details of prior response to ECT and other treatments, and documentation of current mental status. A medical history and physical examination should be obtained, with focus on cardiovascular, pulmonary, and neurological systems, as well as outcomes of prior anesthesia administration. The medical inquiry should also include a review of dental problems and an inspection of the mouth, looking for loose teeth and noting the presence of dentures or other appliances.

No "routine" pre-ECT medical evaluation should be required for all patients. Rather, laboratory testing and consultations should be used to identify the presence and severity of medical risk factors noted in the medical history and examination. Recommendations can then be made in order to optimize the patients' medical status and/or modify the treatment procedure to minimize medical risk. This kind of collaborative approach between the ECT psychiatrist, medical consultants, and anesthesia provider is more meaningful than simply asking for "clearance" from a medical consultant before ECT (3,89).

It is common practice to request a minimum screening battery of tests, including a complete blood count, serum electrolytes, and an electrocardiogram. Spine radiographs are not routinely required, because the use of muscle-paralyzing agents minimizes the risk of musculoskeletal injuries. However, spine radiographs may be useful in selected patients with evidence of spine disease or severe osteoporosis. Similarly, an electroencephalogram or neuroimaging studies (brain computed tomography or magnetic resonance imaging) should be considered when other clinical information suggests a relevant neurological disorder might be present.

The pre-ECT evaluation should document the patient's cognitive status, including capacity to engage in an informed consent process. Cognitive assessment should include, at a minimum, evaluation of orientation and memory (anterograde and retrograde). More detailed neuropsychological assessment is useful in patients with pre-existing cognitive impairment or dementia, so that the cognitive effects of ECT can be more carefully monitored in these patients (3). The Mini-Mental State Exam (MMSE) (90) is the most commonly used bedside rating scale for tracking global cognitive change. The MMSE, however, may not be very sensitive to changes in anterograde or retrograde amnesia (91). Other instruments are available for more formally measuring anterograde amnesia (92–98) and retrograde amnesia for autobiographical events (99,100). However, none of these latter scales is used in routine clinical practice. It is a notable gap that no ECT-specific bedside cognitive assessment instrument has yet been developed (101).

ELECTROCONVULSIVE THERAPY PROCEDURE

Location of Treatment: Inpatient versus Outpatient

An index course of ECT can be administered on an inpatient or outpatient basis, or can be initiated in one setting and changed to another as clinically indicated.

ECT should be initiated on an inpatient basis if the underlying psychiatric condition warrants hospitalization. This is generally the case for patients who are acutely psychotic, actively suicidal, or otherwise severely incapacitated. Inpatient ECT is also indicated for patients at substantial risk for serious medical complications and for those with significant cognitive impairment.

Recommendations for ambulatory ECT have been reviewed in a task force report (102). Candidates for outpatient ECT must be able and willing to comply with the behavioral instructions and restrictions for each treatment. These include following prescribed dietary, toileting, and grooming instructions before each treatment, complying with specific medication instructions, and avoiding activities such as driving, which are likely to be impaired by potential adverse cognitive effects of ECT, especially on the day of treatment. There must also be an available caregiver to accompany the patient home from treatment, help ensure compliance with the treatment plan and behavioral restrictions, and report to the treatment team any adverse effects of ECT or changes in medical condition.

Patient Management and Monitoring During Treatment

Details of the ECT procedure have been reviewed elsewhere (3,103). ECT is generally carried out in a dedicated ECT suite or a postanesthesia care area in a hospital setting. The ECT team typically consists of the ECT psychiatrist, the anesthesia provider, and the ECT nurse(s). Informed consent is obtained prior to initiating a course of ECT. Patients are required to fast overnight prior to treatment the next morning. Once in the treatment area, intravenous access is obtained and monitoring equipment placed as appropriate.

Monitoring of the electrocardiogram, blood pressure, and heart rate should begin prior to anesthesia induction and continue until the patient is awake and until any ECT-related hemodynamic or cardiovascular changes have stabilized (104). Automatic, noninvasive blood pressure measurement is preferred. Oxygen saturation monitoring by pulse oximetry should also be performed during the entire treatment.

Oxygenation with 100% O_2 using positive-pressure ventilation should be maintained from the onset of anesthesia until return of spontaneous respirations.

Seizure duration should be monitored during each treatment, both by observation of motor activity and monitoring of at least one channel of electroencephalography (EEG) activity. Although generalized seizures are usually at least 15 seconds in duration, brief seizures may be due to insufficient or markedly suprathreshold stimulation (3,105,106). Elderly patients tend to have higher initial seizure thresholds and shorter seizure durations than younger patients (106). There is little evidence that seizure duration *per se* correlates with ECT outcome (106,107). Seizures that are longer than 3 minutes in duration should be terminated pharmacologically with additional anesthetic or a benzodiazepine such as intravenous diazepam.

Preliminary evidence suggests that seizures accompanied by higher amplitude rhythmic spike-and-wave activity and followed by greater postictal EEG suppression are associated with better clinical outcome (108–112). However, various other factors can impinge upon ictal and postictal EEG expression, including patient age, treatment number, initial seizure threshold, and medication status.

In recent years, investigators have been trying to predict seizure adequacy and clinical response by other specific attributes of the EEG (113–116). Although there have been a number of promising leads, none of these measures can currently be used alone to reliably predict treatment response or to make specific treatment decisions. However, EEG characteristics can be used in conjunction with clinical factors in making decisions about stimulus dosing or changes in electrode placement.

ELECTROCONVULSIVE THERAPY DEVICES AND STIMULUS PARAMETERS

ECT devices presently marketed in the United States are constant-current devices that use a brief pulse square-wave stimulus. The use of a sine-wave stimulus, which is significantly less efficient at depolarizing neurons and produces considerably greater short-term cognitive deficits, is no longer recommended (3).

Device output can be measured in units of charge (millicoulombs [mC]) or energy (joules), with the latter measurement varying with impedance. In the United States, maximal device output is limited to 576 mC, or approximately 100 joules, at an impedance of 220 ohms. Versions of these devices marketed in Canada, Europe, and elsewhere can deliver at least double this maximal output. It has been argued that for rare patients with very high intrinsic seizure thresholds, the maximal US device output may not be sufficient to produce a seizure (117,118). In addition, there are accumulating data that the dosage of right unilateral ECT must be substantially suprathreshold (e.g., about six-times seizure threshold) for it to reliably equal bilateral ECT in efficacy. For patients with very high initial seizure thresholds, the efficacy of unilateral ECT may be compromised by existing limitations on device output, even when generalized seizures are obtained (3,119–123).

ELECTRODE PLACEMENT

Electrode placement and stimulus dose have independent and interactive effects on treatment outcome and cognitive side effects. Decisions about electrode placement should be made in conjunction with decisions about stimulus intensity (124,125).

Bilateral ECT generally refers to the standard bifrontotemporal positioning of the stimulus electrodes, with each electrode placed approximately 1 inch above the midpoint of a line connecting the external canthus and the tragus. It remains the gold standard against which other electrode placements are judged, but is also associated with more short-term and long-term cognitive side effects than right unilateral ECT.

The extent and duration of retrograde memory deficits for autobiographical events are greater in patients receiving bilateral compared with unilateral ECT (126–129), and the likelihood of developing a transient delirium during an ECT series is greater with bilateral electrode placement (130–132).

Although various electrode placements have been used historically for unilateral ECT, the d'Elia placement (133) maximizes interelectrode distance and appears to be optimal in regards to seizure elicitation and efficacy. This placement involves one electrode in the standard frontotemporal position and the other about 1 inch lateral to the vertex of the skull. Since right-handed and most left-handed patients have language functions lateralized to the left hemisphere, right unilateral ECT is usually administered independent of handedness.

Although there has been much historical debate as to the relative effectiveness of unilateral compared with bilateral ECT (3,113), much of this literature was confounded by less than optimal electrode placement or dosing strategies for unilateral ECT.

Several other bilateral placements have been proposed. A bifrontal placement involving greater separation of the stimulating electrodes compared with an earlier form of bifrontal placement has been reported in several case series to have efficacy equal to or greater than standard bifrontotemporal placement, with fewer cognitive side effects (134–136). Another clinical series has also been reported using an asymmetric placement, with a frontal position on the left side and a standard frontotemporal position on the right side (137). The number of patients in these series remains small, however, and cognitive measures have been limited, necessitating further research on these alternative bilateral placements. A multisite, prospective study comparing

right unilateral, bilateral, and bifrontal electrode placements is currently in progress (CH Kellner, personal communication, 2005).

STIMULUS DOSING

In general, three methods have been used for determining stimulus dosing (3,138). The first is an empirical titration process, involving an initial stimulation at a low stimulus intensity that is likely to be subthreshold, followed by sequential restimulation at higher stimulus intensities until a generalized seizure is obtained (139). Patients can show marked variability in electrical threshold required for seizure elicitation, with 50-fold variations in seizure threshold reported (140,141).

On the other hand, in one large multisite study, 90% of patients treated with right unilateral ECT had seizure thresholds less than 100 mC, suggesting that for most patients seizure thresholds falls within a much narrower range (141). In addition, as Abrams and others have pointed out, seizure threshold is to some extent a moving target, varying with a number of patient and treatment variables, including the particular stimulus parameters being used (113).

Much has been written in recent years about the role of seizure threshold and stimulus dose, and their relation to treatment response and cognitive side effects. Stimulus dose relative to seizure threshold has been reported to affect the rate of clinical improvement with both unilateral and bilateral electrode placements, with more rapid response noted at higher relative stimulus intensities (30,36,120,132). The degree to which stimulus intensity exceeds seizure threshold, and not the absolute stimulus dose administered, is critical in determining the ultimate outcome with unilateral but not bilateral ECT (30,132,142), as well as the magnitude of cognitive side effects in both unilateral and bilateral ECT (132,143).

For many years it was assumed that all seizures, once initiated, were equally efficacious, and that the goal of ECT should be to initiate the seizure using the lowest possible stimulus dose, in order to minimize cognitive side effects (119). However, it has become apparent that a strong dose-response relationship exists for unilateral ECT. Very low-dose unilateral ECT, administered just above seizure threshold, was found to be ineffective, with response rates as low as 17% reported (30,109,132,135). Low-to-moderate dose unilateral ECT, administered at doses of 50% to 150% above seizure threshold, was moderately effective, with response rates from 30% to 35% (30,132).

However, when unilateral ECT was administered at markedly suprathreshold doses (e.g., 500% above or six-times threshold), it was fully equal to bilateral ECT in efficacy (30,143). One group reported a continued positive dose-response relationship for unilateral ECT at doses of eight to 12-times threshold, but the increase in cognitive side effects became steeper at these very high dosage multiples (143).

This same group reported a prospective study in which patients were randomly assigned to receive high-dose unilateral ECT at eight-times seizure threshold, or low-dose bilateral ECT at 50% above or 1.5-times threshold. There were no significant differences between the groups, in terms of treatment response or cognitive side effects, immediately following ECT and over a 1-month period of naturalistic follow-up (144).

Therefore, when using the process of stimulus-dose titration to determine subsequent stimulus dosing, the following general recommendations have been made (3):

■ When using unilateral ECT in treating major depressive disorder, stimulus dose should exceed initial threshold by at least 2.5-fold, with greater efficacy likely at higher doses of six-to-eight-times initial seizure threshold and relatively modest differences in cognitive side effects.

■ With bilateral ECT, lower doses in the range of 50% above or 1.5-times initial seizure threshold may be fully effective, with maximal recommended doses in the range of 150% above or 2.5-times seizure threshold. Higher doses are unlikely to enhance efficacy and may aggravate cognitive side effects.

The second method of stimulus dosing involves use of a formula or algorithm taking into account one or more factors that correlate with seizure threshold. The simplest formulas adjust stimulus intensity according to the patient's age (145) or to half the patient age (146). More complex formulas take into account other predictive factors, such as electrode placement, gender, anesthetic dose, and concomitant medications. However, all known demographic and treatment variables account for only about 40% of the variability in initial seizure thresholds (106,141,147–149). Thus, errors in the formula-based estimates may result in barely suprathreshold stimulation for some patients, which may result in ineffective treatment with right unilateral ECT or markedly suprathreshold stimulation for other patients, which can aggravate cognitive side effects with right unilateral or bilateral ECT (107,150).

The last method involves administration of a fixed electrical dosage. It has been argued that high fixed-dose stimulation maximizes the likelihood of response to right unilateral ECT (143,151). Although this may be true for the modal patient, the same errors described in the formula-based method may occur to an even greater degree. With bilateral ECT, use of a high fixed-dosing strategy should be reserved for patients with serious concomitant medical illness, for whom avoidance of subconvulsive stimulation and rapid initial response is an urgent priority.

Although some disagreement exists in the literature as to the optimum approach to stimulus dosing, there is general agreement that dosing should be individualized,

whether by stimulus dose titration or by formula methods, except in emergency situations. The American Psychiatric Association Task Force on ECT has recommended stimulus dose titration as the preferred method, with formula-based dosing as an acceptable alternative (3).

While most patients can be effectively treated despite current US device output limitations (576 mC), a subgroup of patients with very high initial seizure thresholds (mostly elderly) may not. For these patients, attention should be paid to medication alterations (including the ECT anesthetic) that may raise seizure threshold or impede seizure propagation, considering techniques to augment seizure induction (152), or switching to bilateral or bifrontal electrode placement if initially receiving unilateral ECT.

Once initial stimulus dosing is determined, dosing of subsequent treatments must take into account changes in seizure threshold that occur over the course of treatment, with increases in the range of 25% to 200% above initial threshold reported (153,154).

FREQUENCY AND NUMBER OF TREATMENTS

Decisions about the frequency of ECT depend on the relative importance of speed of response versus avoidance of cognitive side effects, and treatment frequency can be varied over the course of ECT.

Daily ECT may be useful early in a treatment course when rapid response is urgent, such as in patients with catatonia, severe mania, high suicide risk, or inanition. However, continued use of daily ECT, particularly with bilateral electrode placement, increases the risk of cognitive impairment.

In the United States, ECT is most commonly performed three times per week, regardless of electrode placement. Studies have shown that with bilateral ECT, twice-weekly treatment results in the same degree of ultimate clinical improvement, though at a slower rate of response. However, twice-weekly bilateral ECT may cause fewer short-term cognitive side effects (155–157).

The cognitive advantages of unilateral ECT usually allow treatment frequency of three times per week without untoward side effects, but treatment frequency can be reduced to twice weekly with bilateral or unilateral ECT if problematic cognitive side effects do occur. On occasion, reducing ECT to once weekly or interrupting the ECT series may be necessary, but continued use of once-weekly ECT may impede efficacy (158,159).

Multiple-monitored ECT (MM ECT) involves the production of more than one adequate seizure under continuous anesthesia during the same treatment session. It was initially developed with the aim of obtaining more rapid improvement with fewer treatment sessions (160). However, it may be associated with higher risk of cardiovascular and cognitive side effects (1), and few controlled comparisons of MM ECT and conventional ECT have been reported (161). Routine use of MM ECT is not currently recommended, though the occasional use of two adequate seizures during the same treatment session may be justified in urgent clinical circumstances (3).

Wide variation is observed in the number of treatments required to achieve maximal clinical benefit. The number of treatments administered should be a function of the rate of clinical improvement as well as the degree of cognitive side effects. Although a typical course of ECT for patients with mood disorders varies between six and 12 treatments, rate and timing of response can vary considerably. While some patients may show complete response after a few treatments, others may not show substantial improvement until receiving 10 or more treatments (36,37,132,162), and some patients may require as many as 20 or more treatments to achieve full response. The practice of prescribing a fixed number of treatments is not recommended.

EVALUATION OF OUTCOME

Evaluation of response of target symptoms should take place between each treatment and preferably at least 24 hours after the last treatment. Although standardized rating instruments may be useful, routine clinical assessment of symptoms and mental status is usually sufficient.

In patients showing slow or minimal clinical improvement after five or six treatments, reassessment should take place regarding the possible presence of undetected psychiatric or medical comorbidity, and decisions made regarding the need for alteration in ECT technique. This may include increases in stimulus intensity, change from unilateral to bilateral electrode placement, alterations in concomitant medications or anesthetics that may be impeding treatment response, or use of medications to augment efficacy (152,163–165).

Patients who show slow but consistent clinical improvement should continue with ECT until they reach a plateau over at least two treatments. Patients should not be considered nonresponsive to ECT unless they have failed to respond to a course of bilateral suprathreshold ECT, usually involving at least 10 treatments. If response remains limited over a prolonged course of ECT (e.g., between 12 and 20 treatments), reassessment and reconsent is advisable, with consideration of expert consultation when available (3).

Repeated courses of ECT are at times needed because of relapse or recurrence of illness, and ECT is often used as a continuation or maintenance treatment. There is no evidence supporting any maximum lifetime limit on the number of ECT treatments (166,167), and there is no evidence that repeated use of ECT leads to permanent structural brain damage (168–172).

Relapse and Recurrence

By convention, relapse refers to the return of the same episode of mental illness within the first 6 months after the onset of remission, and recurrence to the return of a new episode beyond this time. Continuation treatment is for prevention of relapse, and maintenance treatment for prevention of recurrence (173). For convenience, continuation and maintenance ECT will be referred to collectively as C/MECT.

Relapse of depression following ECT is a major clinical problem (174). Naturalistic studies show that relapse rates during the 6 to 12 months following ECT exceed 50%, and are particularly high in the first few months following initial response (29,30,132,175–181).

Although earlier studies from the 1960s suggested that antidepressants could reduce relapse rates from 50% to approximately 20% (182–184), ECT was often used as a first-line treatment at that time, and antidepressants were often given concurrently with ECT (162,174). Thus, patients were not typically resistant to multiple medications prior to receiving ECT, as is often the case today (3,31), and some may have been responding in part to concomitant antidepressants, which were often continued following ECT.

Retrospective data now exist suggesting that, overall, patients who have failed to respond to TCAs prior to ECT relapse at twice the rate of nonresistant patients, and that standard adequate post-ECT pharmacotherapy makes little difference in the relapse rate of these medication-resistant patients (29). Thus, relapse rates may be particularly high in medication-resistant patients, especially in the first few months after recovery (63,162,185–187). There is also evidence that elderly patients with psychotic depression are at greater risk for relapse or recurrence than nonpsychotic patients (180).

Furthermore, the typical practice of putting patients on the same class of medications to which they failed to respond prior to ECT, at least in the case of heterocyclic antidepressants, is not likely to significantly alter these high relapse rates (29,180). Thus, other strategies for relapse prevention are needed.

A randomized, double-blind, placebo-controlled trial has been published comparing 6-month relapse rates in ECT responders assigned to three different continuation treatment strategies: nortriptyline alone, nortriptyline plus lithium carbonate, and placebo (188). The relapse rate for the placebo group was 84%, 60% for nortriptyline, and 39% for nortriptyline plus lithium. Virtually all of the relapses on nortriptyline plus lithium occurred within the first 5 weeks of ECT termination, while relapse continued throughout the 6-month treatment period in the other groups. Medication-resistant patients and those with greater residual depressive symptoms following ECT had a more rapid relapse.

Thus, evidence exists that nortriptyline plus lithium may be a safe and effective combination that can significantly reduce relapse rates of depression, including for the elderly and those with psychotic depression. Information on optimum lithium blood levels for relapse prevention is limited, but in the above study, lithium levels between

0.5 and 0.9 mEq/L were targeted, with a mean of 0.59 mEq/L.

If pharmacotherapy is being used as a continuation treatment following ECT, it is reasonable to initiate medication immediately following, or even during, the index course of ECT, with the aim of reducing the very high early relapse rates. A multisite, double-blind, placebo-controlled study, which includes geriatric patients, is currently in progress examining whether concurrent use of ECT and nortriptyline or venlafaxine will improve acute response to ECT and diminish early relapse, compared with a group receiving ECT plus placebo. All remitters will then be randomized to receive nortriptyline plus lithium, or venlafaxine plus lithium for a 6-month continuation phase (Sackeim, personal communication, 2005). The results of this study will shed light on whether the newer antidepressant venlafaxine plus lithium is as effective as nortriptyline plus lithium in reducing relapse in a generally medication-resistant group of patients.

ECT is typically stopped as soon as a patient has responded. It has been suggested, though not empirically tested, that a tapering of ECT (e.g., weekly ECT for several weeks) may help reduce early relapse in patients receiving continuation pharmacotherapy after ECT, if they have relapsed rapidly following a previous ECT course (174).

The literature on C/MECT consists primarily of retrospective case reports and case series (189–201) and surveys of clinical practice (202). In one of the few prospective studies published, 27 patients with a mean age of 65 were assigned to a continuation ECT protocol (203). No psychotropic medication was used. Forty-seven percent of patients not completing the protocol relapsed, compared with 8% of those completing the continuation ECT protocol.

A multisite prospective trial, with patients being randomly assigned to nortriptyline plus lithium or continuation ECT for relapse prevention after response to an index course of ECT (58), has recently been completed. The results demonstrate both are relatively safe and moderately effective in preventing depressive relapse (C.H. Kellner, personal communication, 2005).

At present, there are no controlled data to guide the use of C/MECT versus other alternatives, or to recommend one C/MECT protocol over another. However, it is common clinical practice to offer C/MECT after initial improvement with an acute ECT series, following one or more relapses despite adequate pharmacotherapy. Other indications include prior history of medication resistance or intolerance, or patient preference (3).

Treatments are typically started on a weekly basis, with the interval between treatments gradually extended to once per month. The rationale is to use a more intensive schedule during the period of greatest risk of relapse. Intervals are often adjusted empirically, based on the patient's response and stability of improvement, with intervals shortened or a short series of treatments inserted if there are symptoms of an impending relapse.

Some patients with severe and frequently relapsing illnesses appear to benefit from prolonged courses of C/MECT (193). Some practitioners eventually taper treatment intervals to less than once per month, or even target the use of C/MECT to periods of greatest risk, as with patients with a seasonal pattern to their illness (204). In the absence of controlled data, the frequency of maintenance treatments should be kept to the minimum that is empirically compatible with maintaining remission. It has been recommended that the overall treatment plan and informed consent be updated at least every 6 months in patients receiving C/MECT.

In the elderly, increasing medical morbidity, functional impairment, and lack of adequate social support may limit ability to comply with maintenance ECT regimens. However, case report literature suggests that C/MECT is an effective and viable option for some older patients with recurrent depression (191,205). The ongoing CORE study will include elderly patients, and should help clarify the safety, tolerability, and efficacy of C/MECT in this population (58).

Electroconvulsive Therapy and Use of Concurrent Medications

The earlier practice of stopping all psychotropic medication before and during a course of ECT is no longer considered necessary. Antipsychotic medications are safe in combination with ECT, and may confer synergistic antipsychotic effects. Evidence now suggests that most antidepressants are safe in combination with ECT, and may either augment antidepressant effect or help to prevent relapse after ECT (163,164). Medications that raise the seizure threshold or impede seizure propagation, and might therefore interfere with the induction or spread of a robust seizure, should be avoided or decreased in dose. These include the anticonvulsants (used as either mood stabilizers or antiepileptics) and the benzodiazepines. Lithium should be withheld if possible during ECT, or given at a dose that produces a low therapeutic level and withheld the day before ECT to avoid the potential risk of increased confusion or prolonged seizures. Cardiac, antihypertensive, and anti-gastric reflux medications are typically continued during a course of ECT. The timing and doses of insulin and oral hypoglycemic agents may need to be adjusted because of the period of fasting prior to each ECT. Theophylline levels should be monitored closely, since high levels during ECT have been associated with status epilepticus (206).

In theory, acetylcholinesterase inhibitors used in the treatment of Alzheimer's disease and other dementias could prolong duration of muscle paralysis induced by succinylcholine. However, initial case report literature (207) and growing clinical experience suggests that these medications may be continued safely during ECT.

SIDE EFFECTS OF ELECTROCONVULSIVE THERAPY

ECT is generally regarded as the safest procedure performed under general anesthesia, with a reported mortality rate of 0.002% (208). The side effects of ECT can be divided into two categories: medical and cognitive. The medical morbidity of ECT derives either from the anesthetic administration or the physiological consequences of the induced seizure. Commonly encountered adverse effects include transient elevations or decreases in blood pressure, or heart rate, and transient arrhythmias (3). Rarely, myocardial infarction has been reported (209). Neurological sequelae of ECT are also rare, but include tardive seizures and nonconvulsive status epilepticus (3,210). The most significant relative medical contraindications to ECT are serious unstable cardiovascular disorders (e.g., acute myocardial infarction, serious arrhythmias, uncompensated congestive heart failure) and the presence of increased intracranial pressure. The autonomic effects of ECT may destabilize the cardiac status in very high-risk patients, and the increase in cerebral blood flow accompanying the seizure may lead to brain herniation in patients with increased intracranial pressure. However, these risks can be modified pharmacologically, and may rarely be outweighed by the risks of severe refractory depression. Common, nonserious side effects of ECT include headache, nausea, and muscle aches (3).

By far the most troubling side effect of ECT is cognitive impairment. Although modern ECT techniques advances in anesthesia delivery have decreased the cognitive impact compared with ECT given in the past, most patients have some adverse cognitive effects. For the vast majority of patients, these effects are mild and acceptable. For a small minority they may be considerably more extensive.

The adverse cognitive effects of ECT may be divided into three types: an acute confusional state, anterograde amnesia, and retrograde amnesia.

The acute confusional state occurs after each treatment, and is a consequence of both the seizure and the anesthetic administration. Initially disoriented, the patient recovers orientation, cognitive, and motor abilities over a period of approximately 5 to 50 minutes (129). The intensity of the ECT treatment (largely a function of electrode placement and stimulus dose), and thus the intensity of the seizure, determines the length and depth of the post-treatment acute confusional state. Most patients are ready to leave the recovery area within 30 minutes.

Elderly patients with extensive subcortical gray and white matter lesions, especially ischemic lesions in the basal ganglia, are at risk for more prolonged interictal delirium during a course of ECT (211,212). Interictal delirium may also be particularly prevalent and prolonged in patients with Parkinson's disease (213,214).

Anterograde amnesia refers to the impairment of new memory retention after ECT. This deficit typically resolves within 1 to 3 weeks after a course of ECT. It is the reason that driving is proscribed and increased supervision may be required for a period after a course of ECT.

Retrograde amnesia remains the most serious adverse cognitive effect of ECT, referring to the forgetting of memories from the time period before the course of ECT. Typically, patients will remember little of events that occurred during the several weeks of a course of ECT, and from a variable time period before that. Commonly, many memories from the previous 1 to 3 months will be lost. The amnesia is most dense for events most proximal to the course of ECT. Memories of some events that are initially forgotten will eventually be recovered, but some of the amnesia may be permanent. The extent of pre-ECT cognitive impairment predicts to some degree the extent of retrograde amnesia, as does the duration of post-ECT disorientation (129). Retrograde amnesia is generally greater for public events than for personal information (126). A small subset of patients will have a much more profound retrograde amnestic syndrome (3). The etiology for such occurrences remains unknown, but probably consists of both patient-related and procedure-related variables. To date, pharmacological efforts to decrease the adverse amnestic effects of ECT have failed to yield clinically useful results.

It should be kept in mind that ECT has beneficial effects on the cognitive problems associated with severe depression (3). MMSE scores typically improve after a course of ECT, and IQ is little changed or slightly increased.

The use of ECT in patients with concurrent dementia and depression is a complex subject. Depression may be difficult to diagnose in patients with moderate-to-advanced stages of dementia, and affective disturbances may manifest themselves at times as agitated or screaming behavior, with or without neurovegetative signs. The presence of a past personal or family history of depression may be useful in the differential diagnosis. Overall, it is estimated that 20% to 25% of patients with dementia have concurrent major depression (215), although this may vary depending on the type of dementia and diagnostic criteria used. One review estimates that about one-third of these patients do not respond to antidepressant medications, and are therefore potential candidates for ECT (215).

However, the use of ECT in patients with dementia is of concern because of possible adverse cognitive impact. Outside of a small case report of literature (216–225), there are minimal outcome data to guide clinicians. The available case reports suggest that ECT can be useful for selected patients with dementia and severe, refractory mood disturbances. There are some reports of increased postictal or interictal delirium, though usually not necessitating termination of ECT. There is no evidence of worsening of dementia related to ECT, and there are some reports of cognitive improvement as depression improves.

Prior to considering ECT in patients with dementia, there should be a thorough evaluation of medical or neurologic factors that may be contributing to affective or behavioral disturbances. In order to minimize cognitive side effects, special attention should be paid to issues of concomitant medications, electrode placement, and treatment frequency. Particular attention also needs to be paid to issues of informed consent or proxy consent, with legal requirements and statutes varying in different jurisdictions. Prospective studies are needed to clarify specific indications, efficacy, and side effects of ECT in patients with dementia.

MECHANISM OF ACTION

Although much is known about the physiology of ECT and induced seizures, the exact mechanism by which ECT exerts its antidepressant and antipsychotic actions remains unknown. It has been widely assumed that ECT works by mechanisms similar to those by which antidepressant medications act, that is, by promoting the increased availability of relevant neurotransmitters, such as serotonin, norepinephrine, and dopamine at the synapse, and subsequent modulation of postsynaptic receptors. However, as with the antidepressants, there is little direct conclusive evidence to support this hypothesis.

Another hypothesis (226) suggests that spread of seizure to diencephalic structures re-regulates the many vegetative functions disturbed in major depression (e.g., appetitive behavior, sleep, diurnal hormonal release patterns). A similar hypothesis suggests that ECT-induced seizures facilitate the release of an unknown neuropeptide or neuromodulator that regulates mood (227).

Sackeim et al. have proposed that the anticonvulsant effects of ECT may be central to its antidepressant properties. However, there has been no confirmation of this theory, as clinical samples show no reliable relationship between increase in seizure threshold over a course of ECT and antidepressant response (228–230).

Finally, Sackeim and colleagues have suggested that seizure initiation in prefrontal brain regions is critical for maximizing therapeutic effect. This notion is supported by the finding that there is a correlation between both decreased cerebral blood flow (231) and increased interictal prefrontal EEG slowing (232), and clinical response to ECT. Most recently, molecular genetic techniques have been applied to ECT or the ECT analog in animals, referred to as *electroconvulsive stimulation*. Knowledge about which genes are turned on or off by the ECT seizure and how they are regulated may lead to a better understanding of the way in which ECT exerts its therapeutic actions.

REFERENCES

1. Abrams R. *Electroconvulsive Therapy.* 3rd Ed. New York: Oxford University Press; 1997.
2. Krueger RB, Sackeim HA. Electroconvulsive therapy and schizophrenia. In: Hirsch SR, Weinberger D, eds. *Schizophrenia.* Oxford: Blackwell; 1995:503–545.
3. American Psychiatric Association. *The Practice of ECT: Recommendations for Treatment, Training and Privileging.* 2nd Ed. Washington, DC: American Psychiatric Press; 2001.
4. Mukherjee S, Sackeim HA, Schnur DB. Electroconvulsive therapy of acute manic episodes: a review of 50 years' experience. *Am J Psychiatry.* 1994;151:169–176.
5. Sackeim HA, Rush AJ. Melancholia and response to ECT [letter]. *Am J Psychiatry.* 1995;152:1242–1243.
6. Freeman C, Basson J, Crighton A. Double-blind controlled trail of electroconvulsive therapy (E.C.T.) and simulated E.C.T. in depressive illness. *Lancet.* 1978;1:738–740.
7. Lambourn J, Gill D. A controlled comparison of simulated and real ECT. *Br J Psychiatry.* 1978;133:514–519.
8. Johnstone EC, Deakin JF, Lawler P, et al. The Northwick Park electroconvulsive therapy trial. *Lancet.* 1980;2:1317–1320.
9. West E. Electric convulsion therapy in depression: a double-blind controlled trial. *Br Med J (Clin Res Ed).* 1981;282:355–357.
10. Brandon S, Cowley P, McDonald C, Neville P, Palmer R, Wellstood-Eason S. Electroconvulsive therapy: results in depressive illness from the Leicestershire trial. *Br Med J (Clin Res Ed).* 1984;288:22–25.
11. Gregory S, Shawcross C, Gill D. The Nottingham ECT Study. A double-blind comparison of bilateral, unilateral and simulated ECT in depressive illness. *Br J Psychiatry.* 1985;146:520–524.
12. Grunhaus L, Schreiber S, Dolberg OT, Polak D, Dannon PN. A randomized controlled comparison of electroconvulsive therapy and repetitive transcranial magnetic stimulation in severe and resistant nonpsychotic major depression. *Biol Psychiatry.* 2003; 53:324–331.
13. Fricchione GL, Kaufman LD, Gruber BL, Fink M. Electroconvulsive therapy and cyclophosphamide in combination for severe neuropsychiatric lupus with catatonia. *Am J Med.* 1990;88:442–443.
14. Rummans TA, Bassingthwaighte ME. Severe medical and neurologic complications associated with near-lethal catatonia treated with electroconvulsive therapy. *Convuls Ther.* 1991;7:121–124.
15. Bush G, Fink M, Petrides G, Dowling F, Francis A. Catatonia. II. Treatment with lorazepam and electroconvulsive therapy. *Acta Psychiatr Scand.* 1996;93:137–143.
16. Abrams R. Electroconvulsive therapy in the medically compromised patient. *Psychiatr Clin North Am.* 1991;14:871–885.
17. Weiner R, Coffey CE, Krystal A. Electroconvulsive therapy in the medical and neurologic patient. In: Greenberg D, ed. *Psychiatric Care of the Medical Patient.* 2nd Ed. New York: Oxford University Press; 2000:419–428.
18. Applegate RJ. Diagnosis and management of ischemic heart disease in the patient scheduled to undergo electroconvulsive therapy. *Convuls Ther.* 1997;13:128–144.
19. Dolinski SY, Zvara DA. Anesthetic considerations of cardiovascular risk during electroconvulsive therapy. *Convuls Ther.* 1997;13: 157–164.
20. Rayburn BK. Electroconvulsive therapy in patients with heart failure or valvular heart disease. *Convuls Ther.* 1997;13:145–156.
21. Folkerts H. Electroconvulsive therapy in neurologic diseases. *Nervenarzt.* 1995;66:241–251.
22. Krystal AD, Coffey CE. Neuropsychiatric considerations in the use of electroconvulsive therapy. *J Neuropsychiatry Clin Neurosci.* 1997;9:283–292.
23. Zwil AS, Pelchat RJ. ECT in the treatment of patients with neurological and somatic disease. *Int J Psychiatry Med.* 1994;24:1–29.
24. Kellner C, Bernstein H. ECT as a treatment for neurologic illness. In: Coffey C, ed. *The Clinical Science of Electroconvulsive Therapy.* Washington, DC: American Psychiatric Press; 1993:183–210.
25. Prudic J, Sackeim HA, Devanand DP. Medication resistance and clinical response to electroconvulsive therapy. *Psychiatry Res.* 1990;31:287–296.
26. Prudic J, Haskett RF, Mulsant B, et al. Resistance to antidepressant medications and short-term clinical response to ECT. *Am J Psychiatry.* 1996;153:985–992.
27. Flint AJ, Rifat SL. The treatment of psychotic depression in later life: a comparison of pharmacotherapy and ECT. *Int J Geriatr Psychiatry.* 1998;13:23–28.
28. Petrides G, Fink M, Husain MM, et al. ECT remission rates in psychotic versus nonpsychotic depressed patients: a report from CORE. *J ECT.* 2001;17:244–253.
29. Sackeim HA, Prudic J, Devanand DP, Decina P, Kerr B, Malitz S. The impact of medication resistance and continuation pharma-

cotherapy on relapse following response to electroconvulsive therapy in major depression. *J Clin Psychopharmacol.* 1990;10:96–104.

30. Sackeim HA, Prudic J, Devanand DP, et al. A prospective, randomized, double-blind comparison of bilateral and right unilateral electroconvulsive therapy at different stimulus intensities. *Arch Gen Psychiatry.* 2000;57:425–434.
31. Flint AJ, Rifat SL. The effect of sequential antidepressant treatment on geriatric depression. *J Affect Disord.* 1996;36:95–105.
32. Folkerts HW, Michael N, Tolle R, Schonauer K, Mucke S, Schulze-Monking H. Electroconvulsive therapy vs. paroxetine in treatment-resistant depression—a randomized study. *Acta Psychiatr Scand.* 1997;96:334–342.
33. Gangadhar B, Kapur R, Kalyanasundaram S. Comparison of electroconvulsive therapy with imipramine in endogenous depression: a double blind study. *Br J Psychiatry.* 1982;141:367–371.
34. Greenblatt M, Grooser GH, Wechsler HA. Differential response of hospitalized depressed patients in somatic therapy. *Am J Psychiatry.* 1964;120:935–943.
35. Medical Research Council. Clinical trial of the treatment of depressive illness. Report to the Medical Research Council by its Clinical Psychiatry Committee. *Br Med J.* 1965;1:881–886.
36. Nobler MS, Sackeim HA, Moeller JR, Prudic J, Petkova E, Waternaux C. Quantifying the speed of symptomatic improvement with electroconvulsive therapy: comparison of alternative statistical methods. *Convuls Ther.* 1997;13:208–221.
37. Segman RH, Shapira B, Gorfine M, Lerer B. Onset and time course of antidepressant action: psychopharmacological implications of a controlled trial of electroconvulsive therapy. *Psychopharmacology (Berl).* 1995;119:440–448.
38. Quitkin FM, McGrath PJ, Stewart JW, Taylor BP, Klein DF. Can the effects of antidepressants be observed in the first two weeks of treatment? *Neuropsychopharmacology.* 1996;15:390–394.
39. Sackeim HA, Devanand DP, Nobler MS. Electroconvulsive therapy. In: Bloom F, Kupfer D, eds. *Psychopharmacology: The Fourth Generation of Progress.* New York: Raven; 1995:1123–1142.
40. Husain M, Rush AJ, Kink M, et al. Speed of response and remission in major depressive disorder with acute ECT: a consortium for research in ECT (CORE) report. *J Clin Psychiatry.* 2004;65(4):485–491.
41. Nobler MS, Sackeim HA. Electroconvulsive therapy: clinical and biological aspects. In: Goodnick PJ, ed. *Predictors of Response in Mood Disorders.* Washington, DC: American Psychiatric Press; 1996:177–198.
42. Black DW, Winokur G, Nasrallah A. A multivariate analysis of the experience of 423 depressed inpatients treated with electroconvulsive therapy. *Convuls Ther.* 1993;9:112–120.
43. Hickie I, Parsonage B, Parker G. Prediction of response to electroconvulsive therapy. Preliminary validation of a sign-based typology of depression. *Br J Psychiatry.* 1990;157:65–71.
44. Hickie I, Mason C, Parker G, Brodaty H. Prediction of ECT response: validation of a refined sign-based (CORE) system for defining melancholia. *Br J Psychiatry.* 1996;169:68–74.
45. Sobin C, Prudic J, Devanand DP, Nobler MS, Sackeim HA. Who responds to electroconvulsive therapy? A comparison of effective and ineffective forms of treatment. *Br J Psychiatry.* 1996;169:322–328.
46. Fink M. Is catatonia a primary indication for ECT? *Convuls Ther.* 1989;5:1–4.
47. Fink M. Catatonia: syndrome or schizophrenia subtype? Recognition and treatment. *J Neural Transm.* 2001;108:637–644.
48. Hawkins JM, Archer KJ, Strakowski SM, Keck PE. Somatic treatment of catatonia. *Int J Psychiatry Med.* 1995;25:345–369.
49. Mann SC, Caroff SN, Bleier HR, Antelo E, Un H. Electroconvulsive therapy of the lethal catatonia syndrome. *Convuls Ther.* 1990;6:239–247.
50. Mann S, Caroff S, Bleier H, Welz W, Kling M, Hayashida M. Lethal catatonia. *Am J Psychiatry.* 1986;143:1374–1381.
51. Rohland BM, Carroll BT, Jacoby RG. ECT in the treatment of the catatonic syndrome. *J Affect Disord.* 1993;29:255–261.
52. Philbrick KL, Rummans TA. Malignant catatonia. *J Neuropsychiatry Clin Neurosci.* 1994;6:1–13.
53. Black DW, Bell S, Hulbert J, Nasrallah A. The importance of axis II in patients with major depression. A controlled study. *J Affective Disord.* 1988;14:115–122.
54. Zimmerman M, Coryell W, Pfohl B, Corenthal C, Stangl D. ECT response in depressed patients with and without a DSM-III personality disorder. *Am J Psychiatry.* 1986;143:1030–1032.
55. Buchan H, Johnstone E, McPherson K, Palmer RL, Crow TJ, Brandon S. Who benefits from electroconvulsive therapy? Combined results of the Leicester and Northwick Park trials. *Br J Psychiatry.* 1992;160:355–359.
56. Pande AC, Grunhaus LJ, Haskett RF, Greden JF. Electroconvulsive therapy in delusional and non-delusional depressive disorder. *J Affective Disord.* 1990;19:215–219.
57. Parker G, Roy K, Hadzi-Pavlovic D, Pedic F. Psychotic (delusional) depression: a meta-analysis of physical treatments. *J Affect Disord.* 1992;24:17–24.
58. Petrides G, Fink M, Husain MM, et al. ECT remission rates in psychotic versus nonpsychotic depressed patients: a report from CORE. *J ECT.* 2001;17:244–253.
59. Mulsant BH, Haskett RF, Prudic J, et al. Low use of neuroleptic drugs in the treatment of psychotic major depression. *Am J Psychiatry.* 1997;154:559–561.
60. Black DW, Winokur G, Nasrallah A. Illness duration and acute response in major depression. *Convuls Ther.* 1989;5:338–343.
61. Kindler S, Shapira B, Hadjez J, Abramowitz M, Brom D, Lerer B. Factors influencing response to bilateral electroconvulsive therapy in major depression. *Convuls Ther.* 1991;7:245–254.
62. O'Connor MK, Knapp R, Husain M, et al. The influence of age on the response of major depression to electroconvulsive therapy: a C.O.R.E. Report. *Am J Geriatr Psychiatry.* 2001;9:382–390.
63. Sackeim HA. The use of electroconvulsive therapy in late life depression. In: Schneider LS, Reynolds III CF, Liebowitz BD, Friedhoff AJ, eds. *Diagnosis and Treatment of Depression in Late Life.* Washington, DC: American Psychiatric Press; 1993:259–277.
64. Sackeim HA. The use of electroconvulsive therapy in late-life depression. In: Salzman C, ed. *Geriatric Psychopharmacology.* 3rd Ed. Baltimore, MD: Williams & Wilkins; 1998:262–309.
65. Tew JDJ, Mulsant BH, Haskett RF, et al. Acute efficacy of ECT in the treatment of major depression in the old-old. *Am J Psychiatry.* 1999;156:1865–1870.
66. Gerson SC, Plotkin DA, Jarvik LF. Antidepressant drug studies, 1964 to 1986: empirical evidence for aging patients. *J Clin Psychopharmacol.* 1988;8:311–322.
67. Alexopoulos GS, Meyers BS, Young R, et al. Recovery in geriatric depression. *Arch Gen Psychiatry.* 1996;53:305–312.
68. Rosenbach ML, Hermann RC, Dorwart RA. Use of electroconvulsive therapy in the Medicare population between 1987 and 1992. *Psychiatr Serv.* 1997;48:1537–1542.
69. Thompson JW, Weiner RD, Myers CP. Use of ECT in the United States in 1975, 1980, and 1986. *Am J Psychiatry.* 1994;151:1657–1661.
70. Thompson J, Blaine J. Use of ECT in the United States in 1975 and 1980. *Am J Psychiatry.* 1987;144:557–562.
71. Kramer B. Use of ECT in California, 1977–1983. *Am J Psychiatry.* 1985;142:1190–1192.
72. McCall WV, Cohen W, Reboussin B, Lawton P. Pretreatment differences in specific symptoms and quality of life among depressed inpatients who do and do not receive electroconvulsive therapy: a hypothesis regarding why the elderly are more likely to receive ECT. *J ECT.* 1999;15:193–201.
73. Rubin EH, Kinscherf DA, Wehrman SA. Response to treatment of depression in the old and very old. *J Geriatr Psychiatry Neurol.* 1991;4:65–70.
74. Zubenko GS, Mulsant BH, Rifai AH, et al. Impact of acute psychiatric inpatient treatment on major depression in late life and prediction of response. *Am J Psychiatry.* 1994;151:987–994.
75. Philibert RA, Richards L, Lynch CF, Winokur G. Effect of ECT on mortality and clinical outcome in geriatric unipolar depression. *J Clin Psychiatry.* 1995;56:390-394.
76. Bosworth HB, Hays JC, George LK, Steffens DC. Psychosocial and clinical predictors of unipolar depression outcome in older adults. *Int J Geriatr Psychiatry.* 2002;17:238–246.
77. Alexopoulos GS, Kiosses DN, Choi SJ, Murphy CF, Lim KO. Frontal white matter microstructure and treatment response of late-life depression: a preliminary study. *Am J Psychiatry.* 2002;159:1929–1932.

78. Alexopoulos GS, Kiosses DN, Klimstra S, Kalayam B, Bruce ML. Clinical presentation of the "depression-executive dysfunction syndrome" of late life. *Am J Geriatr Psychiatry.* 2002;10:98–106.

79. Alexopoulos GS, Meyers BS, Young RC, et al. Executive dysfunction and long-term outcomes of geriatric depression. *Arch Gen Psychiatry.* 2000;57:285–290.

80. Kalayam B, Alexopoulos GS. Prefrontal dysfunction and treatment response in geriatric depression. *Arch Gen Psychiatry.* 1999;56:713–718.

81. Hickie I, Scott E, Wilhelm K, Brodaty H. Subcortical hyperintensities on magnetic resonance imaging in patients with severe depression—a longitudinal evaluation. *Biol Psychiatry.* 1997;42: 367–374.

82. Simpson S, Baldwin RC, Jackson A, Burns AS. Is subcortical disease associated with a poor response to antidepressants? Neurological, neuropsychological and neuroradiological findings in late-life depression. *Psychol Med.* 1998;28:1015–1026.

83. Simpson S, Talbot PR, Snowden JS, Neary D. Subcortical vascular disease in elderly patients with treatment resistant depression. *J Neurol Neurosurg Psychiatry.* 1997;62:196–197.

84. Simpson SW, Jackson A, Baldwin RC, Burns A. 1997 IPA/Bayer Research Awards in Psychogeriatrics. Subcortical hyperintensities in late-life depression: acute response to treatment and neuropsychological impairment. *Int Psychogeriatr.* 1997;9:257–275.

85. Coffey CE, Figiel GS, Djang WT, Cress M, Saunders WB, Weiner RD. Leukoencephalopathy in elderly depressed patients referred for ECT. *Biol Psychiatry.* 1988;24:143–161.

86. Steffens DC, Conway CR, Dombeck CB, Wagner HR, Tupler LA, Weiner RD. Severity of subcortical gray matter hyperintensity predicts ECT response in geriatric depression. *J ECT.* 2001;17:45–49.

87. Robinson RG. Poststroke depression: prevalence, diagnosis, treatment, and disease progression. *Biol Psychiatry.* 2003;54:376–387.

88. Currier MB, Murray GB, Welch CC. Electroconvulsive therapy for post-stroke depressed geriatric patients. *J Neuropsychiatry Clin Neurosci.* 1992;4:140-144.

89. McCall WV. Cardiovascular risk during ECT: managing the managers [editorial]. *Convuls Ther.* 1997;13:123–124.

90. Folstein MF, Folstein SE, McHugh PR. "Mini-mental state." A practical method for grading the cognitive state of patients for the clinician. *J Psychiatr Res.* 1975;12:189–198.

91. Sobin C, Sackeim HA, Prudic J, Devanand DP, Moody BJ, McElhiney MC. Predictors of retrograde amnesia following ECT. *Am J Psychiatry.* 1995;152:995–1001.

92. Wechsler D. *Wechsler Adult Intelligence Scale.* 3rd ed. San Antonio, TX: Psychological Corporation; 1997.

93. Randt CT, Brown RE. *Randt Memory Test.* Bayport, New York: Life Science; 1983.

94. Buschke H. Selective reminding for analysis of memory and learning. *J Verbal Learning Verbal Behav.* 1973;12: 543–550.

95. Zervas IM, Jandorf L. The Randt Memory Test in electroconvulsive therapy: relation to illness and treatment parameters. *Convuls Ther.* 1993;9:28–38.

96. Lezak MD. *Neuropsychological Assessment.* 3rd Ed. New York: Oxford University Press; 1995.

97. Sivan AB. *Benton Visual Retention Test.* 5th Ed. San Antonio, TX: Psychological Corporation; 1992.

98. Sackeim HA. Memory and ECT: from polarization to reconciliation. *J ECT.* 2000;16:87–96.

99. Lisanby SH, Maddox JH, Prudic J, Devanand DP, Sackeim HA. The effects of electroconvulsive therapy on memory of autobiographical and public events. *Arch Gen Psychiatry.* 2000;57:581–590.

100. McElhiney M, Moody B, Sackeim H. *The Autobiographical Memory Interview—Short Form.* New York: New York State Psychiatric Institute; 1997.

101. Kellner CH. The cognitive effects of ECT: bridging the gap between research and clinical practice [editorial]. *Convuls Ther.* 1996;12:133–135.

102. Fink M, Abrams R, Bailine S, Jaffe R. Ambulatory electroconvulsive therapy: report of a Task Force of the Association for Convulsive Therapy. *Convuls Ther.* 1996;12:42–55.

103. Abrams R. *Electroconvulsive Therapy.* New York: Oxford University Press; 2002.

104. Folk JW, Kellner CH, Beale MD, Conroy JM, Duc TA. Anesthesia for electroconvulsive therapy: a review. *J ECT.* 2000;16:157–170.

105. Riddle WJ, Scott AI, Bennie J, Carroll S, Fink G. Current intensity and oxytocin release after electroconvulsive therapy. *Biol Psychiatry.* 1993;33(11–12):839–841.

106. Sackeim HA, Devanand DP, Prudic J. Stimulus intensity, seizure threshold, and seizure duration: impact on the efficacy and safety of electroconvulsive therapy. *Psychiatr Clin North Am.* 1991;14:803–843.

107. Shapira B, Lidsky D, Gorfine M, Lerer B. Electroconvulsive therapy and resistant depression: clinical implications of seizure threshold. *J Clin Psychiatry.* 1996;57:32–38.

108. Folkerts H. The ictal electroencephalogram as a marker for the efficacy of electroconvulsive therapy. *Eur Arch Psychiatry Clin Neurosci.* 1996;246:155–164.

109. Krystal AD, Weiner RD, Coffey CE. The ictal EEG as a marker of adequate stimulus intensity with unilateral ECT. *J Neuropsychiatry Clin Neurosci.* 1995;7:295–303.

110. Luber B, Nobler MS, Moeller JR, et al. Quantitative EEG during seizures induced by electroconvulsive therapy: relations to treatment modality and clinical features. II. Topographic analyses. *J ECT.* 2000;16:229–243.

111. Nobler MS, Luber B, Moeller JR, et al. Quantitative EEG during seizures induced by electroconvulsive therapy: relations to treatment modality and clinical features. I. Global analyses. *J ECT.* 2000;16:211–228.

112. Suppes T, Webb A, Carmody T, et al. Is postictal electrical silence a predictor of response to electroconvulsive therapy? *J Affect Disord.* 1996;41:55–58.

113. Abrams R. Stimulus titration and ECT dosing. *J ECT.* 2002;18: 3–9,14–15.

114. Krystal AD, Weiner RD, Lindahl V, Massie R. The development and retrospective testing of an electroencephalographic seizure quality-based stimulus dosing paradigm with ECT. *J ECT.* 2000;16:338–349.

115. Krystal AD, Holsinger T, Weiner RD, Coffey CE. Prediction of the utility of a switch from unilateral to bilateral ECT in the elderly using treatment 2 ictal EEG indices. *J ECT.* 2000;16:327–337.

116. Krystal AD, Weiner RD. EEG correlates of the response to ECT: a possible antidepressant role of brain-derived neurotrophic factor. *J ECT.* 1999;15:27–38.

117. Krystal AD, Dean MD, Weiner RD, et al. ECT stimulus intensity: are present ECT devices too limited? *Am J Psychiatry.* 2000;157: 963–967.

118. Lisanby SH, Devanand DP, Nobler MS, Prudic J, Mullen L, Sackeim HA. Exceptionally high seizure threshold: ECT device limitations. *Convuls Ther.* 1996;12:156–164.

119. Cronholm B, Ottoson J-O. Ultrabrief stimulus technique in electroconvulsive therapy. II. Comparative studies of therapeutic effects and memory disturbances in treatment of endogenous depression with the Elther ES electroshock apparatus and Siemens Konvulsator III. *J Nerv Ment Dis.* 1963;137:268–276.

120. Robin A, De Tissera S. A double-blind controlled comparison of the therapeutic effects of low and high energy electroconvulsive therapies. *Br J Psychiatry.* 1982;141:357–366.

121. Swartz CM, Larson G. ECT stimulus duration and its efficacy. *Ann Clin Psychiatry.* 1989;1:147–152.

122. Swartz CM, Manly DT. Efficiency of the stimulus characteristics of ECT. *Am J Psychiatry.* 2000;157:1504–1506.

123. Rasmussen KG, Zorumski CF, Jarvis MR. Possible impact of stimulus duration on seizure threshold in ECT. *Convuls Ther.* 1994;10: 177–180.

124. Lisanby S, Luber B, Osman M, et al. The effect of pulse width on seizure threshold during electroconvulsive shock (ECS). *Convuls Ther.* 1997;13:56.

125. Devanand DP, Lisanby SH, Nobler MS, Sackeim HA. The relative efficiency of altering pulse frequency or train duration when determining seizure threshold. *J ECT.* 1998;14:227–235.

126. Lisanby SH, Maddox JH, Prudic J, Devanand DP, Sackeim HA. The effects of electroconvulsive therapy on memory of autobiographical and public events. *Arch Gen Psychiatry.* 2000;57:581–590.

127. Sackeim HA. Memory and ECT: from polarization to reconciliation. *J ECT.* 2000;16:87–96.

128. McElhiney MC, Moody BJ, Steif BL, et al. Autobiographical memory and mood: effects of electroconvulsive therapy. *Neuropsychology.* 1995;9:501–517.

129. Sobin C, Sackeim HA, Prudic J, Devanand DP, Moody BJ, McElhiney MC. Predictors of retrograde amnesia following ECT. *Am J Psychiatry*. 1995;152:995–1001.
130. Daniel W, Crovitz H. Recovery of orientation after electroconvulsive therapy. *Acta Psychiatr Scand*. 1982;66:421–428.
131. Daniel W, Crovitz H. Disorientation during electroconvulsive therapy. Technical, theoretical, and neuropsychological issues. *Ann NY Acad Sci*. 1986;462:293–306.
132. Sackeim HA, Prudic J, Devanand DP, et al. Effects of stimulus intensity and electrode placement on the efficacy and cognitive effects of electroconvulsive therapy. *N Engl J Med*. 1993;328:839–846.
133. d'Elia G. Unilateral electroconvulsive therapy. *Acta Psychiatr Scand*. 1970;215(Suppl):1–98.
134. Lawson JS, Inglis J, Delva NJ, Rodenburg M, Waldron JJ, Letemendia FJ. Electrode placement in ECT: cognitive effects. *Psychol Med*. 1990;20:335–344.
135. Letemendia FJ, Delva NJ, Rodenburg M, et al. Therapeutic advantage of bifrontal electrode placement in ECT. *Psychol Med*. 1993;23:349–360.
136. Bailine SH, Rifkin A, Kayne E, et al. Comparison of bifrontal and bitemporal ECT for major depression. *Am J Psychiatry*. 2000;157: 121–123.
137. Swartz CM. Asymmetric bilateral right frontotemporal left frontal stimulus electrode placement for electroconvulsive therapy. *Neuropsychobiology*. 1994;29:174–178.
138. Farah A, McCall WV. Electroconvulsive therapy stimulus dosing: a survey of contemporary practices. *Convuls Ther*. 1993;9:90–94.
139. Sackeim HA, Decina P, Kanzler M, Kerr B, Malitz S. Effects of electrode placement on the efficacy of titrated, low-dose ECT. *Am J Psychiatry*. 1987;144:1449–1455.
140. Sackeim HA. What's new with ECT. *Am Soc Clin Psychopharm Prog Notes*. 1997;8:27–33.
141. Boylan LS, Haskett RF, Mulsant BH, et al. Determinants of seizure threshold in ECT: benzodiazepine use, anesthetic dosage, and other factors. *J ECT*. 2000;16:3–18.
142. Sackeim HA, Decina P, Portnoy S, Neeley P, Malitz S. Studies of dosage, seizure threshold, and seizure duration in ECT. *Biol Psychiatry*. 1987;22:249–268.
143. McCall WV, Reboussin DM, Weiner RD, Sackeim HA. Titrated moderately suprathreshold vs fixed high-dose right unilateral electroconvulsive therapy: acute antidepressant and cognitive effects. *Arch Gen Psychiatry*. 2000;57:438–444.
144. McCall WV, Dunn A, Rosenquist PB, Hughes D. Markedly suprathreshold right unilateral ECT versus minimally suprathreshold bilateral ECT: antidepressant and memory effects. *J ECT*. 2002;18:126–129.
145. Abrams R, Swartz CM. *ECT Instruction Manual for the Thymatron DG*. Chicago: Somatics, Inc.; 1989.
146. Petrides G, Fink M. The "half-age" stimulation strategy for ECT dosing. *Convuls Ther*. 1996;12:138–46.
147. Colenda CC, McCall WV. A statistical model predicting the seizure threshold for right unilateral ECT in 106 patients. *Convuls Ther*. 1996;12:3–12.
148. Coffey CE, Lucke J, Weiner RD, Krystal AD, Aque M. Seizure threshold in electroconvulsive therapy: I. Initial seizure threshold. *Biol Psychiatry*. 1995;37:713–720.
149. Krueger RB, Fama JM, Devanand DP, Prudic J, Sackeim HA. Does ECT permanently alter seizure threshold? *Biol Psychiatry*. 1993; 33:272–276.
150. Enns M, Karvelas L. Electrical dose titration for electroconvulsive therapy: a comparison with dose prediction methods. 1995;11: 86–93.
151. McCall W, Farah B, Reboussin D, Colenda C. Comparison of the efficacy of titrated, moderate dose and fixed, high-dose right unilateral ECT in elderly patients. *Am J Geriatr Psychiatry*. 1995;3: 317–324.
152. Datto C, Rai AK, Ilivicky HJ, Caroff SN. Augmentation of seizure induction in electroconvulsive therapy: a clinical reappraisal. *J ECT*. 2002;18:118–125.
153. Coffey CE, Lucke J, Weiner RD, Krystal AD, Aque M. Seizure threshold in electroconvulsive therapy (ECT) II. The anticonvulsant effect of ECT. *Biol Psychiatry*. 1995;37:777–788.
154. Sackeim HA. The anticonvulsant hypothesis of the mechanisms of action of ECT: current status. *J ECT*. 1999;15:5–26.

155. Gangadhar BN, Janakiramaiah N, Subbakrishna DK, Praveen J, Reddy AK. Twice versus thrice weekly ECT in melancholia: a double-blind prospective comparison. *J Affect Disord*. 1993;27: 273–278.
156. Lerer B, Shapira B, Calev A, et al. Antidepressant and cognitive effects of twice-versus three-times-weekly ECT. *Am J Psychiatry*. 1995;152:564–570.
157. Shapira B, Tubi N, Drexler H, Lidsky D, Calev A, Lerer B. Cost and benefit in the choice of ECT schedule. Twice versus three times weekly ECT. *Br J Psychiatry*. 1998;172:44–48.
158. Janakiramaiah N, Motreja S, Gangadhar BN, Subbakrishna DK, Parameshwara G. Once vs. three times weekly ECT in melancholia: a randomized controlled trial. *Acta Psychiatr Scand*. 1998;98: 316–320.
159. Kellner CH, Monroe RR, Jr., Pritchett J, Jarrell MP, Bernstein HJ, Burns CM. Weekly ECT in geriatric depression. *Convuls Ther*. 1992;8:245–252.
160. Maletzky BM. *Multiple-Monitored Electroconvulsive Therapy*. Boca Raton, Fl: CRC Press; 1981.
161. Maletzky B. Conventional and multiple-monitored electroconvulsive therapy. A comparison in major depressive episodes. *J Nerv Ment Dis*. 1986;174:257–264.
162. Sackeim HA, Prudic J, Devanand DP. Treatment of medication-resistant depression with electroconvulsive therapy. In: Tasman A, Goldfinger SM, Kaufmann CA, eds. *Annual Review of Psychiatry*. Volume 9. Washington, DC: American Psychiatric Press; 1990: 91–115.
163. Nelson JP, Benjamin L. Efficacy and safety of combined ECT and tricyclic antidepressant drugs in the treatment of depressed geriatric patients. *Convuls Ther*. 1989;5:321–329.
164. Lauritzen L, Odgaard K, Clemmesen L, et al. Relapse prevention by means of paroxetine in ECT-treated patients with major depression: a comparison with imipramine and placebo in medium-term continuation therapy. *Acta Psychiatr Scand*. 1996;94:241–251.
165. Klapheke MM. Combining ECT and antipsychotic agents: benefits and risks. *Convuls Ther*. 1993;9:241–255.
166. Lippman S, Manshadi M, Wehry M, et al. 1,250 electroconvulsive treatments without evidence of brain injury. *Br J Psychiatry*. 1985;147:203–204.
167. Devanand DP, Verma AK, Tirumalasetti F, Sackeim HA. Absence of cognitive impairment after more than 100 lifetime ECT treatments. *Am J Psychiatry*. 1991;148:929–932.
168. Weiner RD. Does ECT cause brain damage? *Behav Brain Sci*. 1984;7:1–53.
169. Coffey CE, Weiner RD, Djang WT, et al. Brain anatomic effects of electroconvulsive therapy. A prospective magnetic resonance imaging study. *Arch Gen Psychiatry*. 1991;48:1013–1021.
170. Devanand DP, Dwork AJ, Hutchinson ER, Bolwig TG, Sackeim HA. Does ECT alter brain structure? *Am J Psychiatry*. 1994;151: 957–970.
171. Zachrisson OC, Balldin J, Ekman R, et al. No evident neuronal damage after electroconvulsive therapy. *Psychiatry Res*. 2000;96: 157–165.
172. Abrams R. And there's no proof of lasting brain damage. *Nature*. 2000;403:826.
173. Prien R, Kupfer D. Continuation drug therapy for major depressive episodes: how long should it be maintained? *Am J Psychiatry*. 1986;143:18–23.
174. Sackeim HA. Continuation therapy following ECT: directions for future research. *Psychopharmacol Bull*. 1994;30:501–521.
175. Karlinsky H, Shulman K. The clinical use of electroconvulsive therapy in old age. *J Am Geriatr Soc*. 1984;32:183–186.
176. Spiker DG, Stein J, Rich CL. Delusional depression and electroconvulsive therapy: one year later. *Convuls Ther*. 1985;1:167–172.
177. Aronson TA, Shukla S, Hoff A. Continuation therapy after ECT for delusional depression: a naturalistic study of prophylactic treatments and relapse. *Convuls Ther*. 1987;3:251–259.
178. Grunhaus L, Shipley JE, Eiser A, et al. Shortened REM latency postECT is associated with rapid recurrence of depressive symptomatology. *Biol Psychiatry*. 1994;36:214–222.
179. O'Leary DA, Lee AS. Seven year prognosis in depression. Mortality and readmission risk in the Nottingham ECT cohort. *Br J Psychiatry*. 1996;169:423–429.

180 Flint AJ, Rifat SL. Two-year outcome of psychotic depression in late life. *Am J Psychiatry.* 1998;155:178–183.

181. Malcolm K, Dean J, Rowlands P, Peet M. Antidepressant drug treatment in relation to the use of ECT. *J Psychopharm.* 1991;5:255–258.

182. Seager CP, Bird RL. Imipramine with electrical treatment in depression: a controlled trial. *J Ment Sci.* 1962;108:704–707.

183. Imlah NW, Ryan E, Harrington JA. The influence of antidepressant drugs on the response electroconvulsive therapy and on subsequent relapse rates. *Neuropsychopharmacology.* 1965;4:438–442.

184. Kay D, Fahy T, Garside R. A seven-month double-blind trial of amitriptyline and diazepam in ECT-treated depressed patients. *Br J Psychiatry.* 1970;117:667–671.

185. Bourgon LN, Kellner CH. Relapse of depression after ECT: a review. *J ECT.* 2000;16:19–31.

186. Grunhaus L, Dolberg OH, Lustig M. Relapse and recurrence following a course of ECT: reasons for concern and strategies for further investigation. *J Psychiatr Res.* 1995;29:165–172.

187. Stoudemire A, Hill CD, Dalton ST, Marquardt MG. Rehospitalization rates in older depressed adults after antidepressant and electroconvulsive therapy treatment. *J Am Geriatr Soc.* 1994;42:1282–1285.

188. Sackeim HA, Haskett RF, Mulsant BH, et al. Continuation pharmacotherapy in the prevention of relapse following electroconvulsive therapy: a randomized controlled trial. *JAMA.* 2001;285:1299–1307.

189. Monroe RRJ. Maintenance electroconvulsive therapy. *Psychiatr Clin North Am.* 1991;14:947–960.

190. Stephens SM, Pettinati HM, Greenberg RM, et al. Continuation and maintenance therapy with outpatient ECT. In: Coffey CE, ed. *The Clinical Science of Electroconvulsive Therapy.* Washington, DC: American Psychiatric Press; 1993:143–164.

191. Loo H, Galinowski A, de C, W, Bourdel MC, Poirier MF. Use of maintenance ECT for elderly depressed patients. *Am J Psychiatry.* 1991;148:810.

192. Dubin WR, Jaffe R, Roemer R, Siegel L, Shoyer B, Venditti ML. The efficacy and safety of maintenance ECT in geriatric patients. *J Am Geriatr Soc.* 1992;40:706–709.

193. Fox HA. Extended continuation and maintenance ECT for long-lasting episodes of major depression. *J ECT.* 2001;17:60–64.

194. Petrides G, Dhossche D, Fink M, Francis A. Continuation ECT: relapse prevention in affective disorders. *Convuls Ther.* 1994;10:189–194.

195. Beale MD, Bernstein H, Kellner C. Maintenance electroconvulsive therapy for geriatric depression: a one-year follow-up. *Clin Gerontol.* 1996;16.

196. Russell JC, Rasmussen KG, O'Connor MK, Copeman CA, Ryan DA, Rummans TA. Long-term maintenance ECT: a retrospective review of efficacy and cognitive outcome. *J ECT.* 2003;19:4–9.

197. Thornton JE, Mulsant BH, Dealy R, Reynolds CF III. A retrospective study of maintenance electroconvulsive therapy in a university-based psychiatric practice. *Convuls Ther.* 1990;6:121–129.

198. Vaidya NA, Mahableshwarkar AR, Shahid R. Continuation and maintenance ECT in treatment-resistant bipolar disorder. *J ECT.* 2003;19:10–16.

199. Scott AI, Weeks DJ, McDonald CF. Continuation electroconvulsive therapy: preliminary guidelines and an illustrative case report. *Br J Psychiatry.* 1991;159:867–780.

200. Andrade C, Kurinji S. Continuation and maintenance ECT: a review of recent research. *J ECT.* 2002;18:149–158.

201. Kramer BA. A naturalistic review of maintenance ECT at a university setting. *J ECT.* 1999;15:262–269.

202. Kramer BA. Maintenance electroconvulsive therapy in clinical practice. *Convuls Ther.* 1990;6:279–286.

203. Clarke TB, Coffey CE, Hoffman GW, Weiner RD. Continuation therapy for depression using outpatient electroconvulsive therapy. *Convuls Ther.* 1989;5:330–337.

204. Kramer BA. A seasonal schedule for maintenance ECT. *J ECT.* 1999;15:226–231.

205. Fox HA. Extended continuation and maintenance ECT for long-lasting episodes of major depression. *J ECT.* 2001;17:60–64.

206. Fink M, Sackeim HA. Theophylline and ECT. *J ECT.* 1998;14:286–290.

207. Zink M, Sartorius A, Lederbogen F, Henn FA. Electroconvulsive therapy in a patient receiving rivastigmine. *J ECT.* 2002;18:162–164.

208. Abrams R. The mortality rate with ECT. *Convuls Ther.* 1997;13:125–127.

209. Zielinski RJ, Roose SP, Devanand DP, Woodring S, Sackeim HA. Cardiovascular complications of ECT in depressed patients with cardiac disease. *Am J Psychiatry.* 1993;150:904–909.

210. Polvsen UJ, Wildschiodtz G, Hogenhaven H, Bolwig TG. Nonconvulsive status epilepticus after electroconvulsive therapy. *J ECT.* 2003;19:164–169.

211. Figiel GS, Coffey CE, Djang WT, Hoffman GJ, Doraiswamy PM. Brain magnetic resonance imaging findings in ECT-induced delirium. *J Neuropsychiatry Clin Neurosci.* 1990;2:53–58.

212. Figiel GS, Krishnan KR, Doraiswamy PM. Subcortical structural changes in ECT-induced delirium. *J Geriatr Psychiatry Neurol.* 1990;3:172–176.

213. Figiel GS, Hassen MA, Zorumski C, Krishnan KR, Doraiswamy PM. ECT-induced delirium in depressed patients with Parkinson's disease. *J Neuropsychiatry Clin Neurosci.* 1991;3:405–411.

214. Kellner CH, Beale MD, Pritchett JT, Bernstein HJ, Burns CM. Electroconvulsive therapy and Parkinson's disease: the case for further study. *Psychopharmacol Bull.* 1994;30:495–500.

215. Rao V, Lyketsos CG. The benefits and risks of ECT for patients with primary dementia who also suffer from depression. *Int J Geriatr Psychiatry.* 2000;15:729–735.

216. Benbow SM. ECT for depression in dementia. *Br J Psychiatry.* 1988;152:859.

217. Carlyle W, Killick L, Ancill R. ECT: an effective treatment in the screaming demented patient [letter]. *J Am Geriatr Soc.* 1991;39:637.

218. Krystal AD, Coffey CE. Neuropsychiatric considerations in the use of electroconvulsive therapy. *J Neuropsychiatry Clin Neurosci.* 1997;9:283–292.

219. Grant JE, Mohan SN. Treatment of agitation and aggression in four demented patients using ECT. *J ECT.* 2001;17:205–209.

220. Nelson JP, Rosenberg DR. ECT treatment of demented elderly patients with major depression: a retrospective study of efficacy and safety. *Convuls Ther.* 1991;7:157–165.

221. Zwil AS, McAllister TW, Price TR. Safety and efficacy of ECT in depressed patients with organic brain disease: review of a clinical experience. *Convuls Ther.* 1992;8:103–109.

222. Weintraub D, Lippmann SB. ECT for major depression and mania with advanced dementia. *J ECT.* 2001;17:65–67.

223. Fisman M, Rabheru K, Sharma V. Response to ECT in depressed, demented patients; possible role of apolipoprotein E(4) as response marker. *Int J Geriatr Psychiatry.* 2001;16:919–920.

224. McDonald WM, Thompson TR. Treatment of mania in dementia with electroconvulsive therapy. *Psychopharmacol Bull.* 2001;35:72–82.

225. Roccaforte WH, Wengel SP, Burke WJ. ECT for screaming in dementia. *Am J Geriatr Psychiatry.* 2000;8:177.

226. Abrams R, Taylor MA. Diencephalic stimulation and the effects of ECT in endogenous depression. *Br J Psychiatry.* 1976;129:482–485.

227. Fink M. How does ECT work? *Neuropsychopharmacology.* 1990;3:77–82.

228. Krystal AD, Coffey CE, Weiner RD, Holsinger T. Changes in seizure threshold over the course of electroconvulsive therapy affect therapeutic response and are detected by ictal EEG ratings. *J Neuropsychiatry Clin Neurosci.* 1998;10:178–186.

229. Delva NJ, Brunet D, Hawken ER, et al. Electrical dose and seizure threshold: relations to clinical outcome and cognitive effects in bifrontal, bitemporal, and right unilateral ECT. *J ECT.* 2000;16:361–369.

230. Scott AI, Boddy H. The effect of repeated bilateral electroconvulsive therapy on seizure threshold. *J ECT.* 2000;16:244–251.

231. Nobler MS, Sackeim HA, Prohovnik I, et al. Regional cerebral blood flow in mood disorders, III. Treatment and clinical response. *Arch Gen Psychiatry.* 1994;51:884–897.

232. Sackeim HA, Luber B, Katzman GP, et al. The effects of electroconvulsive therapy on quantitative electroencephalograms. Relationship to clinical outcome. *Arch Gen Psychiatry.* 1996;53:814–824.

Hospice and Palliative Care

16

Ladislav Volicer

Although the primary goal of healthcare is curing an illness and restoring health, this goal cannot always be achieved. Everybody dies eventually, and another important goal for healthcare is to make dying as painless and dignified as possible. Therefore, it is important to include hospice and palliative care in our healthcare continuum. Most psychiatric diseases are not themselves a direct cause of death, but psychiatric patients develop the same spectrum of comorbid conditions as individuals without a psychiatric history. In addition, patients suffering from progressive degenerative dementias are often cared for by psychiatrists. These dementias can be considered terminal diseases, because there is no treatment that can stop or reverse their progression. Therefore, hospice and palliative care are very important options for management of these individuals.

Geriatric psychiatrists play an important role in optimal end-of-life care for individuals with dementia. Although psychiatric issues are more common in the earlier stages of dementia, some of them may persist even in an advanced stage. The most important issue is depression, which may be difficult to diagnose in severe dementia because of the patient's inability to provide adequate history, as well as the considerable symptom overlap with other medical conditions. Depression should be suspected when a patient with dementia exhibits agitation, excessive complaints of pain, resistance to care, or changes in neurovegetative function (e.g., sleep, appetite, activity, or energy levels). Sometimes a diagnosis in advanced dementia is made on the basis of a good response to a trial of antidepressant treatment. Involvement of a geriatric psychiatrist may also be needed to provide support to caregivers of patients with dementia. There is a high incidence of depression in family caregivers, and even professional staff needs support when facing end-of-life decisions.

THE GOALS OF HOSPICE AND PALLIATIVE CARE

The hospice movement started in England and was originally intended for individuals suffering from incurable cancer. However, it was soon recognized that a similar approach might also be appropriate for individuals suffering from other terminal diseases, and criteria for inclusion of such individuals were developed (1). The goal of hospice is to provide appropriate medical care that blends two complementary systems of therapy—curative and palliative. Even if therapies do not produce a cure, they may still be partially successful in establishing disease control.

Palliative care can be provided independently or as a part of hospice care, and the context of treatment may depend on restrictive Medicare criteria for hospice benefit eligibility. The World Health Organization defines palliative care as:

An approach that improves the quality of life of patients and their families facing life-threatening illness, through prevention, assessment, and treatment of pain and other physical, psychosocial, and spiritual problems.

Palliative care:

- Provides relief from pain and other distressing symptoms.
- Affirms life and regards dying as a normal process.
- Intends neither to hasten nor postpone death.
- Offers a support system to help patients live as actively as possible until death.
- Offers a support system to help family cope during the patient's illness and in their own bereavement.
- Uses a team approach to address the needs of patients and their families including bereavement counseling, if indicated.

■ Will enhance the quality of life, and may also positively influence the course of a patient's illness (2).

Many palliative care programs are hospital-based, whereas the traditional hospice is based in patients' homes, although it may also include a short-term hospitalization. Hospice care is often provided in a nursing home or assisted-living facility because these settings are considered patients' homes. Involvement in a hospice program requires a blanket informed consent for all hospice services, while palliative programs may require consent for individual medical interventions. While hospice programs are regulated by National Hospice and Palliative Care Organization standards of practice and Medicare conditions of participation, palliative care programs are not currently regulated (although are often located in Joint Commision for Accreditation of Health Organizations-accredited facilities). Thus, palliative care programs may be more flexible in meeting patients' needs on a long-term basis than hospice programs.

ELIGIBILITY CRITERIA FOR HOSPICE

Involvement of an individual with life-threatening illness in hospice programs is limited by the requirement that the individual must be certified as terminally ill by hospice medical staff and the individual's attending physician. Terminal illness is defined as a medical prognosis that the patient's life expectancy is 6 months or less if the terminal illness runs its normal course. To be included in a hospice, the patient has to waive the right to receive standard Medicare benefits related to the terminal illness, including all treatments for the purposes of curing the illness. Hospice coverage is divided into four discrete election periods, where, during each period, the beneficiary must be certified as terminally ill. The fourth and last period has an indefinite duration, unless or until the beneficiary no longer meets the eligibility requirement of a prognosis of 6 months or less to live (3). General guidelines for determining if a patient is appropriate for hospice care (4) are summarized in Table 16-1.

These general guidelines are usually sufficient for patients with terminal cancers, but do not provide sufficient guidance for individuals with other diseases. Specific guidelines were developed for heart disease, pulmonary disease, dementia, HIV, liver disease, renal disease, stroke and coma, and amyotrophic lateral sclerosis (4,5). For a psychiatrist, the most important are guidelines related to dementia. Dementia is a common condition in elderly individuals—particularly those over the age of 85—and AD is overwhelmingly the most common cause of dementia. Although the exact prevalence is not known, it is estimated that over 4 million people in the United States have AD, and that the prevalence in the age group over 85 nears 50% (6,7). Additional causes of dementia increase this number even further. Advanced dementia should be considered a

TABLE 16-1

HOSPICE ELIGIBILITY CRITERIA

General guidelines for determining whether a patient is appropriate for hospice care require that:

- The patient's condition is life-limiting and the patient and/or family has been informed about this
- The patient and/or family has elected treatment goals directed towards relief of symptoms, rather than cure of the underlying disease
- The patient has either documented clinical progression of the disease or recent impairment of nutritional status related to the terminal process

Documentation of clinical progression may include:

- Evidence documented by physician assessment, laboratory, radiologic, or other studies, or by nursing assessment in home-bound patients
- Multiple emergency room visits or inpatient hospitalizations over the prior 6 months
- Recent decline in functional status documented by Karnofsky Performance Status (5) of ≤50% or dependence in at least three of six activities of daily living

Documentation of recent impairment of nutritional status may include:

- Unintentional, progressive weight loss >10% over the prior 6 months
- Serum albumin <2.5 mg/dL (only in connection with other conditions)

Adapted from References 4 and 5.

terminal disease similar to incurable cancer, because there is no treatment available that can cure or reverse its course. Therefore, hospice care emphasizing comfort and quality of life instead of maximal survival may be appropriate for these patients (8,9). The hospice guidelines related to dementia are summarized in Table 16-2.

It is important to realize that these guidelines are not based on hard clinical data. It was reported by Schonwetter et al. that only 44% of individuals with dementia who died less than 6 months after enrollment in a hospice program actually satisfied the Medicare criteria (1). Thus, strict application of these criteria would deprive many individuals and their families of hospice benefits. In fact, later studies from the same group concluded that Medicare guidelines were not valid predictors of survival in hospice patients with dementia (10). Survival in patients with advanced dementia is difficult to predict because the death is most commonly caused by an intercurrent infection, and even some patients with very advanced dementia do not develop these infections, or survive them even when treated palliatively.

The difficulty with prediction of 6-month survival leads to under-utilization of hospice care for individuals with dementia. In nursing homes, where over 60% of residents suffer from dementia, only 7.3% of residents enrolled in hospice had a primary diagnosis of AD or dementia (11).

TABLE 16-2
HOSPICE GUIDELINES FOR DEMENTIA PATIENTS

The patient should be at or beyond stage 7 of the Functional Assessment Staging Scale (FAST) (9) and show all the following characteristics:

- Unable to ambulate without assistance
- Unable to dress without assistance
- Unable to bathe properly
- Having urinary and fecal incontinence occasionally or more frequently over the past weeks, as reported by knowledgeable informant or caregiver
- Unable to speak or communicate meaningfully, i.e., ability to speak is limited to approximately six or fewer intelligible and different words, in the course of an average day or in the course of an intensive interview

The patient should have one of the following comorbid medical complications, which should be of sufficient severity to warrant medical treatment, documented within the past year, whether or not the decision was made to treat the condition. These conditions include:

- Aspiration pneumonia
- Pyelonephritis or other upper urinary tract infection
- Septicemia
- Decubitus ulcers, multiple, stage 3–4
- Fever recurrent after antibiotics
- Nutritional impairment
- Difficulty swallowing food or refusal to eat, sufficiently severe that the patient cannot maintain sufficient fluid and calorie intake to sustain life, with patient or surrogate refusing tube feedings or parenteral nutrition
- Patients who are receiving tube feedings must have unintentional, progressive weight loss >10% over the past 6 months. Serum albumin <2.5 gm/dL may be a helpful prognostic indicator, but should not be used by itself

Adapted from References 4 and 9.

In addition, 24.2% of these residents with dementia were discharged from hospice before they died. However, 32.7% of residents with a primary diagnosis of cancer who were enrolled in a hospice were also demented.

There is a need to modify eligibility criteria for hospice care, or to develop programs that recognize that individuals with advanced dementia should receive palliative care regardless of expected length of survival. Researchers at the University of Chicago developed the Palliative Excellence in Alzheimer Care Efforts program, which incorporates advance care planning, patient-centered care, family support, and a palliative care focus from the diagnosis of dementia through its terminal stages (12). This program is coordinated through the primary care geriatrics practice, and patients and caregivers are interviewed every 6 months. The nurse coordinator reviews these interviews and provides feedback to physicians.

Another approach is the development of an acute palliative-care service that provides care for patients with a variety of diagnoses including advanced dementia (13).

Such a unit may provide more appropriate care than a standard acute-care hospital unit, where patients with advanced dementia often receive enteral tube feeding and invasive and complex diagnostic tests, and are resuscitated in the event of sudden death (14).

Hospices need to adjust to the special needs of individuals with dementia. They must recognize and respect the long trajectory of the degenerative diseases that require constant care with little outside help. They need to develop skills in evaluating pain and discomfort in cognitively impaired individuals who cannot communicate their symptoms. They also need to develop communication strategies appropriate for this patient population (15) and special programs, such as music therapy (16) and expressive puppetry (17). Another program useful for individuals with advanced dementia is *Snoezelen*. Snoezelen is a multisensory environment, originally developed for children with handicaps (18). A portable part of this environment, consisting of a projector with a record player, may be brought directly to the patient's room. The projector uses wheels with multicolored oils to project moving images on a screen, wall, or ceiling, accompanied by relaxing music. Use of Snoezelen before dental procedures has been shown to decrease resistive behavior (19). Similar approaches may also be useful for individuals with chronic psychiatric conditions who are involved in a hospice program.

Hospice benefits are important not only for the individual with dementia, but also for his or her family. In fact, a survey showed that caregivers were twice as likely to say that hospice would benefit them than they were to say it would benefit the patient (20). The most important features for the caregivers were continued follow-up evaluation and emphasis on helping to avoid hospitalization. Hospice family caregivers are at high risk for both psychological and physical health disorders (21), and the hospice team should be able to assess and treat these problems. Hospice is also important during the bereavement period, when family members require additional support. This support is not typically provided if a resident dies in a nursing home, because most nursing homes lack the resources to provide bereavement support (22).

EFFECTIVENESS OF THERAPEUTIC INTERVENTIONS IN THE ELDERLY

Age by itself should not be used as a criterion for decisions regarding medical care. However, elderly individuals often suffer from multiple medical conditions, which may limit the effectiveness of therapy for each individual one. For instance, use of nonsteroidal anti-inflammatory drugs for treatment of arthritis may limit effectiveness of some antihypertensive medications. Psychiatric conditions may also complicate medical interventions because of drug interactions and possible lack of adherence to a medication regime. In general, dementia is the most important condition that should be taken into consideration when decisions need to be made regarding medical care in the elderly.

Treatment of individuals with advanced progressive dementia should weigh the possible benefits for the patient against the burden imposed by such treatment. Many medical interventions cause discomfort, and a patient who understands the rationale for such interventions is better able to tolerate the discomfort than one who does not. Patients with advanced dementia do not recognize the need for therapeutic interventions, do not always cooperate with treatment, or may actively oppose it. Even minor routine procedures, such as blood drawing or blood pressure measurement may precipitate behavioral disturbances. Accordingly, the burden of therapeutic interventions on patients with advanced dementia is larger than the burden on cognitively intact individuals.

Decisions regarding treatment strategies should also consider that advanced dementia is a terminal disease. Reduced life expectancy is related to both age and dementia severity. Younger demented individuals show the greatest increase in the mortality rate: it is 10 times higher in women and seven times higher in men 65 to 74 years old, four times higher in women and three times higher in men 75 to 84 years old, and two times higher in both men and women over the age of 85 (23,24). In addition, 48-month survival probability in a cohort of community residents of at least 65 years of age is 0.85 for cognitively intact individuals, 0.69 for the mildly impaired, and 0.51 for severely impaired individuals. When adjusted for other health and social covariates, severely demented individuals are twice as likely to die as those who are cognitively intact (25).

Decreased life expectancy should be taken into account in the management of chronic illnesses in this patient population. Preventive measures, such as restricted diets and screening procedures, are often inappropriate in individuals with progressive dementia. Similarly, treatment of chronic conditions, such as hypertension and diabetes, should be conservative and directed toward prevention of potentially serious side effects, such as postural hypotension that may lead to falls and hip fractures.

Cardiopulmonary Resuscitation

Cardiopulmonary resuscitation (CPR) performed in a hospital provides immediate survival for 41% of patients and survival to discharge for 13% (26). However, in the presence of dementia, successful CPR is three times less likely, almost as low as in metastatic cancer. CPR is much less successful if it occurs in a nursing home setting. Among resuscitated nursing home residents, immediate survival was 18.5%, with only 3.4% surviving to hospital discharge (27). In another study, the immediate survival was lower in nursing homes than in other settings (10.4% versus 18.5%), and no nursing home patients survived to hospital discharge, while 5.6% patients from other settings survived (28).

The benefits of successful resuscitation are further diminished by several factors. CPR is a stressful experience for those who survive, often associated with injuries such as broken ribs, and often necessitating mechanical respiration. The intensive care unit environment produces additional confusion and, almost invariably, delirium. Most patients who survive CPR are more cognitively impaired than they were before the arrest (29). Furthermore, the CPR experience is often sufficiently traumatic for the patient's families that a *do not resuscitate* directive is requested, preventing repetition of the CPR (30). Other residents of long-term care facilities who witness the CPR procedure are frequently upset as well.

Transfer to an Acute Care Setting

Transfer of elderly individuals to an emergency room or hospital exposes them to serious risks. Hospitalized elderly individuals often develop physical, mental, and functional decline characterized in part by confusion, anorexia, incontinence, and falls (31). These symptoms are usually managed by medical interventions, such as psychotropic medications, restraints, nasogastric tubes, and Foley catheters, subjecting the patient to possible complications of thrombophlebitis, pulmonary embolus, aspiration pneumonia, urinary tract infection, and septic shock. Shortly after hospital admission of elderly individuals, deterioration can occur in mobility, transfer, toileting, feeding, and grooming, with few if any of these functions improving significantly by discharge (32). Risk factors for such functional decline include cognitive impairment, previous functional impairment, low social activity level, and decubitus ulcers. Research has shown that in individuals with three or four of the risk factors, 63% to 83% suffer functional decline, while 41% to 67% either die in the hospital or have to be placed in a nursing home (33). These findings highlight the substantial risks posed to elderly individuals during acute care hospitalization, particularly those with advanced dementia. As a result, careful consideration should be given to the decision to hospitalize.

Transfer from a long-term care facility to an acute-care setting is most often due to an infection and/or breathing difficulties (34). Pneumonia is a leading cause of infection among patients in long-term care facilities, and its median reported incidence is 1 per 1,000 patient-days (35). Risk of pneumonia is increased in residents who are bedridden, have a debilitating neurological disease, or who require tube feeding (36). Other risk factors include older age, male gender, swallowing difficulty, and inability to take oral medication (37). Since many of these risk factors are not amenable to intervention, the rate of recurrent pneumonia is high. Patients discharged from a hospital after pneumonia have five times the risk for recurrent pneumonia than patients admitted for other conditions (38), and 43% of nursing home residents who survive an episode of pneumonia develop another episode within 12 months (35).

The mortality rate from pneumonia is increased by altered mental status (39), and cognitive impairment increases the mortality risk almost seven times (40). Most studies have found that mortality is also increased in patients with impaired functional status, even if living in the community (41). Among residents of long-term care facilities, mortalities of the least functionally impaired patients at 12 and 24 months were 33% and 48% respectively, while the mortality rates of the most functionally impaired were 65% and 77% (35).

Transfer of long-term care facility residents to an acute-care hospital may not be optimal for management of infections and other conditions. A recent study that reviewed hospital records of 100 unscheduled transfers to a hospital found that 36% of emergency room transfers and 40% of hospital admissions were inappropriate (42). These numbers increased to 44% of emergency room transfers and 45% of hospital admissions when advance directives were considered. The rate of hospitalization varies widely among patients from different long-term care facilities (43) and, if all hospitalizations are considered, cannot be predicted by any particular patient characteristic (44). Approximately 40% of hospitalizations occur within 3 months of admission to long-term care facilities. In hospitalizations that occur after 6 months, severe functional impairment, impairment in activities of daily living, decubitus ulcers, feeding tubes, and primary diagnoses of congestive heart failure or respiratory disease are associated with acute-care transfer (45). Additionally, nursing homes with special care units, greater physician-to-patient ratios, and physician extenders (e.g., nurse practitioner, physician assistant) are less likely to hospitalize their residents (46).

Acute-care hospitalization is often not necessary for optimal treatment of pneumonia in nursing home residents; immediate survival and mortality rates are comparable, regardless of whether the treatment is received in the long-term care facility or the hospital (47,48). Long-term outcomes are, in fact, better for residents treated in a nursing home. The 6-week mortality rate is 18.7% in nonhospitalized residents and 39.5% in hospitalized residents, despite no significant differences between the hospitalized and nonhospitalized groups before diagnosis (49). Similarly, 2 months after the onset of pneumonia, a greater proportion of hospitalized individuals had declined in their functional status or died (50). The improved outcome in nonhospitalized residents was present, however, only in those with a lower respiratory rate during the episode, and best seen in residents who were independent or mildly dependent at baseline.

The available data indicate that transfer to an emergency room or hospital has significant risks and relatively few benefits for elderly individuals. This management strategy should be used only when it is consistent with the overall goals of care, and not as a default option. The transfer to an emergency room or hospital is especially problematic in an individual with advanced dementia. A declining rate of acute-care hospitalization for demented long-term care residents has been reported (51), and may reflect improved assessment or a changing treatment philosophy.

Antibiotic Therapy

Antibiotic therapy is quite effective in treatment of an isolated episode of pneumonia or other systemic infection. In most patients, it is preferable to limit antibiotic therapy to oral preparations, which are at least equally if not more effective than parenteral antibiotics (52,53). Intravenous therapy can be quite difficult in cognitively impaired individuals if they do not understand the need for it, or if they try to remove the intravenous catheters, necessitating the use of physical restraints or psychotropic drugs to prevent removal. In patients with poor oral intake, intramuscular administration of antibiotics when feasible, e.g., cephalosporins, offers a reasonable alternative.

The effectiveness of antibiotic therapy may be limited by the recurrent nature of infections in advanced dementia. Dementia severity increases the mortality after pneumonia because of aspiration and weight loss (54). Antibiotic therapy does not prolong survival in cognitively impaired patients who are unable to ambulate alone or with assistance, and who are mute (55). Similarly, Luchins and colleagues found no significant difference in survival rates between very advanced dementia patients (characterized in their study as at, or past, FAST stage 7C) who were or were not treated with antibiotics (9,56).

In addition, antibiotics might not play a significant role in the maintenance of comfort in some demented individuals. A study using an observational scale for measurement of discomfort (57) found there were no differences in patients' discomfort level increases during the first 3 to 5 days of an infection, whether treated or not treated with antibiotics (58). Likewise, there was no significant difference in the mean discomfort level as the infection resolved. Similar findings were observed in another study, although the starting levels of discomfort were somewhat different (59). Analgesics, antipyretics, and oxygen, if necessary, provide comfort in the absence of antibiotics.

Antibiotic use may cause significant adverse effects. Patients may develop gastrointestinal upset, diarrhea, allergic reactions, hyperkalemia, and rarely, agranulocytosis. Diagnostic procedures such as blood drawing and sputum suctioning, which are necessary for the rational use of antibiotics, can cause discomfort and confusion in demented individuals who do not understand the rationale. In addition, diagnostic procedures fail to indicate the source of the infectious episode in 30% of cases (55). Furthermore, most infections are recurrent in demented individuals, because the underlying causes, such as swallowing difficulties and aspiration, persist (60). A decision on whether to use antibiotics in advanced dementia should take into consideration the recurrent nature of infections, the adverse effects produced by antibiotics and the accompanying diagnostic procedures, and the potential lack of any significant enhancement of patient comfort.

Tube Feeding

Nutritional problems are common in elderly individuals, especially in those who are homebound or reside in an institution (61). These problems may result in protein-calorie undernutrition and increase the risk of dying. The causes of this undernutrition in nursing homes include inability or unwillingness to eat caused by neurogenic dysphagia, anorexia resulting from a brain disease, depression, anorexigenic drugs, poor dental status, the loss of taste and smell, and an environment that may not be conducive to eating. Risk factors for low body weight and weight loss include eating dependency, decubiti, and chewing problems, while depressed behavior and two or more chronic diseases increase the risk of weight loss alone (62).

Chewing and swallowing problems in elderly individuals are sometimes managed by tube feeding. A study of 5,266 nursing home residents over the age of 65 with chewing and swallowing difficulties found that 10.5% had a feeding tube (63). Tube-fed residents had a significantly higher 1-year mortality rate that those without tubes. One quarter of the residents who survived one year had the feeding tube removed, indicating that the placement was temporary during recovery from an acute process. Feeding tubes should be used with caution in elderly individuals because they can pose a significant burden. In a survey of patients rating discomfort levels of procedures, the nasogastric tube was considered the most uncomfortable, followed by mechanical ventilation and physical restraints (64). Tube feeding also deprives the patient of the taste of food, the pleasure of eating, and contact with caregivers during the feeding process.

Eating difficulties are particularly common in individuals with advanced dementia. Apraxia prevents patients from using utensils correctly, and ultimately disrupts their ability to eat unassisted. In addition, patients intermittently refuse food because of depression, dislike of hospital food, or inability to perceive hunger. As the dementia progresses, patients develop swallowing difficulties, often choking on solids as well as liquids. Choking and food refusal are often exhibited simultaneously (65). Eating apraxia can be managed by hand feeding, and food refusal may be improved by administration of antidepressants (66) or appetite stimulants (67). Swallowing difficulties and choking may be minimized by adjustment of diet texture and by replacing thin liquids with thick ones (e.g., yogurt instead of milk) (68). Nevertheless, some practitioners consider tube feeding necessary for appropriate nutrition and the prevention of aspiration (69).

Two excellent reviews recently summarized available evidence considering the risks and benefits of tube feeding in individuals with advanced dementia (70,71). Both reviews found no evidence that long-term feeding tubes

were beneficial. Tube feeding does not necessarily prev aspiration of nasopharyngeal secretions and/or regur tated gastric contents, nor does it always prevent aspirati pneumonia; in fact, in some circumstances tube-feedi may actually increase the incidence of aspiration pneum nia. Moreover, nasogastric tubes may promote sinus a middle ear infections, and gastrostomy tubes may cau cellulitis, abscesses, necrotizing fasciitis, and myosit Feeding tubes themselves can cause physical discomf and other local, pleuropulmonary, or abdominal comp cations (70). Contaminated feeding solutions may cau gastrointestinal symptoms and bacteriuria. Insertion o nasogastric tube may provoke a fatal arrhythmia during t procedure, and percutaneous endoscopic gastrostomy tu placement may prompt a perioperative death. The con mon need for restraints and the increased production urine and stool in patients receiving tube feedings add tionally fosters the development of pressure ulcers. There no evidence that tube feeding promotes the healing pressure ulcers, improves functional status, prevents ma nutrition, or increases survival in individuals wi advanced dementia (70). It is because of this imbalan between the burdens and benefits of long-term tube fee ing that many physicians, supported by both secular ar religious ethicists, often recommend against the use tube feeding in patients with advanced dementia (71). C the other hand, short-term tube feeding limited to sever weeks may be justified in individuals recovering from stroke or an acute infection.

Despite these findings, feeding tubes are still used in large proportion of individuals with advanced dementi In a study of hospitalized dementia patients, 50% receive tube feeding after admission (72), with no measurab influence on survival. The prevalence of tube feeding nursing home residents with advanced dementia has wic regional variation, ranging from 7.5% in Maine to 40.1 in Mississippi (73), indicating that factors other than clin cal considerations influence its use. Major factors assoc ated with increased tube feeding in nursing homes (74) a listed in Table 16-3. The high incidence of feeding tub could also be due to fiscal incentives for the nursir homes, because tube-fed residents generate a higher dai reimbursement rate from Medicaid but require les expensive care (75).

Even if tube feeding has been instituted in a severel demented individual, it may be discontinued. It is possib to convert tube feeding to hand feeding and, in some case patients may be able to feed themselves again (76). should also be realized that voluntary food refusal is ofte initiated even by cognitively intact individuals. One surve reported that patients chose to stop eating and drinkin because they were ready to die, saw continued existence a pointless, and considered their quality of life poor. Eighty five percent of these patients died within 15 days of stop ping food and fluids, and nurses rated their deaths a "good" (77).

TABLE 16-3
FACTORS ASSOCIATED WITH INCREASED TUBE FEEDING

Large facility size
Elevated proportion of Medicaid beds
Presence of full-time speech therapist
High proportion of licensed nursing staff
Absence of a dementia unit
High prevalence of pressure ulcers
Elevated proportion of residents lacking advance directives
Elevated proportion of residents with total functional dependence

Adapted from Reference 74.

THE NEED FOR PALLIATIVE CARE OUTSIDE OF HOSPICE

Involvement of hospice in management of individuals suffering from progressive degenerative dementias is limited by two factors. First, the hospice eligibility is limited to the expected last 6 months of life. However, end-of-life issues should be considered early after the diagnosis, when the individual may still be able to make decisions regarding legal matters and medical care. Also, the progression of dementia has been described as an *ongoing funeral* for the family members, who therefore need bereavement support during the entire course of the disease. The second factor is the unpredictability of disease progression that limits involvement in hospice, even for individuals with advanced dementia who would benefit from care that avoids aggressive medical interventions. The following case will describe some of the issues and their management.

CASE EXAMPLE

Mr. B, a 71-year-old gentleman and former school principal, retired 2 years ago and spent his time enjoying his hobbies. Over time he became less interested in his projects, and had difficulty remembering which project he was currently working on. His wife became concerned about his condition after Mr. B got lost when shopping in the neighborhood he grew up in, and had to be brought home by the police. Mr. B's wife insisted that he see a physician.

Examination by Dr. Smith showed that Mr. B suffered from high blood pressure, controlled by a diuretic and an angiotension converting enzyme inhibitor, and was otherwise healthy except for deficits in short-term memory and abstract thinking. Laboratory tests were within normal limits, but neuropsychological evaluation found deficits in multiple areas of cognitive functioning. Dr. Smith made a diagnosis of probable Alzheimer's Disease and explained to Mr. B and his wife that there was currently no treatment

---

available to stop or reverse the course of the disease. He also made it clear that Mr. B eventually would lose his capacity to make decisions about his finances and medical care as the disease progressed. Therefore, he urged Mr. B to appoint a proxy who could take over his finances, and to discuss which medical treatments he would want in different stages of the disease.

With the progression of dementia, all individuals eventually lose their decision-making capacity. It is very often at that point when difficult decisions regarding end-of-life care have to be made. The decisions would be made more easily if the patient had earlier executed a living will specifying which treatments he or she would prefer. Unfortunately, most living wills are very general, do not provide guidance regarding specific treatment procedures, and do not take into account the slowly progressive nature of dementing diseases that makes it unclear when the living-will decisions should be applied. Therefore, in most situations specific decisions have to be made by a patient's proxy. Ideally, this proxy should be appointed by the patient and should have had a discussion about wishes and philosophy before the patient became demented. In this situation, the proxy can decide on the basis of *substituted judgment*, putting him or herself into the patient's shoes. Substituted judgment is also promoted by a living will that can be interpreted by the proxy and used to make specific decisions.

CASE EXAMPLE, continued

Mr. B decided that he would not want to be resuscitated if he were in the severe stage of dementia, but did not want to make any other decisions. However, he appointed his wife as his healthcare proxy for making additional decisions. Mr. B was started on an acetylcholinesterase inhibitor with subsequent mild improvement in his memory. During the next 2 years, Mr. B's dementia slowly progressed. He developed severe short-term memory deficits and aphasia. Later, he became incontinent and resisted his wife's efforts to clean him, because he did not understand what had to be done. He also had delusions that his wife was a stranger, and on several occasions asked her to leave his house. Mrs. B eventually decided to place Mr. B in a nursing home.

During the admission process, Mrs. B was asked about advance directives regarding Mr. B's treatment. She produced the living will and discussed various scenarios with staff. After being told about the potential risks and benefits of CPR in a nursing home setting, Mrs. B decided that Mr. B should not be resuscitated if his heart or breathing were to stop.

The next time the treatment team met with Mrs. B, other options related to Mr. B's medical management were discussed. These options included transfer of Mr. B to a hospital for treatment of systemic infections, such as pneumonia, use of tube feeding if Mr. B experienced eating difficulties, and use of antibiotics for treatment of systemic infections in the nursing home.

Treatment decisions should be made before a significant change or crisis occurs, and should involve the healthcare proxy, involved family members and/or friends, and the clinical treatment team. The treatment team should include the physician or physician extender (e.g., nurse practitioner), a nursing staff representative, and the assigned social worker, who usually acts as the meeting moderator. The presence of a chaplain is useful for discussing concerns regarding religious and ethical matters. A family conference is a good opportunity to answer all concerns expressed by the proxy and others close to the patient regarding his or her condition and treatment. During the conference, the treatment team should clarify the prognosis and describe options for management of complications and intercurrent diseases. Risks and benefits of all the management strategies, as well as alternatives, should be clearly explained according to the published evidence. The patient's expressed decisions about therapy, to the extent that they are known and documented, should be reviewed at the beginning of the meeting. The discussion may be framed as an opportunity for determining which goals of care are most important—prolongation of life, maintenance of function, or maintenance of comfort (78).

The decisions regarding treatment limitations are often very difficult, and the proxy and other involved caregivers will usually need guidance from the treatment team. Otherwise, they may feel overwhelmed and guilty if they decide to forego some treatment modalities. Although recommendations to the proxy should come from the attending physician, they should be based on input from the entire treatment team. It should be recognized that nursing staff are moral agents who should be consulted before treatment decisions are made, because they have to live with the residents and execute these decisions.

Some staff members may not understand the importance of palliative care in advanced dementia, and may express reservations or outright objections to it. These concerns can be addressed by programs that educate staff about the meaning of palliative care, the scientific and ethical dimensions of various treatments, and the importance of respecting patient and/or proxy wishes. However, if a staff member objects to palliative care and refuses to respect the decision of the patient or proxy (e.g., such as not being fed), it may be appropriate to reassign them to another resident and substitute someone more comfortable with the situation. It is important to develop a clinical team that is dedicated to the palliative care philosophy in order to provide a unified message to caregivers.

CASE EXAMPLE, continued

Mrs. B reported that Mr. B did not make any decisions regarding other treatment options. She felt the most important goal of care, given his present mental and physical state, was maintenance of function, with comfort

second and prolongation of life third. The treatment team recommended to Mrs. B that Mr. B should be treated in the nursing home and not transferred to an acute care hospital if he were to develop pneumonia or other life-threatening infections. The team assured her that Mr. B would be transferred if it were necessary for increased comfort, for instance, if he developed an acute abdominal problem that required surgical treatment, or suffered a fracture that required surgical attention. After weighing the risks and benefits for Mr. B related to a transfer to an acute care setting, Mrs. B agreed with the team's recommendations.

Another issue discussed with Mrs. B was the management of eating difficulties. The team explained to her that although Mr. B did not have any problems eating at the time, he could start refusing food or having difficulties swallowing food and liquids as the dementia progressed. It was explained to her that the treatment team would always continue feeding Mr. B using hand feeding, and would modify the diet composition and texture as necessary to deal with any such difficulties. The team also reviewed with Mrs. B the potential risks and benefits of tube feeding, and she decided that it probably would not be the best option for her husband if the situation presented itself.

Mr. B's dementia slowly progressed. He became unable to walk even with assistance, and lost the ability to communicate meaningfully with others. He became unable to chew and had to be fed pureed food and liquid dietary supplements. Mr. B also started to choke on thin liquids and had to receive all liquids thickened by the addition of yogurt or commercial food thickener. He developed two episodes of aspiration pneumonia that were successfully treated in the nursing home by intramuscular administration of antibiotics.

During Mrs. B's next annual meeting with the treatment team, the team asked her what she felt was the most important goal of care at that point. She decided that in view of the progression of dementia into a terminal stage, the main goal of care should be comfort and maintenance of function, as opposed to prolongation of life. The team described to her the implications of this approach—that if Mr. B developed pneumonia again, the medical treatment would not include antibiotics but would be limited to antipyretics, analgesics, and supplemental oxygen. She concurred with this approach.

Mr. B's condition remained stable for another 6 months. He continued having swallowing difficulties and sometimes choked on food and liquids. He had several episodes of mild fever, but they resolved with the use of acetaminophen. One episode resulted in tachypnea, but Mr. B was kept comfortable with morphine and oxygen. Eventually, Mr. B became unable to open his mouth and swallow. He was provided comfort care that included morphine for pain and maintenance of moist oral mucosa. After several days in this state, Mr. B lapsed into a coma and died peacefully with his wife at his side. A memorial service was held for Mr. B at the nursing home, attended by Mrs. B and nursing home staff. The social worker continued to contact Mrs. B from time to time to discuss how she could be of assistance.

A CAREGIVER'S EXPERIENCE

SALLY CALAHAN

In December 1985, when we received the diagnosis of Alzheimer's disease we were told that the disease was terminal. Knowing how strongly my mother believed in hospice, they were the first people I called. Hospice said, "Call back when she's actively dying."

After several years of heartbreaking decisions I called hospice again in 1992. When I told the director of nurses at the nursing home that the local hospice was willing to evaluate my mother, she asked me to contact three different hospices. Some of the staff that had cared for and loved my mother for so many years did not want hospice. Others were not open to the previous wishes of my mother, who was fiercely independent when she was well, whom they had never met. Some were not willing to honor the doctor's order not to hospitalize. Some were not willing to stop aggressive feeding. Some balked at not doing diagnostic tests and withholding antibiotics. Even though hospice's palliative philosophy supported my mother's wishes perfectly, this resistance resulted in a 3½-week delay until the state's nursing home ombudsman removed the barriers.

It was a family meeting called by the first hospice that clarified that I was to make decisions and our mother was to be allowed to die. The four of my mother's five children in attendance agreed that aggressive feeding was to stop. Although we discussed withholding antibiotics, we did not finalize that decision then. It was the first official acceptance, at least on the part of her children, that my mother was terminally ill and that a palliative care plan was needed to honor her values and wishes.

Toward the end of the first benefit period, hospice recommended that they withdraw since my mother had improved. While their leaving had little impact on my mother's care, I sorely missed their educational efforts with staff and their support of me as primary family caregiver and legal surrogate.

Several months later, my mother's primary nurse suggested that I call hospice again. This time, a different and extraordinary hospice team was in place within 24 hours. This hospice made it clear that they were "guests" in the nursing home. Their role was to educate and support and not to dictate care. During the 13 months that they were involved they conducted extensive staff training and provided incredible support to me. Their concern for my fragile state after almost a decade of dealing with the relentless ravages of Alzheimer's led them to drive to my place of work every week. The young social worker used my journal poems, which had became a repository for the sea of emotion and conflict that were an integral part of my caregiver-surrogate experience, as a vehicle to clarify my mother's end-of-life wishes. While often horrified by the poems, I recognized the importance of getting the issues out in the open so we could separate fact from feeling and review options against my mother's wishes in a supportive, nonjudgmental environment.

Hospice understood that the length of the grieving process and the difficult moral challenges I faced threatened to swallow me whole. Hospice supported my work with a priest whom was invaluable in challenging me to think of my mother in her highest potential and love her enough to let her go. Hospice helped me rediscover my mother's voice and taught me how to use it as she intended.

Our choice of hi-touch over hi-tech care was met with a variety of reactions, ranging from full acceptance to open hostility. End-stage decisions were the point at which my mother's children circled the wagons to protect her rights—particularly and specifically her right to die. We agonized over the chameleon terms *force feeding, comfort versus curative,* and *heroic measures* as hospice gently taught the staff how to transition their loving care from aggressive and curative to palliative.

Hospice recognized and respected the staff's feelings of loss as they taught them about the ethical imperative of respecting patient wishes—a patient whom they could never know because the mind thief named Alzheimer had stolen her away years before the staff met her. Hospice brought a dignified and peaceful end to the agonizingly long journey through the losses of Alzheimer's. But hospice did not reach every staff member. It was not until the following year that ANA and AGS position papers clearly and directly refuted the words of the two nurses who told me that we were "killing her," twice in the last 18 hours of my mother's life.

Although the essence of who she was died decades ago, without hospice my mother might be still alive. Hospice's expertise and gentle guidance gave me the courage to let my mother die. Hospice shifted the weighty view of my surrogacy from executioner to liberator. Hospice knew how to ferret out my previous mother's values and wishes about the end of her life. Hospice provided angels brave enough to enter the land beyond exhaustion where I had struggled for so many years.

While each journey is uniquely personal, and palliative care is not appropriate for all people, such care was the essence of my well mother's end-of-life wishes. Hospice was a perfect fit for my baby-in-the-bed mother who was bedfast, mostly mute, and totally dependent for 5 or 6 years before her death. God bless hospice.

REFERENCES

1. Schonwetter RS, Soendker S, Perron V, Martin B, Robinson BE, Thal AE. Review of Medicare's proposed hospice eligibility criteria for select noncancer patients. *Am J Hosp Palliat Care.* 1998; 155–158.
2. World Health Organization. Palliative care. Available at: www.who. int/hiv/topics/palliative. Accessed in 2003.
3. Office of Inspector General. Publication of the Medicare advisory bulletin on hospice benefits. *Fed Regist.* 1995;60:55721–55722.
4. National Hospice Organization. Medical guidelines for determining prognosis in selected non-cancer diseases. *Hosp J.* 1996;11: 47–63.
5. Karnofsky DA, Abelmann WH, Craver LF, Burchenal JH. The use of nitrogen mustards in the palliative treatment of cancer. *Cancer.* 1948;1:634–656.

6. Markesbery WR, ed. *Neuropathology of Dementing Disorders.* 1st ed. New York, NY: Oxford University Press; 1998.

7. Evans DA, Funkenstein HH, Albert MS, et al. Prevalence of Alzheimer's disease in a community population of older persons. Higher than previously reported. *JAMA.* 1989;262:2551–2556.

8. Volicer L, Hurley A, eds. *Hospice Care for Patients with Advanced Progressive Dementia.* New York, NY: Springer Publishing Co.; 1998.

9. Reisberg B. Functional assessment staging (FAST). *Psychopharmacol Bull.* 1988;24:653–659.

10. Schonwetter RS, Han B, Small BJ, Martin B, Tope K, Haley WE. Predictors of six-month survival among patients with dementia: an evaluation of hospice Medicare guidelines. *Am J Hosp Palliat Care.* 2003;20:105–113.

11. Miller SC, Gozalo P, Mor V. *Use of Medicare's Hospice Benefit by Nursing Facility Residents.* US Department of Health and Human Services; Washington, DC; 2000.

12. Shega JW, Levin A, Hougham GW, et al. Palliative Excellence in Alzheimer Care Efforts (PEACE): a program description. *J Palliat Med.* 2003;6:315–320.

13. Santa-Emma PH, Roach R, Gill MA, Spayde P, Taylor RM. Development and implementation of an inpatient acute palliative care service. *J Palliat Med.* 2003;5:93–100.

14. Ahronheim JC, Morrison RS, Baskin SA, Morris J, Meier DE. Treatment of the dying in the acute care hospital: advanced dementia and metastatic cancer. *Arch Intern Med.* 1996;156: 2094–2100.

15. Thompson PM. Communicating with dementia patients on hospice. *Am J Alz Dis Other Dementia.* 2003;17:299–302.

16. Hilliard RE. The use of music therapy in meeting the multidimensional needs of hospice patients and families. *J Palliat Care.* 2001;17:161–166.

17. Boon T. Expressive puppetry in hospice care. *Caring.* 2001;20: 38–40.

18. Brown EJ. Snoezelen. In: Volicer L, Bloom-Charette L, eds. *Enhancing Quality of Life in Advanced Dementia.* Philadelphia: Taylor & Francis; 1999:168–185.

19. Volicer L, Mahoney E, Brown EJ. Nonpharmacological approaches to the management of the behavioral consequences of advanced dementia. In: Kaplan M, Hoffman S, eds. *Behaviors in Dementia: Best Practices for Successful Management.* Baltimore, MD: Health Professions Press; 1998:155–176.

20. Casarett D, Takesaka J, Karlawish J, Hirschman KB, Clark CM. How should clinicians discuss hospice for patients with dementia? Anticipating caregivers' preconceptions and meeting their information needs. *Alzheimer Dis Assoc Disord.* 2002;16:116–122.

21. Haley WE, LaMonde LA, Han B, Narramore S, Schonwetter R. Family caregiving in hospice: effects on psychological and health functioning among spousal caregivers of hospice patients with lung cancer or dementia. *Hosp J.* 2001;15:1–18.

22. Murphy K, Hanrahan P, Luchins D. A survey of grief and bereavement in nursing homes: the importance of hospice grief and bereavement for the end-stage Alzheimer's disease patient and family. *J Am Geriatr Soc.* 1997;45:1104–1107.

23. Katzman R, Hill LR, Yu ESH, et al. The malignancy of dementia: predictors of mortality in clinically diagnosed dementia in a population survey of Shanghai, China. *Arch Neurol.* 1994;51:1220–1225.

24. Ostbye T, Hill G, Steenhuis R. Mortality in elderly Canadians with and without dementia: a 5-year follow-up. *Neurology.* 1999;53: 521–526.

25. Kelman HR, Thomas C, Kennedy GJ, Cheng J. Cognitive impairment and mortality in older community residents. *Am J Public Health.* 1994;84(8):1255–1260.

26. Ebell MH, Becker LA, Barry HC, Hagen M. Survival after in-hospital cardiopulmonary resuscitation. A meta-analysis. *J Gen Int Med.* 1998;13:805–816.

27. Finucane TE, Harper GM. Attempting resuscitation in nursing homes: policy considerations. *J Am Geriatr Soc.* 1999;47:1261–1264.

28. Benkendorf R, Swor RA, Jackson R, Rivera-Rivera EJ, Demrick A. Outcomes of cardiac arrest in the nursing home: destiny or futility? *Prehosp Emerg Care.* 1997;1:68–72.

29. Applebaum GE, King JE, Finucane TE. The outcome of CPR initiated in nursing homes. *J Am Geriatr Soc.* 1990;38:197–200.

30. Tresch DD, Neahring JM, Duthie EH, Mark DH, Kartes SK, Aufderheide TP. Outcomes of cardiopulmonary resuscitation in nursing homes: can we predict who will benefit? *Am J Med.* 1993;95:123–130.

31. Gillick MR, Serrell NA, Gillick LS. Adverse consequences of hospitalization in the elderly. *Soc Sci Med.* 1982;16:1033–1038.

32. Hirsch CH, Sommers L, Olsen A, Mullen L, Winograd CH. The natural history of functional morbidity in hospitalized older patients. *J Am Geriatr Soc.* 1990;38:1296–1303.

33. Inouye SK, Wagner DR, Acampora D, et al. A predictive index for functional decline in hospitalized elderly medical patients. *J Gen Int Med.* 1993;8:645–652.

34. Volicer L, Hurley AC, Blasi ZV. Characteristics of dementia end-of-life care across care settings. *Am J Hosp Palliat Care.* 2003; 20:191–200.

35. Muder RR, Brennen C, Swenson DL, Wagener M. Pneumonia in a long-term care facility. A prospective study of outcome. *Arch Intern Med.* 1996;156:2365–2370.

36. McDonald AM, Dietsche L, Litsche M, et al. A retrospective study of nosocomial pneumonia at a long-term care facility. *Am J Infec Cont.* 1992;20:234–238.

37. Loeb M, McGeer A, McArthur M, Walter S, Simor AE. Risk factors for pneumonia and other lower respiratory tract infections in elderly residents of long-term care facilities. *Arch Intern Med.* 1999;159:2058–2064.

38. Hedlund JU, Ortquist AB, Kalin M, Scalia-Tomba G, Giesecke J. Risk of pneumonia in patients previously treated in hospital for pneumonia. *Lancet.* 1992;340:396–397.

39. Naughton BJ, Mylotte JM, Tayara A. Outcome of nursing home-acquired pneumonia: derivation and application of a practical model to predict 30 day mortality. *J Am Geriatr Soc.* 2001;48: 1292–1299.

40. Medina-Walpole AM, McCormick WC. Provider practice patterns in nursing home-acquired pneumonia. *J Am Geriatr Soc.* 1998;46: 187–192.

41. Covinsky KE, Palmer RM, Counsell SR, Pine ZM, Walter LC, Chren MM. Functional status before hospitalization in acutely ill older adults: validity and clinical importance of retrospective reports. *J Am Geriatr Soc.* 2000;48:164–169.

42. Saliba D, Kington R, Buchanan J, et al. Appropriateness of the decision to transfer nursing facility residents to the hospital. *J Am Geriatr Soc.* 2000;48:154–163.

43. Thompson RS, Hall NK, Szpiech M. Hospitalization and mortality rates for nursing home-acquired pneumonia. *J Fam Pract.* 1999; 48:291–293.

44. Barker WH, Zimmer JG, Hall WJ, Ruff BC, Freundlich CB, Eggert GM. Rates, patterns, causes, and costs of hospitalization of nursing home residents: a population-based study. *Am J Publ Health.* 1994;84:1615–1620.

45. Fried TR, Mor V. Frailty and hospitalization of long-term stay nursing home residents. *J Am Geriatr Soc.* 1997;45:265–269.

46. Intrator O, Castle NG, Mor V. Facility characteristics associated with hospitalization of nursing home residents: results of a national study. *Med Care.* 1999;37:228–237.

47. Fried TR, Gillick MR, Lipsitz LA. Whether to transfer? Factors associated with hospitalization and outcome of elderly long-term care patients with pneumonia. *J Gen Int Med.* 1995;10:246–250.

48. Mylotte JP, Naughton B, Saludades C, Maszarovics Z. Validation and application of the pneumonia prognosis index to nursing home residents with pneumonia. *J Am Geriatr Soc.* 1998;46: 1538–1544.

49. Thompson RS, Hall NK, Szpiech M, Reisenberg LA. Treatments and outcomes of nursing-home-acquired pneumonia. *J Am Board Fam Pract.* 1997;10:82–87.

50. Fried TR, Gillick MR, Lipsitz LA. Short-term functional outcomes of long-term care residents with pneumonia treated with and without hospital transfer. *J Am Geriatr Soc.* 1997;45:302–306.

51. Mor V, Intrator O, Fries BE, et al. Changes in hospitalization associated with introducing the Resident Assessment Instrument. *J Am Geriatr Soc.* 1997;45:1002–1010.

52. Hirata-Dulas CA, Stein DJ, Guay DR, Gruninger RP, Peterson PK. A randomized study of ciprofloxacin versus ceftriaxone in the treatment of nursing home-acquired lower respiratory tract infections. *J Am Geriatr Soc.* 1991;39:1040–1041.

53. Peterson PK, Stein D, Guay DR, et al. Prospective study of lower respiratory tract infections in an extended-care nursing home program: potential role of oral ciprofloxacin. *Am J Med.* 1988;85: 164–171.

54. Van der Steen JT, Ooms ME, Mehr DR, Van der Wal G, Ribbe MW. Severe dementia and adverse outcomes of nursing home-acquired pneumonia: evidence for mediation by functional and pathophysiological decline. *J Am Geriatr Soc.* 2002;50:439–448.

55. Fabiszewski KJ, Volicer B, Volicer L. Effect of antibiotic treatment on outcome of fevers in institutionalized Alzheimer patients. *JAMA.* 1990;263:3168–3172.

56. Luchins DJ, Hanrahan P, Murphy K. Criteria for enrolling dementia patients in hospice. *J Am Geriatr Soc.* 1997;45:1054–1059.

57. Hurley AC, Volicer BJ, Hanrahan P, Houde S, Volicer L. Assessment of discomfort in advanced Alzheimer patients. *Res Nurs Health.* 1992;15:369–377.

58. Hurley AC, Volicer B, Mahoney MA, Volicer L. Palliative fever management in Alzheimer patients: quality plus fiscal responsibility. *Adv Nurs Sci.* 1993;16:21–32.

59. Van der Steen JT, Ooms ME, Van der Wal G, Ribbe MW. Pneumonia: the demented patient's best friend? Discomfort after starting or withholding antibiotic treatment. *J Am Geriatr Soc.* 2002;50: 1681–1688.

60. Volicer L, Brandeis G, Hurley AC. Infections in advanced dementia. In: Volicer L, Hurley A, eds. *Hospice Care for Patients with Advanced Progressive Dementia.* New York, NY: Springer Publishing Company; 1998:29–47.

61. Rudman D, Feller AG. Protein-calorie undernutrition in the nursing home. *J Am Geriatr Soc.* 1989;37:173–183.

62. Blaum CS, Fries BE, Fiatarone MA. Factors associated with low body mass index and weight loss in nursing home residents. *J Gerontol Med Sci.* 1995;50(3):M162–M168.

63. Mitchell SL, Kiely DK, Lipsitz LA. Does artificial enteral nutrition prolong survival of institutionalized elders with chewing and swallowing problems? *J Gerontol Med Sci.* 1998;53(3):M207– M213.

64. Morrison RS, Ahronheim JC, Morrison GR, et al. Pain and discomfort associated with common hospital procedures and experiences. *J Pain Sympt Manag.* 1998;15:91–101.

65. Volicer L, Seltzer B, Rheaume Y, et al. Eating difficulties in patients with probable dementia of the Alzheimer type. *J Ger Psych Neurol.* 1989;2:169–176.

66. Volicer L, Rheaume Y, Cyr D. Treatment of depression in advanced Alzheimer's disease using sertraline. *J Ger Psych Neurol.* 1994;7: 227–229.

67. Volicer L, Stelly M, Morris J, McLaughlin J, Volicer BJ. Effects of dronabinol on anorexia and disturbed behavior in patients with Alzheimer's disease. *Intern J Geriat Psychiat.* 1997;12: 913–919.

68. Frisoni GB, Franzoni S, Bellelli G, Morris J, Warden V. Overcoming eating difficulties in the severely demented. In: Volicer L, Hurley A, eds. Hospice Care for Patients with Advanced Progressive Dementia. New York, NY: Springer Publishing Co; 1998:48–67.

69. Golden A, Beber C, Weber R, Kumar V, Musson N, Silverman M. Long-term survival of elderly nursing home residents after percutaneous endoscopic gastrostomy for nutritional support. *Nurs Home Med.* 1997;5:382–389.

70. Finucane TE, Christmas C, Travis K. Tube feeding in patients with advanced dementia: a review of the evidence. *JAMA.* 1999;282: 1365–1370.

71. Gillick MR. Sounding board: rethinking the role of tube feeding in patients with advanced dementia. *N Engl J Med.* 2000;342: 206–210.

72. Meier DE, Ahronheim JC, Morris J, Baskin-Lyons S, Morrison RS. High short-term mortality in hospitalized patients with advanced dementia: lack of benefit of tube feeding. *Arch Intern Med.* 2001;161:594–599.

73. Ahronheim JC, Mulvihill M, Sieger C, Park P, Fries BE. State practice variations in the use of tube feeding for nursing home residents with severe cognitive impairment. *J Am Geriatr Soc.* 2001;49: 148–152.

74. Mitchell SL, Kiely DK, Gillick MR. Nursing home characteristics associated with tube feeding in advanced cognitive impairment. *J Am Geriatr Soc.* 2003;51:75–79.

75. Mitchell SL, Buchanan JL, Littlehale S, Hamel MB. Tube-feeding versus hand-feeding nursing home residents with advanced dementia: a cost comparison. *J Am Med Dir Assoc.* 2003;4: 27–33.

76. Volicer L, Rheaume Y, Riley ME, Karner J, Glennon M. Discontinuation of tube feeding in patients with dementia of the Alzheimer type. *Am J Alzheim Care.* 1990;5:22–25.

77. Ganzini L, Goy ER, Miller LL, Harvath TA, Jackson A, Delorit MA. Nurses' experiences with hospice patients who refuse food and fluids to hasten death. *N Engl J Med.* 2003;349:359–365.

78. Gillick M, Berkman S, Cullen L. A patient-centered approach to advance medical planning in the nursing home. *J Am Geriatr Soc.* 1999;47:227–230.

Spirituality and Geriatric Psychiatry

17

Len Sperry

Judging by the number of professional articles, chapters, and books addressing the topic, it seems that an increasing number of adults are searching for ways of incorporating spirituality in their daily lives. Survey research indicates that 94% of Americans believe in God, 9 out of 10 pray, 97% believe their prayers are answered, and two of five report having life-changing spiritual experiences (1). Thus, it should not be too surprising that patients expect geriatric psychiatrists and other clinicians to incorporate the spiritual dimension in treatment. There have been some articles and a few books addressing general issues in aging and spirituality (1–5), but relatively few addressing specific late-life considerations. Understandably, geriatric psychiatrists want to know why spirituality is important in clinical practice, and how they can utilize this important perspective. Consider these case examples:

> **CASE EXAMPLE**
>
> Mr. I was an 89-year-old man admitted to a rehabilitation facility following surgery for a hip fracture. He was noted to be crying frequently on the unit, and staff thought that he was depressed. The psychiatric consultant agreed with this diagnosis, and started Mr. I on an antidepressant. However, a visiting rabbi noted that as an observant Jew, Mr. I was upset that he could not attend synagogue on the upcoming holiday of Rosh Hashanah. The rabbi arranged for Mr. I to receive kosher food and to attend a service for residents at the facility. Staff noticed dramatic improvement in Mr. I's mood and progress in physical therapy, even before the antidepressant had time to kick in.

> **CASE EXAMPLE**
>
> Mr. P was an 85-year-old African American resident at a nursing home. He was a former deacon of his church and would have regular visits from church members to read scriptures and pray. His physician became concerned when Mr. P reported seeing visions of several diseased relatives. Mr. P stated that he was comforted by these "visions from Heaven," but his physician wondered whether Mr. P was having visual hallucinations. Mr. P's social worker attended a similar denominational church as Mr. P and wanted to pray with him, but wondered whether it would be appropriate.

SPIRITUALITY DEFINED

Spirituality may be one of the most misunderstood words in the English language. It conjures up images ranging from monastic practices, such as meditation and fasting, to New Age paraphernalia such as crystals, drum beating, and other forms of spiritual practices. Actually, spirituality is far more basic than any of this: it represents how individuals think, feel, act, and interact in their efforts to find, conserve, and transform the sacred in their lives. It has to do with our deepest desire, a desire difficult to define that everyone experiences but cannot satisfy, since this desire is always and continually stronger than any satisfaction. Thus, spirituality is primarily about what we do with that desire. The concept of spirituality is distinct from *religion*, which is the search for significance through the sacred and within the context of a shared belief system, i.e., through dogma, communal ritual, and liturgy (6). Thus, the disciplines and habits we choose to live by will either lead to a greater integration or to disintegration within our bodies, minds, and souls; and, further, they can either lead to a greater integration or disintegration in the way we are related to God, others, and the cosmic world (7).

Accordingly, spirituality is not something on the fringes of life, nor is it an option that only a few pursue or want to process in psychiatric treatment (8). Rather, everyone has a spirituality that is reflected in everyday thoughts, feelings, and actions. Viewed from this perspective, *spirituality* is not marginal to the treatment process or primarily the domain of spiritually sensitive therapists. Rather, spiritual considerations are basic to any treatment process (9).

It has been noted that the experience of spirituality changes over the course of life. Unlike early adulthood, when spirituality is focused outward, spiritual growth in middle and late life calls for a turning inward, toward a more interior or contemplative life. In fact, developing such an inner life is crucial for meeting the challenges and realizing the potential of late life. Unless this interior life develops, there is little hope that elderhood will advance beyond the growing despair and selfish concerns attached to gradual declines. Conversely, elders who are able to return to the centers of life with new wisdom become role models for younger persons, and especially for the middle-aged, who often see the proximate approach of their later years as a threat to their human integrity and worth (10).

SPIRITUALITY AND PSYCHIATRIC PRACTICE

Four interrelated dimensions characterize the context of spirituality in clinical practice: patients' needs and expectations, professional expectations and demands, psychiatrists' professional and personal commitment to spirituality/religious sensitivity, and the changing treatment context.

Patients' Needs and Expectations

It has been observed that as Americans have become less at home in the religious traditions that have previously provided them with a source of spiritual power and influence, they have become increasingly spiritually homeless (1). Subsequently, they are searching for a sense of healing and spiritual direction from sources outside religious traditions. These sources include psychotherapy, alternative medicine, as well as traditional medicine and psychiatry. According to Steere (1), these individuals seek healing not simply for physical or emotional pain but also for a sense of wholeness and wellness. They are seeking spiritual direction that can bring meaning, purpose, and a

sense of inner fulfillment to their lives. Furthermore, because many of these individuals may manifest psychiatric symptoms and impaired functioning, they are also seeking a cure. For Steere (1), this three-pronged search for healing, spiritual direction, and cure "provides the background for a rapprochement between psychotherapy and spirituality" and propels these seekers into psychiatric treatment.

What are the expectations of psychiatric patients regarding spiritual issues in treatment? At this time there is relatively little published research that bears on this question. A recently reported study of 79 adults and elderly undergoing psychiatric treatment in New South Wales provides some preliminary data (11). The study reported that 79% of these patients rated spirituality as very important in their lives, and 82% thought their psychiatrist or therapist should be aware of their spiritual needs and beliefs. Of those surveyed, 67% believed that their spirituality helped them cope with their psychiatric illness and life stressors. A surprisingly large number— 69%—believed that their spiritual needs should be incorporated in the treatment process. Although this was a relatively small study, these findings can likely be generalized to represent many clients' expectations of their clinicians.

Professional Expectations and Demands

The relationship between spirituality and psychiatry is not new. Until the eighteenth century, the practice of spiritual, psychological, and even physical healing was associated with the role of the priest, hence the designation *priest-healer*. Ellenberger contends that dynamic psychiatry emerged in 1775 in the wake of the famous clash between two well-known personalities, the physician Messmer and the exorcist Gassner (12). Gassner was a priest whose fame in healing through exorcism was fatefully pitted against the psychological methods of Messmer in a contest to treat the same patient. Gassner's loss symbolized the split of religion from psychiatry, and the denigration of religion in the psychotherapeutic context. This denigration was further reinforced by the later work of Freud and other influential psychiatrists. As a result, religion came to be viewed at best as irrelevant and at worst as detrimental to mental health (13).

However, this attitude has begun to change in recent decades. The reason appears to be a combination of Western culture's hunger for the spiritual and an increasing number of studies suggesting that religion and spirituality can positively impact mental health and psychological well-being. The result is that psychiatrists are beginning to reverse both their skepticism and resistance to the involvement of religious and spiritual issues in psychiatric treatment.

As a profession, psychiatry has become increasingly cognizant of its need to become more culturally sensitive to patient needs and expectations, resulting in several bold initiatives. First, the American Psychiatric Association (APA) issued its policy statement on religiosity entitled "Guidelines Regarding Possible Conflict Between Psychiatrist's Religious Commitment and Psychiatric Practice" (14). It had two provisions: the first was that psychiatrists should maintain respect for their patients' religious beliefs and spirituality. Accordingly, psychiatrists would need sufficient information on these beliefs to properly address them in the course of treatment. The second provision was that psychiatrists should not impose their own religious beliefs or spirituality on their patients nor substitute such beliefs or spiritual practices in place of accepted diagnostic or therapeutic practices.

Then, with the publication of the fourth edition of the *Diagnostic and Statistical Manual of Mental Disorders* (DSM-IV), the APA included the V-code *religious or spiritual problems* in its diagnostic nomenclature (15). Furthermore, effective in January, 1995, the Residency Review Committee of the Accreditation Council for Graduate Medical Education explicitly required that all psychiatry residency and fellowship programs address religious and spiritual factors (16). Specifically, these programs were mandated to educate residents about religious and spiritual factors relevant to understanding and relating to patients. In 1996, the *Model Curriculum for Psychiatric Residency Training Programs: Religion and Spirituality in Clinical Practice: A Course Outline* became available (17). As a result, recently trained psychiatrists will have at least some formal training in religious and spiritual issues (13).

Professional and Personal Commitment to Spirituality

Whether they want the role or not, London contends that psychiatrists and psychotherapists have, by default of religious institutions, become today's "secular priests" (18). Whether they agree with this assessment or not, most practicing clinicians have had the experience of being asked for spiritual advice by patients. Clinicians may also experience some of the same spiritual hunger that others seek to satisfy. They want meaning and fulfillment in their lives, personally and professionally. They seek to achieve some measure of balance, given the waves of changes that are reshaping the landscape of healthcare. They may engage in spiritual practices like prayer, meditation, and the like. Yet, most have had no formal training in incorporating the spiritual dimension into clinical practice. Many wonder whether this role of attending to some or all of the spiritual dimension, which in the past seemed to have been discouraged, should be a legitimate part of the practice of clinical psychiatry (19).

While religion and spirituality have been found to be important in the lives of many older individuals, it has been claimed that geriatric psychiatrists neglect the spiritual and religious issues of their patients. Unfortunately, there has been very little published data to support or reject this claim. An Australian survey of the attitudes and clinical practice patterns of geriatric psychiatrists provides some interesting observations (20). First, it was found that 43% of respondents had no formal religious affiliation and only 25% had participated in a religious service in the preceding month. Nevertheless, despite the fact that many did not consider themselves to have a religious or denominational affiliation, 85% believed that there was a link between religion/spirituality, and health. Accordingly, 64% reported that they had referred a patient to a pastoral counselor or chaplain. The conclusion drawn was that while geriatric psychiatrists thought that religion and spirituality were relevant in the assessment and treatment of older patients, they had little or no training in spiritual assessment and intervention.

While there appears to be a growing awareness among psychiatrists about the importance and clinical value of spirituality and religious issues in the treatment process, it should be noted that there remains a wide variation of opinion among practicing psychiatrists about the place of spirituality and religious considerations in the treatment process. While some psychiatrists dismiss or even disparage such considerations, others actively foster incorporation of them into the treatment process. Thurrell describes this variation in the context of the American Psychiatric Association's ethics statement in response to both of these extremes (21).

Professional and Personal Stance on Spirituality

The practice of geriatric psychiatry is influenced not only by one's training and patients' needs and expectations, but also by the expectations and demands of the psychiatry profession itself. The inevitable question is: what are the implications concerning spirituality of psychiatry's demands for both the professional and personal lives of geriatric psychiatrists? In terms of their professional lives, the main implication is that usual and customary care requires sensitivity to spiritual and religious factors in the clinical practice (14). In terms of their personal lives, it does not mean that geriatric psychiatrists expect to change their basic beliefs or ideology about religion and the spiritual domain. More specifically, it means that they can maintain their status as agnostics, atheists, or as nominal or devout adherents to a specific faith or spiritual path.

There are four possible stances regarding professional and personal sensitivity to religious and spiritual factors, outlined in Table 17-1. For example, because psychiatry as a profession is on record supporting religious and spiritual sensitivity as part of usual and customary care, a geriatric psychiatrist will ideally adopt stance C or D, indicating

TABLE 17-1

RELATIONSHIP OF PROFESSIONAL AND PERSONAL COMMITMENT TO SPIRITUAL/RELIGIOUS SENSITIVITY

		Personal Commitment	
		Low	High
Professional Commitment	Low	A	B
	High	C	D

Key:
A = Agnostic or disinterested personal stance, value-free or "scientific" professional stance;
B = Personal spiritual commitment, but value-free or "scientific" professional stance;
C = Agnostic or disinterested personal stance; but sensitive to patients' spiritual/religious issues;
D = Personal spiritual commitment, and sensitive to patients' spiritual/religious issues.

high professional commitment but variable personal commitment to incorporating spiritual or religious sensitivity into their practice. Stances A and B, on the other hand, indicating low professional commitment but variable personal commitment to incorporating spiritual or religious perspectives into their practice are out of step with the prevailing professional standard. Obviously, the stance adopted by a geriatric psychiatrist is purely an individual matter. It is clear, however, that minimal standards require that a clinician exhibit at least a modicum of sensitivity to religious and spiritual factors in their professional practice, irrespective of his or her own personal beliefs and behaviors. Later sections will highlight these stances and offer several case examples.

The Changing Treatment Context

Steere contends that increasing numbers of the "spiritually homeless" have so strained our current two-tiered health care system, comprised of private and public sectors, that a "third tier" is evolving. He envisions the third tier will be comprised of psychiatrists and therapists "who choose to continue to develop and provide this dimension of spiritual presence in their work. They will do so realizing an economically driven system cannot and should not be expected to sustain it. They will do so in response to the demands for it among the spiritually homeless . . . and . . . out of their own need for a sense of spiritual presence that will not diminish or disappear" (1, p. 280).

Because managed care focuses more on achieving a cure than the process of healing, it necessarily bypasses much of the spiritual dimension of medical and psychiatric care.

This is not to say that managed care organizations are impervious to the spiritual dimension, but they may be more disposed to a referral to pastoral counseling rather than incur the expense of a psychiatrist treating a diagnosed "religious or spiritual problem" (V62.89). A major limitation here is that unlike other diagnostic codes, DSM V-codes have no criteria.

It remains to be seen to what extent, if any, third-party payers will sanction and support psychiatric involvement with the spiritual dimension. It likely will depend on the patient's accessibility and ability to pay for such service, and perhaps on the geriatric psychiatrist's level of professional commitment to spiritual and religious sensitivity.

SPIRITUALITY, HEALTH AND AGING

Longevity, Positive Health Outcomes, and Well-Being

Several studies on the health benefits of religious faith have been reported in the past several decades. Interestingly, most of these studies were undertaken with older adults. A review of these empirical studies reveals several important findings:

- Older adults with strong religious faith tend to live longer than those with lesser religious faith (22,23). It appears that faith may provide some risk reduction from cancer and cardiovascular disease in the elderly, probably because those who practice their faith tend to lead healthier lifestyles.
- Older adults with strong religious faith tend to exhibit a stronger sense of well-being than their less religious peers (24). This may be attributed to the cohesiveness of their family life.
- Older adults with strong religious faith are less likely to suffer from depression following stressful life events, and if they become depressed are more likely to rebound faster than their less religious peers (25,26).
- Older adults with strong religious faith who suffer from any physical illness typically do better and have healthier outcomes than those with lesser religious faith (27).

A closer analysis of these various research studies suggests that religious faith is a necessary but not sufficient condition for increased levels of overall health and well-being. Involvement in a faith-based community appears necessary to obtain the maximal health benefits. The data also suggest that these health benefits are unlikely to result if the individual's sole purpose of belief or worship was to achieve health benefits.

Perhaps the most provocative finding is that the individual's image of God is a significant factor. Thus, those whose image of God is understanding, loving, forgiving, or merciful are more likely to have positive health benefits than those whose image of God is uncaring, distant, angry, punishing, or vengeful. It seems that positive God images encourage the believer to engage in loving behavior and service. On the other hand, negative God images are more likely to be associated with unquestioning devotion and obedience of a believer to a powerful religious leader, and involvement with a faith community that is more likely to be isolated from one's family and the broader community. Koenig suggests that this does not reflect healthy behavior, and thus fewer positive health benefits are likely (28). Fortunately, psychotherapy can modify negative God images (29).

Negative Spiritual Perspectives and Health Outcomes

Most longitudinal studies have consistently found links between active religious and spiritual involvement and increased longevity and/or improved health outcomes (22,23,30). However, a few studies have suggested that a patient's religion or spirituality can serve as a source of distress or conflict, and thereby result in poor or negative health outcomes. For instance, a recently reported 2-year follow-up study of older hospitalized patients found that spiritual distress such as feeling abandoned by God or questioning God's love for them increased their risk of dying by as much as 28%, even after controlling for depressed mood and quality of life (31). Interestingly, such distressing religious beliefs also predicted a decline in the activities of daily living among those who survived. It was surmised that negative emotions associated with feeling abandoned or unloved by God contributed to the higher mortality risks. Alternatively, it may have been that those older individuals who voiced distress and dissatisfaction could have alienated themselves from support by family and friends, which resulted in social isolation. In and of itself, social isolation can increase the risk of earlier mortality and negative health outcomes.

Spirituality and Dementia

There is growing consensus that spirituality is of great importance for not only caregivers, but also for those who suffer from a dementia, such as Alzheimer's disease (AD). In fact, some would contend that those with dementia are still capable of high levels of spiritual well-being even in the later stages of the disease (32). Unfortunately, it appears that the spirituality and religious needs of dementia patients and their caregivers, families, and friends may not be adequately respected nor addressed in clinical settings, in part because health care personnel are not aware of their potential importance.

Those who have worked closely with dementia patients believe that spiritual care should encompass the full experience of the disease, from early to later stages (33). In fact,

"it is often at the end of life that the spiritual experiences of those with dementia are the most profound" (32). Accordingly, they contend that the loss of cognitive capacity does not reflect a loss of spiritual capacity, and those with dementia are still capable of high levels of spiritual well-being. For example, relatively preserved sensory abilities permit persons with dementia to continue to be spiritual beings even when they no longer have the cognitive capacity to effectively articulate their thoughts and emotions. Overlearned ritualistic behaviors can also be preserved into latter stages of dementia. Anecdotal reports tell of demented individuals who have not spoken for years spontaneously singing the words of a religious hymn or otherwise participating in a worship service. Consider the following case examples:

> **CASE EXAMPLE**
>
> Ms. L was a 93-year-old nursing home resident with advanced dementia. She spent most of the day sitting in her wheelchair and making repetitive, incoherent vocalizations. One day the music therapist brought Ms. L into the class, despite the complaints of other residents. He noticed that her verbalizations reminded him of a church hymn. He started playing the music to the hymn on his piano, and to everyone's amazement Ms. L—who had never spoken to any staff or residents since arriving at the facility—suddenly began singing the words in a clear voice. Tears streamed down her face as she sang. Although she reverted back to her incoherent vocalizations afterward, staff now had a spiritual avenue to engage her and provide some soothing.

> **CASE EXAMPLE**
>
> Mr. C was an 84-year-old resident at an assisted living facility and an observant Jew. He attended the morning Jewish service every day without fail, and helped lead the part of the service in which the Torah scrolls were taken out to be read. One day his physician Dr. B attended the morning service, and was amazed to see how adept Mr. C was at saying the prayers and participating in the service. Even though the Hebrew words would sometimes fail him, Mr. C carried the melodies and shook his body in prayer along with the other worshippers. Dr. B knew from Mr. C's dementia work-up that he suffered from moderate cognitive impairment and had difficulty with most daily tasks. Despite this impairment, Mr. C fervently and competently participated in detailed rituals that had been a part of his life since learning them as a boy in Poland.

A few obvious implications for chaplains and geriatric psychiatrists can be noted. First, chaplains would do well to design religious services as multisensory experiences which emphasize noncognitive pathways (e.g., visual symbols, touch, incense, and music) over cognitive pathways (e.g., sermons, readings, etc.). Second, geriatric psychiatrists should become more sensitive to the spiritual and religious needs of dementia patients irrespective of the progression of the disease. Third, geriatric psychiatrists might intentionally address such needs in their treatment planning. Practically speaking, this might mean more attention to collaboration with and referral to chaplains and other spiritual/religious personnel regarding these patients.

COMMENTARY

Rabbi Abraham J. Twerski, MD
Founder and Medical Director Emeritus,
Gateway Rehabilitation Center, Pittsburgh, PA
Associate Professor of Psychiatry, University of Pittsburgh School of Medicine, Pittsburgh, PA

Sperry notes the value of spirituality in Alzheimer's disease (AD).

My mother had AD, and when I visited her, we were served tea. Before she drank the tea, my mother recited the traditional blessing for food. She was clearly meditating and concentrating on each word. Then she smiled and sipped the tea. A moment later, not remembering that she had already recited the blessing, she repeated it, again with profound feeling. When the glass was half empty, she repeated the blessing for a third time.

According to Orthodox Jewish law, pronouncing the name of God when it is not part of a proper ritual is forbidden. Repeating the blessing would have a violation for someone with an intact memory. However, I am certain that God was most pleased with my mother's expression of gratitude.

My mother's smile after she recited the blessing can only be seen as an expression of happiness. She was not conscious of other things that might have made her happy, but maintaining the relationship with God that she had nurtured for 90 years was a source of joy.

Spirituality for Dementia Caregivers

There is also an increasing literature on spirituality for caregivers involved with dementia patients, given the enormous burden that they face in their positions. Besides dramatically altering family dynamics, dementia often taxes caregivers to the point of compromising their own health and well-being. In addition, dementia can also pose significant legal, occupational, financial, and housing challenges to caregivers and family members (34,35).

Several in-depth interview studies with dementia caregivers describe the impact of the caregivers' spirituality and religion on their lives. It appears that those caregivers who hold a spiritual perspective on life (i.e., have spiritual beliefs that are incorporated into their philosophy of life) fared much better than those who had no such beliefs or for

whom such beliefs cause considerable distress or conflict. Caregivers with such a spiritual perspective and integrated beliefs reported that they coped better with stressors and experienced less depression than those caregivers who felt angry or distant from God, or questioned their faith or religious and spiritual beliefs. Not surprisingly, the latter caregivers were more likely to experience clinical depression and tended to perceive caregiving to be an insurmountable burden for them (36). Furthermore, it appears that among caregivers who maintained a spiritual perspective, those who were employed at least part-time and who made a determined effort to seek outside social support throughout the course of their caregiving, tended to report less depression that those caregivers with a spiritual perspective who were not employed or had less social support (37).

CASE EXAMPLE

Mr. S's mother Harriet was 98 years old and suffered from severe dementia. He cared for her at home for as long as he could, but when she became bedridden and required placement of a feeding tube, he had her admitted to a nearby nursing home. Mr. S was guilt-ridden and on the verge of a depression until his pastor began visiting the nursing home to see his mother and also to counsel Mr. S and pray with him. He began to appreciate what he felt was the role of a loving and merciful God in giving his mother such a long and fruitful life, and enabling him to be at her side as much as possible.

CASE EXAMPLE

Ms. W was devastated when her father began developing Parkinson's disease, and as his body and mind failed, she felt increasingly depressed. She began seeing a therapist for her depression and anxiety shortly after her father was hospitalized for aspiration pneumonia and subsequently placed in a nursing home. She was reluctant to see a psychiatrist and take medication, and instead sought advice from her Rabbi. Although he also suggested that she consult a psychiatrist, he instructed her to begin lighting Sabbath candles every Friday evening, and to recite several specific psalms when she visited her father. Ms. W found these rituals incredibly comforting and rejuvenating, and it allowed her to feel less depressed about the situation.

Some implications of the important role of spirituality for geriatric psychiatrists can be noted. First, recognize that spiritual and religious issues are often involved with dementia caregivers and their families. Second, just as there is clinical utility in doing a spiritual history of dementia patients, it is also useful to assess the spiritual perspective and beliefs of caregivers. Third, geriatric psychiatrists might also consider referring a spiritually distressed caregiver to an appropriate spiritual or religious professional.

INCORPORATING SPIRITUALITY IN CLINICAL PRACTICE

In a previous section, different stances or types of professional and personal commitment to religious/spiritual sensitivity were described. In this section, various ways in which psychiatrists can incorporate the spiritual dimension in their professional practice are discussed. Four levels, outlined in Table 17-2, will be described which incorporate the following therapeutic interventions:

- Spiritual history and assessment
- Processing of patients' religious and spiritual issues and/or utilizing spiritual practices with patients
- Referral and/or collaboration with spiritual or religious personnel

These levels are also related to the stances of professional and personal commitment to religious/spiritual sensitivity outlined in Table 17-1. They portray both the psychiatrists' professional level of incorporation as well as their personal commitment to religious/spiritual sensitivity which is reflected in their unique religious beliefs, spiritual practices, and specific religious affiliations—or lack thereof. Keep in mind that the case examples provided of a particular psychiatrist's personal commitment are highly individual and do not necessarily characterize the level of professional incorporation for all clinicians.

Level I: No Incorporation

At this level, geriatric psychiatry practice does not incorporate any of the three therapeutic interventions mentioned

TABLE 17-2

LEVELS OF PROFESSIONAL INCORPORATION OF SPIRITUAL/RELIGIOUS DIMENSION IN CLINICAL PRACTICE

I. NONE	No spiritual assessment
	No processing of spiritual/religious issues
	No referral to spiritual/religious personnel—even if indicated
II. LIMITED	Spiritual assessment
	No or very brief, single processing of spiritual/religious issues
	Referral—if indicated
III. MODERATE	Spiritual assessment
	Some processing of spiritual/religious issues
	Collaboration with spiritual/religious personnel, if indicated
IV. MAXIMAL	Spiritual assessment
	Full processing of spiritual/religious issues
	Collaboration with spiritual/religious personnel, if indicated

Adapted from reference 8.

above. No spiritual assessment, not even a brief spiritual history, is undertaken, no processing of religious/spiritual factors or issues is undertaken, and there is no referral or collaboration with religious/spiritual personnel. This level of incorporation is inconsistent with the stated position of organized psychiatry regarding "usual and customary care." However, this level is perhaps the most common in clinical practice.

Level II: Limited Incorporation

At this level, the clinician does include at least one and sometimes two of the three therapeutic interventions. At a minimum, the geriatric psychiatrist undertakes a spiritual assessment, typically consisting of a brief, screening spiritual history. She may also, based on the spiritual assessment, make a referral to appropriate religious/spiritual personnel if it is indicated, or perhaps herself attempt a brief, single spiritual intervention.

What would level II look like in actual practice? Lipp describes this level in his own practice as a consulting psychiatrist (38). He describes himself as neither religious nor a prayerful person, and contends that all patients are entitled to respectful treatment. He emphasizes that psychiatrists do not need to be religious in order to help patients draw strength from their religious beliefs or spiritual practices. Accordingly, he asks distressed patients: "Have you ever found comfort in prayer?" and if the answer is affirmative, he asks: "Do you think prayer might be helpful now?" (38, p. 314). Lipp continues:

> If the patient agrees, I sit quietly while the patient says the prayer, whether aloud or silently. When the patient is through, I thank the patient for including me in the prayer, if that seems appropriate. Given a willing patient, this technique has without exception resulted in greater calmness for the patient and a closer therapeutic relationship between the patient and myself. (38, p. 314–315)

If the patient is not interested in prayer, Lipp would not pursue the matter. It is noteworthy that Lipp "allows" the patient to pray in his presence rather than suggesting or prescribing it. It appears that his involvement in the practice is purely passive.

At this level of incorporation, the psychiatrist's commitment to understanding and respecting a patient would involve a brief inquiry about spiritual and religious matters in the same way one would ask about work history or sexual matters in the course of completing a comprehensive psychiatric evaluation.

Level III: Moderate Incorporation

At this level, geriatric psychiatry practice includes all three therapeutic interventions. In addition to the spiritual assessment, which is typically more detailed than a brief or screening spiritual history, the geriatric psychiatrist is able and willing to engage in some processing of relevant spiritual/ religious factors that have emerged from the assessment. This often means that the clinician will not only incorporate spiritual/religious factors in the case formulation but also religious or spiritual interventions in the treatment process. If indicated, collaboration occurs with appropriate religious/spiritual personnel. In Level III the geriatric psychiatrist plays a more active role in coordinating the role of religious or spiritual treatment interventions, as opposed to deferring them to a referral, as in Level II.

Matthews, an academic internist, provides a description of a Level III incorporation of spirituality into medical and psychiatric practice (39). A practicing Christian physician, Matthews contends that physicians and other health providers must be concerned about the patient's religious beliefs and spiritual issues because of demonstrated health consequences of religiosity and spirituality. Accordingly, he utilizes a simple spiritual assessment in all initial encounters with patients. It involves three basic questions (39, p. 274):

1. Is religion or spirituality important to you?
2. Do your religious or spiritual beliefs influence the way you look at your problems and the way you think about your health?
3. Would you like me to address your religious or spiritual beliefs and practices with you?

If patients answer no to the first question, the physician would ask if religion or spirituality were ever important to them. Matthews reasons that because research indicates that rejection of religion is associated with higher rates of substance-related disorders and a decline in self-satisfaction and happiness, this information may be a useful prognostic indicator. A positive answer to the third question is followed up to ascertain the patient's preferences and expectations.

Matthews asserts that doing a spiritual assessment expresses interest and respect for the patient's spirituality and religious convictions. While this assessment does not obligate the physician to pursue spiritual matters—a referral to a chaplain or clergy may suffice—he believes that physicians should, when appropriate, combine medical and spiritual interventions. His hope is that physicians will become "proficient in spiritual interventions like praying with patients, spiritual counseling and scripture-sharing" in order to more fully attend to a patient's physical and spiritual needs (39, p. 275). For example, when he treats a depressed patient, Matthews believes in combining "prayer and Prozac" (39, p. 101).

In short, his account suggests that he incorporates a spiritual assessment in evaluating the patient, and not only processes these issues in the course of treatment but also utilizes prayer as an adjunctive therapy. In his written account, Matthews implies that his personal commitment is as high as his professional commitment to religious/ spiritual sensitivity, representing Stance D as outlined in Table 17-1. Parenthetically, his account does not indicate

whether he espouses an integrative spiritual and professional philosophy or utilizes spiritual practices in his personal life.

Level IV: Maximal Incorporation

At this level, geriatric psychiatry practice fully incorporates all three therapeutic factors. Typically, following a more detailed spiritual assessment, the geriatric psychiatrist is able to formulate religious/spiritual dynamics along with relevant psychological and social dynamics as well as biological factors. If indicated, collaboration occurs with appropriate religious/spiritual personnel. Geriatric psychiatrists functioning at this level have sufficient training and experience to process relevant spiritual/religious dynamics as well as incorporate spiritual interventions, such as prayer, in the treatment process. At this time, there are relatively few clinicians who have the training and experience to practice at this level of incorporation. Generally speaking, those that do are usually also highly committed to their own personal development on the spiritual journey.

What would Level IV look like in actual practice? Gersten describes his spiritually oriented practice of psychiatry and chronicles his daily effort to incorporate personal spiritual beliefs and practices into his professional practice of psychiatry (40). Gersten notes that he follows the spiritual teachings of Sathya Sai Baba and tries to reflect them in every waking moment: eating a meal, driving his car, writing a report, or seeing patients. Thus, as he arises he says a prayer of dedication of his upcoming day. He prays while showering, before eating breakfast, and while getting into his car. Similarly, at the end of the day as he drives home, he might chant a mantra for a while before listening to his favorite music. Before retiring he describes reading from a spiritual book before falling asleep in a prayerful frame of mind.

While at his hospital office, and before seeing a patient, he tries to remember to dedicate the session to God. During the session "I imagine that God is sitting in one of the chairs, helping and guiding the session. Sometime when I get stuck, I silently ask, 'God, what does this person need right now?' Immediately I get a thought, feeling or image that guides the session . . ." (40, p. 27). He details an initial and a follow-up appointment with a patient. Gersten describes his approach to evaluating a patient's life: mental, social, relational, family, job, stressors, finances, and health status. He indicates that he probes deeply into subtle manifestations of comorbid illnesses and metabolic difficulties, and inquires about creative outlets, special talents, religious upbringing, as well as current spiritual beliefs and practices. He wants to have a holistic view of the patient's life so that he can better understand their symptoms in this context.

His treatment approach includes medication when indicated and psychotherapeutic discussion of the patient's psychological and spiritual concerns. Imagery exercises and spiritual practices are incorporated when appropriate.

He believes that traditional psychiatry emphasizes the "dark side, our shadows, our unconscious, and it does not lead toward the light side, the bright side. It is essential to deal with both sides . . . Spiritual psychiatry releases the person to something that has God and spirituality in its psychiatric equation" (40, p. 40). Thus, he advocates a "balanced equation" wherein the patient's weaknesses and strengths are identified and emphasizes the development of those strengths. Furthermore, Gersten believes that the spiritually-oriented psychiatrist's role is to help patients identify their spirituality in order to help them heal themselves physically and mentally. He notes that spiritually oriented psychiatry is "about God, faith and hope. It is also about right action. It is not about what feels good at the moment. . . It is about love. It is about the therapeutic role of service. It is about how one can lead the most meaningful, happiest life—whether one is rich or poor, sick or healthy" (40, p. 21).

In short, Gersten's account suggests a professional stance in which he incorporates a spiritual assessment in evaluating patients and formulating cases in terms of biological, psychological, and spiritual dynamics, after which he therapeutically processes these dynamics and utilizes spiritual practices. There is little question that his personal and professional stance are consistent with stance D in Table 17-1. In addition, Gersten describes the evolution of a philosophy of psychiatry and psychiatric practice that is consistent with his own religious/spiritual philosophy of life and spiritual practices.

SPIRITUAL APPLICATIONS IN GERIATRIC PSYCHIATRY

The greater the commitment to religious/spiritual sensitivity and the level of incorporation of the spiritual dimensions into psychiatric practice, the broader the range of applications. Several of these interventions will be described in more detail: spiritual assessment, religious/spiritual diagnosis, healing prayer, and spiritual practices.

The Spiritual Assessment

The spiritual assessment is now considered an essential component of a psychiatric evaluation. A model of this can be found in Table 17-3. Although there is no standardized format or protocol for such an assessment, a comprehensive discussion can be found in Module Two of the *Model Curriculum for Psychiatric Residency Training Programs: Religion and Spirituality in Clinical Practice: A Course Outline* (17). As noted earlier, the use of a spiritual assessment is part of Levels II-IV of spiritual/religious consideration in psychiatric care. Such as assessment is not limited, however, to an initial evaluation, but will guide the differential diagnosis as well as treatment planning.

TABLE 17-3
THE SPIRITUAL ASSESSMENT

BASIC SCREENING QUESTIONS

Is spirituality (or religion) an important part of your life?
    If yes→ how?
    If no→ was it ever?→ how?

Do spiritual beliefs influence your life (i.e., your problems and the way you think about yourself and your health)?
    If yes→ how?
    If no→ why not?

Are you part of a religious or spiritual community?
    If yes→ how are you involved?
    If no→ why not?

Are there any spiritual needs or concerns you would like me to address?

    If yes→ which ones?→ follow up on preferences and expectations
    If no→ why is that?

ADDITIONAL ASSESSMENT QUESTIONS

"How did you learn about spiritual and religious matters when you were growing up?"
"What is your image or concept of God or a higher power?"
"What is the role of prayer in your life?"
"What spiritual beliefs and values are important to you?"
"What religious rituals or spiritual practices are important to you?"

Religious and Spiritual Diagnoses in DSM-IV-TR

As individuals are encouraged to discuss spiritual matters, a clinician's skill in differentiating healthy from pathological religious experiences becomes important. Three common diagnostic considerations are: *voices and visions*, the *dark night of the soul*, and *spiritual emergencies*. Barnhouse provides some criteria for differentiating the hallucinations of the psychotic individual from the voices and visions related to mystical experiences in the nonpsychotic (41). She suggests asking in detail what the individual "thinks an appropriate response to the voices and visions might be. Psychotic responses are highly idiosyncratic, usually having to do with the self, other being involved only in a paranoid way. Normal responses are in the direction of healthier self-understanding, better relations with others or constructive action of some sort" (41, p. 102).

Differentiating clinical depression from the dark night of the spiritual seeker can also be challenging. The *dark night of the soul* refers to a period of spiritual desolation in which the individual feels abandoned by God. Both depression and this dark night may include such features as hopelessness, helplessness, emptiness, loss of self-confidence, and decreased motivation. May offers three differentiating criteria: functioning, sense of humor, and compassion (42). In the dark night, impairment of work and relationships is not noted as it is in major depression. A healthy sense of humor is retained in the dark night as contrasted with anhedonia in major depression and the cynical, bitter humor of dysthymia. Finally, May notes that compassion for others is enhanced during the dark night, which contrasts with the self-absorption observed in clinical depressions.

The term *spiritual emergency* is being used to describe a range of intense conditions involving various emotional and somatic symptoms. Gersten attempts to differentiate "legitimate" spiritual emergencies from the manifestations of mania, dissociative disorders, and borderline personality disorder (40). The DSM-IV-TR focuses more on "spiritual crises" as brief reactive responses to specific religious and spiritual experiences and provides the V-Code: *religious or spiritual problem (V62.89)* (43). This diagnostic category is used when a treatment focus involves a religious or spiritual problem. Such problems include: distressing experiences that could involve the loss of or questioning of one's religious beliefs or convictions; problems that are associated with conversion to a new faith; and questioning of spiritual values that may or may not be associated with an organized religious institution such as a church or synagogue.

Healing Prayer and Other Spiritual Practices

Healing prayer was once "one of the chief therapeutic tools of the nineteenth-century physician, but more recently prayer has been squeezed out of the therapeutic setting by chemicals, machines, and heroic surgical procedures" (38, p. 314). Today, prayer has been reintroduced in clinical context. Whether the clinician prays directly with a patient—as illustrated by Gersten (40) and Matthews (39), or prays for guidance on diagnostic or treatment matters within the session—as illustrated by Gersten, or simply allows the patient to pray within the session—as illustrated in the description of Lipp's practice (38), prayer may be the most common spiritual practice in psychiatry, second only to spiritual assessment.

Spiritual practices are focused activities that have as their purpose to foster spiritual qualities which can result in a balanced and disciplined lifestyle. In addition to healing prayer, other spiritual practices include: contemplation and meditation, fasting, reading sacred writings, forgiveness and repentance, worship and ritual, fellowship, service, seeking spiritual direction, and moral instruction (44,45). In particular, Richards and Bergin have described how clinicians can utilize these spiritual practices within the context of psychotherapy (45).

CASE EXAMPLE: FROM SPIRITUAL ASSESSMENT TO TREATMENT

Evelyn, was an 82-year-old Caucasian, widowed female referred by her internist, Dr. B to a geriatric psychiatry clinic for an evaluation. He had become increasingly exasperated with this patient throughout the 8 months she had been under his care. She would present regularly with varying somatic complaints that eluded diagnosis and were unresponsive to various medication trials. Previously, Evelyn had been a long time patient of Dr. A, an internist in the same group practice with Dr. B, but was transferred upon his retirement.

The psychiatric evaluation was prompted by Evelyn's overdose of various prescription medications. This convinced Dr. B that she needed to be admitted to a psychiatric ward, a view strongly advocated by her daughter Ruth. Evelyn had been living with Ruth's family on and off for the past 3 years after her husband had passed away. Living with her daughter was reportedly marked by ongoing conflict in which the daughter would demand that her mother leave and get her own apartment, go to a nursing home, or more recently, be admitted to a psychiatric facility.

Dr. S, the geriatric psychiatrist at the clinic, completed a comprehensive evaluation of Evelyn, including a spiritual assessment. Evelyn exhibited depressive symptoms and personality dysfunction, and while her cognitive and memory functions were largely intact, she demonstrated poor judgment and limited insight. The social and developmental history noted that she had been an only child, an average student in school, and a former senior-class homecoming queen. After high school she was never gainfully employed, in part because she married at an early age and then gave birth to her only child—her daughter Ruth. After 2 years of marriage her husband "just left one night" and was never heard from again. She was quickly swept off her feet, however, by her newfound lover James, whom she referred to as her "soul mate." They had been married for over 48 years when he died of cancer. She was devastated at the loss of her fun-loving and admiring partner, who provided her a standard of living which she no longer could afford since they had limited savings. She noted that James had called her his "princess" and would not allow her to work or volunteer outside the home. During their long marriage Evelyn had no desire to do anything but indulge the fantasy of being a "kept woman" even though she did have a daughter which she admitted was an "inconvenience." Because she had never worked, she was not entitled to Social Security payments and was forced to subsist on Medicare and Medicaid.

While she was angry about this, she was even more angry at God. During the course of the spiritual assessment, Evelyn had indicated that she was now a "confirmed atheist." When asked what she meant by this, she stated that while she was a very religious person when younger, she now hated God for taking James away from her, and she felt abandoned because God had not answered her prayers to be delivered from the humiliation of having to "live like a disgusting peon." She found living with her daughter's family intolerable, but she could not afford a luxury condo and could not tolerate the prospect of going to a nursing home and living among "all those sick, gorked-out old people." Her suicide gesture appeared to have been prompted by her exasperated daughter calling her a "nut case" and insisting that she be "locked up in a psych ward with all the other old loonies." Evelyn considered her daughter's behavior "completely unforgivable" and refused to consider the prospects of returning to live with her.

The diagnostic formulation included major depressive disorder overlying a dysfunctional personality with narcissistic, histrionic, and borderline features. Central to the clinical formulation were Evelyn's frustrated sense of entitlement (i.e., that her life had changed for the worst and God had not answered her prayer demands), her smoldering anger channeled into somatic symptoms, and her intense feelings of abandonment by James and by God.

Pending a more permanent disposition, a social worker was able to find Evelyn a short-term placement in a group home in a suburban neighborhood with relatively high functioning older adults. The plan was for her to participate in a day program 4 days a week where she would be involved in milieu treatment, reminiscence exercises, group therapy, and individual and family therapy sessions. Part of the treatment agreement was that Evelyn would engage in at least 4 hours of volunteer activity a week. In addition, Dr. S involved the clinic's chaplain. Together, the chaplain and Evelyn began processing the spiritual aspects of her anger and abandonment issues with God and associated forgiveness issues, while Dr. S helped her deal with the psychological aspects of her anger and her personality dynamics. In time, Evelyn was able to transition back to living with her daughter's family, and increased her hours of volunteer work, which she found quite gratifying.

In the case of Evelyn R., the geriatric psychiatry team appeared to have exhibited a high level of professional commitment to spiritual/religious sensitivity, consistent with stance C in which the physician has a low level of personal commitment but a high degree of professional commitment to integrating spiritual or religious considerations into assessment and treatment. Furthermore, the treatment plan that was implemented reflected a moderately high level of incorporation of the religious/spiritual dimension, consistent with Level III. In this case, the identification and integration of spiritual/religious issues was instrumental in helping her to overcome her disgust and hopelessness and find a pathway back to a more meaningful living situation. Her outcome resulted from the synergistic effects of standard psychiatric treatment and spiritual/religious interventions.

Spirituality in Geriatric Psychiatry: A Commentary

Rev. Theodore M. Hesburgh
President Emeritus, University of Notre Dame
Notre Dame, Indiana

Monika Hellwig
President, Association of Catholic Colleges & Universities
Washington DC

From a believer's perspective, Sperry's chapter on spirituality and geriatric psychiatry is good news. It is good

news that increasingly the American Psychiatric Association is acknowledging both the significance and the variety of the spiritual dimension in human lives, the particular importance that spirituality has in aging, and now even the realization that the spiritual is not dependent on any particular level of cognitive ability. This resonates with the believer's understanding of the intrinsic dignity of the human person, made in the divine image, destined for communion with the divine, at a level of being that is not dependent on intellectual ability, physical beauty, or health and strength.

The definition that spirituality has to do with the sacred in one's life, and therefore with one's deepest desire, and what one does with that desire, seems to me a very good definition. Without predetermining belief content, this definition begins with the human longing for meaning, validation, welcome, and communion. Spirituality thus defined seems to be common territory for religion and psychiatry, consisting of the need for vision, hope, and commitment in human life (the time honored theological trio of faith, hope, and charity). The preconditions for integration and focus of vision, hope, and commitment certainly include openness to truth and relationships, and this again is common territory for religion and psychiatry.

Is spirituality more particularly important in the health and well-being of an aging person and an aging population? Although an age-appropriate spiritual development is important at any age, it is probably true that the challenge is sharper for the old. It is sharper because the finitude of one's existence is more evident, because diminishments of various kinds are inescapable, and because autonomy is threatened by illness and approaching death.

Particularly noteworthy in Sperry's paper is the understanding that spirituality is not dependent on ability to articulate, and therefore is a reality even for Alzheimer's patients in a late stage of deterioration. To the extent that spirituality as cultivated by all religions emphasizes love, trust, and peace of mind, care for Alzheimer's patients, as proposed in the article, seems both appropriate and requisite. What is proposed has some implications for all who are aging. Dependence on competence and energy to achieve, to make a mark, to get things done, has to yield to a much deeper sense of self and of one's significance. *Doing* as the key to one's meaning and purpose has to yield to *being*. Plans for the future have to give way to a sense of peace about what has been, and a willingness to let it pass away. Diminishment has to be accepted and the prospect of death welcomed.

What is the role of the psychiatrist in this? The psychiatrist will presumably only deal directly with those for whom the process of aging is for some reason not going well. In such a case an important question for the psychiatrist will be whether religion and pastoral care by religious professionals can help to restore mental health and decrease emotional distress. The question becomes acute in cases where religious beliefs are such as to inspire terror and fear of death. It is important to note, however, that from the pastoral perspective of the priest, minister, rabbi, imam, or guru, the question appears the other way around. Concerned for the desired spiritual well-being of aging members of the religious community, the religious leader may wonder whether psychiatric intervention is likely to help or add confusion. This is especially so if the psychiatrist is not a believer, not well informed about the patient's faith tradition, or even badly misinformed. This last is, alas, all too possible, especially with the non-Western traditions. The situation is further complicated by the fact that all the great traditions have not only their classic versions but all manner of popular versions that often focus more on superstitious practices than authentic spirituality.

Perhaps the last word that should be said is that in our time it is of greatest importance that religious pastors should learn more about what the psychiatrist is trying to do, and that psychiatrists should learn more about the religious traditions.

REFERENCES

1. Steere D. *Spiritual Presence in Psychotherapy: A Guide for Caregivers*. New York: Brunner/Mazel; 1997.
2. Levin J, ed. *Religion in Aging and Health: Theoretical Foundations and Methodological Frontiers*. Thousand Oaks, CA: Sage; 1994.
3. Kimble M, McFadden S, Ellor J, Seeber J, eds. *Aging, Spirituality and Religion: A Handbook*. Minneapolis, MN: Fortress Press; 1995.
4. Schacter-Shalomi Z, Miller R. *From Age-ing to Sage-ing: A Profound New Vision of Growing Older*. New York: Warner Books; 1995.
5. Thomas L, Eisenhandler S, eds. *Religion, Belief and Spirituality in Late Life*. New York: Springer; 1999.
6. Pargament K. The bitter and the sweet: an evaluation of the costs and benefits of religiousness. *Psychological Inquiry: An International Journal of Peer Commentary and Review*. 2002;13(1):168–181.
7. Rolheiser R. *The Holy Longing: The Search for a Christian Spirituality*. New York: Doubleday; 1999.
8. Sperry L. *Spirituality in Clinical Practice: Incorporating the Spiritual Dimension in Psychotherapy and Counseling*. New York: Brunner/ Routeledge; 2001.
9. Sperry L, Shafranske E, eds. Introduction to spiritually-oriented psychotherapy. In: Sperry L, Shafranske E, eds. *Spiritually-Oriented Psychotherapy*. Washington, DC: American Psychological Association; 2005.
10. Bianchi E. *Aging as a Spiritual Journey*. New York: Crossroads; 1982.
11. D'Souza R. Do patients expect psychiatrists to be interested in spiritual issues? *Australian Psychiatry*. 2002;10(1):44–47.
12. Ellenberger H. *The Discovery of the Unconscious: The History and Evolution of Dynamic Psychiatry*. New York: Basic Books; 1970.
13. Larson D, Milano M. Making the case for spiritual intervention in clinical practice. *Mind/Body Medicine: A Journal of Clinical Behavioral Medicine*. 1997;2(1):20–30.
14. American Psychiatric Association Ethics Committee. Guidelines regarding possible conflicts between psychiatrist's religious commitment and psychiatric practice. *Am J Psychiatry*. 1990;147:542.
15. American Psychiatric Association. *Diagnostic and Statistical Manual of Mental Disorders*, 4th Ed. Washington DC: American Psychiatric Association; 1994.
16. Accreditation Council for Graduate Medical Education. *Special Requirements for Residency Training in Psychiatry*. Accreditation Council for Graduate Medical Education; 1994:11–12.
17. Larson D, Lu F, Swyers J. *Model Curriculum for Psychiatric Residency Training Programs: Religion and Spirituality in Clinical Practice: A Course Outline*. Rockville, MD: National Institute of Healthcare Research; 1996.
18. London P. *The Modes and Morals of Psychotherapy*, 2nd Ed. New York: Hemisphere; 1985.
19. Coyle B. Twelve myths of religion and psychiatry: lessons for training psychiatrists in spiritual sensitive treatments. *Mental Health, Religion & Culture*. 2001;4(2):149–174.
20. Paymen V. Do psychogeriatricians "neglect" religion? An antipodean survey. *Int Psychogeriatr*. 2000;12(2)135–144.
21. Thurrell R. Religion and spirituality in the lives of psychiatrists and their patients. *Psychiatric Annals*. 2000;30(8)556–559.
22. Strawbridge W, Cohen R, Shema S, Kaplan G. Frequent attendance at religious services and mortality over 28 years. *Am J Public Health*. 1997;876:947–961.
23. Hummer R, Rogers G, Nam C, Ellison C. Religious involvement and US adult mortality. *Demography*. 1999;36:1–13.
24. Oleckno W, Blacconiere M. Relationship of religiosity to wellness and other health related behaviors and outcomes, *Psychol Rep*. 1991;68:819–826.
25. Koenig H, George L, Peterson B. Religiosity and remission of depression in medically ill older patients. *Am J Psychiatry*. 1998;155:536–542.
26. Larson D, Sherrill K, Lyons J. Associations between dimensions of religious commitment and mental health reported in the American Journal of Psychiatry and Archives of General Psychiatry. *Am J Psychiatry*. 1992;149:557–559.
27. Matthews D, McCullough M, Larson D. Religious commitment and health status: a review of the research and implications for family medicine. *Archives of Family Medicine*. 1998;7:118–124.
28. Koenig H. *The Healing Power of Faith*. New York: Simon & Schuster; 1999.
29. Cheston S, Piedmont R, Eanes B, Lavin L. Changes in client's image of God over the course of outpatient therapy. *Counseling and Values*. 2003;47(2):96–108.
30. Oman D, Reed D. Religion and mortality among the community-dwelling elderly. *Am J Public Health*. 1998;881: 1469–1475.
31. Pargament K, Koenig H, Tarakeshwar N, Hahn J. Religious struggles as a predictor of mortality among medically ill elderly patients: a two-year longitudinal study. *Arch Intern Med*. 2001;161:181–1885.
32. Stuckey J, Post S, Ollerton S, Fallcreeek S. A community dialogue: Alzheimer's disease, religion and the ethics of respect for spirituality. *Alzheimer's Care Quarterly*. 2002;3(1):199–208.
33. Bell V, Troxel D. Spirituality and the person with dementia: a view from the field. *Alzheimer's Care Quarterly*. 2001;2(1):31–45.
34. Ernst RL, Hay JW, Fenn C, et al. Cognitive function and the costs of Alzheimer's Disease. *Arch Neurol*. 1997;54:687–693.
35. Smith A, Harnkness J. Spirituality and meaning: a qualitative inquiry with caregivers of Alzheimer's disease. *Journal of Family Psychology*. 2002;13(1–2):87–108.
36. Shah A, Snow A, Kunik M. Spiritual and religious coping in caregivers of patients with Alzheimer's disease. *Clinical Gerontologist*. 2001;24(3–4):127–136.
37. Robinson K, Kay J. The relationship between spiritual perspective, social support, and depression in caregiving and noncaregiving wives. *Scholarly Inquiry for Nursing Practice*. 1994;8(4): 375–389.
38. Lipp M. *Respectful Treatment: The Human Side of Medical Care*. 2nd Ed. New York: Elsevier; 1986.
39. Matthews D. *The Faith Factor: Proof of the Healing Power of Prayer*. New York: Viking; 1998.
40. Gersten D. *Are You Getting Enlightened or Losing Your Mind? How to Master Everyday and Extraordinary Spiritual Experiences*. New York: Random House/Three Rivers Press; 1998.
41. Barnhouse R. How to evaluate patients' religious ideation. In: Robinson L, ed. *Psychiatry and Religion: Overlapping Concerns*. Washington, DC: American Psychiatric Press; 1986:89–106.
42. May G. *Care of Mind, Care of Soul: A Psychiatrist Explores Spiritual Direction*. San Francisco: HarperCollins; 1992.
43. American Psychiatric Association. *Diagnostic and Statistical Manual of Mental Disorders*, 4th Ed. Text revision. Washington DC: American Psychiatric Association; 2000.
44. Simpkinson A, Simpkinson C. *Soul Work: A Field Guide for Spiritual Seekers*. San Francisco: HarperCollins; 1998.
45. Richards P, Bergin A. *A Spiritual Strategy for Counseling and Psychotherapy*. Washington, DC: American Psychological Association; 1997.

Ethical Issues in Geriatric Psychiatry

18

Jason Borenstein   *Kenneth W. Goodman*

One measure of a civil society is how well it cares for its most vulnerable members. While vulnerability is a complex concept, everyone should recognize its central features: a person is vulnerable if she is at greater risk than others of being harmed or wronged. It can be risky to infer that an individual is vulnerable merely because he has been classified as a member of a certain group. Some elders, for instance, are vulnerable and some are not—or at least not to the same degree. Some behavioral health patients are vulnerable and some are not. Some children, pregnant women, and poor people are vulnerable, although in different degrees and in different ways.

It should not be controversial to suggest that society must take steps to protect its vulnerable citizens, but it is less clear when, how, and, precisely, which members on which occasions should enjoy these protections. It is this uncertainty that has, over a generation, shaped thinking in bioethics. Indeed, ethics and aging have emerged as a subspecialty among those who work in bioethics; likewise ethics and psychiatry. Because some—but not all—of the ethical issues that arise with elders are similar or the same as those that arise with psychiatric patients, there will be some overlap between the two domains. This increases the importance of these issues.

The issues addressed here will probably be familiar to most with an interest in bioethics (although the implications and conclusions might not be). Included in the discussion are issues such as consent and refusal (to treatment and research), end-of-life care, privacy and confidentiality, resource allocation, human-subjects research, genetics, and the role and utility of institutional ethics committees.

VALID CONSENT AND REFUSAL

> **CASE EXAMPLE**
>
> Mr. R., 76, has worsening dementia and has been worked up for recent pulmonary problems. Before his physician has a chance to communicate test results to his patient and discuss treatment options, Mr. R.'s son speaks to the physician and asks about the diagnosis. The physician tells the son his father has been diagnosed with small-cell cancer of the lung. The son insists that his father not be told this diagnosis, suggesting that, "If you tell Dad he has cancer he will drop over and die in front of you. I know him—he just could not bear that news."
>
> The physician agrees to keep the diagnosis a secret, and he and the son then begin to plan for Mr. R.'s treatment, which initially will include radiation therapy.

Respect for autonomy has come to be regarded as a moral cornerstone. Autonomy, typically defined as *self-rule* or *self-determination*, refers to the ability of competent individuals to make decisions over their own lives. In order for autonomy to be meaningful, a person's decisions have to be respected even when the decisions conflict with what others believe to be reasonable or optimal. Autonomy includes, but is not limited to, having the freedom to make decisions about health care, finances, and living arrangements. It follows that competent patients have the right to decide which medical procedures are appropriate for them. It requires of health care professionals that they respect patients by providing accurate and complete information.

The emphasis on autonomy in health care settings has helped to redefine the relationship between physicians and patients. Traditionally, the physician played a more authoritarian or paternalistic role in that he or she would generally decide for the patient what the best course of action would be. Yet over the course of the past several decades, patients have become more actively involved in making decisions concerning their own health care. It should be noted that while this is a widespread trend, it is not a universal phenomenon; it is greatly accelerated in some Western societies.

Valid—or, more familiarly, *informed*—consent encapsulates the notion that patients should have control over their own bodies and should be given the opportunity to accept or refuse a proposed intervention. While some patients might view the consent process as a barrier that interferes with receiving treatment, it is intended to provide protection from unwanted interference and harm. Valid consent is generally regarded as having three main components: patients must have mental capacity, must be adequately informed, and must decide to accept or refuse treatment voluntarily (1).

Capacity and Competence

The terms *capacity* and *competence* are often used interchangeably. Yet this practice overlooks an important distinction. Namely, it is better to think of capacity as referring to cognitive ability and competence to be a legal determination of capacity. A judge, for instance, will make a ruling about a person's competence based on expert testimony by a psychiatrist about that person's cognitive ability. Yet despite the importance of the distinction, for convenience and clarity, we will use the term competence in what follows.

Competence has been defined to mean several different things in the medical literature (2). There are longstanding debates concerning what being competent entails. It has proved difficult to identify criteria for determining whether an individual is competent to make a decision. Some clinicians have assessed competence by determining whether a person's decisions are consistent with what is deemed to be rational. If a patient agrees with the health care team's recommendations, for example, then the patient might be considered competent to make decisions. This notion of competence has obvious pitfalls, including that it does not fully account for cultural differences. It also makes the health care team the only source of rationality, which might be a mistake. To suggest that, "if you disagree with me, you have a behavioral malady," is often arrogant and insensitive. On the other hand, decisions that are out of the rational norm (not necessarily as measured by the health care team) might be evidence of a cognitive shortcoming.

Assessing competence has also been closely tied to a patient's diagnosis. There are several illnesses associated with aging that can compromise a patient's ability to accept or refuse treatment, thus complicating the consent process. For instance, a patient with dementia will appear lucid at one point, but later might lose decision-making capacity because many forms of dementia are typically degenerative. On occasion, patients do change their minds with regard to treatment decisions. Some of these decisions might be viewed skeptically by health care providers if they are a product of depression, anxiety, pressure from family members, or of a personality change resulting from illness. For instance, if a patient suffers from Parkinson's disease, clinicians might rely on the diagnosis as a marker that the patient is not competent. Parkinson's patients increasingly become unable to retain the information provided to them during the course of the disease (3). However, it is dangerous to label patients as incompetent merely because of a diagnosis. Patients suffering from the early stages of Parkinson's disease might retain the ability to consent to treatment. Indeed, one of the great contributions of psychiatry to current ethical debate about valid consent is the fact that competence/capacity is frequently episodic.

Debates continue within medical communities about whether patients with conditions such as dementia are capable of making rational decisions (4). Since dementia typically impairs memory and can interfere with judgment and abstract thinking, a patient will likely become incompetent over time. Yet clinicians disagree about the point at which dementia patients lose the capacity to make decisions. Similarly, health care teams struggle to predict the onset of Alzheimer's disease, and how that disease is going to manifest itself over time (5). Moreover, the effects of delirium can complicate the consent process (6).

Generally, what needs to be examined in a competence assessment is whether an individual can handle the responsibility of making decisions relating to his personal life, finances, and health care. Some relevant indicators include whether the person can communicate choices, understand information given to him/her, and appreciate the consequences of a decision. Even these criteria may be said to oversimplify things, and the "understand-and-appreciate" model of competence is itself inadequate to the task (7).

An elderly patient's capacity to consent can fluctuate, which makes it crucially important that competence is understood to be variable and episodic (8). If given additional time, some patients can become better able to make decisions. Appelbaum suggests that we should not underestimate the ability of individuals suffering from mental illness to make decisions for themselves (9). Appelbaum cautions that looking to surrogate decision-makers for assistance is not always the best option.

Contrarily, respecting autonomy does not necessarily equate to abiding by a patient's current wishes. If the patient suffers from an illness that is not properly diagnosed, the consent process might be meaningless. For instance, if an elderly patient refuses to accept treatment, it is crucially important that the health care team determines whether that decision is a by-product of the patient's illness before treatment is withheld. Further, the health care team might be required to circumvent a patient's current wishes in order to protect the patient from self-harm.

Psychiatric patients might lack the ability to consent to voluntary hospitalization. The illness that might cause a person to seek treatment might simultaneously make that individual incapable of consenting to it. Appelbaum and colleagues examined this issue and noted that most subjects did recognize that restrictions were placed on their ability to leave, which is arguably the most important insight related to voluntary hospitalization (10).

Adequate Information

Before giving consent, a patient must be adequately informed about the medical procedures or treatments in question. This includes, but is not limited to, being informed by the health care team of the risks and potential benefits of a given treatment, the likelihood of the treatment's success, and alternatives to the treatment. As a practical matter, the communication of risks, benefits, and alternatives has evolved into a legal instrument, the consent form. Alas, this evolution in many cases decouples the clinician-as-communicator from the patient. Patients obtain, sometimes read, and then sign these forms. Yet, executing such a document should not be a substitute for open and ongoing communication between clinician and patient. Further, mere hospitalization does not necessarily entail that a patient cannot understand the information needed to make a rational decision. For instance, a study by Appelbaum and Grisso suggests that hospitalized patients and elderly community residents perform similarly in their capacity to understand information presented to them (11).

Moreover, consent forms suffer from a number of shortcomings. Many are poorly written; some are too technical; others are both. This can impede the ability of patients to understand what they are reading despite the fact that they are perfectly competent to consent to or refuse treatment. The point of such a form should be to use understandable language, giving a patient enough information on which to base a decision. It is not even clear if the current inclination to render consent forms as legal documents would actually protect an individual or institution in malpractice cases. One might imagine a complex document being read to a lay jury; if the jurors find the form overly complex or otherwise difficult to understand, in what sense has a clinician or institution served itself? Further, not all patients are native speakers of the form's language.

For these reasons, the communication of information necessary for valid consent should be an ongoing process—one in which a patient feels comfortable to ask questions and to seek additional information, if needed. A nursing home environment, for instance, can erode an elderly person's ability to make decisions if they are not encouraged to be involved in decision-making (12). The opportunity to provide information should be in non-

threatening settings—which is perhaps somewhat more difficult to achieve if one regards signing a consent form as akin to signing a contract. In fact, *any* patient contact is an opportunity to bolster the consent process.

One tool for assisting clinicians in determining whether patients adequately understand the information presented to them is the MacArthur Competence Assessment Tool-Technique (13). It provides guidelines for an interview process whereby an assessment can be made to determine if a patient understands information as presented. Important considerations include whether the patient can repeat relevant information and explain what will happen during the course of proposed treatment.

In practice, the appropriate procedures for obtaining consent are not always followed. One study of the consent process in a group of delirium patients found no documented informed consent in 19% of the cases examined, and that 47% of the patients who signed consent forms had significant degrees of cognitive impairment (6). Further, there was no documentation that risks were discussed with the patients or the patients' surrogates for about half of the procedures recommended by physicians. Even if risks were discussed, the patient charts would not reveal this fact (and, as some plaintiff's lawyers will make clear, the absence of documentation of an event is—at trial—tantamount to the event not occurring). Moreover, some physicians apparently fail to take appropriate steps, including trying to identify a surrogate, when there are questions about a patient's capacity and, indeed, they were able to identify clinically incompetent patients 65% of the time (12).

Voluntariness

Competent, informed patients should not be forced, otherwise coerced, or tricked into making decisions about their health care, including consenting to or refusing treatment. In other words, their decisions must be voluntary. Determining whether a person is being coerced is not always easy; a patient can be coerced in subtle ways by undue pressure from the family or the health care team.

Age and illness may make elderly patients especially vulnerable to being coerced by the health team and/or family members. Elders can be vulnerable by virtue of illness or lack of education. Poverty and restricted freedom of movement can be contributing factors as well. Some elders—and especially those with a variety of behavioral maladies—are especially susceptible to undue influence.

It is not uncommon for some elderly patients to (appear to) prefer to give over decision-making responsibility to family members or friends. Yet it should not be assumed that all elders desire to forgo decision-making power. Further, families do not necessarily act in the best interests of their relatives. When a patient starts to lose the capacity to make health care decisions, the patient's family might put forward a treatment plan that is in its own best interest. For instance, the dementia-related difficulties for caregivers might lead a family to press for inappropriate sedation or even premature termination of health care. For this reason, the health care team needs to be aware of whether the decision being made is based on the patient's or the family's preferences. Family members sometimes disagree about what the best course of action is for their elderly relative, which can place the health care team in the unenviable position of resolving the discrepancy. Institutional ethics committees are often useful resources in such cases.

Debates ensue about whether veracity or truth-telling is an absolute moral obligation. Clinicians have argued that a therapeutic exception or privilege is necessary or appropriate in cases in which sharing information might jeopardize the health of the patient. Some patients, it is suggested, might contemplate suicide if they are diagnosed with a severe, debilitating illness, and so some clinicians might be apprehensive about sharing such a diagnosis. Indeed, hesitancy to be truthful is often caused more by the clinician's discomfort than it is by *bona fide* concern that a patient will actually come to grief because of the news. In most circumstances, health care professionals have a moral obligation to provide their patients with accurate and complete information (although the timing and manner in which the information is presented is crucial). But this is not absolute. A patient's family might not want a psychiatrist to tell their relative that he or she has Alzheimer's disease or other maladies (14), and psychiatrists themselves know that disclosure of bad news to patients can be counterproductive.

This is an exquisitely difficult problem for clinicians. In some cases, disclosure of bad news will cause great distress—only for the news to be forgotten quickly, requiring another disclosure, which will again cause distress. In these instances, it can be permissible to withhold information from a patient. But there is no evidence base against which to evaluate such a strategy. It might be the case that demented patients detect deception, which could be atherapeutic. The best course is to use deception as sparingly as possible.

It should now be clear why the term *valid consent* is preferable to the more traditional *informed consent*. Adequate information about risks, benefits, and alternatives is a necessary but insufficient condition for a successful consent process. A patient might be informed but incompetent, or informed but coerced—which would subvert or *invalidate* any consent obtained. Valid consent emerges not as a legal duty or social courtesy, but a boldface moral obligation without which self-determination is feckless or meaningless.

It should also be clear that if patients choose to refuse a treatment or intervention, then the validity of that choice will be measured by the same three criteria, i.e., adequacy of information, cognitive capacity, and voluntariness.

From this it follows that refusal of a potentially beneficial treatment by an incompetent patient may be invalid. To make this crucial observation is not to provide ethical warrant for forcing treatment on incapacitated patients (which can be permissible) as much as it is to note that the tools of applied ethics entail conclusions that might be broader than expected. In the case of valid refusal, caution—in conjunction with respect for meaningful self-determination—should guide us in cases both of *invalid* consent and of *invalid* refusal.

Consider the problem raised by patients who refuse to eat or take medication. If the refusal is valid, then it should be honored. This is the appropriate stance even if the refusal leads to a worsening of a patient's condition, or even death. The boldface moral requirement to obtain valid consent is empty unless valid refusals are honored. In cases in which a patient lacks capacity to consent or refuse, refusal of food and medication may be overridden. But such a course is risky. Forced interventions are fraught with problems that range from erosion or destruction of a therapeutic relationship to consequences opposite those intended, as demonstrated by cases of nosocomial pneumonia brought on by forced feeding in nursing homes.

Actions that override refusals by incapacitated patients should therefore be considered as a last resort, used sparingly, and ended as rapidly as is medically feasible.

Surrogates, Proxies, and Guardians

It should be obvious that we have special difficulties and extraordinary challenges when a patient is incompetent. While the manner in which information is provided can be improved, and coercion can be stopped, incompetence cannot always be eliminated. Indeed, it is precisely because of the epidemiology of cognitive incapacity in geriatric and psychiatric populations that the problem of consent is so important, difficult, and interesting.

In cases in which a patient has lost decision-making ability, clinicians must turn to surrogate decision makers—generally family or friends—to consent to or refuse treatment. Ideally, a surrogate is selected by a patient in advance of incapacity. In fact, designation of a health care surrogate is a common feature of hospital admission; it is the most common kind of advance directive, ahead of living wills directing end-of-life care.

The role of the surrogate is especially important in geriatrics and behavioral health, in part because of the ease with which self-determination can be overlooked. In the best case, a surrogate becomes the agent for protecting that right to self-determination, and does this by making decisions that the patient would have made were he or she competent. In other words, the surrogate guides the health care team by consenting and refusing as the patient herself would have consented or refused. This role (called *substituted judgment*) is the gold standard when one must make a health care decision for another. Unfortunately, it can be very difficult to meet this standard. When the decisions are complex and the stakes are high, it is no straightforward matter to stand in someone else's shoes. Many surrogates simply do not know what the patient would have chosen. Moreover, whether or not a surrogate does know, it is inappropriate for a surrogate to allow her own preferences to be expressed. In other words, it is not about the surrogate's wishes—it is about the incompetent patient; anything else would subvert the patient's right to self-determination.

When substituted judgment is, by virtue of irremediable ignorance, impossible, surrogates are to apply one of two other standards. The first of these requires that a surrogate make decisions that are in the patient's best interests (again setting aside her own preferences). This is much easier said than done: one's best interests in health care decisions are sometimes difficult to determine. Even life itself might not be in one's best interests if it involves suffering without respite, unconsciousness without end, or indignity without resolution. The other standard for deciding for an incompetent other is the "reasonable person" standard. Introduced in law, the standard is based on the idea that most people value pretty much the same things, and that any reasonable person would, all things being equal, act or decide in such-and-such a way in a given situation.

The same three standards are available to others similarly situated, that is, to proxies and guardians. A proxy is a substitute decision-maker who assumes that role in cases in which a patient has not chosen a surrogate. Most jurisdictions list the order of eligible proxies, usually ranging from spouses and children at the top, to close friends at the bottom.

In cases in which no one from the list is available or willing—or in cases of intractable family disputes—health care organizations and others may petition a court to appoint a guardian. In such cases, courts might seek expert testimony about the nature or level of the cognitive incapacity. Courts will usually demand that there is a "sufficient showing" that the person in question is unable to manage life decisions before a guardian is appointed. This may involve detailing how a functional impairment has interfered with the ward's ability to make rational decisions. Each state is empowered to appoint decision-makers for incompetent individuals, although the circumstances and procedures for appointing guardians vary by state.

It should be emphasized that court-appointed guardians have nearly complete authority to make decisions for their wards. (Exceptions generally include abortion, ECT, sterilization, etc.) It is not necessary to confer with family members or others to confirm the appropriateness of a guardian's decisions—the guardian is presumed in the absence of conflict, negligence, or incompetence to have taken steps to ensure that criteria for surrogate decision making have been followed. It is common in some hospitals and nursing homes to be ignorant of guardianship powers, and this can lead to unnecessary conflict. All other things being equal, a guardian's instructions should be regarded as the patient's.

Advance Directives

For all of these reasons, many clinicians and institutions are keen to have competent patients select surrogates—while they are still able to do so. The use of advance directives (including the appointment of surrogates) is supposed to assist in the process of determining a patient's wishes to ensure they are followed if he or she loses decision-making capacity. Ideally, a patient's wishes would be expressed in writing in order to eliminate confusion about what that person desires, although it can be difficult to anticipate the types of situations and complications that may arise in the future. Hence, an advance directive should be as clear as possible, covering a variety of possible situations. With regard to health care, the author of a directive might want to consider what types of medical procedures would be desired if he or she had Alzheimer's disease, Parkinson's disease, or were in a persistent vegetative state.

An *instructional directive* is a type of advance directive in which the author specifies the types of medical procedures desired in future situations. Instructional directives are typically, but not always, in written form. Psychiatric advanced directives can be written with the intent of expressing what a patient wants in case of incompetence during the course of a psychiatric illness. A living will is a type of instructional directive, because it is created to direct a health care team to use, not start, or halt procedures keeping a patient alive when such efforts are regarded as burdensome.

Instructional directives are imperfect. They are frequently either not specific enough to cover the large variety of scenarios that can occur or they attempt to cover so many scenarios that they are daunting and produce the illusion of comprehensiveness (15). Because of the language used, it is not always clear when a directive should be followed. There can be genuine uncertainty about whether the directive should be implemented if there are reasons to believe it no longer accurately reflects what the patient would want.

Nevertheless, the moral imperatives to obtain valid consent for treatment and to honor valid refusal of treatment by patients who have lost capacity are best met by advance directives that name surrogate decision-makers and/or express patient preferences regarding potentially burdensome treatment. The general, overarching problem with directives is that most patients do not have them (16).

In the case study that began this section, a patient with worsening dementia and a cancer diagnosis has a son who insists that the diagnosis be kept from the patient. While the motives for such deception are often benign, the risks can be great. For one thing, patients with complex medical cases often require treatment and care by many professionals. To ensure the deception will succeed, it is necessary in such cases to enlist potentially many hospital and other staffers in the ruse. Such an enterprise will be difficult to undertake at many institutions. Worse, failure—the patient finds out anyway (in one case in our experience, from a radiation technician who failed to get the message)—might erode trust, engender confusion, and make clinicians and others feel worse for mounting a charade that failed. For these reasons, systematic deception is problematic and should be considered only in extraordinary cases.

PRIVACY, CONFIDENTIALITY, AND THE DUTY TO WARN

> **CASE EXAMPLE**
>
> Ms. C., 78, has burgeoning symptoms of Alzheimer's disease. In two of the last five times that she has driven to her bridge club, she became disoriented and drove randomly, never reaching her destination. Both times a police officer found her in her car by the side of the road and made arrangements for her to be returned home.
>
> Her psychiatrist learns of these episodes during a subsequent visit, and suggests that Ms. C. should consider no longer driving. She responds, "If you take away my driver's license you might as well put me in jail. It will destroy my independence and ruin my life."

When a patient is ill, the default setting for many health care teams is to inform families about relatives' conditions. This can be a mistake in the absence of a patient's permission to do so. That is, it might not be ethically or legally appropriate because of the duty of health care professionals to keep medical information in confidence. This information might include details about diagnosis, prognosis, history of illness, drug use, family history, and sexual activity. *Confidentiality* refers to the duty to share entrusted information responsibly. Health care providers have a responsibility to avoid disclosing personal and medical information that has been entrusted to them without the patient's consent. The Health Insurance Portability and Accountability Act of 1996 (HIPAA) was enacted to help protect information in patient medical records. HIPAA establishes federal standards regulating how electronic data is transmitted and shared. In principle, storing medical records electronically can give physicians, insurance companies, and other parties easier access to medical records. Yet HIPAA guidelines are in place to protect patients from losing control over their information (17). It is striking in ordinary practice how elders—especially those with behavioral maladies—are reckoned to have a lower interest in their privacy than others. There is apparently no evidence to support this belief. It is patronizing, and it perpetuates the stigma of elders as uninterested in the social and moral rights that accompany activities of daily living.

Concerns of justice and of the common good sometimes can supercede the duty to keep information confidential. In most circumstances, health care providers must obtain a patient's consent before sharing that patient's information with other parties. Yet there are rare circumstances, such as where a court order has been issued, where a physician may be legally obligated to disclose a patient's information without his or her consent. Similarly, a physician has a duty to warn the affected individual(s) and/or the authorities if it is believed that a patient poses a threat of harm. With regard to demented and/or behaviorally disordered patients, it is a fairly common problem that they may be unwilling to stop driving a car even though they are not fully capable of operating one (2). Patients can be reluctant to give up their licenses because they fear that they will lose their independence. As we know, however, a demented patient's mental capacity can fluctuate, which can make that person a danger to herself and to others if behind a wheel of a car. This type of situation elicits the tension between the obligation to keep information in confidence and the obligation to prevent patients from causing harm.

Whether physicians, psychologists, and others have a duty to notify authorities if a patient has a physical or mental impairment that may interfere with driving ability varies depending on relevant state law. According to the American Medical Association, there are circumstances in which it is ethically appropriate for physicians to report a patient to the Department of Motor Vehicles if they believe that the individual poses "a strong threat to patient and public safety" (18). Physicians should be careful that they do not erode the trust established between themselves and their patients. They ought not assume that because an elderly patient is diagnosed with a progressive illness that the patient can no longer drive. But the debilitating effects of such illnesses will likely interfere at some point.

Similar but distinct issues arise with genetic information. The ongoing development of predictive genetic testing or screening for Alzheimer's disease not only underscores the importance of privacy and confidentiality protections for information that may be about more than one patient, it also means that clinicians will need to balance those protections against the need or at least desirability of disclosing to unaffected potential patients and others the results of such tests (19). We have our collective work cut out for us as we attempt to manage the following questions, among others:

- Why test in the first place?
- When and to whom should test results be disclosed?
- How should a proband's privacy be weighed against the possibility of harm caused by ignorance among unaffected family members?
- What kind of counseling is available to patients and family members?

What emerges from these considerations should be a view that holds privacy as vital but not absolute. That is, the practice of health care—especially in the case of vulnerable populations—requires that we learn better how to balance various needs and duties.

One of the great challenges associated with the collection of genetic information is preventing the use of that information to discriminate against or stigmatize patients. As if it were not bad enough that the maladies that shape geriatric psychiatry are often stigmatizing, the increasing availability of information about genetic predispositions to these maladies suggests that we must proceed with the greatest caution in collecting, studying and sharing genetic data.

In the case that appears at the outset of this section, an Alzheimer's patient insists she be allowed to continue to drive, despite her psychiatrist's concern that she poses a risk to other motorists. This puts the psychiatrist in a position of either acceding to her wishes and thus allowing her and other motorists to be endangered, or violating her confidentiality and reporting her incapacity to motor vehicle authorities. As we saw, privacy and confidentiality are not absolute. They must be assessed against a background of other values, often involving public health and safety. Optimally, the patient can be persuaded to relinquish her license and car; moral suasion can be effective in such cases, especially if the functions supported by driving (e.g., shopping, visiting friends, keeping doctors' appointments) can be achieved by other means. In the worst case, patients who pose public health risks will enjoy fewer confidentiality protections than others, and it can be permissible to violate confidentiality to achieve these ends. Caution is urged, however: one of the consequences of demoting the values of privacy and confidentiality is that once a patient knows her secrets are no longer safe, she might be disinclined to disclose them in the future. This can be a problem: disclosure of personal information by trusting patients is among the psychiatrists' most powerful and precious tools.

ACCESS TO CARE

> ### CASE EXAMPLE
>
> Mr. W., 78, has severe dementia, which you have been managing quite well. His Medicare coverage is through a provider that reduces reimbursement levels so they fall beneath the threshold acceptable to your practice group. You believe you can continue to help him, but are under pressure by colleagues not to.
>
> "You will cause a drain on the practice," one colleague tells you. "Just tell him and his family you can no longer provide professional services at sub-Medicare levels. Most of our patients are affluent, and this patient is an outlier …"

While few would publicly argue in favor of neglecting either elders—especially those with psychiatric problems—it is an unhappy fact that many members of these groups do not enjoy access to adequate medical treatment (20). This is a moral failure of the first magnitude.

Arguments in favor of rationing care by age usually address high technology and high cost interventions—which are generally not the case in geriatric psychiatry. There is, in fact, no good argument in favor of failing to provide at least a minimum level of basic care to all persons (21), especially in affluent societies. Even if one could, on utilitarian grounds, attempt to defend age-based rationing or neglect, the brute fact that the number of elders is growing dramatically turns those arguments on their heads.

Ageism or, generally, bias against elders, is usually pejorative and used to label a morally blameworthy practice (14). Yet there can be compelling scientific and/or ethical reasons for treating patients differently because of their age. It is reasonable, for example, to refuse to perform heart transplant surgery on a patient in the late stages of Alzheimer's disease, because it is unlikely that the patient will experience a significant benefit from the procedure and valuable resources can be more effectively used elsewhere.

The debate over age-based rationing and resource allocation is as fraught and controversial as any in bioethics (22). What is often overlooked in these debates is that chronological age itself is a poor predictor of success or utility of clinical interventions (23). In the absence of evidence that would demonstrate—or even support—the notion that care for elders is not effective or is futile, then any attempt to use age alone as a test for access to care is biased without justification.

Even in end-of-life care, justifications for limiting treatment are not based on age alone but on the inevitability of death. Note as a moral bright spot that end-of-life care challenges have been met—not with refusal to treat—but by the evolution of a specialized form of care, namely hospice (24).

The selection of treatments can be at least as vexing as rationing. Care for elders with dementia, for instance, can pose exquisitely difficult clinical questions. Does medication or treatment improve the patient's quality of life, or simply make her more manageable for caregivers? Does a drug relieve a symptom at the expense of reducing capacity to consent? Is a patient cured of one malady only to be sedated into incoherence?

A more immediate challenge arises in contexts in which continuity of care is imperiled. While physicians are often lectured, inspired, or hectored about their professional duty to treat, such a duty is often modulated by considerations of reimbursement and other economic factors. It is widely agreed, however, that once a therapeutic relationship has been established, it should be very difficult to end it for economic reasons and without a patient's voluntary concurrence. In the scenario at the outset of this section, the psychiatrist is caught between the demands of colleagues and the obligation to continue to take care of his patient. In some circumstances, unilateral termination of a therapeutic relationship can constitute patient abandonment. This is firstly a moral failure and secondly a variation from professional rules that could expose the physician to liability and license revocation.

Fortunately, the growth of the world's geriatric population is having the salutary effect of stimulating research into optimal interventions. After all, it is scientific or clinical uncertainty that so often leave health care teams grasping at the lesser of evils. Therefore, the needs of more and better research are many, and the challenges great.

HUMAN SUBJECTS RESEARCH

It has generally been acknowledged that elder populations are underrepresented in research. Low participation rates of elder subjects can be partly accounted for by the physical and mental impairments associated with aging. These impairments can make it difficult for geriatric patients to understand the nature and purpose of a research protocol (25). A significant problem associated with studying diseases like dementia is that potential subjects who are needed for the protocols are frequently unable to consent to enroll. Further, enrolled subjects might lose decision-making capacity during the course of a study, which makes it difficult to ascertain whether subjects desire to continue. Advanced directives might be able to help resolve conflicts by specifying the conditions under which an individual would want to be a research subject, but this type of measure is rarely used.

When conducting human subjects research, psychiatric or otherwise, obtaining proper consent is crucially important (26). The consent process must be carefully and thoroughly undertaken before a subject, elderly or otherwise, is enrolled in a research protocol. There is a long history of documented cases in which proper consent was not obtained, and research subjects were thereby mistreated. Ideally, the decision to participate in research must be made voluntarily by a competent individual. Researchers should inform every subject of the potential benefits and risks associated with the research. In the absence of a prospective subject's capacity to consent, an appropriate surrogate must be identified.

Recognizing the complexities associated with psychiatric research, the National Bioethics Advisory Commission released a report in 1998 titled *Research Involving Persons with Mental Disorders that May Affect Decisionmaking Capacity*, recommending guidelines for the use of mentally impaired subjects in research (27). Although the NBAC's report has been criticized for impeding psychiatric research (26), it does emphasize the importance of protecting human subjects against abuse. The authors of the report recognized the importance of classifying research into different categories depending on the degree of risk involved and the likelihood that the subject will receive some type of benefit from participation. "Greater than minimal risk" became a catch phrase differentiating research that might endanger subjects from research that is unlikely to do so (28).

The ability of Alzheimer's and other patients to consent to research can be markedly impaired even during the early stages of the disease (29). The procedure for recruiting Alzheimer's patients typically involves obtaining consent from the subject along with consent from the surrogate. If seeking to enroll Alzheimer's patients for greater than minimal risk research in which subjects are unlikely to benefit from the research, it may be necessary for potential subjects to consent explicitly before allowing them to enroll (30).

One analysis of problems associated with enrolling dementia patients in research protocols revealed that approximately half of eligible subjects could not participate because of complications associated with the consent process; 19% of surrogates did not adequately understand the nature of the research protocol; and there was no available surrogate in 32% of the cases studied (31).

Subjects should not be excluded if they do not appear competent during the initial attempt at obtaining consent. It has been suggested that a waiting period between the time the consent forms are discussed and signed might assist elderly subjects to make a truly informed decision and, further, that a tryout period might be useful to get patients used to what is involved in being research subjects (32). Other methods that could be attempted to improve the capacity of subjects suffering from mental illness include the use of computer programs or videotapes (33).

Subjects and their surrogates might have the perception that no other treatment is available and so might act out of desperation. This feeling can be especially pronounced when the subject suffers from Alzheimer's disease (34). Participants and their surrogates might thus operate under the therapeutic misconception whereby they incorrectly assume that because they are being asked to enroll in research they will receive some kind of (direct) benefit. However, the intent of a research protocol is to find out whether a particular intervention works in the first place; it might not benefit the subject directly. A protocol that investigates the different stages of Alzheimer's disease, for instance, might one day help researchers develop improved therapies, but the subjects might not experience any direct benefit from participation.

There is a related misconception that because subjects are being monitored there is little or no risk (34). Patients and surrogates cannot assume that because a physician asks them to be involved in a research protocol that it is guaranteed to be safe. Further, the duty of physicians to patients and their role as researchers may generate conflicts of interest, which could be detrimental to potential subjects (35).

Unfortunately, decisions regarding research participation are rarely discussed in families. Thus, the wishes of an incompetent person concerning participation are probably not known, which can lead the surrogate to make a decision that does not match what the patient wants. Surrogates may be confused about who is responsible for making the decision to enroll in research, even though they have been appointed as decision-makers (34). Further, it is not always clear how to identify a subject's surrogate. It has been suggested that guidelines identifying surrogates can be delineated within the research protocol (28). To be sure, it is essential that a surrogate for clinical decisions generally be the surrogate for decisions regarding research participation.

As in clinical contexts, a surrogate should make decisions that are consistent with the incompetent person's values and past choices. But this does not always happen. Surrogates have exhibited a willingness to enroll patients in research protocols even though they believe that the patients might not want to participate (26). Further, the decisions of surrogates to enroll patients in research have been found to reflect what the surrogates would want for themselves, and that surrogates have admitted that they were more likely to enroll the patients as subjects than the patients themselves (although there was a general reluctance to enroll patients in high risk protocols) (36).

Responsibility for protecting subjects rests with investigators and institutional review boards, (IRBs). Researchers should be aware of the surrogate's motives and level of familiarity with the incompetent patient's wishes and values. Vigilance here is crucial given the importance of both the research and the vulnerability of the subjects.

Placebos and Wash-Out Studies

There are longstanding disputes concerning the scientific need and ethical appropriateness of using placebo controls in medical research (37,38). Relatedly, some protocols are specifically designed to exacerbate the subject's symptoms for research purposes (39).

Some of the main objections to the use of placebos in psychiatric research include that a patient's illness may get worse by halting medication, and that there is a widespread misconception that patients will receive a direct benefit from participating in research. In a wash-out period, medication or treatment is temporarily withheld to give investigators an unconfounded clean slate with which to test a study drug. Significant disagreement accompanies the question of potential harm to patients placed on placebos, as well as the length of time needed to return to baseline levels. Some argue that if an available treatment has already shown promise, then the continued use of placebos might be unnecessary and hence unethical.

While there are many interesting and important ethical issues that arise in human subjects research in general, those itemized here are of special concern in (potentially) impaired populations. The scientific and ethical merits of research protocols must be assessed by IRBs. IRBs examine research protocols before subjects are enrolled to ensure that ongoing research is conducted in an ethical manner and that the consent process is adequate. While education of IRB members has expanded and improved, comparatively little attention is devoted to the special needs of geriatric populations, especially for behavioral research; this track record ought to be improved (39). The American Geriatrics Society encourages geriatric specialists to serve on IRBs in order to protect the interests of elderly subjects (40).

SPECIAL ISSUES

Challenges faced by the psychiatrist or other health professional who cares for geriatric patients have never been more interesting—or difficult. Some of these challenges arise in non-elder populations; some do not. In most cases, it is safe to say that the geriatric psychiatrist faces more of these challenges than others.

Artificial Hydration and Nutrition

Maladies that range from swallowing disorders to various kinds of unconsciousness can prevent patients from feeding themselves or being fed with assistance. In these cases, nutrition and hydration can be maintained by nasogastric (NG) tubes, intravenous (IV) lines, or percutaneous endoscopic gastrostomy (PEG) tubes. These devices are generally best thought of as temporary interventions until such time as normal feeding behavior can be restored. This is especially true in cases of permanent unconsciousness in which the goals of treatment are often obscure. The reasons for this are straightforward: depending on the underlying malady, artificial hydration and nutrition alone are almost certainly not going to restore cognitive function. In many or most cases, maintaining an unconscious state with no prospects for cognitive improvement has little value to most patients.

Terminating or not starting artificial sustenance can be controversial, however. In some cases this is because family members and others regard NG, IV, and PEG tubes as embodying the kind of loving support that is normally associated with *feeding*. Our language unfortunately reinforces this: we call them feeding tubes, where this connotes something more akin to placing a spoon in a loved-one's mouth than use of a medical device to replace a failed physiologic function or behavior. Psychiatrists and others should take care not to give the impression that artificial hydration and nutrition are anything other than medical interventions whose most appropriate uses are temporary and in service of an outcome other than not dying. Moreover, great care should also be taken in responding to queries about the affective symptoms of terminating a PEG tube, for instance. For patients in a persistent vegetative state, for example, experts in the field believe that there are no sensations of hunger or other discomfort. Knowing this can help family members come more easily to terms with their loved one's impending demise.

Indeed, it is generally the case that dying patients have no or few sensations of hunger and that artificial hydration and nutrition can serve no better purpose than prolonging the dying process and perhaps maximizing suffering caused by other processes.

Use of Restraints

On a day-to-day basis, decisions whether to restrain patients can provide the most difficult and emotionally trying challenges in all geriatric care. The most benign or positive motivation for use of restraints—physical or chemical—is well known and generally well motivated. It is simply the concern that in the absence of restraints a patient will injure himself or someone else. That said, restraints can be dehumanizing, devastating for patient and family members, and even atherapeutic. Accrediting agencies have established high thresholds for the use of restraints, and in some jurisdictions regulatory bodies are wary of restraint overuse. Psychiatrists should check state laws and nursing home regulatory bodies to identify limitations on the use of restraints.

Restraints should be considered when there is no alternative to preventing injury. It follows that other interventions that achieve the same goals are preferred. It is important to emphasize that chemical restraints should generally be disdained, the same as straps and other physical restraints.

When restraints are used, they should be in place for as short a time as possible, and patients who are restrained should be monitored carefully and frequently. Restraints should not be used for the sake of staff members or for institutional convenience. High quality health care requires that vulnerable patients not be subjected to interventions undertaken for others' sake.

Electroconvulsive Therapy (ECT)

Lay misunderstanding of ECT can produce hurdles to effective patient management. Common misconceptions about ECT may make it difficult for patients and surrogates to consent to its use in cases in which it would be effective. In such cases, well-informed psychiatrists should devote extra time to educating patients and family members about the intervention, its uses, and its limitations.

Absent valid consent, ECT should nevertheless be considered for incapacitated patients, but this intervention—much like the use of restraints—may prove counterproductive. Exceptions arise when ECT may be potentially lifesaving, as it can be in cases of serious incapacity or catatonia. In general, ECT use should be carefully negotiated with patients and families, and include the following elements:

- Thorough discussion of risks, benefits, and alternatives, incorporating an explanation of the procedure, with as much underlying science as possible, and including examples of successful applications.
- Gentle correction of misconceptions about the procedure.
- Reassurance that the patient will be closely monitored and cared for.

ETHICS COMMITTEES AND CULTURAL DIVERSITY

The past two decades have seen extraordinary growth in the use and utility of institutional ethics committees. Such committees, often created in order to comply with the standards of the Joint Commission for the Accreditation of Health Care Organizations, are widely recognized as having three primary functions: education (of clinicians, communities and the committee members themselves), policy creation and review, and case consultations. In the practical experience of many ethics committee members, challenges raised by cognitive incapacity—especially in geriatric cases—loom as the most frequent and difficult. While the relationship between psychiatric and ethical expertise is still being explored (41), it should be uncontroversial to suggest that adequate and focused training in geriatric psychiatry is essential for any ethics committee that would presume to provide policies and consultations in the kinds of cases that commonly arise in this domain.

This can be crucially important in cases in which culture or ethnicity are at issue. For instance, ethnicity may play a role in the selection and function of a surrogate (42), and diverse cultures and patient populations present clinicians with challenges related to communication, consent, confidentiality and the role of family members. While increasing one's cultural competency—and so acquiring improved capacity to recognize cultural variations that impinge on clinical and research contexts—it is clear that a well-tuned ethics committee can be invaluable in resolving conflicts and suggesting strategies for managing cases in which values conflict. For additional information, see the chapter in this book on cultural issues.

Like clinical practice, ethics provides few algorithms that can be applied without reflection. It does not prevent tragedy or even sadness. It is fallible. What a robust ethics process can offer, however, is a resource for addressing what many clinicians and researchers regard as their most profound professional challenges. As we saw in the case of valid consent, the tools of applied ethics provide their greatest utility as part of a process. Applied ethics is not about passing moral judgment in a series of discrete events. Rather, it has the goal of guiding health care teams and others in cases in which values matter, and what is needed is a process to guide us and give those values practical meaning in increasingly complex clinical contexts.

REFERENCES

1. Culver CM, Gert B. Ethical issues in oncology. *Psych Med.* 1987;5:389–404.
2. Spar JE. Competency and related forensic issues. In: Coffey CE, Cummings JL, eds. *The American Psychiatric Press Textbook of Geriatric Neuropsychiatry.* 2nd Ed. Washington DC: American Psychiatric Press; 2000:945–963.
3. Dymek MP, Atchison P, Harrell L, Marson DC. Competency to consent to medical treatment in cognitively impaired patients with Parkinson's disease. *Neurology.* 2001;56(1):17–24.

4. Post S. Dementia care ethics. In: Weisstub DN, Thomasma DC, Gauthier S, Tomossy GF, eds. *Aging: Decisions at the End of Life.* Boston: Kluwer Academic Publishers; 2001:177–190.

5. Palmer K, Backman L, Winblad B, Fratiglioni L. Detection of Alzheimer's disease and dementia in the preclinical phase: population based cohort study. *BMJ.* 2003;326:245.

6. Auerswald KB, Charpentier PA, Inouye SK. The informed consent process in older patients who developed delirium: a clinical epidemiologic study. *Am J Med.* 1997;103(5):410–418.

7. Culver C, Gert B. The inadequacy of incompetence. *Milbank Q.* 1990;68(4):619–643.

8. Fazel S. Competence. In: Jacoby R, Oppenheimer C, eds.. *Psychiatry in the Elderly.* 3rd Ed. New York: Oxford University Press, 2002;941–950.

9. Appelbaum PS. Psychiatric research and the incompetent subject. *Psychiatr Serv.* 1997;48(7):873–874.

10. Appelbaum BC, Appelbaum PS, Grisso T. Competence to consent to voluntary psychiatric hospitalization: a test of a standard proposed by APA. *Psychiatr Serv.* 1998;49(9):1193–1196.

11. Appelbaum PS, Grisso T. Capacities of hospitalized, medically ill patients to consent to treatment. *Psychosomatics.* 1997;38(2):119–125.

12. Barton CD, Mallik HS, Orr WB, Janofsky JS. Clinicians' judgment of capacity of nursing home patients to give informed consent. *Psychiatr Serv.* 1996;47(9):956–960.

13. Grisso T, Appelbaum PS, Hill-Fotouhi C. The MacCAT-T: a clinical tool to assess patients' capacities to make treatment decisions. *Psychiatr Serv.* 1997;48:1415–1419.

14. Hughes JC. Ethics and the psychiatry of old age. In: Jacoby R, Oppenheimer C, eds. *Psychiatry in the Elderly.* 3rd Ed. New York: Oxford University Press, 2002;863–895.

15. Goodman K. End-of-life algorithms. *Psychol Public Policy Law.* 1998;4:719–727.

16. Johnston S, Pfeifer M, McNutt R. The discussion about advanced directives. *Arch Intern Med.* 1995;155:1025–1030.

17. Cushman R. Privacy/Data Protection Project. Available at http://privacy.med.miami.edu. Accessed June 7, 2005.

18. American Medical Association. Code of Ethics, E-2.24 Impaired drivers and their physicians. 2000. Available at http://www.ama-assn.org/ama/pub/category/8464.html. Accessed June 7, 2005.

19. Greely HT. Special issues in genetic testing for Alzheimer disease. *Genet Testing.* 1999;3:115–119.

20. Wetle T. Age as a risk factor for inadequate treatment. *JAMA.* 1987;258:516.

21. Buchanan A. The right to a decent minimum of health care. *Philosophy & Public Affairs.* 1984;13(1):55–78.

22. Callahan D. *Setting Limits: Medical Goals in an Aging Society.* New York: Simon and Schuster, 1987.

23. Tadd W, Bayer A. Commentary: medical decision making based on chronological age—cause for concern. *J Clin Ethics.* 2000;11:328–333.

24. Post SG, Whitehouse PJ. The moral basis for limiting treatment: hospice and advanced progressive dementia. In: Volicer L, Hurley A, eds. *Hospice Care for Patients with Advanced Progressive Dementia.* New York: Springer, 1998:117–131.

25. Thomasma DC. Community consent for research on the impaired elderly. In: Weisstub DN, Thomasma DC, Gauthier S, Tomossy GF, eds. *Aging: Decisions at the End of Life.* Boston: Kluwer Academic Publishers, 2001;207–226.

26. Roberts LW, Roberts B. Psychiatric research ethics: an overview of evolving guidelines and current ethical dilemmas in the study of mental illness. *Biol Psychiatry.* 1999;46:1025–1038.

27. National Bioethics Advisory Commission (NBAC). Research involving persons with mental disorders that may affect decision making capacity. 1998. Available at http://www.georgetown.edu/research/nrcbl/nbac/capacity/TOC.htm. Accessed June 7, 2005.

28. Karlawish JHT. Research involving cognitively impaired adults. *N Engl J Med.* 2003;348(14):1389–1392.

29. Kim SYH, Caine ED, Currier GW, Leibovici A, Ryan JM. Assessing the competence of persons with Alzheimer's disease in providing informed consent for participation in research. *Am J Psychiatry.* 2001;158(5):712–717.

30. Alzheimer's Association. Position statements: ethical issues in dementia research. 1997. Available at http://www.alz.org/AboutUs/PositionStatements/overview.asp. Accessed June 7, 2005.

31. Baskin SA, Morris J, Ahronheim JC, Meier DE, Morrison RS. Barriers to obtaining consent in dementia research: implications for surrogate decision-making. *J Am Geriatr Soc.* 1998;46(3):287–290.

32. Rikkert MG, van den Bercken JH, ten Have HA, Hoefnagels WH. Experienced consent in geriatrics research: a new method to optimize the capacity to consent in frail elderly subjects. *J Med Ethics.* 1997;23(5):271–276.

33. Appelbaum PS. Missing the boat: competence and consent in psychiatric research. *Am J Psychiatry.* 1998;155(11):1486–1488.

34. Sugarman J, Cain C, Wallace R, Welsh-Bohmer KA. How proxies make decisions about research for patients with Alzheimer's disease. *J Am Geriatr Soc.* 2001;49(8):1110–1119.

35. Whitehouse P. Ethical issues. In: Coffey CE, Cummings JL. *The American Psychiatric Press Textbook of Geriatric Neuropsychiatry.* 2nd Ed. Washington, DC: American Psychiatric Press, 2000;935–944.

36. Sachs GA, Stocking CB, Stern R, Cox DM, Hougham G, Sachs RS. Ethical aspects of dementia research: informed consent and proxy consent. *Clin Res.* 1994;42(3):403–412.

37. Roberts LW, Lauriello J, Geppert C, Keith SJ. Placebos and paradoxes in psychiatric research: an ethics perspective. *Biol Psychiatry.* 2001;49:887–893.

38. Charney DS. The use of placebos in randomized clinical trials of mood disorders: well justified, but improvements in design are indicated. *Biol Psychiatry.* 2000;47:687–688.

39. Rosenstein DL. IRB review of psychiatric medication discontinuation and symptom-provoking studies. *Biol Psychiatry.* 1999;46:1039–1043.

40. AGS Ethics Committee; AGS Research Committee. The responsible conduct of research. *J Am Geriatr Soc.* 2001;49:1120–1122.

41. Leeman CP. Psychiatric consultations and ethics consultations. *Gen Hosp Psychiatry.* 2000;22:270–275.

42. Hornung CA, Eleazer GP, Strothers HS III, et al. Ethnicity and decision-makers in a group of frail older people. *J Am Geriatr Soc.* 1998;46:280–286.

Psychiatric Disorders

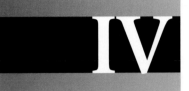

Memory Disorders

19

Yonas Endale Geda   *Selamawit Negash*
Ronald C. Petersen

Concerns about memory are commonly encountered in clinical practice. Hence, it is important for clinicians to have a clear understanding of what constitutes a memory complaint. Once the problem is clearly identified, the next step is to generate a working hypothesis regarding the neuroanatomic structures implicated, then clarify the underlying mechanism of the disorder, and finally initiate appropriate treatment.

What Exactly Is Meant by "Memory Problem"?

Patients and their family members often present to the clinician with a memory complaint. But what constitutes a memory problem? The clinician has to clarify whether the patient is referring to problems of attention/concentration, anomia, or a true memory problem of learning and recall. It is quite common to hear patients say, "I am having a memory problem: I cannot remember the names of my grandchildren." Is this a memory problem or possibly anomia, a language problem?

In order to address this question, let us consider examples of classic amnestic syndromes from the literature. One such syndrome involves anterograde amnesia, which is the inability to acquire new information that occurs in the context of intact attention/concentration, language, and other related cognitive functions. This was very well exemplified by the case record of H.M. In 1957, Scoville and Milner reported that following bilateral anterior temporal lobe resection for intractable epilepsy, H.M. developed the inability to acquire new information (anterograde amnesia) (1). Apart from the anterograde amnesia, he had intact cognitive functions such as language, attention, and executive functions. This clinically relevant, novel, and detailed longitudinal observation shed light on the neuroanatomic localization of memory dysfunction (2).

Another classic memory disorder is Korsakoff's syndrome, in which one has intact cognitive functions, except for problems of learning and recall (3). The person may be able to interact well with the clinician, have an intact sense of direction (visuospatial function), and have no problems with language, but he or she has problems with acquisition of new information. This would become readily apparent when the patient was unable to learn new information on bedside testing. The underlying neurological process implicated in this disorder is that of a failure of consolidation or the inability to form permanent memory traces.

The above examples characterize the concept of anterograde amnesia. Another related term is retrograde amnesia in which, for instance, following a motor vehicle accident or seizure, a patient may complain of having difficulty recalling recent events a few days, weeks, or months prior to the event. Retrograde amnesia may or may not coexist with anterograde amnesia.

Information Processing Model and Localization of Memory Problems

One way of understanding memory disorders is to put them in the context of an information processing model. Mesulam has proposed a set of five large-scale neurocognitive networks which are partially segregated but still overlapping (4). He has identified crucial structures in each neurocognitive network that he refers to as the epicenter of that network. For instance, the hippocampus is the epicenter for memory network and damage to this network can lead to memory disorder. The other four neurocognitive networks and their respective epicenters are:

1. Right-hemisphere-dominant spatial orientation network, with epicenters in dorsal parietal lobe, frontal eye fields, and posterior cingulate;

2. Left-hemisphere-dominant language network, with epicenters in Broca's and Wernicke's areas;
3. Ventral occipitotemporal network for face and object recognition, with epicenters in lateral temporal and temporopolar cortex; and
4. Executive function and comportment network, with epicenters in dorsolateral prefrontal and orbitofrontal cortex, respectively (4,5).

In order to process material to be remembered by a person with intact attention, the external world, as perceived by the sensory organs, is kept "online" by the primary sensory cortex, which, in turn transfers the information to unimodal association, and then to multimodal association cortices. The online holding of information is also referred to as *immediate memory* or *working memory*. For example, when one glances at a telephone directory and starts dialing the number, this information is most likely held in working memory. The online holding of memory function can be assessed clinically by using the digit-span test. This test is typically normal in patients with amnestic syndrome.

However, when the person rehearses the telephone number to memory, the information is passed from the association cortex such as the dorsolateral prefrontal cortex, via the perforant pathway of the entorhinal cortex, to the hippocampal formation and limbic system. This constitutes the anatomical basis for major aspects of the consolidation process. It is worth noting that information is not stored passively in the limbic system; rather, it undergoes a dynamic processing in the limbic system and is then transferred back to the association areas where the neural network for permanent memory exists. As a result of this dynamic interaction, there is a constant remodeling of more permanent information.

Therefore, when a patient presents with problems of encoding or acquisition of information, the structures primarily implicated are the medial temporal lobe/temporolimbic structures such as the hippocampus, entorhinal cortex, perforant pathway, mammillary bodies, thalamus, hypothalamus, basal forebrain, and the interconnecting structures. Bilateral lesions (such as bilateral degeneration of the hippocampus) would give rise to an amnestic syndrome, but unilateral lesions can give rise to verbal or nonverbal processing difficulties.

What Is the Mechanism of Memory Disorders?

It is important for the clinician to understand the temporal profile of the illness, combined with relevant history such as head trauma, epilepsy, psychiatric disorders (such as major depression or severe anxiety disorders), cancer, vascular diseases, etc., in order to generate a plausible explanation for the mechanism of the memory problem.

Acute Memory Loss

If the memory loss is of acute onset, various neurological and psychiatric etiologies should be entertained. A vascular etiology is an important consideration in a person presenting with an acute memory loss. The vertebrobasilar system supplies most of the medial temporal lobe structures, hence, one should look for any stroke involving these structures. For instance, an ischemic insult to the thalamus or certain medial temporal lobe structures can lead to acute memory loss.

Other causes that can present with acute memory loss include hemorrhages (particularly from aneurysms involving the anterior communicating artery), migraines, hypoglycemia, toxic exposure, drug ingestion, and psychogenic disorders. Another important cause to consider is transient global amnesia (TGA). In TGA, patients present with anterograde amnesia for a brief period of time. There is a variable degree of retrograde amnesia in the setting of an otherwise normal neurological examination. The etiology of the disorder is not clear.

Episodic acute memory loss should also alert the clinician to the possibility of a seizure disorder. An electroencephalogram (EEG) and relevant investigations, such as magnetic resonance imaging (MRI) of the head with emphasis on temporal lobe structures, may help to delineate this. In addition to the above neurological conditions, psychiatric problems should also be considered.

One psychiatric condition that needs to be considered is psychogenic amnesia. Patients with this problem may complain of a loss of autobiographical information such as their personal identity, which is typically very resistant to loss. They may complain of retrograde amnesia with little or no anterograde amnesia. On testing, their performance may be variable. They may fail relatively easy tests (such as recognition), while performing relatively normally on other tests (such as free recall). One has to make a deliberate effort to look for organic causes before concluding that the person has psychogenic amnesia.

Subacute Memory Loss

A complaint of memory loss over a period of days to weeks should alert the clinician for possible etiologies including infectious, inflammatory, toxic, or metabolic causes. For instance, the treatable condition herpes simplex encephalitis should be considered in cases of subacute memory loss with associated seizures or other relevant clinical data. Inflammatory conditions such as multiple sclerosis, sarcoidosis, or Sjögren's syndrome should be considered in the appropriate context. Also, limbic encephalitis, meningeal carcinomatosis, and psychiatric etiologies should be considered based on the relevant clinical and investigational data.

Chronic Memory Loss

A memory complaint of insidious onset with gradual progression should alert one for a neurodegenerative disorder such as Alzheimer's disease (AD). However, other

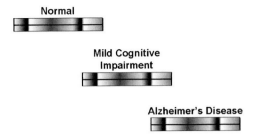

Figure 19-1 Conceptual model of mild cognitive impairment. (Reprinted with permission from Peterson R, et al, 1999. (7)

explanations such as a slowly growing tumor like a meningioma can present with memory problems. Psychiatric conditions such as a major depressive disorder should be entertained. Patients with depression have difficulty with concentration; hence, it is effortful for them to learn new information. However, once learned, they can access or recall better than patients with AD. Another example is Parkinson's disease in which the patient will have delayed learning of new material. Such patients will have problems, but they can recall the learnt material relatively better than patients with AD, who are neither able to learn nor recall.

Mild Cognitive Impairment

The importance of an early diagnosis and treatment of a disease is apparent. This is particularly true of AD, a disease that in the United States alone is projected to afflict as many as 14 million people by the year 2050. Even though life is priceless, the economic impact of AD is quite remarkable: it costs about $40,000 per year to care for a patient with dementia. Hence, the prevention of this disease is not only of academic interest, but is of major public health interest as well (6).

The clinician is often asked by older persons with memory concerns if their symptoms mean that they are developing AD. Indeed, the presence of memory complaints could be an early manifestation of AD, or it could be a manifestation of depression or represent the "worried well" state of normal aging. Even if the memory problem is due to a neurodegenerative disorder, it may not necessarily be AD.

Researchers have increasingly focused on the gray zone between normal aging and dementia. Various names have been given to this concept, one of which is *mild cognitive impairment* (MCI) (7). MCI can be viewed as a transitional state between normal aging and dementia as depicted in Figure 19.1. The case record of a typical patient with amnestic MCI will be discussed in order to illustrate the concept of MCI.

CASE EXAMPLE

A 70-year-old right-handed man presented with an insidious-onset and gradually worsening forgetfulness for recent events and future engagements. For example, over the past few weeks, he had forgotten to keep an important appointment with his personal physician. His family and close friends were beginning to notice these changes and brought them to his attention. He had difficulty identifying the onset of these symptoms but felt that they had gradually become worse in recent months. Otherwise, he was living independently and had no difficulty carrying out activities of daily living, such as handling his own finances, cooking, and driving. He denied depression, stress, or other complicating medical issues. He requested an appointment with a neurologist to determine if this memory problem should be pursued further. Psychometric testing revealed memory impairment, particularly on measures of learning and delayed recall beyond what was felt to be normal for age; but other cognitive domains such as language and visuospatial skills were relatively intact. Magnetic resonance imaging of his head revealed mild hippocampal atrophy.

This patient probably has amnestic MCI. He is becoming slightly more forgetful, and this is noticeable to his family and friends. The most salient feature of the history concerns forgetfulness of insidious onset that gradually progressed over a year or so. All other cognitive domains (i.e., language, comportment-executive function, and visuospatial skills) were intact. The individual did not have a decline in function. This likely represented an early disease process involving the medial temporal lobe, since meaningful information could no longer be stored in an efficient manner or recalled well.

Patients with MCI typically have memory impairment over and above what is expected for their age and educational level, yet they are not demented. They function independently in the community and are not significantly impaired. The diagnosis of MCI is clinical, but neuropsychological testing and neuroimaging studies can aid in clarifying the diagnosis (Table 19-1).

MRI studies have shown that hippocampal volumes of MCI subjects fall midway between those of normal controls and subjects with very mild AD (8). Magnetic resonance spectroscopy studies have also shown that the myoinositol-to-creatinine ratio is elevated in MCI subjects compared to elderly normal controls (9).

TABLE 19-1

CLINICAL CRITERIA FOR AMNESTIC MILD COGNITIVE IMPAIRMENT

1. Memory complaint, preferably corroborated by an informant
2. Essentially normal general cognition
3. Largely normal activities of daily living
4. Objective memory impairment for age
5. Not demented

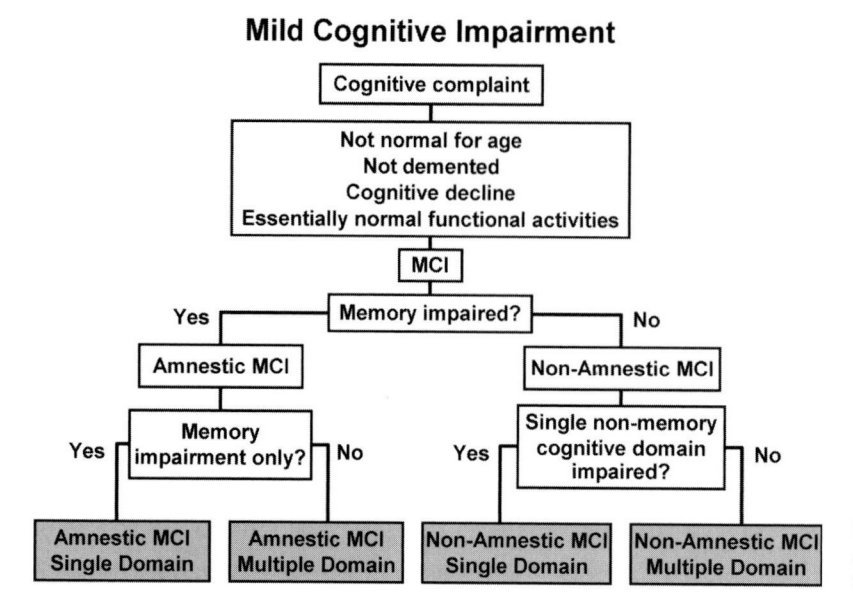

Figure 19-2 Classification of clinical subtypes of mild cognitive impairment. (Reprinted with permission from Petersen RC, 2004). (13)

Recently, MCI has come to be recognized as a heterogeneous entity (10,11). Although most research has focused on the amnestic type of MCI, as the field has advanced it has become apparent that other clinical subtypes exist as well (12,13). As depicted in Figure 19-2, the concept of MCI has been expanded more recently to include at least three more subtypes. *Multiple domain amnestic MCI* pertains to individuals who, in addition to a memory deficit, also have impairments in at least one other cognitive domain such as language, executive function, or visuospatial skills. *Multiple domain non-amnestic MCI*, on the other hand, pertains to individuals who have impairments in multiple cognitive domains, but not including memory. *Single domain non-amnestic MCI*, which is the least common subtype, pertains to individuals with impairment in a single nonmemory domain such as language, executive function, or visuospatial skills. Other cognitive domains including memory are essentially normal. Individuals in this subtype likely have a different outcome from those with memory impairment. It is also important to note that individuals in all of these subtypes of MCI have minimal impairments in functional activities that do not represent a significant change in function from a prior level, and they also do not meet the criteria for dementia.

In addition to the clinical subtypes, there can also be multiple etiologies or causes for each subtype. Therefore, if one selected the single domain amnestic MCI subtype with a presumed degenerative etiology, this would likely represent a prodromal form of AD. However, one could also add the subtype of the multiple domain amnestic MCI, since this subtype has a high likelihood of progressing to AD as well (14). In contrast, the other subtypes emphasizing impairments in nonmemory domains such as comportment-executive function or visuospatial skills, may have a higher likelihood of progressing to a non-AD

dementia, such as FTD in the former, or dementia with Lewy bodies in the latter (15). Therefore, the combination of clinical subtypes and putative etiologies can be useful in predicting the ultimate type of dementia to which these diseases will evolve.

The discussion of the gray zone between normal aging and dementia is not complete without reviewing the genesis of the research work that gave birth to the concept of MCI (16). Reisberg and colleagues were the first to use the term mild cognitive impairment (17). They used the Global Deterioration Scale (GDS), which has a scale of one to seven, with one being normal and seven signifying severe dementia. Subjects that scored GDS of three were classified as having MCI. This approach is in contrast to studies at the Mayo Clinic, which use clinical criteria to arrive at a diagnosis of MCI (7).

The study of early memory concerns with aging dates back to the 1962 publication of Kral on benign and malignant senescent forgetfulness (18). Since then, various experts have published in this area. In 1986, the National Institute of Mental Health convened an experts panel in which Crook and colleagues coined the term *age-associated memory impairment* (AAMI) (19). AAMI has stimulated a tremendous research interest in this area. One shortcoming of AAMI is that, depending on the memory item selected, up to 90% of those older than 50 would be labeled as impaired (20). This is a rather large proportion of the elderly population. Hence, AAMI essentially refers to the normal aging process, whereas MCI refers to a disease process. Likewise, terms such as *benign senescent forgetfulness, age-consistent memory impairment*, and *aging-associated cognitive decline* refer to normal aging. Terms such as *malignant senescent forgetfulness*, MCI, and *mild neurocognitive decline* refer to an abnormal state (21–23).

Evaluation of Memory Problems

Like all medical evaluations, the assessment of memory problems involves history. This includes the important step of gathering collateral history from family members or acquaintances (with the consent of the patient), physical examination, relevant investigations, appropriate consultation, and synthesis of the data to arrive at a diagnosis and initiate relevant treatment.

History

The clinician should inquire about forgetfulness for recent events and future engagements. One may want to ask about generally well-known and widely discussed political, cultural, or sporting events. The clinician can get an idea about the patient's baseline interests and hobbies from the patient and family, and make inquiries about recent experiences. For example, if the patient is a known sports fan, then inquiring about recent games might be informative. Also, finding out about important engagements missed due to forgetfulness, such as a luncheon meeting or a critical doctor appointment, could be helpful.

Corroborating data from the family is helpful, not only in determining comparison with baseline function of the patient, but also to validate the history provided by the patient. Patients with memory problems may give little detail about recent events and tend to be very vague.

Sometimes it is helpful for the clinician to keep in mind the major cognitive domains while eliciting history. That is, the clinician can inquire about memory, language, visuospatial, executive-comportment function, human-face recognition, and object recognition networks. Such an approach will ensure that cognitive domains other than memory are not involved to a significant degree. For example, after inquiring about recent events, one may want to ask for any loss of sense of direction (such as getting lost in one's neighborhood or having difficulty finding the bathroom in one's own house).

In addition to gathering clinical data on cognitive domains, the clinician should also make sure the patient is functioning independently by inquiring about instrumental activities of daily living, such as balancing a checkbook or making travel reservations.

Finally, it is important to inquire about the temporal profile of the illness. If the memory problem is of insidious onset and gradual progression, then one should think of possible underlying neurodegenerative processes. If there has been a more precipitous onset, vascular contributions should be considered.

Physical Examination

Physical examination, which obviously is part and parcel of a physician's clinical evaluation, can render important clinical data. For instance, rigidity, bradykinesia, and tremor in an individual complaining of memory problems may be indicative of Parkinson's disease or any other parkinsonian syndrome. Aphasia and right hemiparesis in a right-handed person presenting with acute memory complaint may be indicative of a left-sided cerebrovascular accident. Fever, nuchal rigidity, and seizure may be suggestive of herpes simplex encephalitis in someone presenting with subacute memory loss.

Mental Status Examination

The mental status examination is an important part of clinical evaluation and aids in the diagnostic process. It also aids the clinician in considering the need for a more detailed neuropsychological evaluation. The clinician can use any of the standard bedside tests, such as Mini Mental State Examination or the Kokmen Short Test of Mental Status (STMS) (24). The clinician has to be familiar with the limitations of these tests. Many tests use the learning of three or four words with a relatively short recall interval. The STMS also has the advantage of assessing learning by taking into account the number of trials the subject requires to learn the several words accurately (25).

A bedside test of memory should consist of items screening for verbal and nonverbal materials learned over several trials and recalled after 15 to 30 minutes of delay. Recent research has shown that in addition to problems of acquisition, delayed recall performance may be a sensitive indicator of early impairment. Based on the bedside testing results, the clinician can recommend a detailed neuropsychological evaluation.

The bedside mental status examination should also screen for problems involving attention or language. If the patient's affect is suggestive of significant depression or anxiety, the mental status examination should be augmented by screening for psychiatric symptoms using a psychiatric inventory such as the Hamilton Depression/Anxiety Rating Scale, Beck Depression/Anxiety Inventory, Geriatric Depression Scale, or similar screening instruments.

Investigations

Neuropsychological Testing

A meticulous history and examination may indicate the need for neuropsychological testing standardized for age and education. Neuropsychological testing is essentially an extension of the bedside mental status exam. In assessing memory problems, both verbal and nonverbal functions need to be addressed. For instance, one commonly employed test is the Rey Auditory Verbal Learning Test in which a patient is given five trials to learn 15 unrelated words. The score of each trial is recorded, which later will be used to generate the learning curve of the patient. Following 30 minutes of delay, the subject is asked to recall the learned material, and should be able to recall 50% or more of the material acquired. This test is an attempt to test the patient's ability to encode

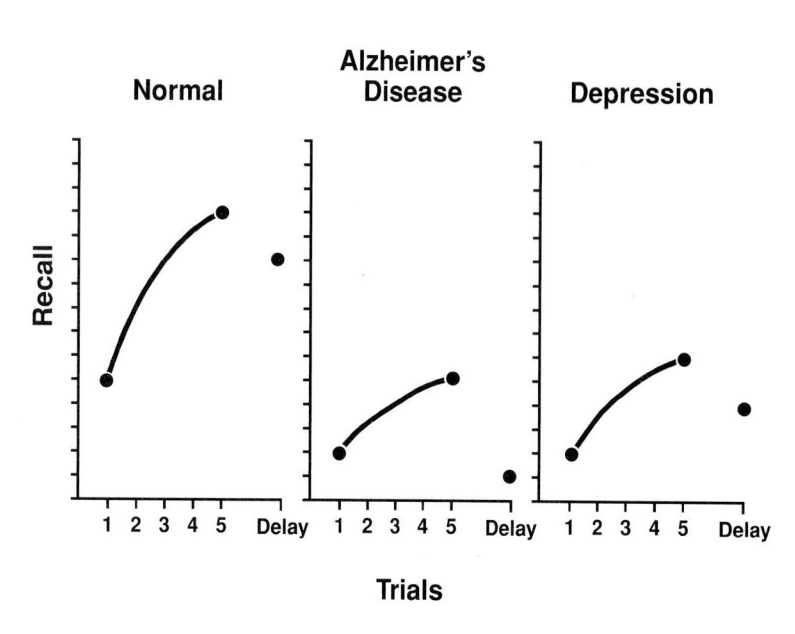

Figure 19-3 Learning curves: normal versus Alzheimer's disease versus depression. (Petersen, 2004. Used with permission.) (11)

learned material and subsequently transfer this from working memory to recent memory. The learning curves generated from such a test have a characteristic pattern. For instance, in patients with AD, the learning curve will be flat (i.e., a curve with a slope approaching zero). In normal individuals, the learning curve will have a positive slope indicating the ability of the individual to learn more with each successive trial. Patients with depression can learn, but show cognitive inefficiency and require more effort than normal individuals. Such a learning curve is somewhat flat, and falls to the right of a normal curve (see Figure 19-3).

In addition to verbal memory, the individual should be tested for retention of nonverbal materials. There are a variety of tests used to assess nonverbal memory. For instance, in the Visual Reproduction subtest of the Wechsler Memory Scale-III, geometric figures are presented and the individual is asked to recall them. Like the verbal memory test, the visual component should be standardized for age and education level in order to make a meaningful interpretation of the results.

As emphasized in the history and examination part of the evaluation, the neuropsychological evaluation should also address nonmemory cognitive domains such as language, attention, and executive function in order to assess their contribution to memory performance.

Neuroimaging

A computed tomography (CT) or MRI scan of the brain should be done in order to visualize the limbic structures in the setting of a memory disorder. An MRI of the brain will be more sensitive in imaging medial temporal lobe structures. A CT of the brain may have a number of artifacts, since the medial temporal lobe structures are located near the calvarium.

In selected cases, one should consider using single positron emission computerized tomography (SPECT) or positron emission tomography (PET) scans. In early stages of the disease, the MRI may not show any gross abnormality, whereas a decreased blood flow pattern on SPECT or decreased glucose utilization on PET could be noted in areas of the brain reported as normal on MRI. Since these tests are expensive, they should be reserved for selected cases. For more information, see the chapter on Neuroimaging in this book.

Electroencephalogram

When a patient presents with episodic memory problems, a seizure disorder should be considered, and EEGs performed while the patient is awake and asleep. Ideally, this study should be done with sleep deprivation. Medial temporal lobe structures such as the amygdala and hippocampus can be prone to seizures; hence, one should look for seizure foci.

Laboratory Tests

The working diagnosis/hypothesis based on history and examination generated by the clinician will guide laboratory tests to be ordered. For instance, if a patient presents with acute-to-subacute cognitive dysfunction and has a history of camping and tick bites, then it is appropriate to screen for Lyme disease. While there are no laboratory tests specific for memory disorders, certain tests that are typically ordered as part of a cognitive impairment workup can be considered in the appropriate clinical context. These include the hematology group; chemistry group; vitamin B12; folate; thyroid function test; sedimentation rate; antinuclear antibody; 24-hour urine for heavy metals; HIV; toxicology screen; and a urine drug-abuse survey that includes alcohol, serum drug screen, paraneoplastic autoantibodies, copper, ceruloplasmin, anticardiolipin antibodies; and arterial blood gas.

Neurological Consultation

The clinician has to decide when to get a neurological consultation based on the clinical and investigation data. For instance, if a patient presents with acute memory loss in the context of risk factors for stroke, a neurological consultation should be considered.

Treatment

It is uncommon to identify a specific etiology for memory disorders. However, if and when identified, a specific treatment should be initiated. For example, if an EEG and clinical examination reveal temporal lobe epilepsy, then the patient should be referred to a neurologist and an appropriate antiepileptic medication should be initiated. Likewise, if depression or anxiety is deemed to be the factor contributing to the cognitive dysfunction presenting with memory complaint, then appropriate treatment such as an antidepressant and/or psychological interventions should be considered.

Treatment of Mild Cognitive Impairment

As the focus of AD research moves toward prevention, numerous clinical trials on MCI are being undertaken (26). According to an evidence-based medicine review, the American Academy of Neurology recommends that MCI is a useful clinical concept worthy of attention. This is because persons with MCI progress to dementia at a rate of 10% to 15% per year, which is in contrast to the normal elderly cohort that convert at 1% to 2% per year (27). Clinical trials involving MCI patients are promising because they are likely to give important information in the detection and intervention of the disease while it is still in a transitional clinical stage. Clinical trials currently underway or recently completed are outlined in Table 19-2. The therapeutic agents being tested are similar to those under consideration for the treatment of Alzheimer's disease, namely: cholinesterase inhibitors, antioxidants, anti-inflammatories, nootropics, and glutamate-receptor modulators.

In their recent reviews, Geda and Petersen (28–30) discussed several clinical trials on MCI including one conducted by the Alzheimer's Disease Cooperative Study (ADCS). The ADCS trial was a randomized, double-blind, placebo-controlled study involving three arms to assess the safety and efficacy of high-dose vitamin E (2000 IU per day) and donepezil (10 mg per day) (29). One of the objectives was to decrease the conversion rate of MCI to AD, from the anticipated 45% down to 30% over the course of 3 years. Seven hundred sixty nine subjects were randomized in the trial, and the annual conversion rate from MCI to AD was approximately 16% per year for all groups combined. Over the course of the study, donepezil reduced the risk of progressing to AD for the first 12 months of the trial, and then the groups came together, indicating no more benefit of donepezil after the first year. Vitamin E had no therapeutic effect. The secondary cognitive measures paralleled the overall group progression rates, with significant differences in memory, language, and an overall cognitive composite measure for the first 12 to 18 months. No unexpected adverse events were observed. This was the first therapeutic trial to demonstrate an ability to delay the clinical diagnosis of AD.

Salloway et al. have also completed a study in which they evaluated the efficacy and safety of the acetylcholinesterase inhibitor donepezil in treating patients with MCI (31). A total of 270 patients with MCI were enrolled in a 24-week, multicenter, randomized, double-blind, placebo-controlled study. The subjects were randomized to receive donepezil (n = 133; 5 mg/day for 42 days, followed by forced dose-escalation to 10 mg/day) or placebo (n = 137). Primary efficacy measures were delayed recall on the New York University and the ADCS Clinician's Global Impression of Change for MCI (ADCS CGIC-MCI). Secondary efficacy measures included the modified Alzheimer's Disease Assessment Scale-Cognitive subscale (ADAS-Cog), the Patient Global Assessment (PGA), as well as additional neuropsychologic measures. Results revealed that although significant treatment effects were not seen in the primary efficacy measures, some secondary measures showed effects favoring donepezil: more donepezil-treated patients showed improvements in ADAS-Cog total scores, in tests of attention and psychomotor speed, and in PGA

TABLE 19-2
CLINICAL TRIALS IN MILD COGNITIVE IMPAIRMENT

Sponsor	Duration	Endpoint	Treatment
ADCS[a]	3 yr	AD	Vitamin E, donepezil
Merck	2–3 yr	AD	Rofecoxib[b]
Novartis	3 yr	AD	Rivastigmine
Janssen	2 yr	Symptoms	Galantamine
Pfizer	6 mo	Symptoms	Donepezil
UCB	1 yr	Symptoms	Piracetam

[a]Alzheimer's Disease Cooperative Study supported by National Institute on Aging, Pfizer, Eisai, and DSM Nutritional Products.
[b] Rofecoxib withdrawn by Merck in 2005.
AD, Alzheimer's disease; ADCS, Alzheimer's Disease Cooperative Study; UCB, proper name of company.

scores. More donepezil-treated patients than placebo-treated patients experienced adverse events, most of which were mild-to-moderate and transient.

The medications currently available for treating memory problems have been developed in the context of AD; as such, there are no specific guidelines for using these medications in MCI. Nonetheless, it is prudent for a clinician working with MCI subjects to be familiar with these treatment options. Most of these medications are cholinomimetics (reversible inhibitors of the acetylcholinesterase enzyme), and were developed based on the rationale that the cholinergic system is involved in learning and has anatomic connections within the limbic system. The first FDA-approved cholinomimetic agent was tacrine (32). It is now rarely used because of its hepatotoxic side effect profile. Currently, there are three FDA-approved cholinomimetics: donepezil, rivastigmine and galantamine (33–35). These medications are not curative but they have been shown to minimize morbidity in AD by improving cognitive functions such as memory, language, and praxis. Recent evidence also suggests that such medications are effective in managing neuropsychiatric and behavioral symptoms in AD patients (36). Side effects of cholinomimetics can be understood by recalling the functions of the cholinergic system. Through their primary action of increased cholinergic activity, these medications can lead to bradycardia, increased gastric acid and pulmonary secretions, and increased gastrointestinal motility. Further considerations pertain to drug-drug interactions; for example, cholinomimetics are known to interact with anesthetics. The US Food and Drug Administration approved memantine, an N-methyl-D-aspartate (NMDA) receptor antagonist to be used in patients with moderate-to-severe dementia. The clinical trials were conducted based on the rationale that glutamate contributes to neurodegenerative disorders by overstimulating the NMDA receptor (37,38).

Apart from the above agents, other medications targeting the monoaminergic system have been considered for symptomatic treatment of cognitive impairment such as seratonin-specific re-uptake inhibitors, adrenergic agents, peptides and nootropics (39). Another group that has attracted research interest is the antioxidants. At least one randomized, placebo-controlled, double-blind, multi-center trial indicates that vitamin E may delay the progression of moderate-to-severe AD (40); but, the research is still underway to determine its efficacy in MCI. A recent meta-analysis indicated that high-dose vitamin E may increase all-cause mortality, and that high-dose vitamin E should be avoided (41).

Thus, while there are several clinical trials being conducted globally, currently there are no pharmacological interventions demonstrated to be efficacious in MCI. As such, one important task of the clinician is to carefully and thoughtfully counsel these patients with regard to the nature of the disease and its progression. This information can be important for both the patient and the caregiver, particularly in planning for the future.

SUMMARY

It is quite common to hear patients and family members complaining of memory problems. However, it is the astute clinician's duty to determine if this indeed constitutes a memory disorder or is due to another condition (such as anomia or another language problem, the so-called worried well, depression, or some other cognitive impairment). Once the clinician has determined that it is a memory problem, appropriate investigations have to be done in order to classify the type of memory problem and look for any underlying etiology.

A memory disorder implies involvement of temporolimbic structures. One prototype memory disorder is amnestic MCI. In this disorder, a patient shows significant departure from baseline including marked forgetfulness for recent events and future engagements, which begins insidiously and progresses gradually. The diagnosis is further corroborated with neuropsychological testing. An MRI typically shows hippocampal atrophy with no significant atrophy of the other parts of the brain. Various clinical trials are underway to develop a medication that is efficacious to treat memory disorders such as amnestic MCI.

ACKNOWLEDGMENTS

We would like to thank Dorla Burton for her superb secretarial assistance. Preparation of this chapter was supported by the following National Institutes of Health grants: KO1MH 68351, UO1AG06786, P50AG16574, and U01AG10483.

REFERENCES

1. Scoville WB, Milner B. Loss of recent memory after bilateral hippocampal lesions. *J Neurol Neurosurg Psychiatry.* 1957;20:11–21.
2. Milner B, Corkin S, Teuber HL. Further analysis of the hippocampal amnesic syndrome: a 14-year follow-up study of H.M. *Neuropsychologia.* 1968;6:215–234.
3. Victor M, Yakovlev P. SS Korsakoff's psychic disorder in conjunction with peripheral neuritis: A translation of Korsakoff's original article. *Neurology.* 1995;5:394–406.
4. Mesulam MM. From sensation to cognition. *Brain.* 1998;121:1013–1052.
5. Mesulam MM. *Principles of Behavioral and Cognitive Neurology.* 2nd Ed. New York: Oxford University Press; 2000.
6. Brookmeyer R, Gray S, Kawas C. Projections of Alzheimer's disease in the United States and the public health impact of delaying disease onset. *Am J Public Health.* 1998;88:1337–1342.
7. Petersen RC, Smith GE, Waring SC, Ivnik RJ, Tangalos EG, Kokmen E. Mild cognitive impairment: clinical characterization and outcome [published erratum appears in Arch Neurol 1999; 56:760]. *Arch Neurol.* 1999;56:303–308.
8. Jack Jr. C, Petersen R, Xu Y, et al. Prediction of AD with MRI-based hippocampal volume in mild cognitive impairment. *Neurology.* 1999;52:1397–1403.

9. Kantarci K, Jack CR, Jr., Xu YC, et al. Regional metabolic patterns in mild cognitive impairment and Alzheimer's disease: a 1H MRS study. *Neurology.* 2000;55:210–217.

10. Petersen R, Doody R, Kurz A, et al. Current concepts in mild cognitive impairment. *Arch Neurol.* 2001;58:1985–1992.

11. Petersen RC. Mild cognitive impairment. *Continuum.* 2004;10: 9–28.

12. Petersen RC. Conceptual Overview. In: Petersen RC, ed. *Mild Cognitive Impairment: Aging to Alzheimer's Disease.* New York: Oxford University Press, Inc.; 2003:1–14.

13. Petersen RC. Mild cognitive impairment as a diagnostic entity. *J Intern Med.* 2004;256(3):183–194.

14. Petersen RC, Ivnik RJ, Boeve BF, Knopman DS, Smith GE, Tangalos EG. Outcome of clinical subtypes of mild cognitive impairment. *Neurology.* 2004;62(Suppl 5), A295.

15. Boeve BF, Ferman TJ, Smith GE, et al. Mild cognitive impairment preceding dementia with Lewy bodies. *Neurology.* 2004;62(Suppl 5), A86.

16. Petersen RC. *Mild Cognitive Impairment: Aging to Alzheimer's Disease.* New York: Oxford University Press; 2003:269.

17. Reisberg B, Ferris SH, de Leon MJ, et al. Stage-specific behavioral, cognitive, and in vivo changes in community residing subjects with age-associated memory impairment and primary degenerative dementia of the Alzheimer's type. *Drug Development Research.* 1988;15:101–114.

18. Kral V. Senescent forgetfulness: benign and malignant. *CMAJ.* 1962;86:257–260.

19. Crook T, Bartus R, Ferris S, Whitehouse P, Cohen G, Gershon S. Age-associated memory impairment: proposed diagnostic criteria and measures of clinical change-report of a National Institute of Mental Health Work Group. *Dev Neuropsychol.* 1986;2:261–276.

20. Smith G, Ivnik RJ, Petersen RC, et al. Age-associated memory impairment diagnoses: problems of reliability and concerns for terminology. *Psychol Aging.* 1991;6:551–558.

21. LaRue A, Spar J, Hill C. Cognitive impairment in late-life depression: clinical correlates and treatment implications. *J Affect Disord.* 1986;11:179–184.

22. Levy R. Aging-associated cognitive decline. *Int Psychogeriatr.* 1994;6:63–68.

23. American Psychiatric Association. *Diagnostic and Statistical Manual of Mental Disorders.* 4th ed. Text Revision (DSM-IV-TR). Washington, DC: American Psychiatric Association; 2000.

24. Kokmen E, Naessens J, Offord K. A short test of mental status: description and preliminary results. *Mayo Clin Proc* 1987;62: 281–288.

25. Tang-Wai DF, Knopman DS, Geda YE, et al. Comparison of the short test of mental status and the mini-mental state examination in mild cognitive impairment. *Arch Neurol.* 2003;60: 1777–1781.

26. Petersen RC. Mild cognitive impairment clinical trials. *Nat Rev.* 2003;2:646–653.

27. Petersen RC, Stevens JC, Ganguli M, Tangalos EG, Cummings JL, DeKosky ST. Practice parameter: early detection of dementia: mild cognitive impairment (an evidence-based review). Report of the Quality Standards Subcommittee of the American Academy of Neurology. [see comments]. *Neurology.* 2001;56:1133–1142.

28. Petersen RC. Mild cognitive impairment clinical trials. *Nat Rev Drug Discov.* 2003;2:646–653.

29. Geda YE, Petersen RC. Clinical trials in mild cognitive impairment. In: Cummings J, ed. *Alzheimer's Disease and Related Disorders.* 2nd Ed. London: Martin Dunitz; 2001.

30. Grundman M, Petersen RC, Ferris SH, et al. Mild cognitive impairment can be distinguished from Alzheimer disease and normal aging for clinical trials. *Arch Neurol.* 2004;61:59–66.

31. Salloway S, Ferris S, Kluger A, et al. Efficacy of donepezil in mild cognitive impairment: a randomized placebo-controlled trial. *Neurology.* 2004;63(4):651–657.

32. Knapp MJ, Knopman DS, Solomon PR, Pendlebury WW, Davis CS, Gracon SI. A 30-week randomized controlled trial of high-dose tacrine in patients with Alzheimer's disease. The Tacrine Study Group. [see comment]. *JAMA.* 1994;271:985–991.

33. Rogers SL, Farlow MR, Doody RS, Mohs R, Friedhoff LT. A 24-week, double-blind, placebo-controlled trial of donepezil in patients with Alzheimer's disease. Donepezil Study Group. [see comment]. *Neurology.* 1998;50:136–145.

34. Rosler M, Anand R, Cicin-Sain A, et al. Efficacy and safety of rivastigmine in patients with Alzheimer's disease: international randomised controlled trial. [see comment] [comment] [erratum appears in BMJ 2001;322(7300):1456]. *BMJ.* 1999;318: 633–638.

35. Wilcock GK, Lilienfeld S, Gaens E. Efficacy and safety of galantamine in patients with mild to moderate Alzheimer's disease: multicentre randomised controlled trial. Galantamine International-1 Study Group. *BMJ.* 2000;321:1445–1449.

36. Cummings JL, Schneider L, Tariot PN, Kershaw PR, Yuan W. Reduction of behavioral disturbances and caregiver distress by galantamine in patients with Alzheimer's disease. *Am J Psychiatry.* 2004;161(3):532–538.

37. Reisberg B, Doody R, Stoffler A, et al. Memantine in moderate-to-severe Alzheimer's disease. [see comment]. *N Engl J Med.* 2003; 348:1333–1341.

38. Tariot PN, Farlow MR, Grossberg GT, et al. Memantine treatment in patients with moderate to severe Alzheimer disease already receiving donepezil: a randomized controlled trial. [see comment]. *JAMA.* 2004;291:317–324.

39. Lockhart BP, Lestage PJ. Cognition enhancing or neuroprotective compounds for the treatment of cognitive disorders: why? when? which? *Exp Gerontol.* 2003;38:119–128.

40. Sano M, Erensto C, Thomas RG, et al. A controlled trial of selegiline, alpha-tocopherol, or both as treatment for Alzheimer's disease. The Alzheimer's Disease Cooperative Study. *N Engl J Med.* 1997;336:1216–1222.

41. Miller ER 3rd, Pastor-Barriuso R, Dalal D, Riemersma RA, Appel LJ, Guallar E. Meta-analysis: high-dosage vitamin E supplementation may increase all-cause mortality. *Ann Intern Med.* 2005;142:37–46.

Alzheimer's Disease

20

David Knopman

The syndrome of dementia is defined as a subacute or insidious decline in cognition from a previously higher level, in which the cognitive and behavioral deficits interfere *significantly* with daily function and independence (1). Alzheimer's disease (AD) is the most common cause of dementia in the elderly. The term *Alzheimer's disease* is used in several senses. Sometimes it is used, incorrectly, as a shorthand for all dementias in the elderly. AD is sometimes used to describe a clinical syndrome of dementia in which anterograde amnesia (short-term memory deficits) is prominent. AD is also used as the name of the pathological condition in which neuritic plaques (NPs) and neurofibrillary tangles (NFTs) occur in the brain. AD can be diagnosed clinically with confidence in a patient with the gradual and progressive impairment of recent memory and dysfunction in at least one other cognitive or behavioral domain (see Table 20-1) (2). The DSM-IV-TR definition is similar (1).

PHENOMENOLOGY OF ALZHEIMER'S DISEASE

Disturbances in recent memory function are at the heart of the typical symptoms that lead to the suspicion and eventual diagnosis of AD. Patients repeat themselves in conversation, re-ask the same question, or forget recent conversations. The symptoms may be so insidious in onset that they may be ignored or misinterpreted by family caregivers or physicians as insignificant, normal aging, or depression. Patients with AD usually ignore their own shortcomings and deny or minimize their deficits (3,4). Symptoms are typically present for 1 to 3 years before family members bring the patient to medical attention. Loss of the ability to carry out key daily tasks such as shopping, handling money, or doing chores around the house may be more powerful triggers than forgetfulness for seeking medical attention. Neuropsychiatric symptoms also are more likely to prompt an evaluation than forgetfulness itself.

Cognitive Deficits in Alzheimer's Disease

A deficit in memory is the hallmark of the cognitive disorder in AD. More precisely, it is a deficit in new learning and encoding of information (5). While the ability to retrieve information from long-term memory is eventually impaired in AD, the important diagnostic feature is the deficit in new learning. It is sometimes referred to as a deficit in short-term memory. Operationally, recall of information after a 5-minute delay is the measure of new learning in AD patients. Orientation for time and place is impaired in patients with AD, at least in part a result of memory impairment.

Difficulties with word-finding and name-finding are frequently seen in AD. Observational studies show that dementia patients exhibit deficits in naming and word fluency at mild stages of disease (6).

Disturbances of visuospatial synthesis are well-recognized symptoms in some AD patients (7,8). Some of these patients with prominent disturbances of visual synthesis often have relatively preserved memory function and relatively preserved insight, and still prove to have AD pathologically. The terms *posterior cortical syndrome* or *visual variant of AD* have been applied to this variant of AD (9).

Impairment of executive functions and attention may be demonstrable neuropsychologically in early AD (10,11), and the consequences of deficits in problem-solving, judgment, foresight, and mental agility lead to loss of competence in daily living (12). Sometimes, impaired judgment, social misbehavior, and other manifestations of a frontotemporal dementia may be as prominent as the memory disorder (13).

The spectrum of changes in behavior and affect in AD are protean, ranging from increased apathy and social withdrawal to disinhibition or irritability (14,15).

TABLE 20-1
CRITERIA FOR THE CLINICAL DIAGNOSIS OF ALZHEIMER'S DISEASE

1. Based on evidence from the history and mental status examination, a disorder characterized by the presence of major impairment of learning and retaining new information, *and* at least one other of the following:
   - Impairment in handling complex tasks;
   - Impairment in reasoning ability;
   - Impaired spatial ability and orientation;
   - Impaired language.
2. The disturbances in #1 significantly interfere with work or usual social activities or relationships with others
3. The disturbances in #1 represent a significant decline from a previous level of functioning
4. The disturbances in #1 are of insidious onset and are progressive, based on evidence from the history or serial mental status examinations.
5. Not occurring exclusively during the course of delirium.
6. The disturbance is not better accounted for by a major psychiatric diagnosis.
7. The disturbance is not better accounted for by a systemic disease or another brain disease.

Adapted from the NINCDS-ADRDA and DSM-IV-TR criteria (1, 2).

EPIDEMIOLOGY OF ALZHEIMER'S DISEASE

Prevalence

The prevalence of dementia and AD increases with advancing age. In 65-to-69 year olds the prevalence of dementia is approximately one per 100 individuals. With each subsequent 5-year increment, the prevalence of dementia and AD doubles (16). Over age 85 years, estimates of the prevalence of dementia vary between 20% to nearly 50%. Beyond age 85, it appears that dementia prevalence continues to rise. Some earlier studies found a decrease above this age, but most recent studies have confirmed that the proportion of individuals with dementia continues to rise over this age.

Incidence

The incidence of dementia, that is, the number of newly diagnosed cases in a certain time interval, also rises dramatically with advancing age (see Figure 20-1) (17,18). Because patients diagnosed with dementia tend to live for several years to as long as a decade or more, incidence rates are considerably lower than prevalence rates.

Conditions that are Associated with Increased Risk

The two most important risk factors for AD are advancing age and a family history of dementia. Several others that are not as potent will be described.

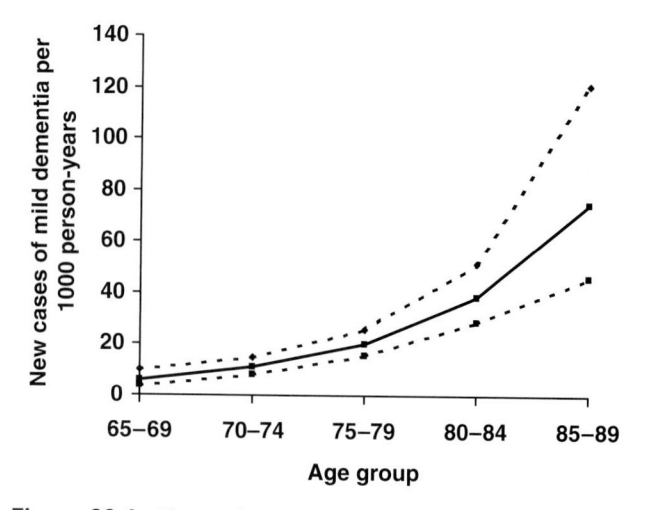

Figure 20-1 The incidence of Alzheimer's disease as a function of age. (Adapted from reference 18.)

Very low educational achievement (less than eighth-grade education) has been a consistently observed but modestly potent risk factor that increases a person's odds of developing AD by two to three fold (19). There may be a threshold effect for education so that beyond an eighth-grade education level, the association is minimal. Even when diagnostic methods are specifically modified to reduce educational or cultural biases, the education effect remains (19).

In a study of a teaching order of Catholic sisters (the "Nun Study"), cognitive performance at age 20 years was predictive of the subsequent development of dementia due to AD roughly 50 years later (20). A study that compared intelligence testing obtained at approximately age 11 years to the subsequent development of dementia also found a relationship between low childhood scores and late-life dementia (21).

The link between educational attainment and risk of late-life dementia is only speculative at this point. One hypothesis is that early life experiences contribute to the development of brain reserve (20). Increased numbers of neurons presumably act as a buffer in ameliorating the deleterious effects of AD pathology. In general, enriched childhood environments will be associated with higher educational attainment, but in addition, it is the sum of all enriching experiences, not the least of which is good childhood nutrition, that protects from the subsequent development of dementia.

From a practical perspective, the association of low education and AD is of little importance to clinicians, because AD strikes individuals of all educational and occupational backgrounds.

Cardiovascular disease confers a small-to-moderate increased risk for AD (22,23). The cardiovascular risk factors associated with AD include atherosclerosis broadly defined, history of stroke, history of midlife hypertension and carotid artery disease.

Elevated homocysteine appears is associated with AD (24). The most compelling study to date measured homocysteine levels in initially nondemented individuals (24). Those individuals who subsequently became demented had higher levels of homocysteine at the baseline measurement. At this point in time, measurement of homocysteine levels is not part of the assessment of AD patients.

The relationship between head injury and AD has been the subject of serious concerns about recall bias among caregivers of diagnosed dementia patients. Because the putative head injury could have occurred 30 years prior to the development of dementia, prospective studies that allow minimization of recall bias have not yet been done. However, because of the link between boxing and AD (25,26), the importance of nonsport related head trauma to AD seems plausible. Mayeux and colleagues have proposed that the risk of head trauma for AD is mediated by the apolipoprotein-epsilon 4 (APOE e4) genotype (27).

Occupational exposure to industrial solvents and agricultural chemicals has not shown consistent increases in risk for AD. The evidence against aluminum as a risk factor for AD (28–31) outweighs suggestions of a possible role for aluminum (32,33). Recent neuropathological studies find no difference between AD and control brains in aluminum content, especially when exquisite attention is paid to analytic techniques (31,34). In case-controlled studies comparing regions with high versus low aluminum levels in drinking water, the risk for AD in the high aluminum region was only trivially increased (30,35,36), except for one study (37).

Protective Factors

Several protective factors have been observed in incidence cohorts. One is estrogen replacement therapy (ERT) (38,39). The ERT story has been thrown into turmoil with the publication of the Women's Health Initiative memory study in which estrogen plus progesterone not only failed to reduce the incidence of dementia, but actually increased it slightly (40). While most of the epidemiological studies examined estrogen alone, the Women's Health Initiative study used estrogen plus progesterone. At this point, the data do not support the use of ERT as a treatment in symptomatic AD patients nor as a prevention strategy in elderly women.

The use of nonsteroidal anti-inflammatory agents (NSAIDs) has also been described (41,42). As with estrogen, clinical trials of NSAIDs in AD patients have not shown benefits (43), but no prevention studies have yet been completed. Moreover, it may be that only some NSAIDs offer protection and not others (44). NSAIDs should not be used as a treatment for symptomatic AD.

The use of statin-type cholesterol lowering drugs has been added to the list of putative protective factors (45–47). However, associations from epidemiological data are not proof of clinical causality, and more research is indicated in this area. Both dietary and supplemental sources of antioxidants have been questioned as protective factors for AD, but the evidence is contradictory, with some positive (48–50), and others negative (51,52).

Cigarette smoking has appeared in the majority of studies as a protective factor for AD (53), although in other studies it has been a risk factor (54–56). Intuitively, it would appear more likely to be a risk factor because of its association with vascular disease. However, the putative mechanism by which smoking could be protective is via stimulation of nicotinic receptors in the brain (57).

ASSESSMENT AND DIAGNOSIS

Conceptually, the differential diagnosis of AD is a two-stage process (see Figure 20-2). The first stage concerns the determination of whether dementia is present. The second stage concerns the differential diagnosis of dementia. AD is a diagnosis of inclusion, but as with any condition, certain diseases that mimic AD should be ruled out. These include drug intoxications, brain structural lesions, major systemic metabolic disturbances, central nervous system infections, vascular dementia, dementia with Lewy Bodies, and frontotemporal lobar degenerations.

The cognitive and functional changes that occur with dementia must be distinguished from a number of other syndromes. The diagnosis of dementia is a clinician's judgment: no laboratory test can make the determination. Ordinary forgetfulness, anxiety disorders, depression, psychotic disorders, aphasia, and severe sensory deprivations could all produce symptoms and signs that could mimic some aspects of dementia. What distinguishes dementia from all of these are the impairments in cognitive functioning in more than one domain in the absence of severe or pervasive disturbances of affect, attention, hearing loss, or visual loss—that themselves could conceivably account for the functional and cognitive deficits. In most instances, these distinctions are relatively easy to make. Because depression, anxiety, thought disturbances, and aphasia can all accompany a dementing illness, the diagnosis of dementia in the presence of major mood disorders or major sensory impairments can be challenging.

Normal aging plays a large role in the differential diagnosis of dementia. Once someone passes into their 70s, accommodation of memory loss is a part of our culture. Consequently, patients, family, and physicians are all too willing to dismiss initial instances of memory loss to aging. Critical analysis of the neuropsychology of normal aging reveals that decreases in rote memory for unrelated words or random digits occur with aging, as well as slowing of many motor and cognitive functions. Needing to ask to have a phone number repeated or forgetting the name of an infrequently encountered acquaintance might be compatible with normal aging, but getting lost in familiar territory or asking the same question repeatedly is not.

Once dementia is established, the differential diagnosis in the elderly involves a small set of commonly observed

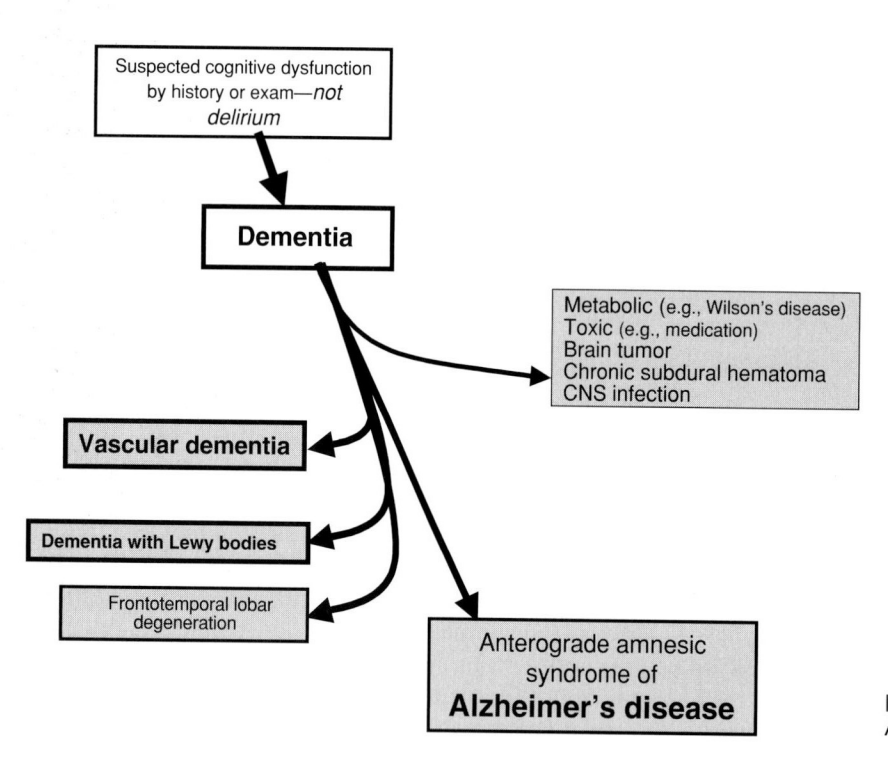

Figure 20-2 The diagnostic approach to Alzheimer's disease.

conditions. There is a much larger set of very uncommon conditions that also enters the differential diagnosis. As AD is the focus of this chapter, we will confine the discussion to the context of the differential diagnosis in late-middle age and in the elderly. AD is the most common of the dementias (58–62), accounting for 50% to 80% in population-based surveys. Vascular dementia and dementia with Lewy bodies are next most common, each approximately one-fifth to one-third as common as AD. The frontotemporal lobar degenerations are considerably less common than AD. Brain diseases associated with potentially surgically remediable conditions such as brain tumors, subdural hematomas, and normal pressure hydrocephalus that present as a dementia that could mimic AD are exceedingly rare. Similarly, central nervous system infections that could mimic AD are exceedingly rare. Systemic metabolic or endocrinologic disorders that produce dementia are also very uncommon.

Many clinical-pathological studies have addressed the diagnostic accuracy of the clinical diagnosis of AD (63–65). The mean sensitivity of the diagnosis of probable AD in these studies was 81% with a range of 49% to 100%. The mean specificity of the diagnosis of probable AD was 70% with a range of 47% to 100% (66). In most instances in routine clinical practice, the diagnostic criteria of the NINCDS-ADRDA Workgroup yield an accurate view of the diagnosis of AD (66). AD is a diagnosis that can be made confidently in most instances. Analysis of diagnostic errors shows that a broad view of the clinical diagnosis of AD will result in a high sensitivity for AD pathology, but at a cost of overinclusiveness and loss of specificity. Difficulties in the diagnosis of non-AD pathologies are beyond the scope of

this chapter, but cases of vascular dementia, Lewy Body disease, frontotemporal lobar degeneration, hippocampal sclerosis, and progressive supranuclear palsy may look very much like AD clinically. See the appropriate chapters in this book for additional information.

Laboratory Evaluations in Suspected Alzheimer's Disease

The American Academy of Neurology guidelines for the laboratory evaluation of dementia include a complete blood count, electrolytes, calcium, blood urea nitrogen, thyroid function tests, and a vitamin B12 level (66,67). Structural neuroimaging is recommended as part of the initial evaluation of a dementia patient. Some procedures should be reserved for specific clinical circumstances (see Table 20-2). The diagnostic yield of pertinent conditions from laboratory evaluations in suspected dementia is low (68).

The diagnosis of AD specifically cannot be verified with a laboratory test at present. A biomarker for AD is desperately needed, but the challenges of proving the value of a biomarker are huge. Several approaches have been advocated.

Structural neuroimaging with magnetic resonance imaging (MRI) is of potential use in the diagnosis of AD. Hippocampal atrophy is increased substantially in AD (69), but there is overlap with nonimpaired elderly. Serial measurements of brain volume on neuroimaging may differentiate normal elderly from those with AD (70). The high degree of technical precision needed to carry out such measurements may not be practical in the routine clinical diagnosis of AD. MRI can detect small infarctions that may

TABLE 20-2
DIAGNOSTIC TESTING IN PATIENTS WITH SUSPECTED ALZHEIMER'S DISEASE

Procedure or Test	Rationale
Neurological history	Cornerstone of diagnosis
Mental status examination	Cornerstone of diagnosis
Neurological examination	Provides evidence for parkinsonism, cerebrovascular disease, or other neurological diseases (e.g., a vertical gaze palsy, chorea, motor neuron disease)
Brain imaging study	MRI preferred, CT acceptable to exclude brain tumors, subdural hematomas, other structural lesions; also to detect covert cerebral infarcts and focal cerebral atrophy such as seen in frontotemporal lobar degenerations
Blood tests: complete blood count, electrolytes, serum calcium, blood urea nitrogen, glucose, vitamin B12, thyroid function	Screen for common medical disorders
Electroencephalography	Not routinely indicated when AD is suspected. Reserve for instances when Creutzfeldt-Jakob disease or seizures are serious considerations
Positron emission tomography or single photon emission tomography	Not routinely indicated when AD is suspected. Reserve for instances when frontotemporal lobar degenerations are serious considerations
Apolipoprotein E genotype	Not routinely indicated when AD is suspected
Lumbar puncture	Not routinely indicated when AD is suspected. Reserve for instances where CNS infections are serious considerations

AD, Alzheimer's disease; CNS, central nervous system; CT, computed tomography; MRI, magnetic resonance imaging.

have been clinically silent (71). It is not clear whether identification of small infarctions has diagnostic value for estimating the burden of vascular pathology relevant to dementia. Although an evidence-based approach cannot justify MRI in all suspected dementia patients, the combination of a visualization of the hippocampal formations with a coronal imaging sequence and the potential to detect small infarctions makes MRI more useful than computed tomography in many instances.

Functional neuroimaging with single positron emission computerized tomography (SPECT) or positron emission tomography (PET) also has promise (72,73). Decreased perfusion of parietal and temporal lobes is thought to be a relatively sensitive and specific marker for AD, but how useful it is in differentiating dementia with Lewy bodies, or vascular dementia from pure AD has not yet been established. In most instances, functional imaging will not be necessary, as the clinical diagnosis coupled with observations from MRI will be more than sufficient to achieve a confident diagnosis. In differentiating AD from frontotemporal dementia, SPECT or PET may offer unique information.

Cerebrospinal fluid markers lack diagnostic precision at present, but there may be instances where abnormalities that appear specific for AD such as depressed levels of amyloid-β-42 (Abeta-42) and increased levels of tau protein (74,75), or the neural thread protein (76), will increase diagnostic certainty slightly. Routine use of assays of cerebrospinal fluid markers cannot be recommended at present, but there might be unique circumstances where they could provide diagnostic assistance.

Genotyping of the APOE gene to confirm or refute the diagnosis of AD generally does not increase certainty over the clinical diagnosis. APOE exhibits three allelic variations in humans. In AD patients, there is a disproportionate representation of the epsilon-4 (e4) allele compared to nondemented populations (77,78). The addition of APOE testing increases diagnostic accuracy for a diagnosis of AD by about 4% if an APOE e4 allele is present (from 90% to 94%), and by 8% for a diagnosis of not-AD if an APOE e4 is absent (from 64% to 72%) (79). The absence of an APOE e4 allele increased specificity from 55% to 70.6% compared to the clinical diagnosis. For some patients, families, and physicians, this increase in diagnostic certainty may be desirable, whereas in most instances it will be unnecessary. APOE testing also raises a number of other management issues such as genetic counseling that may complicate, rather than complement, the initial diagnostic approach (80).

ETIOLOGY OF ALZHEIMER'S DISEASE

Genetics

Family history of dementia is an important risk factor for the subsequent development of AD (81,82). A large multicenter study that involved nearly 1,700 patients found that the lifetime risk to first-degree relatives of clinically diagnosed AD patients was approximately 15% by age 80 years and 39% by age 96 years (81). Other studies have suggested that risk of AD conferred by positive family history decreases with advancing age, so that by age 85 years, family

TABLE 20-3		
GENES IMPLICATED IN ALZHEIMER'S DISEASE		
Protein	**Chromosome**	**Inheritance Pattern**
Alzheimer precursor protein	21	Autosomal dominant
Presenilin I	14	Autosomal dominant
Presenilin II	1	Autosomal dominant
Apolipoprotein E	19	Risk factor
Unknown	10	Risk factor

history of AD ceases to be a risk factor (83). In addition, bearing a child with Down's syndrome is associated with an increased risk for AD in the mothers if they were under age 35 at the birth of the Down's syndrome child (84).

Twin studies have shown an increased rate of AD in monozygotic twins compared to dizygotic twins (85). In a Finnish study, concordance rates were 31.3% and 9.3% respectively for MZ and DZ twins.

There are two patterns of genetic risk for AD (see Table 20-3). One is through autosomal dominant transmission of mutations in one of three genes. The other pattern of genetic risk for AD is mediated by susceptibility genes, of which only one, the APOE gene, has been identified with certainty.

About 30% to 40% of early-onset AD has been shown to be due to mutations in either the Alzheimer precursor protein (also called amyloid precursor protein-APP) located on chromosome 21, the presenilin-1 (PS1) gene located on chromosome 14, and its homologue presenilin-2 (PS2) located on chromosome 1 (86,87). Only a few hundred families have been identified worldwide with mutations in one of these three genes.

The families with mutations in these genes have shown considerable consistency. The age of onset of affected individuals is in the 30-to-50-year range, with only some of the PS1 families showing a slightly later age of onset (88). The clinical features of the dementia are generally indistinguishable from sporadic AD (89). Neuropathologically, the PS1, PS2, and APP genetic forms of AD appear similar by neuropathological analysis except that the genetic forms of AD show greater severity (90). All of the genetic forms of AD also result in overproduction of the Abeta peptide (91).

The families with APP mutations were the first to be identified (92). Five mutations have been observed in APP (93). The link between AD and Down's syndrome anticipated the finding of the APP gene on chromosome 21. The extra dose of a chromosome 21 with the APP gene appears to accelerate the neuropathology of AD in Down's syndrome patients, such that they demonstrate the pathology of AD roughly 30 years earlier than individuals with a normal number of chromosome 21's (94).

The PS1 gene mutations were the next to be linked to autosomal dominant AD (95). A large number of muta-

tions have been found (93). PS1 is the most common gene involved in autosomal dominant AD.

PS2 mutations were first identified in one ethnic group, those of German descent who had emigrated to the western United States and Canada after residing in the Volga region of Russia in the 18th to 19th centuries (96). The PS2 gene is approximately 70% homologous to the PS1 gene. PS2 mutations are much less common than ones in PS1.

Late-Onset Familial Alzheimer's Disease

Late-onset familial Alzheimer's disease refers to the type of disorder seen in individuals over age 65 or 70 years (there is no precise dividing point) who have positive family histories of dementia. The genetic risk of late-onset AD decreases with advancing age in some studies (82,83). Late-onset familial AD is mediated through susceptibility genes. APOE was the first of these genes to be identified. APOE is a lipid-carrying protein present in serum and tissues (97). In humans it is found in three allelic variations that differ from one another by two amino acid substitutions at positions 112 and 158. In Caucasian populations, the e3 allele is most common while the other two variations e2 and e4 are less common (98). In other ethnic groups, such as those of African descent, more individuals possess the e4 allele than in individuals of European descent (99). The APOE e4 allele had been known for some time to be associated with cardiovascular disease when Roses, Poirier, and their colleagues independently showed that the e4 allele was substantially over-represented among AD patients (77,78). The homozygous state carries the most risk, mainly between the ages of 60 and 80 (99). The heterozygous state is associated with a lower risk, expressed in that same age range. Beyond these ages, the risk of AD associated with APOE e4 declines. That the APOE e4 allele is a risk factor and not a typical autosomal dominant disease-causing gene is illustrated by the roughly 50% cumulative incidence of AD in APOE e4 homozygotes in population studies (100–102). The role of APOE in the pathogenesis of AD will be considered in the section on pathogenesis. Its role in diagnosis has already been discussed.

Linkage to a gene or genes on chromosome 10 has been observed as a risk factor for late-onset AD (103). Prospects for the discovery of the specific gene on chromosome 10 are good, but the process is arduous.

PATHOPHYSIOLOGY OF ALZHEIMER'S DISEASE

Gross Pathology

The brain of a patient dying with AD usually shows gross atrophy, particularly of the posterior half of the brain. However, the degree of atrophy is not correlated with dementia severity. Brain weight is almost invariably reduced, roughly 20% on average (104). The cerebellum and brainstem are typically unremarkable.

On coronal sections, the naked eye can easily appreciate atrophy involving the cerebral cortex surrounding the sylvian fissure, as well as the hippocampal formations. The ventricular system is diffusely enlarged, but most notably posteriorly and in the temporal lobes (105).

Microscopic Pathology

There are several microscopic findings that define AD histologically. These include NPs and NFTs. Much has been learned recently about the formation of these two lesions. Less conspicuous findings include granulovacuolar degeneration, Hirano bodies, and amyloid angiopathy.

Neuritic Plaques

NPs contain an amyloid protein core surrounded by extensive degenerating neurites. The degenerating neurites often contain organelles, Abeta peptide, paired helical filaments, as well as other substances (105). They are typically located throughout the depth of the neocortex. NPs are found in the posterior neocortex, especially the temporal and parietal regions, and in somewhat less abundance frontally (106). In the earliest stages of symptomatic AD, diffuse plaques, which lack the degenerating neurites, are much more common than NPs, suggesting that diffuse plaques represent an earlier stage in the formation of NPs (107). The relationship between NP abundance in the neocortex and dementia severity is not a powerful one. Several studies have found a moderately strong relationship (Pearson correlation coefficient ~0.5) between dementia severity and abundance of NP (108,109), while others have not detected a correlation or found it to be weak (110).

The Role of Amyloid Precursor Protein and Abeta Peptide

The Abeta peptide is thought by most researchers in the field to be the pathogenic molecule in AD (93). It is a 40 to 42 or 43 amino-acid fragment of the APP. APP is a transmembrane protein that undergoes proteolytic cleavage at several specific locations.

APP is cleaved by three secretases. Relative overactivity of the β- or γ-secretases, or underactivity of the α-secretase, leads to excess production of Abeta. The finding that patients with familial AD due to mutations in the presenilin genes had elevated levels of Abeta in their brains suggested that presenilin was somehow involved in the trafficking of APP (111). Mutations in the presenilin gene are assumed to produce a gain in function of γ-secretase, thereby generating the higher loads of Abeta observed in models of presenilin mutants (112).

β-secretase, one of the key enzymes involved in the cleavage of the APP, has been sequenced (113). β-secretase is a membrane-bound aspartyl protease that is localized in the Golgi apparatus and endosomes. α-secretase has not yet been definitively identified.

The Abeta1-42 form is more amyloidogenic and is present earliest in plaque formation (114). It is very important to maintain the distinction between the Abeta peptides and the insoluble amyloid product. The amyloid that is found in senile plaques may represent an inert end-product, while the soluble Abeta1-42 oligomers represent the actual pathogenic molecule (115). One hypothesis proposes that the Abeta species induces an inflammatory response in the AD brain and also acts to promote oxidative injury (116). Others have claimed that APP itself could be pathogenetically important (117), while a minority believes that APP and Abeta are not the key molecules in AD (118). In further support of the role of Abeta is the APOE e4 allele dose-effect on the amount of Abeta seen in AD brain. Those individuals who are homozygous for the APOE e4 allele have more Abeta deposition than those with other genotypes (119).

Neurofibrillary Tangles and Their Regional Distribution

NFTs are intraneuronal inclusions that contain hyperphosphorylated tau protein. The regional specificity of NFTs differs from that of NPs. The burden of NFTs is better correlated with disease severity than is NP count (106,110, 120,121). Braak and Braak have shown that there is an orderly progression beginning in middle age from localization of NFTs in the hippocampal regions (120), then on to the perihippocampal and entorhinal regions, and then finally to neocortical association areas. Stages V and VI of the Braak and Braak system is associated with a high likelihood of AD.

The extent of the NFT invasion of the hippocampus and neocortex, plus the cell loss observed in the association areas of the neocortex, suggests that the mechanism by which cellular dysfunction leads to clinical symptoms is via interruption of hippocampal-neocortical circuits and neocortical-neocortical circuits (106,120). If the hippocampus acts as a mediator for consolidating recent memory, then the disconnection of the hippocampus from the neocortex will lead to rapid forgetting. The delinking of various neocortical association areas will lead to less ability to engage and coordinate neocortical activity in response to a particular task.

The Tau Protein

NFTs are composed of paired helically-arranged filaments that, in turn, are composed predominantly of the microtubule-associated protein tau (122). Tau appears in several different forms (isoforms) that are a result of alternative splicing during transcription from the gene located on chromosome 17 (123). Tau undergoes phosphorylation at several sites along its length. In NFTs, tau is excessively phosphorylated. Hyperphosphorylation leads to the aggregation of tau molecules into paired helical filaments, and then on to the insoluble NFTs. In AD, it is not clear what induces tau hyperphosphorylation and NFT formation, but the most likely mechanism may be induction by elevated levels of Abeta peptide (124). Tau phosphorylation could be a primary event in the pathogenesis of AD, but the sequence of pathological alterations in AD brain suggests that Abeta pathology precedes tau pathology (125).

Histological Diagnosis of Alzheimer's Disease

The most widely used neuropathological diagnostic criteria for AD, the Consortium to Establish a Registry for Alzheimer's Disease (CERAD) neuropathological criteria, are based on the numbers of plaques with cores in the neocortex (126). More recently, a follow-up conference elaborated on the initial criteria by citing a role for NFTs in the diagnosis of AD using the Braak and Braak staging system (120,127). The 1997 National Institute on Aging-Reagan Institute criteria state that there is a high likelihood of AD when both the NP abundance is frequent, according to CERAD criteria, and the NFT pathology falls into Braak and Braak stages V or VI (127). An intermediate likelihood of AD exists when the NP burden is moderate by CERAD criteria, and Braak and Braak stages III or IV NFT pathology is present.

Amyloid Angiopathy

Amyloid angiopathy is commonly found in the brains of patients dying of AD (128–130). The small-to-medium-sized vessels in the leptomeninges and superficial cortex are typically involved. On microscopic cross-section, the media of the vessel wall is thickened and hyalinized as a result of amyloid deposition. The vascular amyloid is of the same composition as the plaque cores, consisting of both the Abeta1-40 and Abeta 1-42 forms of the amyloid protein. In rare instances, AD patients experience intracerebral hemorrhages due to the amyloid angiopathy, but in the majority of patients the amyloid presence in the vasculature does not appear to have a clinical correlate.

Neurotransmitter and Neuropeptide Abnormalities

Deficits in choline acetyltransferase, a key enzyme in the synthetic pathway for acetylcholine, have consistently been noted in the neocortex of patients with moderate to severe AD (131,132). In patients with mild cognitive impairment (MCI), the cholinergic system is upregulated in the hippocampus and frontal cortex compared to nondemented subjects (133). The major pathway for cholinergic innervation of the neocortex and hippocampus originates with neurons in the nucleus basalis, septum, and diagonal band. These regions are challenged during the MCI stage of AD,

and eventually undergo cellular dysfunction, NFT formation, and finally cell death (134,135). However, the cholinergic deficit is an epiphenomenon caused by, rather than being the cause of, pathological mechanisms central to AD.

In younger AD patients, mild deficits in other classic neurotransmitters, such as norepinephrine and serotonin, occur. However, serotonergic and noradrenergic deficits are inconsistent and not correlated with AD severity (136). Serotonergic deficits in a subset of patients might account for the appearance of agitated behavior (137). Decreased levels of glutamate are seen in the hippocampus as well as the neocortex in AD (138), reflecting the dysfunction and eventual demise of both subcortical projection neurons and cortical-cortical projection neurons (139).

TREATMENT OF ALZHEIMER'S DISEASE

The management of AD patients utilizes a combination of pharmacologic and nonpharmacological approaches, which should be initiated simultaneously (see Figure 20-3). Primary treatments for AD include the acetylcholinesterase inhibitors and glutaminergic antagonists. Medications may also be needed to treat the secondary symptoms of AD, such as depression, anxiety, agitation, delusions, hallucinations, and other neuropsychiatric manifestations. Nonpharmacological management includes extensive education of the caregiver and other involved family members; facilitation of access to community services such as day care, respite care, homemaker and related services; review of safety issues such as driving, access to firearms, medication administration; and review of legal and financial issues. Referral to the Alzheimer Association is essential.

PHARMACOTHERAPY

The number of potential therapeutic targets for AD continues to grow. Prevention, disease-modification, or cure are future goals of anti-AD therapies. At the present time, only palliative therapies, exemplified by the acetylcholinesterase inhibitors (AChEIs) and memantine, are available (see Table 20-4).

Acetylcholinesterase Inhibitors

AChEIs represented the only FDA-approved primary treatment option for AD as of 2003. Based on theoretical and empiric grounds, AChEI therapy is a reasonable palliative approach (140).

Donepezil, rivastigmine, and galantamine have been shown to have cognitive and other clinical benefits in mild to moderate AD patients (141–146). The consistent efficacy of different AChEIs shows that the entire class has similar effects on the symptoms of AD. In clinical trials of the AChEIs, the primary outcome measures have been the

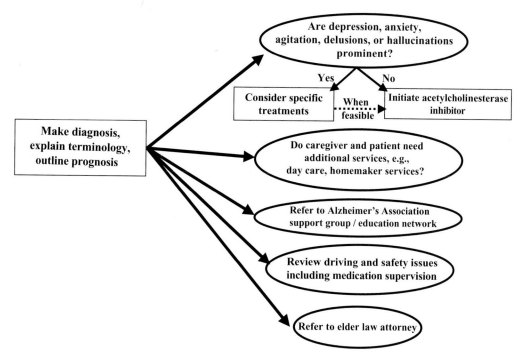

Figure 20-3 A flow chart for the initial management of Alzheimer's disease.

Alzheimer's Disease Assessment Scale-Cognitive sub-scale (ADAS-cog) and some form of a global rating scale (147–149). Compared to placebo groups, the ADAS-cog change over 24 to 30 weeks has ranged from slightly less than three points to about five points. For the global assessments, the 24 to 30 week ratings have yielded about 0.25 to 0.50 points improvement (where three points would be the maximal improvement) compared to the placebo groups. The Mini Mental State Examination (MMSE) improves relative to placebo, ranging between one and two points.

The size of the AChEIs effect can be estimated from various 6-month clinical trials, open-label long-term extension studies (150,151), and a 1-year study (152). Uncontrolled open-label extension studies have also been reported, but they probably overestimate drug benefits.

There are considerable differences in pharmacology between the various AChEIs, but not in plasma half-life, mechanism of cholinesterase inhibition, and mechanism

of degradation. Gastrointestinal (GI) side effects, such as nausea, diarrhea, and anorexia, have been the most frequent use-limiting adverse events, suggesting these drugs should be taken with food. The GI side effects appear to be dose-dependent.

Practical issues in the use of AChEIs include knowing the circumstances in which to avoid their use. Although there are few identifiable interactions with other drugs, the use of AChEIs in patients on high-dose NSAIDs or warfarin may carry a slightly greater risk because of the concern over the possibility of GI bleeding. AChEIs should not be prescribed for AD patients when the family of the patient cannot guarantee the reliability of administration. AD patients must be assumed to be unreliable, and families and physicians must assure that a method for safe medication-taking is in place.

Based on clinical trial data alone, the AChEIs should be used in patients with mild to moderate AD. In practice, they are often also used in AD patients in the severe stages

TABLE 20-4
DRUGS FOR THE TREATMENT OF ALZHEIMER'S DISEASE

Drug	Mechanism of Action	Starting Dose	Maximum Dose
Donepezil	Acetylcholinesterase inhibitor	5 mg once/day	10 or 15 mg once/day
Galantamine	Acetylcholinesterase inhibitor	4 mg twice/day*	8 or 12 mg twice/day[†]
Rivastigmine	Acetylcholinesterase inhibitor	1.5 mg twice/day	6 mg twice/day
Memantine	Glutamate modulator	5 mg once/day	10 mg twice/day

* Available in immediate release and also a once-a-day preparation (8 mg/day)
[†] 16 or 24 mg/day (once-a-day preparations)

of the disease. There may be some rationale for their institution in severe AD, such as a patient who, despite all of the other features of severe dementia, might still be cared for at home or still interacts with family members. On the other hand, to the extent that AChEIs have any efficacy in delaying the progression of severe dementia, one could question the value of prolonging a phase of the disease in which quality of life is so poor and dignity compromised.

There is no consensus on when to stop AChEIs. One strategy might be to use them for 6 to 12 months and then discontinue them; but that makes little sense, especially if a patient has declined negligibly over that time frame. Instead, AChEIs should be continued until patients reach the stage of severe dementia or when accelerated decline would have no further impact on quality of life.

Vitamin E

Vitamin E is an anti-oxidant. Based on the rationale that oxidative injury might be one of the intermediary mechanisms of the disease, there has been interest in vitamin E as a therapy for AD. While an earlier study of high doses of vitamin E appeared to show modest benefits for moderately severe AD patients (153), concerns about safety of higher doses have been raised. Moreover, a study of vitamin E in patients with mild cognitive impairment failed to show benefits (Peterson R. Personal communication, 2005). The concerns raised about excess mortality with high doses of vitamin E, coupled with the demonstration of lack of efficacy in mild cognitive impairment, has dampened enthusiasm for using vitamin E as a therapy for AD patients.

Memantine

Memantine became available in the United States in 2004, and is indicated for use in patients with moderate to severe AD. It demonstrated clinical benefit in both cognitive and functional parameters, compared to placebo. Memantine antagonizes glutamate-gated N-methyl-D-asparate receptor channels. In patients with moderately severe AD, memantine was superior to placebo on a clinician's global rating of change and on change in an activities-of-daily-living measure (154). It did not bring about improvements in function or cognition in this study, but memantine-treated patients had less symptomatic worsening over the 6 months of the trial. Results from trials in patients with mild AD are not yet available, but the drug holds promise, perhaps as an adjunctive treatment with AChEIs.

Strategies Aimed at β-Amyloid Processing

Inhibition of either β- or γ-secretase activity is an obvious strategy for reducing Abeta production. Initial human studies of β- and γ-secretase inhibitors are in early phase II investigations. Important questions about safety must, of course, first be answered. Ultimately, if these agents prove to be safe, trials to show efficacy will have to be conducted.

Whether these will involve studies in symptomatic AD patients, those at risk for AD (MCI-type trials), or simply aged individuals (i.e., a prevention strategy) remains to be seen.

MANAGEMENT OF BEHAVIORAL DISTURBANCES IN DEMENTIA

Treatment of Depression

Depressed mood commonly occurs in dementia patients (155,156). Depressive symptoms may be part of the initial presentation of the dementia syndrome, or they may occur later in patients with established dementia (155). Major depression is uncommon in AD (15,157). The depression that occurs in dementia patients may manifest in the usual ways, with tearfulness and overt verbalizations of sadness. Patients may state that they feel that life is not worth living or that they would rather be dead. However, apathy is not necessarily a symptom of depression in a demented patient, since apathy and loss of initiative are also integral features of dementia.

Families are generally better in identifying depressive symptomatology than the patient (158). Demented patients, either because of their lack of insight, their memory impairment, or both, may be unable to report on their own behavior that had occurred yesterday, or last week. Treating depression on the strength of the caregiver's observations, without necessarily obtaining affirmation from the patient, is the preferred approach in such a situation.

Treatment of depression is covered elsewhere in this textbook in chapters on depression associated with dementia, as well as on major depression and related disorders. The principles of treating depression in AD patients are not fundamentally different than those in nondemented individuals.

Management of Agitation

Agitation is the collective term for a number of disruptive behaviors that occur over the course of dementia due to AD (15,155). Agitation includes physical aggressiveness, verbal irritability, hallucinations, delusions, hyperactivity such as wandering, tearfulness, and overt anxiety. Agitation is a major source of burden to caregivers of dementia patients.

Managing behavioral disorders may require both pharmacologic and nonpharmacologic techniques. To minimize physical or verbal abusiveness, caregivers can often be taught to avoid the circumstances that seem to trigger outbursts of anger. Hallucinations and anxiety may both be exacerbated by lack of social interactions; health professionals may encourage family caregivers to change the living arrangement or add day-care to the weekly schedule in lieu of medicating those behaviors.

When any form of agitation occurs in an AD patient, it is possible that the disruptive behavior is being caused by some underlying physical ailment. For example, an unrecognized urinary tract infection or a worsening of congestive heart failure can increase disruptive behaviors. Other medical conditions that could precipitate agitation include pain from joint disease, skin breakdown, or dental problems; constipation; dehydration; or a decompensation of another underlying illness such as emphysema.

Hallucinations and delusions may not require active treatment if they are not disruptive, anxiety provoking, or frightening. Sometimes, it is only the caregivers who are (understandably) bothered by the bizarre comments of the patient. Once the nature of the delusions or hallucinations is explained to the caregivers, they usually become much more tolerant of the patient's behavior. Isolated verbal aggressiveness, without physical aggressiveness, depression, anxiety, or paranoia, may be difficult to treat pharmacologically. As with delusions and hallucinations, promotion of insight by the caregiver may be sufficient to ameliorate the problem.

Pharmacological treatment of agitation is also dealt with elsewhere in this textbook, in the chapter on agitation and psychosis associated with dementia. There are a wide variety of medications that have been advocated for use in agitation, including the newer generation of antipsychotics.

Sleep Disturbances

Disturbances of nocturnal sleep are common in AD and are a source of considerable caregiver burden and stress. Although there are effective medications for treating sleep disturbances, disruptive nighttime sleep in a dementia patient is often due to daytime sleeping or other variations in the sleep-wake cycle. Moreover, the daytime sleeping may be allowed or encouraged by the caregiver out of desperation, but without regard to the nighttime conse-

quences. Another common cause of nocturnal awakening is an early bedtime relative to the caregiver. When sleep disturbances are due to either of these causes, use of sedatives is likely to be ineffective. Management of sleep disorders, therefore, often involves service interventions to manage the daytime and early evening behavior. That in turn may require the use of such social services as day-care or home health aides. Involving a patient in day-care may keep the patient occupied and more active during the daytime, and hence more likely to sleep at night.

For sleep disorders due to disordered sleep patterns independent of daytime sleeping, trazodone was the first choice in an expert consensus survey, with the short-acting benzodiazepines being remote second-line choices (159). Pharmacologic treatment is covered elsewhere in this text, in the chapter on sleep disorders.

COURSE OF ALZHEIMER'S DISEASE

Natural History and Survival

The natural history of AD varies considerably from one individual to the next, but there are some approximate values that can be applied to the different phases of the illness (see Figure 20-4). The average length of time from onset of symptoms until diagnosis is about 2 to 3 years. The average duration of time from diagnosis to nursing home placement (a marker of severe dementia) is roughly 3 to 6 years (160,161). Alzheimer patients spend an average of 3 years in nursing homes prior to death (162). The total duration of AD is 9 to 12 years on average, from symptom onset to death.

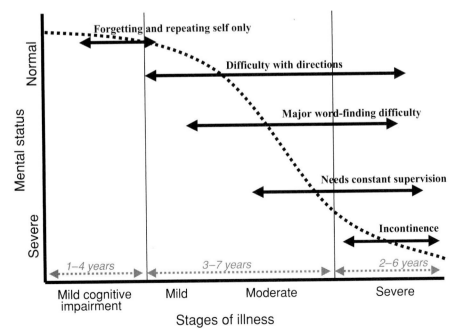

Figure 20-4 A schematic view of the major symptoms and milestones in the clinical course of Alzheimer's disease (based on a graphic of Steven Gracon, DVM).

In patients whose initial MMSE scores ranged from 10 to 26, the average rate of decline per year is about three points (163). The variability is considerable, as indicated by a standard deviation of approximately 4 (164). The rate of decline obeys a curvilinear relationship to the cognitive test scores (165). Faster rates of decline occur in the mid-portions of the scales, and slower rates occur among milder and more severe patients. Moreover, a decline over one 6-month or 1-year period does not predict the rate of decline over a subsequent time interval.

There are few predictors of rate of progression, but parkinsonian signs, hallucinations, and delusions have been shown to be associated with more rapid decline (166). This set of observations is consistent with findings that patients with dementia with Lewy bodies have a faster rate of decline than comparably demented AD patients (167).

Mortality in AD averages less than 10% per year (168). Median survival for patients with AD is roughly 5 to 6 years (168–170). Causes of death in AD include pneumonia, sepsis, and other common causes of mortality in the elderly, such as cardiovascular disease and stroke (171).

Presymptomatic Phase

At the present time, it is not possible to identify presymptomatic individuals who are at risk to develop AD, except for those very rare individuals from families with known autosomal dominant AD. Several studies have shown that, in retrospect, individuals destined to develop AD are cognitively inferior, as a group, to those not destined to develop AD (172,173). The group differences, however, are not distinctive enough to be of use in prediction in individual instances.

Studies that have combined PET imaging and assessment of genetic susceptibility for AD conferred by apolipoprotein E (APOE) genotype have shown that nondemented individuals who are homozygous for the e4 allele have a pattern of reduced parietal lobe metabolism that is seen in patients with established AD (174,175). These intriguing findings support the belief that biochemical dysfunction is occurring in presymptomatic AD. However, at this time, an abnormal PET scan in a nondemented individual has no proven predictive value for subsequent AD.

Mild Cognitive Impairment

Individuals destined to become demented due to AD often first develop difficulties with short-term memory and learning new information, but otherwise function normally. This state is referred to as amnesic MCI (172). A person with MCI may remain in that state for several years, but approximately 15% of MCI patients per year deteriorate and qualify for a diagnosis of AD (172). MCI is an important condition to recognize because it is a risk-state for subsequently developing AD.

Diagnostic criteria for MCI include a memory complaint, objective evidence of impaired recent memory, intact daily function, and intact nonmemory cognitive functions (172). The lack of significant impairment in functioning in daily affairs is perhaps the major distinction between early dementia and MCI. Individuals with MCI defined as above show memory impairment comparable to AD patients, but have scores on most nonmemory neuropsychological tests that are comparable to normal elderly individuals (176).

Several predictors of conversion from MCI to AD have been observed. One is an increasing level of dysfunction in daily affairs as reported by an informant, but not by the patient (177). Hippocampal atrophy on MRI, together with neuropsychological features, hold considerable promise for identifying MCI patients who are at risk to progress to AD within a few years (178,179). A study of patients with a syndrome nearly identically defined as MCI showed that PET imaging abnormalities of the Alzheimer type (i.e., parietal hypometabolism) was usually seen in MCI patients who converted to AD during the follow-up period (180). For more information, see the chapter on memory disorders in this textbook.

Mild Alzheimer's Disease

The syndrome of mild AD (Clinical Dementia Rating [CDR] Scale stage I [181] or Global Deterioration Scale stages III or IV [182]), is characterized by clear-cut deficits in recent memory, deficits in at least one of the other cognitive domains, and loss of functional independence. Functional loss might take the form of difficulties with financial affairs, difficulties with geographic orientation in patients' own homes and other familiar places, or an inability to do tasks such as those in one's job or around the home. Patients' ability to recall information from the past is often only minimally impaired at this stage of the illness. Changes in personality frequently are part of the presentation of mild AD. Personality changes may include increased apathy, social withdrawal, disinhibition, or irritability. Depression also is common, and can exacerbate cognitive deficits (155). Paranoia and obsessions may become evident, although these are more likely to occur in later stages of the disease. Frank delusions and hallucinations occasionally occur in mild AD.

Patients with mild AD score between 20 and 26 on the MMSE. Memory performance may be the most abnormal portion of the cognitive examination. Patients may recall nothing after a short delay. A mild AD patient may have largely intact conversational comprehension and spontaneous speech. However, mild AD patients and their families report word-finding difficulties, which can be observed with naming tests that use less common objects. Abstract reasoning deficits may be detectable with more difficult tasks that require mental agility to manipulate sequential tasks. However, prior intellectual and occupational achievement strongly affect how well a mild AD patient will do with naming or abstract reasoning. Most patients with mild AD have some constructional difficulties. On more detailed neuropsychological testing, deficits in visuospatial processing are often observed.

The motor neurological examination is typically normal in patients with mild AD. Some subtle extrapyramidal signs may be seen.

Moderate Alzheimer's Disease

Patients with moderate AD (CDR stage 2) not only are dependent on others for higher-level daily living activities, such as managing finances, shopping, or transportation, but may on occasion need to be reminded to bathe and to dress appropriately. Moderate AD patients may fail to recognize acquaintances who are not part of the patient's daily retinue. Patients at this stage of AD should no longer operate motor vehicles or devices such as lawn movers, power saws, or probably even stoves and microwaves. Neuropsychiatric disturbances may become prominent. Delusions and hallucinations are common. Patients often no longer recognize their own homes. Irritability and paranoia are common symptoms of moderate AD. Disrupted sleep may also occur.

On mental status examinations with the MMSE, moderately severe AD patients will score between 10 and 19. Patients at this stage have word- and name-finding deficits that are obvious in conversation. New information or recent events are often almost instantly forgotten. Motor apraxia may be evident at this stage of AD, though it is rarely prominent.

If patients with moderate AD have reasonably competent caregivers, they can often remain in the family residence. If not, moderate AD patients may need supervised living situations. Some assistance almost always becomes needed for solo caregivers in the later stages of moderate AD.

Even at this stage of the illness, the motor neurological examination may be normal except for signs of mild rigidity or bradykinesia.

Severe Alzheimer's Disease

Patients with severe AD (CDR stage 3) need 24-hour supervision. They have negligible memory for events, conversations and unfortunately, even close family members. They have substantial word-finding difficulties. Their spontaneous speech is impoverished. They may be virtually mute, or they may use jargon-filled speech that conveys no meaningful information (183). They need extensive assistance with bathing, dressing, eating, and toileting. They are more likely than milder patients to become aggressive when offered assistance with undressing or toileting, although some severe patients are very docile. Despite their fragmentary cognition, severely demented patients may experience depression, anxiety, and fear. They typically score below 10 on the MMSE (183,184).

A minority of AD patients experience generalized seizures (185), often in the severe stage of the disease. Patients may also exhibit marked rigidity, bradykinesia, gait and balance difficulties, and masked facies.

PSYCHOSOCIAL, LEGAL, AND ETHICAL ISSUES

Dealing with the Patient Who is Still Driving

Revocation of driving privileges in dementia patients is one of the most contentious issues in the management of AD patients. There is no question that dementia patients experience an increased rate of crashes compared to their age-matched peers (186). Dementia patients are more likely to become lost. Dementia patients seem to voluntarily reduce the number of miles they drive (187). As a consequence, the absolute number of crashes and other vehicular misadventures committed by dementia patients is low.

Some authorities believe that once patients have been diagnosed with dementia they should stop driving. Others take the opposite view, stating that the diagnosis of mild AD or some other form of dementia should never, by itself, lead to revocation of a person's right to drive (188). The American Academy of Neurology has issued guidelines that state that patients with dementia severity of CDR = 1 or greater pose a significant safety risk and should therefore be carefully evaluated (189).

Unfortunately, there is no consensus on best methods for assessing driving safety. Neurological assessment or standard neuropsychological assessments appear to have inadequate predictive value (190). AD patients are impaired in the various functions that contribute to safe driving, such as in understanding traffic signs (191). Road testing is the most accurate (190,192), but it is not available in all communities. Specific performance features of unsafe drivers that were readily distinguished from safer ones were: impaired overall judgment, drifting attention, unawareness of how driving was affecting other drivers (e.g., unexpected braking), and inappropriate speed (unsafe drivers usually drive too slowly) (192). Use of a driving simulator that lets the subjects drive until they crash has shown that even mild AD patients experienced a much higher rate of crashes than nondemented elderly (193).

Clinicians who lack driving simulators or facilities for road testing must rely on their own judgment. The opinion that a patient should cease driving will be based on a history of unsafe driving practices, evidence of impulsiveness, visuospatial impairment, and other pertinent clues from the history or mental status examination.

The Caregiver as the Co-patient

Most caregivers of dementia patients are either spouses or adult children. Spouse caregivers are nearly as elderly as the typical dementia patient, and they may have their own medical problems. Child caregivers often have their own families, and may live at some distance from their demented parent. Both suffer from high rates of depression and stress (194,195). Especially in the case of spouse caregivers, social isolation is a frequent occurrence.

There are several key aspects of the care of dementia patients where physicians can be of particular assistance to caregivers (196). Caregivers need to be offered education about the phenomena that they are or will be encountering. Physicians cannot provide most of the education about dementia in one office visit. Moreover, the specific problems that confront caregivers change over the course of the disease (197). Regularly scheduled follow-up appointments to discuss new problems are essential. Referral to the local chapter of the Alzheimer Association should be standard practice. Physicians should also be proactive in referring the patient and caregiver to community services such as day-care or home care. Caregivers need honest appraisals of current therapies. With all of the sources of medical information today, from the mass media that often gives stories about AD front-page coverage, to innumerable websites, many family caregivers have more raw facts than do physicians. Yet it is the skilled clinician who can put the headlines and hype into perspective and keep the caregivers grounded in legitimate expectations. Finally, physicians should never forget that caregivers are partners in decision-making for the care of dementia patients.

Caregiver education, support, and empowerment, if properly tailored, can have tangible benefits for patients and their families. A recent clinical trial showed that intense, direct support for caregivers by trained health professionals can delay nursing home placement and increase a sense of well-being in caregivers (198).

Sharing the Diagnosis and Prognosis with Patient and Family

The diagnosis of AD should be freely shared, without excessive apology or fear, with the family. There should be no delay out of a fear of mentioning the word "Alzheimer's." Telling the patient is a more controversial point. Some clinicians feel that patients with AD do not wish to hear the diagnosis. Both physicians and families fear that the patient may become seriously depressed if told. However, most patients with moderate to severe dementia will show no visible reaction to the diagnosis. Many patients will simply deny that they have a problem. Other experts take the view that mild AD patients are entitled to hear their diagnosis. It may be justifiable to withhold the diagnosis from a patient with moderate or severe dementia, however (199,200). The benefits of disclosing the diagnosis to the mild patient are several. First, the family can use the word "Alzheimer's" without fear of producing anxiety on the part of the patient. Second, use of the diagnostic term can provide some leverage for family care-

givers to bring about changes in behavior. For example, family members can demand that a patient stop driving based on the diagnosis of AD. Third, in mild patients, sharing the diagnosis can allow them to express their wishes about important family matters or end-of-life issues.

REFERENCES

1. American Psychiatric Association. *Diagnostic and Statistical Manual of Mental Disorders.* 4th Ed. Text Revision (DSM-IV-TR). Washington, DC: American Psychiatric Association; 2000.
2. McKhann G, Drachman D, Folstein M, et al. Clinical diagnosis of Alzheimer's disease: report of the NINCDS-ADRDA Work Group under the auspices of Department of Health and Human Services Task Force on Alzheimer's Disease. *Neurology.* 1984;34: 939–944.
3. Starkstein SE, Sabe L, Chemerinski E, Jason L, Leiguarda R. Two domains of anosognosia in Alzheimer's disease. *J Neurol Neurosurg Psychiatry.* 1996;61:485–490.
4. Grut M, Jorm AF, Fratiglioni L, et al. Memory complaints of elderly people in a population survey: variation according to dementia stage and depression. *J Am Geriatr Soc.* 1993;41: 1295–1300.
5. Petersen RC, Smith GE, Ivnik RJ, Kokmen E, Tangalos EG. Memory function in very early Alzheimer's disease. *Neurology.* 1994;44:867–872.
6. Faber-Langendoen K, Morris JC, Knesevich JW, et al. Aphasia in senile dementia of the Alzheimer type. *Ann Neurol.* 1988;23: 365–370.
7. Mendez MF, Mendez MA, Martin R, Smyth KA, Whitehouse PJ. Complex visual disturbances in Alzheimer's disease. *Neurology.* 1990;40:439–443.
8. Giannakopoulos P, Gold G, Duc M, et al. Neuroanatomic correlates of visual agnosia in Alzheimer's disease: a clinicopathologic study. *Neurology.* 1999;52:71–77.
9. Mendez MF, Ghajarania M, Perryman KM. Posterior cortical atrophy: clinical characteristics and differences compared to Alzheimer's disease. *Dement Geriatr Cogn Disord.* 2002;14:33–40.
10. Kopelman MD. Frontal dysfunction and memory deficits in the alcoholic Korsakoff syndrome and Alzheimer-type dementia. *Brain.* 1991;114:117–137.
11. Albert MS, Moss MB, Tanzi R, Jones K. Preclinical prediction of AD using neuropsychological tests. *J Int Neuropsychol Soc.* 2001;7:631–639.
12. Marson DC, Cody HA, Ingram KK, Harrell LE. Neuropsychologic predictors of competency in Alzheimer's disease using a rational reasons legal standard. *Arch Neurol.* 1995;52:955–959.
13. Johnson JK, Head E, Kim R, Starr A, Cotman CW. Clinical and pathological evidence for a frontal variant of Alzheimer disease. *Arch Neurol.* 1999;56:1233–1239.
14. Mega MS, Cummings JL, Fiorello T, Gornbein J. The spectrum of behavioral changes in Alzheimer's disease. *Neurology.* 1996;46: 130–135.
15. Devanand DP, Jacobs DM, Tang MX, et al. The course of psychopathologic features in mild to moderate Alzheimer disease. *Arch Gen Psychiatry.* 1997;54:257–263.
16. Hy LX, Keller DM. Prevalence of AD among Whites: a summary by levels of severity. *Neurology.* 2000;55:198–204.
17. Gao S, Hendrie HC, Hall KS, Hui S. The relationships between age, sex, and the incidence of dementia and Alzheimer disease: a meta-analysis. *Arch Gen Psychiatry.* 1998;55:809–815.
18. Jorm AF, Jolley D. The incidence of dementia: a meta-analysis. *Neurology.* 1998;51:728–733.
19. Stern Y, Tang MX, Denaro J, Mayeux R. Increased risk of mortality in Alzheimer's disease patients with more advanced educational and occupational attainment. *Ann Neurol.* 1995;37:590–595.
20. Snowdon DA, Kemper SJ, Mortimer JA, et al. Linguistic ability in early life and cognitive function and Alzheimer's disease in late life. Findings from the Nun Study. *JAMA.* 1996;275:528– 532.
21. Whalley LJ, Starr JM, Athawes R, et al. Childhood mental ability and dementia. *Neurology.* 2000;55:1455–1459.

22. Carmelli D, Swan GE, Reed T, et al. Midlife cardiovascular risk factors, ApoE, and cognitive decline in elderly male twins. *Neurology*. 1998;50:1580–1585.

23. Hofman A, Ott A, Breteler MM, et al. Atherosclerosis, apolipoprotein E, and prevalence of dementia and Alzheimer's disease in the Rotterdam Study. *Lancet*. 1997;349:151–154.

24. Seshadri S, Beiser A, Selhub J, et al. Plasma Homocysteine as a Risk Factor for Dementia and Alzheimer's Disease. *N Engl J Med*. 2002;346:476–483.

25. Jordan BD, Relkin NR, Ravdin LD, et al. Apolipoprotein E epsilon4 associated with chronic traumatic brain injury in boxing. *JAMA*. 1997;278:136–140.

26. Roberts GW, Allsop D, Bruton C. The occult aftermath of boxing. *J Neurol Neurosurg Psychiatry*. 1990;53:373–378.

27. Mayeux R, Ottman R, Maestre G, et al. Synergistic effects of traumatic head injury and apolipoprotein-epsilon 4 in patients with Alzheimer's disease. *Neurology*. 1995;45:555–557.

28. Graves AB, White E, Koepsell TD, et al. The association between aluminum-containing products and Alzheimer's disease. *J Clin Epidemiol*. 1990;43:35–44.

29. Hachinski V. Aluminum exposure and risk of Alzheimer disease. *Arch Neurol*. 1998;55:742.

30. Salib E, Hillier V. A case-control study of Alzheimer's disease and aluminum occupation. *Br J Psychiatry*. 1996;168:244–249.

31. Bjertness E, Candy JM, Torvik A, et al. Content of brain aluminum is not elevated in Alzheimer disease. *Alzheimer Dis Assoc Disord*. 1996;10:171–174.

32. Crapper DR, Krishnan SS, De Boni U, Tomko GJ. Aluminum: a possible neurotoxic agent in Alzheimer's disease. *Trans Am Neurol Assoc*. 1975;100:154–156.

33. Good PF, Perl DP, Bierer LM, Schmeidler J. Selective accumulation of aluminum and iron in the neurofibrillary tangles of Alzheimer's disease: a laser microprobe (LAMMA) study. *Ann Neurol*. 1992;31:286–292.

34. Lovell MA, Ehmann WD, Markesbery WR. Laser microprobe analysis of brain aluminum in Alzheimer's disease. *Ann Neurol*. 1993;33:36–42.

35. Forster DP, Newens AJ, Kay DW, Edwardson JA. Risk factors in clinically diagnosed presenile dementia of the Alzheimer type: a case-control study in northern England. *J Epidemiol Community Health*. 1995;49:253–258.

36. Martyn CN, Barker DJ, Osmond C, et al. Geographical relation between Alzheimer's disease and aluminum in drinking water. *Lancet*. 1989;1:59–62.

37. McLachlan DR, Bergeron C, Smith JE, Boomer D, Rifat SL. Risk for neuropathologically confirmed Alzheimer's disease and residual aluminum in municipal drinking water employing weighted residential histories. *Neurology*. 1996;46:401–405.

38. Paganini-Hill A, Henderson VW. Estrogen replacement therapy and risk of Alzheimer disease. *Arch Intern Med*. 1996;156:2213–2217.

39. Tang MX, Jacobs D, Stern Y, et al. Effect of oestrogen during menopause on risk and age at onset of Alzheimer's disease. *Lancet*. 1996;348:429–432.

40. Shumaker SA, Legault C, Thal L, et al. Estrogen plus progestin and the incidence of dementia and mild cognitive impairment in postmenopausal women: the Women's Health Initiative Memory Study: a randomized controlled trial. *JAMA*. 2003;289:2651–2662.

41. Breitner JC, Gau BA, Welsh KA, et al. Inverse association of anti-inflammatory treatments and Alzheimer's disease: initial results of a co-twin control study. *Neurology*. 1994;44:227–232.

42. Stewart WF, Kawas C, Corrada M, Metter EJ. Risk of Alzheimer's disease and duration of NSAID use. *Neurology*. 1997;48:626–632.

43. Aisen PS, Schafer KA, Grundman M, et al. Effects of rofecoxib or naproxen vs placebo on Alzheimer disease progression: a randomized controlled trial. *JAMA*. 2003;289:2819–2826.

44. Weggen S, Eriksen JL, Das P, et al. A subset of NSAIDs lower amyloidogenic Abeta42 independently of cyclooxygenase activity. *Nature*. 2001;414:212–216.

45. Jick H, Zornberg GL, Jick SS, Seshadri S, Drachman DA. Statins and the risk of dementia. *Lancet*. 2000;356:1627–1631.

46. Wolozin B, Kellman W, Ruosseau P, Celesia GG, Siegel G. Decreased prevalence of Alzheimer disease associated with 3-hydroxy-3-methyglutaryl coenzyme A reductase inhibitors. *Arch Neurol*. 2000;57:1439–1443.

47. Rockwood K, Kirkland S, Hogan DB, et al. Use of lipid-lowering agents, indication bias, and the risk of dementia in community-dwelling elderly people. *Arch Neurol*. 2002;59:223–227.

48. Masaki KH, Losonczy KG, Izmirlian G, et al. Association of vitamin E and C supplement use with cognitive function and dementia in elderly men. *Neurology*. 2000;54:1265–1272.

49. Morris MC, Evans DA, Bienias JL, et al. Dietary intake of antioxidant nutrients and the risk of incident Alzheimer disease in a biracial community study. *JAMA*. 2002;287:3230–3237.

50. Engelhart MJ, Geerlings MI, Ruitenberg A, et al. Dietary intake of antioxidants and risk of Alzheimer disease. *JAMA*. 2002;287: 3223–3229.

51. Mendelsohn AB, Belle SH, Stoehr GP, Ganguli M. Use of antioxidant supplements and its association with cognitive function in a rural elderly cohort: the MoVIES Project. Monongahela Valley Independent Elders Survey. *Am J Epidemiol*. 1998;148: 38–44.

52. Laurin D, Foley DJ, Masaki KH, White LR, Launer LJ. Vitamin E and C supplements and risk of dementia. *JAMA*. 2002;288: 2266–2268.

53. Brenner DE, Kukull WA, van Belle G, et al. Relationship between cigarette smoking and Alzheimer's disease in a population-based case-control study. *Neurology*. 1993;43:293–300.

54. Ott A, Slooter AJ, Hofman A, et al. Smoking and risk of dementia and Alzheimer's disease in a population- based cohort study: the Rotterdam Study. *Lancet*. 1998;351:1840–1843.

55. Galanis DJ, Petrovitch H, Launer LJ, et al. Smoking history in middle age and subsequent cognitive performance in elderly Japanese-American men. The Honolulu-Asia Aging Study. *Am J Epidemiol*. 1997;145:507–515.

56. Prince M, Lewis G, Bird A, Blizard R, Mann A. A longitudinal study of factors predicting change in cognitive test scores over time, in an older hypertensive population. *Psychol Med*. 1996;26:555–568.

57. Whitehouse PJ, Kalaria RN. Nicotinic receptors and neurodegenerative dementing diseases: basic research and clinical implications. *Alzheimer Dis Assoc Disord*. 1995;9(Suppl 2):3–5.

58. Bachman DL, Wolf PA, Linn R, et al. Prevalence of dementia and probable senile dementia of the Alzheimer type in the Framingham Study. *Neurology*. 1992;42:115–119.

59. Evans DA, Funkenstein HH, Albert MS, et al. Prevalence of Alzheimer's disease in a community population of older persons. Higher than previously reported. *JAMA*. 1989;262:2551–2556.

60. Hendrie HC, Osuntokun BO, Hall KS, et al. Prevalence of Alzheimer's disease and dementia in two communities: Nigerian Africans and African Americans. *Am J Psychiatry*. 1995;152: 1485–1492.

61. White L, Petrovitch H, Ross GW, et al. Prevalence of dementia in older Japanese-American men in Hawaii: the Honolulu-Asia Aging Study. *JAMA*. 1996;276:955–960.

62. Canadian Study of Health and Aging Working Group. Canadian study of health and aging: study methods and prevalence of dementia. *CMAJ*. 1994;150:899–913.

63. Holmes C, Cairns N, Lantos P, Mann A. Validity of current clinical criteria for Alzheimer's disease, vascular dementia and dementia with Lewy bodies. *Br J Psychiatry*. 1999;174:45–50.

64. Jobst KA, Barnetson LP, Shepstone BJ. Accurate prediction of histologically confirmed Alzheimer's disease and the differential diagnosis of dementia: the use of NINCDS-ADRDA and DSM-III-R criteria, SPECT, X-ray CT, and apo E4 in medial temporal lobe dementias. Oxford Project to Investigate Memory and Aging. *Int Psychogeriatr*. 10:271–302.

65. Lim A, Tsuang D, Kukull W, et al. Clinico-neuropathological correlation of Alzheimer's disease in a community-based case series. *J Am Geriatr Soc*. 1999;47:564–569.

66. Knopman DS, DeKosky ST, Cummings JL, et al. Practice parameter: diagnosis of dementia (an evidence-based review). *Neurology*. 2001;56:1143–1153.

67. Practice parameter for diagnosis and evaluation of dementia. (summary statement) Report of the Quality Standards Subcommittee of the American Academy of Neurology. *Neurology*. 1994;44:2203–2206.

68. Siu AL. Screening for dementia and investigating its causes. *Ann Intern Med*. 1991;115:122–132.

69. Jack CR Jr, Petersen RC, Xu YC, et al. Medial temporal atrophy on MRI in normal aging and very mild Alzheimer's disease. *Neurology.* 1997;49:786–794.

70. Fox NC, Freeborough PA, Rossor MN. Visualisation and quantification of rates of atrophy in Alzheimer's disease. *Lancet.* 1996;348:94–97.

71. Longstreth WT Jr, Bernick C, Manolio TA, et al. Lacunar infarcts defined by magnetic resonance imaging of 3660 elderly people: the Cardiovascular Health Study. *Arch Neurol.* 1998;55:1217–1225.

72. Jagust W, Thisted R, Devous MD, et al. SPECT perfusion imaging in the diagnosis of Alzheimer's disease: a clinical-pathologic study. *Neurology.* 2001;56:950–956.

73. Silverman DH, Small GW, Chang CY, et al. Positron emission tomography in evaluation of dementia: regional brain metabolism and long-term outcome. *JAMA.* 2001;286:2120–2127.

74. Galasko D, Chang L, Motter R, et al. High cerebrospinal fluid tau and low amyloid beta42 levels in the clinical diagnosis of Alzheimer disease and relation to apolipoprotein E genotype. *Arch Neurol.* 1998;55:937–945.

75. Andreasen N, Vanmechelen E, Van de Voorde A, et al. Cerebrospinal fluid tau protein as a biochemical marker for Alzheimer's disease: a community based follow up study. *J Neurol Neurosurg Psychiatry.* 1998;64:298–305.

76. Kahle PJ, Jakowec M, Teipel SJ, et al. Combined assessment of tau and neuronal thread protein in Alzheimer's disease CSF. *Neurology.* 2000;54:1498–1504.

77. Corder EH, Saunders AM, Strittmatter WJ, et al. Gene dose of apolipoprotein E type 4 allele and the risk of Alzheimer's disease in late onset families. *Science.* 1993;261:921–923.

78. Poirier J, Davignon J, Bouthillier D, et al. Apolipoprotein E polymorphism and Alzheimer's disease. *Lancet.* 1993;342:697–699.

79. Mayeux R, Saunders AM, Shea S, et al. Utility of the apolipoprotein E genotype in the diagnosis of Alzheimer's disease. Alzheimer's Disease Centers Consortium on Apolipoprotein E and Alzheimer's Disease. *N Engl J Med.* 1998;338:506–511.

80. McConnell LM, Koenig BA, Greely HT, Raffin TA. Genetic testing and Alzheimer disease: has the time come? Alzheimer Disease Working Group of the Stanford Program in Genomics, Ethics & Society. *Nat Med.* 1998;4:757–759.

81. Lautenschlager NT, Cupples LA, Rao VS, et al. Risk of dementia among relatives of Alzheimer's disease patients in the MIRAGE study: what is in store for the oldest old? *Neurology.* 1996;46:641–650.

82. Heston LL, Mastri AR, Anderson VE, White J. Dementia of the Alzheimer type. Clinical genetics, natural history, and associated conditions. *Arch Gen Psychiatry.* 1981;38:1085–1090.

83. Silverman JM, Smith CJ, Marin DB, Mohs RC, Propper CB. Familial patterns of risk in very late-onset Alzheimer disease. *Arch Gen Psychiatry.* 2003;60:190–197.

84. Schupf N, Kapell D, Lee JH, Ottman R, Mayeux R. Increased risk of Alzheimer's disease in mothers of adults with Down's syndrome. *Lancet.* 1994;344:353–356.

85. Raiha I, Kaprio J, Koskenvuo M, Rajala T, Sourander L. Alzheimer's disease in Finnish twins. *Lancet.* 1996;347:573–578.

86. Blacker D, Tanzi RE. The genetics of Alzheimer disease: current status and future prospects. *Arch Neurol.* 1998;55:294–296.

87. Tanzi RE, Bertram L. New frontiers in Alzheimer's disease genetics. *Neuron.* 2001;32:181–184.

88. Bird TD, Levy-Lahad E, Poorkaj P, et al. Wide range in age of onset for chromosome 1-related familial Alzheimer's disease. *Ann Neurol.* 1996;40:932–936.

89. Lampe TH, Bird TD, Nochlin D, et al. Phenotype of chromosome 14-linked familial Alzheimer's disease in a large kindred. *Ann Neurol.* 1994;36:368–378.

90. Lippa CF, Saunders AM, Smith TW, et al. Familial and sporadic Alzheimer's disease: neuropathology cannot exclude a final common pathway. *Neurology.* 1996;46:406–412.

91. Mann DM, Iwatsubo T, Nochlin D, et al. Amyloid (Abeta) deposition in chromosome 1-linked Alzheimer's disease: the Volga German families. *Ann Neurol.* 1997;41:52–57.

92. Goate A, Chartier-Harlin MC, Mullan M, et al. Segregation of a missense mutation in the amyloid precursor protein gene with familial Alzheimer's disease. *Nature.* 1991;349:704–706.

93. Hardy J. Amyloid, the presenilins and Alzheimer's disease. *Trends Neurosci.* 1997;20:154–159.

94. Wisniewski KE, Wisniewski HM, Wen GY. Occurrence of neuropathological changes and dementia of Alzheimer's disease in Down's syndrome. *Ann Neurol.* 1985;17:278–282.

95. Sherrington R, Rogaev EI, Liang Y, et al. Cloning of a gene bearing missense mutations in early-onset familial Alzheimer's disease. *Nature.* 1995;375:754–760.

96. Rogaev EI, Sherrington R, Rogaeva EA, et al. Familial Alzheimer's disease in kindreds with missense mutations in a gene on chromosome 1 related to the Alzheimer's disease type 3 gene. *Nature.* 1995;376:775–778.

97. Boyles JK, Zoellner CD, Anderson LJ, et al. A role for apolipoprotein E, apolipoprotein A-I, and low density lipoprotein receptors in cholesterol transport during regeneration and remyelination of the rat sciatic nerve. *J Clin Invest.* 1989;83:1015–1031.

98. Hallman DM, Boerwinkle E, Saha N, et al. The apolipoprotein E polymorphism: a comparison of allele frequencies and effects in nine populations. *Am J Hum Genet.* 1991;49:338–349.

99. Farrer LA, Cupples LA, Haines JL, et al. Effects of age, sex, and ethnicity on the association between apolipoprotein E genotype and Alzheimer disease. A meta-analysis. APOE and Alzheimer Disease Meta Analysis Consortium. *JAMA.* 1997;278:1349–1356.

100. Hyman BT, Gomez-Isla T, Briggs M, et al. Apolipoprotein E and cognitive change in an elderly population. *Ann Neurol.* 1996;40:55–66.

101. Myers RH, Schaefer EJ, Wilson PW, et al. Apolipoprotein E epsilon4 association with dementia in a population-based study: the Framingham study. *Neurology.* 1996;46:673–677.

102. Henderson AS, Easteal S, Jorm AF, et al. Apolipoprotein E allele epsilon 4, dementia, and cognitive decline in a population sample. *Lancet.* 1995;346:1387–1390.

103. Ertekin-Taner N, Graff-Radford N, Younkin LH, et al. Linkage of plasma Abeta42 to a quantitative locus on chromosome 10 in late-onset Alzheimer's disease pedigrees. *Science.* 2000;290:2303–2304.

104. Koo EH, Price DL. The neurobiology of dementia. In: Whitehouse, PJ, ed. *Dementia.* Philadelphia: F.A. Davis Company; 1993:55–91.

105. Terry RD, Masliah E, Hansen LA. Structural basis of the cognitive alterations in Alzheimer Disease. In: Terry, RD, Katzman R, Bick KL, eds. *Alzheimer Disease.* New York: Raven Press, Ltd.; 1994:179–196.

106. Arnold SE, Hyman BT, Flory J, Damasio AR, Van Hoesen GW. The topographical and neuroanatomical distribution of neurofibrillary tangles and neuritic plaques in the cerebral cortex of patients with Alzheimer's disease. *Cereb Cortex.* 1991;1:103–116.

107. Morris JC, Storandt M, McKeel DW J., et al. Cerebral amyloid deposition and diffuse plaques in "normal" aging: evidence for presymptomatic and very mild Alzheimer's disease. *Neurology.* 1996;46:707–719.

108. Price JL, Davis PB, Morris JC, White DL. The distribution of tangles, plaques and related immunohistochemical markers in healthy aging and Alzheimer's disease. *Neurobiol Aging.* 1991;12:295–312.

109. Haroutunian V, Perl DP, Purohit DP, et al. Regional distribution of neuritic plaques in the nondemented elderly and subjects with very mild Alzheimer disease. *Arch Neurol.* 1998;55:1185–1191.

110. Arriagada PV, Growdon JH, Hedley-Whyte ET, Hyman BT. Neurofibrillary tangles but not senile plaques parallel duration and severity of Alzheimer's disease. *Neurology.* 1992;42:631–639.

111. Wolfe MS, Xia W, Ostaszewski BL, et al. Two transmembrane aspartates in presenilin-1 required for presenilin endoproteolysis and gamma-secretase activity. *Nature.* 1999;398:513–517.

112. Duff K, Eckman C, Zehr C, et al. Increased amyloid-beta42(43) in brains of mice expressing mutant presenilin 1. *Nature.* 1996;383:710–713.

113. Vassar R, Bennett BD, Babu-Khan S, et al. Beta-secretase cleavage of Alzheimer's amyloid precursor protein by the transmembrane aspartic protease BACE. *Science.* 1999;286:735–741.

114. Citron M, Diehl TS, Gordon G, et al. Evidence that the 42- and 40-amino acid forms of amyloid beta protein are generated from

the beta-amyloid precursor protein by different protease activities. *Proc Natl Acad Sci U S A.* 1996;93:13170–13175.

115. Walsh DM, Klyubin I, Fadeeva JV, Rowan MJ, Selkoe DJ. Amyloid-beta oligomers: their production, toxicity and therapeutic inhibition. *Biochem Soc Trans.* 2002;30:552–557.

116. Yan SD, Chen X, Fu J, et al. RAGE and amyloid-beta peptide neurotoxicity in Alzheimer's disease. *Nature.* 1996;382:685–691.

117. Neve RL, Robakis NK. Alzheimer's disease: a re-examination of the amyloid hypothesis. *Trends Neurosci.* 1998;21:15–19.

118. Terry RD. The pathogenesis of Alzheimer disease: an alternative to the amyloid hypothesis. *J Neuropathol Exp Neurol.* 1996;55:1023–1025.

119. Pastor P, Roe CM, Villegas A, et al. Apolipoprotein E e4 modifies Alzheimer's disease onset in an E280A PS1 kindred. *Ann Neurol.* 2003;54:163–169.

120. Braak H, Braak E. Neuropathological staging of Alzheimer-related changes. *Acta Neuropathol.* (Berl) 1991;82:239–259.

121. Haroutunian V, Purohit DP, Perl DP, et al. Neurofibrillary tangles in nondemented elderly subjects and mild Alzheimer disease. *Arch Neurol.* 1999;56:713–718.

122. Grundke-Iqbal I, Iqbal K, Tung YC, et al. Abnormal phosphorylation of the microtubule-associated protein tau (tau) in Alzheimer cytoskeletal pathology. *Proc Natl Acad Sci USA.* 1986;83:4913–4917.

123. Spillantini MG, Goedert M. Tau protein pathology in neurodegenerative diseases. *Trends Neurosci.* 1998;21:428–433.

124. Lewis J, Dickson DW, Lin WL, et al. Enhanced neurofibrillary degeneration in transgenic mice expressing mutant tau and APP. *Science.* 2001;293:1487–1491.

125. Price JL, Morris JC. Tangles and plaques in nondemented aging and "preclinical" Alzheimer's disease. *Ann Neurol.* 1999;45:358–368.

126. Mirra SS, Hart MN, Terry RD. Making the diagnosis of Alzheimer's disease. A primer for practicing pathologists. *Arch Pathol Lab Med.* 1993;117:132–144.

127. Hyman BT. New neuropathological criteria for Alzheimer disease. *Arch Neurol.* 1998;55:1174–1176.

128. Ellis RJ, Olichney JM, Thal LJ, et al. Cerebral amyloid angiopathy in the brains of patients with Alzheimer's disease: the CERAD experience, part XV. *Neurology.* 1996;46:1592–1596.

129. Greenberg SM, Vonsattel JP. Diagnosis of cerebral amyloid angiopathy. Sensitivity and specificity of cortical biopsy. *Stroke.* 1997;28:1418–1422.

130. Greenberg SM. Cerebral amyloid angiopathy: prospects for clinical diagnosis and treatment. *Neurology.* 1998;51:690–694.

131. DeKosky ST, Harbaugh RE, Schmitt FA, et al. Cortical biopsy in Alzheimer's disease: diagnostic accuracy and neurochemical, neuropathological, and cognitive correlations. Intraventricular Bethanecol Study Group. *Ann Neurol.* 1992;32:625–632.

132. Davis KL, Mohs RC, Marin D, et al. Cholinergic markers in elderly patients with early signs of Alzheimer disease. *JAMA.* 1999;281:1401–1406.

133. DeKosky ST, Ikonomovic MD, Styren SD, et al. Upregulation of choline acetyltransferase activity in hippocampus and frontal cortex of elderly subjects with mild cognitive impairment. *Ann Neurol.* 2002;51:145–155.

134. Rasool CG, Svendsen CN, Selkoe DJ. Neurofibrillary degeneration of cholinergic and noncholinergic neurons of the basal forebrain in Alzheimer's disease. *Ann Neurol.* 1986;20:482–488.

135. Saper CB, German DC, White CL. Neuronal pathology in the nucleus basalis and associated cell groups in senile dementia of the Alzheimer's type: possible role in cell loss. *Neurology.* 1985;35:1089–1095.

136. Bierer LM, Haroutunian V, Gabriel S, et al. Neurochemical correlates of dementia severity in Alzheimer's disease: relative importance of the cholinergic deficits. *J Neurochem.* 1995;64:749–760.

137. Palmer AM, Stratmann GC, Procter AW, Bowen DM. Possible neurotransmitter basis of behavioral changes in Alzheimer's disease. *Ann Neurol.* 1988;23:616–620.

138. Francis PT, Cross AJ, Bowen DM. Neurotransmitters and neuropeptides. In: Terry, RD, Katzman R, Bick KL, eds. *Alzheimer Disease.* New York: Raven Press, Ltd.; 1994:247–261.

139. Terry RD, Masliah E, Salmon DP, et al. Physical basis of cognitive alterations in Alzheimer's disease: synapse loss is the major correlate of cognitive impairment. *Ann Neurol.* 1991;30:572–580.

140. Doody RS, Stevens JC, Beck C, et al. Practice parameter: management of dementia (an evidence-based review). Report of the Quality Standards Subcommittee of the American Academy of Neurology. *Neurology.* 2001;56:1154–1166.

141. Rogers SL, Farlow MR, Doody RS, Mohs R, Friedhoff LT. A 24-week, double-blind, placebo-controlled trial of donepezil in patients with Alzheimer's disease. *Neurology.* 1998;50:136–145.

142. Burns A, Rossor M, Hecker J, et al. The effects of donepezil in Alzheimer's disease—results from a multinational trial. *Dement Geriatr Cogn Disord.* 1999;10:237–244.

143. Corey-Bloom J, Anand R, Veach J, for the ENA 713 B352 Study Group. A randomized trial evaluating the efficacy and safety of ENA 713 (rivastigmine tartrate), a new acetylcholinesterase inhibitor, in patients with mild to moderately severe Alzheimer's disease. *Int J Geriatric Psychopharmacol.* 1998;1:55–65.

144. Rosler M, Anand R, Cicin-Sain A, et al. Efficacy and safety of rivastigmine in patients with Alzheimer's disease: international randomised controlled trial. *BMJ.* 1999;318:633–640.

145. Raskind MA, Peskind ER, Wessel T, Yuan W. Galantamine in AD: a 6-month randomized, placebo-controlled trial with a 6-month extension. *Neurology.* 2000;54:2261–2268.

146. Tariot PN, Solomon PR, Morris JC, et al. A 5-month, randomized, placebo-controlled trial of galantamine in AD. *Neurology.* 2000;54:2269–2276.

147. Rosen WG, Mohs RC, Davis KL. A new rating scale for Alzheimer's disease. *Am J Psychiatry.* 1984;141:1356–1364.

148. Knopman DS, Knapp MJ, Gracon SI, Davis CS. The Clinician Interview-Based Impression (CIBI): a clinician's global change rating scale in Alzheimer's disease. *Neurology.* 1994;44:2315–2321.

149. Schneider LS, Olin JT, Doody RS, et al. Validity and reliability of the Alzheimer's Disease Cooperative Study—Clinical Global Impression of Change. The Alzheimer's Disease Cooperative Study. *Alzheimer Dis Assoc Disord.* 1997;11(Suppl 2):S22–32.

150. Rogers SL, Friedhoff LT. Long-term efficacy and safety of donepezil in the treatment of Alzheimer's disease: an interim analysis of the results of a US multicentre open label extension study. *Eur Neuropsychopharmacol.* 1998;8:67–75.

151. Farlow M, Anand R, Messina J, Hartman R, Veach J. A 52-week study of the efficacy of rivastigmine in patients with mild to moderately severe Alzheimer's disease. *Eur Neurol.* 2000;44:236–241.

152. Mohs RC, Doody RS, Morris JC, et al. A 1-year, placebo-controlled preservation of function survival study of donepezil in AD patients. *Neurology.* 2001;57:481–488.

153. Sano M, Ernesto C, Thomas RG, et al. A controlled trial of selegiline, alpha-tocopherol, or both as treatment for Alzheimer's disease. The Alzheimer's Disease Cooperative Study. *N Engl J Med.* 1997;336:1216–1222.

154. Reisberg B, Doody R, Stoffler A, et al. Memantine in moderate-to-severe Alzheimer's disease. *N Engl J Med.* 2003;348:1333–1341.

155. Levy ML, Cummings JL, Fairbanks LA, et al. Longitudinal assessment of symptoms of depression, agitation, and psychosis in 181 patients with Alzheimer's disease. *Am J Psychiatry.* 1986;153:1438–1443.

156. Forsell Y, Winblad B. Major depression in a population of demented and nondemented older people: prevalence and correlates. *J Am Geriatr Soc.* 1998;46:27–30.

157. Weiner MF, Edland SD, Luszczynska H. Prevalence and incidence of major depression in Alzheimer's disease. *Am J Psychiatry.* 1994;151:1006–1009.

158. Teri L, Wagner AW. Assessment of depression in patients with Alzheimer's disease: concordance among informants. *Psychol Aging.* 1991;6:280–285.

159. Treatment of special populations with the atypical antipsychotics. Collaborative Working Group on Clinical Trial Evaluations. *J Clin Psychiatry.* 1998;59(Suppl 12):46–52.

160. Heyman A, Peterson B, Fillenbaum G, Pieper C. Predictors of time to institutionalization of patients with Alzheimer's disease: the CERAD experience. Part XVII. *Neurology.* 1997;48:1304–1309.

161. Severson MA, Smith GE, Tangalos EG, et al. Patterns and predictors of institutionalization in community-based dementia patients. *J Am Geriatr Soc.* 1994;42:181–185.

162. Welch HG, Walsh JS, Larson EB. The cost of institutional care in Alzheimer's disease: nursing home and hospital use in a prospective cohort. *J Am Geriatr Soc.* 1992;40:221–224.

163. Schneider LS. Tracking dementia by the IMC and the MMSE. *J Am Geriatr Soc.* 1992;40:537–538.

164. Knopman D, Gracon S. Observations on the short-term "natural history" of probable Alzheimer's disease in a controlled clinical trial. *Neurology.* 1994;44:260–265.

165. Morris JC, Edland S, Clark C, et al. The consortium to establish a registry for Alzheimer's disease (CERAD). Part IV. Rates of cognitive change in the longitudinal assessment of probable Alzheimer's disease. *Neurology.* 1993;43:2457–2465.

166. Chui HC, Lyness SA, Sobel E, Schneider LS. Extrapyramidal signs and psychiatric symptoms predict faster cognitive decline in Alzheimer's disease. *Arch Neurol.* 1994;51:676–681.

167. Olichney JM, Galasko D, Salmon DP, et al. Cognitive decline is faster in Lewy body variant than in Alzheimer's disease. *Neurology.* 1998;51:351–357.

168. Heyman A, Peterson B, Fillenbaum G, Pieper C. The consortium to establish a registry for Alzheimer's disease (CERAD). Part XIV: demographic and clinical predictors of survival in patients with Alzheimer's disease. *Neurology.* 1996;46:656–660.

169. Wolfson C, Wolfson DB, Asgharian M, et al. A reevaluation of the duration of survival after the onset of dementia. *N Engl J Med.* 2001;344:1111–1116.

170. Helmer C, Joly P, Letenneur L, Commenges D, Dartigues JF. Mortality with dementia: results from a French prospective community-based cohort. *Am J Epidemiol.* 2001;154:642–648.

171. Beard CM, Kokmen E, Sigler C, et al. Cause of death in Alzheimer's disease. *Ann Epidemiol.* 1996;6:195–200.

172. Petersen RC, Smith GE, Ivnik RJ, et al. Apolipoprotein E status as a predictor of the development of Alzheimer's disease in memory-impaired individuals. *JAMA.* 1995;273:1274–1278.

173. Elias MF, Beiser A, Wolf PA, et al. The preclinical phase of Alzheimer disease: a 22-year prospective study of the Framingham cohort. *Arch Neurol.* 2000;57:808–813.

174. Reiman EM, Caselli RJ, Yun LS, et al. Preclinical evidence of Alzheimer's disease in persons homozygous for the epsilon 4 allele for apolipoprotein E. *N Engl J Med.* 1996;334:752–758.

175. Small GW, Mazziotta JC, Collins MT, et al. Apolipoprotein E type 4 allele and cerebral glucose metabolism in relatives at risk for familial Alzheimer disease. *JAMA.* 1995;273:942–947.

176. Petersen RC, Smith GE, Waring SC, et al. Mild cognitive impairment: clinical characterization and outcome. *Arch Neurol.* 1999;56:303–308.

177. Tabert MH, Albert SM, Borukhova-Milov L, et al. Functional deficits in patients with mild cognitive impairment: prediction of AD. *Neurology.* 2002;58:758–764.

178. Jack CR, Petersen RC, Xu YC, et al. Prediction of AD with MRI-based hippocampal volume in mild cognitive impairment. *Neurology.* 1999;52:1397–1403.

179. Visser PJ, Verhey FR, Hofman PA, Scheltens P, Jolles J. Medial temporal lobe atrophy predicts Alzheimer's disease in patients with minor cognitive impairment. *J Neurol Neurosurg Psychiatry.* 2002;72:491–497.

180. Berent S, Giordani B, Foster N, et al. Neuropsychological function and cerebral glucose utilization in isolated memory impairment and Alzheimer's disease. *J Psychiatr Res.* 1999;33: 7–16.

181. Hughes CP, Berg L, Danziger WL, Coben LA, Martin RL. A new clinical scale for the staging of dementia. *Br J Psychiatry.* 1982;140:566–572.

182. Reisberg B, Ferris SH, de Leon MJ, Crook T. The Global Deterioration Scale for assessment of primary degenerative dementia. *Am J Psychiatry.* 1982;139:1136–1139.

183. Peavy GM, Salmon DP, Rice VA, et al. Neuropsychological assessment of severely demented elderly: the severe cognitive impairment profile. *Arch Neurol.* 1996;53:367–372.

184. Volicer L, Hurley AC, Lathi DC, Kowall NW. Measurement of severity in advanced Alzheimer's disease. *J Gerontol.* 1994;49: M223–226.

185. Mendez MF, Catanzaro P, Doss RC, Arguello R, Frey WH II. Seizures in Alzheimer's disease: clinicopathologic study. *J Geriatr Psychiatry Neurol.* 1994;7:230–233.

186. Drachman DA, Swearer JM. Driving and Alzheimer's disease: the risk of crashes. *Neurology.* 1993;43:2448–2456.

187. Stutts JC. Do older drivers with visual and cognitive impairments drive less? *J Am Geriatr Soc.* 1998;46:854–861.

188. Lundberg C, Johansson K, Ball K, et al. Dementia and driving: an attempt at consensus. *Alzheimer Dis Assoc Disord.* 1997;11:28–37.

189. Dubinsky RM, Stein AC, Lyons K. Practice parameter: risk of driving and Alzheimer's disease (an evidence-based review): report of the Quality Standards Subcommittee of the American Academy of Neurology. *Neurology.* 2000;54:2205–2211.

190. Fox GK, Bowden SC, Bashford GM, Smith DS. Alzheimer's disease and driving: prediction and assessment of driving performance. *J Am Geriatr Soc.* 1997;45:949–953.

191. Carr DB, LaBarge E, Dunnigan K, Storandt M. Differentiating drivers with dementia of the Alzheimer type from healthy older persons with a Traffic Sign Naming test. *J Gerontol A Biol Sci Med Sci.* 1998;53:M135–139.

192. Hunt LA, Murphy CF, Carr D, et al. Reliability of the Washington University Road Test. A performance-based assessment for drivers with dementia of the Alzheimer type. *Arch Neurol.* 1997;54:707–712.

193. Rizzo M, McGehee DV, Dawson JD, Anderson SN. Simulated car crashes at intersections in drivers with Alzheimer disease. *Alzheimer Dis Assoc Disord.* 2001;15:10–20.

194. Gwyther LP, George LK. Caregivers for dementia patients: complex determinants of well-being and burden. *Gerontologist.* 1986;26:245–247.

195. Schulz R, O'Brien AT, Bookwala J, Fleissner K. Psychiatric and physical morbidity effects of dementia caregiving: prevalence, correlates, and causes. *Gerontologist.* 1995;35:771–791.

196. Gwyther LP. Social issues of the Alzheimer's patient and family. *Am J Med.* 1998;104:17S-21S; discussion 39S-42S.

197. Steele CD. Management of the family. In Burns A, Levy R, eds. *Dementia.* London: Chapman and Hall Medical. 1994:541– 552.

198. Mittelman MS, Ferris SH, Shulman E, Steinberg G, Levin B. A family intervention to delay nursing home placement of patients with Alzheimer disease. A randomized controlled trial. *JAMA.* 1996;276:1725–1731.

199. Drickamer MA, Lachs MS. Should patients with Alzheimer's disease be told their diagnosis? *N Engl J Med.* 1992;326:947–951.

200. Maguire CP, Kirby M, Coen R, et al. Family members' attitudes toward telling the patient with Alzheimer's disease their diagnosis. *BMJ.* 1996;313:529–530.

Vascular Dementia

21

Helen Lavretsky   Helena C. Chui

The contribution of cerebrovascular disease (CVD) and stroke to cognitive impairment and behavioral disturbances has long been recognized (1,2). The understanding of this relationship has evolved considerably since the 1960s, however, when it was widely believed that CVD was a rare cause of dementia and that senile dementia was responsible for most cases of dementia in the elderly (3). A decade later, research found that some people develop dementia due not to arteriosclerosis of brain vasculature, but rather as a consequence of a series of strokes affecting different brain regions, and the term *multi-infarct dementia* was introduced (4). In the 1990s, it also became clear that several other mechanisms (e.g., ischemic white matter lesions, lacunes) may underlie cerebrovascular damage which culminates in cognitive decline; therefore, the broader term *vascular dementia* (VaD) was adopted (5). VaD may be the second most common type of dementia following Alzheimer's Disease (AD), accounting for up to 20% of dementia cases (6,7). Similar to AD, VaD is commonly associated with behavioral disturbances (8,9).

DEFINITION AND CLASSIFICATION

VaD may be defined as a clinical syndrome of acquired intellectual impairment resulting from brain injury due to a cerebrovascular disorder. Clinicians wishing to formally diagnose VaD have several sets of criteria available, although four dominate. These include diagnostic criteria from the National Institute of Neurological Disorders and Stroke-Alzheimer Neurological Disorders and the Association Internationale pour la Recherche et L'Enseignment en Neurosciences (NINDS-AIREN) (5), the Alzheimer's Disease Diagnostic Treatment Centers (ADDTC), the International Classification of Mental and Behavioral Disorders, 10th Edition (ICD-10) (10), and the American Psychiatric Association Diagnostic and Statistical Manual of Mental Disorders, 4th Edition, Text Revision (DSM-IV-TR) (11).

Each set of diagnostic criteria requires identification of a so-called vascular profile in clinical presentation, along with neuroimaging of vascular lesions. Although the criteria are not interchangeable, they share common features. All require that dementia be present and assume that cognitive impairment was caused by cerebral infarcts (12). The criteria for dementia are modeled after those of AD, and are based on the consensus of experts. The probability of VaD diagnosis may be affected by which criteria are used; for example, Chui and colleagues (13) found that the DSM-IV-TR and modified Hachinski Ischemia Score (HIS) criteria were the most liberal, ADDTC and the original HIS were intermediate (14), and NINDS-AIREN criteria were the most conservative. Wetterling and colleagues found that overlap of VaD diagnoses using the DSM-IV-TR and the ICD-10 criteria was about 50% (15). Diagnostic criteria for VaD are summarized in Table 21-1.

VaD may be classified by underlying CVD or stroke according to location (cortical, deep or periventricular white matter, basal ganglia, thalamus), size (volume), vascular distribution (large, small, or microvessel), severity (chronic ischemia versus infarction), and etiology (embolism, atherosclerosis, arteriosclerosis, cerebral amyloid angiopathy, and hypoperfusion) of the lesions (16,17). Even small, deep, strategic infarcts may produce dementia due to a more global effect on cortical deactivation. Recent observations suggest that the risk of subsequent dementia is sharply increased in patients with lacunar strokes rather than macroinfarction (18). Indeed, diffuse white matter changes, microinfarction (<20 mL volume) or microvascular disease, hypoperfusion rather than macroinfarction, functional tissue loss, and strategic site of lesion appear to be significant predictors of cognitive decline or dementia in patients with CVD (18).

Another major classification of VaD divides cortical from subcortical disease. Cortical VaD results from single or multiple infarcts to cerebral cortex. Associated neurologic impairment is most often characterized by hemiplegia or

TABLE 21-1

GENERAL DIAGNOSTIC CRITERIA FOR VASCULAR DEMENTIA

Major diagnostic criterion sets for vascular dementia suggest the following requirements:

1. Dementia involving memory impairment and one (or more) of the following cognitive disturbances: aphasia (language disturbance), apraxia (impaired ability to carry out motor activities despite intact motor function), agnosia (impaired ability to recognize or identify objects despite intact sensory function), and executive dysfunction (i.e., deficits in planning, organizing, abstracting) with significant, resultant impairment of social and functional capabilities;
2. Evidence of cerebrovascular disease provided by patient history (e.g., vascular risk factors), the presence of focal neurologic findings (e.g., gait disturbance, unsteadiness and frequent falls, urinary incontinence, frontal lobe impairment, psychomotor retardation, extrapyramidal symptoms, and pseudobulbar palsy), and/or the results of brain imaging (e.g., single or multiple cortical, subcortical, or white matter lesions) that are believed to be related to the cognitive impairment; and
3. A causal relationship between elements 1 and 2, as determined based on a temporal relationship between stroke and dementia, an abrupt or stepwise decline in cognitive function or a fluctuating course, and/or brain imaging findings documenting damage to brain structures relevant to cognitive function.

NINDS-AIREN Diagnostic criteria further specify the probability of diagnosis as unlikely, possible, probable, and definite, based on the availability of confirming history and evidence of cerebrovascular disease that is judged to be etiologically related to the dementia.

NINDS-AIREN, National Institute of Neurological, Communicative Disorders and Stroke-Alzheimer Neurological Disorders Stroke-Association Internationale pour la Recherche et l'Enseignement en Neurosciences.
Adapted from References 5, 54, and 55.

paresis contralateral to the lesion. The exact form of cognitive impairment due to cortical injury depends on whether the dominant or nondominant hemisphere is affected (most individuals are left hemisphere dominant), and then on the particular lobe(s) affected: frontal, parietal, occipital, or temporal. Subcortical VaD is most commonly due to lacunar strokes that occur in the basal ganglia (putamen, caudate nucleus, globus pallidus, and several brainstem nuclei), thalamus, and internal capsule. Risk factors include older age, history of prior stroke, hypertension, diabetes mellitus, tobacco use, elevated levels of homocysteine and fibrinogen, and other conditions that can cause brain hypoperfusion such as obstructive sleep apnea, congestive heart failure, cardiac arrhythmias, and orthostatic hypotension (19,20).

Clinically, the dementia associated with subcortical lacunar infarction is characterized by slowing of information processing, memory deficits, impaired executive functions, gait dysfunction, and alterations in personality and affect. Common findings from neurological examination of subcortical VaD include parkinsonism with gait disturbances, dysarthria, pseudobulbar palsy, and incontinence (19). Apathy, depression, and psychosis are particularly common in subcortical VaD. In fact, such behavioral changes may initially be more prominent than cognitive changes.

Binswanger's disease, also known as *subcortical arteriosclerotic encephalopathy* or *ischemic periventricular leukoencephalopathy*, is a slowly progressive subcortical VaD associated with chronic hypertension. It is due to widespread, incomplete infarction of white matter due to critical stenosis of medullary arterioles and hypoperfusion (19). Symptoms of Binswanger's disease include motor and cognitive slowing, forgetfulness, dysarthria, mood changes, urinary problems, and short-stepped gait. These manifestations probably result from ischemic interruption of parallel circuits from the prefrontal cortex to the basal ganglia and corresponding thalamocortical connections. Characteristic magnetic resonance imaging (MRI) findings are white matter hyperintensities in periventricular and deep white matter regions (seen in T2-weighted images).

Another less common form of subcortical VaD is *cerebral autosomal dominant arteriopathy with subcortical infarcts and leukoencephalopathy* (CADASIL), a dominant, inherited disorder usually striking in the mid-40s and causing recurrent strokes and eventual VaD. Associated histopathology is fairly consistent, typically demonstrating granular thickening of cerebral arterioles. CADASIL has been localized to chromosome 19, and the notch 3 gene has been implicated in its etiology. Clinically, CADASIL may progress over 20 years and involve transient ischemic attacks and strokes, focal neurologic symptoms, headaches, mood disorders, and seizures, in addition to dementia. Neuropsychiatric symptoms and changes in personality and cognition frequently predominate over focal ischemic symptoms in the victims of this rare disorder (21). Frequency of asymptomatic, new subcortical infarcts and leukoencephalopathy found on diffusion-weighted MRI may serve as a surrogate marker of disease progression (22).

Familial cerebral amyloid angiopathies can result from genetic mutations and are characterized by the deposition of beta amyloid protein in cerebral blood vessels, resulting in recurrent lobar hemorrhages, ischemic strokes, and evolving dementia. Other disorders potentially leading to vascular cognitive impairment and dementia include mitochondrial disorders, familial occipital calcifications, sickle cell disease, and Fabry's disease (23).

The concept of *mixed dementia* must be included under a broad classification of VaD. Virtually 90% of the elderly with late-onset dementia exhibit neuropathological features consistent with AD, VaD, or dementia with Lewy bodies (DLB), alone and in combination. Longitudinal studies suggest a strong association between vascular factors predisposing to CVD and AD. Stroke or severe transient ischemic attacks are three times more likely to increase the risk for acquiring AD. Vascular risk factors such as hypertension, atrial fibrillation, carotid thickening, aortic sclerosis, and diabetes mellitus can substantially increase the risk for AD in people older than 60. Furthermore, cerebrovascular and neurodegenerative pathologies may be additive in the way they influence clinical presentation. In a proposed common pathway, brain vascular injury or systemic vascular disease may initiate hypoperfusion, resulting in cerebral changes that in turn can yield VaD or AD, depending upon the duration and degree of insult (17).

In addition to vascular injury, altered cholesterol synthesis is another common risk factor for both AD and VaD (24). The enzymatic conversion of cerebral cholesterol to 24S-hydroxycholesterol, or cerebrosterol, which readily crosses the blood-brain barrier, is the major pathway for its elimination (24). Like other oxysteroids, 24S-hydroxycholesterol normally is efficiently converted into bile acids or excreted in bile in its sulfated and glucuronidated form. Concentrations of 24S-hydroxycholesterol in plasma and cerebrospinal fluid are significantly higher in both AD and VaD during early stages of the disease compared to healthy subjects. Variations in genetic background, time of disease onset, and severity of dementia are potential sources of variance.

Behavioral and neuropsychiatric disturbances in vascular and mixed dementias include a wide range of symptoms and syndromes, ranging from impairments in mood and motivation to agitation and psychosis. To date there have been relatively few studies attempting to elucidate differences in the behavioral symptoms between AD and VaD (25).

VaD VERSUS AD

Dementia resulting from CVD certainly lies along a continuum, a fact that adds to the complexity of differential diagnosis. The term *vascular cognitive impairment* (VCI) refers to this continuum of cognitive disorders of vascular origin, and describes a heterogeneous syndrome of cognitive impairment in which cerebrovascular or cardiovascular causes are implicated (26). Three broad clinical subtypes are included: VCI that does not meet dementia criteria, mixed AD/VaD, and VaD. These can be further classified radiographically as showing any cortical or subcortical infarctions, or predominantly white matter changes. Jorm and colleagues reported that the presence of cerebrovascular risk factors, such as previous stroke and focal neurological signs, may help distinguish VaD from AD (27).

Despite the relative heterogeneity of VaD pathology and diagnostic criteria used, there are measurable group differences in neuropsychological deficits in AD and VaD (28–31). Although frontal system pathology is common in AD, VaD, and many other degenerative dementias, VaD disproportionately affects frontal systems (32–35). Subcortical

lesions in VaD indirectly affect frontal cortical metabolism, particularly if they include lacunar infarctions of the basal ganglia and thalamus. Aneurysm of the anterior communicating artery is another cause of executive dysfunction, resulting in not only cognitive but also functional impairment with respect to activities of daily living (36,37).

The two groups do not differ significantly on language tests, unless discrete language centers are impaired by stroke. No differences have been observed in constructional abilities, memory registration, conceptual function, visual perception, and attention and tracking. There is insufficient evidence to draw conclusions on the cognitive domains of general intelligence, nonverbal long-term memory, orientation, and tactile perception. VaD patients generally have more psychomotor retardation and motor dysfunction compared to AD patients, which can be attributed to disruption of motor association pathways (31).

EPIDEMIOLOGY

Given the higher prevalence range for AD and the more variable range for DLB, VaD in all of its forms is generally viewed as the second most common form of dementia, likely accounting for 10% to 20% of dementia cases (3,4). However, estimates of the prevalence of VaD have varied widely due to differences in sampling methods, assessment techniques, and diagnostic paradigms, as well as true differences among populations. In community-based studies, the proportion of dementia patients considered to have VaD have ranged from 9% in the Framingham study (34) to greater than 50% in Japanese and Chinese studies (38,39). In two autopsy case series, AD was the primary basis for dementia in 25% of cases, while "arteriosclerosis" was the basis in 18% of cases (40,41).

Other epidemiological studies have looked at community samples to determine general rates of dementia, including variance by race and gender (42,43). For example, the East Baltimore Mental Health Survey was conducted in 1981 as part of the Epidemiological Catchment Area Program (42). This survey provided an opportunity to assess the prevalence of dementia in a community-based, cross-sectional sample. Detailed clinical evaluation resulted in an overall prevalence of dementia of 4.5% in individuals 65 and older. Results found community prevalence rates of 2% for AD, 2% for VaD, and 0.5% for mixed dementia. Greater rates of dementia were seen in females, non-Caucasians, and individuals with lower educational levels. As the level of education increased in the sample, the prevalence of AD increased and that of VaD decreased (42).

ASSESSMENT OF VaD

The general dementia workup, described elsewhere in this text, will apply to individuals with potential VaD. Diagnosis of VaD relies upon establishing a history of vascular risk

TABLE 21-2
THE HACHINSKI ISCHEMIC SCALE

Give the patient the number of points indicated for the presence of each feature:

Feature	Points
Abrupt onset	2
Stepwise deterioration	1
Fluctuating course	2
Nocturnal confusion	1
Relative preservation of personality	1
Depression	1
Somatic complaints	1
Emotional incontinence	1
History or presence of hypertension	1
History of strokes	2
Evidence of associated atherosclerosis	1
Focal neurological symptoms	2
Focal neurological signs	2

Scoring:
0 to 4 Dementia more consistent with Alzheimer's disease
5 to 6 Diagnosis unclear based on scale
≥7 More consistent with vascular dementia

Adapted from Reference 14.

factors, the presence of focal neurologic signs, and vascular lesions on neuroimaging. Careful neurological examination is particularly important when brain damage due to CVD or stroke has resulted in very subtle and previously undetected neurological signs. Official nomenclature of stroke does recognize asymptomatic or "silent" strokes, despite the fact that they produce subtle neurological signs and symptoms (44–47). Many of the factors that point to a diagnosis of VaD have been integrated into the useful HIS clinical scale (48). The scale, listed in Table 21-2, assigns a score to each variable, so that higher scores are more consistent with VaD. Much of the information on the HIS scale can be obtained with a clinical interview.

Routine blood values are part of every dementia workup, but there are no laboratory tests specific to VaD. Likewise, there are no specific genetic tests for AD, despite the fact that an increased frequency of the apolipoprotein E-4 (APOE-4) allele has been reported in both AD and VaD, particularly in middle-aged and older persons with atherosclerosis (49–52). Because APOE-4 is involved in the growth, maintenance, and repair of myelin and neuronal membranes during development and after injury, it may also be involved in ischemic white matter disease, seen commonly in both VaD and AD. Despite this association, genetic testing is not routinely recommended in dementia assessment, since it will not necessarily improve diagnostic certainty.

Both clinical history and neuropsychological testing will help distinguish VaD from AD, based on many of the differences discussed earlier, and particularly the greater tendency to see frontal lobe and executive function disturbances in VaD. Another key component to assessment is differentiating between cortical and subcortical VaD. As noted earlier, subcortical VaD typically associated with lacunar infarcts is a common but not always immediately recognized form of VaD (53). Many of the key differences are presented in Table 21-3, based on work by Cummings and Mabler (54,55).

Structural neuroimaging studies, such as computed tomography (CT) and MRI, are necessary to identify CVD and previous stroke. However, it is not always possible to establish an absolute link between CT or MRI findings and VaD, especially with findings such as cerebral atrophy, ventricular enlargement, and smaller or more diffuse cortical damage. One of the most controversial MRI findings is the presence of white matter hyperintensities, or *leukoariosis*. White matter hyperintensities are common subcortical findings, appearing in the brains of 30% to 80% of older individuals, including those with VaD and AD. Although their exact nature is not certain, they are believed to represent small areas of ischemic damage. Even when present, however, they are not always associated with cognitive impairment (56). Functional scans, including positron emission tomography (PET) and functional MRI, are evolving as more useful means to establish dementia diagnosis, but more research is needed to refine their use for VaD.

PSYCHIATRIC SYMPTOMS IN VASCULAR DEMENTIA

Psychiatric symptoms are common in all forms of VaD and in mixed dementias. They stem from a variety of sources, including primary cerebrovascular damage to neural circuits and nuclei that control mood and behavior (especially frontal lobe, subcortical, and limbic structures), comorbid medical and psychiatric disorders, and the effects of medications. In a case-control study, the most frequent psychiatric symptoms as reported by caregivers of patients with VaD were irritability (57.3%), apathy (44.4%), insomnia (43.6%), agitation (40.7%), impatience (37%), and emotional lability (28.3%) (57). Other common psychological and behavioral manifestations of VaD include depression, anxiety, catastrophic reaction, aggression, agitation, psychosis, and disturbances of sleep, appetite, and sexual functioning (58–64). Regardless of exact prevalence, these psychological and behavioral disturbances are common to both VaD and AD patients, especially when matched by age and dementia severity (65). Several of these disorders will be highlighted. For more information, see the appropriate chapters in this textbook.

Depression

The link between depressive disorders and other behavioral symptoms and CVD has been recognized since the mid 19th century (1). As long ago as 1843, Durand-Fardel

TABLE 21-3

CORTICAL VERSUS SUBCORTICAL DEMENTIA

Feature	Cortical Dementia	Subcortical Dementia
Memory	+++Memory impairment	++Memory impairment
Cognition	Aphasia, apraxia, and agnosia ++Executive dysfunction	Slowed cognitive processing Disruptions in arousal and attention +++Executive dysfunction
Motor Behavior	Apraxia Later onset and less prominent motor disturbances	Prominent psychomotor retardation Dysarthric speech, gait disturbances, Parkinsonism and other movement disorders
Motivation	++Apathy	+++Apathy
Mood	++Depression	+++Depression
Pathology	Primary damage to neocortex and hippocampus	Primary damage to deep gray matter and white matter structures, including the thalamus, basal ganglia, brain stem nuclei, and frontal lobe projections

Data derived from References 54 and 55.

reported irritability and depression to be common acute sequelae of strokes (66). In 1926, Guilarovsky suggested that the predominance of affective symptoms in the elderly was due to "cerebro-arteriosclerotic" changes (67). Later, Mayer-Gross, Slater, and Roth suggested that sustained depressive symptoms occurred in patients with atherosclerosis more often than by chance alone (67).

Depression following vascular injury to the cerebral hemispheres is now a well-recognized clinical entity, and is seen in 20% to 50% of individuals in the first year post-stroke (68–70). Minor depression has been reported in 10% to 30% of patients following stroke (70–72). Although these rates seem high, Primeau concluded from a review of the literature that depression may be as common in patients with stroke as in the elderly with other physical illnesses (73). In VaD, severe depression occurs in about 25% of cases and clinically significant depression occurs in about 60%, which is over four times the occurrence rate seen in AD (6). Several studies have suggested that the increased depression seen in VaD might be related to impairment in frontal and frontal-subcortical circuits (74,75).

There is growing evidence that depression may also affect brain vasculature and increase the likelihood of stroke in patients with vascular risk factors or disease (76,77). One study found that depressed elderly with hypertension were two to three times more likely to suffer from stroke than nondepressed, hypertensive patients (77). These data support the idea of aggressive treatment of depression in VaD as a potential preventative strategy.

The location of a stroke may influence the course of depression, with subcortical basal ganglia and brainstem lesions associated with significantly shorter-duration depressions than cortical lesions (78). Several studies have replicated the relationship between lesion location and post-stroke depression (69,70,79). Robinson and Szetela found an inverse correlation between severity of depression and the distance of the lesion from the left frontal pole in patients with subacute stroke (80). Major depression was significantly more frequent among patients with left anterior lesions than any other lesion location. However, there is some disagreement on the role of laterality in development of depression. Bolla-Willson and colleagues found no relationship between left anterior lesions and depression (81). They attributed this discrepancy to the fact that their study excluded patients with any language disorder. Herrmann and colleagues studied a group of German stroke patients selected as having a single demarcated unilateral infarct (82). They found no significant difference in depression-rating scores between patients with right and left hemisphere infarcts, and no correlation between severity of depression and the anterior location of infarct. Starkstein has suggested that the etiology of depression may differ in right versus left hemisphere stroke (83). One of his studies indicated that lesions of the left basal ganglia resulted in significantly greater depression than lesions of the right basal ganglia or of the left or right thalamus (84). The relevance of cortical-subcortical connections was demonstrated by Sultzer and colleagues, who reported that cortical metabolic dysfunction identified by PET scans in VaD patients was related to subcortical ischemic lesions identified on MRI (85).

Although the location of cerebrovascular damage is certainly important in the pathophysiology of depression, it may not be an exclusive etiological factor. The heterogeneity in the distribution of vascular lesions makes it difficult to attribute depressive symptoms to any particular lesion, or to develop a unifying pathogenetic model. Other factors, including individual and family history of depression, personal vulnerability, life stresses before and after stroke, and physical and social impairment due to post-stroke neurological deficits may also contribute to the development of depression (86).

Apathy

Apathy often occurs following stroke and is related in large degree to lesion location (59,87–93). Apathy is defined as diminished motivation not attributable to decreased levels of consciousness, cognitive impairment, or emotional distress. Motivation denotes that aspect of behavior concerned with the initiation, direction, and intensity of goal-directed behavior (90–92). Diminished motivation may affect motor (e.g., lack of initiative), cognitive (e.g., lack of interest), and emotional aspects of behavior (e.g., flat affect, indifference) (90–92). Motivational circuitry of the brain includes such important structures as the nucleus accumbens, ventral pallidum, and ventral tegmental area. These structures give to and receive projections from the amygdala, hippocampus, basal ganglia, motor cortex, and anterior cingulate. These circuits provide different components of motivation, including motivational working memory, cognitive coloring, and reward memory. Any interruption within these circuits will produce disorders of motivation.

Contrary to common beliefs, apathy is not a depressive equivalent (94,95). Like depression, apathy has validity as both a syndrome and a dimension of behavior (90–92). Diagnosis of apathy depends on detecting simultaneous diminution in goal-related actions, thoughts, and emotional responses. *Abulia* is a more profound state of psychomotor retardation and apathy characterized by flat affect, reduced motor responses, fixed gaze, blank face, perseveration, and lack of awareness of having the condition (96). Abulia can result from strokes that disrupt fronto-subcortical pathways, such as anterior cingulate and capsular lesions (59).

Differentiating the syndromes of apathy and depression is sometimes difficult because of overlapping or coexisting clinical features. For example, anhedonia, psychomotor retardation, and bradyphrenia (slowed thinking) may be features of both depression and apathy. During clinical interviews, however, the emotional responses of depressed patients may be more unpleasant, negative, and dysphoric, while apathetic patients tend to show attenuated positive and negative responses (92).

Mania

Mania may arise after stroke and represent a secondary mood disorder, or may be a continuation of a long-standing bipolar disorder that has become destabilized by cerebral damage. Mania is characterized by elevated mood, increased irritability, motor hyperactivity, sleep and appetite disturbance, increases in energy and libido, and inappropriate social and sexual behavior. Mood-congruent delusions and hallucinations may occur. There are very little data pertaining specifically to VaD, although some studies indicate prevalence rates of 1% to 2% (97). Manic-like symptoms appear to be associated more frequently with right-sided lesions, particularly right thalamic lesions (41,98–100).

Anxiety Disorders

Although anxiety disorders are common in VaD, with prevalence rates ranging from 17% to 38%, they have received far less attention than depression. This may be due to the fact that there is a less reliable relationship between stroke localization and symptoms of anxiety. Anxiety is most frequently experienced during the first year after stroke (101). Several studies have suggested a significant relationship between generalized anxiety disorder (GAD) and CVD (102–104). GAD after stroke is a common and long-lasting affliction that substantially interferes with social life and functional recovery. In a population-based cohort of 80 patients with acute stroke, the prevalence of GAD was about 28%, and this number did not change over 3 years of follow-up (105). At 1 year, only 23% of patients with GAD had recovered, and those who did not recover were at risk for development of chronic anxiety. Comorbidity with major depression was high and seemed to worsen the prognosis of depression. At the acute stage after stroke, GAD plus depression was associated with left hemispheric lesions. Anxiety disorder without depression may be associated with right posterior lesions in stroke patients and, in general, anxiety appears to be more common with cortical rather than subcortical lesions (99,106).

Obsessive and compulsive symptoms, or frank obsessive-compulsive disorder (OCD), may develop in VaD following basal ganglia strokes and striatal lesions, with predominance of combined bilateral or unilateral lesions of the caudate and putamen nuclei (107). Binswanger's disease has been associated with greater obsessive and compulsive behaviors than AD. The demented subjects with obsessive compulsive symptoms typically have no awareness of their behaviors, unlike patients with idiopathic OCD (108).

Emotional Lability

Emotional lability after stroke has a number of names, including pathological crying (or laughing, in some cases), emotional incontinence, and pseudobulbar palsy. These states mimic depression and are often diagnosed as such, even though patients will deny feeling sad and will not manifest other symptoms of depression. Ross has suggested that spontaneous weeping is a form of *aprosodia*, or inability to express emotion (109).

Agitation and Psychosis

Various forms of agitation, including anger, irritability, hostility, and aggression are common after stroke and in VaD (41). Agitation is seen more commonly following damage to areas of the brain that have the greatest involvement in behavioral control, including the frontal and temporal lobes, and limbic structures such as the amygdala, hypothalamus, and cingulum (41). Reductions in key neurotransmitters such as serotonin, gamma amino butyric acid and acetylcholine may also lead to increased impulsivity and agitation.

Psychosis is also seen frequently in VaD, usually associated with agitation, and may be characterized by delusions (seen in 8% to 50% of affected individuals), delusional misidentifications (19% to 30%), and visual hallucinations (14% to 60%) (110). Psychotic symptoms have been associated with lesions in temporo-parietal and temporo-parietal-occipital cortical regions, deep gray matter, and frontal white matter ischemic lesions (111).

TREATMENT OF VASCULAR DEMENTIA

Once VaD has been diagnosed, a first step in treatment is to prevent, to the greatest degree possible, further cerebrovascular damage. Known vascular risk factors to be controlled include hypertension, diabetes mellitus, smoking, alcohol abuse, atrial fibrillation, obesity, and hyperlipidemia. All can be effectively controlled in the presymptomatic or mildly symptomatic stages. In particular, anticoagulation can prevent embolic strokes due to atrial fibrillation. In a study of low-dose aspirin and low-intensity oral anticoagulation in men at risk for cardiovascular disease, test scores measuring verbal fluency and mental flexibility were significantly better in patients taking antithrombotic medications (especially aspirin) than those taking placebo (112). Caution with anticoagulant therapy is needed in those individuals at risk for cerebral hemorrhage. Reduction in cholesterol levels using statin medications has been used as a preventive technique for cardiovascular disease, and may play a role in reducing the incidence of stroke and VaD (21,113,114).

Acetylcholinesterase Inhibitors

Beyond prevention of stroke, growing evidence suggests that the same medications used in AD to maintain or boost acetylcholine (ACh) levels in the brain may play an important role in temporarily improving and/or stabilizing cognitive, functional, and behavioral impairment seen in VaD (115–119). Underlying these findings is the cholinergic hypothesis that proposes that a relative deficiency of ACh that develops in AD is largely responsible for symptoms of cognitive impairment. It has been proposed for VaD as well, and supported in part by animal models and postmortem studies showing that vascular lesions may also produce significant cholinergic dysfunction in the brain (120,121).

Medications currently on the market to boost ACh levels work by inhibiting acetylcholinesterase (AChE), the main enzyme responsible for ACh metabolism. These include donepezil, rivastigmine, and galantamine. Several double-blind, placebo-controlled studies examining the use of AChE inhibitors in VaD have shown significant improvement in treating symptoms of both cognitive and functional impairment, with good tolerability (117–119). Dosing strategies for each agent are the same as for AD. Donepezil starts at 5 mg/day and is titrated after 4 weeks to 10 mg/day (maximum dose can be increased to 15 mg/day). Rivastigmine starts at 1.5 mg twice a day and is titrated in 1.5 mg increments every 2 to 4 weeks to 6 mg twice a day. Galantamine (extended-release) starts at 8 mg a day and is titrated after 4 weeks to 16 mg a day (maximum dose can be increased to 24 mg a day). The most common side effects are gastrointestinal, which are often transient and can sometimes be reduced by administering the medication with food. The AChE inhibitors should be avoided in patients with active bradyarrhymias, peptic ulcer disease, and excessive pulmonary secretions.

Glutamate Receptor Antagonists

The benefits of the glutamate receptor (N-methyl-D-aspartate) antagonist, memantine, developed for AD patients, may also extend to VaD (122). Several double-blind clinical trials in patients with mild-to-moderate VaD have found both cognitive and functional improvement or stabilization on memantine (123,124). The combination of memantine with an AChE inhibitor in VaD has not yet been studied, but may hold promise given findings in patients with AD (125).

Ginkgo Biloba

The herbal medication ginkgo biloba is commonly used in the treatment of early stage AD and VaD, and clinical trials have suggested a benefit in treating dementia as well (126). The potential neuroprotective benefits of ginkgo biloba may be due to its multiple roles as an antioxidant, a neuronal membrane stabilizer, an inhibitor of platelet-activating factor, a stimulator of hippocampal choline uptake, an inhibitor of beta-amlyoid deposition, and/or an inhibitor of age-related loss of muscarinergic cholinoceptors and alpha-adrenoreceptors (126). Gingko biloba is generally well tolerated, but it can increase the risk of bleeding if used in combination with warfarin, antiplatelet agents, and certain other herbal medications. Potential side effects include nausea, diarrhea, headaches, dizziness, palpitations, restlessness, weakness, and skin rash. Dosing ranges from 120 to 240 mg per day, in divided doses.

Neuroprotective and Neuroenhancing Agents

A number of medications considered to have either protective or enhancing effects on cerebral function have been used to treat VaD. Unfortunately, none of these agents have well-established efficacy for VaD, and are therefore not routinely recommended for treatment. Calcium channel blockers such as nimodopine and nicardipine may play a beneficial role in enhancing cerebral blood flow, especially for small vessel VaD (127). Ergoloid mesylates are an ergot derivative thought to work as a cerebral vasodilator that may also have antioxidant properties. Past studies suggested both cognitive and behavioral benefits of ergoloid mesylates for VaD patients, although much of the research consisted of small samples without consistent diagnostic methods (128,129). Doses range from 1.5 to 12 mg/day, though the typical dose is 3 to 6 mg/day, split into three doses. Ergoloid mesylates are typically well tolerated, with the most common side effects being nausea and headache.

Nootropic (acting on the mind) agents are a group of amino acid compounds that include piracetam and oxiracetam. These agents have been tested and marketed by several European pharmaceutical companies that claim they can improve cognition by increasing cerebral metabolism, increasing the number of cholinergic receptors, and enhancing noradrenergic and dopaminergic function. More extensive and less well-documented claims can be found on the internet. Cytidinediphosphocholine (CDP-choline) activates the biosynthesis of structural phospholipids in neuronal membranes and has been demonstrated to have positive short-term effects on memory and behavior in VaD (127). However, there is no substantial evidence to recommend it.

REFERENCES

1. Lavretsky H, Kumar A. Depressive disorders and cerebrovascular disease. In: Chiu E, Ames D, Katona C, eds. *Vascular Disease and Affective Disorders*. London: Martin Dunitz Ltd.; 2002:127–147.
2. Roman GC. Historical evolution of the concept of vascular dementia. In: Bowler JV, Hachinski V, eds. *Vascular Cognitive Impairment: Preventable Dementia*. London: Oxford University Press; 2003:12–32.
3. Bonelli RM. Editorial comment—how to treat vascular dementia? *Stroke*. 2003;34(10):2331–2332.
4. Hachinski VC, Lassen NA, Marshall J. Multi-infarct dementia. A cause of mental deterioration in the elderly. *Lancet*. 1974;2 (7874):207–210.
5. Roman GC, Tatemichi TK, Erkinjuntti T, et al. Vascular dementia: diagnostic criteria for research studies. Report of the NINDS-AIREN International Workshop. *Neurology*. 1993;43(2):250–260.
6. Feinberg TE, Farah MJ. *Behavioral Neurology and Neuropsychology*. New York: McGraw-Hill; 1997.
7. Rocca WA, Hofman A, Brayne C, et al. The prevalence of vascular dementia in Europe: facts and fragments from 1980–1990 studies. EURODEM-Prevalence Research Group. *Ann Neurol*. 1991;30(6):817–824.
8. Ballard C, Stephens S, McLaren A, et al. Neuropsychological deficits in older stroke patients. *Ann NY Acad Sci*. 2002;977:179–182.
9. Bowler JV, Hachinski V. Vascular dementia. In: Feinberg TE, Farah MJ, eds. *Behavioral Neurology and Neuropsychology*. New York: McGraw-Hill; 1997;589–603.
10. World Health Organization. *The International Classification of Mental and Behavioral Disorders. Clinical Description and Diagnostic Guidelines*. Geneva; WHO; 2003.
11. *American Psychiatric Association: Diagnostic and Statistical Manual of Mental Disorders*. 4th ed. Text Revision. Washington, DC: American Psychiatric Association; 2000.
12. Rockwood K, Shea C. Behavioral and psychological symptoms in vascular cognitive impairment. In: Bowler JV, Hachinski V, eds. *Vascular Cognitive Impairment: Preventable Dementia*. London: Oxford University Press; 2003:110–125.
13. Chui HC, Mack W, Jackson JE, et al. Clinical criteria for the diagnosis of vascular dementia: a multicenter study of comparability and interrater reliability. *Arch Neurol*. 2000;57(2):191–196.
14. Hachinski VC, Iliff LD, Zilhka E, et al. Cerebral blood flow in dementia. *Arch Neurol*. 1975;32(9):632–637.
15. Wetterling T, Kanitz RD, Borgis KJ. Comparison of different diagnostic criteria for vascular dementia (ADDTC, DSM-IV, ICD-10, NINDS-AIREN). *Stroke*. 1996;27(1):30–36.
16. Chui HC, Victoroff JI, Margolin D, Jagust W, Shankle R, Katzman R. Criteria for the diagnosis of ischemic vascular dementia proposed by the State of California Alzheimer's Disease Diagnostic and Treatment Centers. *Neurology*. 1992;42(3, pt 1):473–480.
17. Kalaria RN. Comparison between Alzheimer's disease and vascular dementia: implications for treatment. *Neurol Res*. 2003;25 (6):661–664.
18. Damasio AR, Graff-Radford NR, Eslinger PJ, Damasio H, Kassell N. Amnesia following basal forebrain lesions. *Arch Neurol*. 1985;42(3):263–271.
19. Roman GC, Erkinjuntti T, Wallin A, Pantoni L, Chui HC. Subcortical ischaemic vascular dementia. *Lancet Neurol*. 2002;1 (7):426–436.
20. Folstein MF. *Neurobiology of Primary Dementia*. Washington, DC: American Psychiatric Press, Inc.; 1998.
21. Adair JC. Is it Alzheimer's? *Hosp Pract (Off Ed)*. 1998;33(8):35–36, 51.
22. O'Sullivan M, Rich PM, Barrick TR, Clark CA, Markus HS. Frequency of subclinical lacunar infarcts in ischemic leukoaraiosis and cerebral autosomal dominant arteriopathy with subcortical infarcts and leukoencephalopathy. *AJNR Am J Neuroradiol*. 2003;24(7):1348–1354.
23. Markus HS. Genetics of vascular dementia. In: Bowler JV, Hachinski V, eds. *Vascular Cognitive Impairment: Preventable Dementia*. London: Oxford University Press; 2003:93–109.
24. Lutjohann D, Papassotiropoulos A, Bjorkhem I, et al. Plasma 24S-hydroxycholesterol (cerebrosterol) is increased in Alzheimer and vascular demented patients. *J Lipid Res*. 2000;41(2):195–198.
25. Bathgate D, Snowden JS, Varma A, Blackshaw A, Neary D. Behaviour in frontotemporal dementia, Alzheimer's disease and vascular dementia. *Acta Neurol Scand*. 2001;103(6):367–378.
26. Erkinjuntti T, Rockwood K. Vascular cognitive impairment. *Psychogeriatrics*. 2001;1:27–38.
27. Jorm AF, Fratiglioni L, Winblad B. Differential diagnosis in dementia. Principal components analysis of clinical data from a population survey. *Arch Neurol*. 1993;50(1):72–77.
28. Cummings JL, Miller B, Hill MA, Neshkes R. Neuropsychiatric aspects of multi-infarct dementia and dementia of the Alzheimer type. *Arch Neurol*. 1987;44(4):389–393.
29. McPherson SE, Cummings JL. Neuropsychological aspects of vascular dementia. *Brain Cogn*. 1996;31(2):269–282.
30. Cummings JL. Frontal-subcortical circuits and human behavior. *J Psychosom Res*. 1998;44(6):627–628.
31. Sachdev PS, Looi JCL. Neuropsychological differentiation of Alzheimer's disease and vascular dementia. In: Hachinski V, Bowler JV, eds. *Vascular Cognitive Impairment: Preventable Dementia*. London: Oxford University Press; 2003:153–175.
32. Gislason TB, Sjogren M, Larsson L, Skoog I. The prevalence of frontal variant frontotemporal dementia and the frontal lobe syndrome in a population based sample of 85 year olds. *J Neurol Neurosurg Psychiatry*. 2003;74(7):867–871.
33. Ishii N, Nishihara Y, Imamura T. Why do frontal lobe symptoms predominate in vascular dementia with lacunes? *Neurology*. 1986;36(3):340–345.

34. Pohjasvaara T, Erkinjuntti T, Vataja R, Kaste M. Dementia three months after stroke. Baseline frequency and effect of different definitions of dementia in the Helsinki Stroke Aging Memory Study (SAM) cohort. *Stroke.* 1997;28(4):785–792.
35. Wolfe N, Linn R, Babikian VL, Knoefel JE, Albert ML. Frontal systems impairment following multiple lacunar infarcts. *Arch Neurol.* 1990;47(2):129–132.
36. Royall DR, Lauterbach EC, Cummings JL, et al. Executive control function: a review of its promise and challenges for clinical research. A report from the Committee on Research of the American Neuropsychiatric Association. *J Neuropsychiatry Clin Neurosci.* 2002;14(4):377–405.
37. Kase CS, Wolf PA, Chodosh EH, et al. Prevalence of silent stroke in patients presenting with initial stroke: the Framingham Study. *Stroke.* 1989;20(7):850–852.
38. Li Y, Meyer JS, Thornby J. Depressive symptoms among cognitively normal versus cognitively impaired elderly subjects. *Int J Geriatr Psychiatry.* 2001;16(5):455–461.
39. Ueda K, Kawano H, Hasuo Y, Fujishima M. Prevalence and etiology of dementia in a Japanese community. *Stroke.* 1992;23(6):798–803.
40. Chui HC. Dementia. A review emphasizing clinicopathologic correlation and brain-behavior relationships. *Arch Neurol.* 1989;46(7):806–814.
41. Tomlinson BE, Blessed G, Roth M. Observations on the brains of demented old people. *J Neurol Sci.* 1970;11(3):205–242.
42. Folstein MF, Bassett SS, Anthony JC, Romanoski AJ, Nestadt GR. Dementia: case ascertainment in a community survey. *J Gerontol.* 1991;46(4):M132–M138.
43. Still CN, Jackson KL, Brandes DA, Abramson RK, Macera CA. Distribution of major dementias by race and sex in South Carolina. *J S C Med Assoc.* 1990;86(8):453–456.
44. Birkett DP. *The Psychiatry of Stroke.* Washington, DC: American Psychiatric Press, Inc.; 1996.
45. Gross CR, Shinar D, Mohr JP, et al. Interobserver agreement in the diagnosis of stroke type. *Arch Neurol.* 1986;43(9):893–898.
46. Kempster PA, Gerraty RP, Gates PC. Asymptomatic cerebral infarction in patients with chronic atrial fibrillation. *Stroke.* 1988;19(8):955–957.
47. National Institute of Neurological Disorders and Stroke. Special report from the National Institute of Neurological Disorders and Stroke. Classification of cerebrovascular diseases III. *Stroke.* 1990;21(4):637–676.
48. Hachinski VC, Iliff LD, Zilhka E, et al. Cerebral blood flow in dementia. *Arch Neurol.* 1975;32:632–637.
49. Roses AD. Apolipoprotein E, a gene with complex biological interactions in the aging brain. *Neurobiol Dis.* 1997;4(3–4):170–185.
50. Hofman A, Ott A, Breteler MM, et al. Atherosclerosis, apolipoprotein E, and prevalence of dementia and Alzheimer's disease in the Rotterdam Study. *Lancet.* 1997;349(9046):151–154.
51. Davignon J, Gregg RE, Sing CF. Apolipoprotein E polymorphism and atherosclerosis. *Arteriosclerosis.* 1988;8(1):1–21.
52. Shimano H, Ishibashi S, Murase T, et al. Plasma apolipoproteins in patients with multi-infarct dementia. *Atherosclerosis.* 1989;79 (2–3):257–260.
53. Aharon-Peretz J, Daskovski E, Mashiach T, Tomer R. Natural history of dementia associated with lacunar infarctions. *J Neurol Sci.* 2002;203–204:53–55.
54. Cummings JL. Vascular subcortical dementias: clinical aspects. *Dementia.* 1994;5(3–4):177–180.
55. Mahler ME, Cummings JL. Behavioral neurology of multi-infarct dementia. *Alzheimer Dis Assoc Disord.* 1991;5(2):122–130.
56. Fein G, Van Dyke C, Davenport L, et al. Preservation of normal cognitive functioning in elderly subjects with extensive white-matter lesions of long duration. *Arch Gen Psychiatry.* 1990;47: 220–223.
57. Harris Y, Gorelick PB, Cohen D, Dollear W, Forman H, Freels S. Psychiatric symptoms in dementia associated with stroke: a case-control analysis among predominantly African-American patients. *J Natl Med Assoc.* 1994;86(9):697–702.
58. Starkstein SE, Cohen BS, Fedoroff P, Parikh RM, Price TR, Robinson RG. Relationship between anxiety disorders and depressive disorders in patients with cerebrovascular injury. *Arch Gen Psychiatry.* 1990;47:246–251.
59. Starkstein SE, Fedoroff JP, Price TR, Leiguarda R, Robinson RG. Apathy following cerebrovascular lesions. *Stroke.* 1993;24:1625–1630.
60. Starkstein SE, Fedoroff JP, Price TR, Leiguarda R, Robinson RG. Catastrophic reaction after cerebrovascular lesions: frequency, correlates, and validation of a scale. *J Neuropsychiatry Clin Neurosci.* 1993;5(2):189–194.
61. Hebert R, Lindsay J, Verreault R, Rockwood K, Hill G, Dubois MF. Vascular dementia: incidence and risk factors in the Canadian study of health and aging. *Stroke.* 2000;31(7):1487–1493.
62. Lyketsos CG, Steinberg M, Tschanz JT, Norton MC, Steffens DC, Breitner JC. Mental and behavioral disturbances in dementia: findings from the Cache County Study on memory in aging. *Am J Psychiatry.* 2000;157(5):708–714.
63. Leroi I, Voulgari A, Breitner JC, Lyketsos CG. The epidemiology of psychosis in dementia. *Am J Geriatr Psychiatry.* 2003;11(1):83–91.
64. Porter VR, Buxton WG, Fairbanks LA, et al. Frequency and characteristics of anxiety among patients with Alzheimer's disease and related dementias. *J Neuropsychiatry Clin Neurosci.* 2003;15 (2):180–186.
65. Aharon-Peretz J, Kliot D, Tomer R. Behavioral differences between white matter lacunar dementia and Alzheimer's disease: a comparison on the neuropsychiatric inventory. *Dement Geriatr Cogn Disord.* 2000;11(5):294–298.
66. Post F. *The Significance of Affective Symptoms in Old Age, a Follow-Up Study of One Hundred Patients.* London, New York: Oxford University Press; 1962.
67. Mayer-Gross W, Slater E, Roth M. *Clinical Psychiatry.* London: Balliere, Tindall & Cassell; 1960.
68. Kumar A, Cummings J. Depression in neurodegenerative disorders and related conditions in Alzheimer's disease and related conditions. In: Gothier S, Cummings J, eds. *Alzheimer's Disease and Related Disorders.* London: Martin Dunitz; 2001:123–141.
69. House A, Dennis M, Mogridge L, Warlow C, Hawton K, Jones L. Mood disorders in the year after first stroke. *Br J Psychiatry.* 1991;158:83–92.
70. Robinson RG, Bolduc PL, Price TR. Two-year longitudinal study of poststroke mood disorders: diagnosis and outcome at one and two years. *Stroke.* 1987;18(5):837–843.
71. Chemerinski E, Robinson RG. The neuropsychiatry of stroke. *Psychosomatics.* 2000;41(1):5–14.
72. Eastwood MR, Rifat SL, Nobbs H, Ruderman J. Mood disorder following cerebrovascular accident. *Br J Psychiatry.* 1989;154:195–200.
73. Primeau F. Post-stroke depression: a critical review of the literature. *Can J Psychiatry.* 1988;33(8):757–765.
74. Looi JC, Sachdev PS. Differentiation of vascular dementia from AD on neuropsychological tests. *Neurology.* 1999;53(4):670–678.
75. Lind K, Edman A, Karlsson I, Sjogren M, Wallin A. Relationship between depressive symptomatology and the subcortical brain syndrome in dementia. *Int J Geriatr Psychiatry.* 2002;17(8):774–778.
76. Ramasubbu R. Relationship between depression and cerebrovascular disease: conceptual issues. *J Affect Disord.* 2000;57(1–3):1–11.
77. Simonsick EM, Wallace RB, Blazer DG, Berkman LF. Depressive symptomatology and hypertension-associated morbidity and mortality in older adults. *Psychosom Med.* 1995;57(5):427–435.
78. Starkstein SE, Robinson RG, Price TR. Comparison of cortical and subcortical lesions in the production of poststroke mood disorders. *Brain.* 1987;110(pt 4):1045–1059.
79. Robinson RG, Price TR. Post-stroke depressive disorders: a follow-up study of 103 patients. *Stroke.* 1982;13(5):635–641.
80. Robinson RG, Szetela B. Mood change following left hemispheric brain injury. *Ann Neurol.* 1981;9(5):447–453.
81. Bolla-Wilson K, Robinson RG, Starkstein SE, Boston J, Price TR. Lateralization of dementia of depression in stroke patients. *Am J Psychiatry.* 1989;146(5):627–634.
82. Herrmann M, Bartels C, Schumacher M, Wallesch CW. Poststroke depression. Is there a pathoanatomic correlate for depression in the postacute stage of stroke? *Stroke.* 1995;26(5):850–856.
83. Starkstein SE, Robinson RG, Honig MA, Parikh RM, Joselyn J, Price TR. Mood changes after right-hemisphere lesions. *Br J Psychiatry.* 1989;155:79–85.

84. Starkstein SE, Robinson RG, Price TR. Comparison of patients with and without poststroke major depression matched for size and location of lesion. *Arch Gen Psychiatry.* 1988;45(3): 247–252.

85. Sultzer DL, Mahler ME, Cummings JL, Van Gorp WG, Hinkin CH, Brown C. Cortical abnormalities associated with subcortical lesions in vascular dementia. Clinical and position emission tomographic findings. *Arch Neurol.* 1995;52(8):773–780.

86. Bush BA. Major life events as risk factors for post-stroke depression. *Brain Inj.* 1999;13(2):131–137.

87. Cummings JL. Frontal-subcortical circuits and human behavior. *Arch Neurol.* 1993;50(8):873–880.

88. Duffy JD, Kant R. Apathy secondary to neurologic disease. *Psychiatr Ann.* 1997;27:39–43.

89. Finset A, Andersson S. Coping strategies in patients with acquired brain injury: relationships between coping, apathy, depression and lesion location. *Brain Inj.* 2000;14(10):887–905.

90. Marin RS. Differential diagnosis and classification of apathy. *Am J Psychiatry.* 1990;147(1):22–30.

91. Marin RS. Apathy and related disorders of diminished motivation. *American Psychiatric Press Review of Psychiatry.* 1996;15: 205–242.

92. Marin RS. Differential diagnosis of apathy and related disorders of diminished motivation. *Psychiatr Ann.* 1997;27:30–33.

93. Okada K, Kobayashi S, Yamagata S, Takahashi K, Yamaguchi S. Poststroke apathy and regional cerebral blood flow. *Stroke.* 1997;28(12):2437–2441.

94. Levy ML, Cummings JL, Fairbanks LA, et al. Apathy is not depression. *J Neuropsychiatry Clin Neurosci.* 1998;10(3):314–319.

95. Marin RS, Fogel BS, Hawkins J, Duffy J, Krupp B. Apathy: a treatable syndrome. *J Neuropsychiatry Clin Neurosci.* 1995;7(1):23–30.

96. Fisher CM. Honored guest presentation: abulia minor vs. agitated behavior. *Clin Neurosurg.* 1983;31:9–31.

97. Lyketsos CG, Lopez O, Jones B, Fitzpatrick AL, Breitner J, DeKosky S. Prevalence of neuropsychiatric symptoms in dementia and mild cognitive impairment: results from the cardiovascular health study. *JAMA.* 2002;288(12):1475–1483.

98. Cummings JL, Mendez MF. Secondary mania with focal cerebrovascular lesions. *Am J Psychiatry.* 1984;141(9):1084–1087.

99. Starkstein SE, Mayberg HS, Berthier ML, et al. Mania after brain injury: neuroradiological and metabolic findings. *Ann Neurol.* 1990;27(6):652–659.

100. Starkstein SE, Bryer JB, Berthier ML, Cohen B, Price TR, Robinson RG. Depression after stroke: the importance of cerebral hemisphere asymmetries. *J Neuropsychiatry Clin Neurosci.* 1991;3(3): 276–285.

101. Astrom M, Asplund K, Astrom T. Psychosocial function and life satisfaction after stroke. *Stroke.* 1992;23(4):527–531.

102. Coyle PK, Sterman AB. Focal neurologic symptoms in panic attacks. *Am J Psychiatry.* 1986;143(5):648–649.

103. Mathew RJ, Wilson WH, Nicassio PM. Cerebral ischemic symptoms in anxiety disorders. *Am J Psychiatry.* 1987;144(2):265.

104. Schultz SK, Castillo CS, Kosier JT, Robinson RG. Generalized anxiety and depression. Assessment over 2 years after stroke. *Am J Geriatr Psychiatry.* 1997;5(3):229–237.

105. Astrom M. Generalized anxiety disorder in stroke patients. A 3-year longitudinal study. *Stroke.* 1996;27(2):270–275.

106. Castillo CS, Starkstein SE, Fedoroff JP, Price TR, Robinson RG. Generalized anxiety disorder after stroke. *J Nerv Ment Dis.* 1993;181(2):100–106.

107. Etcharry-Bouyx F, Dubas F. Obsessive-compulsive disorders in association with focal brain lesions. In: Bogousslavsky J, Cummings JL, eds. *Behavior and Mood Disorders in Focal Brain Lesions.* Cambridge: Cambridge University Press; 2000:304–326.

108. Lawrence RM. Is the finding of obsessional behaviour relevant to the differential diagnosis of vascular dementia of the binswanger type? *Behav Neurol.* 2000;12(3):149–154.

109. Ross ED. The aprosodias. Functional-anatomic organization of the affective components of language in the right hemisphere. *Arch Neurol.* 1981;38(9):561–569.

110. Ballard C, Neill D, O'Brien J, McKeith IG, Ince P, Perry R. Anxiety, depression and psychosis in vascular dementia: prevalence and associations. *J Affect Disord.* 2000;59(2):97–106.

111. Edwards-Lee T, Cummings JL. Focal lesions and psychosis. In: Bogousslavsky J, Cummings JL, eds. *Behavior and Mood Disorders in Focal Brain Lesions.* Cambridge: Cambridge University Press; 2000:419–436.

112. Richards M, Meade TW, Peart S, Brennan PJ, Mann AH. Is there any evidence for a protective effect of antithrombotic medication on cognitive function in men at risk of cardiovascular disease? Some preliminary findings. *J Neurol Neurosurg Psychiatry.* 1997; 62(3):269–272.

113. Jick H, Zornberg GL, Jick SS, Seshadri S, Drachman DA. Statins and the risk of dementia. *Lancet.* 2000;356(9242):1627–1631.

114. Amarenco P, Lavallee P, Touboul PJ. Statins and stroke prevention. *Cerebrovasc Dis.* 2004;17(suppl 1):81–88.

115. Black S, Roman GC, Geldmacher DS, et al. Efficacy and tolerability of donepezil in vascular dementia: positive results of a 24-week, multicenter, international, randomized, placebo-controlled clinical trial. *Stroke.* 2003;34(10):2323–2330.

116. Small G, Erkinjuntti T, Kurz A, Lilienfeld S. Galantamine in the treatment of cognitive decline in patients with vascular dementia or Alzheimer's disease with cerebrovascular disease. *CNS Drugs.* 2003;17(12):905–914.

117. Wilkinson D, Doody R, Helme R, et al. Donepezil in vascular dementia: a randomized, placebo-controlled study. *Neurology.* 2003;61(4):479–486.

118. Erkinjuntti T, Kurz A, Gauthier S, Bullock R, Lilienfeld S, Damaraju CV. Efficacy of galantamine in probable vascular dementia and Alzheimer's disease combined with cerebrovascular disease: a randomised trial. *Lancet.* 2002;359(9314):1283–1290.

119. Moretti R, Torre P, Antonello RM, Cazzato G, Bava A. Rivastigmine in subcortical vascular dementia: an open 22-month study. *J Neurol Sci.* 2002;203–204:141–146.

120. Amenta F, Di Tullio MA, Tomassoni D. Arterial hypertension and brain damage—evidence from animal models (review). *Clin Exp Hypertens.* 2003;25(6):359–380.

121. Gottfries CG, Blennow K, Karlsson I, Wallin A. The neurochemistry of vascular dementia. *Dementia.* 1994;5(3–4):163–167.

122. Winblad B, Jelic V. Treating the full spectrum of dementia with memantine. *Int J Geriatr Psychiatry.* 2003;18(suppl 1):S41–S46.

123. Orgogozo JM, Rigaud AS, Stoffler A, Mobius HJ, Forette F. Efficacy and safety of memantine in patients with mild to moderate vascular dementia: a randomized, placebo-controlled trial (MMM 300). *Stroke.* 2002;33(7):1834–1839.

124. Wilcock G, Mobius HJ, Stoffler A. A double-blind, placebo-controlled multicentre study of memantine in mild to moderate vascular dementia (MMM 500). *Int Clin Psychopharmacol.* 2002;17 (6):297–305.

125. Tariot P, Farlow M, Grossberg G, et al. Memantine/donepezil dual-therapy is superior to placebo/donepezil therapy for treatment of moderate to severe Alzheimer's disease. Presented at: American Geriatrics Society's 2003 Annual Scientific Meeting. May 14–18, 2003; Baltimore, MD.

126. Sierpina VS, Wollschlaeger B, Blumenthal M. Ginkgo biloba. *Am Fam Physician.* 2003;68(5):923–926.

127. Roman GC. Vascular dementia revisited: diagnosis, pathogenesis, treatment, and prevention. *Med Clin North Am.* 2002;86(3): 477–499.

128. Schneider LS, Olin JT. Overview of clinical trials of Hydergine in dementia. *Arch Neurol.* 1995;51:787–798.

129. Thompson T, Filley C, Mitchell D, et al. Lack of efficacy of Hydergine in patients with Alzheimer's disease. *New Eng J Med.* 1990;323:445–448.

22

Dementia with Lewy Bodies

Ian G. McKeith

Dementia with Lewy bodies (DLB) was only fully recognized about a decade ago, and is now thought to be the second most prevalent cause of degenerative dementia in older people (1). It is therefore a relative newcomer to many clinicians, for whom it poses significant difficulties in diagnosis. DLB has previously carried a variety of diagnostic labels, including diffuse Lewy body disease (2), Lewy body dementia (3), the Lewy body variant of Alzheimer's disease (4), senile dementia of Lewy body type (5), and dementia associated with cortical Lewy bodies (6). The importance of recognizing DLB relates particularly to its pharmacological management, with reports of good responsiveness to acetylcholinesterase inhibitors (AChEIs) (7), extreme sensitivity to the side effects of neuroleptics (8,9), and limited responsiveness to levo-dopa.

CASE EXAMPLE

Mrs. A, a 74-year-old retired teacher, was initially referred at age 71 for psychiatric assessment because she was distressed by seeing people in her garden. She thought they were spying on her through the windows of her dining room. Mrs. A's husband described her as an active and cheerful woman who had become physically and mentally slower over the previous 18 months. Now she could not concentrate on simple tasks, such as reading a book or cooking a meal, and was prone to falling asleep in her chair often throughout the day. Her memory was also less reliable, and she sometimes had difficulty finding things in her cupboards and drawers. She also had difficulty setting the table and folding sheets. Mr. A was exasperated that some days she was much better than others, and wondered if she was simply lazy or not trying.

On examination, Mrs. A described the visual hallucinations in great detail and appeared to have some insight into their unreality. Her mood was normal, but she did seem mildly apathetic and slow to respond. Her Mini-Mental State Examination (MMSE) score was 27/30, losing two points for serial sevens and one point because she was unable to copy pentagons. There were no abnormal physical signs. A diagnosis of early dementia with an associated delirium (due to a presumed urinary tract infection) was made. She was prescribed antibiotics and her hallucinations improved after about 2 weeks.

She was next seen in the emergency room 6 months later, after an unobserved fall fractured her right radius and ulna. Her husband thought Mrs. A's cognitive impairment was worsening, although it was still very variable from day to day. At her best, she was virtually independent and could hold a good, well-informed conversation. At her worst, she was very muddled about where she was and misidentified her husband as her father. He also commented on her walking more slowly. On examination, she had a mild postural instability, gait disorder, parkinsonian syndrome, and body and facial bradykinesia, but no tremor. These motor features progressed over the next year. The introduction of levodopa helped her rigidity and akinesia, but also seemed to precipitate the reoccurrence of visual hallucinations on a daily basis. Mrs. A also started to have nocturnal problems, having 1 to 2 hours of restless sleep and then waking with hallucinations and distress, during which she thrashed about the bed and shouted. This was improved by clonazepam 0.5 mg at night.

Reassessment revealed Mrs. A had an MMSE of 17/30, and was unable to copy, do serial sevens, or orient herself accurately in time or place. Her short-term recall was surprisingly good, remembering two of the three items. Her Unified Parkinson's Disease Rating Scale motor score was 26 and her Neuropsychiatric Inventory score was 28, with positive responses for hallucinations (visual modality only), delusions, apathy, anxiety, and sleep disturbance. Brain magnetic resonance imaging (MRI) showed only mild cortical atrophy, with relatively intact hippocampal volume and mild generalized white matter lesions. Seen a week later for physical review in the fracture clinic, her MMSE had improved to 23/30.

A diagnosis of probable DLB was made and Mrs. A was started on an AChEI, which she tolerated in full dose with no apparent side effects other than a fine action tremor in both hands. Her daytime sleepiness, visual hallucinations, and general cognitive function improved markedly after 6 weeks of treatment.

A year later, her husband called in a distressed state to say that Mrs. A had been generally stable over the year but had suddenly deteriorated, becoming immobile, mute, and doubly incontinent. Two weeks earlier, she had been prescribed a medication for anxiety and restlessness, while staying at her daughter's vacation house, by a doctor who did not ask the family about her diagnosis. The new medication turned out to be an atypical antipsychotic, and when this was discontinued Mrs. A slowly improved over several months, but never reached her pre-vacation level of function.

At final assessment, she was still mobile with the assistance of her husband, but had severe truncal rigidity and flexion. Her speech was indistinct and hypophonic, but it was apparent that she was sometimes able to retain new information. She still reached out at times towards hallucinatory people or objects, but when confronted (e.g., by the examiner), she was usually unable to focus attention upon them. Mrs. A subsequently died of bronchopneumonia following another fall and fractured femur. Neuropathological autopsy revealed subcortical and cortical Lewy bodies, with high amyloid plaque density but few neurofibrillary tangles.

PHENOMENOLOGY

DLB is recognized by progressive signs and symptoms of dementia, with marked impairments in visuospatial, attentional, and executive functions. Episodic recall can be relatively preserved in the early stages, in contrast to Alzheimer's disease (AD), in which memory failure is often the presenting complaint. Fluctuating cognition, recurrent visual hallucinations, and extrapyramidal motor symptoms are the core features distinguishing DLB clinically, although these features are now known to be absent in a significant minority of cases (10), leading to difficulties in diagnosis. The onset tends to be insidious, although reports of a period of increased confusion or prominent hallucinations may give the impression of a sudden onset. The course is generally progressive, with cognitive test scores declining about 10% per annum, similar to AD (11). Cognitive fluctuations may contribute to large variability in repeated test scores (e.g., five MMSE points difference over the course of

a few days or weeks) (12), making it difficult to be sure of the severity of cognitive impairment by a single examination. Survival times from onset until death are also similar to AD (13), although a minority of DLB patients have a very rapid disease course (14,15).

Cognition

The profile of neuropsychological impairments in patients with DLB differs from that of AD and other dementia syndromes (16), reflecting the combined involvement of cortical and subcortical pathways and relative sparing of the hippocampus. Patients with DLB perform better than those with AD on tests of verbal memory (17), but worse on visuospatial performance tasks (18) and tests of attention (19). Thus, on the MMSE a DLB patient may be well orientated and score two or three points out of three for delayed recall, but be unable to copy pentagons or write a sentence. Fluctuations in cognitive function, which may vary over minutes, hours, or days, occur in 50% to 75% of patients and are associated with shifting levels of attention and alertness. The assessment of fluctuating cognitive impairment poses considerable difficulty to most clinicians, and has repeatedly been cited as a reason for low clinical ascertainment of DLB (12,20). Newly proposed caregiver and observer-rated scales may be particularly helpful in this regard (21). Questions such as, "Are there episodes when his or her thinking seems quite clear and then becomes muddled?" were originally thought to be useful probes (22), although two recent studies (23,24) found most caregivers responded positively to such questions regardless of diagnostic subtype. More reliable predictors of DLB diagnosis are objective questions about daytime sleepiness, episodes of staring blankly or incoherent speech, and qualitative assessment of the range of fluctuation (e.g., best versus worst). Recording variation in attentional performance using a computer-based test system offers an independent method of measuring fluctuation that is also sensitive to drug treatment effects (25).

Neuropsychiatric Features

Almost any neuropsychiatric feature may occur in DLB (26), and consequently many cases present to geriatric psychiatry rather than to memory clinics or standard dementia services. Visual hallucinations are the most characteristic symptom, occurring in up to 80% of cases. Their presence early in the presentation (27) and their persistence help distinguish visual hallucinations from the transient perceptual disturbances that occur in dementias of other etiology, or during delirium. Persistent visual hallucinations in a patient with dementia are a strong predictor of a DLB diagnosis. Well-formed, detailed, and animate figures are experienced, provoking emotional responses varying through fear, amusement, or indifference, usually with some insight into the unreality of the episode once it is over. Auditory hallucinations also occur in about 20% of cases and, together with olfactory and tactile hallucinations, may lead to initial diagnoses of late-onset psychosis (28) or temporal-lobe epilepsy (17). Delusions are also common in DLB, and are usually based on recollections of hallucinations and perceptual disturbances. They consequently have a complex and bizarre content that contrasts with the mundane and often poorly formed persecutory ideas encountered in AD patients, which are based on forgetfulness and confabulation. The combination of prominent psychotic symptoms and cognitive impairment in DLB may generate significant anxiety, agitation, and behavioral disturbance.

Sleep disorders have more recently been recognized as common in DLB, with daytime somnolence and nocturnal restlessness (29), sometimes as prodromal features. Rapid eye movement (REM) sleep-wakefulness dissociations may explain several features of DLB that are characteristic of narcolepsy (REM-sleep behavior disorder, daytime hypersomnolence, visual hallucinations, and cataplexy) (30). Sleep disorders may contribute to the fluctuations typical of DLB, and their treatment may improve fluctuations and quality of life (24). Finally, apathy and depression (31) are also frequently encountered, and their assessment is complicated not only by each other, but also by facial and body bradykinesia and attentional dysfunction.

Parkinsonism

Extrapyramidal symptoms (EPS) are reported in 25% to 50% of DLB cases at diagnosis, and 75% to 80% develop some EPS during the natural course. The profile of EPS in DLB is generally similar to that in age-matched, nondemented Parkinson's disease (PD) patients (32), with greater postural instability and facial impassivity but less tremor (33). Rate of motor deterioration is about 10% per annum, similar to PD (34), but levo-dopa responsiveness is reduced, possibly due to additional intrinsic striatal pathology and dysfunction (35).

Other Common Clinical Features

Repeated falls may be due to posture and/or gait and balance difficulties, particularly in patients with parkinsonism. Syncopal attacks with complete loss of consciousness and muscle tone also occur. These may be secondary to orthostatic hypotension and/or carotid sinus hypersensitivity, which are more common in DLB than AD or age-matched controls (36). Or they may represent one extreme of fluctuating attention and cognition. Early onset of urinary incontinence has been reported in DLB compared with AD (37), reflecting involvement of autonomic systems.

EPIDEMIOLOGY

There is very little systematically collected information about the prevalence, incidence, and associated risk factors for DLB. A community study of individuals 85 and older in Finland found 5% met consensus criteria for DLB (3.3% probable, 1.7% possible), representing 22% of all demented cases (38). This is similar to other clinical estimates (39,40), and consistent with estimates of Lewy body (LB) prevalence (15%) in a dementia case register followed to autopsy (41). Little is known about risk factors for LB disease except for male gender and age of onset, which is on average 10 years later for DLB (mean 75 years in most studies) than for PD.

ASSESSMENT AND DIAGNOSIS

The clinical diagnosis of DLB rests on obtaining a detailed history of symptoms from the patient and an informant, a mental status examination, appropriate cognitive testing, and a neurological examination (1). Systemic and pharmacological causes of delirium need to be rigorously excluded. The diagnosis of probable or possible DLB is then made by the application of internationally used consensus criteria (Table 22-1), which require the core features of fluctuating cognitive impairment, recurrent visual hallucinations, and parkinsonism. The specificity of a clinical diagnosis of probable DLB (two or more core features present) is high at >80%, but sensitivity is generally limited to around 50% (42). The use of the more lenient possible DLB criteria that require the presence of only one core feature increases case detection rates at the cost of reduced diagnostic accuracy, and may be useful in clinical practice for screening purposes (43).

DIFFERENTIAL DIAGNOSIS

The main differential diagnoses of DLB are AD, vascular dementia, Parkinson's disease with dementia (PDD), atypical parkinsonian syndromes such as progressive supranuclear palsy, multiple symptom atrophy, corticobasal degeneration, and also Creutzfeldt-Jacob disease (1). There are as yet no clinically applicable electrophysiological, genotypic, or cerebrospinal fluid markers to support a DLB clinical diagnosis (44), but neuroimaging investigations may be helpful. Changes associated with DLB include preservation of hippocampal and medial temporal lobe volume on MRI (45,46), and occipital hypoperfusion on single positron emission computerized tomography (SPECT) (47,48). Other features such as generalized atrophy (46), white matter changes (49), and rates of progression of whole brain atrophy (50) appear to be unhelpful in differential diagnosis. Dopamine transporter loss in the caudate and putamen, a marker of

TABLE 22-1

CONSENSUS GUIDELINES FOR THE CLINICAL DIAGNOSIS OF PROBABLE AND POSSIBLE DEMENTIA WITH LEWY BODIES

1. Central feature

Progressive cognitive decline of sufficient magnitude to interfere with normal social and occupational function. Prominent or persistent memory impairment may not necessarily occur in the early stages, but is usually evident with progression. Deficits on tests of attention and of frontal-subcortical skills and visuospatial ability may be particularly prominent.

2. Core features (two core features essential for a diagnosis of probable, one for possible DLB)
- Fluctuating cognition with pronounced variations in attention and alertness
- Recurrent visual hallucinations that are typically well-formed and detailed
- Spontaneous features of parkinsonism

3. Supportive features
- Repeated falls
- Syncope
- Transient loss of consciousness
- Neuroleptic hypersensitivity
- Systematized delusions
- Hallucinations in other modalities
- Rapid eye movement sleep behavior disorder
- Depression

4. Features less likely to be present
- History of stroke
- Any other physical illness or brain disorder sufficient enough to interfere with cognitive performance

DLB, dementia with Lewy bodies.
Adapted from Reference 1.

nigrostriatal degeneration, can be detected by dopaminergic SPECT. In preliminary studies, this finding has shown specificity and sensitivity of 85% or higher, and may be particularly helpful (51,52).

One issue which repeatedly causes difficulty in diagnosing DLB is uncertainty about its relationship with idiopathic PD, a disorder in which dementia may eventually develop in up to 75% of cases. PD is similar to DLB (53,54) with respect to fluctuating neuropsychological function (55), neuropsychiatric features (56), and extrapyramidal motor features (32). These clinical similarities reflect a common pathological endpoint. An arbitrary *1-year rule* that proposes that the onset of dementia within 12 months of the onset of parkinsonism qualifies as DLB, and more than 12 months of parkinsonism before the onset of dementia qualifies as PDD, is frequently used to distinguish between the two disorders. This is certainly helpful in individual clinical case diagnosis and management, but is hard to justify from a neurobiological point of view because there do not appear to be major neuropatho-

logical differences between them. Labels such as PDD and DLB may in fact do little more than describe the order of onset of symptoms within a single diagnostic entity, called *LB disease*. Given our new insights into these disorders, one can easily justify using this unifying label of LB disease as the primary diagnosis, qualified by a secondary descriptive epithet, for example, LB disease with parkinsonism, or LB disease with dementia, or LB disease with parkinsonism and dementia. Clinicians need to decide which is the most appropriate label for each patient, and carefully explain the terminology to the patient and his or her caregivers (57).

PATHOLOGY AND ETIOLOGY

The original delineation of DLB from other dementing disorders was made on the basis of neuropathological findings, i.e., the presence of cortical LB at autopsy, so it is of interest to note that although guidelines for assessment of LB pathology exist (1), no formal criteria for the pathological diagnosis of DLB have been established to date. It is generally accepted that most cases show alpha (α)-synuclein-positive LBs and Lewy neurites, together with abundant Alzheimer-type pathology, predominantly in the form of amyloid plaques. Tau-positive inclusions and neocortical neurofibrillary tangles sufficient to meet Braak stages V or VI (sufficient to qualify for a diagnosis of concomitant AD) occur in only a minority (10% to 25%) of cases. Alzheimer pathology of any type is not a prerequisite for the existence of dementia, however, since older patients with pure LB disease (no plaques or tangles) may present clinically with cognitive impairment and other neuropsychiatric features. Cortical LB density is not robustly correlated with either the severity or duration of dementia (58,59), although associations have been reported with LB and plaque density in midfrontal cortex (60). Lewy neurites and neurotransmitter deficits are suggested as more likely correlates of clinical symptoms (59,61). α-synuclein immunoreactive deposits with many of the characteristics of LB have also been reported in a high proportion of AD cases, particularly in the amygdala (62). In this context they may represent an end-stage phenomenon, with secondary accumulation of aggregated synuclein in severely dysfunctional neurons that are already heavily burdened by plaque and tangle pathology (63). Whatever the explanations for this considerable overlap in pathological lesions in DLB and AD, it is clear that clinical separation of cases is going to be less than 100% precise. The presence of Alzheimer pathology in DLB appears to modify the typical clinical presentation, making these cases harder to differentiate clinically (10), with the core DLB features either scant or absent, and the clinical picture more closely resembling AD. There are recent reports that triplication of the α-synuclein gene (SNCA) can cause DLB, PD, and PDD, whereas gene duplication is associated only with motor PD, suggesting a gene dose effect (64). However, SNCA multiplication is not found in most LB disease patients (65).

TREATMENT

When treating a patient with DLB, it is helpful first to develop a problem list of cognitive, psychiatric, and motor disabilities, and then ask the patient and caregiver to identify the symptoms they find most disabling or distressing (66). Functional disability in DLB is generally greater than in AD patients with similar severity of cognitive impairment. Most of the additional burden is due to motor impairments that cause difficulty with mobility, feeding, and toileting. A multidisciplinary approach including adequate physical, speech, and occupational therapy is therefore essential.

Nonpharmacologic strategies are an important way of treating people with dementia and an integral part of the management of DLB, not least because of the poor tolerance of some commonly used psychotropic medications. Established methods include explanation, education, reassurance, orientation and memory prompts, attentional cues, and targeted behavioral interventions. No formal recommendations have yet been made about specific strategies that are most effective in DLB, nor has there been an evaluation of the system changes and costs needed to support them.

The clinician should explain, before any medications are prescribed, that treatment gains in target symptoms may be associated with worsening of symptoms in other domains. The specific risks for DLB patients for severe neuroleptic sensitivity reactions should be mentioned in all cases, and it is prudent to mark patient records with an alert to reduce the possibility of inadvertent neuroleptic prescribing or dosing, particularly in primary care or emergency room settings.

The single most important aspect of pharmacological management of DLB is to recognize the potentially fatal consequences to these patients of administration of antipsychotic agents. Abnormal hypersensitivity to the adverse effects of traditional neuroleptics (e.g., haloperidol) occurs in about 50% of DLB patients, and is associated with a two-to-three-fold increased mortality secondary to the onset of rigidity, sedation, and increased confusion (8). Atypical antipsychotics used at low doses may be safer in this regard, but sensitivity reactions have been documented with most, including risperidone (9), olanzapine (67), and clozapine (68), and they should be used with great caution (44). Recent reports that quetiapine may be less likely to cause severe sensitivity reactions than other atypicals are encouraging (69–71), but need to be confirmed by controlled trials. Benzodiazepines, particularly low dose clonazepam (0.5–1.0 mg) may be useful to treat insomnia and nocturnal hallucinations (72), although increased confusion and falls may occur.

The effectiveness of levodopa on motor symptoms in DLB is less than in uncomplicated PD (73). This relative refractoriness to treatment may be partly related to intrinsic striatal neuritic degeneration that is not seen in uncomplicated PD (36). The clinician should aim for the lowest effective dose of levodopa monotherapy (74), because higher doses or use of other antiparkinsonian agents are likely to be associated with increased confusion and hallucinations.

Evidence is accumulating that AChEI drugs are effective and relatively safe in the treatment of neuropsychiatric and cognitive symptoms in DLB, but the number of patients studied is still relatively small and larger trials are needed. There are reports of similar efficacy with each of the currently available agents, but insufficient data to yet determine whether one agent is to be preferred over others (75). Apathy, anxiety, impaired attention, hallucinations, delusions, sleep disturbance, and cognitive changes are the most frequently cited treatment-responsive symptoms. Visual hallucinations in DLB are associated with greater deficits in cortical acetylcholine (76), and predict better response to AChEIs (77). In addition to the usual gastrointestinal side effects associated with this drug class, increased cholinergic activity in DLB patients may cause hypersalivation, rhinorrhea, and lacrimation (78), and exacerbate postural hypotension and falls (79). Short-term (6 month) improvements are generally reported as significantly greater than those achieved in AD (80,81). Dosing and titration rates in DLB are similar to those recommended for AD. There are at present only limited open-label data available of long-term AChEI treatment effects in DLB (82), but the benefits do seem to be sustained, with symptomatic deterioration (sometimes rapid) occurring when treatment is suddenly withdrawn (83). Dosing information may be found in Appendix A of this textbook.

COURSE AND PROGNOSIS

The most striking aspect of DLB is the fluctuant nature of the symptoms, which occur with a background of progressive intellectual, motor, and general physical decline. Early reports suggested the decline was more rapid than in AD, with a reduced survival time until death. Controlled studies have not lent much support to this view, with mean rates of annual decline of about 10% in both cognitive and parkinsonism scores. These mean values, however, probably conceal considerable heterogeneity, and some patients with DLB do seem to have a very rapid disease course (14,15). Whether there are any specific features, other than the inappropriate administration of neuroleptic medication, associated with more rapid disease progression or poorer survival is not yet known.

PSYCHOSOCIAL ISSUES

The giving and receiving of a diagnosis of dementia is a complicated process for all parties, even when the message is a relatively straightforward one, for example a diagnosis of AD, which is followed up with adequate information and educational materials. DLB is by contrast an unfamiliar term to most people, although this situation is improving quickly because of the internet and newly established support groups such as the Lewy Body Dementia Association Inc. (www.lewybodydementia.org). In countries with less developed dementia services, these complications are even greater, and there is a pressing need for suitable educational materials to be developed and disseminated through appropriate international and regional organizations. Not only are the educational, treatment, and care needs of DLB patients subtly different from other people with dementia, they are sometimes omitted as a diagnostic category from treatment guidelines and prescribing protocols, so that DLB patients and their families are denied access to treatments (such as AChEIs), from which they might derive considerable benefits. Increasing awareness and more intervention studies focused on DLB are urgently needed. If DLB is recognized and treated appropriately, much can be done to help people with this common disorder, which was not even listed in the textbooks a decade ago.

REFERENCES

1. McKeith IG, Galasko D, Kosaka K, et al. Consensus guidelines for the clinical and pathologic diagnosis of dementia with Lewy bodies (DLB): report of the Consortium on DLB International Workshop. *Neurology.* 1996;47:1113–1124.
2. Kosaka K, Yoshimura, Ikeda K, Budka H. Diffuse type of Lewy body disease: progressive dementia with abundant cortical Lewy bodies and senile changes of varying degree—a new disease? *Clin Neuropathol.* 1984;3(5):185–192.
3. Gibb WRG, Esiri MM, Lees AJ. Clinical and pathological features of diffuse cortical Lewy body disease (Lewy body dementia). *Brain.* 1987;110:1131–1153.
4. Hansen L, Salmon D, Galasko D, et al. The Lewy body variant of Alzheimer's disease: a clinical and pathologic entity. *Neurology.* 1990;40:1–8.
5. Perry RH, Irving D, Blessed G, Fairbairn A, Perry EK, et al. Senile dementia of Lewy body type. A clinically and neuropathologically distinct form of Lewy body dementia in the elderly. *J Neurol Sci.* 1990;95:119–139.
6. Byrne EJ, Lennox G, Godwin-Austen LB, et al. Dementia associated with cortical Lewy bodies. Proposed diagnostic criteria. *Dementia.* 1991;2:283–284.
7. McKeith I, Del Ser T, Spano P, et al. Efficacy of rivastigmine in dementia with Lewy bodies: a randomised, double-blind, placebo-controlled international study. *Lancet.* 2000;356:2031–2036.
8. McKeith I, Fairbairn A, Perry R, Thompson P, Perry E. Neuroleptic sensitivity in patients with senile dementia of Lewy body type. *BMJ.* 1992;305:673–678.
9. Ballard C, Grace J, McKeith I, Holmes C. Neuroleptic sensitivity in dementia with Lewy bodies and Alzheimer's disease. *Lancet.* 1998;351:1032–1033.
10. Merdes AR, Hansen LA, Jeste DV, et al. Influence of Alzheimer pathology on clinical diagnostic accuracy in dementia with Lewy bodies. *Neurology.* 2003;60(10):1586–1590.
11. Ballard C, O'Brien J, Morris CM, et al. The progression of cognitive impairment in dementia with Lewy bodies, vascular dementia and Alzheimer's disease. *Int J Geriatr Psychiatry.* 2001;16(5):499–503.

12. Mega MS, Masterman DL, Benson DF, et al. Dementia with Lewy bodies: reliability and validity of clinical and pathologic criteria. *Neurology.* 1996;47:1403–1409.
13. Walker Z, Allen RL, Shergill S, Mullan E, Katona C. Three years survival in patients with a clinical diagnosis of dementia with Lewy bodies. *Int J Geriatr Psychiatry.* 2000;15:267–273.
14. Armstrong TP, Hansen LA, Salmon DP, et al. Rapidly progressive dementia in a patient with the Lewy body variant of Alzheimer's disease. *Neurology.* 1991;41:1178–1180.
15. Lopez OL, Wisniewski S, Hamilton RL, Becker JT, Kaufer DI, DeKosky ST. Predictors of progression in patients with AD and Lewy bodies. *Neurology.* 2000;54(9):1774–1779.
16. Collerton D, Burn D, McKeith I, O'Brien J. Systematic review and meta-analysis show that dementia with Lewy bodies is a visual-perceptual and attentional-executive dementia. *Dement Geriatr Cogn Disord.* 2003;16(4):229–237.
17. McKeith IG, Perry RH, Fairbairn AF, Jabeen S, Perry EK. Operational criteria for senile dementia of Lewy body type (SDLT). *Psychol Med.* 1992;22:911–922.
18. Walker Z, Allen RL, Shergill S, Katona CL. Neuropsychological performance in Lewy body dementia and Alzheimer's disease. *Brit J Psychiatry.* 1997;170:156–158.
19. Sahgal A, Galloway PH, McKeith IG, Edwardson JA, Lloyd S. A comparative study of attentional deficits in senile dementias of Alzheimer and Lewy body types. *Dementia.* 1992;3:350–354.
20. Litvan I, MacIntyre A, Goetz CG, et al. Accuracy of the clinical diagnoses of Lewy body disease, Parkinson's disease, and dementia with Lewy bodies. *Arch Neurol.* 1998;55:969–978.
21. Walker MP, Ayre GA, Cummings JL, et al. The Clinician Assessment of Fluctuation and the One Day Fluctuation Assessment Scale. Two methods to assess fluctuating confusion in dementia. *Brit J Psychiatry.* 2000;177:252–256.
22. Ballard CG, Mohan RNC, Patel A, Bannister C. Idiopathic clouding of consciousness—do the patients have cortical Lewy body disease? *Int J Geriatr Psychiatry.* 1993;8:571–576.
23. Bradshaw J, Saling M, Hopwood M, Anderson V, Brodtmann A. Fluctuating cognition in dementia with Lewy bodies and Alzheimer's disease is qualitatively distinct. *J Neurol Neurosurg Psychiatry.* 2004;75:382–387.
24. Ferman T, Smith GE, Boeve BF, et al. DLB fluctuations: specific features that reliably differentiate from AD and normal aging. *Neurology.* 2004;62(2):181–187.
25. Wesnes KA, McKeith IG, Ferrara R, et al. Effects of rivastigmine on cognitve function in dementia with Lewy bodies: a randomised placebo-controlled international study using the Cognitve Drug Research computerised assessment system. *Dement Geriatr Cogn Disord.* 2002;13(3):183–192.
26. Del Ser T, McKeith I, Anand R, Cicin-Sain A, Ferrara R, Spiegel R. Dementia with Lewy bodies: findings from an international multicentre study. *Int J Geriatr Psychiatry.* 2000;15:1034–1045.
27. Ballard C, Holmes C, McKeith I, et al. Psychiatric morbidity in dementia with Lewy bodies: a prospective clinical and neuropathological comparative study with Alzheimer's disease. *Am J Psychiatry.* 1999;156(7):1039–1045.
28. Birkett DP, Desouky A, Han L, et al. Lewy bodies in psychiatric patients. *Int J Geriatr Psychiatry.* 1992;7:235–240.
29. Boeve BF, Silber MH, Ferman TJ, REM sleep behavior disorder in Parkinson's Disease and dementia with Lewy bodies. *J Geriatr Psychiatry Neurol.* 2004;17(3):146–157.
30. Boeve BF, Silber MH, Ferman TJ, Lucas JA, Parisi JE. Association of REM sleep behavior disorder and neurodegenerative disease may reflect an underlying synucleinopathy. *Mov Disord.* 2001;16:622–630.
31. Klatka LA, Louis ED, Schiffer RB. Psychiatric features in diffuse Lewy body disease: findings in 28 pathologically diagnosed cases. *Neurology.* 1996;46:A180.
32. Aarsland D, Ballard C, McKeith I, Perry RH, Larsen JP. Comparison of extrapyramidal signs in dementia with Lewy bodies and Parkinson's disease. *J Neuropsychiatry Clin Neurosci.* 2001;13:374–379.
33. Burn DJ, Rowan EN, Minett T, et al. Extrapyramidal features in Parkinson's disease with and without dementia and dementia with Lewy bodies: a cross-sectional comparative study. *Mov Disord.* 2003;18(8):884–889.

34. Ballard C, O'Brien J, Swann A, et al. One year follow-up of parkinsonism in dementia with Lewy bodies. *Dement Geriatr Cogn Disord.* 2000;11:219–222.

35. Duda JE, Giasson BI, Mabon ME, Lee VM, Trojanowski JQ. Novel antibodies to synuclein show abundant striatal pathology in Lewy body diseases. *Ann Neurol.* 2002;52(2):205–210.

36. Ballard C, Shaw F, McKeith I, Kenny R. High prevalence of neurovascular instability in neurodegenerative dementias. *Neurology.* 1998;51:1760–1762.

37. Del-Ser T, Munoz DG, Hachinski V. Temporal pattern of cognitive decline and incontinence is different in Alzheimer's disease and diffuse Lewy body disease. *Neurology.* 1996;46:682–686.

38. Rahkonen T, Eloniemi-Sulkava U, Rissanen S, Vatanen A, Viramo P, Sulkava R. Dementia with Lewy bodies according to the consensus criteria in a general population aged 75 years or older. *J Neurol Neurosurg Psychiatry.* 2003;74(6):720–724.

39. Shergill S, Mullen E, D'Ath P, Katona C. What is the clinical prevalence of Lewy body dementia? *Int J Geriatr Psychiatry.* 1994;9: 907–912.

40. Stevens T, Livingston G, Kitchen G, Manela M, Walker Z, Katona C. Islington study of dementia subtypes in the community. *Brit J Psychiatry.* 2002;180:270–276.

41. Holmes C, Cairns N, Lantos P, Mann A. Validity of current clinical criteria for Alzheimer's disease, vascular dementia and dementia with Lewy bodies. *Brit J Psychiatry.* 1999:45–51.

42. Litvan I, Bhatia KP, Burn DJ, et al. Movement Disorders Society Scientific Issues Committee report: SIC Task Force appraisal of clinical diagnostic criteria for parkinsonian disorders. *Mov Disord.* 2003;18(5):467–486.

43. Luis CA, Barker WW, Gajaraj K, et al. Sensitivity and specificity of three clinical criteria for dementia with Lewy bodies in an autopsy-verified sample. *Int J Geriatr Psychiatry.* 1999;14:526–533.

44. McKeith I, Mintzer J, Aarsland D, et al. Dementia with Lewy bodies. *Lancet Neurol.* 2004;3:19–28.

45. Barber R, Gholkar A, Scheltens P, Ballard C, McKeith IG, O'Brien JT. Medial temporal lobe atrophy on MRI in dementia with Lewy bodies. *Neurology.* 1999;52:1153–1158.

46. Barber R, Ballard C, McKeith IG, Gholkar A, O'Brien JT. MRI volumetric study of dementia with Lewy bodies. A comparison with AD and vascular dementia. *Neurology.* 2000;54:1304–1309.

47. Lobotesis K, Fenwick JD, Phipps A, et al. Occipital hypoperfusion on SPECT in dementia with Lewy bodies but not AD. *Neurology.* 2001;56:643–649.

48. Colloby SJ, Fenwick JD, Williams ED, et al. A comparison of 99m Tc-HMPAO SPECT changes in dementia with Lewy bodies and Alzheimer's disease using statistical parametric mapping. *Eur J Nucl Med Mol Imaging.* 2002;29(5):615–622.

49. Barber R, Gholkar A, Scheltens P, Ballard C, McKeith IG, O'Brien JT. MRI volumetric correlates of white matter lesions in dementia with Lewy bodies and Alzheimer's disease. *Int J Geriatr Psychiatry.* 2000;15:911–916.

50. O'Brien JT, Paling S, Barber R, et al. Progressive brain atrophy on serial MRI in dementia with Lewy bodies, AD, and vascular dementia. *Neurology.* 2001;56(10):1386–1388.

51. Walker Z, Costa DC, Ince P, McKeith IG, Katona CL. In-vivo demonstration of dopaminergic degeneration in dementia with Lewy bodies. *Lancet.* 1999;354:646–647.

52. O'Brien JT, Colloby SJ, Fenwick J, et al. Dopamine transporter loss visualized with FP-CIT SPECT in dementia with Lewy bodies. *Arch Neurol.* 2004;61(6):919–925.

53. Emre M. Dementia associated with Parkinson's disease. *Lancet Neurol.* 2003;2(4):229–237.

54. Aarsland D, Andersen K, Larsen JP, Lolk A, Kragh-Sorensen P. Prevalence and characteristics of dementia in Parkinson disease: an 8-year prospective study. *Arch Neurol.* 2003;60(3):387–392.

55. Ballard CG, Aarsland D, McKeith I, et al. Fluctuations in attention: PD dementia vs DLB with parkinsonism. *Neurology.* 2002;59(11): 1714–1720.

56. Aarsland D, Ballard C, Larsen JP, McKeith I. A comparative study of psychiatric symptoms in dementia with Lewy bodies and Parkinson's disease with and without dementia. *Int J Geriatr Psychiatry.* 2001;16:528–536.

57. McKeith IG. Dementia with Lewy bodies (DLB) and other difficult diagnoses. *Int Psychogeriatr.* 2004;16(2):123–127.

58. Harding AJ, Halliday GM. Cortical Lewy body pathology in the diagnosis of dementia. *Acta Neuropathologica.* 2001;102: 355–363.

59. Gómez-Tortosa E, Newall K, Irizarry MC, et al. Clinical and quantitative pathological correlates of dementia with Lewy bodies. *Neurology.* 1999;53: 1284–1291.

60. Samuel W, Galasko D, Masliah E, Hansen LA. Neocortical Lewy body counts correlate with dementia in the Lewy body variant of Alzheimer's disease. *J Neuropathol Exp Neurol.* 1996;55(1): 44–52.

61. Perry EK, Piggott MA, Johnson M, et al. Neurotransmitter correlates of neuropsychiatric symptoms in dementia with Lewy bodies. In: Bedard M-A, Agid Y, Chouinard S, et al., eds. *Mental and Behavioral Dysfunction in Movement Disorders.* Totowa, NJ: Humana Press Inc.; 2003: 285–294.

62. Hamilton RL. Lewy bodies in Alzheimer's disease: a neuropathological review of 145 cases using alpha-synuclein immunohistochemistry. *Brain Pathol.* 2000;10:378–384.

63. Lippa CF, McKeith I. Dementia with Lewy bodies: improving diagnostic criteria. *Neurology.* 2003;60:1571–1572.

64. Singleton A, Gwinn-Hardy K. Parkinson's disease and dementia with Lewy bodies: a difference in dose? *Lancet.* 2004;364(9440): 1105–1107.

65. Johnson J, Hague SM, Hanson M, et al. SNCA multiplication is not a common cause of Parkinson disease or dementia with Lewy bodies. *Neurology.* 2004;63(3):554–556.

66. Barber R, Panikkar A, McKeith IG. Dementia with Lewy bodies: diagnosis and management. *Int J Geriatr Psychiatry.* 2001;16: S12–S18.

67. Walker Z, Grace J, Overshot R, et al. Olanzapine in dementia with Lewy bodies: a clinical study. *Int J Geriatr Psychiatry.* 1999;14(6): 459–466.

68. Burke WJ, Pfeiffer RF, McComb RD. Neuroleptic sensitivity to clozapine in dementia with Lewy bodies. *J Neuropsychiatry Clin Neurosci.* 1998;10(2):227–229.

69. Fernandez HH, Wu CK, Ott BR. Pharmacotherapy of dementia with Lewy bodies. *Expert Opin Pharmacother.* 2003;4(11): 2027–2037.

70. Terao T, Shimomura T, Izumi Y, Nakamura J. Two cases of quetiapine augmentation for donepezil-refractory visual hallucinations in dementia with Lewy bodies. *J Clin Psychiatry.* 2003;64(12): 1520–1521.

71. Baskys A. Lewy body dementia: the litmus test for neuroleptic sensitivity and extrapyramidal symptoms. *J Clin Psychiatry.* 2004;65: 16–22.

72. Boeve BF, Silber MH, Parisi JE, et al. Synucleinopathy pathology and REM sleep behavior disorder plus dementia or parkinsonism. *Neurology.* 2003;61:40–45.

73. Bonelli SB, Ransmayr G, Steffelbauer M, Lukas T, Lampl C, Deibl M. L-dopa responsiveness in dementia with Lewy bodies, Parkinson disease with and without dementia. *Neurology.* 2004;63 (2):376–378.

74. Burn DJ, McKeith IG. Current treatment of dementia with Lewy bodies and dementia associated with Parkinson's disease. *Mov Disord.* 2003;18(6):S72–S79.

75. Aarsland D, Mosimann UP, McKeith IG. Role of cholinesterase inhibitors in Parkinson's disease and dementia with Lewy bodies. *J Geriatr Psychiatry Neurol.* 2004;17(3):164–171.

76. Perry EK, McKeith I, Thompson P, et al. Topography, extent, and clinical relevance of neurochemical deficits in dementia of Lewy body type, Parkinson's disease and Alzheimer's disease. *Ann NY Acad Sci.* 1991;640:197–202.

77. McKeith IG, Wesnes KA, Perry E, Ferrara R. Hallucinations predict attentional improvements with rivastigmine in dementia with Lewy bodies. *Dement Geriatr Cogn Disord.* 2004;18: 94–100.

78. Thomas AJ, Burn DJ, Rowen EN, et al. Efficacy of donepezil in Parkinson's disease with dementia and dementia with Lewy bodies. *Int J Geriatr Psychiatry* (In Press).

79. McLaren AT, Allen J, Murray A, Ballard CG, Kenny RA. Cardiovascular effects of donepezil in patients with dementia. *Dement Geriatr Cogn Disord.* 2003;15(4):183–188.

80. Samuel W, Caligiuri M, Galasko D, et al. Better cognitive and psychopathologic response to donepezil in patients prospectively diagnosed as dementia with Lewy bodies: a preliminary study. *Int J Geriatr Psychiatry.* 2000;15(9):794–802.

81. Aarsland D, Laake K, Larsen JP, Janvin C. Donepezil for cognitive impairment in Parkinson's disease: a randomised controlled study

[erratum appears in: *J Neurol Neurosurg Psychiatry.* 2002;73(3):354]. *J Neurol Neurosurg Psychiatry.* 2002;72(6): 708–712.

82. Grace J, Daniel S, Stevens T, et al. Long-term use of rivastigmine in patients with dementia with Lewy bodies: an open-label trial. *Int Psychogeriatr.* 2001;13(2):199–205.

83. Minett TS, Thomas A, Wilkinson LM, et al. What happens when donepezil is suddenly withdrawn? An open label trial in dementia with Lewy bodies and Parkinson's disease with dementia. *Int J Geriatr Psychiatry.* 2003;18:988–993.

Frontotemporal Dementia

23

Andrew Kertesz

Frontotemporal dementia (FTD) is a new name for clinical Pick's disease (PiD). Many would prefer to continue using the eponymic term because of its obvious symmetry to Alzheimer's disease (AD) for the sake of lay audiences and for historical accuracy. Arnold Pick described the clinical picture of frontotemporal atrophy a century ago (1). Pick's initial case of a progressive aphasic patient with behavioral disturbances had only gross examination without any microscopic data, but the clinical description and its relationship to focal atrophy is the basis of the syndrome. Gans suggested the eponymic term and considered a predilection for the phylogenetically younger frontal and temporal lobes in the etiology (2). Subsequently, PiD was defined on the basis of histology, initially described by Alzheimer (3). Onari and Spatz re-examined a series of cases from Pick and others, emphasizing this histological picture associated with focal atrophy (4). Several of Pick's descriptions were concerned with progressive aphasia and apraxia, but subsequently the dramatic behavioral deficits were emphasized (5–10). Schneider described several stages of PiD: first, a disturbance of judgement and asocial behavior, followed by aphasia, and later with more generalized dementia (6). He also distinguished rapid and slow forms. The temporal lobe variety of PiD presenting with progressive aphasia was described quite early, and these descriptions are similar to those of primary progressive aphasia (PPA) (1,11,12). In his review of PiD (13), Caron stated that the most common form is characterized by early development of aphasia, and others have also emphasized early speech disturbance or aphasia in PiD (14,15). Most series of PiD were based on postmortem examination, and often the clinical features were incompletely described because of the retrospective nature of these studies. This gave rise to the notion that

PiD is difficult to diagnose *in vivo*. It also became apparent that cases of clinical PiD with frontal lobe and temporal lobe symptomatology may not show the typical histological picture on autopsy (16). A dichotomy of nosology arose because some people use the term PiD on the basis of histological criteria, while others use PiD to describe the clinical picture of focal atrophies, as Pick did originally.

With the development of neuroimaging, frontotemporal atrophy was demonstrated with increasing frequency in vivo, first with air studies, then computed tomography in the 1970s, and magnetic resonance imaging (MRI) and single photon emission computed tomography (SPECT) more recently. The *in vivo* diagnosis of PiD continued to be made sporadically on the basis of dramatic behavioral symptomatology supported by neuroimaging. However, instead of shifting the diagnosis of PiD back to the clinic, the *in vivo* studies applied new labels such as frontal lobe dementia (FLD), PPA, and frontotemporal degeneration as distinct entities, while reserving the diagnosis of PiD to increasingly restricted histological criteria. This gave rise to the paradox that PiD, a former clinical entity, could only be diagnosed by pathologists. Further development in pathological descriptions contributed to the proliferation of an astonishing variety of terms (Table 23-1).

In order to alleviate the nosological dichotomy and use a historically correct term, yet retain the well-established eponym, we suggested the term *Pick complex* to encompass all the related entities, both clinically and pathologically (17). In a recent consensus conference, the use of FTD for the overall syndrome was found to be most common, although it has continued to be used for the behavioral presentation as well (18). The major presentations of FTD

TABLE 23-1

GLOSSARY OF PICK COMPLEX

1. Circumscribed cerebral atrophy
2. Pick's disease (PiD)
3. Progressive subcortical gliosis (PSG)
4. Corticodentatonigral degeneration
5. Progressive supranuclear palsy (PSP)
6. Frontal lobe dementia (FLD)
7. Primary progressive aphasia (PPA)
8. Corticobasal degeneration (CBD)
9. Dementia lacking distinctive histology (DLDH)
10. Semantic dementia
11. Frontotemporal dementia (FTD)
12. Frontotemporal lobar degeneration (FTLD)
13. FTD-motor neuron disease (FTD-MND)
14. Motor neuron disease inclusion dementia (MNDID)
15. Argyrophilic grain disease
16. Spongiform encephalopathy of long duration
17. Atypical presenile dementia
18. Hereditary dysphasic dementia
19. Pallido-ponto-nigral degeneration
20. Disinhibition dementia amyotrophy parkinsonism

are discussed separately, but it should be remembered that they are overlapping manifestations of the same disease.

FRONTOTEMPORAL DEMENTIA— BEHAVIORAL VARIANT

In the second half of the 1980s, two European groups described FLD as a distinct entity and contrasted the clinical features with AD (19–22). They estimated its relative incidence to be 15% to 20% of degenerative dementias. Both groups recognized that even though some of the cases had Pick bodies and the majority did not, the clinical syndrome was the same. They called the pathology without Pick bodies *dementia of the frontal lobe type*, consisting of neuronal loss and gliosis in the frontal cortex, with or without spongiform changes or ballooned neurons (19). At the same time, Knopman et al. described a similar clinicopathological picture as dementia lacking distinctive histology (23). More recently, the most common neuropathology is found to be associated with the tau-negative ubiquitin-positive inclusions characteristic of motor neuron disease (MND) (24,25).

The groups who described dementia of the frontal lobe type changed the terminology to *frontotemporal degeneration*, and summarized the consensus criteria for diagnosis (26). The term frontotemporal degeneration, or frontotemporal dementia (27), does not include the frequent subcortical involvement, parietal pathology, and extrapyramidal symptomatology. Furthermore, it does not distinguish between the clear-cut behavioral presentation of FLD and aphasic presentation of PPA, which is one of the most valuable contributions of the recent descriptions of the

clinical picture in these conditions. It does reflect, however, the frequent combination of frontal and anterior temporal atrophy originally described by Pick. Articles have recently appeared with terms like *frontal* and *right* and *left temporal variant of FTD* to distinguish the behavioral and aphasic presentation. The clinically more descriptive term *FTD-behavioral variant* (FTD-bv) is probably preferable.

The predominantly behavioral changes often begin with apathy and disinterest, which may be mistaken for depression. On the other hand, the symptoms of disinhibition may suggest a manic psychosis or a personality disorder (28). Cases of PiD with behavioral manifestations, therefore, are more likely to be presented to a psychiatrist than to a neurologist. Those who are more interested in behavioral disorders are less likely to report the language disorder in great detail, often describing the progressive nonfluent aphasia as mutism (29). Neurologists, on the other hand, may see the primarily aphasic or movement disorder more often and may underreport the multifaceted behavioral syndrome often accompanying the language disturbance, or appearing somewhat later.

Behavioral terminology is undergoing constant change and is difficult to standardize or define. The psychiatric descriptions from the French-Swiss literature (30) bear little resemblance to those of the Swedish (29), English (22), or American papers (23). Sometimes the symptoms resembled the so-called Klüver-Bucy syndrome, which is produced in monkeys by bilateral ablation of the temporal neocortex, the amygdala, or the orbitofrontal cortex, consisting of hyperorality, hypersexuality, and compulsive touching (32). Severe disinhibition syndrome may be seen with nondominant temporal lobe atrophy (32). It is difficult to separate the contribution of the temporal and frontal lobes in most cases. Considering the frequent temporal involvement in the pathology, FTD is a logical revision of the previous term—FLD. Since this symptomatology is highly complex and requires experience to recognize, early cases often remain puzzling for first-time observers. Even dementia authorities claimed at one time or another that AD and PiD are similar clinically and cannot be distinguished reliably by clinical or neuropsychological methods (33–35). In fact, the clinical syndrome of PiD is striking and is best illustrated with an actual case.

CASE EXAMPLE

Mr. W, a 65-year-old, previously shy and reserved accountant, began making out of character remarks, wondering aloud how his daughter and son-in-law were having sex. He would grab strangers, start talking to them, or make remarks about somebody having nice legs. He was uncharacteristically aggressive with his dog by throwing things at him, and also laughed without reason on several occasions. Mr. W bought groceries his family did not need and tried making love to his wife during shopping, and sometimes said things that were completely irrelevant to the questions asked. He bought $2,000 worth of windows they did not need on a phone solicitation. Mr. W displayed no emotion when his wife committed suicide (she had a depressive illness, aggravated by her husband's significant personality changes). He exhibited stereotypic slapping of his hands and repetitive banging of walls. The initial diagnosis was obsessive-compulsive disorder.

When seen 2 years after the onset of his illness, Mr. W appeared healthy but distant and disengaged. He was oriented, except for the date, which he remembered later. His assessment was limited by restlessness—he would not stay put for very long and walked out of the office several times. His speech was normal, although he tended to be laconic and speak in short sentences. He remembered recent events, but had to be asked about details.

As time passed Mr. W would not get out of bed or shave. He became less talkative than previously, and repeated questions in an echolalic fashion. He would eat a whole tub of ice cream for breakfast, or a whole handful of candy at once. Sometimes he would put so much food in his mouth that he choked. He became incontinent, or would come out of the bathroom with his pants still down. Despite the symptoms, Mr. W's memory remained reasonably good. He could recall what people were talking about, who was there, what people said, or what he heard in the news. He was hospitalized because of restlessness, pacing, and repetitive noisiness. Sedation and a course of electroconvulsive therapy seemed to temporarily reduce some of his behavioral disturbance.

MRI showed remarkably demarcated frontal lobe atrophy, with more atrophy on the right side (Figure 23-1). Mr. W died approximately 8 years after the onset of his illness, and his brain showed severe frontotemporal atrophy with the gyri having a knife-edge appearance. Histology showed marked neuronal loss, gliosis, and linear spongiosis in the superficial cortical layers. Ballooned neurons (Pick cells) but no typical Pick bodies were seen, and numerous tau-positive inclusions were found in the oligodendroglia, with considerable subcortical involvement. This pathology was considered to have features of both PiD and corticobasal degeneration, but most resembled the features described in hereditary tauopathies (see *Genetics* below).

The definition of FLD consists of a mixture of clinical, imaging, and pathological criteria. The Lund and Manchester Groups achieved a consensus concerning the main features of what they began to call *frontotemporal degeneration* (26). The core diagnostic features of frontotemporal degeneration were loss of personal hygiene and social awareness, disinhibition, mental rigidity, hyperorality, perseveration, distractibility, utilization behavior, loss of insight, indifference, remoteness, inertia, and aspontaneity. Reduction of speech, output, and finally mutism were considered common. Revised criteria were later created at a consensus meeting (Table 23-2) (36).

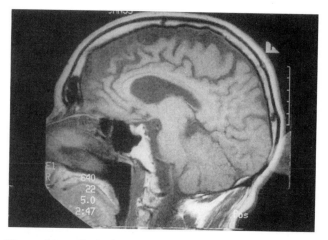

Figure 23-1   Sagittal magnetic resonance imaging showing well-demarcated frontal atrophy.

Neuropsychological test results in FLD patients are variable (20,22,37–39). Frontal lobe patients are often impulsive, cursory, or amotivational, and answer only laconically and at times echolalically. Performance is often inconsistent and patchy. Recognition memory appears better than recall, and the patient tends to benefit from multiple-choice alternatives. Orientation and episodic memory is relatively preserved. The family members' complaint of forgetfulness is more like "forgetting to remember," which may not manifest itself during formal testing. The most common frontal lobe deficits are perseveration on the Wisconsin Card Sorting Task, impaired word fluency, trail-making, and picture arrangement from the Wechsler Adult Intelligence Scale or WAIS-R. Some patients reach floor effect, while others are uncooperative and testing is incomplete. Some patients, however, have normal or near-normal scores on the frontal lobe function test, despite a severe behavioral disturbance. Although drawings in FTD-bv patients may be impoverished due to amotivational performance, visuospatial function is generally intact. The patients may be perseverative in drawing, and copying can be compulsively faithful to detail. At times artistic talent seems to emerge, while other functions deteriorate (40). Visuospatial tasks requiring executive function, such as trail-making, are impaired at an early stage, but block design and Raven's Coloured Progressive Matrices may be preserved. At times, echopraxia and utilization behavior are observed during neuropsychological testing. While memory loss and spatial deficit are characteristic of AD, these functions are relatively preserved in FTD-bv (32,41–43). Screening tests of dementia do not distinguish between AD and FTD, but behavioral quantitation does.

Further distinctions have been made between clinical subtypes of FTD, such as apathetic, disinhibited, and stereotypic (44). The disinhibited type mainly involves the orbitofrontal region. In the apathetic type, the dorsal lateral convexity appears to be affected more, and the stereotypic

TABLE 23-2
REVISED CRITERIA FOR FTD DIAGNOSIS

Core Diagnostic Features	Supportive Diagnostic Features
Insidious onset and gradual progression	Decline in personal hygiene and grooming
Early decline in social interpersonal conduct	Mental rigidity and inflexibility
Early impairment in personal conduct	Distractibility and impersistence
Early emotional blunting	Hyperorality and impersistence
Early loss of insight	Perseverative and stereotyped behavior
	Utilization behavior

type appears to have more extrapyramidal involvement and striatal pathology. Occasionally patients present with failing executive function, usually a job failure or disorganization of homemaking, without the behavioral abnormality. Not all patients can be easily subcategorized, and these distinctions tend to become blurred as the disease progresses.

Quantitation of behavior has been attempted by Gustafson and Nielson in order to separate PiD from AD (45). The Manchester Group also assessed the symptoms of FLD in a retrospective study, to correlate the clinical diagnosis with autopsy findings (46). Their results distinguished FLD and AD with a high degree of success. Lopez et al. found more symptoms of major depression, agitation, irritability, lability of mood, disinhibition, inertia, and social withdrawal in FTD patients when compared to AD patients, who displayed more signs of delusional psychosis (47). Gregory and Hodges reviewed the psychiatric symptomatology in FTD patients who had at least five of the core diagnostic features (28). Only 50% of the patients were diagnosed as FTD at presentation, and one-third received an initial psychiatric diagnosis such as schizophrenia, psychosis, depression with obsessive/compulsive features, alcohol dependency, and psychogenic memory impairment. Miller et al. evaluated the presence or absence of the Lund/Manchester items in 30 patients with FTD retrospectively (48). The patients were selected on the basis of SPECT scans. Discriminant function showed a loss of hygiene, hyperorality, stereotypic, and perseverative behavior. Miller and colleagues emphasized the "loss of self" manifesting in dramatic alterations of personality and behavior, particularly with right temporal atrophy (49).

There are numerous existing behavioral inventories serving a more general purpose of exploring abnormal behavior in geriatric, psychiatric, or a general demented population (50–54). Geriatric scales often combine cognition, behavior and activities of daily living to measure the global extent of decline, but do not discriminate specific behavior syndromes. Psychiatric behavioral scales also dilute the few frontal behaviors with symptoms of other psychiatric illness.

We constructed a 24-item *frontal behavioral inventory* (FBI) to target the most specific behaviors for optimum diagnostic accuracy for FTD, to be used at the initial inter-

view or for retrospective diagnosis (55). These items were selected from the core diagnostic features of the Lund/Manchester criteria and the most common symptoms in our FTD-bv patients. The inventory was designed as a series of structured questions scripted so both the normal and abnormal negative aspects of the behaviors were included, giving the caregiver a choice (Table 23-3). If the caregiver seemed to hesitate or did not understand, the question was rephrased. Each item was scored on a scale from zero to three, where 0 = none, 1 = mild or occasional, 2 = moderate, and 3 = severe or most of the time.

The items were grouped as negative behaviors such as apathy, aspontaneity, indifference, inflexibility, concreteness, personal neglect, distractibility, inattention, loss of insight, logopenia, verbal apraxia, and alien hand. These last three items were included to capture specific motor and speech behaviors that may be associated with FTD. The second group of behaviors contained items of disinhibition such as perseveration, irritability, jocularity, irresponsibility, inappropriateness, impulsivity, restlessness, aggression, hyperorality, hypersexuality, utilization of behavior, and incontinence. Minor modifications and additions have been standardized (56).

Significantly higher FBI scores are seen in the frontal group compared with the two control groups on the ANOVA (Figure 23-2). FBI scores discriminated reliably between FTD and the control groups, with little overlap between them. This suggested cut-off points to operationalize the behavioral diagnosis of FTD. A sensitive cut-off point is 27, including all FTD scores. There was only one false positive among depressive dementias. These patients could be identified by the vegetative symptoms of depression and positive depression inventories (57). All AD patients and most depressive patients scored below 24. A conservative or specific cut-off point of 30 excluded most non-FTD patients. These cut off points may serve as FBI criteria in grouping patients behaviorally for future studies.

Further standardization using discriminant function correctly classified 92.7% of FTD patients versus all others, but 19% of vascular dementia (VaD) patients were misclassified as FTD (56). Vascular patients, however, are differentiated by their sudden onset, stepwise evolution, and evidence of strokes on neurological examination and

TABLE 23-3
FRONTAL BEHAVIORAL INVENTORY

Name: _____ Age: ____ Diagnosis: _____ Date: _____

Caregiver: _____ Examiner: _____

Frontal Behavioral Inventory

Explain to the caregiver that you are looking for a change in behavior and personality. Ask the caregiver these questions in the absence of the patient. Elaborate if necessary. At the end of each question, ask about the extent of the behavioral change, and then score it according to the following: 0 = none; 1 = mild, occasional; 2 = moderate; 3 = severe, most of the time.

1. Apathy: Has the patient lost interest in friends or daily activities, or is he or she interested in seeing people and doing things?

    _____

2. Aspontaneity: Does the patient start things on his or her own, or does he or she have to be asked?

    _____

3. Indifference, emotional flatness: Does the patient respond to occasions of joy or sadness as much as ever, or has he or she lost emotional responsiveness?

    _____

4. Inflexibility: Can the patient change his or her mind with reason, or does he or she appear stubborn or rigid in thinking lately?

    _____

5. Personal neglect: Does the patient take as much care of his or her personal hygiene and appearance as usual, or, for example, does the patient neglect to wash or change his or her underwear?

    _____

6. Disorganization: Can the patient plan and organize complex activity, or is he or she easily distractible, impersistent, or unable to complete a job?

    _____

7. Inattention: Does the patient pay attention to what is going on, or does he or she seem to lose track or not follow at all?

    _____

8. Loss of insight: Is the patient aware of any problems or changes, or does he or she seem unaware of them or deny them when discussed?

    _____

9. Logopenia: Is the patient as talkative as before, or has his or her amount of speech decreased significantly?

    _____

    Negative Behavior Score: _____

    _____

10. Perseverations, obsessions: Does the patient repeat or perseverate actions or remarks? Are there any obsessive routines or behaviors, or has he or she always been a creature of habit?

    _____

11. Irritability: Has the patient been irritable or short-tempered, or is the patient reacting to stress or frustration as he or she always has?

    _____

12. Excessive jocularity: Has the patient been making jokes excessively or offensively or at the wrong time, or has he or she always had a jocular manner or a quirky sense of humor?

    _____

13. Poor judgment: Has the patient been using good judgment in decisions or in driving, or has he or she acted irresponsibly, neglectfully, or in poor judgment?

    _____

14. Hoarding: Has the patient started to hoard objects or money excessively, or have his or her saving habits remained unchanged?

    _____

15. Inappropriateness: Has the patient kept social rules, or has he or she said or done things outside what are acceptable? Has he or she been rude, or childish?

    _____

16. Impulsivity: Has the patient acted or spoken without thinking about consequences, on the spur of the moment, or is he or she able to think matters through?

    _____

17. Restlessness: Has the patient been restless or pacing, or is his or her activity level normal?

    _____

18. Aggression: Has the patient shown aggression, or shouted at anyone or hurt anyone physically, or is there no change in this respect?

    _____

19. Hyperorality: Has the patient been excessively drinking or eating anything in sight, or developing food fads, or even putting objects in his or her mouth, or has the patient always had a large appetite?

    _____

(continued)

TABLE 23-3
continued

20. Hypersexuality: Has the patient's sexual behavior been unusual or excessive? This could include remarks or undressing, or is there no change in this respect?

_____

21. Utilization behavior: Does the patient seem to need to touch, feel, examine, or pick up objects within reach and sight, or can the patient keep his or her hands to him or herself?

_____

22. Incontinence: Has the patient wet or soiled him or herself, or does the patient have problems that can be explained by urinary tract infection or childbirth/prostate problems?

_____

Disinhibition Score: _____   Total Score: _____

neuroimaging. In patients with low overall scores (below the cut-off of 27), progressive aphasics can be discriminated by their clinical features and high scores on verbal apraxia and logopenia. Some depressed patients achieve high scores on apathy, aspontaneity, and disorganization questions, and some manic patients achieve high disinhibition scores, but the age of onset and the clinical course of the illness is distinctive. In a further study with the behavioral inventory, we demonstrated that only 75% of FTD and AD patients can be distinguished using cognitive tests, while 100% discrimination was achieved by adding the FBI to the discriminant function (58).

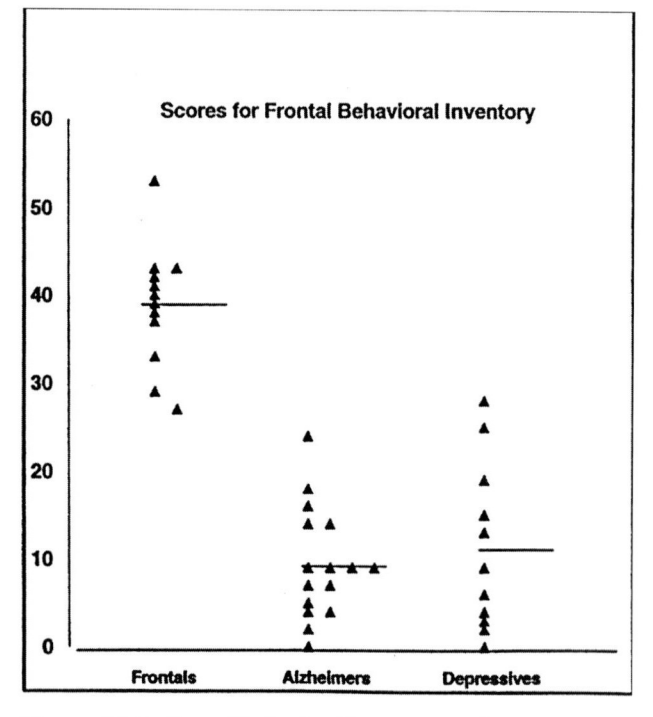

Figure 23-2 Frontal behavioral inventory total scores in three populations. Horizontal bars are means. Differences between frontotemporal dementia and the other two groups are significant (p < 0.01).

Direct behavioral assessment of FTD patients uses items to detect motor or cognitive perseveration, verbal intrusions, disinhibition, loss of spontaneity, imitation, and utilization behavior. Attempts have been made to formalize these frontal lobe signs in an executive interview (59) or the _Frontal Assessment Battery_ (60). Some of the items from these tests are often incorporated into a neurological examination and are complementary to the FBI.

In summary, the diagnosis of FTD-bv depends on a good history from a caregiver. The emergence of food fads, gluttony, rudeness, poor judgment, indifference, hoarding, and childish joking in a presenile individual with relatively retained memory and spatial cognition should ring an alarm bell. The quantitation of behavioral abnormality and confirmation with neuroimaging is desirable. AD patients are older, have major memory and visuospatial deficit, and diffuse atrophy. Exclusion of VaD and manic depressive illness is essential.

PRIMARY PROGRESSIVE APHASIA

A series of patients with progressive language deficit, before other cognitive domains were involved, was described and subsequently named PPA by Mesulam (61,62). Detailed modern case reports of PiD with progressive aphasia appeared at the same time (63,64). The term PPA has been widely used, although similar patients were reported under variations of this terminology, such as progressive aphasia without dementia (65), progressive nonfluent aphasia (66), and pure progressive aphemia (67). Although both Pick (1) and Alzheimer (68) described their original patients as being significantly aphasic, the significance of language impairment in dementia has not been emphasized and documented systematically until recently (69–72). Pick's conclusion was that "a more or less circumscribed type of aphasia could result from a single circumscribed atrophic process" (1).

The initial presentation of PPA is often anomia, or word-finding difficulty. In this respect, PPA patients are not much different from AD patients, except they have relatively preserved memory and nonverbal cognition. AD patients, by the time they show word-finding difficulty, already have significant memory loss and disorientation, and constructional, visuospatial, and other cognitive impairment. The relatively isolated language disturbance in the first 2 years of the illness, suggested by Mesulam as the operational definition of PPA, more or less distinguishes the two groups of patients (62). However, some of the pathologically proven cases have behavioral or extrapyramidal features that appear before the 2 year deadline. Although the 2 year "purity" criteria may be arbitrary and exclude patients who in fact have the disease, it seems useful to predict Pick complex pathology, which includes PiD, corticobasal degeneration (CBD), dementia lacking distinctive histology (DLDH), or FTD-motor neuron disease (FTD-MND) (73).

The more typical clinical picture progresses from anomia to a nonfluent type of aphasia with increasing word-finding difficulty. Logopenia is defined as a phenomenon where the word-finding difficulty is prominent, but the phrase length is still longer than four words and syntax is preserved (74). Decreasing speech output involves spontaneous speech first, and repetition is affected to a lesser extent initially (75). Sometimes the aphasic disturbance resembles Broca's aphasia, with grammatical errors and phonemic paraphasias. The relative preservation of comprehension is typical, and nonverbal intelligence and episodic memory is demonstrably maintained (58,74–77). Broca's aphasia with agrammatism is more characteristic of stroke patients, but it may be seen in PPA as a transient stage, usually progressing with increasing word-finding difficulty to mutism. The course is variable and may be quite prolonged, but sometimes patients who develop pathology in the basal ganglia or motor neurons progress quickly and develop difficulty with swallowing and choking; the course may be as short as 2 years from onset to death (17,78,79).

Naming errors were analyzed in PPA by Weintraub et al. (80). They found more phonemic paraphasias, fewer circumlocutions and perceptual errors than similar patients with AD. Snowden et al. combined all their cases of progressive language disorders with lobar atrophy (77). In addition to five nonfluent cases with preserved comprehension and five cases of fluent (semantic) aphasias, they also found a group of mixed cases where progressive loss of speech output was also associated with loss of comprehension. Writing was relatively preserved in some of the patients (75,77). Transcortical motor, anomic, Broca's, and global aphasic patterns were described in four patients with various degrees of left hemispheric dysfunction on SPECT and a variable rate of decline on the Western Aphasia Battery (WAB) (81). In a study of 67 patients with PPA, most were classified as relatively fluent anomic aphasic on the WAB initially (58), but on a follow-up visit nonfluent cases predominated. The fluency/nonfluency distinction depended on the stage at which patients were examined. In contrast, AD patients remained anomic and

fluent until late in the course of the disease. PPA patients had significantly lower aphasia quotients than comparably staged AD patients. Some of the nonverbal control tests were relatively preserved in early PPA, such as the drawing of pentagons, a clock, or Raven's Coloured Progressive Matrices. About half of the patients followed at a yearly interval developed the behavioral abnormality of FTD, and a significant number (N = 15) developed the extrapyramidal symptoms resembling CBD.

Some patients present with stuttering or slow dysprosodic speech and verbal apraxia, which includes articulatory difficulty and phonological paraphasias. Cortical dysarthria, anarthria, aphemia, or pure motor aphasia are alternate terms to describe the phenomena when writing and comprehension are relatively preserved (67). The articulatory impairment is characterized by particular difficulty with initial consonants, such as omission, repetition, and substitution. Although this is often called verbal apraxia, it may occur with or without buccofacial or limb apraxia (82,83). These patients are less likely to be mistaken for AD patients. A progressive limb apraxia can be a prominent feature (84), indicating a clinical overlap between PPA and the apraxic-extrapyramidal syndrome of CBD.

Several patients, well after 10 years of illness, continue to function normally at home even though they are completely mute. One of our younger patients, who managed to take care of her children and her household, was considered hysterical by the psychologist, speech pathologist, and neurologist before neuroimaging showed severe frontal atrophy and the patient was diagnosed as having probable PiD (17). A frontal biopsy confirmed the diagnosis, with Pick bodies and swollen neurons, and autopsy 12 years after the onset of her illness confirmed these findings. Another patient, who managed to carry on working well into the fifth year of his illness, was referred because of possible depression to a psychiatrist, who recognized his problem as PPA (17).

Mutism has been considered characteristic of PiD, and tends to be the end-stage of all forms of FTD, even those that start with behavioral abnormalities rather than language disturbance (22,29). Decreased speech output and mutism are core symptoms in the description of FTD, and there is a great deal of overlap between the descriptions of language deficit, FTD, PPA, and PiD. End-stage mutism also occurs in AD, but usually in a patient who already has a global dementia with loss of comprehension and basic functions of daily living (69). Unlike global aphasia or severe AD, in PPD, FTD, and PPA mutism occurs with relative preservation of comprehension.

SEMANTIC DEMENTIA (APHASIA)

A distinct, fluent form of PPA that is different from the more common nonfluent variety was described as *semantic dementia* by Snowden et al. (85). These patients progressively lost the meaning of words, but retained fluency and were able to carry out a conversation. Subsequent descriptions of this entity adopted this term (86), although these patients are not demented in the usual sense. *Semantic aphasia* was a term used by Head for a two-way disturbance of comprehension and naming (87). The picture is similar to transcortical sensory aphasia in which articulation, phonology, and syntax remain intact, but the patient does not comprehend well and has word-finding difficulty. *Transcortical sensory aphasia* was commonly used for describing patients with degenerative disease, and this particular syndrome also appears in AD. However, patients with semantic dementia or primary progressive fluent aphasia differ significantly from the fluent aphasics of AD, because they have a relatively preserved episodic memory and autobiographical memory, with loss of semantic memory in a rather selective fashion. Some very interesting studies showed that these patients retain information that has immediate relevance to their environment or to their person, yet lose the meaning of other common things (88). The behavior can be so dissociative that some of these patients are considered hysterical. The following case example illustrates the initially isolated syndrome, which almost invariably becomes associated with the behavioral abnormality of FTD.

CASE EXAMPLE

Mr. W, a 46-year-old engineer, initially developed word-finding difficulty, but later a peculiar loss of the meaning of things appeared. He would ask, for example, "What is 'shoe-polish,' 'ice age,' or 'asbestos?'" when these words came up in conversation. At meetings he did not understand everything that was being said, and had to ask his coworkers to elaborate. Mr. W remained competent for visuospatial tasks, blueprints, and most nonverbal problem-solving tasks; therefore, his language problems were initially overlooked at work and Mr. W was still employed as a professional engineer when he was referred for a neurological assessment.

Initially his speech output was normal, except for the mild word-finding problem and semantic substitutions; for instance, he called a bicycle helmet a "safety hat." When tested, Mr. W named about half of the objects, and described the use and showed by gesture some of those he could not name. However, for several items he could not even do that; he not only did not know what an egg beater was, he could not show how to use it. The meaning of some things seemed to have become lost, even when the object was in front of him. Technically, he had visual agnosia for these items as well. When he read words with irregular spelling he did not recognize, he would regularize them; for example yacht was read "yatcht." He developed an auditory agnosia, or impaired recognition of voices on the telephone. In contrast to his progressive semantic aphasia, also labelled as semantic

dementia, Mr. W remembered events such as his recent move to London and his daughter's recent graduation. He continued to drive a car, pay his bills, and carry out carpentry.

Two years after his initial visit, Mr. W developed a set of behavioral symptoms that was quite distressing to his wife, to the extent that it was she who was admitted to a psychiatric unit with a depressive breakdown. He insisted on altering his basement to put up his huge jigsaw puzzle pictures, despite her efforts to dissuade him. He also developed compulsive routines and food fads, such as eating Chinese food every time they passed a food court in a mall, a fondness for bananas, and having donuts instead of a proper lunch. He was childish about trying to get the largest donut, and pouted if he got a small one. He put a great deal of plum sauce on rice and excessive maple syrup on pancakes, and went back for several helpings of Chinese food. On several occasions he drove to his favorite donut shop in Toronto, where he used to live, 200 kilometers away.

On Mr. W's last visit his speech was still relatively fluent and phonologically and grammatically intact, but he had a great deal of trouble comprehending single words, even common ones such as pencil, cup, and comb. He could not point to these objects even when he had only six to choose from. On the other hand, he had no problem pointing to letters, numbers, or colors. These abstractions, although meaningful, do not have the same semantic content that objects do.

Attempts to stop Mr. W's compulsive roaming and driving were met with stubborn resistance and anger. Eventually, they took his car keys away. He resorted to hot-wiring his ignition, and on another occasion was ready to drive away in someone else's car when he found the key in the ignition. The police were called and Mr. W ended up in the closed ward of the psychiatric hospital. Using his superior visuospatial skills, he watched staff punch in the door code and quickly learned the code and escaped; eventually handle covers had to be used to control this. He then used windows for exit. He took food away from other people, and even when he was tied to a chair, he would get up with the chair on his back and move around. Mr. W's verbal output became restricted to, "Oh no, oh yes," and he also began choking on food such as meat.

Standardized language testing is useful to diagnose and follow the course of illness of both PPA and semantic dementia. Of particular importance is an examination of spontaneous speech for fluency and content to document comprehension and naming, preferably with low and high-frequency items and repetition. Examining reading and writing is also important, particularly a list of irregular words to detect transcortical alexia (reading without meaning). Additional psycholinguistic testing is of considerable interest in exploring the processing deficit, particularly in progressive fluent aphasia or semantic dementia (77,86, 88–90).

CORTICOBASAL DEGENERATION/ PROGRESSIVE SUPRANUCLEAR PALSY

There have been several case descriptions of PiD where the patients had prominent extrapyramidal features (8,91,92). Ferraro and Jervis stated that extrapyramidal symptoms were common in PiD (9). Sometimes unilateral rigidity and parkinsonism were the first symptoms to attract attention. It was recognized that subcortical changes occur in PiD, even without extrapyramidal symptomatology (93,94). Constantinidis et al. (16) described extrapyramidal involvement particularly in group B PiD (pathology with ballooned neurons), and Mann et al. described extrapyramidal involvement in eight out of 12 FTD patients (95). Changes in the basal ganglia, especially in the striatum and the substantia nigra, in addition to cortical pathology, occurred in the majority of 30 cases in one review (96).

When Rebeiz et al. described corticodentatonigral degeneration, they recognized the similarity of the pathology to PiD (97). The clinical syndrome of unilateral rigidity, prominent apraxia, gaze palsy, reflex myoclonus, and the alien hand syndrome was relabelled *corticobasal* or *corticobasal ganglionic degeneration* (98,99). Including the original description, most of the literature concerning this condition acknowledges the clinical and pathological overlap between CBD and PiD (100–103).

CBD suffers from a similar dichotomy as PiD, in that the pathological and clinical descriptions do not fully overlap. There are some case reports describing patients presented clinically as CBD and as defined by unilateral rigidity, apraxia, and alien hand syndrome, but who have the pathological findings of PiD with Pick bodies (104). Other cases pathologically typical of CBD have a frontal type of dementia without the extrapyramidal features (100,105–108). CBD pathology can also be seen with a clinical picture of PPA (17,103,109–113). We suggested that the clinical syndrome of prominent apraxia, unilateral extrapyramidal syndrome and alien hand phenomenon should be designated as *corticobasal degeneration syndrome* (CBDS) (114).

The rather focused interest in the extrapyramidal syndrome led to the idea that behavioral changes and dementia occur only in a minority of CBD cases (115). When the publications are specifically reviewed, however, cognitive decline, especially executive deficit, language disturbances, and personality and behavioral changes are common. Even the first patient described with this syndrome started to show personality changes and a progressive language disorder a year after her motor symptoms appeared (97). Gibb and colleagues' first patient also had progressive aphasia (98).

Neuropathologically selected CBD series showed an even greater incidence of cognitive deficit, frontal lobe symptomatology, and progressive aphasia (116–119). In one series from a brain bank, the most common presenta-

tion was dementia, and six of these had the clinical diagnosis of AD (117). Yet some others reiterated the perceived low frequency of cognitive impairments (118). Our experience with CBDS showed significant overlap between CBDS and the syndromes of FTD/Pick complex (120). All of our 35 patients with clinical CBDS had either a language disorder or a behavioral and personality change characteristic of FTD. At times, the movement disorder and the progressive aphasia or behavioral disorder developed simultaneously, but in the majority of cases the cognitive disorder came first (N = 20). Similarly, in all the primary movement presentations (N = 15), aphasic or behavioral change developed sooner or later, indicating that CBD should be considered part of the Pick complex. In eleven of our 35 cases with autopsy, six had CBD pathology (one was considered to have features of *progressive supranuclear* palsy [PSP]), three cases had PiD, one had MND-type inclusions, and one had DLDH.

Patients with axial dystonia, bradykinesia, falls, dysphagia, and vertical gaze palsy are considered typical of PSP, but the overlap with CBDS has been increasingly recognized. Many CBD patients also have vertical gaze palsy, and some have falls and symmetrical extrapyramidal syndrome (121). Two of our CBDS series patients with CBD pathology, for instance, received the clinical diagnosis of PSP at one time or another. Some studies comparing the neuropsychological features of PSP and CBD found no significant difference between them (122), and the pathological features are also considered to be overlapping to a great extent (123). Biochemical and genetic evidence also supports the relationship (124,125). They are both considered to be predominantly four-repeat tauopathies. There is continuing controversy as to what extent PSP and CBD can be differentiated, although pathological criteria for each have recently been validated (126). The evidence is overwhelming that CBD/PSP is also part of the Pick complex, and subcortical involvement is much too frequent to restrict the disease to cortical degeneration.

MOTOR NEURON DISEASE AND FRONTOTEMPORAL DEMENTIA

Recently a great deal of interest has been shown in the association of dementia with MND (78,127). It became evident that cases of dementia with MND have ubiquitin-positive, tau-negative inclusions in the cortex, which have been previously described in the motor neurons in *amyotrophic lateral sclerosis* (ALS) (128,129), subsequently named *motor neuron disease inclusion dementia* (130). Cognitive and behavioral impairment has been observed in ALS, and some estimate it to be as high as 50% (131,132). *Creutzfeldt-Jakob disease* has also been described with MND, but now it appears that many of these cases were not instances of prion protein disease, but rather pathology resembling FTD with spongiform changes in the superficial cortical layers

(133). There are a significant number of cases of FTD and PPA patients developing MND (78,79).

Recently, the ubiquitin-positive, tau-negative inclusions have been found in FTD without clinical MND, even in the familial form (134). In fact, a majority of cases that were previously described as having DLDH have these rather distinct inclusions, also called FTD with MND type inclusions, or FTD-MND (24,25). In the familial cases, intranuclear inclusions of similar histochemistry have recently been discussed (135).

NEUROPATHOLOGY

The Pick complex neuropathology is initially asymmetrical, and this is the reason for the variations in clinical presentation, but at postmortem the findings are bilateral as a rule. The underlying neuronal loss, gliosis, and superficial linear spongiosis in affected cortical areas is common to all histological subtypes. Ballooned neurons, or Pick cells, occur with variable frequency in all varieties. They appear swollen pink on H & E stain, lack Nissl substance (neuronal achromasia) of the cytoplasm, and express phosphorylated neurofilaments. There is tau reactivity in the oligodendroglial cells and astrocytic processes. The superficial layer spongiosis is seen in layers II and III of the cortex, in contrast to the spongiform change of Creutzfeldt-Jakob disease, which tends to be throughout the cortex. Various distinctive features, such as Pick bodies, astrocytic plaques in CBD, tufted astrocytes in PSP, and ubiquitin-positive, tau-negative inclusions in MND-type dementia have been described, but they can also occur with each of the other clinical varieties. Cases lacking any of these distinctive features are often labelled DLDH, but many turn out to have the MND-type inclusions (FTD-MND). These inclusions are found in more than half of the FTD cases on autopsy, and form the largest single pathological variety of Pick complex (24,25). They appear similar in location and morphology to Pick bodies, but differ in their histochemical characteristics.

There is substantial overlap between all pathological varieties, although their distinctiveness is also argued (136). As mentioned before, the clinical varieties of Pick complex do not predict the overall pathological spectrum. Nevertheless, there is a prominence of CBD pathology in the extrapyramidal and aphasic presentation, the FTD-MND type with the behavioral presentation and semantic dementia, and Pick body dementia with all of them. Progressive subcortical gliosis is clinically and pathologically similar to PiD, and remains so far only a doubtful pathological distinction (137,138). About 30 cases have been described in the literature (139,140).

BIOCHEMISTRY

Abnormally phosphorylated and aggregated tau proteins are biochemical markers of various forms of degenerative dementia, including AD, PiD, CBD, PSP, the Parkinsonism-dementia of Guam, dementia pugilistica, etc., collectively called *tauopathies*. However, tau mutations have been discovered only in FTD with parkinsonism linked to chromosome 17 (FTDP-17). Neurofibrillary tangles of AD contain all six human tau isoforms. Abnormally phosphorylated tau forms three bands on Western blot studies with a molecular weight of 55, 64, and 69 kdalton in AD. PiD has a 64-kdalton and 55-kdalton band, and CBD and PSP have 69-kdalton and 64-kdalton doublets. The amounts of abnormal tau can be low in FTD, and sometimes even absent. At times FTD has a tau triplet, as in AD (141). Sometimes different band compositions are obtained from different parts of the brain (142). In some studies, two bands were seen in brainstem neurons and triplets in the hippocampal neurons in PSP.

Normal tau proteins contribute to axonal transport by binding to microtubular protein (143,144). Six tau isoforms are created by the differential splicing of exon 10, making three or four repeats of the microtubular binding domain of tau. Three-repeat (3R) tau predominates in PiD, and four-repeat (4R) tau is more common in CBD and PSP. Lately 4R tau is found with equal frequency in some cases of PiD, so the biochemical differences are not as sharp as was previously thought (145). Tau-negative hereditary dysphasic disinhibition dementia and some sporadic cases of DLDH with prominent language and behavioral deficit have been recently attributed to the loss of normal tau in the brain, with the same effect as the tauopathies with tau-positive pathology (146).

GENETICS

Wilhelmsen et al. (147) discovered linkage to chromosome 17 q21–22 in a large family with variable symptomatology of FTD, aphasia, parkinsonism, and amyotrophy (148). A consensus conference summarized the clinical features and pathology of 12 families linked to chromosome 17, resembling the sporadic cases. Although each family was initially described under different terminology (see Table 23-1 for some of them), the term FTDP-17 was accepted (149). The microtubular associated protein tau was suspected as the candidate gene for mutation, and a year later several tau mutations were discovered (144,150, 151).

To date, about 20 tau mutations in more than 50 families have been identified. The exon 10 splice mutations alter the ratio of 4R to 3R tau isoforms, most often resulting in pathology resembling CBD or PSP. The phenotypes range from FTD and PiD to CBD, and often the same mutation results in different clinical presentation (152). Similarly, the same mutation, for example, the common P301L, may produce pathology with Pick bodies, CBD, or DLDH. The missense mutations disrupt the interaction between tau and microtubules, and unbound tau becomes abnormally phosphorylated and polymerized into filaments and inclusions. Mutations in exons 9, 12, and 13 result in either accumulation of all six isoforms of tau-forming tangles or in a predominance of 3R tau and Pick body dementia. Although different tau mutations differentially alter biochemical properties of tau isoforms (153), these mutations do not predict the clinical presentations. They do, however, predict the overall clinical morphological picture resembling sporadic FTD or Pick complex.

Tau polymorphisms, from the two main haplotypes of tau, were also studied. H_1 haplotype is over represented in both PSP and CBD (124) and in FTD (154). The increase of H_2 haplotype with an interaction with ApoE4 in FTD and anomic aphasia was suggested by Short et al. (155), perhaps representing the AD patients included in the sample. The search for another genetic locus for the large number of tau negative families is underway. So far linkage to chromosome 3 (156) and chromosome 9 (157) has been demonstrated, but no mutations have been found. The chromosome 9 linkage was shown with familial ALS associated with FTD.

TREATMENT

There is evidence that cholinergic receptor binding is decreased in PiD in affected cortical regions (158–160). Serotonin and imipramine binding has been found to be decreased in the hypothalamus, frontal, and temporal lobes associated in PiD (161). The decreased serotonin binding could correlate with the overeating, cravings for bananas, sweet cravings, and weight gain observed in some patients with PiD/FTD/Pick complex. Other behavioral impairments, such as depression, irritability, and apathy, with relative preservation of memory are also compatible with serotoninergic dysfunction (162). Selective serotonin-reuptake inhibitors have been tried in an open-label application in FTD patients, improving some of the obsessive symptoms (163). Trazodone has been found effective in improving behavior in FTD in a placebo cross-over design (164). Acetylcholinesterase inhibitors have not been tried systematically, and anecdotal reports of worsening or improvement are not reliable. Small doses of atypical neuroleptics are effective to cope with the restlessness, roaming, and asocial behavior. Much of the current treatment is only symptomatic; to date no drugs have shown disease-modifying properties.

CONCLUSIONS

FTD or PiD is a relatively common but still underdiagnosed presenile dementia. Estimated prevalence ranges from 6% to 25%, with a ratio of 1:4 to AD and 1:1 to early onset dementia (under age 65) (165). The lack of reliable prevalence data stems from the difficulty in identification

of cases and a negative bias in autopsy series from brain banks affiliated with Alzheimer centers. The high estimates come from centers interested in the disease, and may represent a positive bias. The familial incidence of FTD is high—approximately 30% to 40% of cases—but tau mutation is found in only about 10% of the families tested in some centers, and so far not in any sporadic cases (166). The detection of increased tau in the cerebrospinal fluid is unreliable and not specific, and so far the diagnosis depends on good clinical acumen and neuroimaging.

Think of FTD when you encounter:

- Disinhibition with indifference appearing in middle age (we are not talking about advanced AD patients)
- Progressive unexplained aphasia
- Patients who ask, "What is steak, shoe polish?" etc.
- Those with a unilateral rigid levitating hand that appears "alien"
- Patients who fall and have vertical gaze palsy
- Dementia with MND

Spend extra time with the caregivers to find out what the presenting symptom was when you see patients in mid-stage, when the diagnosis is complicated by more generalized dementia or mutism. Caregivers of FTD patients also need extra time for counseling, particularly as the disease progresses and results in social, family, and personality breakdown.

REFERENCES

1. Pick A. Über die Beziehungen der senilen Hirnatrophie zur Aphasie. *Prag Med Wochenschr.* 1892;17:165–167.
2. Gans A. Betrachtungen über Art und Ausbreitung des krankhaften Prozesses in einem Fall von Pickscher Atrophie des Stirnhirns. *Ztschr fur die gse Neurol u Psychiatr.* 1922;80:10–28.
3. Alzheimer A. Über eigenartige Krankheitsfälle des späteren Alters. *Z Gesamte Neurol Psychiatr.* 1911;4:356–385.
4. Onari K, Spatz H. Anatomische Beitrage zur Lehre von der Pickschen umschriebenen Grosshirnrinden-Atrophie ("Picksche Krankheit"). *Z Gesamte Neurol Psych.* 1926;101:470–511.
5. Schneider C. Über Picksche Krankheit. *Monatsschr Psychiatr Neurologie.* 1927;65:230–275.
6. Schneider C. Weitere Beitrage zur Lehre von der Pickschen Krankheit. *Z Gesamte Neurol Psych.* 1929;120:340–384.
7. Thorpe FT. Pick's disease (circumscribed senile atrophy) and Alzheimer's disease. *J Ment Sci.* 1932;78:302–314.
8. Lowenberg K. Pick's disease—a clinicopathologic contribution. *Arch Neurol Psychiatr.* 1936;36:768–789.
9. Ferraro A, Jervis GA. Pick's disease—clinicopathologic study with report of two cases. *Arch Neurol Psychiatr.* 1936;36:739–767.
10. Nichols IC, Weigner WC. Pick's disease—a specific type of dementia. *Brain.* 1938;61:237–249.
11. Pick A. Zur symptomatologie der linksseitigen Schlafenlappenatrophie. *Monatsschr Psychiatr Neurologie.* 1905;16:378–388.
12. Rosenfeld M. Die partielle Grosshirnatrophie. *J Psychol Neurol.* 1909;14:115–130.
13. Caron M. *Étude Clinique de la Maladie Pick.* Paris: Vigot; 1934.
14. Kosaka K. On aphasia of Pick's disease: a review of our own 3 cases and 49 autopsy cases in Japan. (In Japanese). *Seishin Igaku.* 1976;18:1181–1189, as quoted by Ohashi (1983).
15. Ohashi H. An aphasiologic approach to Pick's disease. In: Hirano A, Miyoshi K, eds. *Neuropsychiatric Disorders in the Elderly.* Tokyo: Igaku-Shoin; 1983;132–135.

16. Constantinidis J, Richard J, Tissot R. Pick's disease—histological and clinical correlations. *Europ Neurol.* 1974;11:208–217.

17. Kertesz A, Hudson L, Mackenzie IRA, Munoz DG. The pathology and nosology of primary progressive aphasia. *Neurology.* 1994;44:2065–2072.

18. Kertesz A, Hillis A, Munoz DG. Frontotemporal dementia and Pick's disease. *Ann Neurol.* 2003;54(Suppl 5):S1–S35.

19. Brun A. Frontal lobe degeneration of non-Alzheimer type. I. Neuropathology. *Arch Gerontol Geriatr.* 1987;6:193–208.

20. Gustafson L. Frontal lobe degeneration of non-Alzheimer type. II. Clinical picture and differential diagnosis. *Arch Gerontol Geriatr.* 1987;6:209–223.

21. Neary D, Snowden JS, Bowen JS, et al. Neuropsychological syndromes in presenile dementia due to cerebral atrophy. *J Neurol Neurosurg Psychiatry.* 1986;49:163–174.

22. Neary D, Snowden JS, Northen B, Goulding P. Dementia of frontal lobe type. *J Neurol Neurosurg Psychiatry.* 1988;51:353–361.

23. Knopman DS, Mastri AR, Frey WH, Sung JH, Rustan T. Dementia lacking distinctive histologic features: a common non-Alzheimer degenerative dementia. *Neurology.* 1990;40:251–256.

24. Munoz DG, Dickson DW, Bergeron C, Mackenzie IRA, Delacourte A, Zhukareva V. The neuropathology and biochemistry of frontotemporal dementia. *Ann Neurol.* 2003;54(Suppl 5):S24–S28.

25. Hodges JR, Davies R, Xuereb J, Kril J, Halliday G. Survival in frontotemporal dementia. *Neurology.* 2003;61:349–354.

26. The Lund and Manchester Groups. Clinical and neuropathological criteria for frontotemporal dementia. *J Neurol Neurosurg Psychiatry.* 1994;57:416–418.

27. Kumar A, Gottlieb G. Frontotemporal dementias. *Am J Geriatr Psychiatry.* 1993;1:95–108.

28. Gregory CA, Hodges JR. Frontotemporal dementia: use of consensus criteria and prevalence of psychiatric features. *Neuropsychiatry Neuropsychol Behav Neurol.* 1996;9:145–153.

29. Gustafson L, Brun A, Risberg J. Frontal lobe dementia of non-Alzheimer type. In: Wurtman RJ, Corkin S, Growdon J, Ritter-Walker E, eds. *Alzheimer's Disease.* New York: Raven Press; 1990;65–71.

30. Tissot R, Constantinidis J, Richard J. Pick's disease. In: Frederiks JAM, ed. *Handbook of Clinical Neurology.* Amsterdan: Elsevier Science BC; 1985;233–246.

31. Cummings JL, Duchen LW. Kluver-Bucy Syndrome in Pick disease: clinical and pathologic correlations. *Neurology.* 1981;31:1415–1422.

32. Miller BL, Boone K, Mishkin F, Swartz JR, Koras N, Kushii J. Clinical and neuropsychological features of frontotemporal dementia. In: Kertesz A, Munoz DG, eds. *Pick's Disease and Pick Complex.* New York: Wiley-Liss, Inc.; 1998;23–32.

33. American Psychiatric Association. *Diagnostic and Statistical Manual of Mental Disorders (DSM-III-R).* Washington, DC: American Psychiatric Association; 1987.

34. Katzman R. Differential diagnosis of dementing illness. *Neurol Clin North Am.* 1986;4:329–340.

35. Knopman DS, Christensen KJ, Schut LJ, et al. The spectrum of imaging and neuropsychological findings in Pick's disease. *Neurology.* 1989;39:362–368.

36. Neary D, Snowden JS, Gustafson L, et al. Frontotemporal lobar degeneration—a consensus on clinical diagnostic criteria. *Neurology.* 1998;51:1546–1554.

37. Miller BL, Cummings JL, Villanueva-Meyer J, et al. Frontal lobe degeneration: clinical, neuropsychological, and SPECT characteristics. *Neurology.* 1991;41:1374–1382.

38. Elfgren C, Brun A, Gustafson L, et al. Neuropsychological tests as discriminators between dementia of Alzheimer type and frontotemporal dementia. *Int J Geriatr Psychiatry.* 1994;9:635–642.

39. Pachana N, Boone KB, Miller BL, Cummings JL, Berman N. Comparison of neuropsychological functioning in Alzheimer's disease and frontotemporal dementia. *J Int Neuropsychol Soc.* 1996;2:505–510.

40. Miller BL, Cummings J, Mishin F, et al. Emergence of artistic talent in frontotemporal dementia. *Neurology.* 1998;51:978–982.

41. Hodges JR, Garrard P, Perry R, et al. The differentiation of semantic dementia and frontal lobe dementia (temporal and frontal variants of frontotemporal dementia) from early Alzheimer's disease: a comparative neuropsychological study. *Neuropsychology.* 1999;13:31–40.

42. Rascovsky K, Salmon DP, Ho GJ, et al. Cognitive profiles differ in autopsy—confirmed frontotemporal dementia and AD. *Neurology.* 2002;58:1801–1808.

43. Kertesz A, Davidson W, McCabe P, Munoz D. Behavioral quantitation is more sensitive than cognitive testing in frontotemporal dementia. *Alzheimer Dis Assoc Disord.* 2003;17(4):223–229.

44. Snowden JS, Neary D, Mann DMA. *Fronto-Temporal Lobar Degeneration: Fronto-temporal Dementia, Progressive Aphasia, Semantic Dementia.* London: Churchill Livingstone; 1996.

45. Gustafson L, Nielson L. Differential diagnosis of presenile dementia on clinical grounds. *Acta Psychiatr Scand.* 1982;65:194–209.

46. Barber R, Snowden JS, Craufurd D. Frontotemporal dementia and Alzheimer's disease: retrospective differentiation using information from informants. *J Neurol Neurosurg Psychiatry.* 1995;59:61–70.

47. Lopez OL, Gonzalez MP, Becker JT, Reynolds CF, Sudilovsky A, DeKosky ST. Symptoms of depression and psychosis in Alzheimer's disease and frontotemporal dementia. *Neuropsychiatry Neuropsychol Behav Neurol.* 1996;9:154–161.

48. Miller BL, Ikonte C, Ponton M, et al. A study of the Lund-Manchester research criteria for frontotemporal dementia: clinical and single-photon emission CT correlations. *Neurology.* 1997;48:937–942.

49. Miller BL, Seeley WW, Mychack P, Rosen HJ, Mena I, Boone K. Neuroanatomy of the self—evidence from patients with frontotemporal dementia. *Neurology.* 2001;57:817–821.

50. Hersch EL, Kral VA, Palmer RB. Clinical value of the London Psychogeriatric Rating Scale. *J Am Geriatr Soc.* 1978;26:348–354.

51. Schwartz GE. Development and validation of the Geriatric Evaluation by Relatives Rating Instrument (GERRI). *Psych Reports.* 1983;53:479–488.

52. Reisberg B, Borenstein J, Salob SP. Behavioral symptoms in Alzheimer's disease: phenomenology and treatment. *J Clin Psychiatry.* 1987;48:9–15.

53. Baumgarten M, Beck R, Gauthier S. Validity and reliability of the Dementia Behavior Disturbance Scale. *J Am Geriatr Soc.* 1990;38:221–226.

54. Cummings JL, Mega M, Gray K, Rosenberg-Thompson S, Carusi DA, Gornbein J. The Neuropsychiatric Inventory: comprehensive assessment of psychopathology in dementia. *Neurology.* 1994;44:2308–2314.

55. Kertesz A, Davidson W, Fox H. Frontal Behavioral Inventory: diagnostic criteria for frontal lobe dementia. *Can J Neurol Sci.* 1997;24:29–36.

56. Kertesz A, Nadkarni N, Davidson W, Thomas AW. The Frontal Behavioral Inventory in the differential diagnosis of frontotemporal dementia. *J Int Neuropsychol Soc.* 2000;6:460–468.

57. Beck AT, Ward CH, Mendelson M, Erbaugh JK. An inventory for measuring depression. *Arch Gen Psychiatry.* 1961;4:561–571.

58. Kertesz A, Davidson W, McCabe P, Takagi K, Munoz D. Primary progressive aphasia: diagnosis, varieties, evolution. *J Int Neuropsychol Soc.* 2003;9:710–719.

59. Royall DR, Mahurin RK, Gray KF. Bedside assessment of the executive cognitive impairment: the executive interview. *Am Geriatr Soc.* 1992;40:1221–1226.

60. Dubois B, Slachevsky A, Litvan I, Pillon B. The FAB—a frontal assessment battery at bedside. *Neurology.* 2000;55:1621–1626.

61. Mesulam M-M. Slowly progressive aphasia without generalized dementia. *Ann Neurol.* 1982;11:592–598.

62. Mesulam M-M. Primary progressive aphasia—differentiation from Alzheimer's disease. *Ann Neurol.* 1987;22:533–534.

63. Holland AL, McBurney DH, Moossy J, Reinmuth OM. The dissolution of language in Pick's disease with neurofibrillary tangles: a case study. *Brain Lang.* 1985;24:36–58.

64. Wechsler AF, Verity A, Rosenstein LD, Fried I, Scheibel AB. Pick's disease: a clinical, computed tomographic, and histologic study with Golgi impregnation observations. *Arch Neurol.* 1982;39:287–290.

65. Kirshner HS, Tanridag O, Thurman L, Whetsell WO Jr. Progressive aphasia without dementia: two cases with focal spongiform degeneration. *Ann Neurol.* 1987;22:527–532.

66. Turner RS, Kenyon LC, Trojanowski JQ, Gonatas N, Grossman M. Clinical, neuroimaging, and pathologic features of progressive nonfluent aphasia. *Ann Neurol.* 1996;39:166–173.

67. Cohen L, Benoit N, Van Eeckhout P, Ducarne B, Brunet P. Pure progressive aphemia. *J Neurol Neurosurg Psychiatry.* 1993;56:923–924.

68. Alzheimer A. On peculiar disease of the cerebral cortex. *Allg Z Psychiatrie.* 1907;64:146.

69. Appell J, Kertesz A, Fisman M. A study of language functioning in Alzheimer patients. *Brain Lang.* 1982;17:73–91.

70. Bayles KA. Language function in senile dementia. *Brain Lang.* 1982;16:265–280.

71. Kertesz A, Appell J, Fisman M. The dissolution of language in Alzheimer's disease. *Can J Neurol Sci.* 1986;13:415–418.

72. Faber-Langendoen K, Morris JC, Knesevich JW, LaBarge E, Miller JP, Berg L. Aphasia in senile dementia of the Alzheimer type. *Ann Neurol.* 1988;23:365–370.

73. Kertesz A, Munoz DG. Primary progressive aphasia and Pick complex. *J Neurol Sci.* 2003;206:97–107.

74. Mesulam MM, Weintraub S. Primary progressive aphasia: sharpening the focus on a clinical syndrome. In: Boller F, Forette F, Khachaturian Z, Poncet M, Christen Y, eds. *Heterogeneity of Alzheimer's Disease.* Berlin: Springer-Verlag; 1992;43–66.

75. Karbe H, Kertesz A, Polk M. Profiles of language impairment in primary progressive aphasia. *Arch Neurol.* 1993;50:193–201.

76. Duffy JR, Petersen RC. Primary progressive aphasia. *Aphas.* 1992;6:1–15.

77. Snowden JS, Neary D, Mann DMA, Goulding PJ, Testa HJ. Progressive language disorder due to lobar atrophy. *Ann Neurol.* 1992;31:174–183.

78. Neary D, Snowden JS, Mann DMA, Northen B, Goulding PJ, Macdermott N. Frontal lobe dementia and motor neuron disease. *J Neurol Neurosurg Psychiatry.* 1990;53:23–32.

79. Caselli RJ, Windebank AJ, Petersen RC, et al. Rapidly progressive aphasic dementia and motor neuron disease. *Ann Neurol.* 1993;33:200–207.

80. Weintraub S, Rubin NP, Mesulam M-M. Primary progressive aphasia: longitudinal course, neuropsychological profile, and language features. *Arch Neurol.* 1990;47:1329–1335.

81. Cappa SF, Perani D, Messa C, Miozzo A, Fazio F. Varieties of progressive non-fluent aphasia. *Ann NY Acad Sci.* 1996;777:243–248.

82. Tyrell PJ, Kartsounis LD, Frackowiak RSJ, Findley LJ, Rossor MN. Progressive loss of speech output and orofacial dyspraxia associated with frontal lobe hypometabolism. *J Neurol Neurosurg Psychiatry.* 1991;54:351–357.

83. Hart RP, Beach WA, Taylor JR. A case of progressive apraxia of speech and non-fluent aphasia. *Aphas.* 1997;11:73–82.

84. Fukui T, Sugita K, Kawamura M, Shiota J, Nakano I. Primary progressive apraxia in Pick's disease: a clinicopathologic study. *Neurology.* 1996;47:467–473.

85. Snowden JS, Goulding PJ, Neary D. Semantic dementia: a form of circumscribed cerebral atrophy. *Behav Neurol.* 1989;2:167–182.

86. Hodges JR, Patterson K, Oxbury S, Funnell E. Semantic dementia: progressive fluent aphasia with temporal lobe atrophy. *Brain.* 1992;115:1783–1806.

87. Head, H. *Aphasia and Kindred Disorders of Speech.* Cambridge: Cambridge University Press; 1926.

88. Snowden JS, Griffiths H, Neary D. Semantic dementia: autobiographical contribution to preservation of meaning. *Cog Neuropsychol.* 1994;11:265–288.

89. Parkin AJ. Progressive aphasia without dementia—a clinical cognitive neuropsychological analysis. *Brain Lang.* 1993;44:201–220.

90. Harasty JA, Halliday GM, Code C, Brooks WS. Quantification of cortical atrophy in a case of progressive fluent aphasia. *Brain.* 1996;119:181–190.

91. von Branmühl A. Ueber Stammganglien veränderungen bei Pickscher Krankheit. *Z Gesamte Neurol Psychiatr.* 1930;124:214.

92. Akelaitis AJ. Atrophy of basal ganglia in Pick's disease. A clinicopathologic study. *Arch Neurol Psychiatr.* 1944;51:27–34.

93. Winkelman NW, Book MH. Asymptomatic extrapyramidal involvement in Pick's disease. *Arch Neurol Psychiatr.* 1944;8:30–42.

94. Munoz-Garcia D, Ludwin SK. Classic and generalized variants of Pick's disease: clinicopathological, ultrastructural, and immunocytochemical comparative study. *Ann Neurol.* 1984;16:467–480.

95. Mann DMA, South PW, Snowden JS, Neary D. Dementia of frontal lobe type: neuropathology and immunohistochemistry. *J Neurol Neurosurg Psychiatry.* 1993;56:605–614.

96. von Bagh K. Anatomic findings in 30 cases of systematic atrophy of cortex (Pick's disease) with special consideration of basal ganglia and long descending nerve tracts, preliminary report. *Arch Psychiatrie.* 1941;114:68.

97. Rebeiz JJ, Kolodny EH, Richardson EP Jr. Corticodentatonigral degeneration with neuronal achromasia. *Arch Neurol.* 1968;18:20–33.

98. Gibb WRG, Luthert PJ, Marsden CD. Corticobasal degeneration. *Brain.* 1989;112:1171–1192.

99. Riley DE, Lang AE, Lewis MB, et al. Cortical-basal ganglionic degeneration. *Neurology.* 1990;40:1203–1212.

100. Clark AW, Manz HJ, White CL III, Lehmann J, Miller D, Coyle JT. Cortical degeneration with swollen chromatolytic neurons: its relationship to Pick's disease. *J Neuropathol Exp Neurol.* 1986;45:268–284.

101. Luthert PJ, Wightman G, Leigh PN, Marsden CD. Corticobasal degeneration: immunohistochemical study. *Neuropathol Appl Neurobiol.* 1992;18:293.

102. Jendroska K, Rossor MN, Mathias CJ, Daniel SE. Morphological overlap between corticobasal degeneration and Pick's disease: a clinicopathological report. *Mov Disord.* 1995;10:111–114.

103. Brown J, Lantos PL, Roques P, Fidani L, Rossor MN. Familial dementia with swollen achromatic neurons and corticobasal inclusion bodies: a clinical and pathological study. *J Int Neuropsychol Soc.* 1996;135:21–30.

104. Lang AE, Bergeron C, Pollanen MS, Ashby P. Parietal Pick's disease mimicking cortical-basal degeneration. *Neurology.* 1992;44:1436–1440.

105. Paulus W, Selim M. Corticonigral degeneration with neuronal achromasia and basal neurofibrillary tangles. *Acta Neuropathol.* 1990;81:89–94.

106. Rey GJ, Tomer R, Levin BD, Sanchez-Ramos J, Bowen B, Bruce JH. Psychiatric symptoms, atypical dementia, and left visual field inattention in corticobasal degeneration. *Mov Disord.* 1995;10:106–110.

107. Frisoni GB, Pizzolato G, Zanetti O, Bianchetti A, Chierichetti F, Trabucchi M. Corticobasal degeneration: neuropsychological assessment and dopamine D2 receptor SPECT analysis. *Europ Neurol.* 1995;35:50–54.

108. Mathuranath PS, Xuereb JH, Bak T, Hodges JR. Corticobasal ganglionic degeneration and/or frontotemporal dementia? A report of two overlap cases and review of literature. *J Neurol Neurosurg Psychiatry.* 2000;68:304–312.

109. Lippa CF, Smith TW, Fontneau N. Corticonigral degeneration with neuronal achromasia. A clinicopathological study of two cases. *J Neurol Sci.* 1990;98:301–310.

110. Dobato JL, Mateo D, de Andres C, Gimenez-Roldan S. Degeneracion ganglionica corticobasal presentandose como un sindrome de afasia progresiva primaria. *Neurologia.* 1993;8:141.

111. Marti-Masso JF, Lopez de Muniain A, Poza JJ, Urtasun M, Carrera N. Degeneracion corticobasal ganglionica: a proposito de siete observaciones diagnosticada clinicamente. *Neurologia.* 1994;9:115–120.

112. Sakurai Y, Hashida H, Uesugi H, et al. A clinical profile of corticobasal degeneration presenting as primary progressive aphasia. *Europ Neurol.* 1996;36:134–137.

113. Mimura M, Oda T, Tsuchiya K, et al. Corticobasal degeneration presenting with nonfluent primary progressive aphasia: a clinicopathological study. *J Neurol Sci.* 2001;183:19–26.

114. Kertesz A, Munoz DG. *Pick's Disease and Pick Complex.* New York: Wiley-Liss, Inc.; 1998.

115. Rinne JO, Lee MS, Thompson PD, Marsden CD. Corticobasal degeneration. *Brain.* 1994;117:1183–1196.

116. Schneider JA, Watts RL, Gearing M, Brewer RP, Mirra SS. Corticobasal degeneration: neuropathologic and clinical heterogeneity. *Neurology.* 1997;48:959–969.

117. Grimes DA, Lang AE, Bergeron CB. Dementia as the most common presentation of corticobasal ganglionic degeneration. *Neurology.* 1999;53:1969–1974.

118. Wenning GK, Litvan I, Jankovic J, et al. Natural history and survival of 14 patients with corticobasal degeneration confirmed at

postmortem examination. *J Neurol Neurosurg Psychiatry*. 1998;64: 184–189.

119. Boeve BF, Maraganore DM, Parisi JE, et al. Pathologic heterogeneity in clinically diagnosed corticobasal degeneration. *Neurology*. 1999;53:795–800.

120. Kertesz A, Martinez-Lage P, Davidson W, Munoz DG. The corticobasal degeneration syndrome overlaps progressive aphasia and frontotemporal dementia. *Neurology*. 2000;55:1368–1375.

121. Litvan I, Goetz C, Lang A. *Corticobasal Degeneration and Related Disorders. Advances in Neurology*. Philadelphia: Lippincott, Williams & Wilkins; 2000.

122. Pillon B, Blin J, Vidailhet M, et al. The neuropsychological pattern of corticobasal degeneration: comparison with progressive supranuclear palsy and Alzheimer's disease. *Neurology*. 1995;45: 1477–1483.

123. Feany MB, Mattiace LA, Dickson DW. Neuropathologic overlap of progressive supranuclear palsy, Pick's disease and corticobasal degeneration. *J Neuropathol Exp Neurol*. 1996;55: 53–67.

124. Houlden H, Baker M, Morris HR, et al. Corticobasal degeneration and progressive supranuclear palsy share a common tau haplotype. *Neurology*. 2001;56:1702–1706.

125. Poorkaj P, Muma NA, Zhukareva V, et al. An R5L τ mutation in a subject with a progressive supranuclear palsy phenotype. *Ann Neurol*. 2002;52:511–516.

126. Dickson D, Bergeron C, Chin SS, et al. Office of rare diseases neuropathologic criteria for corticobasal degeneration. *J Neuropathol Exp Neurol*. 2002;61:935–946.

127. Mitsuyama Y. Presenile dementia with motor neuron disease in Japan: clinicopathological review of 26 cases. *J Neurol Neurosurg Psychiatry*. 1984;47:953–959.

128. Okamoto K, Hirai S, Yamazaki T, Sun X, Nakazato Y. New ubiquitin-positive intraneuronal inclusions in the extra-motor cortices in patients with amyotrophic lateral sclerosis. *Neurosci Lett*. 1991;129:233–236.

129. Wightman EM, Anderson VER, Martin J, et al. Hippocampal and neocortical ubiquitin-immunoreactive inclusions in amyotrophic lateral sclerosis with dementia. *Neurosci Lett*. 1992;139:269–274.

130. Jackson M, Lennox G, Lowe J. Motor neurone disease-inclusion dementia. *Neurodegeneration*. 1996;5:339–350.

131. Lomen-Hoerth C, Anderson T, Miller B. The overlap of amyotrophic lateral sclerosis and frontotemporal dementia. *Neurology*. 2002;59:1077–1079.

132. Strong MJ, Lomen-Hoerth C, Caselli RJ, Bigio EH, Yang W. Cognitive impairment, frontotemporal dementia, and the motor neuron diseases. *Ann Neurol*. 2003;54(Suppl 5):S20–S23.

133. Salazar A, Masters C, Gajdusek DC, Gibbs CJ Jr. Syndromes of amyotrophic lateral sclerosis and dementia: relation to transmissible Creutzfeldt-Jakob disease. *Neurology*. 1982;32:4-A167.

134. Kertesz A, Kawarai T, Rogaeva E, et al. Familial frontotemporal dementia with ubiquitin-positive, tau-negative inclusions. *Neurology*. 2000;54:818–827.

135. Woulfe J, Kertesz A, Munoz DG. Frontotemporal dementia with ubiquitinated cytoplasmic and intranuclear inclusions. *Acta Neuropathol*. 2001;102:94–102.

136. Feany MB, Dickson DW. Neurodegenerative disorders with extensive tau pathology: a comparative study and review. *Ann Neurol*. 1996;40:139–148.

137. Neumann MA. Pick's disease. *J Neuropathol Exp Neurol*. 1949;8: 255–282.

138. Neumann MA, Cohn R. Progressive subcortical gliosis: a rare form of presenile dementia. *Brain*. 1967;90:405–418.

139. Verity MA, Wechsler AF. Progressive subcortical gliosis of Neumann: a clinicopathological study of two cases with review. *Arch Gerontol Geriatr*. 1987;6:245–261.

140. Bergeron C, Pollanen MS, Weyer L, Black SE, Lang AE. Unusual clinical presentations of cortical-basal ganglionic degeneration. *Ann Neurol*. 1996;40:893–900.

141. Delacourte A, Sergeant N, Wattez A, Robitaille Y. The biochemistry of the cytoskeleton in Pick complex. In: Kertesz A, Munoz DG, eds. *Pick's Disease and Pick Complex*. New York: Wiley-Liss, Inc.; 1998;243–258.

142. Schmidt ML, Huang R, Martin JA, et al. Neurofibrillary tangles in progressive supranuclear palsy contain the same tau epitopes identified in Alzheimer's disease PHFtau. *J Neuropathol Exp Neurol*. 1996;55:534–539.

143. Poorkaj P, Bird TD, Wijsman E, et al. Tau is a candidate gene for chromosome 17 frontotemporal dementia. *Ann Neurol*. 1998;43:815–825.

144. Spillantini MG, Crowther RA, Kamphorst W, Heutink P, Van Swieten JC. Tau pathology in two Dutch families with mutations in the microtubule-binding region of tau. *Am J Pathol*. 1998;153: 1359–1363.

145. Zhukareva V, Mann D, Pickering-Brown S, et al. Sporadic Pick's disease: a tauopathy characterized by a spectrum of pathological tau isoforms in gray and white matter. *Ann Neurol*. 2002;51:730–739.

146. Zhukareva V, Vogelsberg-Ragaglia V, Van Deerlin V, et al. Loss of brain tau defines novel sporadic and familial tauopathies with frontotemporal dementia. *Ann Neurol*. 2001;49:165–175.

147. Wilhelmsen KC, Lynch T, Pavlou E, Higgins M, Nygaard TG. Localization of disinhibition dementia parkinsonism amyotrophy complex to 17q21–22. *Am J Hum Genet*. 1994;55:1159–1165.

148. Lynch T, Sano M, Marder KS, et al. Clinical characteristics of a family with chromosome 17-linked disinhibition-dementia-parkinsonism-amyotrophy complex. *Neurology*. 1994;44: 1878–1884.

149. Foster NL, Wilhelmsen K, Sima AFA, et al. Frontotemporal dementia and parkinsonism linked to chromosome 17: a consensus conference. *Ann Neurol*. 1997;41:706–715.

150. Hutton M, Lendon CL, Rizzu P, et al. Association of missense and 5'-splice-site mutations in tau with the inherited dementia FTDP-17. *Nature*. 1998;393:702–705.

151. Clark LN, Poorkaj P, Wszolek Z, et al. Pathogenic implications of mutations in the tau gene in pallido-ponto-nigral degeneration and related neurodegenerative disorders linked to chromosome 17. *Proc Natl Acad Sci*. 1998;95:13103–13107.

152. Bird TD, Nochlin D, Poorkaj P, et al. A clinical pathological comparison of three families with frontotemporal dementia and identical mutations in the tau gene (P301L). *Brain*. 1999;122:741–756.

153. Hong M, Zhukareva V, Vogelsberg-Ragalia V, et al. Mutation-specific functional impairments in distinct tau isoforms of hereditary FTDP-17. *Science*. 1998;282:1914–1917.

154. Hughes A, Mann D, Pickering-Brown S. Tau haplotype frequency in frontotemporal lobar degeneration and amyotrophic lateral sclerosis. *Exp Neurol*. 2003;181:12–16.

155. Short RA, Graff-Radford NR, Adamson J, Baker M, Hutton M. Differences in tau and apolipoprotein E polymorphism frequencies in sporadic frontotemporal lobar degeneration syndromes. *Arch Neurol*. 2002;59:611–615.

156. Brown J, Ashworth A, Gydesen S, et al. Familial non-specific dementia maps to chromosome 3. *Hum Mol Genet*. 1995;4: 1625–1628.

157. Hosler BA, Siddique T, Sapp PC, et al. Linkage of familial amyotrophic lateral sclerosis with frontotemporal dementia to chromosome 9q21–q22. *JAMA*. 2000;284:1664–1669.

158. Yates CM, Simpson J, Maloney AFJ, Gordon A. Neurochemical observations in a case of Pick's disease. *Neurol Sci*. 1980;48: 257–263.

159. Hansen LA, DeTeresa R, Tobias H, Alford M, Terry RD. Neocortical morphometry and cholinergic neurochemistry in Pick's disease. *Am J Pathol*. 1988;131:507–518.

160. White P, Goddhardt MJ, Keet JP, et al. Neocortical cholinergic neurons in elderly people. *Lancet*. 1977;1:668–670.

161. Sparks DL, Markesbery WR. Altered serotonergic and cholinergic synaptic markers in Pick's disease. *Arch Neurol*. 1991;48:796–799.

162. Mann JJ, McBride PA, Stanley M. Postmortem monoamine receptors and enzyme studies in suicide. *Ann NY Acad Sci*. 1986;487:114–121.

163. Swartz JR, Miller BL, Lesser IM, Darby AL. Frontotemporal dementia: treatment response to serotonin selective reuptake inhibitors. *J Clin Psychiatry*. 1997;58:212–216.

164. Lebert F, Pasquier F. Trazodone in the treatment of behaviour in frontotemporal dementia. *Hum Psychol Pharmacol Clin Exp*. 1999;14:279–281.

165. Ratnavalli E, Brayne C, Dawson K, Hodges JR. The prevalence of frontotemporal dementia. *Neurology*. 2002;58:1615–1621.

166. Bird T, Knopman D, van Swieten J, et al. Epidemiology and genetics of frontotemporal dementia/Pick's disease. *Ann Neurol*. 2003;54(Suppl 5):S29–S31.

Delirium in the Elderly

24

David J. Meagher   *John W. Norton*   *Paula T. Trzepacz*

DELIRIUM: A GROWING HEALTH CARE CHALLENGE IN THE ELDERLY

Delirium is the term currently applied to all acute disturbances of global cognitive function (1) and has superseded terms such as acute confusional state, toxic encephalopathy, acute brain failure, and postoperative or intensive care psychosis. It is a complex neuropsychiatric disorder that occurs across the age range, but is particularly prevalent and problematic in the elderly and those who have preexisting brain impairment. Delirium is a common problem in all health care settings, with a point prevalence in general hospital patients of 10% to 30%. Among the elderly, 10% to 15% have delirium on admission, and a further 10% to 40% develop it during the course of their hospital stay (2). Overall, more than 2 million Americans develop delirium annually, with rates steadily increasing in tandem with the rise in mean age of the general population. It is clear that delirium will assume greater importance as health care systems attempt to provide for our increasingly aged population. Moreover, the need to improve our understanding and treatment of delirium is further emphasized by studies that indicate a substantial excess of morbidity and mortality, which is relatively independent of underlying physical illness. This suggests that the traditional concept of delirium as a transient and highly reversible disorder is no longer appropriate.

DELIRIUM: A COMPLEX NEUROPSYCHIATRIC SYNDROME

Delirium is characterized by widespread cognitive disturbance, but also includes a range of noncognitive symptoms (Table 24-1) (3,4). Impaired attention is a key diagnostic indicator and can allow discrimination from demented patients when tested using the Digit Span Backwards and Digit Cancellation Test (5). Inattention, however, does not explain the full constellation of physical, biological, and psychological symptoms that occur in delirium. Most patients have impaired orientation, memory, and visuospatial ability, as well as a range of noncognitive symptoms (sleep-wake cycle impairment, thinking and language difficulties, disturbed perception, affective lability, and a variety of motoric presentations). Delirious patients have difficulty making sense out of their environment, which used to be classically referred to as "clouding of consciousness." Patients can develop hallucinations, delusions, and illusions—perceptual disturbances often of a visual nature but which can also involve other sensory modalities. Delusions are typically persecutory in nature and poorly formed rather than complex. It is important to be aware that patients in delirium can pose a danger to themselves due to fear or paranoia, and that appropriate measures must be taken to reduce the risk of deliberate or inadvertent self-harm. In one study, 7% of delirious patients attempted some form of self-harm during an episode (6). Sleep disturbances may involve disintegration of the normal sleep-wake cycle and can include napping, nocturnal awakenings, sleeplessness, and nightmares. Affective lability is more pronounced than in mood disorders and is often mood-incongruent—anxiety, sadness, or hypomania may occur and complicate accurate diagnosis.

THE VARIABLE CLINICAL COURSE OF DELIRIUM

No single symptom is characteristically unique to delirium. The symptom constellation represents dysfunction of nearly all cortical regions supporting higher cortical functions. However, the temporal co-occurrence of these symptoms supports a delirium diagnosis.

Temporal course characteristically involves an acute onset (from hours to a few days) and fluctuating course (waxing and waning symptom severity over a 24-hour

TABLE 24-1
DELIRIUM SYMPTOMS AND FREQUENCY

Cognitive impairment (100%)
Inattention
Disorientation
Impaired memory (short term, long term, verbal, visual)
Visuoconstructional ability
Executive function

Psychomotor disturbance (38–96%)
Hyperactivity
Hypoactivity
Mixed

Sleep-wake cycle disturbance (25–96%)
Sleeplessness
Reversal of normal cycle
Fragmentation

Psychosis (17–68%)
Perceptual disturbances (illusions, hallucinations)
Delusions
Thought disorder (tangentiality, loose associations)

Affective/mood changes (43–63%)
Abnormal mood
Labile mood
Incongruous affect
Anger/irritability

Impaired language (41–93%)
Word-finding difficulty
Dysgraphia
Altered semantic content

Adapted from References 3,4.

period). Symptoms often worsen at night, which places responsibility on nursing staff to record alterations in mental status and inform treating clinical teams, especially when a patient appears recovered and more lucid in the morning. In nonhospitalized elderly, the onset of delirium may be less dramatic and gradually evolves, or may be confounded by a concurrent dementia.

Delirium onset often includes a prodromal state involving alterations of alertness and sleep-wake cycle, malaise, restlessness, anxiety, irritability, or nightmares (7,8). Subsyndromal delirium is associated with electroencephalography (EEG) slowing and is clinically significant, with a prognosis intermediate between delirious and nondelirious patients (7,9). Many cases of delirium are transient, particularly when they occur in the context of a concussion, postictal state, or postoperatively. Delirium is a frequent occurrence as one emerges from coma, though less so when the coma is drug-induced (10). Delirium in children is similar to that in adults, but with fewer delusions and hallucinations (11,12). Diagnosis of delirium in those who are mentally retarded is more difficult due to baseline impairments in cognition, but is suggested by any acute deterioration in cognition.

The duration of delirium and of its individual components is highly variable. Rudberg and colleagues studied delirium duration in hospitalized elderly and found that it lasted only 1 day in two-thirds of cases (13). Similarly, other studies of cancer populations indicate that the majority of cases of delirium are reversible, and that it should not be considered an acceptable part of the terminal process (14,15). In contrast, however, the traditional concept of delirium as a brief, transient, and highly reversible condition is not supported by longitudinal studies that indicate markedly elevated rates of dementia in the aftermath of a delirium episode (16,17), although the role of underlying etiologies and pre-existing cognitive deficits has not been clearly delineated.

EPIDEMIOLOGY

Delirium can occur at any age, but is particularly common in the very young and the very old. Most epidemiologic studies focus on elderly populations who are at higher risk of delirium due to the changes that occur in the brain with aging, such as decreased cholinergic activity, that result in a reduced brain reserve. The frequent occurrence of central nervous system (CNS) disorders (e.g., stroke, hypertensive and diabetic vessel changes, tumor) in the elderly further increases their vulnerability to delirium. Up to two thirds of cases of delirium occur superimposed on pre-existing cognitive impairment (18), with delirium approximately three times more common in patients with dementia compared to nondemented controls (19,20). The risk of delirium appears greatest for vascular dementia and late-onset Alzheimer's disease, where neuronal disturbance is particularly widespread.

Improving our understanding and treatment of delirium will be a considerable health care challenge in the coming years, because the world's population is aging at a dramatic rate. In the United States, by 2050 almost 25% of the elderly will be over 85 (21). This is particularly worrisome because dementia affects 5% to 8% of those over age 65, 15% to 20% of those over 75, and 25% to 50% of those older than 85 (22).

Most studies of the incidence and prevalence of delirium report general hospital populations consisting of either referral samples or consecutive admissions to a given service, with relatively less information regarding the rate of delirium in the general population. In addition, not all studies employ sensitive and specific diagnostic and measurement techniques. Fann's review found an incidence range from 3% to 42%, and a prevalence range from 5% to 44% in hospitalized patients (2). Up to 60% of nursing home patients older than 65 may be delirious in cross-sectional evaluation (23). In addition, 10% to 15% of the elderly are delirious when admitted to a hospital, and another 10% to 40% are diagnosed with delirium during hospitalization. As a generalization, approximately one-in-five general hospital patients has delirium at some time during the stay.

NEUROPATHOPHYSIOLOGY

Delirium is clearly a brain disorder, yet its specific neuropathology is not well understood. Somehow, a great diversity of etiologies can result in delirium with its characteristic symptoms, supporting the notion that certain neural pathways and regions are particularly affected despite the great diversity of pathophysiological, pharmacological, and structural insults that can cause this syndrome. In addition, the constellation of symptoms distinguishes delirium from other neuropsychiatric disorders including dementia, with which it most overlaps.

A hypothesis of a *final common neural pathway* has been proposed to explain how delirium symptoms result from the many different etiologies directly or indirectly affecting brain function (24–26). Structural and functional neuroimaging case reports and case series support a role for certain brain regions, in particular prefrontal cortex, basal ganglia, nondominant parietal cortex, fusiform cortex, and anterior thalamus (especially the right side). Interestingly, many of these areas also play a key role in attentional mechanisms. Electrophysiological evidence also supports a role for subcortical regions and thalamus. Some etiologies of delirium may alter neurotransmission via their effects on general metabolism and oxygenation of the brain, whereas others may antagonize or interfere with specific receptors and neurotransmitters or neurological function.

It has been proposed that the delirium final common neural pathway involves reduced cholinergic and increased dopaminergic activity (26)—even though other neurotransmitters may be involved—in such a manner that these two are ultimately affected to produce the characteristic symptoms. A wide variety of medications and their metabolites have anticholinergic activity and have been reported to cause delirium. This anticholinergicity can be postsynaptic, indirectly through noncholinergic presynaptic actions, or through more potent anticholinergic metabolites of a parent drug, such as norfentanyl and normeperidine. Delirium induced by anticholinergic drugs is associated with generalized EEG slowing, and is reversed by treatment with physostigmine or some neuroleptics (27,28).

A number of physiological and structural causes of delirium may actually be acting through anticholinergic effects. Age-associated changes in cholinergic function and plasticity might explain increased delirium incidence with advanced age. It is well-appreciated that patients with Alzheimer's and vascular dementias have an increased risk for delirium, and these are disorders known to cause reduced brain cholinergic activity. Lewy body dementia involves significant loss of cholinergic neurons in the nucleus basalis, and its symptoms mimic delirium—fluctuating symptom severity, confusion, visual hallucinations, delusions—along with EEG slowing. These delirium-like symptoms have responded to donepezil (29). Thiamine deficiency, hypoxia, and hypoglycemia appear to reduce acetylcholine levels by altering oxidative metabolism of glucose and the production of acetyl coenzyme A (CoA), which is critical as the rate-limiting step in acetylcholine synthesis (26). Elevated serum levels of drugs with anticholinergic activity are associated with delirium in postoperative or post-electroconvulsive therapy patients (30,31). Brain structural insults—stroke and traumatic brain injury—are less appreciated as being associated with decreased cholinergic activity, in which a low cholinergic state occurs acutely following the event during the same time frame when delirium occurs (32). Thus, there is considerable support for an anticholinergic mechanism for many diverse etiologies of delirium.

Cholinergic neurotransmission may be altered in many ways, including via multiple effects on oxidative metabolism. Metabolic pathways for the oxidation of glucose in the production of adenosine triphosphate (ATP) involve oxygen, vitamins (cofactors for enzymes), and substrates related to neurotransmission (e.g., amino acids and CoA). Acetylcholine is synthesized from the enzymatic reaction (via choline acetyltransferase) involving CoA being combined with choline. The citric acid cycle produces CoA and requires oxygen and glucose to produce it. During delirium and the stress of medical illness, these important nutrients on which the brain is so dependent may not be as available due to poor perfusion, poor nutrition, etc., and a deficiency of CoA will lead to decreased acetylcholine production.

Cholinergic neurons are rich in thiamine, which is necessary for their proper function. Cholinergic neurons with long axons may be at higher risk for damage during low oxygenation states, when limited energy reserves of neurons are progressively stressed during delirium (33). Brown further hypothesizes that calcium influx floods hypoxic neurons secondary to depletion of ATP, which then accelerates activity of tyrosine hydroxylase, with subsequent increased dopamine production and release, causing delirium symptoms (33). This may also be a mechanism for more sustained damage following a delirious episode, if the duration of neuronal depolarization is prolonged and ischemic damage results.

An absolute or relative excess of dopaminergic activity also appears to play a role in delirium. Intoxication with dopaminergic drugs (34), and cocaine binges, (35) cause delirium. Dopamine may also play a role in alcohol withdrawal (36), opiate intoxication, hypoxia (37), and hepatic encephalopathy (38).

Dopamine agonists, active at D1 and D2 receptors, have been shown to cause EEG slowing and behavioral arousal in rats (39), findings similar to those seen in rats treated with atropine (40,41). Dopamine can affect release of acetylcholine at presynaptic receptors, where stimulation of D1 receptors can facilitate acetylcholine release, whereas D2 stimulation can reduce acetylcholine release (42). Blockade of D2 receptors may decrease this reduction effect. Neuroleptics, which are antidopaminergic agents, are used to treat delirium with apparent improvement in symptoms. This supports a role for dopamine in delirium, including delirium caused by anticholinergic drugs (27,43).

RECOGNIZING DELIRIUM

Poor recognition remains the single greatest obstacle to both clinical and research efforts in delirium. It is commonplace for delirium to be either missed or recognized late, with over one-third of cases not detected in clinical practice. Johnson et al. studied consecutive elderly general hospital admissions, and noted that delirium was explicitly recognized in 5% and documented as a syndrome in 18%, with variable but poor recognition of individual delirium symptoms as well as diagnosis (44). Missed cases were diagnosed as dementia (25%), a functional psychiatric disorder (25%), or with no diagnosis documented (50%). In a study of elderly emergency room patients with delirium, Lewis et al. found that altered mental status was noted in only 13% of cases, and almost one-third of delirious cases were discharged directly home (45). Nonidentification is particularly frequent in older patients, where hypoactive presentations are common and frequently misdiagnosed as depression (46) or dementia (44). Delirium in the elderly can develop more slowly due to progressive medication accumulation or gradual worsening of underlying medical conditions.

Explicit recognition of delirium is associated with shorter inpatient stays and lower mortality (47). Nondetection may result in a poorer outcome, due to failure to appreciate and correct underlying causes, as well as the consequences of not addressing delirium symptoms because of the patients' resistance or impaired ability to cooperate with treatment, such as traumatic removal of in-dwelling vascular and other lines and catheters (due to agitation), and bed sores in hypoactive patients. Improving detection rates requires education of clinical staff regarding key indicators of delirium and the use of tools to assist diagnosis.

Delirium recognition is often based on a cognitive-only assessment—disorientation alone, or perhaps the Mini Mental State Examination. These fail to distinguish delirium from dementia and do not detect the full range of symptoms. Screening is helpful if followed up by more specific evaluation, and if it is not assumed that cognitive deficits in the elderly are expected or due to dementia. The *clinical rule of thumb* is that it is delirium until proven otherwise.

The Confusion Assessment Method (CAM) is a 4-item screening instrument based on Diagnostic and Statistical Manual-III-R (DSM-III-R) criteria that assists in delirium recognition and diagnosis, and can be readily applied in routine clinical settings by nonpsychiatric medical and nursing staff (48). It is important not to rely upon the presence of disorientation or other highly fluctuant features in the recognition of delirium. Inattention, a cardinal symptom of delirium but not dementia, should be routinely tested for at the bedside, particularly in high-risk elderly populations. The *serial sevens* or *months of the year backwards* tests are suitable. Rockwood et al. found that delirium educational programs emphasizing these issues and aimed at house staff substantially improve detection rates (47).

DELIRIUM AND PSYCHIATRIC DIFFERENTIAL DIAGNOSIS

Delirium commonly occurs comorbidly with dementia in older persons (*acute on chronic cognitive disturbance*), where accurate differentiation from pure dementia is particularly challenging. As a general rule, dementia is characterized primarily by memory impairment and follows a chronic deteriorating course, whereas delirium is characterized primarily by an impairment of attentional processes and tends to be acute in onset and fluctuant in nature. This distinction is somewhat blurred by the high comorbidity. In addition, dementia of the multi-infarct or Lewy body variety can present acutely, and the latter is highly fluctuant. Moreover, the latter stages of dementia have been likened to a chronic delirious state because of the breadth and severity of higher cortical impairments. The precise nature of the relationship between delirium and dementia remains unresolved with, on one hand, the suggestion that delirium may be a harbinger for silent dementia, while on the other, the possibility that delirium may contribute to dementia risk by virtue of some inherent neurotoxicity. In either case, it is clear that experiencing an episode of delirium is associated with a marked increase in the rate of subsequent diagnosis of dementia (17).

The most difficult differential diagnosis for delirium is dementia (Table 24-2). However, delirium can usually be distinguished from dementia with careful history taking, examination, and investigation. Attention and level of consciousness tend to remain intact in uncomplicated dementia. Sleep disturbances in dementia tend to involve nocturnal disruption, compared to the often extensive disturbances of sleep-wake cycle that characterize delirium. A new nocturnal disturbance may indicate an incipient delirium. Psychotic symptoms are similar in that visual hallucinations predominate in either disorder, though delusions tend to be stereotyped in dementia of the Alzheimer's type, and poorly formed and often persecutory in delirium. Overall, it is evident that the symptoms of delirium tend to dominate the clinical picture when it co-occurs with dementia (49). To this end, the Delirium Rating Scale (50), Delirium Rating Scale Revised-98 (51), and the Cognitive Test for Delirium (52,53) can assist in the identification of delirium, even when it occurs in the context of an underlying dementia.

TABLE 24-2
DISTINGUISHING DELIRIUM FROM DEMENTIA

	Delirium	Dementia
Onset	Acute/subacute	Typically insidious
Medical status	Acute precipitating factor present	Often absent
Course	Fluctuating	Progressive
Consciousness	Impaired and fluctuant	Clear until later stages
Principal cognitive deficit	Inattention	Short-term memory
Sleep	Gross disruption of sleep-wake cycle	Nocturnal disruption
Psychomotor disturbance	Almost invariable	Often absent
Psychotic symptoms	Delusions not fixed, visual hallucinations	Delusions often stereotyped, visual hallucinations
Bedside testing	DRS $\geq$ 10 DRS-98 $\geq$ 18 CTD < 19	DRS < 10 DRS-98 < 18 CTD > 19 (until late stages)
Generalized EEG slowing	80%	33%

CTD, Cognitive Test for Delirium; DRS, Delirium Rating Scale; DRS-98, Delirium Rating Scale Revised-98; EEG, electroencephalogram.

In difficult diagnostic cases, when ictal causes are suspected, EEGs can be helpful (Table 24-3). Most dementias are not associated with much slowing of the dominant posterior rhythm until late in the disease progression. In contrast, generalized background EEG slowing (more than one Hertz from an individual's baseline) is common in delirium (80% versus 33%), with a higher percentage on quantitative EEG indicative of delirium (54). Older patients may have ischemia-related new-onset seizures that can present as delirium during postictal states or complex partial status epilepticus. In such cases the EEG may evidence epileptiform activity in addition to generalized slowing.

A targeted medical evaluation, including laboratory and radiological tests where indicated, can usually uncover one or more etiologies related to a delirium episode, whereas most dementias are not associated with new or acute identifiable medical etiologies. The broad range of neuropsychiatric symptoms that occurs in delirium overlaps with other psychiatric disorders and results in a complex differential diagnosis (Fig. 24-1). The early behavioral changes of delirium are often mistaken for adjustment reactions to adverse events, particularly in patients who have experienced major trauma or have cancer. Hypoactive delirium is frequently mistaken for depression (6). In fact, many symptoms of depression can occur in delirium (e.g., psychomotor slowing, sleep disturbances, irritability). However, in major depression, symptom onset tends to be less acute and mood disturbances typically dominate the clinical picture, with any cognitive impairments of depression resembling a mild dementia, called *pseudodementia*. Delirium can be precipitated by dehydration or malnutrition in severely depressed patients who are unable to maintain food or fluid intake. The distinction of delirium from depression is particularly important because, in addition to delayed treatment, some antidepressants have anticholinergic activity that can aggravate delirium. Conversely, the overactive, disinhibited profile of some delirious patients can closely mimic similar disturbances encountered in patients with agitated depression or mania. The most severe mania, *Bell's mania*, includes cognitive impairment and mimics delirium.

Abnormalities of thought and perception can occur in both delirium and schizophrenia, but are more fluctuant and fragmentary in delirium. The often fleeting delusions in delirium contrast with the more fixed and complex nature of those in schizophrenia, and first rank symptoms are uncommon (55). Unlike schizophrenia, hallucinations in delirium tend to be visual rather than auditory. Consciousness, attention and memory are generally less impaired in schizophrenia, with the exception of the pseudo-delirious picture that can occur due to marked perplexity in the acute stage of illness. Careful physical examination, coupled with EEG and/or an instrument such as the DRS, generally distinguishes delirium from these functional disorders.

TABLE 24-3
EEG EVALUATION IN DELIRIUM

Normal background can be seen in psychiatric illness
Diffuse slowing can be seen in dementia and delirium
Triphasic waves are seen in hepatic encephalopathy
Periodic complexes are seen with Creutzfeldt-Jacob disease
Focal slowing suggests a structural lesion in that area
Focal sharp waves are seen in a seizure disorder
Absence of activity is seen in deep coma
Intermittent spike and wave is seen in subclinical status epilepticus
Excessive fast (beta wave) activity is seen with benzodiazepine use

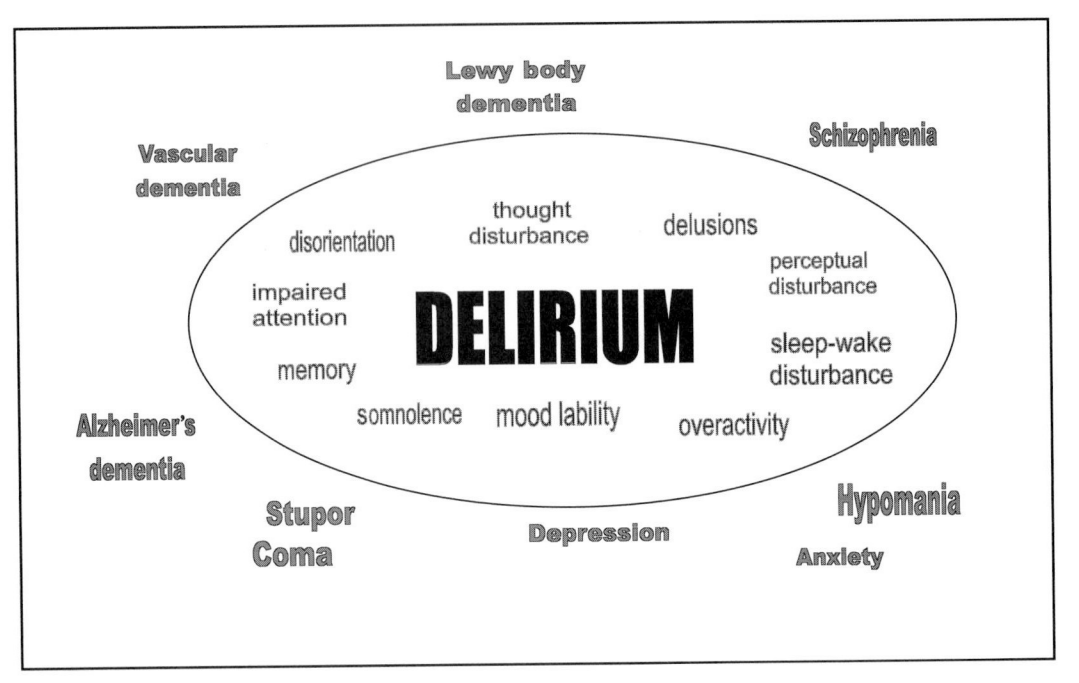

Figure 24-1 The neuropsychiatric differential diagnosis of delirium reflects its broad symptom profile.

DELIRIUM IS ASSOCIATED WITH POORER OUTCOMES

While it is generally recognized that virtually any brain disease increases the risk for a delirium episode, it has been less appreciated that a delirium episode is associated with poorer longitudinal functional outcomes. Comorbid delirium increased hospital length of stay (LOS) by 114% in elderly patients (56), 300% in critical care patients (57), and 250% in hip surgery patients (58). The elderly are at particular risk of decreased independent living status and increased institutionalization following hospital discharge after a delirium episode (59–61). Incident delirium occurring within nursing home settings is linked to a poor 6-month outcome, with behavioral decline, initiation of physical restraints, greater risk of hospitalization, and increased mortality (62). Even after adjusting for age, sex, marital status, living location, comorbidity, illness severity, and dementia, McCusker et al. found that a delirium episode in elderly patients was associated with significantly greater morbidity at 12-month follow-up (63).

Delirium can adversely affect outcome in a variety of ways—decreased capacity to give informed consent, inability to comply with medical management and rehabilitation, medication refusal, difficulty with self-care, reduced ambulation, disruptive behavior, and complications such as falls, fractures, and decubiti (64). Interestingly, subsyndromal delirium is also associated with increased LOS of the index admission and poorer post-discharge function and mortality, even after adjusting for age, sex, marital status, previous living arrangement, comorbidity, dementia

status, and clinical or physiological severity of illness (7). Numerous studies have reported an increased mortality associated with an index episode of delirium, both during and after the admission. Most study designs have parameters that complicate possible attribution of increased mortality to delirium *per se* versus medical comorbidity, pre-existing dementia, inability to comply with treatments, etc. This literature remains controversial. Recent research that controls for some baseline factors like medical comorbidity and physical and/or cognitive functioning suggests there may indeed be an independent risk for increased mortality attributable to the delirium (61,65–70). Thus, it is likely that delirium symptoms are directly related to excess persistent morbidity, with some clinicians advocating that the state of delirium may in itself be neurotoxic (71).

RISK FACTORS FOR DELIRIUM

While delirium is more common in the very young and very old, any patient exposed to adequate insult may develop delirium. It is generally felt that the aged brain is more vulnerable, in part related to structural/degenerative changes and reduced neurochemical flexibility. However, children are also considered at higher risk for delirium, possibly related to ongoing microstructural and neurochemical brain development. For example, there is continued pruning of synaptic bulbs and maturation of the cholinergic system into mid-adolescence, in particular in layer III of the prefrontal cortex. This layer is an associative area that interconnects with other brain association regions and is important for executive cognitive functions. It develops slowly throughout childhood, is highly cholinergic, and is particularly affected in late life by Alzheimer's neuropathological changes. Perhaps immaturity or degeneration of this prefrontal cholinergic layer is relevant to vulnerability for delirium.

The degree of delirium risk relates to a variety of patient, environmental, and iatrogenic factors (Table 24-4). Being hospitalized increases the risk of delirium due to alterations of sleep-wake cycles and exposure to medications and infections, among other risk factors. Models of causation indicate that risk factors interact in a cumulative fashion and combine with a patient's baseline vulnerability for greater predictability (72,73). O'Keeffe and Lavan found that delirium risk increased in direct proportion to one or more of three factors—chronic cognitive impairment, severe illness, and elevated serum urea nitrogen (72). If baseline vulnerability is low, patients are highly resistant to developing

delirium, but if vulnerability is high, minor insults can precipitate delirium. Inouye et al. developed a model that included four *predisposing* factors (cognitive impairment, severe illness, visual impairment, dehydration) and five *precipitating* factors (polypharmacy, catheterization, use of restraints, malnutrition, and any iatrogenic event) that predicted a 17-fold variation in relative risk of developing delirium (73). It remains unclear whether certain patients are vulnerable to particular precipitating factors, or if particular risk factor combinations are especially deliriogenic. Moreover, the temporal relationship between exposure to factors and heightened delirium risk is not known.

Serum albumin is a transporter for many drugs. Hypoalbuminemia is common in ill older patients, with the possibility of resultant increases in unbound, free drug and bioavailability, even within measured therapeutic ranges, and increased risk for delirium (74,75).

Increased blood-brain barrier permeability, secondary to causes such as uremia and hypocholesterolemia, increases delirium risk by allowing entry of substances into the brain, such as medications and toxins, which would not ordinarily penetrate the blood-brain barrier. Van der Mast described postoperative physiological perturbations from physical stress and immune activation that increase delirium risk by altering blood-brain barrier permeability, as well as causing increased limbic-hypothalamic-pituitary-adrenocortical axis activity and low thyroid hormone syndrome (76).

Primary prevention by modification of risk factor exposure is possible. Medication exposure, for example, is implicated in 20% to 40% of delirium cases. Benzodiazepines, opiates, and drugs with anticholinergic activity have a particular association with delirium (33,77). Many drugs unexpectedly contribute to delirium by virtue of underappreciated anticholinergic effects. Tune et al. found that 10 of the 25 most utilized drugs in the elderly had sufficient anticholinergic activity, particularly when combined, to cause cognitive impairment in normal elderly subjects (Table 24-5) (78). Careful consideration must therefore be given to the rationale for using drugs in those at risk of delirium.

TABLE 24-4
RISK FACTORS FOR DELIRIUM

Patient factors
Age (children and elderly)
Pre-existing cognitive impairment
Previous delirium episode
Central nervous system disorder

Environmental factors
Sensory extremes
Visual deficits
Hearing deficits
Immobility
Novel environment
Stress
Sleep deprivation

Medical factors
Severe medical comorbidity
Organ insufficiency
Dehydration
Infection
Hypoxemia
Metabolic disturbances
Low serum albumin
Hypothermia
Fracture
Burns
HIV/AIDS

Surgical factors
Peri-operative
Emergency procedure
Longer duration of operation
Particular procedures (e.g., emergency hip surgery)

Drug Exposure
Polypharmacy
Psychoactive drug use
Drug/alcohol dependence
Specific agents (e.g., anticholinergics)

TABLE 24-5
MEDICATIONS WITH UNDERAPPRECIATED ANTICHOLINERGIC EFFECTS COMMONLY USED IN THE ELDERLY

Cimetidine
Prednisolone
Theophylline
Digoxin
Furosemide
Nifedipine
Ranitidine
Isosorbide dinitrate
Warfarin
Dipyridamole

Adapted from Reference 78.

Inouye and colleagues demonstrated a significant reduction in the number and duration of delirium episodes with a multicomponent intervention involving sensory deficit correction, attention to hydration, and implementation of protocols to address disorientation, sleep-disturbance, and immobilization (79).

Prophylactic medication treatment of at-risk patients, e.g., preoperative patients, is under investigation. Low dose neuroleptic treatment may be an effective means of preventing delirium or reducing its severity in high-risk populations. Kalisvaart et al. used low-dose haloperidol in elderly patients for 3 days before and after hip surgery, and found lower incidence and shorter duration of delirium where it occurred (80). The potential usefulness of atypical antipsychotic agents in this regard requires study. Other work has focused on the usefulness of enhancing cholinergic activity as a means of reducing delirium incidence. Citicoline (81) and donepezil (82) have been studied, but have not been associated with significant benefits compared to placebo in reducing delirium incidence. Secondary prevention through early identification and treatment of delirium may be associated with superior outcome, but direct evidence is lacking.

Recent studies have investigated genetic factors in delirium vulnerability and suggest associations between dopamine transporter gene and neuropeptide-Y gene polymorphisms, and vulnerability to alcohol-withdrawal delirium (83,84).

Thiamine deficiency—perhaps linked to poor dietary habits—was identified as a risk factor for delirium in oncology patients (85) and nonalcoholic elderly patients (86).

CLINICAL ASSESSMENT OF SUSPECTED DELIRIUM

The patient with delirium is often overlooked, especially when the presentation is hypoactive, which is common in the elderly. Cognitive decline is often missed in the quiet or "good" patient, and the treatment team must not presume that patients who are not a management problem on the ward are necessarily well. Although some form of motoric disturbances is almost invariable in delirium (4), the classic stereotype of delirium as it occurs in alcohol withdrawal (*delirium tremens*), with marked agitation and florid psychosis is not the norm, with most cases having a mixed or hypoactive profile (87). It is therefore important not to equate delirium with agitation. More consistent detection of delirium occurs when the focus is on a change in cognitive status rather than just outward behaviors.

Delirium involves a global disruption of cognitive processes. A reduced ability to attend to and interact with the external environment is a central feature. This so-called *clouding of consciousness* is a qualitative concept that is difficult to clearly define, so the diagnosis of delirium is based on more consistently measurable aspects of cognition, such as diminished level of consciousness, attention, and concentration as minimum hallmarks. Disorientation has been used as a key indicator of delirium, but is a highly fluctuant feature with periods of relative lucidity (typically in the morning and coinciding with ward rounds), which can mask the diagnosis and hamper detection. Inattention is readily tested by the serial sevens, or in patients with less education, by asking them to state either the months of the year or days of the week in reverse. Delirious patients typically have impaired visuospatial function, which has been suggested as a useful means of distinguishing delirium from dementia in intensive care unit patients (53), and can be tested by the ability to copy designs such as overlapping pentagons or clock-drawing.

The cornerstone of detection of delirium and accurately identifying underlying etiological factors involves a thorough physical examination, which helps to focus the myriad of potential causes. Given the many causes and significant impact on outcome, delirium may be considered a medical emergency, and all cases require robust investigation.

Clues Regarding Delirium Etiology from Vital Signs Abnormalities

Vital signs may reveal fever or hypothermia due to infection, opiate intoxication, exposure, or an abnormality of thyroid function. Tachycardia may relate to a cardiac condition, hypovolemia, severe anemia, anticholinergic toxicity, and alcohol or benzodiazepine withdrawal. Bradycardia may be due to hypothyroidism, cold exposure, opiate intoxication, cholinergic excess, or a primary cardiac abnormality, including myocardial infarction. Hypertension may indicate neuroleptic malignant syndrome, pheochromocytoma, cocaine or amphetamine exposure, thyroid storm, and delirium tremens, among others. Hypotension suggests possible sepsis, opiate intoxication, myocardial infarction, bradyarrhythmia, and alpha blockade by a medication, among possible etiologies.

Neurological Findings Useful in Delirium

Examination of the eye may reveal pupil dilatation due to hyperthyroidism, afferent pupillary defects, amphetamine or cocaine intoxication, or sympathomimetic agents. Constricted pupils may indicate cholinergic excess, opiate intoxication, or hypothermia. Patients who present with ptosis may be in a myasthenic crisis, have an anticholinergic toxicity, or a third cranial nerve palsy. The latter also causes the eye to deviate laterally and downward. Ophthalmoplegia can suggest Wernicke-Korsakoff syndrome or impairment of the third, fourth, or sixth cranial nerves.

Abnormalities of the other cranial nerves suggest damage to the brainstem or lesions above the brainstem acting posteriorly. It is important to look for an asymmetric facial droop. If the entire side of the face is involved, it suggests a lesion at the brainstem, whereas involvement of only the lower face indicates a contralateral lesion at the internal capsule or above. Patients can also have other cranial neuropathies, such as bilateral sixth nerve palsies that reduce lateral gaze, which is most often due to increased intracranial pressure. Patients can have a fourth nerve palsy due to trauma, and report viewing objects as being on top of one another; also, their head tilts toward the involved side and the eye is deviated upward on primary gaze.

Motor examination can also help to localize the level of cerebral lesions. A hemiparesis contralateral to the lesion will involve the face and arms more than legs with a middle cerebral artery lesion, and *vice versa* with an anterior cerebral artery lesion. If all three body parts are similarly involved, the lesion is subcortical. Tone is diminished contralateral to a stroke in acute phases, but over time increases, with emergence of hyperreflexia and a positive Babinski sign. Transient hemiparesis may follow a focal seizure contralateral to the weakness, a phenomenon termed *Todd's paralysis*. Asterixis and myoclonus represent bicortical damage in a manner termed *release phenomenon*. Paratonia reflects bifrontal damage and can occur in conjunction with other frontal lobe release signs such as grasp, suck, snout, and palmomental reflexes. Patients may also have a hyperactive jaw jerk, reflecting damage to both frontal lobes.

Patients with ataxia, nystagmus, and problems with rapid alternating movements may have cerebellar lesions. Abnormalities with posterior column function (position and vibration sense) can lead to falls. This occurs with neurosyphilis as well as deficiencies of vitamin B12 or folate.

Gait can also provide clues to underlying causation in delirium. A wide-based unsteady gait is typical of cerebellar or brainstem lesions. Spastic or scissoring gait may reflect bifrontal lesions, whereas a hemiparetic gait is seen with a contralateral motor strip lesion. Parkinsonian gait reflects basal ganglia involvement. Some patients may appear magnetized to the floor and have trouble initiating movement, a so-called apraxic gait, seen with lesions of the left parietal lobe and frontal lobes. Patients may neglect one side as they walk, suggesting a lesion in the contralateral parietal lobe.

Physical Examination

The physical examination may also provide clues regarding delirium etiology. Adenopathy may suggest malignancy or infection, including HIV. Lung sounds evaluate the possibility of pneumonia, pneumothorax, or bronchoconstriction. Heart sounds can suggest an arrhythmia or valvular heart disease. The abdominal examination can evaluate for pancreatitis, hepatic dysfunction, splenic lesions, ileus, and appendicitis. The pelvic exam may reveal ovarian or pelvic pathology. Examination of the lower extremities may suggest congestive heart failure or deep venous thrombosis. Skin lesions can suggest HIV, syphilis, Kaposi's sarcoma, or connective tissue disease, among others.

TABLE 24-6
POTENTIAL CATEGORIES FOR ETIOLOGIES OF DELIRIUM

Drug-related: prescribed/illicit, intoxication/withdrawal
Endocrine: metabolic
Traumatic
Epilepsy
Cerebrovascular/Cardiovascular
Tumor
Infection
Organ failure
Not otherwise specified: heavy metal/insecticide poisoning, heatstroke, radiation injury

---

ETIOLOGIES

When evaluating a patient with delirium, the practitioner must consider a broad differential diagnosis of potential causes and should not conclude that the most obvious etiology is the only cause. A systematic workup allows for a more complete diagnosis that accounts for the typically multifactorial nature of causation. Although the physical and neurological examination can be helpful in tailoring the workup, it is important to remember that most cases of delirium typically involve more than one contributory etiology. Table 24-6 depicts the mnemonic, DETECTION, which can aid recall of categories to consider as contributory etiologies. The following are conditions to consider in the older delirium patient:

- *Intracerebral lesions* include subdural and epidural hematoma or intracranial bleed. These often present with headache. The patient may have varying alterations in consciousness with somnolence, and focal neurological findings. A high index of suspicion must be maintained in patients with coagulopathies, at risk of falls, and with basal ganglia disorders. Cerebral abscess is a particular concern in the immunocompromised and is suggested by fever, focal neurological findings, headaches, and seizures. Sinus thrombosis may occur in patients who are dehydrated or hypercoagulable. Tumors often present with altered cognition and headaches. Brain trauma that does not lead to bleeding can also cause delirium due to the presence of white matter shearing injuries, which in severe cases can produce dementia.
- *Infection* may be peripheral or central. The symptoms of a central nervous system infection include fever, nuchal rigidity, cranial neuropathy, headache, altered cognition, and seizures (including subclinical status epilepticus). Lumbar puncture should be withheld until a space-occupying lesion has been ruled out, usually by neuroimaging. Sinusitis can lead to delirium in the elderly. Patients who have slow virus infections may present with myoclonus and confusion, which requires EEG and CSF analysis to clarify the picture.

- *Epilepsy* may cause delirium ictally or during the postictal state. Patients with subclinical, complex, or partial-status epilepticus may be particularly hard to diagnose, because they are able to carry out simple tasks and the condition can be misattributed to nonneurological causes. They may have atypical movements and automatisms including lip smacking, eye blinking, or pelvic motions. An EEG can reveal diffuse slowing (postictal state) or spike and wave activity (status). Benzodiazepine treatment will produce an improvement in epilepsy, whereas benzodiazepines cause more confusion with other causes of delirium. Catatonia and sedative-hypnotic withdrawal typically improve with benzodiazepines.

- *Ischemia* may involve focal or global hypoperfusion. The differential diagnosis for stroke is extensive, but cardiac, arteriosclerotic, and hypercoagulable etiologies must be considered. Focal ischemic events tend to cause delirium only when they are large and located in the brainstem or right hemisphere. Patients with global hypoperfusion often develop hypoxic ischemic encephalopathy and may display myoclonus, reflecting cortical involvement.

- *Endocrine abnormalities* may be present. Hypothyroidism is characterized by lateral thinning of the eyebrows, constipation, weight gain, cold intolerance, and periorbital edema. Patients with hypoparathyroidism present with signs of tetany, hyperactive reflexes, and seizures. Hyperthyroidism is characterized by tachycardia, heat intolerance, tremor, diarrhea, or weight loss. Patients with hyperparathyroidism may seem slowed, constipated, depressed, and confused. Impaired adrenal function (Addison's) can present with confusion in a patient with a history of hyperpigmentation, bradycardia, hypotension, and hypoglycemia. Patients who have hyperadrenal states (Cushing's) may have fat deposits, shiny skin, hyperglycemia, hypertension, and edema around the face.

- *Metabolic etiologies* often present with nonlocalized signs. The major systems involved include pulmonary, hepatic, and renal dysfunction. Secondary problems involving acid-base balance and electrolyte disturbances may also alter cognition. Asterixis occurs with uremic and hepatic insufficiency. Drug metabolism and elimination is further altered in the elderly by these major organ system pathologies, and may secondarily cause physical signs that are unique to that particular drug's toxic profile.

- *Collagen vascular disorders* include systemic lupus erythematosus, rheumatoid arthritis, temporal arteritis, scleroderma, and giant cell arteritis. These conditions often present with rashes, muscle or joint pain, and renal problems. Delirium may reflect cerebral vasculitis, treatment exposure, or both. Elevated erythrocyte sedimentation rate is typical and flags the need for more specific tests as indicated (e.g., autoantibodies).

- *Medications* are a frequent cause of delirium, with anticholinergic agents, opiates, and benzodiazepines commonly implicated. Any medication that has been added since the development of delirium should be scrutinized, because almost every medication class can cause or aggravate delirium, especially in overdose, increased blood-brain barrier permeability conditions, or hypoalbuminemia. When drug interactions occur in the elderly, even modest exposure to relatively benign medications may cause delirium, because the elderly are more susceptible to both pharmacokinetic and pharmacodynamic adverse effects. Medication withdrawal states may also contribute to delirium, and in the case of longer half-life agents, symptoms may appear after a long delay following discontinuation. Use of over-the-counter and "natural" drugs needs to be queried in addition to prescribed drugs.

- *Illicit/recreational drugs* should always be a consideration, and toxicology screens are helpful. Though ethanol is probably the most commonly abused drug in the elderly, there is currently a cohort effect with the aging of adults who were more likely to abuse illicit drugs such as marijuana and cocaine, so other drugs also need to be considered. Low or absent ethanol levels may be the cause of withdrawal delirium in a dependent patient. Cocaine, amphetamines, and crystal methamphetamine can cause stroke, cardiac ischemia, and hypertensive crisis. Benzodiazepines can cause respiratory and cognitive impairment. Opiates may produce small, reactive pupils. Marijuana and hallucinogens do not produce abnormal physical findings, except for conjunctival irritation with marijuana.

- *Alcohol-related* delirium may coexist with a dementia. Wernicke-Korsakoff syndrome consists of the triad of ophthalmoplegia, ataxia, and confusion in the acute (Wernicke's) phase, with Korsakoff's characterized by a persistent amnestic disorder. This is due to thiamine deficiency and occurs in patients with AIDS, malnutrition, and chronic alcohol use. The syndrome affects diencephalic and medial temporal lobe structures. Alcoholic dementia affects about 10% of chronic drinkers and is associated with atrophy of the medial temporal lobe structures, corpus callosum, mammillary bodies, hippocampus, and the frontal lobe. The presence of concurrent subdural or epidural hematomas should always be considered in drinkers, along with other lifestyle-associated illnesses such as AIDS, hepatitis, and syphilis.

- *Psychiatric etiologies* can produce states that mimic delirium or perhaps are psychiatric causes of delirium. Severe mania presents with disorientation, distractibility, rapid speech, irritability, sleeplessness, and grandiose ideation. Depressed patients resemble those with hypoactive delirium due to reduced responsiveness, apparent unawareness, some cognitive impairment, and social withdrawal but, typically, depressed mood dominates rather than the affective instability typical of delirium. Acute psychosis in schizophrenics can present with the marked perplexity and impaired attention that produces a pseudo-delirium. EEG can assist in the differentiation of these primary psychiatric causes of confusion from other medical causes (Table 24-3).

■ *Other etiologies* that interfere with normal biological rhythms or environmental homeostasis can contribute to the development of delirium. Being in an intensive care environment, lack of sleep, the postoperative state, cataracts or other visual abnormalities that diminish visual cues, hearing loss, or a mere shift to a new environment in elderly and/or patients with mental retardation or dementia can all be associated with the emergence of delirium, though these etiologies are not causative by themselves. Environmental toxins such as lead or arsenic can produce dementia, but may present initially with delirium. These etiologies tend to have normal physical examination, EEG, and laboratory workup (except for toxins).

■ *Sleep disorders* can cause daytime confusion that resembles delirium. Narcolepsy involves sudden onset of daytime sleep, cataplexy, and vivid hallucinations upon entering (hypnagogic) and coming out of (hypnopompic) sleep. Patients with obstructive sleep apnea tend to be obese, suffer excessive snoring, and may have periods in which they stop breathing at night, with excessive sleepiness during the day.

INVESTIGATIONS

The wide range of possible etiologies for delirium makes it important that a systematic history and physical examination guides the investigation, to avoid unnecessary and unhelpful tests. Interviews of family and caregivers and a careful review of the current and recent medical records are critically important sources of information, because a delirious patient cannot give an informed or reliable history. At times, pharmacies need to be contacted for accurate medication histories. Sometimes, even the hospital roommate offers observations that are invaluable. At the same time, it is important to bear in mind that delirium is typically multifactorial and the identification of a single etiology should not bring an end to diagnostic efforts. Some of the more commonly performed investigations that should be considered in all delirious patients are shown in Table 24-7, along with other potential investigations that are applicable to particular suspected etiologies.

MANAGEMENT OF THE DELIRIOUS PATIENT

Delirium is a brain disorder that deserves treatment as such, even while a thorough investigation to determine its

TABLE 24-7
WORK-UP OF SUSPECTED DELIRIUM

1. **Careful history and physical examination**
2. **Collateral history**
   Baseline cognition
   Presence of sensory impairments
   Exposure to risk factors
   Review of medications, procedures, tests, intraoperative data

3. **First-line investigations**
   Complete blood count
   Electrolytes, Mg, Ca, PO_4
   LFTs
   Urinalysis
   Electrocardiogram
   Erythrocyte sedimentation rate
   Blood glucose
   Chest radiograph
   Urinalysis

4. **Second-line investigations (as indicated)**
   Drug screen
   Blood cultures
   Cardiac enzymes
   Blood gases
   Serum folate/B12
   Electroencephalography
   Cerebrospinal fluid examination
   Computed tomography of the brain
   Magnetic resonance imaging of the brain
   Prolactin level
   HIV antibodies
   Syphilis serology
   Urinary porphyrins

underlying etiologies is occurring. Delirium should be considered an urgent situation and, in some cases, a medical emergency. Delirium requires a coordinated biopsychosocial approach to assessment and treatment for both the brain disorder and any other organ system perturbation associated with the impairment. The delirious patient provides a considerable test of the cohesiveness of medical-nursing relationships, and their ability to utilize relatives and caregivers in the ongoing assessment of delirium severity and the provision of an optimal environment for recovery. Treatment involves addressing the specific symptoms of delirium, ensuring safety of the patient and of his or her environment, minimizing aggravating factors, and identifying and treating underlying causes. Rapid treatment is important because of the high associated morbidity and mortality from both the delirium itself and its underlying causes. Diagnosis and treatment should occur concurrently, and regular re-evaluation of progress is important. The key role played by nursing staff and relatives in monitoring the delirious patient's clinical course must be recognized, particularly given that many patients are most impaired outside of usual physician working hours.

Supportive and Environmental Measures

Facilitating adequate sleep, nutrition and fluid intake, encouraging optimal stimulation, maximizing the patient's ability to interact with surroundings (e.g., ensuring the use of hearing aids, glasses, and dentures), and to comply with treatment are central to good delirium management. However, environmental manipulations are underutilized and often applied only in response to behavioral disturbance rather than to the degree of cognitive impairment (88). Greater use of environmental strategies in hyperactive patients may relate to the tendency to equate severe delirium with hyperactive features, despite some evidence that these patients may have better outcomes than those with hypoactive presentations, perhaps due to more reversible underlying causes or treatment differences (89). Recovered patients report that simple but firm communication, reality orientation, a visible clock, and the presence of a relative all contribute to a heightened sense of control during delirium (90). Many supportive measures (e.g., attention to noise, lighting, mobility levels, adequate pain management) reflect basic features of a good therapeutic environment and should be a routine feature of care settings. Other measures (e.g., reorientation efforts including large clocks, calendars with the days marked off, and family photos) may address particular delirium symptoms and require specific recognition within individual patient treatment plans. Particularly agitated or paranoid patients may require sitters to prevent inadvertent self-harm—delirious patients have been known to jump out of hospital windows to their deaths. Delirium nurse specialists and special delirium hospital units are part of an effort to limit risk factors, enhance recognition, and encourage standardized treatment (91).

Family members or usual caregivers can facilitate efforts to reassure and orient patients. Clear explanation about the delirium is important, because upset or ill-informed caregivers can exacerbate patient distress. Delirium is often associated with terminal stages of illness and can shape enduring memories of loved ones as crazy or disturbed, unless explained and managed sensitively. Breitbart et al. studied the delirium experience in recovered patients, their families, and nurses, and found that greater distress levels were associated with presence of delusions, perceptual disturbances, and loss of functionality (14). Clarification of the cause and meaning of symptoms, combined with recognition of treatment goals, allows for better management of what is a distressing experience for both the patient and loved ones. In addition to assisting care during hospitalization, relatives frequently play crucial roles in planning and monitoring post-discharge care.

DRUG TREATMENT

The goal of drug treatment of delirium is to achieve effective symptom control while minimizing undesirable effects.

There is no drug with a Food and Drug Administration (FDA) indication for the treatment of delirium. Double-blind, randomized, placebo-controlled studies of efficacy and safety are lacking; therefore, current pharmacotherapies are empirical or anecdotal. No medication has been explored or discovered that has been specifically targeted for use in delirium, and current treatments are borrowed from the pharmacopeia for other psychiatric disorders. It is important to remember that medications can either treat or cause delirium, and are implicated as significant etiological factors in over one-third of cases. While sedatives can reduce agitation, they may worsen cognitive impairment, complicate ongoing mental status assessment, impair the ability to understand or cooperate with treatment, and even worsen delirium. Intensive care units rely heavily on medications such as fentanyl and midazolam to manage patients, both of which can induce delirium. The rationale for drug treatment should be explicit: is the primary goal to specifically remedy delirium, or to target problem behavior?

Neuroleptics (Antipsychotics)

Neuroleptics remain the cornerstone of pharmacological treatment of delirium, despite the lack of clinical placebo-controlled efficacy and safety trials. Neuroleptics may ameliorate a range of delirium symptoms, are effective in patients with both hyperactive and hypoactive clinical profile and, with careful use, improve cognition (92). Onset of action is rapid, with improvement usually evident within hours or days, so improvement often occurs prior to treatment of underlying causes. The apparent effectiveness of antipsychotics does not relate closely to their inherent sedative properties, nor does it follow the time frame associated with an antipsychotic effect in schizophrenia (93).

Neuroleptics are preferred to benzodiazepines in delirium related to causes other than sedative-hypnotic or alcohol withdrawal. Chlorpromazine and haloperidol have similar efficacy (93), but haloperidol is preferable due to having only one active metabolite and much less potential for anticholinergic, sedative, and hypotensive effects. Haloperidol can be administered orally, intramuscularly, or intravenously, although the intravenous route has not been approved by the FDA, and more recently has been increasingly reported as causing prolongation of QTc interval and torsades de pointes, and tachyarrhythmia (multifocal ventricular tachycardia), even in younger adults (94). Patients receiving intravenous haloperidol need to be on a cardiac-monitored bed and their magnesium and calcium levels kept in the normal range. Although high potency antipsychotics like haloperidol have an increased risk of extrapyramidal side effects, the actual reported incidence in studies of delirium is surprisingly low, except in high-risk populations such as those with Lewy body dementia or AIDS, and may reflect an inherent protective effect of the central nervous system's low cholinergic state that often underlies delirium. Parenteral droperidol has been used when a faster onset of action (about 15 minutes) or greater sedation is required, but its use is no longer recommended due to its serious cardiovascular adverse events profile (including hypotension and QTc prolongation).

Dose is determined by the route of administration, age, level of agitation, side effect propensity, and therapeutic setting. Low-dose oral haloperidol (1 to 10 mg/day in divided doses) produces symptomatic improvement in most patients (43,93,95). Drug treatment of highly disturbed patients derives from studies of patients with general agitation, rather than delirium in particular. Successful control of agitation has not been clearly linked to improved outcome in delirium, but is inferred from evidence linking poorer outcome to complications of unchecked illness, such as interference with treatment and immobility (89).

Atypical antipsychotic agents are increasingly joining the delirium armamentarium. To date, use of olanzapine (5 to 20 mg), risperidone (1.5 to 4 mg), and quetiapine (up to 750 mg) has been supported by case reports, retrospective case series, or open-label case control convenience samples (96–99), or by open-label prospective trials using standardized measures (100–104). Doses in the elderly should always begin at the lower end of the dosage range and be carefully titrated. Case reports suggest that poor response to haloperidol can be associated with improvement of delirium after switching to an atypical agent (105–107). Lower degrees of extrapyramidal effects and studies of neuropsychological effects of atypicals in normal elderly volunteers suggest advantages over traditional agents (108). In addition, the increasing availability of atypicals in intramuscular formulations makes them increasingly attractive therapeutic options for clinicians. Recent concerns, however, regarding a possible increased risk of cerebrovascular events in elderly patients with dementia treated with atypical antipsychotics suggest a need for greater caution in their use, particularly in view of the high rate of concomitant dementia in patients with delirium (109,110). Other work suggests the risk of stroke is no higher in elderly patients receiving atypical compared to typical antipsychotics (111), and that medication choice should be guided by a careful consideration of the overall benefit-risk ratio (112).

Benzodiazepines

Benzodiazepines are first-line treatment for delirium related to seizures or withdrawal from ethanol or sedative-hypnotics, and are avoided in other causes of delirium. They are also a useful adjunctive treatment in patients who are intolerant of antipsychotics, because they permit use of lower antipsychotic doses (113) and have the significant advantage of potential rapid reversal with flumazenil. Therapeutic aims should be explicit, since anxiolytic, sedative, and hypnotic effects occur with increasing doses. Lorazepam has several advantages due to its sedative prop-erties, rapid onset and short duration of action, reduced risk of accumulation, absence of active metabolites, and more predictable bioavailability compared to other benzodiazepine agents when given intramuscularly. Lower doses are necessary in the elderly, those with hepatic disease, or those already receiving drugs that undergo extensive hepatic oxidative metabolism (e.g., cimetidine, isoniazid).

Other Drug Therapies

Disturbances of cholinergic metabolism are implicated in delirium due to hypoxia, traumatic brain injury, hypoglycemia, and drug-related etiologies. Physostigmine can reverse anticholinergic delirium, but its side effects and short half-life have limited use in routine clinical treatment; anticholinergic delirium is generally treated conservatively by removal of the offending agent. A more recent study of physostigmine administered in the emergency department to patients with suspected muscarinic toxicity resulted in reversal of delirium in 55% of cases, with a single adverse event (brief seizure) in one patient (114). Other procholinergic agents currently used to counter cholinergic deficits in dementia have theoretical potential. A possible role for donepezil in the treatment of delirium occurring postoperatively, in Lewy body dementia, and in alcohol dementia is supported by case reports (115–117). However, Liptzin did not find a significant benefit of donepezil used prophylactically in high-risk cases of elderly patients undergoing surgery, perhaps reflecting its long half-life and delayed impact on cholinergic activity (82). A randomized placebo-controlled trial of citicoline in nondemented hip surgery patients, given 1 day prior to and each of 4 days after surgery, indicated fewer cases of delirium in the citicoline group (17% versus 12%), but the difference was not statistically significant (81). Smoking has been identified as a protective factor against delirium, but the usefulness of nicotine replacement therapies in prophylaxis against delirium is untested (118).

Trazodone and mianserin are antidepressant compounds with antagonistic actions at 5HT-2 receptors. Open studies of low-dose therapy in delirium indicate rapid reduction of noncognitive symptoms in particular. This effect was apparently independent of mood-altering actions, but may be related to sedative activity (119–121). A single intravenous dose of ondansetron, a 5-HT3 antagonist, was reported to reduce agitation in 35 post-cardiotomy delirium patients (122). Antagonism of presynaptic 5-HT3 receptors on cholinergic neurons can increase release of acetylcholine (123).

POST-DELIRIUM MANAGEMENT

Many patients experiencing delirium are discharged before full resolution of symptoms and, unfortunately, continued monitoring and management are often not part of post-discharge planning. Problems with attention and orientation are particularly persistent (124). Further episodes may be prevented by addressing risk factors such as medication exposure and sensory impairments. There has been little study of the psychological aftermath of delirium, but recent work suggests around 50% of sufferers can recall the episode (14). Depression and post-traumatic stress disorder has been described, but most dismiss the episode once it has passed, often despite lingering concerns that the episode heralds a first step towards loss of mental faculties and independence (90). Other patients experience *silent delirium* and are ashamed or afraid to admit to symptoms. Explicit recognition and discussion of the meaning of delirium can facilitate adjustment, and can also allow more detailed discussion of how best to minimize future risk. A follow-up visit can facilitate post-delirium adjustment by clarifying the transient nature of delirium symptoms in contrast to dementia (125), as well as providing any ongoing medication adjustments.

CONCLUSIONS

Delirium is a complex neuropsychiatric syndrome that is common in medical and surgical populations, especially in the elderly, in the intensive care setting, and in those with pre-existing brain disorders. The recognition of its high morbidity and mortality, and its relevance in an increasingly aged society, has stimulated greater interest in improving our understanding of its accurate diagnosis and management. A high index of suspicion, with careful attention to alterations in cognition, assisted by routine screening for inattention, is key to improved detection. Delirium is underrecognized and often misdiagnosed as depression or dementia. Comorbidity with dementia in the elderly is a particular challenge, though the delirium symptoms dominate the presentation and the patient is best managed as having delirium until proven otherwise.

Delirium requires a careful medical differential diagnosis for its underlying causes. A wide variety of pathophysiological mechanisms funnel into *a final common neural pathway* to produce a characteristic syndrome that has been proposed as a low cholinergic state in the brain, accompanied by a relative excess of dopaminergic activity. Differential diagnosis of causation requires a systematic approach, and efforts to identify causative factors do not end when a single etiology has been uncovered.

Management requires close cooperation between family and clinical staff to provide an optimal recovery environment. Treatment for delirium as an independent neuropsychiatric disorder needs to occur concurrently with investigation for and treatment of its underlying etiologies. Both hypoactive and hyperactive presentations of delirium require equivalent medical attention and treatment. Medications, particularly antipsychotic agents, seem clinically effective in relieving delirium symptoms based on empirical and anecdotal reports, but given the lack of definitive efficacy and safety studies, they must be used prudently. Post-delirium recovery is facilitated by explicit recognition of the episode and education of the patient and relatives, as well as efforts to reduce exposure to future risk factors.

REFERENCES

1. American Psychiatric Association. *Diagnostic and Statistical Manual of Mental Disorders*. 4th ed. Washington, DC: American Psychiatric Association; 1994.
2. Fann JR. The epidemiology of delirium: a review of studies and methodological issues. *Semin Clin Neuropsychiatry*. 2000;5:86–92.
3. Meagher DJ, Trzepacz PT. Delirium phenomenology illuminates pathophysiology, management, and course. *J Geriatr Psychiatry Neurol*. 1998;11:150–157.
4. Meagher DJ. The significance of motoric symptoms and subtypes in delirium. New Research Abstracts. American Psychiatric Association Annual Meeting. May 2003; San Francisco.
5. O'Keeffe ST, Gosney MA. Assessing attentiveness in older hospitalized patients: global assessment vs. test of attention. *J Am Geriatr Soc*. 1997;45:470–473.
6. Nicholas LM, Lindsey BA. Delirium presenting with symptoms of depression. *Psychosomatics*. 1995;36:471–479.
7. Cole M, McCusker J, Dendukuri N, Han L. The prognostic significance of subsyndromal delirium in elderly medical inpatients. *J Am Geriatr Soc*. 2003;51:754–760.
8. Harrell R, Othmer E. Postcardiotomy confusion and sleep loss. *J Clin Psychiatry*. 1987;48:445–446.
9. Matsushima E, Nakajima K, Moriya H, et al. A psychophysiological study of the development of delirium in coronary care units. *Biol Psychiatry*. 1997;41:1211–1217.
10. McNicoll L, Pisani MA, Zhang Y, et al. Delirium in the intensive care unit: occurrence and clinical course in older patients. *JAGS*. 2003;51:591–598.
11. Turkel SB, Braslow K, Tavare CJ, Trzepacz PT. The Delirium Rating Scale in children and adolescents. *Psychosomatics*. 2003;44:126–129.
12. Turkel SB, Trzepacz PT, Tavare J. Comparison of delirium symptoms across the life cycle [abstract]. *Psychosomatics*. 2004;45:162.
13. Rudberg MA, Pompeii P, Foreman MD, et al. The natural history of delirium in older hospitalized patients: a syndrome of heterogeneity. *Age Ageing*. 1997;26:169–174.
14. Breitbart W, Gibson C, Tremblay A. The delirium experience: delirium recall and delirium-related distress in hospitalized patients with cancer, their spouses/caregivers and their nurses. *Psychosomatics*. 2002;43:183–194.
15. Ljubisavljevic V, Kelly B. Risk factors for development of delirium among oncology patients. *Gen Hosp Psychiatry*. 2003;25(5):345–352.
16. Kolbeinsson H, Jonsson A. Delirium and dementia in acute medical admissions of elderly patients in Iceland. *Acta Psychiatr Scand*. 1993;87:123–127.
17. Rockwood K, Cosway S, Carver D, et al. The risk of dementia and death after delirium. *Age Ageing*. 1999;28:551–556.
18. Wahlund LA, Bjorlin GA. Delirium in clinical practice: experiences from a specialized delirium ward. *Dement Geriatr Cogn Disord*. 1999;10:389–392.
19. Erkinjuntti T, Wikstrom J, Parlo J, et al. Dementia among medical inpatients: evaluation of 2000 consecutive admissions. *Arch Intern Med*. 1986;146:1923–1926.
20. Jitapunkul S, Pillay I, Ebrahim S. Delirium in newly admitted elderly patients: a prospective study. *Q J Med*. 1992;83:307–314.
21. Jackson SA. The epidemiology of aging. In: Hazzard WR, Blass JP, Ettinger WH, et al., eds. *Principles of Geriatric Medicine and Gerontology*. New York: McGraw-Hill; 1999:203.
22. American Psychiatric Association. Practice guidelines for treatment of patients with Alzheimer's disease and other dementias of late life. *Am J Psychiatry*. 1997;154(suppl):1–39.

23. Sandberg O, Gustafson Y, Brannstrom B, et al. Prevalence of dementia, delirium and psychiatric symptoms in various care settings for the elderly. *Scand J Soc Med.* 1998;26:56–62.

24. Trzepacz PT. Update on the neuropathogenesis of delirium. *Dement Geriatr Cogn Disord.* 1999;10:330–334.

25. Trzepacz PT. Is there a final common neural pathway in delirium? Focus on acetylcholine and dopamine. *Semin Clin Neuropsychiatry.* 2000;5:132–148.

26. Trzepacz PT, Meagher DF, Wise M. Neuropsychiatric aspects of delirium. In: Yudofsky SC, Hales RE, eds. *American Psychiatric Publishing Textbook of Neuropsychiatry and Clinical Neurosciences.* 4th ed. Washington, DC: American Psychiatric Publishing; 2002:525–564.

27. Itil T, Fink M. Anticholinergic drug-induced delirium: experimental modification, quantitative EEG, and behavioral correlations. *J Nerv Ment Dis.* 1966;143:492–507.

28. Stern TA. Continuous infusion of physostigmine in anticholinergic delirium: a case report. *J Clin Psychiatry.* 1983;44:463–464.

29. Kaufer DI, Catt KE, Lopez OL, et al. Dementia with Lewy bodies: response of delirium-like features to donepezil. *Neurology.* 1998; 51:1512–1513.

30. Mondimore FM, Damlouji N, Folstein MF, et al. Post-ECT confusional states associated with elevated serum anticholinergic levels. *Am J Psychiatry.* 1983;140:930–931.

31. Tune LE, Dainloth NF, Holland A, et al. Association of postoperative delirium with raised serum levels of anticholinergic drugs. *Lancet.* 1981;2:651–653.

32. Yamamoto T, Lyeth BG, Dixon CE, et al. Changes in regional brain acetylcholine content in rats following unilateral and bilateral brainstem lesions. *J Neurotrauma.* 1988;5:69–79.

33. Brown TM. Drug-induced delirium. *Semin Clin Neuropsychiatry.* 2000;5:113–125.

34. Ames D, Wirshing WC, Szuba MP. Organic mental disorders associated with bupropion in three patients. *J Clin Psychiatry.* 1992;53:53–55.

35. Wetli CV, Mash D, Karch SB. Cocaine-associated agitated delirium and the neuroleptic malignant syndrome. *Am J Emerg Med.* 1996;14:425–428.

36. Sander T, Harms H, Podschus J, et al. Alleleic association of a dopamine transporter gene polymorphism in alcohol dependence with withdrawal seizures or delirium. *Biol Psychiatry.* 1997;41:299–304.

37. Broderick PA, Gibson GE. Dopamine and serotonin in rat striatum during in vivo hypoxic-hypoxia. *Metab Brain Dis.* 1989;4: 143–153.

38. Knell AJ, Davidson AR, Williams R, et al. Dopamine and serotonin metabolism in hepatic encephalopathy. *BMJ.* 1974;1: 549–551.

39. Ongini E, Caporali MG, Massotti M. Stimulation of dopamine D-1 receptors by SKF 38393 induces EEG desynchronization and behavioral arousal. *Life Sci.* 1985;37:2327–2333.

40. Leavitt M, Trzepacz PT, Ciongoli K. Rat model of delirium: atropine dose-response relationships. *J Neuropsychiatry Clin Neurosci.* 1994;6:279–284.

41. Trzepacz PT, Leavitt M, Ciongoli K. An animal model for delirium. *Psychosomatics.* 1992;33:404–415.

42. Ikarashi Y, Takahashi A, Ishimaru H, et al. Regulation of dopamine D1 and D2 receptors on striatal acetylcholine release in rats. *Brain Res Bull.* 1997;43:107–115.

43. Platt MM, Breitbart W, Smith M, et al. Efficacy of neuroleptics for hypoactive delirium. *J Neuropsychiatry Clin Neurosci.* 1994;6: 66–67.

44. Johnson JC, Kerse NM, Gottlieb G, et al. Prospective versus retrospective methods of identifying patients with delirium. *J Am Geriatr Soc.* 1992;40:316–331.

45. Lewis LM, Miller DK, Morley JE, et al. Unrecognized delirium in emergency department geriatric patients. *Am J Emerg Med.* 1995;13:142–145.

46. Armstrong SC, Cozza KL, Watanabe KS. The misdiagnosis of delirium. *Psychosomatics.* 1997;38:433–439.

47. Rockwood K, Cosway S, Stolee P, et al. Increasing the recognition of delirium in elderly patents. *JAGS.* 1994;42:252–256.

48. Inouye SK, van Dyke CH, Alessi CA, et al. Clarifying confusion: the Confusion Assessment Method. *Ann Intern Med.* 1990;113: 941–948.

49. Trzepacz PT, Mulsant BH, Dew MA, et al. Is delirium different when it occurs in dementia? A study using the Delirium Rating Scale. *J Neuropsychiatry Clin Neurosci.* 1998;10:199–204.

50. Trzepacz PT, Baker RW, Greenhouse J. A symptom rating scale for delirium. *Psychiatry Res.* 1988;23:89–97.

51. Trzepacz PT, Mittal D, Torres R, et al. Validation of the Delirium Rating Scale—Revised-98: comparison to the Delirium Rating Scale and Cognitive Test for Delirium. *J Neuropsychiatry Clin Neurosci.* 2001;13:229–242.

52. Hart RP, Best AM, Sessler CN, et al. Abbreviated Cognitive Test for Delirium. *J Psychosom Res.* 1997;43:417–423.

53. Hart RP, Levenson JL, Sessler CN, et al. Validation of a cognitive test for delirium in medical ICU patients. *Psychosomatics.* 1996;37:533–546.

54. Jacobson SA, Jerrier S. EEG in delirium. *Semin Clin Neuropsychiatry.* 2000;5:86–93.

55. Cutting J. The phenomenology of acute organic psychosis: comparison with acute schizophrenia. *Br J Psychiatry.* 1987;151: 324–332.

56. Schor JD, Levkoff SE, Lipsitz LA, et al. Risk factors for delirium in hospitalized elderly. *JAMA.* 1992;267:827–831.

57. Kishi Y, Iwasaki Y, Takezawa K, et al. Delirium in critical care unit patients admitted through an emergency room. *Gen Hosp Psychiatry.* 1995;17:371–379.

58. Berggren D, Gustafson Y, Eriksson B, et al. Postoperative confusion following anesthesia in elderly patients treated for femoral neck fractures. *Anesth Analg.* 1987;66:497–504.

59. George J, Bleasdale S, Singleton SJ. Causes and prognosis of delirium in elderly patients admitted to a district general hospital. *Age Ageing.* 1997;26:423–427.

60. Cole MG, Primeau FJ. Prognosis of delirium in elderly hospital patients. *CMAJ.* 1993;149:41–46.

61. Inouye SK, Rushing JT, Foreman MD, et al. Does delirium contribute to poor hospital outcome? *J Gen Intern Med.* 1998;13: 234–242.

62. Murphy KM. The baseline predictors and 6-month outcomes of incident delirium in nursing home residents: a study using the minimum data set. *Psychosomatics.* 1999;40:164–165.

63. McCusker J, Cole M, Abrahamowicz M, et al. Delirium predicts 12-month mortality. *Arch Int Med.* 2002;162:457–463.

64. Gustafson Y, Berggren D, Brahnstrom B, et al. Acute confusional states in elderly patients treated for femoral neck fracture. *J Am Geriatr Soc.* 1988;36:525–530.

65. Curyto KJ, Johnson J, TenHave T, et al. Survival of hospitalized elderly patients with delirium: a prospective study. *Am J Geriatr Psychiatry.* 2001;9:141–147.

66. Minagawa H, Uchitomi Y, Yamawaki S, et al. Psychiatric morbidity in terminally ill cancer patients: a prospective study. *Cancer.* 1996;78:1131–1137.

67. Lawlor PG, Gagnon B, Mancini IL, et al. Occurrence, causes and outcome of delirium in patients with advanced cancer. *Arch Intern Med.* 2000;160:786–794.

68. Ely EW, Shintani A, Truman B, et al. Delirium as a predictor of mortality in mechanically ventilated patients in the intensive care unit. *JAMA.* 2004;291:1753–1762.

69. Kakuma R, Galbaud du Fort G, Arsenault L, et al. Delirium in older emergency department patients discharged home: effect on survival. *J Am Geriatr Soc.* 2003;51:443–450.

70. Kelly KG, Zisselman M, Cutillo-Schmitter T, et al. Severity and course of delirium in medically hospitalized nursing facility residents. *Am J Geriatr Psychiatry.* 2001;9:72–77.

71. Meagher DJ. Delirium episode as a sign of undetected dementia among community dwelling elderly subjects. *J Neurol Neurosurg Psychiatry.* 2001;70:812–827.

72. O'Keeffe ST, Lavan JN. Predicting delirium in elderly patients: development and validation of a risk-stratification model. *Age Ageing.* 1996;25:317–321.

73. Inouye SK, Charpentier PA. Precipitating factors for delirium in hospitalized elderly patients: predictive model and interrelationships with baseline vulnerability. *JAMA.* 1996;275:852–857.

74. Trzepacz PT, Francis J. Low serum albumin and risk of delirium [letter]. *Am J Psychiatry.* 1990;147:675.

75. Dickson LR. Hypoalbuminemia in delirium. *Psychosomatics.* 1991;32:317–323.

76. van der Mast RC, Fekkes D. Serotonin and amino acids: partners in delirium pathophysiology? *Semin Clin Neuropsychiatry.* 2000;5:125–131.

77. Marcantonio ER, Juarez G, Goldman L, et al. The relationship of postoperative delirium with psychoactive medications. *JAMA.* 1994;272(b):1518–1522.

78. Tune L, Carr S, Hoag E, et al. Anticholinergic effects of drugs commonly prescribed for the elderly: potential means for assessing risk of delirium. *Am J Psychiatry.* 1992;149:1393–1394.

79. Inouye SK, Bogardus ST, Charpentier PA, et al. A multicomponent intervention to prevent delirium in hospitalized older patients. *New Engl J Med.* 1999;340:669–676.

80. Kalisvaart K, Prophylactic haloperidol cuts delirium. American Association of Geriatric Psychiatry, Annual Meeting. 2003; Honolulu.

81. Diaz V, Rodriguez J, Barrientos P, et al. Use of procholinergics in the prevention of postoperative delerium in hip fracture surgery in the elderly. A randomized controlled trial. *Rev Neurol.* 2001; 33:716–719.

82. Liptzin B. Donepezil in the prevention and treatment of postoperative delirium following elective prthopedic surgery. *Am J Ger Psychiatry.* In press.

83. Wernicke C, Smolka M, Gallinat J, Winterer G, Schmidt LG, Rommelschpacher H. Evidence for the importance of the human dopamine transporter gene for withdrawal symptomatology of alcoholics in a German population. *Neurosci Lett.* 2002;333: 45–48.

84. Gorwood P, Limosin F, Batel P, Hamon M, Ades J, Boni C. The A9 allele of the dopamine transporter gene is associated with delirium tremens and alcohol-withdrawal seizure. *Biol Psychiatry.* 2003;53:85–92.

85. Seear M, Lockitch G, Jacobson B, et al. Thiamine, riboflavin and pyridoxine deficiency in a population of critically ill children. *J Pediatr.* 1992;121:533–538.

86. O'Keeffe ST, Tormey WP, Glasgow R, et al. Thiamine deficiency in hospitalized elderly patients. *Gerontology.* 1994;40:18–24.

87. Meagher DJ, Trzepacz PT. Motoric subtypes of delirium. *Semin Clin Neuropsychiatry.* 2000;5:76–86.

88. Meagher DJ, O'Hanlon D, O'Mahony E, et al. Use of environmental strategies and psychotropic medication in the management of delirium. *Br J Psychiatry.* 1996;168:512–515.

89. O'Keeffe ST, Lavan JN. Clinical significance of delirium subtypes in older people. *Age Ageing.* 1999;28:115–119.

90. Schofield I. A small exploratory study of the reaction of older people to an episode of delirium. *J Adv Nurs.* 1997;25:942–952.

91. Simon L, Jewell N, Brokel J. Management of acute delirium in hospitalized elderly: a process improvement project. *Geriatr Nursing.* 1997;18:150–154.

92. American Psychiatric Association. Practice guidelines for the treatment of patients with delirium. *Am J Psychiatry.* 1999; 156(suppl):1–20.

93. Breitbart W, Marotta R, Platt MM, et al. A double-blind trial of haloperidol, chlorpromazine, and lorazepam in the treatment of delirium in hospitalized AIDS patients. *Am J Psychiatry.* 1996;153:231–237.

94. O'Brien JM, Rockwood RP, Suh KI. Haloperidol-induced torsades de pointes. *Ann Pharmacother.* 1999;33:1046–1050.

95. Nakamura J, Uchimura N, Yamada S, et al. Does plasma free-3-methoxy-4-hydroxyphenyl(ethylene)glycol increase the delirious state? A comparison of the effects of mianserin and haloperidol on delirium. *Int Clin Psychopharmacol.* 1997;12(a): 147–152.

96. Schwartz TL, Masand PS. Treatment of delirium with quetiapine. Primary Care Companion. *J Clin Psychiatry.* 2000;2:10–12.

97. Torres R, Mittal D, Kennedy R. Use of quetiapine in delirium: case reports. *Psychosomatics.* 2001;42:347–349.

98. Sipahimalani A, Masand PS. Use of risperidone in delirium: case reports. *Ann Clin Psychiatry.* 1997;9:105–107.

99. Masand PS, Sipahimalani A. Olanzapine in the treatment of delirium. *Psychosomatics.* 1998;39:422–430.

100. Horikawa N, Yamazaki T, Miyamoto K, et al. Treatment for delirium with risperidone: results of a prospective open trial with 10 patients. *Gen Hosp Psychiatry.* 2003;25:289–292.

101. Breitbart W, Tremblay A, Gibson C. An open trial of olanzapine for the treatment of delirium in hospitalized cancer patients. *Psychosomatics.* 2002;43:175–182.

102. Kim KY, Bader GM, Kotlyar V, Gropper D. Treatment of delirium in older patients with quetiapine. *J Geriatr Psychiatry Neurol.* 2003;16:29–31.

103. Skrobik Y, Bergeron N, Dumont M, Gottfried SB. Olanzapine versus haloperidol: treating delirium in a critical care setting. *Intensive Care Med.* 2004;30:444–449.

104. Mittal D, Jimerson NA, Neely E, et al. Risperidone in the treatment of delirium: results from a prospective open label trial. *J Clin Psychiatry.* 2004;65:662–667.

105. Passik SD, Cooper M. Complicated delirium in a cancer patient successfully treated with olanzapine. *J Pain Symptom Manage.* 1999;17:219–223.

106. Leso L, Schwartz TL. Ziprasidone treatment of delirium. *Psychosomatics.* 2002;43:61–62.

107. Al-Samarrai S, Dunn J, Newmark T, Gupta S. Quetiapine for treatment-resistant delirium. *Psychosomatics.* 2003;44:350–351.

108. Beuzen JN, Taylor N, Wesnes K, Wood A. A comparison of the effects of olanzapine, haloperidol and placebo on cognitive and psychomotor functions in healthy elderly volunteers. *J Psychopharmacol.* 1999;13:152–159.

109. Katz IR, Jeste DV, Mintzer JE, et al. Comparison of risperidone and placebo for psychosis and behavioral disturbances associated with dementia: a randomized double-blind trial. *J Clin Psychiatry.* 1999;60:107–115.

110. Brodaty H, Ames D, Snowdon J, et al. A randomised-controlled trial of risperidone for the treatment of aggression, agitation, and psychosis of dementia. *J Clin Psychiatry.* 2003;64: 134–143.

111. Herrmann N, Mamdani M, Lanctot KL. Atypical antipsychotics and risk of cerebrovascular accidents. *Am J Psychiatry.* 2004;161: 1113–1115.

112. Insau P, Lawley D. CSM guidance on antipsychotic use. Care of the elderly in psychosis. *Geriatric Medicine.* 2004;14(suppl):6–7.

113. Menza MA, Murray GB, Holmes VF, Rafuls WA. Decreased extrapyramidal symptoms with intravenous haloperidol. *J Clin Psychiatry.* 1987;48:278–280.

114. Schneir AB, Offerman SR, Ly BT, et al. Complications of diagnostic physostigmine administration to emergency department patients. *Ann Emerg Med.* 2003;42:14–19.

115. Wengel SP, Burke WJ, Roccaforte WH. Donepezil for postoperative delirium associated with Alzheimer's disease. *J Am Geriatr Soc.* 1999;47:379–380.

116. Wengel SP, Roccaforte WH, Burke WJ. Donepezil improves symptoms of delirium in dementia: implications for future research. *J Geriatr Psychiatry Neurol.* 1998;11:159–161.

117. Burke WJ, Roccaforte WH, Wengel SP. Treating visual hallucinations with donepezil. *Am J Psychiatry.* 1999;156:1117–1118.

118. Culp K, Tripp-Reimer T, Wadle K, et al. Screening for acute confusion in elderly long-term care residents. *J Neuroscience Nurs.* 1997;29:86–100.

119. Uchiyama M, Tanaka K, Isse K, et al. Efficacy of mianserin on symptoms of delirium in the aged: an open trial study. *Prog Neuropsychopharmacol Biol Psychiatry.* 1996;20:651–656.

120. Nakamura J, Uchimura N, Yamada S, et al. The effect of mianserin hydrochloride on delirium. *Human Psychopharmacology.* 1995;10: 289–297.

121. Okamato Y, Matsuoka Y, Sasaki T, et al. Trazadone in the treatment of delirium. *J Clin Psychopharmacol.* 1999;19:280–282.

122. Bayinder O, Akpinar B, Can E, et al. The use of the 5-HT$_3$ antagonist ondansetron for the treatment of post-cardiotomy delirium. *J Cardiothorac Vasc Anesth.* 2000;14:288–292.

123. Kennedy JS, Zagar A, Bymaster F, et al. The central cholinergic system profile of olanzapine compared with placebo in Alzheimer's disease. *Int J Geriatr Psychiatry.* 2001;16(suppl 1): S24–S32.

124. Levkoff SE, Liptzin B, Evans D, et al. Progression and resolution of delirium in elderly patients hospitalized for acute care. *Am J Geriatr Psychiatry.* 1994;2:230–238.

125. Easton C, MacKenzie F. Sensory-perceptual alterations: delirium in the intensive care unit. *Heart Lung.* 1988;17:229–237.

Major Depression and Related Disorders in Late Life

25

Darren J. Thompson   Soo Borson

Depression in older adults leads to enormous individual and family burden and has far-reaching medical, social, and economic consequences. Overall increases in utilization of health care resources are associated with depression in late life, independent of mental health services and after controlling for medical disorders (1–4), and functional deficits and loss of quality of life compound the suffering caused by the mood disorder itself (5,6). Depression is also associated with increased mortality from both suicide (7) and medical illness (8,9). Depression in older adults is a group of heterogeneous clinical disorders that can challenge diagnostic acumen and requires a broad scope of therapeutic intervention, as illustrated in the following case example:

CASE EXAMPLE

The son-in-law of Mr. R, an 83-year-old man, frantically calls from out of state about his father-in-law, whom he fears is dying. He has observed a change in his father-in-law's usual personality and behavior—he has become withdrawn, seems to be declining quickly, and will not leave his apartment in a local senior assisted-living facility to get help. Mr. R refuses to come for an evaluation. The psychiatrist makes an emergency home visit, finding the patient's daughter and a part-time caregiver, who speaks very limited English, hovering around him. Mr. R sits on the sofa, minimally responsive, eyes downcast, clean but poorly groomed, mumbling a few words to be polite. He admits to being depressed when asked directly, but does not speak unless addressed. The walls of his one bedroom

---

apartment in this well-appointed newer retirement complex are empty, and nowhere in evidence is a hint of what his life has been—no memorabilia, photographs, or other signs of personal history. His bed is neatly made and the environs are clean but sterile.

Mr. R's medical history includes significant cardiovascular disease, hypertension, a coronary bypass graft some years earlier, and a remote stroke, but he has not seen his internist or had any revision in his medication regimen in over a year. His blood pressure is 90/60, pulse 84, and he is unable to lift himself off the sofa unless pulled up by two people. His mouth is very dry and his mentation sluggish, though he is generally oriented and understands the reason for the visit after it has been explained, and he accepts a drink of water. Once on his feet he is able to walk slowly, but would lose his balance and fall unless supported.

The home visit breaks the stalemate of care avoidance that had lasted for several years, and sets the stage for Mr. R's consent to an inpatient admission. There the presence of a major depression was easily observed in symptoms of marked anhedonia, fatigue and loss of initiative, feelings of worthlessness and desire for death, and signs of broken sleep, psychomotor retardation, and fluid depletion. Cognitive screening was mildly abnormal with a Mini-Mental State Examination (MMSE) score of 26/30, and executive dysfunction was apparent on a clock-drawing task. Urinary tract infection was present and brain magnetic resonance imaging (MRI) disclosed periventricular and scattered multiple, sometimes confluent, deep white-matter lesions. Treatment was initiated with trimethoprim/sulfamethoxazole for his urinary tract infection, citalopram 10 and then 20 mg daily for his depression, and initial intravenous fluids followed by insistent oral hydration. His blood pressure returned to normal levels within 2 days and he became more alert but still minimally interactive. Within 2 weeks his mood had brightened, his sleep had improved remarkably, he ate without prompting and responded agreeably to friendly approaches, and his family commented that he was himself again. A troubling lack of initiative remained, however, and he was content to do little unless stimulated. His gait remained somewhat impaired.

Mr. R's chronic major depressive episode was complicated by the dysexecutive syndrome commonly associated with extensive cerebral microvascular disease, and by his family's inability to appropriately take charge of decisions for him when he began to fail. It was later discovered that he had been depressed for several years since the death of his wife, but neither he nor his family had sought treatment on his behalf, feeling unsure about whether it was right to force him, and also uncertain as to whether his condition was normal in a man of his advanced age. Once he had recovered enough to leave the hospital, his family, at the urging of psychiatric staff, decided to place him in a nursing home affiliated with his former assisted-living facility. Though his mood had brightened strikingly with antidepressant treatment and good general medical and nursing care, his executive dysfunction remained functionally limiting. He required ongoing external stimulation, structure, and basic support for nutrition, hydration, and social activity, and was happy to let others make decisions for him, though he never developed much insight into what they did or why they had to do it.

Late-life depression is underrecognized, particularly in primary care settings, general hospitals, and nursing homes (10). As illustrated by this case, family members can miss the depression too, until it has advanced to a critical and potentially life-threatening stage. In this example, the threat to life came not from active suicidal intent, but from the interaction of depression, brain disease, and physical vulnerability, and from a well-meaning family's desire to avoid offending its former patriarch. Such clinical and pathogenetic ambiguities are not rare in old people. This chapter seeks to provide a conceptual framework, based on current empirical knowledge, for recognition, assessment, and care of these challenging conditions.

PHENOMENOLOGY

Mood disorders are relatively common in late life, and often have special clinical presentations and consequences compared with depressive disorders in the younger patient population. Although DSM-IV-TR diagnostic criteria for major depression, minor depression, and dysthymia are the same for all age groups (11), symptom expression can be age-dependent (Table 25-1). The tendency of depressed

TABLE 25-1

SPECIAL CLINICAL FEATURES ENCOUNTERED IN LATE-LIFE DEPRESSION

Depression without sadness
Lack of feeling or emotion
Prominent cognitive complaints
Prominent somatic complaints (e.g., preoccupation with bowel function)
Unexplained health worries
Heightened pain experience/complaints
Multiple primary care visits without resolution of the problem
Irritability
Social withdrawal, avoidance of social interaction
Prominent loss of interest and pleasure in activities
Signs of functional impairment or otherwise unexplained functional decline

older adults to report more somatic and cognitive symptoms than affective symptoms (12) has long been a source of diagnostic confusion for clinicians, and many patients are irritable and socially withdrawn without subjective complaints of feeling depressed. Depression without sadness (13) is one variant in which anhedonia, a lack of feelings or emotions, or medically unexplained somatic complaints or anxiety replace or exceed the hallmark mood change. Recognizing the variety of depression's clinical manifestations in older adults is particularly important, as the feeling of hopelessness, not sadness, is most strongly associated with suicidal ideation (14).

Depression at any age can be debilitating. Of particular concern in the elderly are problems with initiative, self-care, household maintenance, travel, understanding and communicating, participating in society, and getting along with others in both elderly community (15) and medical patient (16) populations. Changes in functional status and signs of functional impairment, such as uncharacteristic lack of attention to personal care or appearance, can be important indicators. When depression and impairment of everyday function occur together, it is often difficult to know in advance which components of disability are caused by mood disorder and which are caused by cognitive disorders, frailties, and medical disease. Trials of a variety of approaches to treatment across all these domains are often necessary to arrive at a plan of care that will provide optimal recovery.

EPIDEMIOLOGY AND RISK FACTORS

The range of mood disorder subtypes seen in elderly patients is broad (17). Classical major depression is generally less frequent in older than in younger adults, with an overall prevalence of about 1% (about 2% for dysthymic disorder) (11,18). However, 15% to 25% of older adults experience depressive symptoms that do not meet criteria for a specific depressive syndrome, but cause distress and interfere with daily functioning (19). Most of these patients would be classified as having minor depression, best conceptualized as a state of often intermittent low mood and lowered quality of life, associated with risk for chronicity and later decline into syndromal major depression.

Several theories have been advanced to explain why major depression seems to be less common in the elderly. Healthy older adults acquire *resilience*, defined as the capacity to adjust to and recover from stressors without loss of equanimity. This resilience may confer some resistance to depression as people age, and partially explain the lower rates of some depressive syndromes. Moreover, a cohort effect may produce variations in prevalence across generations that are not directly related to age, but rather to shared experience (20) or generational temperament. The prevalence of major depression has been increasing in the more recently born, perhaps indicating that the prevalence of late-life depression might rise as these cohorts age. However, the most popular explanatory models look for flaws in the diagnostic approaches used in epidemiological research, suggesting insensitivity to depressive variants, or seek confounding elements from disability, comorbidities, or features misattributed to personality disorder or dementia. Other factors could include selective attrition of depressed elderly from community populations, owing to higher levels of disability and higher mortality rates. Moreover, interviewing methods used in population studies may contribute to underidentification of depression in elderly adults, who may be reluctant or unable to recall or report emotional symptoms that younger patients might be more willing or able to relate (21).

Although major depression may be less common in the older population than in the younger, certain subgroups are particularly vulnerable, including medically ill, disabled, and institutionalized elderly. High scores on global measures of medical burden are associated with a tripling of the risk of incident depressive disorders over 1 year in community-based studies (22) and continue to elevate risk longer term, even after controlling for past history of depression, spousal death, demographic factors, and other potential psychosocial risk factors (23). In primary care clinics, depression has been identified in 17% to 37% of medically ill elderly (24), 30% of whom met criteria for major depression and the remainder for clinically important depressive symptoms. In medically hospitalized elderly, major depression occurred in 11% and depressive symptoms in 25% (25) and, in long-term care, the corresponding percentages were 12% and 30% (26).

The specificity of depression in medically ill older adults continues to engender confusion and controversy, but serious medical disease is a generally acknowledged risk factor. Older adults with malignancies, neurologic and endocrine disorders (such as Parkinson's disease [PD], stroke, Alzheimer's disease [AD], pancreatic cancer, and hypothyroidism) are thought to be particularly at risk,

although figures vary across studies. Approximately one-fourth of cancer inpatients (27), one-quarter to over one-half of poststroke patients (28,29), up to one-third of individuals with AD (30), and up to one-half of those with PD suffer from depressive disorders at sometime during the course of disease (31). Cardiovascular disease, including coronary heart disease and congestive heart failure, can be another important medical determinant of depression. Approximately one-third of patients develop major depression at some time during the 12 months following a myocardial infarction (32). In the absence of medical illness and other psychosocial risk factors, the presence of disability alone (measured by activities of daily living limitations) increases the risk of incident depression by a factor of four over 1 year in older adults living at home (33).

Demographic factors and life events are also associated with geriatric depression. These include low socioeconomic status and social support, marital separation and divorce, and recent adverse and unexpected life events including bereavement (17). Lack of social contact is associated with increased risk of onset of depression in some, but not all, longitudinal analyses (34). Neurotic personality characteristics interact with stressful life events and medical illness to increase risk of depressive outcome (35).

New widowhood is a particularly potent precipitating factor for depression. By age 65, over half of all women and over a tenth of all men have been widowed at least once (36), and the rates rise dramatically for both women and men thereafter. A large cohort study involving 12,522 spouse pairs followed for 14 to 23 years found a significantly increased mortality rate in bereaved men and women after adjusting for age, education, and health status, with the highest relative risk occurring 7 to 12 months following spousal loss (37), when the risk of incident depression is highest. Twenty-four percent of widows and widowers develop clinically significant depression during this period, 9% during the first 2 years, and 3% during the first 3 years (23,38,39).

Caregiving for a frail, physically ill, dependent, or demented older adult is a significant risk factor for depression, with prevailing rates in most studies between 38% to 67% (40). Women report more depressive symptoms than men, relinquish the caregiving role later, and receive less informal support from friends and family members (41). Adult children caregivers are typically daughters dealing with juggling multiple roles such as parenting and jobs, and they frequently face conflict with their siblings over caregiving issues, resulting in high caregiver burden and depression (42).

Living in a nursing home is an important correlate of depression prevalence. The prevalence of depression in long-term care greatly exceeds that found in geriatric community populations, with reported rates ranging from 30% to 50%, with 15% meeting criteria for major depression and the remainder experiencing less severe but clinically significant depressive symptoms (43). The 1-year incidence among new admissions ranges from 12% to 25% (44).

Depression is often considered an expected or a natural consequence of the chronic diseases and disability that lead to nursing home placement, and the environmental changes and existential factors the individual must bear in such a move. However, unlike normal grief responses, depressions in long-term care patients are typically persistent and associated with greater cognitive and functional decline, pain problems, self-care deficits, malnutrition, and mortality (45,46).

SUICIDE AND LATE-LIFE DEPRESSION

Suicide rates in the elderly are strikingly high, particularly in older Caucasian men, in whom the rate per 100,000 population in 1989 was 43.5, far higher than in the general (12.2) or overall older population (20.1) or women of similar age (5.9) (47). Suicide rates rose 9% between 1980 and 1992 and continue to rise, particularly for men between 80 to 84 years of age (48). Psychological autopsy studies point to psychiatric disorder as the common substrate underlying late-life suicide, most commonly a first episode of major depression (7). The majority of patients have visited their physicians within a few months of their death, but were not diagnosed or appropriately treated for depression (49). Other important risk factors for suicide include severe forms of depression, e.g., psychotic depression, alcoholism (which itself can be a response to depression), recent loss or bereavement, being divorced or widowed, the development of disability, and the abuse of sedatives, hypnotics, and analgesics (50).

ASSESSMENT

Most elderly people with depression and other psychiatric disorders are seen not by psychiatrists but only by their primary care physicians, and usually on a regular basis (51). However, geriatric depression is often underrecognized and under treated, in part because of the frequent presence of several different medical disorders all commanding attention as possible causes of the patient's symptoms. This may help to explain why 65% of depressed patients received more than five medications compared to 35.6% of nondepressed patients in one study (17). Standardized rating scales can be clinically useful in the initial assessment of depression. Routine clinical screening with instruments assessing global cognition such as MMSE, and interviewer-rated or self-rated depression scales, such as the Hamilton Rating Scale for Depression (HAM-D) and various forms of the Geriatric Depression Scale (GDS), may help to reduce the rate of underrecognized late-life depression and misattribution to dementia.

Identifying depression in the nursing home setting can be assisted by screening and assessment scales as well, provided they have been validated in long-term care

patients. The 30-item GDS has been shown to have 84% sensitivity and 91% specificity for individuals with MMSE scores of 15 or greater (52), and shorter versions carry most of the discriminating power of the original. Nursing home staff use of instruments such as the HAM-D or the Cornell Scale for Depression in Dementia has been reported to increase detection of depression from about 32% to 50% (53). The routinely collected Minimum Data Set has not been shown to be an adequate tool for screening nursing home residents for clinical forms of depression (54).

Variations in life experiences, medical status and history, personality and cognitive functioning, and relevant psychosocial factors are the norm in older populations. Accordingly, evaluation of patients with suspected depression depends on careful weighing of biological, psychological, and social factors that could play a role in shaping the clinical presentation. Figure 25-1 maps the general approach and domains essential to consider.

Table 25-2 lists some of the more important comorbid medical conditions to assess as possible mediating and moderating factors in depressed older patients, based on expert consensus guidelines (50). It is also important to consider recent loss, disability, and environmental problems, such as emotional, financial, or physical abuse or neglect of a frail, vulnerable older person by caregivers or relatives. Moreover, it is necessary to identify new functions or responsibilities the individual has had to assume as a result of loss, of separation from significant others, or of spousal disability.

Comorbid psychiatric disorders should also be considered, since they are not uncommon in late-life depression and may mask the mood disorder (55). The three most common psychiatric comorbidities are alcohol use disorders (15% to 30% in major depression, three to four times that of nondepressed elderly) (56), generalized anxiety and phobic disorders (57), and personality disorders, the most common being in the cluster C category (avoidant, dependent, and obsessive-compulsive) (58,59). Psychotic depression is relatively frequent in psychiatric samples, ranging from a prevalence of 3.6% of older depressed outpatients to a high of 20% to 45% among elderly people hospitalized for depression (60), and should be suspected in cases of severe depression.

In current psychiatric practice and research, two principal approaches define depression:

1. Depressive symptoms
2. More specific depressive illnesses or disorders defined in terms of duration, number, and type of depressive symptoms

Most nonpsychiatrists typically regard depression in terms of the first construct, whereas psychiatrists tend to apply the second (61). Other terms, describing observed clinical syndromes or presumptive etiopathologies, have also been used to distinguish among the subtypes.

TABLE 25-2

IMPORTANT COMORBID CONDITIONS TO CONSIDER IN LATE-LIFE DEPRESSION

Most important	Current alcohol/substance-use disorder, including withdrawal
	Medications that can cause or mimic mood disorders
	Dementia, including Alzheimer's disease
Important	Prescribed medications—accidental or intentional misuse; unintended consequences
	Chronic pain or its treatment
	Nutritional or metabolic problems (e.g., poorly controlled diabetes, B12 or folate deficiency, malnutrition, thyroid or other endocrine dysfunction)
	Cerebral disorders—recent head injury, vascular or any neurodegenerative disease
	Cardiovascular disorders—occult myocardial infarction, hypotensive episodes,
	Congestive heart failure
	Chronic pulmonary insufficiency—poorly controlled or chronic asthma, chronic obstructive pulmonary disease
	Cancer
	Physical, verbal, or emotional abuse by caregivers/relatives

Adapted from Reference 50.

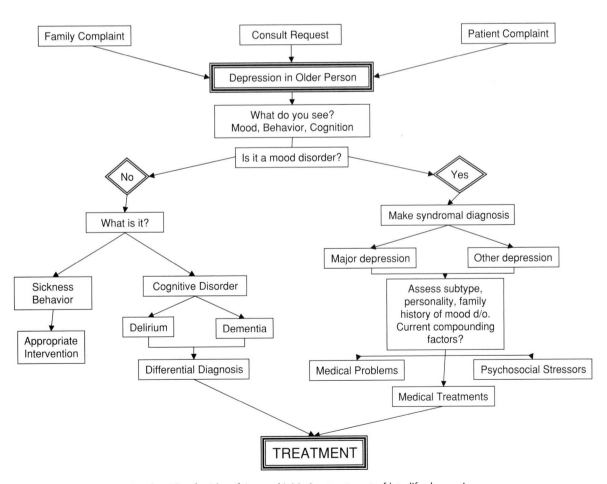

Figure 25-1 An algorithm for identifying and initiating treatment of late-life depression.

FORMS OF DEPRESSIVE DISORDERS

Major Depression

Major depressive disorder is diagnosed using the same DSM-IV-TR criteria for both the younger and older patient population. Some depressed elderly patients may present with a symptom cluster similar to their younger counterparts, but others, as illustrated previously, do not; DSM-IV-TR does not distinguish late-life variants. Disturbances in sleep, sexual functioning, and appetite are not always reliable indicators of depression in older adults because these functions can be affected by normal aging, by medications, by a variety of physical illnesses, and by social situations (62). Older depressed patients are more likely to experience weight loss and are less likely to report suicidal thoughts (63).

Early-Onset Versus Late-Onset Depression

An important distinction among older individuals with major depression concerns the age of onset of their first depressive episode. The onset may occur in earlier adulthood with a recurrent course into older age (*early onset depression*, or EOD), or the onset of the first episode may be late in life (*late-onset depression*, or LOD), generally set at about age 50 in most studies. This dichotomous classification has limitations due to indistinct or insidious onset of symptoms, difficulty establishing when a depressive syndrome was fully formed, and problems of memory and recall bias. Despite these problems, the concept of LOD as a fundamentally different disease entity from EOD has gained considerable empirical ground. Elderly patients with EOD have been found to have more first-degree relatives with depression, suggesting stronger genetic loading, compared to those with LOD. On the other hand, those with LOD have more chronic physical illness, and may have less complete responses to treatment, a more chronic course with a poorer prognosis, and increased mortality (64–68). Elderly individuals with LOD are more likely to have brain imaging findings indicative of brain disease, such as ventriculomegaly and white-matter hyperintensities (WMH) (60); are less likely to have psychiatric comorbidity, such as personality disorder, substance abuse, or panic disorder; and are more likely to present with loss of interest and apathy than individuals with EOD (69,70).

Depression with Reversible Dementia

Depression in late life (whether EOD or LOD) is often associated with cognitive impairments. Historically, these cognitive deficits had been regarded as benign and reversible, referred to as *pseudodementia* or depression with reversible dementia. It is now recognized that many such patients experience persisting cognitive impairment after amelioration of depression, or are in the process of developing a diagnostically distinguishable dementia (71) that is unmasked by the presence of depression. There is evidence that depressive symptoms may represent early manifestations or prodromal signs of dementia (72,73), and this is more likely to be the case with more severe depression that is associated with psychomotor retardation or psychosis (71). Furthermore, a lifetime history of depressive symptoms and depression diagnoses has been observed to be associated with an increased risk of developing AD (73), although this finding has not been universally replicated. Thus, many clinicians prefer to avoid the term pseudodementia.

Vascular Depression

Some depressions can be etiologically linked to cerebrovascular disease (CVD), both typical acute neurological syndromes due to cortical strokes and more chronic microvascular, usually subcortical, syndromes. The presumed etiology sometimes represents a frontostriatal disconnection state, and the clinical presentation includes executive dysfunction, reduced interest in activities (apathy), more cognitive impairment, psychomotor retardation, and impaired insight, but limited or absent feelings of guilt (12,74). Gait impairment and incontinence are also common results of CVD in such patients, and executive dysfunction is the cognitive deficit most associated with impairments in instrumental activities of daily living. Executive dysfunction has prognostic significance, implying poorer outcome of treatment, higher risk of relapse, and recurrence of major depression (5,75). Depression-executive dysfunction syndrome of late life is a related concept used to describe a syndrome of pronounced frontostriatal-limbic dysfunction (76) with prominent disability, psychomotor retardation, and reduced interest in activities, but limited vegetative symptoms and depressive ideation. Whether this syndrome is a more phenomenologically accurate term than vascular depression, and whether it will encapsulate the latter designation, is not yet clear.

Poststroke Depression

Patients who suffer new-onset depressive syndromes (major and minor) 3 to 6 months after a stroke have more vegetative features and larger lesion volumes than patients who first met criteria for depression 12 to 24 months later, suggesting a stronger biological pathogenesis for more proximal-onset cases (77). Later-onset cases appear to be more influenced by social and physical impairments, suggesting potentially remediable psychosocial and functional deficits contributing to depression that develops 1 year or longer after a stroke (77).

Depression with Psychosis

Psychotic depressions are not unique to older adults, but are psychiatric emergencies in this population. These depressions respond not at all to placebos, poorly to anti-depressants used alone (60), and more often to combinations of antidepressant and antipsychotic medications (78). Hospitalization is typically indicated and electroconvulsive therapy (ECT) is the treatment of first choice when agitation, starvation, dehydration, or suicidality threatens survival. Psychotic features in late-life major depression occur in about 4% of depressed older outpatients, but up to 45% of hospitalized older depressives. Patients with psychotic depression may display many types of delusions, most commonly delusional guilt, jealousy, paranoia, or somatization. They frequently complain bitterly of somatic symptoms without medical explanation, and can express profound nihilistic beliefs and hopelessness, but hallucinations are relatively infrequent (17). Psychotic depressions frequently recur; the risk of suicide is not necessarily higher than in nonpsychotic depression, but the extreme degrees of agitation and hour-to-hour fluctuation in clinical symptoms that can accompany this clinical presentation may promote unpredictable, impulsive acts.

Nonmajor Depressive Disorders

There has been limited consensus on the definitions of nonmajor depressive disorders. Epidemiologic studies have used the terms subsyndromal, subclinical, and subthreshold to collectively describe the depressive states that fall below the threshold for case-level depression (79). DSM-IV-TR, on the other hand, uses a categorical approach to describe nonmajor depression and lists dysthymic disorder, adjustment disorder, mood disorder due to a general medical condition, substance-induced mood disorder, dementia with depressed mood, and depressive disorder not otherwise specified, which includes minor depressive disorder (11). Data are sparse on the clinical course and outcome of this broad category, largely because of the lack of consensus on definitions. On the whole, nonmajor depression can be associated with significant functional impairment and disability, impaired quality of life, and increased use of health services and medications (16,80). Some authors emphasize that nonmajor depression represents a depressive continuum between euthymia and major depression (81). In fact, older adults with subsyndromal depression were found in one study to be significantly more likely to meet criteria for major depression at 1-year follow-up than were those in the nondepressed group (81).

Dysthymia in late life has been found to have quite different clinical characteristics than dysthymia in young adults. For example, axis II disorders occur in a minority of elderly patients with dysthymic disorder, it has a predominantly late age at onset, a larger male representation, and a relatively low frequency of comorbid psychiatric disorders (58,82). Late-life dysthymic disorder is often associated with medical illness, disability, institutionalization, chronicity, progression to major depression, and poor

response to antidepressant medication treatment (83). Dysthymic symptoms such as anhedonia, blunted affect, lack of energy, and other somatic complaints are often overlooked or discounted by health care providers who erroneously assume they are a normal part of aging, particularly in the context of medical illness and residence in a nursing facility (82). Minor depressive disorder is listed as a "potential category" in DSM-IV-TR and is qualitatively identical to major depression except that only two to four symptoms are needed to make the diagnosis (11). The individual can express sadness or depression, or can express the loss of interest and pleasure in activities without feeling depressed (depression without sadness).

Bereavement and Depression

Many elderly experience a great deal of loss, not only in the form of death (e.g., spouse, friends, relatives, loved pets), but also in other spheres of life such as loss of physical ability, financial income, social status, mobility, life ambitions, and independence. Conjugal bereavement is a common life event for older adults. It can be associated with a range of reactions including denial, disbelief, sadness, anger, despair, guilt, and a sense of yearning for the deceased. Typically, uncomplicated bereavement-related dysphoria is often triggered by thoughts or reminders of the deceased, and the sadness tends to present intermittently, in waves, interspersed by periods of more upbeat mood and an intact ability to socialize and function normally. If present, functional impairment is often transient and mild.

Bereavement is frequently associated with symptoms of a major depressive episode, with subsyndromal depressive symptoms, or with posttraumatic distress (84). For example, insomnia, anorexia, and weight loss are frequent depressive symptoms accompanying bereavement. DSM-IV-TR notes that the diagnosis of major depressive episode is generally not made unless the symptoms continue to be present 2 months after the loss, and outlines symptoms that assist in differentiating bereavement from major depression (11). These include:

- Guilt about things other than actions taken or not taken by the survivor at the time of the death
- Thoughts of death other than the survivor feeling that he or she would be better off dead or should have died with the deceased person
- Morbid preoccupation with worthlessness
- Marked psychomotor retardation
- Prolonged and marked functional impairment
- Hallucinatory experiences other than thinking that he or she hears the voice of, or transiently sees the image of, the deceased person

Chronic Caregiving Depression

Caregivers, particularly those caring for demented spouses, often experience clinically significant depressive symptoms and can develop depressive disorders (85–87). Caregivers, especially aging spouses, simultaneously bear heightened responsibility, new physical demands, challenges to assimilating their own aging process, risk of social isolation, and grief about the cognitive and/or physical loss of the loved one they once knew. Caregivers frequently do not recognize the extent of their depression, despite bearing often overwhelming stress and experiencing disabling symptoms such as insomnia, poor energy, anhedonia, and social withdrawal. They may express their distress in a more indirect somatic manner. The presenting depressive symptom of a depressed caregiver is often simply feeling burned out. However, some caregivers, even when suffering from profound depression, may not complain of feeling even slightly burdened.

By denying their strain, caregivers may protect themselves from feeling that they have betrayed their spouse or family member, fearing that discussing their problems is tantamount to complaining about their loved one, a sign of disloyalty. Discussing their difficulties and depressive feelings may represent failure, not only as a caregiver, but also as a spouse, friend, confidant, parent, and able society member. Thus, some may feel that their self-worth is at stake. Caregivers may believe that requesting help will place too high a burden on family or friends. Furthermore, they may feel paralyzed by feelings of ambivalence and guilt towards their loved one, placing themselves in a position of being unable to ask for any outside assistance at all. With the onset of depressive symptoms, such as impaired sleep and energy, the quality of caregiving often precipitously declines. Taken together, this frequently necessitates others to aid in both the recognition of depression and in the active decision-making process, such as judging the degree of outside help needed.

Caregiver depression is often recognized, and may be treated, by clinicians who treat the care recipient. Inquiry into caregiver depression and burden can be approached directly by asking about psychiatric and physical symptoms, level of support, health maintenance, and other aspects concerning quality of life, such as the amount of time spent alone, ability to participate in enjoyable activities, and capacity to maintain or form meaningful social relationships. Frequently, however, the clinician may need to approach this subject very creatively, and in a fashion that is attuned to the caregiver's emotional and relational style, to avoid undue shame, guilt, or denial. Optimal treatment may require the care recipient and the caregiver to be treated simultaneously, and because other members of the family are often actively involved in the therapeutic process, the clinician may need to serve the role as family psychiatrist or family geriatrician.

Depression and Medical Illness

There is a reciprocal relationship between medical illness burden and geriatric depression. Increased medical burden increases depressive symptoms, and long-term depressive symptoms increase medical burden (88) and mortality (89). For example, depression lowers self-rated health and intensifies physical symptoms, including amplifying the perception of pain, and chronic pain worsens depression (90). Physical symptoms can mimic or mask depression, as is the case in hypoactive delirium characterized by psychomotor retardation, social withdrawal, reduced speech, and nonspecific dysphoria (91). Similarly, depressive symptoms can be misattributed to medical disorders, particularly loss of interest, changes in appetite and sleep, weight loss, poor concentration, and low energy.

Distinguishing medical from depressive symptoms can be very difficult. What matters most in clinical practice is considering the possibility that symptoms that are apparently part of one condition, such as depression or heart failure, could be caused by the other. For research purposes, at least four approaches have been used for the identification of depressive symptoms in the medically ill elderly. The *exclusive approach* excludes neurovegetative symptoms (changes in sleep, energy, appetite, weight) as part of the depressive syndrome. The *inclusive approach* assumes that all symptoms that could be caused by depression should be counted toward a depression diagnosis. The *substitutive approach* replaces neurovegetative symptoms (that could be due to medical causes) with depressive ideas (e.g., hopelessness). The *best-estimate approach* demands that a clinical judgment is required for each symptom as to whether the symptom is caused by a medical illness or depression (10,92–94). The prevalence of major depression in the elderly varies twofold depending on whether an exclusive or an inclusive approach is used (95), and there is no clinical consensus on which to take. The major hazard of the best-estimate method is the level of nonpsychiatric medical knowledge and experience required of the clinician.

Differential Diagnosis

Once depression has been established in the older adult, the clinician has the challenge of distinguishing amongst a broad differential diagnostic inventory to help guide treatment. Applying the DSM-IV-TR, the list includes major depressive disorder, dysthymic disorder, minor depressive disorder, adjustment disorder with depressed mood, personality disorder, anxiety disorder, bipolar depression, bereavement, mood disorder due to a general medical condition, substance-induced mood disorder, dementia with depressed mood, and depressive disorder not otherwise specified (11). It is also important to consider age of onset and prior history of depressions, as this may have implications for nonpsychiatric etiologies and for treatment.

To aid in differentiating depression in older adults, the clinician often needs to take a symptom inventory from both the patient and from those close to him or her. Additionally, a thorough social, medical, and family history is required. A strong family history of depression, for example, may help in distinguishing EOD from LOD. Recent significant life events, including loss, may lead the clinician to consider the diagnoses of adjustment disorder or of bereavement. The clinician needs to rule out substance abuse and dependence, including alcohol, illicit drugs, prescription, and over-the-counter medications. It is not unusual for older adults to take medications provided by family members, so it is imperative to inquire directly along these lines. Certain medical illnesses, disability and medical burden, and medications can precipitate or exacerbate depression, and need to be reviewed by the assessing clinician.

Cerebral Abnormalities

Neuroimaging studies have added to our understanding of late-life depression, demonstrating, most importantly, that structural brain abnormalities are more frequent in patients with LOD than EOD. Findings thought to be important in the etiopathogenesis of many cases of LOD include signal hyperintensities in white-matter tracts (i.e., WMH), especially when found in deep white-matter pathways linking subcortical with cortical (generally frontal) regions. Such changes are difficult to appreciate on computed tomography and are best seen with MRI and newer imaging methods such as diffusion tensor imaging. Although some WMH are found in up to 92% of elderly control subjects (96), their severity correlates with late-life depression (97,98). Depression is particularly common with higher grades of WMH in the frontal lobes, even after controlling for vascular risk factors such as hypertension, diabetes, or ischemic heart disease (99), but some association has also been found between depression and periventricular location of WMH (100). Perhaps the most compelling argument from MRI studies comes from some of the earliest work in the field, describing a specific association between WMH and first-episode LOD (74,101).

WMH are most often considered by radiologists to represent ischemic lesions, including small, neurologically silent subcortical infarcts (102), and one postmortem study supports the idea that ischemic rather than "other" WMH are specifically associated with LOD (103). Clinicians must be aware that while many vascular risk factors are associated with increased WMH, precipitous or chronic hypotension contributes significantly to their development (103). One report documents an abnormal pattern of reduced nocturnal blood pressure in LOD patients with evidence of silent cerebral infarction (104). In addition to WMH, brain atrophy is also associated with LOD (105), and both smaller prefrontal lobe brain volumes and greater WMH volume independently increase the odds of developing depression (106–108). The normal right-left frontal lobe asymmetry may be attenuated in older adults with a depressive disorder (109), and LOD patients may have disproportionately smaller right frontal

lobes compared with older adults with EOD and elderly controls (110).

Functional imaging investigations extend the structural findings, most often showing signs of prefrontal cortical dysfunction (111,112). One study observed that older adults with LOD had significantly lower bilateral anterior frontal cerebral perfusion than age and gender-matched controls (113). The exact role of the frontal lobes in the pathogenesis of depression remains unclear. However, the frontal lobes modulate certain aspects of mood, neuroendocrine, and cognitive functions that are often impaired during depression (114).

Studies of neurological patients provided the initial inspiration for psychiatric theories, and later investigations, of possible neural substrates of depression in both early and later life. Neurological diseases characterized by subcortical degeneration and resulting damage to frontal lobe inputs are classically associated with depression. These include PD, Huntington's disease, caudate strokes, and progressive supranuclear palsy. Imaging studies have corroborated the importance of specific circuits in depression in such patients, and proposed a unified theory of the neurobiology of depression that encompasses functional anatomic pathways, neuroendocrine dysregulation, and neurotransmitter impairments as part of a coordinated pattern of adaptive failure (115,116).

TREATMENT

The treatment recommendations given in Table 25-3 represent a distillation of clinical experience and published literature on treatment of late-life depression, much of it contributed by specialists in geriatric psychiatry. Since most patients with depressions in later life never see a psychiatrist—let alone a geriatrically trained one—most depressed elderly patients who receive any treatment do so in the context of primary care, where medication-only approaches are often the initial, and may be the only, strategy. Under dosing, too-short medication trials, difficulty making accurate appraisals of response to treatment, and lack of familiarity with what can be expected from alternative and augmentation strategies are continuing problems. Clear practice recommendations that can be applied across settings and provider types are important. The Prevention of Suicide in Primary Care Elderly—Collaborative Trial algorithm was developed with the aim of decreasing suicidal ideation in older primary care patients by improving physician recognition and treatment of late-life depression (117). The treatment algorithm stresses the use of pharmacotherapy in primary care because of its pragmatic utility in primary care settings. Particular focus is on issues of tolerability, target doses of antidepressant medications, duration of antidepressant trials, and strategies for treating patients with partial response. A second published treatment algorithm was developed in a stage-wise manner, the Duke Somatic

TABLE 25-3

THE TREATMENT OF LATE-LIFE DEPRESSIONS: BEST PRACTICES FOR MULTIPLE CLINICAL PRESENTATIONS

For major depressive disorder	Combine antidepressant medication and psychotherapy (CBT, IPT, PST, DBT, BDT, supportive). Some patients may require only one modality. Match the therapy to patient and family preferences, and when possible, also utilize psychosocial interventions.
For more severe major depression including partial remission	Augment basic treatment, above, with other medications or therapies to boost response; may consider ECT.
For major depression with psychosis	Combine antidepressant and antipsychotic medications, or use ECT.
For dysthymia and persisting minor depression	Use psychotherapy; consider antidepressant medication if clinical syndrome warrants. Some patients may respond well to one modality alone or psychosocial support (i.e., family counseling, psychoeducation, peer-led support groups, visiting nurse services, or seniors day programs/seniors centers.). Be aware of CBASP, a psychotherapeutic approach to characterological chronic depressions.
For medical illness and disability-related depression	Optimize management of medical illness; consider potential for adverse interactions between antidepressants and medical diseases or drugs used in their treatment. Combine antidepressants with psychotherapeutic approaches tailored to patient preference and tolerance. Maximize psychosocial support interventions.
For bereavement-related depression	Treat as for major depression, above, if meets diagnostic criteria. Otherwise use psychotherapeutic or psychosocial interventions (i.e., IPT, PST, BDT, bereavement counseling, bereavement groups, self-help groups, and family counseling), adding medications if required.
For caregiving-related depression	Treat as for major depression, above, if meets diagnostic criteria. Use psychosocial interventions such as family counseling, psychoeducation, peer-led support groups, skills training, self-care, and physical and social changes to the home environment.
For depression in nursing home patients	Same as for specific clinical syndromes, above. For more severe or persistent depression not requiring ECT or hospitalization, combine antidepressants, psychotherapy, and psychosocial strategies. For less severe depression, stand-alone antidepressant, psychotherapy, or psychosocial interventions (such as recreational activities and/or peer-volunteer intervention groups supervised by trained staff) may be initiated. Group CBT and an activity-based psychosocial approach are the only nonpharmacological therapies studied for depression in this setting (for those without severe cognitive impairment). Daily bright light therapy can be a stand-alone or augmentation option where feasible.
Medication augmentation strategies	Use caution, clearly define treatment end-points before starting, and anticipate higher rates of neuropsychiatric, physical, and functional side effects. Older adults are vulnerable to pharmacodynamic and drug-disease/drug-drug interactions that may not be predictable on the basis of published research.

BDT, brief dynamic therapy; CBASP, cognitive behavioral analysis system of psychotherapy; CBT, cognitive behavioral therapy; DBT, dialectical behavior therapy; ECT, electroconvulsive therapy; IPT, interpersonal therapy; PST, problem-solving therapy.

Treatment Algorithm for Geriatric Depression. Five stages of care, based on treatment history and including recommendations for cases of partial response and nonresponse (118), can be easily adopted in both primary and specialty care. A third approach, Improving Mood-Promoting Access to Collaborative Treatment (IMPACT), developed by Unützer and colleagues (119), emphasizes the role of a trained depression clinical specialist, supervised by a psychiatrist, as a provider of primary mental health care in the general medical outpatient setting. This approach is significantly more effective than usual care for treatment of late-life major depression, dysthymia, or both (119), and a series of follow-up studies document its value in reducing pain associated with arthritis and improving a number of other functional outcomes.

Specific Treatment Modalities

The treatment of geriatric depression arguably requires the most comprehensive biopsychosocial approach of any of the psychiatric illnesses. Extensive ancillary information (e.g., laboratory tests, collateral information from a family member, neuroimaging data) may be required to make an accurate diagnosis and to arrive at an adequate treatment plan for individual patients. A combination of pharmacotherapy and psychotherapy (84), supplemented with psychosocial and environmental enrichments for more disabled patients, should be considered the best overall approach, and can be modified toward greater or lesser intensity as clinical conditions dictate.

Pharmacotherapy

Antidepressant medications improve depressive symptoms in approximately 50% to 60% of all elderly patients regardless of the class of medication prescribed, with placebo response rates of 30% to 40% (120) when depression is not psychotic in character or clinically severe enough to require hospitalization. However, in a recent study comparing citalopram versus placebo in the old-old (mean age 79.6 years), flexibly dosed medication was no more effective than placebo (121), and sites reported widely varying rates of response to active medication (18–82%) and to placebo (16–80%), with some sites reporting markedly better placebo than drug response rates. The reason for such wide site-to-site variation is unknown, but likely resulted from variations in the severity and clinical characteristics of patients enrolled (though all met the same diagnostic criteria), as well as in the psychotherapeutic qualities of study personnel.

It is important to note that age-related changes will influence pharmacokinetics and predispose the elderly to adverse side effects; of particular note is the risk of *serotonin syndrome*, particularly partial forms, when serotonergic agents have been prescribed. Chronic medical illness and medication use should also be carefully considered, because polypharmacy is frequent in elderly patients and can result in drug interactions that worsen side effects. Care should be taken with initial dosing titration schedules. Although end therapeutic doses do not greatly differ from those necessary in younger patients, it takes longer for drugs to reach steady-state levels in the aged, and plasma levels can be lower at any given dose (122,123).

Historically, the tricyclic antidepressants (TCAs) have been widely and successfully used to treat late-life depression, although as medications have evolved their popularity gave way to the use of selective serotonin-reuptake inhibitors (SSRIs) for ease of use, especially in nonspecialty settings. TCAs are more likely to cause adverse effects due to anticholinergic properties (e.g., mental dulling, confusion or forgetfulness, constipation, tachycardia, urinary retention, decreased vision.). The TCAs are sometimes the only drugs that prove effective for individual patients, however, and should not be dismissed. They are also considerably cheaper than newer agents for patients who must purchase medications out of pocket. Clinicians should remember that although TCAs are more difficult to use than drugs with lower side-effect profiles, many older patients will do well with carefully titrated doses, and many can be maintained with relatively infrequent contact. Low-dose TCAs have a place in the management of chronic pain in older adults, though similar cautions apply. Among the TCAs, nortriptyline and desipramine are less anticholinergic and sedating, and nortriptyline induces the least orthostatic hypotension at therapeutic plasma levels (124), with therapeutic concentrations similar to those needed for younger patients (125). TCAs should be used with caution in patients with underlying cardiac or prostatic disease, glaucoma, cognitive impairment, suicidality, and in those who are frail and at risk for falling.

The SSRIs have emerged as the drugs of choice for initial treatment of late-life depressions because of their more favorable side-effect profile, but they are not more effective than TCAs, as reported in a meta-analysis (126). In a larger, randomized, controlled comparative study of nortriptyline and paroxetine involving a mixed population of older depressed inpatients and outpatients, there was no significant difference in efficacy between these two agents, but the nortriptyline group was twice as likely to drop out because of side effects (127). Common adverse effects associated with SSRIs include gastrointestinal distress, agitation, akathisia, insomnia, pseudoparkinsonism, and sexual dysfunction. Hyponatremia due to inappropriate antidiuretic hormone secretion, a risk with many classes of central nervous system active drugs, is an important complication of treatment with SSRIs, occurring in up to 20% of older adults treated with SSRIs and venlafaxine (128). Hyponatremia risk and severity is increased in patients who are also taking diuretics. Serum sodium should be periodically monitored throughout therapy, as delayed onset has been reported.

Other psychotropic agents such as venlafaxine, mirtazapine, bupropion, the monoamine oxidase inhibitors (MAOIs), or psychostimulants may be considered as standalone agents or in part of an augmentation strategy. Allard and colleagues (129) reported the safety and efficacy of venlafaxine in one randomized, double-blind trial for geriatric depression. However, one study reported that venlafaxine was less well-tolerated in frail nursing home residents compared with sertraline (130). Two randomized controlled trials comparing mirtazapine with paroxetine and amitriptyline reported equal efficacy for geriatric depression (131,132). There is some evidence to support the efficacy of MAOIs in late-life depression (133), but they have not been systematically studied in the old-old. Clinicians have generally used the MAOIs as third-line agents for refractory geriatric depression because of fear of potentially fatal hypertensive crises from food and drug interactions. Psychostimulants appear to activate the anergic, apathetic patient who has become physically and psychologically overwhelmed by intense or prolonged physical illness (134), but it is unclear whether this represents a true antidepressant response. Psychostimulants are generally quite well-tolerated, but several adverse effects have been reported including insomnia, nausea, tremor, appetite changes, palpitations, tachycardia, blood pressure fluctuations, confusion, agitation, restlessness, and exacerbation of psychosis. A summary of recommended antidepressant agents in the elderly appears in Table 25-4.

Psychotherapy

Fifteen years ago, the National Institutes of Health consensus statement on the treatment of geriatric depression

TABLE 25-4

RECOMMENDED ANTIDEPRESSANTS FOR LATE-LIFE DEPRESSION[a]

Agent	Half-Life in Adults (hours)	Dosing Range (mg/day)
Tricyclic Antidepressants		
Desipramine	14.3–24.7	10–100
Nortriptyline	15–39	10–100
SSRIs		
Citalopram	33–37	20–60
Escitalopram	22–32	10–20
Fluoxetine	4–6 days	10–60
		90 (weekly dosing)
Paroxetine	15–22	10–60
		25–75 (CR)
Sertraline	22–32	25–200
SNRIs		
Duloxetine	11–16	30–90
Venlafaxine	3–7	37.5–375
Others		
Bupropion	12–30	100–450
Mirtazapine	25–40	7.5–45
Nefazodone	1.9–5.3	100–400

[a] This table is condensed from Table 25-3 in Appendix A. Please refer to Appendix A for additional details on each medication and a complete list of all antidepressant, psychostimulant, and other psychotropic medications that may be used in the treatment of major depression and related disorders.
CR, continuous release; SNRIs, selective serotonin/norepinephrine reuptake inhibitors; SSRIs, selective serotonin-reuptake inhibitors.

ranked psychotherapy third in a line of treatment options, behind antidepressant medication and ECT, indicating that there was insufficient evidence to recommend psychotherapy as a first-line treatment (135). There is a clear disparity in the number of geriatric psychotherapy and medication investigations, illustrated by a review of the literature between 1997 and 2002 revealing 700 medication trials versus only nine psychotherapy trials (136). There is insufficient research information on the efficacy of psychotherapy for treatment of late-life dysthymia and minor depression, early versus late-onset depression, depression with cognitive impairment, and in special patient populations such as the medically ill frail elderly and older adults from minority groups.

Of the intervention studies available, stand-alone cognitive-behavioral therapy (CBT) and problem-solving therapy (PST), and combined antidepressant medication with interpersonal therapy (IPT), has the largest base of evidence in support of efficacy for late-life major depression in ambulatory older adults (84,137). One study comparing CBT with desipramine in elderly patients with major depression suggested that CBT, and the combination of CBT with desipramine, was more efficacious than desipramine alone (138). For chronic, recurrent major depression in late life (i.e., early onset depression), IPT plus pill-placebo was found to be more effective than pill-placebo in preventing the recurrence of major depression (139). In the IMPACT trial, including patients aged 60 and older with major depression, dysthymia, or both, collaborative care management was significantly more effective

than usual care (119). In this study, the intervention group was assigned to depression care managers who were supervised by a psychiatrist and a primary care expert, and received education, care management, and support of antidepressant management by the patient's primary care clinician or brief PST for depression.

There is emerging evidence supporting the use of CBT and PST for late-life dysthymia (140,141), IPT and PST for late-life minor depression (141,142), and brief dynamic therapy (BDT) for geriatric major depression (143). Similarly, there is also early evidence to support PST in elderly patients suffering from major depression with executive dysfunction (144), and combined dialectical behavior therapy (DBT) group skills training with antidepressant medications in a mixed elderly population suffering early onset or late-onset geriatric major depression (145). The cognitive behavioral analysis system of psychotherapy (CBASP) is a therapeutic technique developed explicitly for treatment of chronic depressions characterized by entrenched, characterological belief in, and patterns of, ineffectiveness in achieving important personal goals (146). CBASP has not yet been studied in older depressed patients, but holds promise for some difficult-to-treat subgroups of neurotic patients whose chronic depressions frustrate their families' and doctors' attempts to help.

Research appears to indicate that matching therapies to patient and family preferences and concerns is an important factor in treatment outcome. For example, in one study of depressed caregivers of patients with dementia, long-term caregivers (more than 44 weeks) were more responsive to CBT than BDT, and those whose patients had more recently been diagnosed with dementia were more responsive to BDT than CBT (147). It was suggested that this difference may be due to the fact that individuals who have been caring for demented family members may be faced with a need to perform more structured problem solving around coping with the care recipients' cognitive decline, whereas newer caregivers may need to cope with and process affect around the diagnosis of dementia (136).

There is ample evidence now to direct clinicians toward the use of psychotherapy as a component of treatment when depression occurs in later life. What kind of psychotherapy, how much, how long, and how best to match patient characteristics to specific treatments are questions for which definitive answers are not yet available. Additional studies would be useful to help guide practice in choice of combination psychotherapy/pharmacotherapy paradigms, and to test the efficacy of psychotherapeutic intervention in the treatment of dysthymia, minor depression, depression with cognitive impairment, frail medically ill depressed elderly, and older adults from specific minority groups. The separation of depressions into EOD versus LOD groups has been useful in understanding clinical variations in older patients, but it is less clear that this distinction helps clinicians to plan and conduct treatment of individual patients. Lessons learned from research based on this dichotomy, however, are useful and sometimes crucial in patient management. The most important lessons relate to the need to incorporate comorbidities, including brain disease, functional disabilities, chronic medical conditions and their treatments, social support factors, and complex quality of life issues into developing individualized treatment plans. For research, depression treatment outcomes need to focus broadly on other functional domains (e.g., better management of illness, quality of life, activities of daily living), and not be limited to measuring decrements in depressive symptoms (136).

Obstacles to Using Psychotherapy in the Elderly
There are several important obstacles that may prevent the older depressed adult from benefiting from psychotherapy. Patient and family obstacles relate to lack of accurate information about the nature and value of psychotherapies, fears about disclosing highly personal information to a person (the therapist) who is not a close family member or friend, perceptions of the mental health field, and fears of being proclaimed mentally ill or crazy if they seek help for depression. Poor or absent insurance coverage, carved out mental health benefits, and inequities in coverage of treatment for psychiatric diagnoses relative to general medical conditions are important, and sometimes decisive, deterrents too. Socioeconomic status, culture, ethnicity, and education are other important contributing factors.

Obstacles also come from the provider side. There is a critical shortage of psychotherapists trained in modern, evidence-based techniques who are specifically interested in treatment of older adults. Many therapists are uncomfortable, or feel devalued, in attempting to work collaboratively with physicians, and some find it unfamiliar to work with families and others involved in helping the elderly. Attitudes about aging also come into play: as one psychoanalyst put it, "It was more fun to treat younger patients and [paraphrasing the original] to maintain my own fantasy of eternal youth" (148). Moreover, formal, in-depth training in geriatric psychotherapy is not widely available, and reimbursement can be difficult, reducing incentives for learning. This situation will likely not improve much unless new research initiatives and funding are made available.

Treatment Resistance

Although there is considerable debate about what constitutes true treatment-resistant geriatric depression, this designation should be reserved for persistently depressed individuals who do not respond to treatment despite receiving a reasonable level of care with both medications and psychotherapy, administered in adequate dose, for an adequate time, by a skilled clinician sensitive to the particular qualities and needs of the patient. For the treatment resistant geriatric patient, more intensive approaches are often required.

Other Somatic Therapies, Primarily Considered in Treatment Resistance
Pharmacological Augmentation
A considerable number of depressed elderly patients develop a chronic course of depression. Compared with the younger age group, depressed patients over the age of 70 appear to experience a more brittle course, characterized by a higher and more rapid rate of recurrence (122). Despite continued advances in antidepressant therapy, two major limitations exist in the elderly. The first is the delayed onset of therapeutic activity characteristic of all antidepressant medications, which is a particular problem in the elderly because of the necessity to start low and go slow. The second is the lack of full remission that the depressed elderly frequently experience, even among those who complete an adequate trial, with evidence showing that only about 50% of patients experience a full response (149). However, there are a limited number of controlled studies involving augmentation techniques in the elderly. One common augmenting technique with anecdotal evidence is to combine two or more antidepressants acting on different neurotransmitter systems or different aspects of neurotransmission. Careful monitoring is needed, because adding a second antidepressant is likely to increase side effects and cause adverse drug interactions in the elderly. Lithium may be used to augment TCAs or SSRIs, but studies have shown only a modest improvement in therapeutic response and a higher likelihood of neuropsychiatric side

effects in this patient population (60). Other augmenting strategies with at least anecdotal support include combining TCAs or SSRIs with mirtazapine, bupropion, venlafaxine, thyroid hormone, pindolol, atypical antipsychotics, psychostimulants, or dopamine-3 agonists such as pramipexole. One study reported the efficacy of augmenting antidepressants with the calcium-channel blocking medication nimodipine in the treatment of vascular depression (150). Despite the lack of full remission and delayed onset of antidepressant effects in older adults, the role of augmenting agents has been limited because this population is frequently unable to tolerate combination therapies due to side effects.

Electroconvulsive Therapy

Although approximately 50% to 60% of elderly patients improve clinically with antidepressant therapy (120), the efficacy of these agents may be lower in subgroups of depressed older adults. For example, WMH and lacunar infarcts seen on brain MRI, especially if large, predict less robust and durable antidepressant response (151), and other modalities frequently need to be considered. ECT is the most important of the nonpharmacological somatic treatments, and is the treatment of choice in certain older patients with severe depression due to poor tolerance of psychotropic medications, psychotic features, significant comorbid medical conditions, or marked disability associated with depression. Indeed, the use of ECT in major depression increases with age, with the elderly constituting a disproportionate share of those receiving this form of treatment (152). However, randomized trials investigating the use of ECT in depressed elderly patients are sparse in general and altogether lacking for depression associated with PD, CVD, and dementia (153), although case series document its successful use in small numbers of patients. Based on decades of safe and successful use, some well-designed small clinical trials, and published uncontrolled experience trials in patients failing other treatment, ECT remains an important treatment option in geriatric psychiatry. Published protocols are available for selecting appropriate patients and for administering and monitoring treatment of older adults (153). For more information, see the chapter on ECT in this textbook.

Repetitive Transcranial Magnetic Stimulation

Repetitive transcranial magnetic stimulation (rTMS) is a newer technology that delivers magnetic pulses through the skull, inducing an electrical current in underlying brain tissue, which in turn depolarizes neurons. The promise of this technique for treating depression lies in its noninvasive nature, avoidance of sedation and anesthesia, and its capacity to stimulate precise areas of the brain. Many investigators are currently studying rTMS as a potential antidepressant treatment. However, few elderly subjects have been studied, with limited data indicating minimal side effects but only modest improvements in mood (154). Cerebral atrophy and increased distance between the skull

and underlying brain tissue that can be present in older patients probably changes the stimulus requirements for effective rTMS treatment of elderly subjects. Currently, the role of rTMS in the elderly remains unclear; in its current form, it cannot be considered an alternative to ECT and has not been found superior to drug therapies.

Vagus Nerve Stimulation

This novel treatment uses an implanted, programmable stimulator that is wrapped around the vagus nerve in the neck to deliver electrical pulses at preset frequency and intensity. No randomized trials have been published. The largest, best-designed open trial thus far included 60 patients, and the oldest completer was 63 years old (155). Results indicated that severe treatment resistance was not overcome by this approach, but that mildly to moderately resistant patients might respond. Side effects include headache, nausea, and vocal hoarseness.

Deep Brain Stimulation

After the introduction of deep brain stimulation (DBS) for treatment of drug-resistant PD, extension of the idea to treatment-resistant depression seemed natural. In the only depression trial of DBS thus far (156), bilateral wires, each ending in four separate stimulus electrodes, were inserted into Brodmann area 25, the subgenual white matter, in six patients aged 37 to 59 with treatment-resistant major depression (all had failed at least four classes of antidepressants, each prescribed at maximum tolerable doses; several augmentation strategies; CBT; and, in five cases, ECT). Four patients were in full remission at 6 months of chronic stimulation. Though no elderly people were included in this first trial, it is described here to familiarize clinicians with the potential of this or modified forms of DBS to treat selected older patients. The only known contraindication is the presence of another electrical stimulating device (e.g., a cardiac pacemaker) or use of diathermy. Readers should also be aware of an emerging literature on DBS for disabling, refractory obsessive-compulsive disorder, which can afflict older patients, especially those vulnerable to psychotic depression.

SPECIAL ISSUES: DEPRESSION ASSOCIATED WITH DIFFICULT LIFE CONDITIONS

Medical Illness

The reasons for association of chronic medical illness with depression likely include a combination of biological mechanisms that have not been fully elucidated, as well as psychological and social predisposing, precipitating, and perpetuating factors. Medical illness can lead to profound alterations in the way one views one's self, personal agency, mortality, future, relationships, and purpose. While it is necessary to identify and treat associated medical conditions, major depressions generally do not remit until adequate psychiatric treatment is added. For instance, depression in a hypothyroid elderly patient rarely responds to thyroid supplementation alone. Conversely, an antidepressant trial is often ineffective before hypothyroidism is corrected (17). Antidepressant medications are often efficacious in elderly patients with depression suffering from common comorbid medical disorders such as stroke, PD, AD, chronic obstructive pulmonary disease, arthritis, ischemic heart disease, and cancer (157,158). There is also some evidence to support the use of psychostimulant medications, such as methylphenidate, for the short-term treatment of depressive symptoms in medically ill elderly patients (159,160). Frequently, a combination of antidepressant medications and well-focused psychotherapy, concurrent with appropriate medical care, provides optimal treatment of depression in the context of significant medical illness. ECT also remains a treatment option for medical illness-related depression, with few contraindications.

Bereavement

Depression precipitated by grief over loss of a spouse or another close relationship can remit spontaneously as the bereaved person makes the necessary emotional and life adjustments. Certainly, all bereaved older adults should be supported with compassionate psychotherapeutic conversations and understanding, but by no means all require treatment by a psychiatrist. Major depressive episodes persisting after the period of acute grief, however, can require antidepressants, psychotherapy, or a combination of both (84). Self-help groups, counseling, individual dynamic psychotherapy, and group therapy can help the grieving older adult, but have not yet been rigorously studied.

Caregiving

A wide variety of services and programs have been developed to assist caregivers, and several have been shown to alleviate caregiving burden and sometimes to reduce associated depressive symptoms. These interventions range from simple peer-led support groups to complex, multifaceted programs involving counseling, skills training, respite, self-care, and physical and social changes to the home environment (42). Psychoeducational interventions assist caregivers to effectively manage problem behaviors and reduce depression (161). The nature and degree of assistance needed depends most importantly on caregiver-related factors, but also on the particular stage of the care recipient's illness, cumulative stressor burden, and caregiver resources (e.g., social support from family and friends, financial flexibility). All caregivers can benefit from enhanced knowledge about the care recipient's illness and available supportive resources, and many benefit from training in general problem-solving skills, including skills that target the management of care recipient

behaviors. Individual and family counseling sessions and the availability of skilled counselors to assist with crises may also reduce depressive symptoms in caregivers (162). The efficacy of individual CBT and BDT in treating caregiver depression has been described earlier. Helping caregivers find their way to the level of help they can most benefit from remains a significant problem in providing optimal services to this population.

Living in Long-Term Care

A wide range of interventions, many outside the scope of strict mental health practice, has been evaluated to treat various depressive mood states in nursing home patients, among them a peer-volunteer intervention supervised by a social worker (163), self-selected pleasurable activities (164), daily bright light (10,000 lux) therapy (165), and daily hour-long outdoor rides in a wheelchair pulled by a staff member on a bicycle (166). The value of these interventions speaks to the relative impoverishment of meaningful, enjoyable activities and social engagement long cited as deficits in institutional life. Formal psychotherapies have not been well explored in this setting, but one study found a significant reduction in depressive symptoms for recipients of group cognitive therapy compared with a marginal decrease in recipients of music therapy (167), and the proven efficacy of psychotherapies for some geriatric depressions in other clinical settings supports a role for psychotherapeutic approaches in long-term care.

Antidepressants are widely used in nursing home practice, most often for depressive symptoms and disorders (SSRIs) but also as part of chronic pain management (most often low-dose TCAs) (168). Clinically relevant outcome studies are sparse, however, and only a few formal studies have evaluated efficacy and tolerability (three randomized, double-blind, placebo-controlled studies and three open-label trials), and with mixed results depending on the agent used and clinical patient factors (169–174). The psychiatric, medical, and cognitive heterogeneity and multiple etiologies of depression in the nursing home population continues to impede finding and effectively treating the depressed patient who can benefit from psychosocial intervention, formal psychotherapy, and/or medications, and it is unlikely that randomized controlled trials will resolve these issues in the near future. Nevertheless, clinical work with depressed nursing home patients can be a profoundly gratifying aspect of geropsychiatric practice, especially when a series of trial and error approaches finally achieves the patient's recovery.

COURSE AND PROGNOSIS

Left untreated, late-life major depression tends to remit spontaneously after 12 to 48 months, but patients with first-episode depression with onset after age 60 have a 70% chance of recurrence within 2 years (175). When recognized and treated, older patients are less likely to receive newer antidepressants than younger patients, and almost half of those on TCAs receive therapeutically inadequate doses (176). Compared with mid-life patients, elderly patients receiving adequate antidepressant treatment tend to have slower resolution of depressive symptoms and a higher relapse rate during continuation therapy, with a median time to remission of 12 weeks (122). Data from naturalistic studies have identified several predictors of relapse and recurrence (123):

- Prior history of frequent episodes.
- High pretreatment severity of depression and anxiety
- Supervening medical illness
- History of myocardial infarction or vascular disease
- Cognitive impairment, particularly frontal lobe dysfunction

Recurrent depressive illness, high severity of depression, psychotic symptoms, long previous episodes, medical illness, and WMH predict a chronic course, with chronicity rates amongst depressed elderly patients ranging from 7% to 40% (17).

Longitudinal studies of elderly people who are cognitively impaired during an episode of depression find that while many improve to normal cognitive functioning with remission, some of these still progress to irreversible dementia over time (71). In epidemiological studies, depressive symptoms often precede the clinical emergence of dementia, possibly reflecting decreased cognitive reserve capacity unmasked by depression (40) or a prodromal phase of dementia (73).

PSYCHOSOCIAL AND CULTURAL ISSUES

Psychosocial factors contribute significantly to the risk of developing late-life depression. Financial problems and negative life events, including the death of a family member, are associated with increased depressive symptoms (177). Involuntary relocation may be a risk factor for depression, but a sense of control, predictability, and quality of the new environment all appear to moderate outcomes (178). The effects of stress on depression may be modified by relationships, including being married and/or other social support (23). Unexpected, undesirable, and off-schedule (non-normative) life events are the most stressful (40) in promoting depression, and availability of a confidante is the single most important protective factor (179). Loneliness is a neglected predisposing factor for depression in older adults (180).

Ethnicity and cultural factors play an important role in the etiology, expression, and treatment of geriatric depression. For example, chronic health conditions are associated with higher levels of expressed depressive symptoms in Hispanic elders. Korean and Chinese elderly tend to somatize their psychological distress, and Mexican immigrants under high acculturative stress have higher levels of depres-

sion and suicidal ideation than others (40). Depressive disorders are relatively underdiagnosed among African Americans, who are more likely to express thoughts of death, but who are not more likely to report sadness, somatic, or vegetative symptoms (13). Among older immigrant populations, inability to speak the language of the adopted country, few opportunities for acculturation, transportation, friends, social support, and the loss of traditional roles can lead to loneliness and depression, and family relationships can be distorted by the elders' need to rely on adult children or even grandchildren to navigate the mainstream culture. Additionally, difficulties accessing health care and health insurance, sometimes a preference for traditional forms of treatment, and the stigma associated with mental and emotional symptoms (including the view that depression brings shame and dishonor to the family) can all be major deterrents to seeking help (40). For more information, refer to the chapter on cultural issues in this textbook.

LEGAL AND ETHICAL ISSUES

The major legal and ethical issues pertinent to late-life depressions arise when severely ill patients lose decisional capacity or refuse potentially effective treatment. Loss of decisional capacity most often arises when depression is combined with dementia, but can occur in patients with severe psychotic depressions who have lost all perspective on their illness and realistic options for recovery. Treatment refusal when not all effective modalities have been tried is a particularly difficult problem, and is most often also associated with psychotic depression, but can occur in patients with very chronic entrenched nonpsychotic depressions with long-lasting pessimism or personality disorder. When patients are suicidal, or are gravely disabled by their illness (have stopped eating, are malnourished or severely dehydrated, are placing themselves in hazardous or inadequately supported environments, or are being abused or neglected by others), involuntary treatment and adult protection laws can be invoked to allow transfer of the patient to a protective, therapeutic environment. Compelling a specific treatment modality (most often pertinent to ECT) is more problematic, posing legal ambiguities and undesirable delays. Clinicians need to know the laws that govern psychiatric treatment in their states, and must be prepared to initiate appropriate actions when dealing with these very difficult situations. Additional information can be found in the chapters on forensic and ethical issues in this textbook.

REFERENCES

1. Callahan CM, Hui SL, Nienaber NA, Musick BS, Tierney WM. Longitudinal study of depression and health services use among elderly primary care patients. *J Am Geriatr Soc.* 1994;42:833–838.

2. Luber MP, Hollenberg JP, Williams-Russo PG. Diagnosis, treatment, comorbidity, and resource utilization of depressed patients in a general medical practice. *Int J Psychiatry Med.* 2000;30:1–13.
3. Luber MP, Meyers BS, Williams-Russo PG, et al. Depression and service utilization in elderly primary care patients. *Am J Geriatr Psychiatry.* 2001;9:169–176.
4. Unützer J, Patrick DL, Simon G, et al. Depressive symptoms and the cost of health services in HMO patients aged 65 years and older. *JAMA.* 277(20):1618–1623.
5. Alexopoulos GS, Vrontou C, Kakuma T, et al. Disability in geriatric depression. *Am J Psychiatry.* 1996;153(7):877–885.
6. Unützer J, Patrick DL, Diehr P, Simon G, Grembowski D, Katon W. Quality adjusted life years in older adults with depressive symptoms and chronic medical disorders. *Int Psychogeriatr.* 2000;12(1):15–33.
7. Conwell Y, Duberstein PR, Cox C, Hermann JH, Forbes NT, Caine ED. Relationships of age and axis I diagnoses of victims of completed suicide: a psychological autopsy study. *Am J Psychiatry.* 1996;153:1001–1008.
8. Penninx BW, Geerlings SW, Deeg DJ, van Eijk JT, van Tilburg W, Beekman AT. Minor and major depression and the risk of death in older persons. *Arch Gen Psychiatry.* 1999;56(10):889–895.
9. Bruce ML, Leaf P, Rozal G, Florio L, Hoff RA. Psychiatry status and 9-year mortality data in the New Haven Epidemiologic Catchment Area Study. *Am J Psychiatry.* 1994;51(5):716–721.
10. Mulsant BH, Ganguli M. Epidemiology and diagnosis of depression in late-life. *J Clin Psychiatry.* 1999;60(Suppl 20):9–15.
11. American Psychiatric Association. *Diagnostic and Statistical Manual of Mental Disorders.* 4th Ed. Text Revision. Washington, DC: American Psychiatric Association; 2000.
12. Alexopoulos GS, Borson S, Cuthbert BN, et al. Assessment of late life depression. *Biol Psychiatry.* 2002;52:164–174.
13. Gallo JJ, Rabins PV. Depression without sadness: alternative presentations of depression in late life. *Am Fam Physician.* 1999;60:820–826.
14. Cooper-Patrick L, Crum RM, Ford DE. Identifying suicidal ideation in general medical patients. *JAMA.* 1994;272(22):1757–1762.
15. Bruce ML, Seeman TE, Merrill SS, Blazer DG. The impact of depressive symptomatology on physical disability: MacArthur Studies of Successful Aging. *Am J Public Health.* 1994;84(11):1796–1799.
16. Wells KB, Stewart A, Hays RD, et al. The functioning and well-being of depressed patients: results from the Medical Outcomes Study. *JAMA.* 1989;262(7):914–919.
17. Alexopoulos GS. Mood disorders. In: Sadock BJ, Sadock VA, eds. *Kaplan & Sadock's Comprehensive Textbook of Psychiatry.* 7th Ed. Philadelphia: Lippincott Williams & Wilkins; 2000;3060–3068.
18. Kramer M, German PS, Anthony JC, Van Korff M, Skinner EA. Patterns of mental disorders among the elderly residents of Eastern Baltimore. *J Am Geriatric Soc.* 1985;33:236–245.
19. Koenig HG, Blazer DG. Epidemiology of geriatric affective disorders. *Clin Geriatr Med.* 1992;8(2):235–251.
20. Henderson AS, Korten AE, Jorm AF, Christensen H, Mackinnon AJ, Scott LR. Are nursing homes depressing? *Lancet.* 1994;344(8929):1091.
21. Snowdon J. Is depression more prevalent in old age? *Aust NZ J Psychiatry.* 2001;35:782–787.
22. Prince MJ, Harwood RH, Thomas A, Mann AH. A prospective population-based cohort study of the effects of disablement and social milieu on the onset and maintenance of late-life depression. The Gospel Oak Project VII. *Psychol Med.* 1998;28:337–350.
23. Schoevers RA, Beekman AT, Deeg DJ, Geerlings MI, Jonker C, Van Tilburg W. Risk factors for depression in later life: results of a prospective community based study (AMSTEL). *J Affect Disord.* 2000;59(2):127–137.
24. Alexopoulos GS. Geriatric depression in primary care. *Int J Geriatr Psychiatry.* 1996;11:397–400.
25. Blazer DG. Epidemiology of late life-depression. In: Schneider LS, Reynolds CF III, Lebowitz BD, et al., eds. *Diagnosis and Treatment of Depression in Late Life: Results of the NIH Consensus Development Conference.* Washington: American Psychiatric Press; 1994;9–19.
26. Parmelee PA, Katz IR, Lawton MP. Depression among institutionalized aged: assessment and prevalence estimation. *J Gerontol.* 1989;44(1):M22–M29.
27. Evans DL. Depression in the medical setting: biopsychological interactions and treatment considerations. *J Clin Psychiatry.* 1999;60(Suppl 4):40–55.
28. Astrom M, Adolfsson R, Asplund K. Major depression in stroke patients. A 3-year longitudinal study. *Stroke.* 1993;24:976–982.
29. Tiller JW. Post-stroke depression. *Psychopharmacology.* 1992;106:S130–S133.
30. Mega MS, Cummings JL, Fiorello T, Gornbein J. The spectrum of behavioral changes in Alzheimer's disease. *Neurology.* 1996;46(1):130–135.
31. Cumming JL. Depression and Parkinson's disease: a review. *Am J Psychiatry.* 1992;149:443–454.
32. Lespérance F, Frasure-Smith N, Talajic M. Major depression before and after myocardial infarction: its nature and consequences. *Psychosom Med.* 1996;58(2):99–110.
33. Prince MJ, Bird AS, Blizard RA, Mann AH. Is the cognitive function of older patients affected by antihypertensive treatment? Results from 54 months of the Medical Research Council's trial of hypertension in older adults. *BMJ.* 1996;312(7034):801–805.
34. Bruce ML. Psychosocial risk factors for depressive disorders in late life. *Biol Psychiatry.* 2002;52:175–184.
35. Ormel J, Oldehinkel AJ, Brilman EI. The interplay and etiological continuity of neuroticism, difficulties, and life events in the etiology of major and subsyndromal, first and recurrent depressive episodes in later life. *Am J Psychiatry.* 2001;158:885–891.
36. Zisook S, Paulus M, Shuchter SR, Judd LL. The many faces of depression following spousal bereavement. *J Affect Disord.* 1997;45(1–2):85–94.
37. Schaefer C, Quesenberry CP, Dui S. Mortality following conjugal bereavement and the effects of a shared environment. *Am J Epidemiol.* 1996;141(12):1142–1152.
38. Bruce ML, Kim KM, Leaf PJ, Jacobs S. Depressive episodes and dysphoria resulting from conjugal bereavement in a prospective community sample. *Am J Psychiatry.* 1990;147:608–611.
39. Turvey CL, Carney C, Arndt S, Wallace RB, Herzog R. Conjugal loss and syndromal depression in a sample of elders aged 70 years and over. *Am J Psychiatry.* 1999;156:1596–1601.
40. Alexopoulos GS, Buckwalter K, Olin J, Martinez R, Wainscott C, Krishnan KR. Comorbidity of late-life depression: an opportunity for research in mechanisms and treatment. *Biol Psychiatry.* 2002;52:543–558.
41. Yee JL, Schulz R. Gender differences in psychiatric morbidity among family caregivers: a review and analysis. *Gerontologist.* 2000;40(2):147–164.
42. Connell CM, Janevic MR, Gallant MP. The costs of caregiving: impact of dementia on family caregivers. *J Geriatr Psychiatry Neurol.* 2001;14(4):179–188.
43. Kim E, Rovner B. Epidemiology of psychiatric disturbance in nursing homes. *Psychiatr Ann.* 1995;25:409–412.
44. Streim JE, Rovner BW, Katz IR. Psychiatric aspects of nursing home care. In: Sadavoy J, Lazarus LW, Jarvik LF, et al., eds. *Comprehensive Review of Geriatric Psychiatry.* Washington: American Psychiatric Press; 1996:907–936.
45. Katz IR, Parmelee PA. Depression in the residential care elderly. In: Schneider LS, Reynolds CF III, Lebowitz BD, et al., eds. *Diagnosis and Treatment of Depression in Late Life: Results of the NIH Consensus Development Conference.* Washington: American Psychiatric Press; 1993:437–461.
46. Katz IR, Parmelee PA. Depression in the residential care elderly, an overview. In: Rubinstein RL, Lawton MO, eds. *Shades of Gray: Depression Among the Frail Elderly.* New York: Springer; 1997:1–25.
47. McIntosh JL. Suicide prevention in the elderly (age 65–99). *Suicide Life Threat Behav.* 1995;25(1):180–192.
48. Centers for Disease Control and Prevention. Suicide among older persons—United States, 1980–1992. *MMWR Morb Mortal Wkly Rep.* 1996;45:3–6.
49. Conwell Y, Olsen K, Caine ED, Flannery C. Suicide in later life: psychological autopsy findings. *Int Psychogeriatr.* 1991;3:59–66.
50. Alexopoulos GS, Katz IR, Carpenter D, Docherty JP. The expert consensus guideline series: pharmacotherapy of depressive disorders in older patients. *Postgrad Med.* 2001;(Special issue):1–82.
51. Regier DA, Farmer ME, Rae DS, et al. One-month prevalence of mental disorders in the United States and sociodemographic

characteristics: The Epidemiologic Catchment Area study. *Acta Psychiatr Scand.* 1993;88(1):35–47.

52. McGivney SA, Mulvihill M, Taylor B. Validating the GDS depression screen in the nursing home. *J Am Geriatr Soc.* 1994;42(5):490–492.

53. Teresi J, Abrams R, Holmes D, Ramirez M, Eimicke J. Prevalence of depression and depression recognition in nursing homes. *Soc Psychiatry Psychiatr Epidemiol.* 2001;36:613–620.

54. Snowden M, Sato K, Roy-Byrne P. Assessment and treatment of nursing home residents with depression or behavioral symptoms associated with dementia: a review of the literature. *J Am Geriatr Soc.* 2003;51(9):1305–1317.

55. Borson S, Unutzer J. Psychiatric disorders of late life. In: Sadock BJ, Sadock VA, eds. *Kaplan & Sadock's Comprehensive Textbook of Psychiatry.* 7th Ed. Philadelphia: Lippincott Williams & Wilkins; 2000:3045–3053.

56. Devanand DP. Comorbid psychiatric disorders in late life depression. *Biol Psychiatry.* 2002;51:236–242.

57. Manela M, Katona C, Livengston G. How common are the anxiety disorders in old age? *Int J Geriatr Psychiatry.* 1996;11:65–70.

58. Devanand DP, Turret N, Moody BJ, et al. Personality disorders in elderly patients with dysthymic disorder. *Am J Geriatric Psychiatry.* 2000;8:188–195.

59. Kunik ME, Mulsant BH, Rifai AH, Sweet RA, Pasternak R, Zubenko GS. Diagnostic rate of comorbid personality disorder in elderly psychiatric inpatients. *Am J Psychiatry.* 1994;151:603–605.

60. Alexopoulos GS, Salzman C. Treatment of depression with heterocyclic antidepressants, monoamine oxidase inhibitors, and psychomotor stimulants. In Salzman C, ed. *Clinical Geriatric Psychopharmacology.* 3rd Ed. Baltimore: Williams & Wilkens; 1998;184–244.

61. Lavretsky H, Kumar A. Clinically significant non-major depression: old concepts, new insights. *Am J Geriatric Psychiatry.* 2002;10(3):239–255.

62. Salzman C. Mood Disorders. In: Coffey CE, Cummings JL, eds. *The American Psychiatric Press Textbook of Geriatric Psychiatry.* 2nd Ed. Washington: American Psychiatric Press, Inc.; 2000:313–328.

63. Blazer DG. Depression in the elderly: myths and misconceptions. *Psychiatr Clin North Am.* 1997;20:111–119.

64. Baldwin RC, Tomenson B. Depression in later life: a comparison of symptoms and risk factors in early and late onset cases. *Br J Psychiatry.* 1995;167:649–652.

65. Coffey CE. Brain morphology in primary mood disorders: implications for ECT. *Psychiatr Ann.* 1996;26:713–716.

66. Coffey CE, Figiel GS, Djang WT, Weiner RD. Subcortical hyperintensity on magnetic resonance imaging: a comparison of normal and depressed elderly subjects. *Am J Psychiatry.* 1990;147:187–189.

67. Katz IR, Miller D, Oslin D. Diagnosis of late-life depression. In: Salzman C. *Clinical Geriatric Psychopharmacology.* 3rd Ed. Baltimore: Williams & Wilkins; 1998:153–183.

68. Nelson JC. Treatment of major depression in the elderly. In: Nelson JC, ed. *Geriatric Psychopharmacology.* New York: Marcel Dekker; 1998:61–98.

69. Lyness JM, Pearson JL, Lebowitz BD, Kupfer DJ. Age of onset of late-life depression. *Am J Geriatr Psychiatry.* 1994;2:4–8.

70. Heun R, Kocker M, Papassotiropoulos A. Distinction of early- and late-onset depression in the elderly by their lifetime symptomatology. *Int J Geriatr Psychiatry.* 2000;15:1138–1142.

71. Alexopoulos GS, Meyers BS, Young RC, Mattis S, Kakuma T. The course of geriatric depression with "reversible dementia": a controlled study. *Am J Psychiatry.* 1993;150:1693–1699.

72. Chen P, Ganguli M, Mulsant B, DeKosky S. The temporal relationship between depressive symptoms and dementia: a community-based prospective study. *Arch Gen Psychiatry.* 1999;56:261–266.

73. Geerlings MI, Schoevers RA, Beekman AT, et al. Depression and risk of cognitive decline and Alzheimer's disease: results of two community-based studies in the Netherlands. *Br J Psychiatry.* 2000;176:568–575.

74. Krishnan KR, Hays JC, Blazer DG. MRI-defined vascular depression. *Am J Psychiatry.* 1997;154:497–500.

75. Alexopoulos GS, Meyers BS, Young RC, et al. Executive dysfunction and long-term outcome of geriatric depression. *Arch Gen Psychiatry.* 2000;57(3):285–290.

76. Alexopoulos GS. The depression-executive dysfunction syndrome of late life: a specific target of D3 agonists? *Am J Geriatr Psychiatry.* 2001;9(1):22–29.

77. Tateno A, Kimura M, Robinson RG. Phenomenological characteristics of poststroke depression. *Am J Geriatr Psychiatry.* 2002;10(5):575–582.

78. Alexopoulos GS, Abrams RC. Depression in Alzheimer's disease. *Psychiatr Clin North Am.* 1991;14(2):327–340.

79. Flint AJ. The complexity and challenge of non-major depression in late life. *Am J Geriatric Psychiatry.* 2002;10(3):229–232.

80. Broadhead WE, Blazer DG, George LK, Tse CK. Depression, disability days, and days from work in a prospective epidemiological survey. *JAMA.* 1990;264:2524–2528.

81. Lyness JM, Caine ED, King DA, Conwell Y, Duberstein PR, Cox C. Depressive disorders and symptoms in older primary care patients: one-year outcomes. *Am J Geriatric Psychiatry.* 2002;10(3):275–282.

82. Devanand DP, Nobler MS, Singer T, et al. Is dysthymia a different disorder in the elderly? *Am J Psychiatry.* 1994;53:175–182.

83. Charney DS, Reynolds CF III, Lewis L, et al. Depression and bipolar support alliance consensus statement on the unmet needs in diagnosis and treatment of mood disorders in late life. *Arch Gen Psychiatry.* 2003;60:664–672.

84. Reynolds CF III, Miller MD, Pasternak RE, et al. Treatment of bereavement-related major depressive episodes in late-life: a controlled study of acute and continuation treatment with nortriptyline and interpersonal psychotherapy. *Am J Psychiatry.* 1999;156(2):202–208.

85. Gallant MP, Connell CM. Predictors of decreased self-care among spouse caregivers of older adults with dementing illness. *J Aging Health.* 1997;9:373–395.

86. Gallagher D, Rose J, Rivera P, Lovett S, Thompson LW. Prevalence of depression in family caregivers. *Gerontologist.* 1989;29:449–456.

87. Dura JR, Stukenberg KW, Kiecolt-Glaser JK. Anxiety and depressive disorders in adult children caring for demented parents. *Psychol Aging.* 1991;6:467–473.

88. Meeks S, Murrell SA, Mehl RC. Longitudinal relationship between depressive symptoms and health in normal older and middle-aged adults. *Psychol Aging.* 2000;15:100–109.

89. Arfken CL, Lichtenberg PA, Tancer ME. Cognitive impairment and depression predict mortality in medically ill older adults. *J Gerontol A Biol Sci Med Sci.* 1999;54:152–156.

90. Schulberg HC, Mulsant BH, Schulz R, Rollman BL, Houck PR, Reynolds CF III. Characteristics and course of major depression in older primary care patients. *Int J Psychiatry Med.* 1998;28(4):421–436.

91. Armstrong SC, Cozza KL, Watanabe KS. The misdiagnosis of delirium. *Psychosomatics.* 1997;38:433–439.

92. Cohen-Cole SA, Stoudemire A. Major depression and physical illness. *Psychiatr Clin North Am.* 1987;10:1–17.

93. Kathol RG, Mutgi A, Williams J, Clamon G, Nayes R Jr. Diagnosis of major depression in cancer patients according to four sets of criteria. *Am J Psychiatry.* 1990;147:1021–1024.

94. Cassem EH. Depression and anxiety secondary to medical illness. *Psychiatr Clin North Am.* 1990;13:597–612.

95. Callahan CM, Hendrie HC, Tierney WM. The recognition and treatment of late-life depression: a view from primary care. *Int J Psychiatry Med.* 1996;26(2):155–171.

96. Awad IA, Johnson PC, Spetzler RF, Hodak JA. Incidental subcortical lesions identified on magnetic resonance imaging in the elderly, II: postmortem pathological correlations. *Stroke.* 1986;17:1090–1097.

97. O'Brien J, Desmond P, Ames D, Schweitzer I, Harrigan S, Tress B. A magnetic resonance imaging study of white matter lesions in depression and Alzheimer's disease. *Br J Psychiatry.* 1996;168:477–485.

98. Coffey CE, Wilkinson WE, Weiner RD, et al. Quantitative cerebral anatomy in depression. A controlled magnetic resonance imaging study. *Arch Gen Psychiatry.* 1993;50:7–16.

99. Firbank MJ, Lloyd AJ, Ferrier N, O'Brien JT. A volumetric study of MRI signal hyperintensities in late-life depression. *Am J Geriatr Psychiatry.* 2004;12(6):606–612.

100. de Groot JC, de Leeuw F-E, Oudkerk M, Hofman A, Jolles J, Breteler MM. Cerebral white matter lesions and depressive

symptoms in elderly adults. *Arch Gen Psychiatry*. 2000;57:
1071–1076.

101. Figiel GS, Krishnan KR, Doraiswamy PM, Rao VP, Nemeroff CB, Boyko OB. Subcortical hyperintensities on brain magnetic resonance imaging: a comparison between late age onset and early onset elderly depressed subjects. *Neurobiol Aging*. 1991;12: 245–247.

102. Miller MD, Lenze EJ, Dew MA, et al. Effect of cerebrovascular risk factors on depression treatment outcome in later life. *Am J Geriatr Psychiatry*. 2002;10(5):592–598.

103. Thomas AJ, Perry R, Barber R, Kalaria RN, O'Brien JT. Pathologies and pathological mechanisms for white matter hyperintensities in depression. *Ann NY Acad Sci*. 2002;977:333–339.

104. Hamada T, Murata T, Omori M, et al. Abnormal nocturnal blood pressure fall in senile-onset depression with subcortical silent cerebral infarction. *Neuropsychobiology*. 2003;47(4):187–191.

105. Rabins PV, Pearlson GD, Aylward E, Kumar AJ, Dowell K. Cortical magnetic resonance imaging changes in elderly patients with major depression. *Am J Psychiatry*. 1991;148:617.

106. Kumar A, Miller D, Ewbank D, et al. Quantitative anatomic measures and comorbid medical illness in late-life major depression. *Am J Geriatr Psychiatry*. 1997;5(1):15–25.

107. Kumar A, Jin Z, Bilder W, Udupa J, Gottlieb G. Late-onset minor and major depression: early evidence for common neuroanatomical substrates detected by using MRI. *Proc Nat Acad Sci USA*. 1998;95:7654–7658.

108. Lai T, Payne ME, Byrum CE, Steffens DC, Krishnan KR. Reduction of orbital frontal cortex volume in geriatric depression. *Biol Psychiatry*. 2000;15:971–975.

109. Kumar A, Bilker W, Lavretsky H, Gottlieb G. Volumetric asymmetries in late-onset mood disorders: an attenuation of frontal asymmetry with depression severity. *Psych Res*. 2000;100: 41–47.

110. Almeida OP, Burton EJ, Ferrier N, McKeith IG, O'Brien JT. Depression with late onset is associated with right frontal lobe atrophy. *Psychol Med*. 2003;33:675–681.

111. Lesser IM, Mena I, Boone KB, Miller BL, Mehringer CM, Wohl M. Reduction of cerebral blood flow in older depressed patients. *Arch Gen Psychiatry*. 1994;51(9):677–686.

112. de Asis JM, Stern E, Alexopoulos GS, et al. Hippocampal and anterior cingulate activation deficits in patients with geriatric depression. *Am J Psychiatry*. 2001;158(8):1321–1323.

113. Navarro V, Gasto C, Lomena F, Mateos JJ, Marcos T. Frontal cerebral perfusion dysfunction in elderly late-onset major depression assessed by 99MTC-HMPAO SPECT. *Neuroimage*. 2001;14 (1 Pt 1):202–205.

114. Fuster JM. Synopsis of function and dysfunction of the frontal lobe. *Acta Psychiatr Scand Suppl*. 1999;395:51–57.

115. Mayberg HS. Modulating dysfunctional limbic-cortical circuits in depression: towards development of brain-based algorithms for diagnosis and optimized treatment. *Br Med Bulletin*. 2003;65: 193–207.

116. Mayberg HS. Limbic-cortical dysregulation: a proposed model of depression. *J Neuropsych Clin Neurosci*. 1997;9:471–481.

117. Mulsant BH, Alexopoulos GS, Reynolds CF III, et al. Pharmacological treatment of depression in older primary care patients: the PROSPECT algorithm. *Int J Geriatr Psychiatry*. 2001;16:585–592.

118. Steffens DC, McQuoid DR, Krishnan KR. The Duke Somatic Treatment Algorithm For Geriatric Depression (STAGED) approach. *Psychopharm Bull*. 2002;36(2):58–68.

119. Unützer J, Katon W, Callahan CM, et al. Collaborative care management of late-life depression in the primary care setting. a randomized controlled trial. *JAMA*. 2002;288(22):2836–2845.

120. Schneider LS, Olin JT. Efficacy of acute treatment for geriatric depression. *Int Psychogeriatr*. 1995;7(Suppl):7–25.

121. Roose SP, Sackeim HA, Krishnan KR, et al. Antidepressant pharmacotherapy in the treatment of depression in the very old: a randomized, placebo-controlled trial. *Am J Psychiatry*. 2004;161 (11):2050–2059.

122. Reynolds CF III, Frank E, Kupfer DJ, et al. Treatment outcome in recurrent major depression: a post hoc comparison of elderly ("young old") and midlife patients. *Am J Psychiatry*. 1996;153 (10):1288–1292.

123. Reynolds CF III, Kupfer DJ. Depression and aging: a look to the future. *Psychiatr Serv*. 1999;50(9):1167–1172.

124. Roose SP, Glassman AH. Cardiovascular effects of tricyclic antidepressants in depressed patients with and without heart disease. *J Clin Psychiatry*. 1989;50(Suppl):1–18.

125. Small GW. Treatment of geriatric depression. *Depress Anxiety*. 1998;8(Suppl 1):32–42.

126. Schneider LS. Pharmacologic consideration in the treatment of late-life depression. *Am J Geriatr Psychiatry*. 1996;4:S51–S65.

127. Mulsant BH, Pollock BG, Nebes R, et al. A twelve-week, double-blind, randomized comparison of nortriptyline and paroxetine in older depressed inpatients and outpatients. *Am J Geriatr Psychiatry*. 2001;9(4):406–414.

128. Kirby D, Harrigan S, Ames D. Hyponatraemia in elderly psychiatric patients treated with selective serotonin reuptake inhibitors and venlafaxine: a retrospective controlled study in an inpatient unit. *Int J Geriatr Psychiatry*. 2002;17(3):231–237.

129. Allard P, Gram L, Timdahl K, Behnke K, Hanson M, Sogaard J. Efficacy and tolerability of venlafaxine in geriatric outpatients with major depression: a double-blind, randomized 6-month comparative trial with citalopram. *Int J Geriatr Psychiatry*. 2004;19(12):1123–1130.

130. Oslin DW, Ten Have TR, Streim JE, et al. Probing the safety of medications in the frail elderly: evidence from a randomized clinical trial of sertraline and venlafaxine in depressed nursing home residents. *J Clin Psychiatry*. 2003;64(8):875–882.

131. Høyberg OJ, Maragakis B, Mullin J, et al. A double-blind multicentre comparison of mirtazapine and amitriptyline in elderly depressed patients. *Acta Psychiatr Scand*. 1996;93:184–190.

132. Schatzberg AF, Kremer C, Rodrigues HE, Murphy GM Jr, Mirtazapine vs. Paroxetine Study Group. Double-blind, randomized comparison of mirtazapine and paroxetine in elderly depressed patients. *Am J Geriatr Psychiatry*. 2002;10(5):541–550.

133. Georgotas A, McCue RE, Cooper TB, Nagachandran N, Chang I. How effective and safe is continuation therapy in elderly depressed patients? *Arch Gen Psychiatry*. 1988;45:929–932.

134. Masand PS, Tesar GE. Use of stimulants in the medically ill. *Psychiatr Clin North Am*. 1996;19(3):515–547.

135. National Institutes of Health consensus conference: diagnosis and treatment of depression in late life. *JAMA*. 1992;268: 1018–1024.

136. Areán PA, Cook BL. Psychotherapy and combined psychotherapy/pharmacotherapy for late life depression. *Biol Psychiatry*. 2002;52:293–303.

137. Rokke PD, Scogin F. Depression treatment preferences in younger and older adults. *J Clin Geropsychol*. 1995;1:243–257.

138. Thompson LW, Coon DW, Gallagher-Thompson D, Sommer BR, Koin D. Comparison of desipramine and cognitive/behavioral therapy in the treatment of elderly outpatients with mild-to-moderate depression. *Am J Geriatr Psychiatry*. 2001;9: 225–240.

139. Reynolds CF III, Frank E, Perel JM, et al. Nortriptyline and interpersonal psychotherapy as maintenance therapies for recurrent major depression: a randomized controlled trial in patients older than 59 years. *JAMA*. 1999;281:39–45.

140. Leung SN, Orrell MW. A brief cognitive behavioral therapy group for the elderly: who benefits? *Int J Geriatr Psychiatry*. 1993;8: 593–598.

141. Williams JW Jr, Barrett J, Oxman T, et al. Treatment of dysthymia and minor depression in primary care: a randomized controlled trial in older adults. *JAMA*. 2000;284(12):1519–1526.

142. Mossey JM, Knott KA, Higgins M, Talerico K. Effectiveness of a psychosocial intervention, interpersonal counseling, for subdysthymic depression in medically ill elderly. *J Gerontol A Biol Sci Med Sci*. 1996;51(4):M172–M178.

143. Thompson LW, Gallagher D, Breckenridge JS. Comparative effectiveness of psychotherapies for depressed elders. *J Consult Clin Psychol*. 1987;55:785–799.

144. Alexopoulos GS, Raue P, Areán P. Problem-solving therapy versus supportive therapy in geriatric major depression with executive dysfunction. *Am J Geriatr Psychiatry*. 2003;11(1):46–52.

145. Lynch TR, Morse JQ, Mendelson T, Robins CJ. Dialectical behavioral therapy for depressed older adults. *Am J Geriatr Psychiatry*. 2003;11(1):33–45.

146. McCullough JP. *Treatment for Chronic Depression*. New York: Guilford Press; 2000.

147. Gallagher-Thompson D, Steffen AM. Comparative effects of cognitive-behavioral and brief psychodynamic psychotherapies for depressed family caregivers. *J Consult Clin Psychol*. 1994;62: 543–549.

148. Plotkin F. Treatment of the older adult: the impact on the psychoanalyst. *J Am Psychoanal Assoc*. 2000;48(4):1591–1616.

149. Lavretsky H, Kumar A. Methylphenidate augmentation of citalopram in elderly depressed patients. *Am J Geriatr Psychiatry*. 2001;9:298–303.

150. Taragano FE, Allegri R, Vicario A, Bagnatti P, Lyketsos CG. A double blind, randomized clinical trial assessing the efficacy and safety of augmenting standard antidepressant therapy with nimodipine in the treatment of 'vascular depression'. *Int J Geriatr Psychiatry*. 2001;16:254–260.

151. Simpson S, Jackson A, Baldwin RC, Burns AS. Subcortical hyperintensities in late-life depression: acute response to treatment and neuropsychological correlates. *Int Psychogeriatrics*. 1997;9 (3):257–275.

152. Thompson JW, Weiner RD, Meyers CP. Use of ECT in the United States in 1975, 1980, and 1986. *Am J Psychiatry*. 1994;151: 1657–1661.

153. Van der Wurff FB, Stek ML, Hoogendijk WL, Beekman AT. Electroconvulsive therapy for the depressed elderly. *Cochrane Database Syst Rev*. 2003;(2):CD003593.

154. George MS, Nahas Z, Kozel FA, Goldman J, Molloy M, Oliver N. Improvement of depression following transcranial magnetic stimulation. *Curr Psychiatry Rep*. 1999;1(2):114–124.

155. Sackeim HA, Rush AJ, George MS, Marangell LB, et al. Vagus nerve stimulation (VNS(tm)) for treatment-resistant depression: efficacy, side effects, and predictors of outcome. *Neuropsychopharmacology*. 2001;25(5):713–728.

156. Mayberg HS, Lozano AM, Voon V, et al. Deep brain stimulation for treatment-resistant depression. *Neuron*. 2005;45(5):651–660.

157. Reynolds CF III. Psychopharmacology: antidepressants and mood stabilizers. In: Sadock BJ, Sadock VA, eds. *Kaplan & Sadock's Comprehensive Textbook of Psychiatry*. 7th Ed. Philadelphia: Lippincott Williams & Wilkins; 2000:3090–3094.

158. Borson S, McDonald GJ, Gayle T, Deffebach M, Lakshminarayan S, VanTuinen C. Improvement in mood, physical symptoms, and function with nortriptyline for depression in patients with chronic obstructive pulmonary disease. *Psychosomatics*. 1992;33(2): 190–201.

159. Wallace AE, Kofoed LL, West AN. Double-blind, placebo-controlled trial of methylphenidate in older, depressed, medically ill patients. *Am J Psychiatry*. 1995;152:929–931.

160. Kaplitz SE. Withdrawn, apathetic geriatric patients responsive to methylphenidate. *J Am Geriatr Soc*. 1975;23:271–276.

161. Clyburn LD, Stones MJ, Hajistavropoulos T, Tuokko H. Predicting caregiver burden and depression in Alzheimer's disease. *J Gerontol B Psychol Sci Soc Sci*. 2000;55:S2–S13.

162. Mittelman MS, Ferris SH, Shulman E, Steinberg G, Levin B. A family intervention to delay nursing home placement of patients with Alzheimer disease: a randomized controlled trial. *JAMA*. 1996;276(21):1725–1731.

163. McCurren C, Dowe D, Rattle D, Looney S. Depression among nursing home elders: testing an intervention strategy. *Appl Nurs Res*. 1999;12:185–195.

164. Rosen J, Rogers JC, Marin RS, Mulsant BH, Shahar A, Reynolds CF III. Control-relevant intervention in the treatment of minor and major depression in a long-term care facility. *Am J Geriatr Psychiatry*. 1997;5:247–257.

165. Sumaya IC, Rienzi BM, Deegan JF II, Moss DE. Bright light treatment decreases depression in institutionalized older adults: a placebo-controlled crossover study. *J Gerontol A Biol Sci Med Sci*. 2001;56(6):M356–M360.

166. Fitzsimmons S. Easy rider wheelchair biking. A nursing-recreation therapy clinical trial for the treatment of depression. *J Gerontol Nurs*. 2001;5:14–23.

167. Zerhusen JD, Boyle K, Wilson W. Out of the darkness: group cognitive therapy for depressed elderly. *J Psychosoc Nurs Ment Health Serv*. 1991;29:16–21.

168. Borson S, Scanlan JM, Doane K, Gray S. Antidepressant prescribing in nursing homes: is there a place for tricyclic antidepressants? *Int J Geriatr Psychiatry*. 2002;17:1140–1145.

169. Katz IR, Simpson GM, Curlik SM, Parmelee PA, Muhly C. Pharmacologic treatment of major depression for elderly patients in residential care settings. *J Clin Psychiatry*. 1990;51 (Suppl):41–47.

170. Streim JE, Oslin DW, Katz IR, et al. Drug treatment of depression in frail elderly nursing home residents. *Am J Geriatr Psychiatry*. 2000;8(2):150–159.

171. Magai C, Kennedy G, Cohen CI, Gomberg D. A controlled clinical trial of sertraline in the treatment of depression in nursing home patients with late-stage Alzheimer's disease. *Am J Geriatr Psychiatry*. 2000;8(1):66–74.

172. Trappler B, Cohen CI. Use of SSRIs in "very old" depressed nursing home residents. *Am J Geriatr Psychiatry*. 1998;6(1):83–89.

173. Oslin DW, Streim JE, Katz IR, et al. Heuristic comparison of sertraline with nortriptyline for the treatment of depression in frail elderly patients. *Am J Geriatr Psychiatry*. 2000;8(2):141–149.

174. Rosen J, Mulsant BH, Pollock BG. Sertraline in the treatment of minor depression in nursing home residents: a pilot study. *Int J Geriatr Psychiatry*. 2000;15:177–180.

175. Zis AP, Grof P, Webster M, Goodwin FK. Prediction of relapse in recurrent affective disorder. *Psychopharmacol Bull*. 1980;16: 47–49.

176. Donohue JC, Tylee A. The treatment of depression: antidepressant prescribing for elderly patients in primary care. *Pharm J*. 1998;260:500–502.

177. Krause N. Stress and isolation from close ties in later life. *J Gerontol*. 1991;46:S183–S194.

178. Ryff CD, Essex MU. The interpretation of life experience and well being: the sample case of relocation. *Psychol Aging*. 1992;7: 507–517.

179. Hays JC, Landerman LR, George LK, et al. Social correlates of the dimensions of depression in the elderly. *J Gerontol B Psychol Sci Soc Sci*. 1998;53:31–39.

180. Walton CG, Shultz CM, Beck CM, Walls RC. Psychological correlates of loneliness in the older adult. *Arch Psychiatr Nurs*. 1991;5:165–170.

Geriatric Bipolar Disorder

26

Brent Forester   Francesca Cannavo Antognini   Andrew Stoll

Bipolar disorder in later life provides both a fascinating presentation of complex neuropsychiatric symptoms and a confounding syndrome that often eludes the efforts of clinicians skilled in diagnosis and treatment. The illness is recurrent, usually presenting for the first time in adolescence or early adulthood. The toll of bipolar disorder on patients and families as a result of complications such as substance abuse, legal problems, and suicide is enormous. Cross-sectional analyses have reported that older adults with bipolar disorder continue to use health services at high rates (1). Despite this, however, there has been little longitudinal study to date on the effects of aging on the course of bipolar disorder. Mania itself may present for the first time after the age of 50, and this later-life onset is often associated with underlying medical or neurological comorbidity. The differential diagnostic assessment of manic symptoms and the complexities of treatment occurring in later life are more extensive than for younger adults, and can include the confounding syndromes of delirium and dementia. All of these factors present complex diagnostic and therapeutic challenges. Complicating the clinician's attempts at treatment is the paucity of controlled studies in the elderly of the now numerous pharmacological interventions at different phases of bipolar disorder, as studied in younger adults.

Imagine the myriad of clinically vexing questions that arise in the evaluation and management of the geriatric bipolar patient. What are the effects of lithium treatment acutely and chronically on an aging brain? How do older adults with acute mania respond to treatments, including lithium, divalproex, and the atypical antipsychotic agents, which are approved to treat acute mania or mixed states in younger adults? What treatments are effective for rapid cycling or maintenance therapy? What is the appropriate pharmacological management of bipolar depression in the elderly, a challenging enough condition to treat successfully in a younger population? What is the evidence-based role of psychotherapeutic treatments of bipolar disorder in later life? Does the clinical course of bipolar disorder universally worsen over time? How does one clinically differentiate the syndromes of mania, delirium, and dementia in a patient with a history of bipolar disorder presenting with mood instability and increased confusion? What are the effects of life-long bipolar disorder on cognitive functioning and, specifically, are patients with bipolar disorder at an increased risk of developing degenerative dementias at a certain age?

Some of these questions will be answered in this chapter through the presentation and discussion of a case that illustrates the recurrent aspect of bipolar disorder through the life cycle and its effects on functioning, quality of life, and morbidity. Epidemiological data will also be presented, followed by a discussion of the differential diagnosis of mania and bipolar depression in later life. A review of the current understanding of pharmacotherapeutic and psychotherapeutic challenges in geriatric bipolar disorder will be followed by recommended clinical guidelines for an integrated treatment approach. Many of these questions will, however, remain unanswered by our experience to date; thus, suggestions for promising avenues for acute and longitudinal research studies will be discussed. As is typical of geriatric psychiatry treatments in general, until the clinical research is adequate, the approach to geriatric bipolar disorder must rely on the extrapolation of data from studies of younger adults with bipolar disorder.

CASE EXAMPLE

Mr. W is a 77-year-old Caucasian divorced male who has been followed at an academic hospital-based geriatric psychiatry clinic over the past year for weekly outpatient psychotherapy and approximately monthly medication management. He has had a number of depressive episodes throughout his adult life, some requiring inpatient treatment, as well as periods of elevated mood with affective and behavioral features consistent with hypomania. Although his diagnosis has appeared unclear to some past treaters, the current clinical impression is that the patient suffers from bipolar II disorder.

History of Illness

Mr. W's depression first became a problem in high school, when he began to experience periods of poor concentration and social withdrawal. These were, however, punctuated by episodes of extreme productivity when he would, for example, stay up all night to work on his school newspaper. Despite what he describes as his natural tendencies toward social avoidance, he recalls being in high gear at other times, at one point successfully running for president of his high school class.

After graduating from a prestigious college and then working at a number of temporary jobs, Mr. W began a graduate program. During this time, however, his mood swings worsened to the extent that he was ultimately unable to continue his studies. Around that time he began to consult a psychiatrist on a regular basis, receiving psychoanalysis 5 times per week. Starting in the early 1970s he also took lithium under the care of a separate psychopharmacologist. After a year or two on the medication, it was discontinued because the patient did not find it helpful. Mr. W remained in analysis for approximately 20 years until the late 70s when he had his first hospitalization for depression and the analyst dropped him. He describes a profound sense of loss, since there was a strong therapeutic transference, with Mr. W at times referring to this doctor as "the only person who ever truly loved me."

Mr. W married in his 30s and taught high school for several years. He reports his marriage gradually deteriorated as financial problems arose. During these years, he was hospitalized several times for major depressive episodes. He also allegedly experienced intervening hypomanic episodes characterized by periods of elation, grandiosity, and irritability. Ultimately, Mr. W was forced to leave his teaching position because of increasingly frequent flare-ups of his illness, thereafter relying on his father's trust for financial support.

Following his first hospitalization, Mr. W sought treatment from two more psychiatrists who also provided psychotherapy. During this time, he was treated with two antidepressants, the names of which he could not recall, but he states that he was on paroxetine for a number of years until shortly before his last hospital admission.

Family History

Mr. W was the son of a wealthy entrepreneur and the fourth of five children, having one younger brother, two older brothers, and an older sister. His mother, a homemaker, suffered from bipolar I disorder and had multiple hospitalizations for mania throughout the patient's childhood and adolescence. Mr. W's father, described by the patient as harsh and remote, abused alcohol, and his older brother, having identified himself as an alcoholic, attained long-term sobriety through Alcoholics Anonymous. The patient reports that one other brother suffered from some form of mental disorder, but he is unable to offer more specifics. All his siblings are deceased with the exception of his sister, with whom he maintains consistent contact.

Current Family and Social Context

Mr. W's marriage, which ultimately ended in divorce, produced two children, a son and a daughter. He describes the son as dysfunctional, since he has had serious difficulty working independently. Mr. W recalls having had a brother with similar problems. He feels his son, who lived with him as an adult for a time, suffers primarily from depression. They are now estranged; the son lives near his mother in a town about an hour away. Mr. W's daughter had lived in another state for a time, but recently returned to the area. When nearby, she takes an active role in monitoring his progress, which he describes as bordering on controlling. Mr. W has had a girlfriend for the past 10 years. He describes the relationship as romantic but nonsexual, due to religious beliefs. He at times perceives his girlfriend, who is a divorced woman with teenage children, as controlling and also financially demanding.

Recent History of Illness

Mr. W was hospitalized for depression and suicidal ideation in the summer of 2002. He had undergone two knee replacements earlier that year, the last of which was complicated by a postoperative pneumonia. Prior to his hospitalization he had lost 40 pounds. At the time of his admission he was placed on venlafaxine XR 300 mg per day by his outpatient psychiatrist. Early in his hospitalization, he was placed on gabapentin 300 mg per day (which appears to have been discontinued shortly thereafter), and the venlafaxine XR was tapered and discontinued. During the course of his hospitalization, bupropion SR, 100 mg in the morning, sertraline 50 mg once a day, and olanzapine 7.5 mg at bedtime were added.

Mr. W was maintained on the above medication regimen throughout his subsequent 2-month participation in a geriatric partial hospitalization program. Neuropsychological testing was performed to evaluate reports of memory and word-finding difficulties. While the results showed no signs of dementia, he did demonstrate fluctuations in attention, effortful concentration, and verbal memory difficulties (measured by his performance on the

California Verbal Learning Test), which were significantly improved by cueing.

Following his discharge from the partial program, Mr. W was seen for outpatient medication management and weekly psychotherapy. During the ensuing 11 months, he continued on varying doses of sertraline, olanzapine, and bupropion. In the first 6 months of treatment, he displayed brief episodes of hypomania, in one therapy session expressing an intention to visit the President at the White House later that week to offer advice on foreign policy. At this time his speech was pressured and his affect euphoric. Such episodes would, within a few days, give way to longer periods of depression, characterized by hopeless mood, anhedonia, sleep difficulties, and social withdrawal. As time went by, Mr. W had fewer hypomanic episodes and his periods of depression became more manageable, although increasingly characterized by cognitive slowing and lethargy. During this period, Mr. W saw a neurologist for evaluation of a tremor, and was advised to have his olanzapine tapered, which was subsequently initiated by his psychiatrist. Mr. W reported for his psychotherapy session a week later in a hypomanic state, with pressured and tangential speech and elevated mood. At this time, his olanzapine had been tapered to half the dose (5 mg). One week later, with the olanzapine taper almost complete, Mr. W presented as euthymic for the first time in many months.

EPIDEMIOLOGY

Most of what we know about the demographics of geriatric bipolar disorder is extracted from data collected in adult populations that include both geriatric and nongeriatric members. Lifetime prevalence rates of bipolar disorder appear to be uniform across cultures and similar between men and women (2). According to Weissman, Leaf, and colleagues, the 1-year prevalence of bipolar disorder among adults 65 and older is 0.4%, which is significantly lower than the 1.4% seen in younger adults (3). In general, across all age groups and illness subtypes, bipolar disorder is a highly recurrent condition, with 85% to 100% of patients experiencing a recurrence after the initial episode (4).

Angst et al. found a relationship between gender and the onset of mania (5). They reported that one of the two lifetime peaks for the onset of mania in women occurs during the fifth decade, at approximately the time of menopause. Among men, an increase in the incidence of mania in the 8th and 9th decades of life has been reported (6,7). Whether these incidence rates are spuriously elevated due to the decreasing size of the reference cohort that occurs with age (which decreases the denominator for an incidence rate, particularly for men) remains a question (8). On the other hand, the high

mortality rate among manic patients from suicide and other causes of death may reduce prevalence rates through selective elimination of those affected (8). For example, in a retrospective chart review study of inpatients with an index episode of mania, Shulman and Tohen reported a 30% probability of remaining alive after 10 years of follow-up, compared with a 75% probability for an age and sex matched group of patients with unipolar depression (9). This latter study highlights the significant morbidity and mortality associated with geriatric bipolar disorder.

As many as 10% of all patients with bipolar disorder develop their illness after the age of 50 (10). New onset of bipolar symptoms in later years may represent a consequence of secondary mania attributable to medical, pharmacological, or other organic dysfunction. In general, later-onset bipolar disorder is associated with a lower rate of familial illness than early onset cases, and a higher rate of medical and neurological comorbidity (11). Patients with a history of unipolar depression may not develop mania until later life, with reports of up to a 15-year interval between the first episode of depression and subsequent mania (11). Goldberg reported a 40% incidence of a later manic switch in patients hospitalized for unipolar major depression and followed for 15 years (12). Misdiagnosis is common in bipolar disorder, particularly bipolar disorder, type II. Eliciting a history of hypomania earlier in life is often difficult, even with information provided by family members or other clinicians.

Finally, onset of bipolar disorder at a later age may be associated with an increased vulnerability to relapse (11). Angst has noted an association between increased age at onset and a decreased inter-episode euthymic interval (13).

DIAGNOSIS

The *Diagnostic and Statistical Manual of Mental Disorders*, 4th Edition, Text Revision (DSM-IV-TR) diagnostic classification system is used for the diagnosis of bipolar disorder in the elderly (14). This includes the diagnosis of bipolar disorder, type I (recurring episodes of mania with or without depression), bipolar disorder, type II (hypomania and recurrent major depression), and cyclothymia (hypomanic symptoms alternating with sub-threshold depression). DSM-IV-TR also identifies bipolar disorder, mixed state and rapid-cycling subtypes as important considerations. See Table 26-1 for an adapted list of DSM-IV-TR criteria for bipolar disorder.

In the elderly bipolar patient, however, the presenting symptoms are often confounded by the presence of comorbid medical or neurological conditions, or by the presence of delirium or dementia. Furthermore, the acute and chronic effects of substance abuse and misuse may also

TABLE 26-1
DSM-IV-TR CRITERIA FOR BIPOLAR DISORDER

I. Bipolar I disorder requires the presence of at least one manic episode in patient's lifetime

  A. Manic episode
1. A distinct period of abnormally and persistently elevated, expansive, or irritable mood lasting at least 1 week.
2. During the period of mood disturbance, three or more of the following symptoms have persisted and been present to a significant degree:
   a. Inflated self-esteem or grandiosity
   b. Decreased need for sleep
   c. More talkative than usual or pressured speech
   d. Flight of ideas or racing thoughts
   e. Distractibility
   f. Increase in goal-directed activity or psychomotor agitation
   g. Excessive involvement in pleasurable activities that have a high potential for painful consequences (e.g., buying sprees, sexual indiscretion)
3. The mood disturbance is sufficient to cause marked impairment in occupational or social functioning, or to necessitate hospitalization, or there are psychotic features.
4. The symptoms are not due to the direct physiological effects of a substance or a general medical condition.

  B. Hypomanic episode
1. A distinct period of abnormally and persistently elevated, expansive or irritable mood, lasting at least 4 days, that is clearly different from the usual nondepressed mood.
2. The episode is associated with an unequivocal change in functioning that is uncharacteristic of the person when not symptomatic.
3. Remainder of manic episode criteria, *except* the episode is not severe enough to cause a marked impairment in social or occupational functioning, or to necessitate hospitalization, and there are no psychotic features.

  C. Mixed episode
1. The criteria are met for both a manic and a major depressive episode (except for duration) nearly every day during at least a 1-week period.
2. The mood disturbance is sufficient to cause marked impairment in occupational or social functioning or to necessitate hospitalization or if there are psychotic features.
3. The symptoms are not due to the direct physiological effects of a substance or a general medical condition.

  D. Bipolar disorder criteria sets include
1. Bipolar I disorder, single manic episode
2. Bipolar I disorder, most recent episode hypomanic
3. Bipolar I disorder, most recent episode manic
4. Bipolar I disorder, most recent episode depressed
5. Bipolar I disorder, most recent episode unspecified

  E. For all bipolar disorder criteria sets the following specifiers may apply
1. Severity/psychotic/remission specifiers
2. With catatonic features
3. With postpartum onset
4. Longitudinal course specifiers (with and without inter-episode recovery)
5. With seasonal pattern
6. With rapid cycling (at least four episodes of a mood disturbance in the last 12 months that meet criteria for either a major depressive, manic, mixed or hypomanic episode)

II. Bipolar II disorder (recurrent major depressive episodes with hypomanic episodes)

Adapted from Reference 14.

cloud the diagnostic picture. Although such substance abuse may involve drugs such as cocaine or heroin, it appears that this current cohort of older adults more commonly misuses or abuses alcohol, benzodiazepines, prescription pain medications, or over-the-counter medications that have anticholinergic side effects, such as diphenhydramine. A thorough assessment of medication use (both over-the-counter and prescription), as well as dietary supplements (including nutritional agents and herbal therapies), must be pursued. For more information, see the chapter on pharmacotherapy.

GERIATRIC MANIA

Diagnosis of mania in later life presents specific clinical challenges. The DSM-IV-TR criteria for diagnosing mania focus on the presence of a mood disturbance with abnormal and persistent elevation of mood, expansiveness, or irritability (14). In contrast to younger patients, who tend to present with elevated or irritable mood, older adults more often display a mixed symptom picture with the concurrent presence of depressive and manic symptoms (15). As with younger bipolar patients, sleep difficulties are often present. Mood incongruent paranoid delusions become more frequent with aging and may occur along with mood congruent delusions (15). Similar to younger bipolar patients, thought disorder symptoms such as incoherence, loose associations, derailment, illogical thinking, and neologism may occur in late-life mania, with severity as great as in schizophrenia (16). Irritability is more common than hyperactivity in older manics, and circumstantiality is often seen instead of flight of ideas (10). Cognitive impairment is more often noted in manic older adults than manic younger adults, perhaps reflecting the increased relevance of medical factors (17). In contrast, older patients with mania are less likely than younger manic patients to show increases in activity, sexual interest, religiosity, and initiating and making plans (18). These differences in the presentation of mania in later life decrease the sensitivity of the DSM-IV-TR criteria as a diagnostic tool for geriatric mania.

The specificity of the DSM-IV-TR criteria for geriatric mania is also limited. As Umapathy and colleagues have noted, diagnostic specificity in detecting bipolar disorder is a problem across the life span (19). Among child and adolescent patients, the challenge is distinguishing bipolar disorder from attention deficit disorder with hyperactivity. In young to middle adulthood, differential diagnosis attempts to distinguish bipolar disorder from other psychotic and mood disorders, substance abuse disorders, and personality disorders.

SECONDARY MANIA

In older adults, the challenge becomes differentiating mania in the context of bipolar disorder from a diagnosis of mood disorder due to a general medical condition with manic features, also known as *secondary mania*. Clinically, individuals with secondary mania may present with neuropsychiatric symptoms very similar to patients whose mania reflects a new onset or a recurrence of bipolar disorder. Secondary mania is associated with a medical or neurological illness, or with an adverse effect of pharmacological treatment (20). It is most often seen with a late onset and is less commonly associated with a family history of mood disorder or with prominent symptoms of delirium (20). Table 26-2 lists the myriad conditions to which secondary mania has most often been attributed.

A retrospective study by Tohen, which assessed 50 manic subjects older than 65, demonstrated the high fre-

TABLE 26-2

CAUSES OF SECONDARY MANIA

Neurologic disorders (8,10,18,20,145–148)	Space-occupying or traumatic lesions, especially right orbitofrontal and right basotemporal localities Epilepsy, especially right temporal focus Alzheimer's disease Vascular dementia Parkinson's disease Pick's disease (frontotemporal dementia) Tourette's syndrome Wilson's disease Encephalitis Chronic alcoholism Multiple sclerosis Right hemisphere cerebrovascular disease
Infections (8,18,20,149)	Viral: influenza, AIDS Rickettsial: Q fever Spirochetes: neurosyphilis
Pharmacological and somatic treatments (8,10,20)	Antidepressants Benzodiazepines Corticosteroids Estrogen Thyroid replacement Amphetamines/cocaine Levodopa Captopril Isoniazid Enalapril Procarbazine Lithium Decongestants ECT Bronchodilators Metoclopramide Procyclidine Stimulants Phencyclidine
Endocrine and Metabolic disturbances (8,10,20)	End-stage renal disease Hemodialysis-related metabolic changes Postoperative metabolic disturbances Anemia Hyperthyroidism B12 deficiency Niacin deficiency

ECT, electroconvulsive therapy. Reprinted with permission from Reference 15.

quency of medical etiologies in late-life mania. In that cohort, neurological disorders were reported in 74% of the manic patients with late onset and 28% of those with early onset (21).

DIFFERENTIATING AMONG MANIA, DEMENTIA, AND DELIRIUM

The evaluation of manic symptoms or episodes in an older adult requires a thorough differential diagnosis in order to determine the most accurate etiology and to help direct appropriate treatment. The diagnoses of mania or major depression with anxious features should be considered when a patient is known to have suffered prior mood disorder episodes. Early stages of dementia may present with symptoms of mania, including irritable mood, emotional lability, sleep disturbance, and impaired social judgment. The co-occurrence of significant signs of confusion, fluctuation of alertness, or evidence of autonomic dysfunction may indicate the presence of delirium and requires a thorough medical and neurological evaluation. For a patient with a history of bipolar disorder, any change in baseline mood symptoms or functioning suggesting a decompensation warrants a workup for a concurrent medical condition.

In the presence of dementia, the diagnosis of mania is particularly problematic. McDonald and Nemeroff highlight the difficulties in distinguishing mania from dementia, delirium, or agitated depression among patients older than 70 with Mini-Mental State Examination scores below 15 on the 30 point scale (22). The following clinical pearls, suggested by Forester et al. (15), may help with the differential diagnosis in patients who present with a combination of manic and cognitive symptoms:

- A rapid decline in cognitive functioning in a demented patient, along with fluctuations in mood, energy, and sleep, may indicate the onset of a manic episode.
- Mixed manic and depressive symptoms are common in older manic patients.
- Focal neurological findings such as aphasia, apraxia, or impaired visuospatial functioning are typically associated with dementia rather than with mania.
- Nighttime agitation and confusion (i.e., sundowning) is more typically associated with dementia or delirium than with mania.
- A negative family history for bipolar disorder may be unreliable, because an older patient's siblings and ancestors may have been diagnosed (or misdiagnosed) prior to the modern diagnostic classification. Prior to the widespread availability of mood-stabilizing agents, clinicians were less sensitive to the presence of bipolar disorder (23).

Table 26-3 lists characteristic features of mania as contrasted with delirium and dementia.

BIPOLAR DEPRESSION

Unfortunately, there has been little in the literature regarding the clinical presentation of geriatric bipolar depression and how it compares to the symptomatic profile in a younger population (11). In addition, it is unclear whether the common clinical perception that symptoms such as hypersomnia, hyperphagia, and psychomotor retardation occur more often in adult bipolar depression as opposed to unipolar depression also holds true for an elderly cohort.

DIAGNOSTIC AIDS: NEUROPSYCHOLOGICAL TESTING AND NEUROIMAGING

There have been a growing number of studies of cognitive function in bipolar patients using neuropsychological test results as the dependent variable. For bipolar adults in general, neurocognitive impairment may be a trait rather than a state variable, or a slowly evolving process that is neither trait nor state. Cavanagh and colleagues reviewed controlled studies showing significant deficits in verbal memory among euthymic bipolar adults, as assessed by the California Verbal Learning Test (24). Other researchers confirm these results, with additional findings of impaired executive function and sustained attention in euthymic bipolar patients. This includes a recent controlled study of 18 euthymic bipolar patients 60 and older that found evidence of executive dysfunction on the Mattis Dementia Rating Scale and the Executive Interview (25). There was no association between the cognitive dysfunction and age of first episode, duration of illness, or use of specific mood stabilizers.

There also appears to be a positive correlation between the degree of cognitive impairment (specifically, verbal learning and memory) and the number and cumulative duration of manic episodes in a given patient (24), a finding that would seem to have implications for geriatric patients with early-onset bipolar disorder. Goodwin and Jamison report studies that yielded differences between early-onset and late-onset bipolar patients on the Aphasia Screening Test, with early-onset patients committing more errors (26). Many hypotheses regarding the causes of cognitive impairment in geriatric bipolar disorder have been offered, including neurodevelopmental abnormalities, toxicity of recurrent mood episodes, cerebrovascular disease, substance abuse comorbidity, and medication side effects (25).

Neuroimaging studies of geriatric bipolar disorder have focused on cerebrovascular changes and cerebral volume loss. Migliorelli and colleagues, using single positron emission computerized tomography scans, found a relative decrease in cerebral blood flow in the right basal temporal cortex of bipolar patients (27). In another study, patients with late-onset mania had a higher proportion of silent cerebral infarcts compared to patients with late-onset unipolar depression (28). Additionally, an increase in subcortical hyperintensities in the inferior half of the frontal lobe in elderly manic patients was reported by McDonald and colleagues (29). Altschuler et al. (30) report studies

TABLE 26-3

DIAGNOSTIC CONSIDERATIONS IN GERIATRIC BIPOLAR DISORDER

Data Source	Mania (DSM-IV TR)	Dementia	Delirium	Secondary Mania
History (150,151)	At least 1-week duration of elevated, expansive or irritable mood and distractibility	Gradual onset	Rapid onset, with fluctuation during course of day	There is close temporal relationship between manic episode and primary medical disorder in 20% of patients (a latent period of months to years may also be observed)
Physical examination (21,152–154)	Not attributable to a medical condition; neurological signs such as ataxia and frontal release signs may be present	Identifiable functional decline; movement disorders are common over time	Evidence of underlying physical illness or medication effect	Evidence of accompanying neurological or other disorders
Family history (20)	Mood disorders	Dementia	Unknown	Is not associated with family history of bipolar disorder
Mental status examination (155,156)	Alert; exhibits two or more of the following: grandiosity, pressured speech, psychomotor agitation, flight of ideas, increased goal-directed activity	Alert; aphasia, apraxia, agnosia; impaired executive functioning	Disturbance of consciousness, orientation, and sleep/wake cycle	Irritable mood, persecutory delusions of mood-incongruent type, grandiose delusions not as common as seen in mania
Attention and concentration	Tangential, flight of ideas, with grandiosity; easily distracted	Decreased ability to register new data, but may respond well to prompting	Easily distracted, ability to maintain and shift focus is impaired	May or may not be relevant, depending on primary condition
Speech	Pressured	Aphasia	Varies	May be pressured but also disorganized, due to primary condition
Sleep	Decreased need is common	No direct association, but sleep/wake cycle reversal is common	Sleep-wake cycle disturbances common: daytime sleepiness/ night-time agitation	Sleep/wake cycle disturbance due to agitation and irritability
Laboratory findings	No specific findings	No specific findings in most common forms of dementia	Lab abnormalities common, associated with underlying medical condition	Lab abnormalities associated with primary condition but mostly non-diagnostic
Neuroimaging and EEG (157)	Increased perfusion in orbital and supragenual medial frontal cortex seen on functional scans. No specific EEG findings	Neuroimaging may reveal cerebral atrophy, but no uniform findings. EEG typically shows diffuse showing	EEG abnormal; frequently generalized slowing. Neuroimaging may reveal cerebral etiology	Neuroimaging may show neurological disorders or head trauma; right-sided lesions of frontal projection pathways are more common

EEG, electroencephalography; URI, upper respiratory infection; UTI, urinary track infection. Adapted from Reference 15.

showing significantly larger amygdala volumes in bipolar patients, as well as larger lateral and third ventricles, which suggest a reduction in the volume of the thalamus or hypothalamus (31). Others report a significant reduction of gray matter in the left subgenual area of the prefrontal cortex (32). A number of these studies were conducted on euthymic bipolar patients, suggesting that these are trait abnormalities (33).

Clearly, further research is needed in the quest to more thoroughly understand the behavioral, cognitive, and neurological manifestations of bipolar disorder in older adults.

PHARMACOLOGICAL TREATMENT

Most of what we know about the treatment of bipolar disorder comes from randomized, controlled clinical trials in adult or mixed-age populations. There are no double-blind, placebo-controlled studies in geriatric bipolar disorder, but there are a number of plausible explanations for this lack of controlled clinical data. Diagnostic overlap between geriatric mania, delirium, and dementia, as well as other clinical syndromes such as secondary mania, not only confound diagnosis but also make assessment of efficacy and tolerability of pharmacological interventions more challenging. Furthermore, Young and colleagues note that the large numbers of patients with geriatric bipolar disorder necessary for prospective clinical trials are not available at single-site academic centers, thereby raising the need for conducting collaborative studies in multiple centers in this population (34). Finally, the pharmaceutical industry has little interest in studying a geriatric population when a drug can obtain a bipolar indication in younger, less medically complex adults.

As with younger adults, the pharmacological approach to the treatment of geriatric bipolar disorder can be broken down into three clinical scenarios:

- Treatment of acute geriatric mania (including subtypes of mixed states and rapid cycling)
- Treatment of geriatric bipolar depression
- Maintenance treatment/prevention of recurrent mania and bipolar depression

This section will consider each one of these scenarios, reviewing the evidence-based literature in geriatric bipolar disorder, commenting on controlled data in younger adults, and making recommendations about clinical choice of agent and dosing.

Geriatric Mania

More is known about the treatment of mania in younger populations than in older ones and, as stated earlier, there are no placebo-controlled, double-blind studies examining the treatment of geriatric mania. Our best current guidelines for treating mania in the elderly, therefore, are derived from uncontrolled studies and the extrapolation of findings reported in younger and mixed-adult populations. Most published reports have focused on somatic approaches, especially the use of antipsychotic medications, benzodiazepines, lithium salts, anticonvulsants, or electroconvulsive therapy. Table 26-4 outlines a pharmacological approach to the treatment of geriatric mania with recommendations for dosing.

As we consider the treatment of geriatric mania, it is important to define not only adequate treatment dose but also duration (34). The appropriate management of geriatric mania begins with the identification of comorbid medical and neurological disorders, and includes the elimination of unnecessary psychotropic medications. In younger patients, polypharmacy is often used from the outset for rapid symptom control. In contrast, monotherapy is usually the first step of treatment in geriatric mania to reduce the potential for the additional side effect burden of combined treatment.

Antipsychotic Medications

In treating older manic adults, conventional antipsychotic medications historically have been used in treating the acute phase of the disorder, when a patient's safety or health might be endangered by awaiting the therapeutic effects of less rapidly-acting approaches. McDonald and Nemeroff (22) suggest an antipsychotic regimen for older patients, emphasizing the use of lower doses in order to limit adverse effects. They recommend initiation of treatment with haloperidol 0.25 mg to 0.5 mg intramuscularly or orally, followed 1 hour later by lorazepam 0.5 mg intramuscularly or orally. Repeated alternating doses can be given on an hourly basis until the patient is calm but not oversedated. In addition to sedation, other side effects to monitor include orthostatic hypotension, extrapyramidal symptoms, and neuroleptic malignant syndrome. The risk of tardive dyskinesia (TD) is heightened with long-term antipsychotic use and is increased in older adults, females, and mood disorder patients. A review by Jeste and colleagues found the cumulative incidence of TD in older adults prescribed conventional antipsychotics approximates 29% after 1 year, 50% after 2 years, and 63% after 3 years (35). The concurrent administration of lorazepam, though useful in limiting the maximum necessary antipsychotic dose, is not without its own complications, which may include unwanted sedation, ataxia, falls, cognitive impairment, withdrawal symptoms (if lorazepam is continued regularly for more than 2 to 3 weeks), and disinhibition (36).

Largely due to the adverse effects associated with conventional antipsychotic medications, atypical antipsychotic agents have been increasingly used in the treatment of younger manic patients. In the elderly, atypical antipsychotic agents may be used alone or in combination with mood stabilizers (37). According to Jeste and colleagues, atypical agents have generally supplanted conventional antipsychotic medications as first-line treatments in geriatric clinical practice (38). All atypicals, except for clozapine, have at least one controlled study in younger adults with mania. Clozapine has one controlled study for maintenance treatment (39). Clozapine, risperidone, olanzapine, quetiapine, ziprasidone, and aripiprazole have been proven beneficial in younger manic patients in controlled

TABLE 26-4

PHARMACOTHERAPY OF GERIATRIC BIPOLAR DISORDER

I. Pharmacotherapy of Geriatric Mania
A. Initial evaluation
1. Complete blood count, electrolytes, liver function tests, urinalysis, thyroid stimulating hormone
2. Orthostatic vital signs, ECG, cognitive assessment, and neurological evaluation
3. Choice of drug should consider tolerability, prior response to treatment, and prior adverse effects of medications
B. First-line treatment—monotherapy with mood stabilizer along with elimination of antidepressant medication
1. Lithium carbonate (300 to 900 mg/day, with serum levels between 0.4 to 0.8 mEq/L; higher levels of 0.8 to 1.0 mEq/L may be needed in some cases). More conservative dosing in presence of renal insufficiency, medications (e.g., diuretics, NSAIDs) that increase concentration/dose ratio, and the presence of brain pathology (e.g., microvascular ischemic disease) (34); OR
2. DVP (500 to 1000 mg/day, blood levels between 40 and 100 μg/mL). May be preferred choice, particularly in patients with pre-existing cognitive impairment; OR
3. Lithium or DVP plus olanzapine (5 to 15 mg/day), quetiapine (100–400 mg/day), risperidone (1–3 mg/day), or aripiprazole (5–15 mg/day)
C. Second-line treatment
1. Carbamazepine: 100–1,000 mg/day in divided doses
2. Other choices: oxcarbazepine, gabapentin, tiagabine, topiramate (dosing ranges not well established)
D. Duration of acute treatment in geriatric mania not determined. In the absence of evidence-based guidelines, clinical experience suggests a minimum duration of 3 to 4 weeks (34), followed by maintenance therapy (see V below)

II. Pharmacotherapy of Refractory Mania/Mixed Symptoms
A. Addition of atypical antipsychotic or another mood stabilizer
1. Combine lithium or DVP with olanzapine, risperidone, quetiapine, or aripiprazole, OR
2. Combine lithium with DVP, OR
3. Clozapine (25–112.5 mg/day)

III. Pharmacotherapy of Bipolar Depression
A. Monotherapy
1. Lithium or lamotrigine (starting at 12.5 mg every day, titrate every 2 weeks to dosages in 100 to 200 mg/day range. If co-administered with DVP, start at 12.5 mg every other day to target dose of 100 mg/day)
B. Combination therapy
1. Lithium or DVP or lamotrigine plus antidepressant
2. Antidepressant selection based on treatment history and potential and/or previous adverse effects

IV. Electroconvulsive Therapy
A. Consider in patients with mania, bipolar depression, or rapid cycling that is refractory to pharmacotherapy, or in those with acute features including suicidality and inadequate food and fluid intake. No systematic data comparing ECT and pharmacotherapy in elderly bipolar patients (34)

V. Pharmacotherapy for Maintenance Therapy of Geriatric Bipolar Disorder
A. Pharmacotherapy that has proven to be efficacious for acute treatment of mania or bipolar depression should be continued for 6 to 12 months. If remission is sustained, long-term treatment with a mood stabilizer remains essential. Slow discontinuation of adjunctive antidepressants, antipsychotics, or antianxiety agents can be attempted under close monitoring. Common maintenance regimens include:
1. Lithium, OR
2. DVP +/− atypical antipsychotic (olanzapine, risperidone, quetiapine, aripiprazole), OR
3. Lamotrigine +/− atypical antipsychotic medication

DVP, Divalproex; ECG, electrocardiogram; ECT, electroconvulsive therapy; NSAIDs, nonsteroidal anti-inflammatory drugs.

or uncontrolled trials, but no controlled trials yet attest to their safety and efficacy in older adults (19). In fact, olanzapine, quetiapine, risperidone, and aripiprazole have all been FDA approved for the treatment of acute mania (both as monotherapy and with either lithium or divalproex). Antimanic efficacy appears to be a class effect of the atypical antipsychotic medications.

Overall, the atypical antipsychotics are associated with less-severe extrapyramidal effects than conventional agents, but many of them can produce adverse effects including weight gain, glucose intolerance, hyperprolactinemia, orthostatic hypotension, gait disturbance, and sedation. Dosing of atypical antipsychotics in the elderly is typically one-half to one-third the daily dose recommended for younger patients, although effective dosing varies with such factors as comorbid medical illness and age (40). McDonald and Nemeroff recommend risperidone 0.5 mg or olanzapine 5.0 mg as acceptable alternatives to haloperidol in the regimen described above (41). Mixed-age patients benefit from using adjunctive risperidone with divalproex or lithium (42,43); however, only one of three patients older than 55 responded in these reports. Olanzapine monotherapy demonstrated superior efficacy compared with placebo for the treatment of mania in mixed-age patients, and a preliminary analysis of manic patients 50 and older suggests efficacy of olanzapine monotherapy (34). Preliminary open label experience with quetiapine in older adults has suggested that it may have a role in the management of geriatric bipolar patients (44). Mean dosing of quetiapine in elderly patient groups, including patients with bipolar disorder, has been around 100 mg/day (44), although present-day dosing suggests that increases up to around 300–400 mg/day, as a split dose, may be more efficacious in some patients.

Shulman reported the use of clozapine in doses ranging from 25 mg to 112.5 mg/day for management of refractory geriatric bipolar mania (45). Aripiprazole in the range of 10 mg to 30 mg/day has been useful in treating mania in younger adults, and it may be that a lower dose range, perhaps 5 mg to 20 mg/day, will be appropriate for geriatric patients (46). Despite apparent efficacy and an improved side-effect profile compared with the conventional antipsychotic agents, the need remains for further controlled data on the optimal use of atypical antipsychotic agents in older adults with mania (47).

Lithium

While many clinicians have come to rely on atypical antipsychotic medications during the acute treatment of geriatric mania, some authorities still include lithium salts among the first-line agents for both acute and longer-term treatment (36). Lithium remains one of the first-line treatments for acute mania in younger adults, and is a proven maintenance treatment for bipolar disorder in the adult population (48). Lithium, olanzapine, and lamotrigine are the only FDA-approved medications for maintenance treatment in bipolar disorder. Available as lithium carbonate or as the liquid lithium citrate, lithium salts have not been studied in the elderly under double-blind conditions, but have been reported effective as acute or prophylactic treatments in several open trials (19). Lithium pharmacokinetics are altered in the aging body. The older adult's decreased volume of distribution for hydrophilic drugs like lithium, combined with reduced renal clearance, can elevate serum lithium levels (47). Reduced clearance also increases the elimination half-life of lithium in the elderly, from the 24 hours typical for younger adults to about 28 to 36 hours. Perhaps even more than in younger patients, lithium treatment of older patients can be associated with discouraging side effects such as polyuria, tremor, mental slowing and memory difficulties, sinus node dysfunction, peripheral edema, hypothyroidism or nontoxic goiter, a worsening of arthritis, nausea, diarrhea, or worsening of acne or psoriasis. These effects may become intolerable even at serum levels well below those regarded as toxic in younger adults. The presence of cognitive impairment or pre-existing tremor increases the likelihood of side effects. Finally, recovery from lithium-induced delirium can be prolonged in older patients (49).

An ongoing review of concomitant medications while prescribing lithium is essential. Lithium's serum level can be raised by many nonsteroidal anti-inflammatory agents, angiotensin-converting enzyme inhibitors, and even more strongly by thiazide diuretics. For these reasons, the pretreatment workup should include a thorough review of current medications, as well as an electrocardiogram, electrolytes, renal function tests (blood urea nitrogen and creatinine levels) and thyroid-stimulating hormone. Serum creatinine levels can be imprecise in an elderly individual, due to decreased skeletal muscle mass and a concomitant decrease in glomerular filtration rate; thus a 24-hour creatinine clearance may be more useful for establishing an accurate baseline measure of renal function (17). If the serum creatinine rises, or if there is concern about the risk of lithium-induced renal insufficiency, a 24-hour creatinine clearance should be obtained.

Lithium treatment can be initiated at a dosage of 150 mg to 300 mg at bedtime. Lithium citrate, the liquid form of lithium, provides a simple means for dose titration or for using lower dosages. If nausea is present, Lithobid or Eskalith CR, the slow release preparations of lithium, may be better tolerated. For patients with diarrhea, the sustained release preparations may exacerbate the problem. Administration of the entire lithium dose at bedtime may reduce daytime sedation. The dose range of lithium typically used is 300 mg to 900 mg/day, in order to achieve serum levels between 0.6 mg and 1.0 mEq/L (8), although lower levels such as 0.4 to 0.8 mEq/L have also been advocated as effective (50). Recent studies have supported lower levels of lithium (0.8 mEq/L) in maintenance treatment (51). Lithium levels and other laboratory parameters should be monitored at regular intervals and in response to such events as dosage changes, changes in sodium or water intake or excretion, or co-administration of medications that affect lithium metabolism.

Interestingly, serum lithium levels may not correlate with brain lithium levels based on preliminary findings from MRI spectroscopy studies (52). More recent work has demonstrated an increased brain-to-peripheral lithium concentration ratio, with increased age potentially increasing vulnerability to neurocognitive toxicity (53). These findings may have clinical implications for an older patient on lithium, and support the use of the lowest possible serum levels necessary to maintain therapeutic effect and avoid toxicity.

Mood-Stabilizing Anticonvulsants

Divalproex Sodium

Divalproex sodium (DVP) is effective for the acute treatment of mania in younger adults, and appears to be at least modestly effective and fairly well-tolerated in elderly manic patients (54,55). Unfortunately, no double-blind, placebo-controlled trials are yet available in elderly cohorts. A mixed-age population of lithium refractory patients and those with neurological abnormalities appears to be particularly responsive to DVP (56). Additional support for the use of DVP in older manic patients derives from the observation that younger patients with mixed states respond better to DVP than to lithium (57).

Sanderson noted a recent trend toward less frequent use of lithium and more frequent use of DVP in the treatment of hospitalized elderly manic patients at a university-affiliated teaching hospital (58). Increased use of DVP was attributed to patient choice, presence of rapid-cycling mood symptoms, intolerance of lithium side effects, or medical concerns such as compromised renal function or thyroid abnormalities. Compared with lithium or carbamazepine, however, DVP treatment was not associated with a decreased average length of stay.

Treatment with DVP can be accompanied by side effects including nausea, tremor, ataxia, asymptomatic serum hepatic transaminase elevations, alopecia, increased appetite, weight gain, sedation, and cognitive impairment. Some older patients with mania often acutely require higher doses and serum levels of DVP, but toxic side effects—including sedation, gait disturbance, and cognitive impairment—may develop. Hepatic and pancreatic toxicity is infrequent among the elderly, although baseline liver and pancreatic function should be assessed. DVP is highly protein-bound, and thus capable of interacting with other highly bound medications such as warfarin (17). In addition, DVP modestly inhibits the cytochrome P450 enzyme system, and strongly inhibits certain glucuronidation enzymes. The inhibition of specific glucuronidation pathways can lead to a clinically significant increase in the levels of lamotrigine.

DVP is available as capsules, sprinkles, or as Depakene syrup, accommodating patients who have difficulty swallowing. A typical starting dose of DVP is 125 to 250 mg at bedtime, with a recommended increase over several days to 250 mg twice a day, and eventually to a range of 500 to 1000 mg/day. Blood levels between 50 and 100 μg/mL are usually optimal (8), although clinical efficacy in the elderly may be obtained with somewhat lower levels. A DVP extended-release formulation, allowing for once-daily dose administration, has been approved for the treatment of migraine headaches. This formulation of divalproex (Depakote ER) may be better tolerated than DVP and have clinical utility in geriatric bipolar disorder, although no randomized, controlled clinical trials are yet available.

Other Mood-Stabilizing Anticonvulsants

Other anticonvulsants have been used in elderly bipolar patients, although with limited support from controlled studies. Carbamazepine, problematic because of its neurological side effects, such as ataxia, cognitive impairment, and drug interactions, has largely been superseded by DVP. More recently, oxcarbazepine has been used as a potentially better-tolerated replacement for carbamazepine. However, there is far less efficacy data in mania for oxcar-

bazepine than for carbamazepine. Serum sodium levels should be monitored for patients on both medications regardless of changes in mental status, due to the approximately 2.5% incidence of hyponatremia. Several other anticonvulsants that claim more tolerable side-effect profiles have elicited interest, including gabapentin, topiramate, tiagabine, zonisamide, lamotrigine, and levetiracetam. Gabapentin co-administered with venlafaxine was reported to control the recurrent depressive symptoms and suicidal ideation in a lithium-intolerant 73-year-old bipolar patient (59). A recent case series of seven patients (59 and older) reported the safe and effective use of gabapentin (dosages of 600 to 1200 mg/day) along with antipsychotic medications and DVP in the treatment of geriatric mania (60). Topiramate was successfully used as adjunctive therapy (along with DVP, olanzapine, and lorazepam) at a dose of 250 mg/day in a 65-year-old male with treatment-resistant bipolar disorder (61). However, as was the case with gabapentin, topiramate and leviteracetam failed in pharmaceutical industry-supported studies of acute mania. Zonisamide appears to hold some promise of efficacy in studies of adults with bipolar disorder, and is well tolerated. Overall, however, these newer anticonvulsants have not yet been sufficiently studied with prospective controlled trials in elderly bipolar mania patients to justify an authoritative recommendation for use.

Changing Prescription Practice

Shulman and colleagues report that among older bipolar patients, the number of new lithium users decreased while the number of DVP users jumped from 1993 to 2001 (62). The authors argue that before lithium is abandoned in favor of DVP, further systematic evaluation of safety, effectiveness, and comparable or superior efficacy is needed (62). This advice is further supported by a recent study by Goodwin comparing lithium to DVP in a large HMO cohort of over 20,000 cases (63). Using a case-control design, lithium was far superior to DVP in terms of preventing suicide attempts.

Newer Agents

In time, it is likely that additional classes of agents will prove efficacious in treating late-life mania. Among medications currently in use for other indications, the acetylcholinesterase inhibitors may warrant further investigation with respect to the treatment of mania. In a case series of 11 younger treatment-resistant bipolar adults that included four manic and five mixed patients, Burt and colleagues found donepezil effective and well-tolerated in doses ranging from 3.75 to 10 mg/day (64). Side effects included insomnia, diarrhea, nausea, and sedation. Further study of the acetylcholinesterase inhibitors as treatments for geriatric mania (or perhaps other phases of the disorder) is warranted.

Electroconvulsive Therapy (ECT)

ECT, a valuable treatment in late-life depressive episodes, also remains an important intervention in the acute treatment of late-life mania. ECT is often reserved for patients who are resistant to medication or who require a rapid symptomatic resolution due to risks of dangerousness or malnutrition. Most responders can then be switched to pharmacologic maintenance, with or without ECT maintenance (15). An important consideration in using ECT in an elderly population is the issue of electrode placement. Bilateral treatments may have efficacy advantages in mania (65), while unilateral placement may be associated with reduced cognitive disturbance (66). McDonald (8) has recommended that suprathreshold stimulus (150% to 400% over the stimulus threshold) using unilateral placement is as effective as bilateral treatments. The co-administration of ECT and lithium should be avoided due to the risk of confusional reactions (11).

Mania may also occur in the context of behavioral agitation in patients with dementia. McDonald and Thompson reported a series of three patients with mania in dementia, refractory to psychotropic medication, who responded to an acute and maintenance course of right-unilateral ECT (67). For more information, see the chapter on ECT in this textbook.

GERIATRIC BIPOLAR DEPRESSION

Bipolar depression is a complex and difficult-to-treat condition that remains seriously understudied. As with the state of evidence-based knowledge with geriatric mania and mixed manic/rapid-cycling subtypes, the pharmacological management of bipolar depression in the elderly has not been adequately studied (42). Nonetheless, there is now a large and accumulating body of evidence in support of the use of lamotrigine and olanzapine plus fluoxetine in the treatment of adult bipolar depression.

The diagnosis of bipolar depression is often overlooked due to its similarity to unipolar depression, and to the frequent difficulty in identifying past hypomanic and manic episodes. The proper management of bipolar depression in younger adult populations is becoming more certain, due in part to the growing quantity of controlled data. Compared to lamotrigine and certain atypical antipsychotic agents, the traditional mood stabilizers lithium and DVP have limited efficacy in bipolar depression, particularly when compared to their strong antimanic effects. Despite the potential risk of a switch into hypomania or mania, the addition of an antidepressant drug to ongoing mood-stabilizer treatment has been the standard of care in the community. Preliminary studies support the use of bupropion or an SSRI in this situation, due to their apparent reduced rate of switch into mania, at least compared to tricyclic antidepressants and monoamine oxidase inhibitors (68).

BIPOLAR DEPRESSION: OVERALL TREATMENT STRATEGY

The goal of treatment for any patient with bipolar depression is relief of the depressive symptoms, but without inducing a switch into mania or an acceleration of cycle frequency. This goal can be achieved through proper mood-stabilizer treatment and by minimal and cautious use of antidepressant agents (69,70). Antidepressants can be considered a necessary evil, since they often provide short-term benefit, but over the long-term almost certainly increase the risk of mania and rapid cycling (71,72). Thus, minimizing the patient's exposure to antidepressants is another important goal. Decreasing the use of antidepressants in bipolar depression is now easier to achieve, since some newer mood stabilizers appear to have stronger antidepressant properties than conventional mood stabilizers. These mood-elevating mood stabilizers, including lamotrigine, some atypical antipsychotics, and omega-3 fatty acids from fish oil, appear to have at least modest antimanic effects and strong antidepressant action.

One way to think about treatment strategies for bipolar depression is to divide patients into categories based on the potential morbidity or lethality of their illness. For example, in patients with mild bipolar depression, where the risk of suicide is limited and there is little vocational and psychosocial disability, there is a larger range of treatment options. Some of the acceptable pharmacological options for mild cases of bipolar depression may have only anecdotal evidence supporting their efficacy. The use of these less-proven treatments may be justified if the side effect burden is less or if other, more conventional treatments, have been tried and failed. In addition, through self-help groups, the burgeoning number of books on the subject, and the Internet, more and more patients themselves are demanding alternative and less-tested treatment options. A risk-benefit analysis performed with the active participation of the patient should be performed and documented, particularly if a nonestablished treatment is to be used.

Patients with severe bipolar depression, with the attendant risks of suicide and psychosocial dysfunction, require more conventional and aggressive therapy, often with multiple agents and psychosocial interventions. Because of the severity of the illness, the use of treatments with established efficacy, even if these agents have less-than-favorable side-effect profiles, are required, at least initially. These more established treatments include ECT or standard mood stabilizers, with or without conventional antidepressants.

Mild to Moderate Bipolar Depression

Patients with cyclothymia or bipolar disorder (DSM-IV-TR type I, II, or not otherwise specified) may present with only mild symptoms of depression. If a patient with mild bipolar depression is already receiving a mood stabilizer, then one of the best strategies is to do nothing (72). If the patient is not receiving medication, a mood stabilizer should be considered to reduce the risk of subsequent mania. Although usually more effective for manic states, introducing lithium, DVP, or carbamazepine will sometimes produce antidepressant effects. Providing support until the depressive episode spontaneously remits is often adequate for mild or even moderate bipolar depression, particularly if the risk of suicide or disability from ongoing depressive symptoms is minimal. Psychotherapy can also be useful (73,74). This avoidance of antidepressants will reduce the likelihood of inducing mania or rapid cycling over the long term.

Intervention with mood-elevating treatments may be indicated for some patients with mild-to-moderate depressive symptoms who cannot tolerate them, or who strongly request antidepressant treatment. Antidepressants may also be indicated if mild depressive symptoms persist. If suicide risk and psychosocial dysfunction is minimal, then safer, although less-proven treatments, may be tried first if desired. These less-established treatment modalities include the use of brief, daily treatment with bright light therapy (75,76), intermittent sleep deprivation (77,78), or omega-3 fatty acids from fish oil. It is important to emphasize that the patient (and often the family) should be informed of the risks and benefits of a range of reasonable treatment options. The combination of a standard mood stabilizer, such as lithium or DVP, with an antidepressant is a common and accepted form of treatment (79).

Severe or Treatment-Refractory Bipolar Depression

If a patient with bipolar disorder is suffering from a moderate to severe episode of major depression or is treatment-refractory, more aggressive pharmacotherapy or ECT is indicated. Aggressive pharmacotherapy usually involves the use of a mood stabilizer with an antidepressant, with or without an augmentation agent. Aggressive antidepressant treatment is indicated because of the high morbidity and mortality in patients with severe bipolar depression. Newer agents, such as lamotrigine, atypical antipsychotic agents, or omega-3 fatty acids appear to induce mania or cycle acceleration less often than conventional antidepressants, and can be added to an existing regimen of an antidepressant and a mood stabilizer to boost the effectiveness of the treatment.

Highly refractory and protracted depressive episodes in bipolar disorder have not been studied systematically in adult populations, much less in a geriatric cohort. Patients with such difficult-to-treat bipolar depressive episodes may require treatment strategies with minimal support in the medical literature, and must make decisions based on clinical judgment or consensus guidelines (79).

Some of these measures include lowering the dose or even discontinuing a mood stabilizer, sleep deprivation, ECT, or combination therapies, including tranylcypromine plus risperidone (80) or venlafaxine plus mirtazapine (81).

Major Depression with Rapid-Cycling

If a patient with current bipolar depression also has rapid cycling, one should generally discontinue any antidepressant treatment, optimize the mood stabilizer(s), and wait. It may take several weeks to months for the patient's mood to stabilize. Continuing with antidepressant therapy in a depressed patient with rapid-cycling bipolar disorder may lift the depressive symptoms acutely, but could be associated with the long-term risk of mood cycle acceleration. Once again, lamotrigine, atypical antipsychotic agents, and the omega-3 fatty acids may be of benefit. In monotherapy, the anticonvulsant mood stabilizers DVP and carbamazepine tend to be more effective than lithium monotherapy in rapid cycling. However, combinations of mood stabilizers are usually required in these patients (79).

MOOD-ELEVATING MOOD STABILIZERS

Although not specifically studied in controlled trials of older adults with bipolar disorder, the mood-elevating mood stabilizers, such as lamotrigine, atypical antipsychotic agents, and perhaps omega-3 fatty acids, appear to have at least modest antimanic effects, but exhibit strong antidepressant action in adult populations. The risk of a switch into hypomania or mania by the mood-elevating mood stabilizers appears to be lower than with the conventional antidepressants.

Lamotrigine

The lack of sedation and generally benign side-effect profile makes lamotrigine a very attractive treatment option for the elderly, although prospective controlled data are not available. Lamotrigine has now been shown to have acute and prophylactic antidepressant effects. In the largest double-blind, placebo-controlled study of bipolar depression to date, Calabrese and colleagues observed that both 50 mg (N = 66) and 200 mg (N = 63) per day of lamotrigine were superior to placebo (N = 63) by week 3 onwards, in an 8-week study of patients with acute bipolar depression (82). In terms of prophylactic antidepressant action, two large, double-blind, placebo-controlled maintenance trials of 18 months duration were performed. The first study examined the prophylactic effects of lamotrigine monotherapy (N = 59) versus lithium monotherapy (N = 46) versus placebo (N = 70) in patients with bipolar disorder type I, who were recently manic or hypomanic (83). Lamotrigine and lithium were equivalent to each other, and both were substantially superior to placebo in delaying the time to a mood episode. When the data were examined more closely, it was observed that lamotrigine strongly delayed the onset of bipolar depression, while lithium and placebo did not. In contrast, lithium was superior to both lamotrigine and placebo in delaying the recurrence of mania or hypomania. The second study was similar in design and results to the first study, except that all of the subjects were recently depressed (84). As observed in the first study, lamotrigine (three different dosages combined statistically for the primary endpoint analysis, N = 221) and lithium (N = 121) were superior to placebo (N = 121) in delaying the time to any mood episode. As before, lamotrigine had robust prophylactic antidepressant action, superior to both lithium and placebo, while lithium bested both lamotrigine and placebo for prophylactic antimanic effects. In September 2003, lamotrigine was approved by the FDA for the maintenance treatment of bipolar type I disorder.

Lamotrigine therapy should be initiated at 12.5 to 25 mg/day, increasing no more than 12.5 to 25 mg/day every 2 weeks, with a target dosage of 200 mg/day in younger adult patients. The lamotrigine dosage of 200 mg/day was the approximate median effective dosage in the more recent controlled studies. Target dosages of lamotrigine for a geriatric population are not known. Starting low and going slow will minimize the risk of benign skin rash and greatly reduce the likelihood of Stevens-Johnson syndrome (SJS). The most significant known drug interaction for lamotrigine involves DVP. Conjugation via glucuronidation is the major route of lamotrigine biotransformation. DVP can double the serum level and half-life of lamotrigine via inhibition of lamotrigine glucuronidation. If lamotrigine is started in a patient already receiving DVP, it is important to reduce lamotrigine dosage titration by approximately 50%. Specifically, lamotrigine in the presence of DVP should be started at 12.5 to 25 mg every other day for 2 weeks, then 12.5 to 25 mg/day for 2 weeks, increasing by 12.5 to 25 mg every 2 weeks to a target dosage of approximately 100 mg/day. More rapid dosage titration when DVP and lamotrigine are used concurrently increases the likelihood of skin reactions.

This same pharmacokinetic interaction will lead to a marked drop in lamotrigine serum levels if DVP is discontinued. When switching from DVP to lamotrigine in patients with bipolar disorder, one reasonable method to accomplish this transition is to begin a gradual taper of the DVP dosage once lamotrigine has reached its target dosage and achieved a steady-state serum concentration (approximately 4 days later). At a DVP dosage of approximately 500 mg/day or less, the inhibition of lamotrigine conjugation is greatly diminished, and the dosage of lamotrigine may be doubled over a 1-week period. Over the same week-long period, the DVP may be tapered and then discontinued.

The opposite strategy is used if DVP is added to ongoing lamotrigine. Upon adding 500 mg/day of DVP, one could expect a doubling of the lamotrigine serum level, so an immediate 50% lamotrigine dose reduction is necessary.

Among the major mood stabilizers, lamotrigine stands out as the best-tolerated medication. There is no appreciable sedation, weight gain, or cognitive dulling. In addition, laboratory studies are not necessary. These features may make lamotrigine in the treatment of older adults particularly attractive. There are no other mood stabilizers with this favorable combination of efficacy and tolerability. Lamotrigine is also neuroprotective in animal models of brain ischemia via its blockade of the sodium channel linked to the excitatory N-methyl-D-aspartate (NMDA) glutamate neurotransmitter system.

Despite its attractive features, lamotrigine has several drawbacks that have limited its use in bipolar disorder. The most important is the frequent occurrence of benign skin rashes and the very rare presentation of more serious and life-threatening dermatological reactions, notably SJS (85,86). SJS is a form of exfoliative dermatitis, generally drug induced, where the epidermis becomes necrotic and sloughs off. Patients require early and aggressive treatment in intensive care or burn units. There is an overall mortality rate of 10% with SJS and 50% with the more severe form, known as toxic epidermal necrolyisis. Early detection and treatment greatly reduces the mortality rate (87). The overwhelming majority of skin rashes are benign, and recede spontaneously even with continued lamotrigine therapy. If a lamotrigine-associated rash develops, many clinicians keep the dose constant or lower it until the rash subsides. Once the rash is gone, the dose titration can resume, but at a slower pace.

The major drawback to lamotrigine is the slow dosage titration required for safe use. This gradual titration reduces the risk of SJS to that of most other drugs, but unfortunately precludes the rapid use of lamotrigine for acute bipolar depression or mixed states. There is a lot of misinformation and confusion over the risk of SJS and other serious dermatologic reactions from lamotrigine. With the currently recommended titration schedule, the risk of SJS is similar to or less than that of carbamazepine, phenobarbital, and many other common drugs. The disproportionate fear of SJS can be traced to the extraordinarily high dosages used initially (100 mg twice a day) after its release in Germany in 1993. Compare this 200 mg/day starting dosage with the current recommended starting dose of 12.5 to 25 mg/day. With a gradual dosage titration, the risk of a serious skin rash may be as low as one case per 100,000 to 500,000 exposures. It is also important to put the risk of actually dying from lamotrigine-associated SJS into perspective. The lifetime risk of dying from bipolar disorder (suicide, accidents, etc.) is somewhere between 10% to 25%. A promptly detected and appropriately managed case of SJS from a recommended lamotrigine dosage titration schedule has a mortality rate probably approaching one to two cases per one million exposures. This rate is no different from many commonly used medications.

Lithium

There are several older controlled studies of bipolar depression using lithium monotherapy, in which lithium was more effective than placebo or the comparison medication

(88,89). However, these studies were performed in the late 1960s and 1970s, when many patients diagnosed with bipolar disorder may have had more classic forms of bipolar disorder type I, with predominantly euphoric manias. More recent studies have demonstrated, in contrast, high rates of psychiatric comorbidity, including substance abuse, and a significant presence of dysphoric or mixed manic states and rapid cycling (90).

Assuming it is effective, lithium has several distinct advantages over other mood stabilizers for the treatment of bipolar depression. For example, lithium is the only mood stabilizer with demonstrated anti-suicide effects (91). Other mood stabilizers may also possess this clinical action but, to date, the data are lacking. Lithium has also been used for more than 30 years in bipolar disorder, and clinicians are familiar with its use. However, lithium has some distinct disadvantages as well. For example, lithium can be neurotoxic or deadly in overdose, an obvious risk when treating depressed and impulsive patients. In addition, despite the strategies developed over the years to mitigate some lithium-associated side effects, the burden of these symptoms may be too great for some patients to bear over the long term. Any patient with bipolar disorder, whether receiving lithium or not, may develop low-grade depressive symptoms. These mild depressive states must be distinguished from the similar-appearing cognitive dulling often seen during lithium therapy, as well as from lithium-induced hypothyroidism.

The optimal serum lithium level for bipolar depression remains unclear. Until more data are published, it is reasonable to use a dosage of lithium to produce serum lithium levels in the usual therapeutic range of 0.5 to 1.0 mEq/L. As demonstrated in the above clinical example, the lower end of this range is often adequate for many older patients.

Divalproex

There are no published studies examining the efficacy of DVP in bipolar depression. Clinically, most experts agree that while DVP is a first-line drug for mania, DVP monotherapy is generally not adequate for pure bipolar depression (79). Generally, any antidepressant, including a monoamine oxidase inhibitor (MAOI), can be added to a patient already receiving DVP. Presumably, as is the case with lithium, DVP would at least partially protect against mania and cycle acceleration induced by the antidepressant. Anecdotally, as with lithium, DVP has been observed to either induce depression or to stabilize or lock the patient's mood in a depressed state. Controlled data regarding DVP in bipolar depression would help to clarify these issues.

Carbamazepine

There is some limited, but positive data regarding the efficacy of carbamazepine in bipolar depression (92), as well as mixed manic states and possibly rapid cycling (93).

Recent findings suggest that carbamazepine's effects in bipolar disorder may diminish over the long term (94), perhaps due, in part, to carbamazepine's induction of the cytochrome system, leading to its own increased metabolism and clearance (autoinduction). Unfortunately, carbamazepine has several distinct drawbacks, most notably drug interaction risk, acting as a potent inducer of the cytochrome P450 enzymes, especially 3A3 and 3A4 (95). Finally, adverse effects on cognition and gait limit its use in an older population.

Atypical Antipsychotic Agents

In 2005, the atypical antipsychotic medication, olanzapine, in combination with the antidepressant fluoxetine (marketed under the brand name Symbyax) became the first FDA-approved medication for the treatment of bipolar depression (96). There are no clinical data published using this agent in geriatric bipolar depression, and clinical experience in this population is limited.

Antidepressant-Associated Mania in Late Life

Switching from depression to mania during pharmacotherapy with tricyclic and other antidepressant agents can occur in older adults, as in younger patients (97,98). While SSRIs and bupropion are favored in younger bipolar-depressed patients to reduce rates of switching, there have been no systematic comparisons of the association of mania with various antidepressants in an older population. MAOIs can benefit younger bipolar-depressed patients (99), and they are effective in geriatric unipolar depression (100), but have not been studied in geriatric bipolar depression. In general, tricyclic antidepressants and MAOIs have higher rates of switching than SSRIs and bupropion. Young and colleagues recently reported a retrospective review of inpatients over the age of 60 with bipolar disorder (98). They found that elderly antidepressant-associated mania patients were more often experiencing their first manic episode and had a later age of onset as compared with elderly patients with manic episodes not associated with antidepressant use. Most of these patients were treated with tricyclic antidepressant medications, since the study sample was selected from admissions prior to 1990 (98). The authors point out that this contrasts with studies showing an association between greater number of prior manic episodes and early age of illness onset among younger adults with antidepressant-associated mania (101).

Exploring this relationship in geriatric bipolar depression patients, investigators from Toronto found a lower-than-expected incidence of antidepressant-induced mania. Schaffer and colleagues identified 1,072 patients 66 and older who were hospitalized for mania or bipolar depression and had received a prescription for an antidepressant medication from 1994 to 2001, along with 3,000 other elderly patients with bipolar disorder who had not received antidepressants (102). Sixty percent of the antidepressants prescribed were SSRIs, 10% were venlafaxine, and 9% were tricyclic antidepressants. Hospital admissions for mania were more likely among non-antidepressant users than antidepressant users. This information contradicts most of the data about younger bipolar patients and the risk of mania with antidepressant medication, and again points out the great need for evidence-based treatment guidelines for geriatric bipolar disorder.

Omega-3 Fatty Acids

Omega-3 fatty acids are a group of nutritionally essential polyunsaturated lipids derived from marine or plant sources. Cold-water, oily ocean fish are one of the few sources of the physiologically active long-chain omega-3 fatty acids, i.e., EPA (eicosapentaenoic acid; 20-carbon, fatty acid chain with 5 double bonds), and DHA (docosahexanoic acid; 22-carbon fatty acid chain with 6 double bonds). Recently, a series of controlled studies have reported efficacy of omega-3 fatty acids (particularly EPA) for the treatment of bipolar disorder, unipolar depression, schizophrenia, and borderline personality disorder (103).

Many brands of omega-3 supplements exist, with large and significant differences among them. EPA appears to be the active mood component of omega-3 supplements. A starting dosage of 0.5 to 1 g twice a day of EPA is now typical. If ineffective, the dosage may be increased gradually over 1 to 3 weeks to 6 g/day of EPA. Omega-3 supplements are very well tolerated and have numerous established health benefits. However, large amounts of any oil may produce occasional diarrhea or oily stools. Taking the supplement with a meal increases omega-3 absorption. The anti-platelet action of high-dose omega-3 oils could theoretically potentiate the anticoagulant effects of blood thinners. However, no well-documented cases of bleeding associated with omega-3s have been reported. There are no known controlled studies of omega-3 fatty acids in geriatric bipolar patients.

Natural Antidepressants

In addition to the omega-3 fatty acids, mood-elevating compounds such as inositol, St. John's wort (*Hypericum perforatums*), and S-adenosyl-L-methionine (SAMe) are becoming increasingly popular. All of these compounds appear to have some antidepressant effects and are well tolerated (104–106). However, SAMe has been associated with a high rate of manic induction (107) and is therefore contraindicated in patients with bipolar disorder. Inositol, the precursor to the second messenger molecule, inositol triphosphate, is currently under study as an antidepressant in bipolar depression (108).

There are little or no data supporting the use of St. John's wort in bipolar depression. There have been isolated case reports of mania induced by St. John's wort (109,110), which is not unexpected, considering its antidepressant qualities. One recently identified downside to St. John's wort is its moderate induction of cytochrome P450 3A4, which would lead to marked reductions in the blood levels of any 3A4 substrate.

MAINTENANCE THERAPY

Little information is available regarding maintenance treatment and prevention of subsequent episodes of late-life mania. DVP and lithium, which are effective maintenance medications in younger adults, are often used in the elderly as well, without rigorous supporting evidence (111). Lamotrigine and olanzapine are FDA approved for the prevention of recurrent episodes of bipolar I disorder (112). There are no controlled data of maintenance therapy using these agents in a geriatric population. Maintenance ECT is an option for patients who show poor response to maintenance medication regimens (19).

THEMES IN PHARMACOTHERAPY

Several themes seem to emerge in this review of pharmacotherapy for geriatric bipolar disorder. There is preliminary evidence that both lithium and DVP can be helpful in the treatment of late-life manic and mixed episodes. The treatment of bipolar depression in the elderly, however, is largely unexplored. There are inconsistent data regarding maintenance efficacy of lithium or DVP for the prevention of recurrent mania or bipolar depression in the elderly. Furthermore, the efficacy of these agents was studied mostly in uncontrolled studies, case reports, and case series, and not randomized, controlled clinical trials.

The acute and maintenance efficacy of other mood stabilizers, antidepressants, and antipsychotic medications has received even less attention, and only case reports and case series can serve as a guide for intervention with these medications. The risk and consequences of medication-related side effects in the elderly reflect age-related changes in pharmacokinetics. Medication-related toxicities are also affected by age-associated pharmacodynamic influences, as well as medical and neurological comorbidities.

Although the widely accepted mantra of starting low and going slow in the titration of medications for geriatric psychiatric conditions holds true for geriatric bipolar disorder, clinicians must be aware that conventional doses are often required to achieve optimum benefit in individual patients. A more gradual dose titration approach may help to limit unwanted side effects in an elderly population. In other words, our older patients with geriatric bipolar disorder may eventually require the same dose of medication as younger adults, it may just take longer to get there.

Table 26-4 shows recommended pharmacological approaches to the treatment of geriatric mania, bipolar depression, and maintenance therapy.

MEDICATION COMPLIANCE

The problem of poor medication compliance, also called medication adherence, among geriatric patients with unipolar depression has been studied, and lamented, by a number of researchers. And while the equally distressing prevalence of inadequate medication compliance among bipolar adults has been amply addressed in the literature, there are no compliance studies that focus specifically on geriatric bipolar patients. This section will therefore focus largely on compliance problems with bipolar adults in general, in the hope that some extrapolation to older adults is applicable, and in fact warranted, given the compliance data for geriatric patients with unipolar depression.

In a disturbing report, Post estimates that up to 75% of relapses in bipolar patients may be associated with noncompliance (93). The problem is longstanding and widely acknowledged. Basco and Rush found that 46% of bipolar clinic patients who were prescribed lithium failed to take their medications as directed (113). Conducting unannounced spot checks on 26 clinic patients, Schwarcz and Silbergeld found that blood-lithium levels in 42% of the patients were too low to be therapeutically effective (114). In an even earlier survey, Jamison and colleagues found that 90% of those who were prescribed lithium had considered discontinuing the medication (115). Eleven years later, these experts, still concerning themselves with the issue of compliance, asserted that nearly one-half of successfully treated lithium patients do not adhere to their prescribed medication regimen (26). Moving beyond the statistics, Craighead and Miklowitz explored the issue of what underlies noncompliance in bipolar patients (116). They cite lack of awareness about the medication's importance, denial of the illness, avoidance of medication because of associated stigma, physical side effects, missing the euphoria of manic episodes, and issues in the doctor-patient relationship. Scott reports on a study comparing doctor and patient perceptions of the reasons for noncompliance (117). The study found that clinicians attributed poor compliance in their bipolar patients to somatic side effects, while the patients themselves identified cognitive changes such as mental confusion and memory loss as the strongest factors in their noncompliance.

In a recent review of antidepressant compliance in older adults, Miller and colleagues focus on ways to maximize compliance, citing cost, concern about side effects, confusion, and poor understanding of the role of medication in illness management as factors in noncompliance (118). Reporting on research by Grossberg and colleagues (119), the authors counterintuitively conclude that elderly noncompliance is an intentional act rather than a consequence of faulty memory. Salzman offers a more forgiving interpretation, observing that compliance for older adults is complicated by the large number of medications taken for conditions related to aging (120). Estimating noncompliance in the elderly as ranging from 40% to 75%, Salzman cites data showing, for example, that when the number of drugs prescribed increases four-fold, noncompliance increases 15-fold. Finally, Salzman stresses the impact of the doctor-patient relationship, noting the statistically significant positive correlation between compliance and patient knowledge about medication. More information may be found in the chapter on Pharmacotherapy in this book.

The likely interaction effects between the factors known to contribute to noncompliance in bipolar patients in general, and those associated with noncompliance in patients with geriatric depression, justify a hypothesis that significant compliance problems exist in geriatric bipolar patients. Empirical research is clearly needed to motivate and inform the development of relevant and successful interventions.

PSYCHOTHERAPY

The efficacy of psychotherapy for geriatric bipolar disorder has not yet been addressed in the psychiatric literature, perhaps due to the appearance, only recently, of nonpharmacological treatments as an object of empirical study for geriatric mental disorders. The field of geriatric psychotherapy has expanded significantly in the last decade (121). This section will focus on important components of psychotherapy in bipolar disorder in general, followed by a discussion about specific psychotherapeutic interventions. For more information, see the chapter on psychotherapy in this textbook.

Psychotherapy with Bipolar Patients: General Principles

It is no secret that psychotherapists are a bit intimidated by the prospect of taking on a bipolar patient. Scott attributes this reluctance to:

- Widely accepted etiological models that highlight genetic and biological aspects of the disorder.
- A persistent belief that bipolar patients function normally between episodes.
- A psychoanalytic view of bipolar patients that historically viewed them as dependent, irritable, and lacking in introspective abilities (117).

The advent of lithium sparked an enormous body of literature on bipolar disorder, now spanning more than 3 decades, including empirical studies revealing that the probability of relapse is affected by a number of factors that are most appropriately addressed in the context of psychotherapy. According to Bloch and colleagues, psychosocial factors may account for 25% to 30% of the variance in the course of bipolar illness (122).

Perhaps the most frequently cited psychosocial trigger of relapse in the bipolar patient is poor medication adherence, which, as noted earlier in this chapter, is a problem for depressed older adults. A number of studies, however, have demonstrated the efficacy of psychotherapy in improving medication compliance (123–125). More recently, researchers have attempted to define the psychotherapeutic factors that are most potent in producing a favorable change in compliance. Miklowitz and colleagues stress the value of psychoeducation, but also underscore the importance of addressing the emotional underpinnings of noncompliance, including "grieving of the lost healthy self" (126). Over the past decade, there is also a growing body of literature implicating stressful events and disruption of biological rhythms, including sleep, as potent triggers of bipolar relapse. In a study spanning 2 years, Ellicott and colleagues found that bipolar patients with high life-events stress scores were 4.5 times more likely to suffer a flare-up of the illness than those with low-to-medium life stress (127). In some promising preliminary studies, interventions in which bipolar patients are taught to monitor and manage stress have been effective in reducing recurrence rates (128–130).

Certain types of family interactions have been associated with relapse in bipolar patients. *Expressed Emotion* (EE), a term coined by Miklowitz and colleagues, collectively refers to three negative attitudes overtly expressed in close relatives of psychiatric patients: criticism, hostility, and emotional over-involvement (126,131). A high-measured level of EE in the family of the bipolar patient has been shown to contribute to poor outcome. Recent studies have demonstrated the efficacy of family interventions focused on reducing EE in lowering relapse rates in bipolar patients (132–134).

Despite the assertion by the group therapist Irving Yalom that having bipolar patients in a therapy group is "one of the worst calamities" that could occur (117), studies of group interventions with bipolar patients over the past 3 decades have yielded positive results, including reduced readmissions and improved medication compliance (124,125,135). More recently, interest in group therapy for mood disorders has been motivated in part by managed-care mandates for more cost-effective treatment. Pollack conducted one of the few studies of inpatient group treatment for bipolar disorder, delineating three therapeutic goals: sharing information about the illness, learning strategies of coping with the disorder, and improving interpersonal relationships (136). Other researchers have reported effective group treatments that have included psychoeducation regarding triggers, confrontation of denial about the illness, and restoration of the patient's identity and capacity for intimacy (137,138). In addition, various theoretical models have been proposed for intervening with bipolar patients, and two in particular have demonstrated promising results: interpersonal psychotherapy, which for bipolar patients has been combined with social rhythm therapy and referred to as IPSRT (128), and cognitive behavior therapy (139,140).

Specific Psychotherapeutic Interventions

The potential value of psychotherapeutic treatment of a geriatric mood disorder is suggested by findings of psychotherapeutic efficacy in geriatric unipolar depression. Researchers stress the relative power of combined psychosocial and pharmacological treatments of older depressed adults (141) when compared to either form of treatment alone. Although there are no similar data for bipolar geriatric patients, it would be a reasonable hypothesis that the same might hold true for them. McQuaid and colleagues (142) offer one of the very few reports of psychotherapy in the treatment of psychosis in geriatric patients. This pilot study employed a novel integrated treatment combining cognitive-behavioral therapy and social skills training, adapted for older adults with schizophrenia. Sessions included a focus on medication compliance, identifying relapse warning signs, developing an emergency plan for coping with these symptoms, and reducing the likelihood of recurrence through self-monitoring. The results, although limited, were promising.

In our academic hospital-based geriatric psychiatry setting, which employs a model of continuity of geriatric psychiatric care from inpatient to partial hospitalization to outpatient, we have treated large numbers of geriatric bipolar patients and have found certain techniques quite useful. The majority of clinicians would agree that individual therapy with a medically unstabilized, actively manic patient of any age is an exercise in futility. However, psychosocial intervention can be accomplished at this stage with a program designed for the patient's family. As noted earlier, Miklowitz designed a program of psychoeducation and support for the family of the bipolar patient that offers promising results (132). Similar interventions can be accomplished with the family of an older patient, the difference being that the family now consists of an elderly spouse and/or grown children. Most families of the bipolar older adult will have ongoing experience with the disorder; grown children may have witnessed it first-hand in their childhood years, with the not-infrequent result being longstanding resentment of the ill parent. This makes support and validation of the adult child's ongoing struggle as caretaker an important part of the intervention. At the same time, the unique features of geriatric mania—for example, agitation and pronounced cognitive slippage—may be presenting for the first time, creating confusion and further distress for the family, and therefore becoming an important component of psychoeducation.

As the patient stabilizes, group therapy becomes a viable inpatient option; because of managed care issues and staff shortages, individual therapy is less frequently utilized in the inpatient setting. The older bipolar patient can benefit tremendously from groups that address medication compliance, illness management, and stress reduction. Psychoeducation is an integral component of such treatment, which also has the advantage of being appealing to the current cohort of older adults. As the bipolar older adult stabilizes, remnants of the irritability, pressured speech, and agitation of the manic episode may still be manifest in group therapy, albeit attenuated. This is readily apparent to other patients in the group, although group members will also acknowledge the magnitude of the bipolar patient's improvement during stabilization. The therapist in such cases maintains a delicate balance between setting limits and validating the bipolar patient as he or she attempts to return to baseline modes of effective communication. Many patients at this stage will acknowledge some awareness of their residual symptoms: "I am talking too much, right, doctor?" At this point the technique of *focused interactive listening* (FIL), a form of listening in which the therapist focuses attentively and carefully to content while also responding with nonverbal cues to mirror the patient's concerns, becomes an important component of treatment for a patient who may be experiencing considerable difficulty feeling heard by peers, staff, or even family (143). As the therapist models FIL within the group setting, while gently setting limits as needed, the other group members often follow suit, allowing the newly stabilized bipolar patient a context of acceptance and support. For the bipolar patient in a depressed state, the initial goal in group therapy becomes gradual encouragement of the patient to speak openly, with others in the group in more advanced stages of stabilization serving as models for productive sharing.

As the patient graduates to partial and outpatient settings, individual therapy becomes more available. At this stage, the patient has usually stabilized. Patients whose most recent episode was manic may be euthymic, while patients originally presenting with depression are experiencing improved mood. The family continues to be seen supportively, and with the patient's return home, some modifications in behavior and communication among family members can be actively rehearsed. Individual sessions with the patient involve an integrated approach with historical exploration to assess the patient's experiences in the early years of his or her illness, which for older adults may have preceded the advent of lithium. The purpose of this is two-fold: to validate the patient's long struggle—and strength—in dealing with the illness, and to provide a retrospective view of what the patient has learned over the course of his illness about triggering factors and management of the condition. Throughout the sessions, the therapist assumes an actively mirroring and reinforcing stance. This assists the patient in repairing the self-fragmentation triggered by the flare-up of the illness, which is superimposed on an elderly self (144) already taxed by the losses

and limitations brought on by aging. This historical review generates an empathic diagnosis (144), which informs further therapeutic intervention to address current difficulties, resulting in an integrative form of psychotherapy that combines a developmental perspective with cognitive interventions modified for older adults (143). This approach has been termed *gerocognitive behavior therapy* (GBT). This integrative model of treatment offers preventive strategies including management of stress, attention to biological rhythms, improved medication compliance, and reparative measures to deal with the interpersonal, social, and practical aftermath of the manic or depressive episode.

More research is needed to generate psychotherapeutic approaches that can be standardized for the treatment of geriatric bipolar disorder. Interest in empirical validation of such techniques will hopefully grow as members of the largest generation in United States history begin to form the next cohort of older adults.

CASE EXAMPLE UPDATE

Mr. W (cited earlier) began outpatient therapy with pronounced feelings of inadequacy and guilt about his relapse and subsequent hospitalization. He also touched on a number of family issues—his estranged son, his divorce, his relationship with his caring but somewhat controlling daughter, and a romantic relationship that he had been in for a number of years. While in a partial hospitalization program, treatment had included periodic sessions with his daughter to offer education and support around the patient's illness. However, once in outpatient treatment, Mr. W strongly expressed a preference for therapy alone. This was respected and interpreted as the patient's attempt to become more autonomous, and also to allow his daughter to "live her own life." The patient agreed to reconsider this plan at a later stage in treatment. In the absence of the structure of the partial program, Mr. W was at a loss for how to prevent and control the hypomanic episodes that were rapidly cycling through longer periods of depression. Mr. W was offered a weekly program of gerocognitive behavior therapy (GBT), beginning with a thorough exploration of his history, with mirroring and FIL as an integral part of the process, even during the evaluation period. It became clear that growing up in an emotionally chaotic and deprived environment, with a bipolar mother who required frequent hospitalization, and a critical, alcoholic father, Mr. W had internalized a belief system about himself that was distorted and self-defeating. As Mr. W looked back on a life that included significant personal achievements, despite multiple episodes of illness, he was gradually able to credit himself with strength and perseverance and grant that his educational and career achievements, as well as his ability to raise a family while struggling with a chronic mental illness, were victories rather than failures. Thus, with the help of active, positive reframing by the therapist, he was able to significantly modify his cognitive distortions and core belief system to achieve a figure/ground reversal in the perception of his life. Cognitive therapy was helpful in challenging and changing his negative core beliefs, and behavioral approaches were useful in building his skills for asserting himself with his daughter and girlfriend and managing stress, while also fine tuning his awareness of the early warning signs of both hypomania and depression. The patient has fortunately been consistently medication compliant, so this was not a necessary focus of treatment.

This period of relative stability continued for several months until, in December of 2003, Mr. W fell while helping a neighbor shovel his car out of a snow bank. The injury resulted in reduced mobility and precipitated a depressive episode severe enough to necessitate an inpatient stay of several weeks. Mr. W's insight regarding his depression was that the increased dependency induced by the fall was reminiscent of periods in his life when his autonomy had been compromised by psychiatric illness. Mr. W was discharged on the following medications: clonazepam 0.5 mg twice a day, lamotrigine 25 mg at bedtime, and sertraline 200 mg in the morning.

Immediately upon discharge from the hospital, Mr. W, with the help of his daughter, moved to an assisted-living facility. Following a 4-week return to the partial hospital program, where he had been treated 15 months earlier, Mr. W resumed his outpatient treatment in the early spring of 2004. Since then he has manifested a steady rate of improvement. He still struggles with periods of depression, but they are more manageable, and his hypomanic episodes have been attenuated to the extent that when his mood lifts he describes more a state of euthymia than being "up." Most importantly, the feelings of shame and inadequacy, which contributed to his suicidal ideation 2 years earlier and precipitated his hospitalization a year ago, have improved to the extent that he now spontaneously acknowledges his strengths and is able to credit himself for even the smallest steps he takes every day to stay well.

His current medications are as follows: lamotrigine 100 mg once a day, clonazepam 0.5 once a day, sertraline 200 mg in the morning, and mirtazapine 30 mg at bedtime. Mr. W has been largely euthymic, with some minor fluctuations in mood, for the past 6 months.

Case Commentary

Mr. W's case history provides an example of the complex presentation of bipolar disorder through the life cycle. Although diagnosed by his clinicians as bipolar disorder type II with periods of hypomania and depression, some of the hypomanic episodes may have met criteria for mania given the duration of symptoms and effects on psychosocial functioning. Cognitive changes in the course of bipolar disorder were evident, since Mr. W presented with memory and word finding difficulties later in life, with neuropsychological evidence of attention and verbal memory difficulties. Furthermore, pharmacological challenges were notable throughout the duration of his treatment. His self-discontinuation of lithium led to periods of affective instability. Mood stabilizers, most recently

lamotrigine, were ultimately helpful, along with appropriate and judicious use of concomitant antidepressant medications. As this case demonstrates, symptom presentation and response to treatment can be quite variable in an older adult with bipolar disorder. Adjunctive ongoing treatment with psychotherapy was essential for long-term mood stability and to maximize psychosocial functioning.

CONCLUSIONS

Bipolar disorder presents complex diagnostic and treatment challenges in later life. Confounding syndromes of delirium and dementia often present difficulties in accurate diagnosis when standard DSM-IV-TR criteria for mania are used. The occurrence of mania in late life can represent recurrent illness, new, late-onset bipolar disorder, or a complication of various other neuropsychiatric conditions. The occurrence of manic symptoms in an older adult must prompt careful evaluation to identify treatable medical conditions. Pharmacological approaches and ECT can be helpful in acute and maintenance treatment of late-life mania as well as bipolar depression. Unfortunately, prospective randomized, controlled trials in all phases of geriatric bipolar disorder are currently lacking. Psychotherapy has much to offer in enhancing treatment compliance, addressing relapse risks, and helping patients cope with the implications of a chronic mental disorder. Controlled clinical research, in partnership with the technologies of genetics, molecular biology, and functional neuroimaging, will provide a better understanding of the neurobiological causes of geriatric bipolar disorder and help promote more specific and effective treatment strategies.

REFERENCES

1. Bartels SJ, Forester B, Miles KM, Joyce T. Mental health service use by elderly patients with bipolar disorder and unipolar major depression. *Am J Geriatr Psychiatry.* 2000;8(2):160–166.
2. Weissman MM, Bland RC, Canino GJ, et al. Cross-national epidemiology of major depression and bipolar disorder. *JAMA.* 1996;276(4):293–299.
3. Weissman MM, Leaf PJ, Tischler GL, et al. Affective disorders in five United States communities. *Psychol Med.* 1988;18(1): 141–153.
4. Angst J, Sellaro R. Historical perspectives and natural history of bipolar disorder. *Biol Psychiatry.* 2000;48(6):445–457.
5. Angst J, Baastrup P, Grof P, Hippius H, Poldinger W, Weis P. The course of monopolar depression and bipolar psychoses. *Psychiatr Neurol Neurochir.* 1973;76(6):489–500.
6. Spicer CC, Hare EH, Slater E. Neurotic and psychotic forms of depressive illness: evidence from age-incidence in a national sample. *Br J Psychiatry.* 1973;123(576):535–541.
7. Sibisi CD. Sex differences in the age of onset of bipolar affective illness. *Br J Psychiatry.* 1990;156:842–845.
8. McDonald WM. Epidemiology, etiology, and treatment of geriatric mania. *J Clin Psychiatry.* 2000;61(suppl 13):3–11.
9. Shulman KI, Tohen M, Satlin A, Mallya G, Kalunian D. Mania compared with unipolar depression in old age. *Am J Psychiatry.* 1992;149(3):341–345.
10. Yassa R, Nair NP, Iskandar H. Late-onset bipolar disorder. *Psychiatr Clin North Am.* 1988;11(1):117–131.

11. Young RC. Bipolar mood disorders in the elderly. *Psychiatr Clin North Am*. 1997;20(1):121–136.
12. Goldberg JF, Harrow M, Whiteside JE. Risk for bipolar illness in patients initially hospitalized for unipolar depression. *Am J Psychiatry*. 2001;158(8):1265–1270.
13. Angst J. The course of affective disorders: II. Typology of bipolar manic-depressive illness. *Arch Psychiatr Nervenkr*. 1978;226(1):65–73.
14. American Psychiatric Association. *Diagnostic and Statistical Manual of Mental Disorders-Text Revision (DSM-IV-TR)*. Washington, DC: American Psychiatric Association; 2000.
15. Forester BP, Antognini F, Sivrioglu EY, Schoos R, Fish DW, Ellison JM. Geriatric mania. *Directions in Psychiatry*. 2004; 24(1)43–55.
16. Harrow M, Grossman LS, Silverstein ML, Meltzer HY. Thought pathology in manic and schizophrenic patients. Its occurrence at hospital admission and seven weeks later. *Arch Gen Psychiatry*. 1982;39(6):665–671.
17. Satlin A, Liptzin B. Diagnosis and treatment of mania. In: Salzman C, ed. *Clinical Geriatric Psychopharmacology*. Baltimore, MD: Lippincott Williams and Wilkins; 1998:310–330.
18. Shulman KI, Herrmann N. The nature and management of mania in old age. *Psychiatr Clin North Am*. 1999;22(3):649–665.
19. Umapathy C, Mulsant BH, Pollock BG. Bipolar disorder in the elderly. *Psychiatric Annals*. 2000;30:473–480.
20. Krauthammer C, Klerman GL. Secondary mania: manic syndromes associated with antecedent physical illness or drugs. *Arch Gen Psychiatry*. 1978;35(11):1333–1339.
21. Tohen M, Castillo J, Pope HG Jr, Herbstein J. Concomitant use of valproate and carbamazepine in bipolar and schizoaffective disorders. *J Clin Psychopharmacol*. 1994;14(1):67–70.
22. McDonald W, Nemeroff CB. Practical guidelines for diagnosing and treating mania and bipolar disorder in the elderly. *Medscape Psychiatry & Mental Health eJournal*. 1998;3(2).
23. Stoll AL, Tohen M, Baldessarini RJ, et al. Shifts in diagnostic frequencies of schizophrenia and major affective disorders at six North American psychiatric hospitals, 1972–1988. *Am J Psychiatry*. 1993;150(11):1668–1673.
24. Cavanagh JT, Van Beck M, Muir W, Blackwood DH. Case-control study of neurocognitive function in euthymic patients with bipolar disorder: an association with mania. *Br J Psychiatry*. 2002;180:320–326.
25. Gildengers AG, Butters MA, Seligman K, et al. Cognitive functioning in late-life bipolar disorder. *Am J Psychiatry*. 2004; 161(4):736–738.
26. Goodwin FK, Jamison KR. Psychotherapy. In: Goodwin FK, Jamison KR, eds. *Manic Depressive Illness*. Oxford: Oxford University Press; 1990:725–745.
27. Migliorelli R, Starkstein SE, Teson A, et al. SPECT findings in patients with primary mania. *J Neuropsychiatry Clin Neurosci*. 1993;5(4):379–383.
28. Kobayashi S, Okada K, Yamashita K. Incidence of silent lacunar lesion in normal adults and its relation to cerebral blood flow and risk factors. *Stroke*. 1991;22(11):1379–1383.
29. McDonald WM, Krishnan KR, Doraiswamy PM, Blazer DG. Occurrence of subcortical hyperintensities in elderly subjects with mania. *Psychiatry Res*. 1991;40(4):211–220.
30. Altshuler LL, Bartzokis G, Grieder T, et al. An MRI study of temporal lobe structures in men with bipolar disorder or schizophrenia. *Biol Psychiatr*. 2000;48(2):147–162.
31. Videbech P. MRI findings in patients with affective disorder: a meta-analysis. *Acta Psychiatr Scand*. 1997;96(3):157–168.
32. Drevets WC, Price JL, Simpson JR Jr, et al. Subgenual prefrontal cortex abnormalities in mood disorders. *Nature*. 1997;386 (6627):824–827.
33. Ferrier IN, Thompson JM. Cognitive impairment in bipolar affective disorder: implications for the bipolar diathesis. *Br J Psychiatry*. 2002;180:293–295.
34. Young RC, Gyulai L, Mulsant BH, et al. Pharmacotherapy of bipolar disorder in old age: review and recommendations. *Am J Geriatr Psychiatry*. 2004;12(4):342–357.
35. Jeste DV, Caligiuri MP, Paulsen JS, et al. Risk of tardive dyskinesia in older patients. A prospective longitudinal study of 266 outpatients. *Arch Gen Psychiatry*. 1995;52(9):756–765.
36. Young RC. Use of lithium in bipolar disorder. In: Nelson JC, ed. *Geriatric Psychopharmacology*. New York: Marcel Dekker, Inc.; 1998:259–272.
37. Beyer J, Siegal A, Kennedy J, et al. Olanzapine, divalproex, and placebo treatment: non-head-to-head comparisons of older-adult acute mania. In: 10th Congress of the International Psychogeriatric Association. Sept. 9–14, 2001; Nice, France. International Psychogeriatrics 2001;13(suppl 2):203–205.
38. Jeste DV, Rockwell E, Harris MJ, Lohr JB, Lacro J. Conventional vs. newer antipsychotics in elderly patients. *Am J Geriatr Psychiatry*. 1999;7(1):70–76.
39. Suppes T, Webb A, Paul B, Carmody T, Kraemer H, Rush AJ. Clinical outcome in a randomized 1-year trial of clozapine versus treatment as usual for patients with treatment-resistant illness and a history of mania. *Am J Psychiatry*. 1999;156(8): 1164–1169.
40. Fuller MA, Sajatovic M. *Drug Information for Mental Health*. Cleveland, OH: Lexi-Comp Inc.; 2001.
41. McDonald WM, Nemeroff CB. The diagnosis and treatment of mania in the elderly. *Bull Menninger Clin*. 1996;60(2):174–196.
42. Niedermier JA, Nasrallah HA. Clinical correlates of response to valproate in geriatric inpatients. *Ann Clin Psychiatry*. 1998; 10(4):165–168.
43. Regenold WT, Prasad M. Uses of intravenous valproate in geriatric psychiatry. *Am J Geriatr Psychiatry*. 2001;9(3):306–308.
44. Yeung PP TP, Schneider LS, Salzman C, Rak JW. Quetiapine for elderly patients with psychotic disorders. *Psychiatric Annals*. 1999;30:197–201.
45. Shulman RW, Singh A, Shulman KI. Treatment of elderly institutionalized bipolar patients with clozapine. *Psychopharmacol Bull*. 1997;33(1):113–118.
46. Keck PE Jr, Marcus R, Tourkodimitris S, et al. A placebo-controlled, double-blind study of the efficacy and safety of aripiprazole in patients with acute bipolar mania. *Am J Psychiatry*. 2003;160(9): 1651–1658.
47. Sajatovic M. Treatment of bipolar disorder in older adults. *Int J Geriatr Psychiatry*. 2002;17(9):865–873.
48. Goldberg JF. Treatment guidelines: current and future management of bipolar disorder. *J Clin Psychiatry*. 2000;61(suppl 13): 12–18.
49. Nambudiri DE, Meyers BS, Young RC. Delayed recovery from lithium neurotoxicity. *J Geriatr Psychiatry Neurol*. 1991;4(1):40–43.
50. Schaffer CB, Garvey MJ. Use of lithium in acutely manic elderly patients. *Clin Gerontol*. 1984;3:58–60.
51. Nemeroff CB, Evans DL, Gyulai L, et al. Double-blind, placebo-controlled comparison of imipramine and paroxetine in the treatment of bipolar depression. *Am J Psychiatry*. 2001;158(6): 906–912.
52. Gonzalez RG, Guimaraes AR, Sachs GS, Rosenbaum JF, Garwood M, Renshaw PF. Measurement of human brain lithium in vivo by MR spectroscopy. *AJNR Am J Neuroradiol*. 1993;14(5):1027–1037.
53. Moore CM, Demopulos CM, Henry ME, et al. Brain-to-serum lithium ratio and age: an in vivo magnetic resonance spectroscopy study. *Am J Psychiatry*. 2002;159(7):1240–1242.
54. McFarland BH, Miller MR, Straumfjord AA. Valproate use in the older manic patient. *J Clin Psychiatry*. 1990;51(11):479–481.
55. Risinger RC, Risby ED, Risch SC. Safety and efficacy of divalproex sodium in elderly bipolar patients. *J Clin Psychiatry*. 1994;55(5):215.
56. Stoll AL, Banov M, Kolbrener M, et al. Neurologic factors predict a favorable valproate response in bipolar and schizoaffective disorders. *J Clin Psychopharmacol*. 1994;14(5):311–313.
57. Bowden CL. Anticonvulsants in bipolar elderly. In: Nelson J, ed. *Geriatric Psychopharmacology*. New York: Marcel Dekker, Inc.; 1998:285–299.
58. Sanderson DR. Use of mood stabilizers by hospitalized geriatric patients with bipolar disorder. *Psychiatr Serv*. 1998;49(9): 1145–1147.
59. Sheldon LJ, Ancill RJ, Holliday SG. Gabapentin in geriatric psychiatry patients. *Can J Psychiatry*. 1998;43(4):422–423.
60. Sethi MA, Mehta R, Devanand DP. Gabapentin in geriatric mania. *J Geriatr Psychiatry Neurol*. 2003;16(2):117–120.
61. Madhusoodanan S, Bogunovic O, Brenner R, Gupta S. Use of topiramate as an adjunctive medication in an elderly patient with treatment-resistant bipolar disorder. *Am J Geriatr Psychiatry*. 2002;10(6):759.

62. Shulman KI, Rochon P, Sykora K, et al. Changing prescription patterns for lithium and valproic acid in old age: shifting practice without evidence. *BMJ*. 2003;326(7396):960–961.

63. Goodwin FK, Fireman B, Simon GE, Hunkeler EM, Lee J, Revicki D. Suicide risk in bipolar disorder during treatment with lithium and divalproex. *JAMA*. 2003;290(11):1467–1473.

64. Burt T, Sachs GS, Demopulos C. Donepezil in treatment-resistant bipolar disorder. *Biol Psychiatry*. 1999;45(8):959–964.

65. Small JG, Small IF, Milstein V, Kellams JJ, Klapper MH. Manic symptoms: an indication for bilateral ECT. *Biol Psychiatry*. 1985;20(2):125–134.

66. Black DW, Winokur G, Nasrallah A. Treatment of mania: a naturalistic study of electroconvulsive therapy versus lithium in 438 patients. *J Clin Psychiatry*. 1987;48(4):132–139.

67. McDonald WM, Thompson TR. Treatment of mania in dementia with electroconvulsive therapy. *Psychopharmacol Bull*. 2001;35(2):72–82.

68. Altshuler L, Suppes T, Black D, et al. Impact of antidepressant discontinuation after acute bipolar depression remission on rates of depressive relapse at 1-year follow-up. *Am J Psychiatry*. 2003;160(7):1252–1262.

69. Zornberg GL, Pope HG Jr. Treatment of depression in bipolar disorder: new directions for research. *J Clin Psychopharmacol*. 1993;13(6):397–408.

70. Potter WZ. Bipolar depression: specific treatments. *J Clin Psychiatry*. 1998;59(suppl 18):30–36.

71. Kukopulos A, Reginaldi D, Laddomada P, Floris G, Serra G, Tondo L. Course of the manic-depressive cycle and changes caused by treatment. *Pharmakopsychiatr Neuropsychopharmakol*. 1980;13(4):156–167.

72. Wehr TA, Goodwin FK. Can antidepressants cause mania and worsen the course of affective illness? *Am J Psychiatry*. 1987;144(11):1403–1411.

73. Callahan AM, Bauer MS. Psychosocial interventions for bipolar disorder. *Psychiatr Clin North Am*. 1999;22(3):675–688.

74. Miklowitz DJ, Hooley JM. Developing family psychoeducational treatments for patients with bipolar and other severe psychiatric disorders. A pathway from basic research to clinical trials. *J Marital Fam Ther*. 1998;24(4):419–435.

75. Wirz-Justice A, Quinto C, Cajochen C, Werth E, Hock C. A rapid-cycling bipolar patient treated with long nights, bedrest, and light. *Biol Psychiatry*. 1999;45(8):1075–1077.

76. Kusumi I, Ohmori T, Kohsaka M, Ito M, Honma H, Koyama T. Chronobiological approach for treatment-resistant rapid cycling affective disorders. *Biol Psychiatry*. 1995;37(8):553–559.

77. Smeraldi E, Benedetti F, Barbini B, Campori E, Colombo C. Sustained antidepressant effect of sleep deprivation combined with pindolol in bipolar depression. A placebo-controlled trial. *Neuropsychopharmacology*. 1999;20(4):380–385.

78. Colombo C, Benedetti F, Barbini B, Campori E, Smeraldi E. Rate of switch from depression into mania after therapeutic sleep deprivation in bipolar depression. *Psychiatry Res*. 1999; 86(3):267–270.

79. American Psychiatric Association. Practice guideline for the treatment of patients with bipolar disorder. *Am J Psychiatry*. 1994;151(suppl 12):1–36.

80. Stoll AL, Haura G. Tranylcypromine plus risperidone for treatment-refractory major depression. *J Clin Psychopharmacol*. 2000;20(4):495–496.

81. Stahl SM. Selecting an antidepressant by using mechanism of action to enhance efficacy and avoid side effects. *J Clin Psychiatry*. 1998;59(suppl 18):23–29.

82. Calabrese JR, Bowden CL, Sachs GS, Ascher JA, Monaghan E, Rudd GD. A double-blind placebo-controlled study of lamotrigine monotherapy in outpatients with bipolar I depression. Lamictal 602 Study Group. *J Clin Psychiatry*. 1999;60(2):79–88.

83. Bowden CL, Calabrese JR, Sachs G, et al. A placebo-controlled 18-month trial of lamotrigine and lithium maintenance treatment in recently manic or hypomanic patients with bipolar I disorder. *Arch Gen Psychiatry*. 2003;60(4):392–400.

84. Calabrese JR, Bowden CL, Sachs G, et al. A placebo-controlled 18-month trial of lamotrigine and lithium maintenance treatment in recently depressed patients with bipolar I disorder. *J Clin Psychiatry*. 2003;64(9):1013–1024.

85. Matsuo F. Lamotrigine. *Epilepsia*.1999;40(suppl 5):S30–S36.

86. Messenheimer J, Mullens EL, Giorgi L, Young F. Safety review of adult clinical trial experience with lamotrigine. *Drug Saf*. 1998;18(4):281–296.

87. Rzany B, Correia O, Kelly JP, Naldi L, Auquier A, Stern R. Risk of Stevens-Johnson syndrome and toxic epidermal necrolysis during first weeks of antiepileptic therapy: a case-control study. Study Group of the International Case Control Study on Severe Cutaneous Adverse Reactions. *Lancet*. 1999;353(9171):2190–2194.

88. Fieve RR, Platman SR, Plutchik RR. The use of lithium in affective disorders. I. Acute endogenous depression. *Am J Psychiatry*. 1968;125(4):487–491.

89. Goodwin FK, Murphy DL, Dunner DL, Bunney WE Jr. Lithium response in unipolar versus bipolar depression. *Am J Psychiatry*. 1972;129(1):44–47.

90. Keller MB. Improving the course of illness and promoting continuation of treatment of bipolar disorder. *J Clin Psychiatry*. 2004;65(suppl 15):10–14.

91. Baldessarini RJ, Tondo L, Hennen J. Effects of lithium treatment and its discontinuation on suicidal behavior in bipolar manic-depressive disorders. *J Clin Psychiatry*. 1999;60(suppl 2):77–84, 111–116.

92. Ballenger JC, Post RM. Carbamazepine in manic-depressive illness: a new treatment. *Am J Psychiatry*. 1980;137(7):782–790.

93. Post RM, Denicoff KD, Frye MA, et al. A history of the use of anticonvulsants as mood stabilizers in the last two decades of the 20th century. *Neuropsychobiology*. 1998;38(3):152–166.

94. Greil W, Kleindienst N. The comparative prophylactic efficacy of lithium and carbamazepine in patients with bipolar I disorder. *Int Clin Psychopharmacol*. 1999;14(5):277–281.

95. Anderson GD. A mechanistic approach to antiepileptic drug interactions. *Ann Pharmacother*. 1998;32(5):554–563.

96. Tohen M, Vieta E, Calabrese J, et al. Efficacy of olanzapine and olanzapine-fluoxetine combination in the treatment of bipolar I depression. *Arch Gen Psychiatry*. 2003;60(11):1079–1088.

97. Bittman BJ, Young RC. Mania in an elderly man treated with bupropion. *Am J Psychiatry*. 1991;148(4):541.

98. Young RC, Jain H, Kiosses DN, Meyers BS. Antidepressant-associated mania in late life. *Int J Geriatr Psychiatry*. 2003;18(5):421–424.

99. Himmelhoch JM, Fuchs CZ, Symons BJ. A double-blind study of tranylcypromine treatment of major anergic depression. *J Nerv Ment Dis*. 1982;170(10):628–634.

100. Georgotas A, McCue RE, Hapworth W, et al. Comparative efficacy and safety of MAOIs versus TCAs in treating depression in the elderly. *Biol Psychiatry*. 1986;21(12):1155–1166.

101. Boerlin HL, Gitlin MJ, Zoellner LA, Hammen CL. Bipolar depression and antidepressant-induced mania: a naturalistic study. *J Clin Psychiatry*. 1998;59(7):374–379.

102. Schaffer A, Mamdani M, Levitt A, Herrmann N. Effect of antidepressant use on admissions to hospital among elderly bipolar patients. In: Poster presented at APA Annual Meeting. May 2003; San Francisco, CA.

103. Stoll AL, Severus WE, Freeman MP, et al. Omega 3 fatty acids in bipolar disorder: a preliminary double-blind, placebo-controlled trial. *Arch Gen Psychiatry*. 1999;56(5):407–412.

104. Abramowicz M, ed. SAMe for depression. *Med Lett Drugs Ther*. 1999;41(1065):107–108.

105. Levine J, Barak Y, Gonzalves M, et al. Double-blind, controlled trial of inositol treatment of depression. *Am J Psychiatry*. 1995;152(5):792–794.

106. Carney MW, Chary TK, Bottiglieri T, Reynolds EH. Switch and S-adenosylmethionine. *Ala J Med Sci*. 1988;25(3):316–319.

107. Lipinski JF, Cohen BM, Frankenburg F, et al. Open trial of S-adenosylmethionine for treatment of depression. *Am J Psychiatry*. 1984;141(3):448–450.

108. Kofman O, Belmaker RH. Ziskind-Somerfeld Research Award 1993. Biochemical, behavioral, and clinical studies of the role of inositol in lithium treatment and depression. *Biol Psychiatry*. 1993;34(12):839–852.

109. Schneck C. St. John's wort and hypomania. *J Clin Psychiatry*. 1998;59(12):689.

110. O'Breasail AM, Argouarch S. Hypomania and St. John's wort. *Can J Psychiatry*. 1998;43(7):746–747.

111. Bowden CL, Calabrese JR, McElroy SL, et al. A randomized, placebo-controlled 12-month trial of divalproex and lithium in treatment of outpatients with bipolar I disorder. Divalproex Maintenance Study Group. *Arch Gen Psychiatry.* 2000;57(5): 481–489.

112. Goldberg JF, Citrome L. Latest therapies for bipolar disorder: looking beyond lithium. *Postgrad Med* 2005;117(2):25–36.

113. Basco MR, Rush AJ. Compliance with pharmacotherapy in mood disorders. *Psychiatric Ann.* 1995;25:78–82.

114. Schwarcz G, Silbergeld S. Serum lithium spot checks to evaluate medication compliance. *J Clin Psychopharmacol.* 1983;3(6): 356–358.

115. Jamison KR, Gerner RH, Goodwin FK. Patient and physician attitudes toward lithium: relationship to compliance. *Arch Gen Psychiatry.* 1979;36(spec no 8):866–869.

116. Craighead WE, Miklowitz DJ. Psychosocial interventions for bipolar disorder. *J Clin Psychiatry.* 2000;61(suppl 13):58–64.

117. Scott J. Psychotherapy for bipolar disorder. *Br J Psychiatry Psychiatr.* 1995;167(5):581–588.

118. Miller MD, Pollack BG, Foglia J, Begley A, Reynolds CG. Maximizing antidepressant compliance in depressed geriatric patients. *Directions in Psychiatry.* 2000;48(6):582–592.

119. Grossberg GT, Manepalli J, Hassan R, Solomon K. Use of psychotropics in the elderly in the United States: an overview. In: Bergemer M, Hasegawa K, Finkel SI, Nishimura T, eds. *Aging and Mental Disorders: International Perspectives.* New York: Springer;1992;212–238.

120. Salzman C. Medication compliance in the elderly. *J Clin Psychiatry.* 1995;56(suppl 1):18–22.

121. Huxley NA, Parikh SV, Baldessarini RJ. Effectiveness of psychosocial treatments in bipolar disorder: state of the evidence. *Harv Rev Psychiatry.* 2000;8(3):126–140.

122. Bloch S, Hafner J, Harari E, et al. *The Family in Clinical Psychiatry.* New York: Oxford University Press USA;1994.

123. Peet M, Harvey N. NIMH workshop report on treatment of bipolar disorder. *Psychopharmacology Bull.* 1991;26:409–427.

124. Shakir SA, Volkmar FR, Bacon S, Pfefferbaum A. Group psychotherapy as an adjunct to lithium maintenance. *Am J Psychiatry.* 1979;136(4A):455–456.

125. Volkmar FR, Bacon S, Shakir SA, Pfefferbaum A. Group therapy in the management of manic-depressive illness. *Am J Psychother.* 1981;35(2):226–234.

126. Miklowitz DJ, Frank E, George EL. New psychosocial treatments for the outpatient management of bipolar disorder. *Psychopharmacol Bull.* 1996;32(4):613–621.

127. Ellicott A, Hammen C, Gitlin M, Brown G, Jamison K. Life events and the course of bipolar disorder. *Am J Psychiatry.* 1990; 147(9):1194–1198.

128. Frank E, Hlastala S, Ritenour A, et al. Inducing lifestyle regularity in recovering bipolar disorder patients: results from the maintenance therapies in bipolar disorder protocol. *Biol Psychiatry.* 1997;41(12):1165–1173.

129. Frank E, Swartz HA, Mallinger AG, Thase ME, Weaver EV, Kupfer DJ. Adjunctive psychotherapy for bipolar disorder: effects of changing treatment modality. *J Abnorm Psychol.* 1999;108(4): 579–587.

130. Satterfield JM. Adjunctive cognitive-behavioral therapy for rapid-cycling bipolar disorder: an empirical case study. *Psychiatry.* 1999;62(4):357–369.

131. Miklowitz DJ, Goldstein MJ, Nuechterlein KH, Snyder KS, Mintz J. Family factors and the course of bipolar affective disorder. *Arch Gen Psychiatry.* 1988;45(3):225–231.

132. Miklowitz DJ, Goldstein MJ. *Bipolar Disorder: A Family-Focused Treatment Approach.* New York: Guilford; 1997.

133. Miklowitz DJ, Simoneau TL, George EL, et al. Family-focused treatment of bipolar disorder: 1-year effects of a psychoeducational program in conjunction with pharmacotherapy. *Biol Psychiatry.* 2000;48(6):582–592.

134. Simoneau TL, Miklowitz DJ, Richards JA, Saleem R, George EL. Bipolar disorder and family communication: effects of a psychoeducational treatment program. *J Abnorm Psychol.* 1999; 108(4):588–597.

135. Davenport YB, Ebert MH, Adland ML, Goodwin FK. Couples group therapy as an adjunct to lithium maintenance of the manic patient. *Am J Orthopsychiatry.* 1977;47(3):495–502.

136. Pollack LE. Improving relationships. Groups for inpatients with bipolar disorder. *J Psychosoc Nurs Ment Health Serv.* 1990; 28(5): 17–22.

137. Cerbone M, Mayo JA, Cuthbertson BA, O'Connell RA. Group therapy as an adjunct to medications in the management of bipolar affective disorder. *Group.* 1992(16):174–187.

138. Kanas N. Group psychotherapy with bipolar patients: a review and synthesis. *Int J Group Psychother.* 1993;43(3):321–333.

139. Cochran SD. Preventing medical noncompliance in the outpatient treatment of bipolar affective disorders. *J Consult Clin Psychol.* 1984;52(5):873–878.

140. Scott J. Cognitive therapy as an adjunct to medication in bipolar disorder. *Br J Psychiatry.* 2001;178(suppl 41):S164–S168.

141. Niederehe G. Psychosocial treatments with depressed older adults: a research update. *Am J Geriatr Psychiatry.* 1996;4(suppl 1):S66–S78.

142. McQuaid JR, Granholm E, McClure FS, et al. Development of an integrated cognitive-behavioral and social skills training intervention for older patients with schizophrenia. *J Psychother Pract Res.* 2000;9(3):149–156.

143. Antognini F. Psychotherapy with depressed older adults. In: Ellison JM, Verma S, eds. *Depression in Later Life: A Multidisciplinary Psychiatric Approach.* New York: Marcel Dekker; 2003;257–295.

144. Muslin HL. *Psychotherapy of the Elderly Self.* New York: Brunner Maezel; 1992.

145. Starkstein SE, Manes F. Mania and manic-like disorders. In: Bogousslavsky J, Cummings JL, eds. *Behavior and Mood Disorders in Focal Brain Lesions.* Cambridge, UK: Cambridge University Press; 2000:202–216.

146. Cummings JL. Frontal-subcortical circuits and human behavior. *Arch Neurol.* 1993;50(8):873–880.

147. Starkstein SE, Robinson RG. Mechanism of disinhibition after brain lesions. *J Nerv Ment Dis.* 1997;185(2):108–114.

148. Jorge RE, Robinson RG, Starkstein SE, Arndt SV, Forrester AW, Geisler FH. Secondary mania following traumatic brain injury. *Am J Psychiatry.* 1993;150(6):916–921.

149. Lyketsos CG, Hanson AL, Fishman M, Rosenblatt A, McHugh PR, Treisman GJ. Manic syndrome early and late in the course of HIV. *Am J Psychiatry.* 1993;150(2):326–327.

150. Mirchandani IC, Young RC. Management of mania in the elderly: an update. *Ann Clin Psychiatry.* 1993;5(1):67–77.

151. Das A, Khanna R. Organic manic syndrome: causative factors, phenomenology and immediate outcome. *J Affect Disord.* 1993;27(3):147–153.

152. Shulman K, Post F. Bipolar affective disorder in old age. *Br J Psychiatry.* 1980;136:26–32.

153. Snowdon J. A retrospective case-note study of bipolar disorder in old age. *Br J Psychiatry.* 1991;158:485–490.

154. Stone K. Mania in the elderly. *Br J Psychiatry.* 1989;155:220–224.

155. Tariot PN. The concept of secondary mania in dementia [slide presentation in FDA dockets]. Available at: http://www.fda.gov/ohrms/dockets/ac/00/slides/3590s1c/sld001.htm. 2003. Accessed June 20, 2005.

156. Evans DL, Byerly MJ, Greer RA. Secondary mania: diagnosis and treatment. *J Clin Psychiatry.* 1995;56(suppl 3):31–37.

157. Starkstein SE, Boston JD, Robinson RG. Mechanisms of mania after brain injury. 12 case reports and review of the literature. *J Nerv Ment Dis.* 1988;176(2):87–100.

Suicide in Older Adults

27

Paul R. Duberstein   *Marnin J. Heisel*   *Yeates Conwell*

Engaging more patients in better treatments for mental disorders will diminish suicide risk, but treatment can only be initiated after health care professionals and their patients appreciate the need for it. Few older patients in need of services receive mental health treatment, and this may be especially true of those at risk for suicide (1). Our fundamental premise is that older adults at risk for suicide pose special challenges, because their risk is more likely than not to be underappreciated by health care providers, family members, and friends. Their mental health symptoms are rarely severe and thus more difficult to detect, and they tend not to seek help from mental health professionals, family, or friends. Their physical disease burden and functional limitations may lead physicians to concentrate on the patients' physical problems and ignore their mental health needs. All of these problems are exacerbated by societal attitudes towards mental health problems (ageism, stigma) and an inadequate and outdated infrastructure for service delivery. The manner in which mental health providers are taught to conceptualize suicide risk needs revision. Novel interventions are needed that will encourage psychiatrists and other mental health professionals to practice in both traditional clinical practices and community settings.

In this chapter, after noting basic epidemiologic facts about suicide, we review clinical characteristics that confer risk for suicide. To illustrate our points we present case material derived from interviews conducted with family members of people who took their own lives. The Diagnostic and Statistical Manual (DSM) multiaxial system provides the organizing frame for the review, as mental disorders (Axis I), personality traits and disorders (Axis II), physical illnesses and functional impairment (Axes III and V), and stressful life circumstances (Axis IV) all confer risk.

Clinical risk factors have traditionally been conceptualized, at least implicitly, as providing a motive for the suicide: "Mr. X wants to kill himself because he is depressed, has bad family relations and was recently diagnosed with cancer". The same clinical characteristic that may increase the appeal of suicide to an older adult may also undermine the ability of family, friends, and service providers to prevent the suicide. For example, major depression increases the motivation for suicide, but is often less severe in older adults and therefore more likely to remain undetected and untreated. Conversely, family members may experience depressive symptoms as discomforting, and so avoid discussion of their older relative's emotional distress. Clinicians are encouraged to conceptualize risk factors as both providing a motive and masking an opportunity for intervention. Clinical implications of our *motive-missed opportunity* formulation approach are relatively straightforward. In addition to asking, "What characteristics of this patient may increase the likelihood of suicide?" clinicians could also ask, "What characteristics of this patient may lead me to miss indicators of suicide risk?" The final section of the chapter concerns approaches to intervention and prevention. The long-term goal of the design and delivery of mental health services is not to bring the suicide rate down to zero—an unrealistic goal—but rather to decrease the probability of missed opportunities.

Three caveats delimit the discussion. First, generalizations about suicide among older people should be made with caution. No firm age cut-off exists at which one becomes older, and the age at which one is considered older varies across cultures and changes from one era to the next. An accepted but arbitrary convention is to use 65 years of age as a cut-off, corresponding to the traditional retirement age in North America. This group, like others, is heterogeneous. Although the risk factors for suicide in a 65-year-old and an 85-year-old may differ, there are few data on this issue (2,3). Second, the conceptualization and measurement of mental disorders in individuals with life-threatening illness remains ambiguous, and the ethics of intervention in that context is debatable (4). Although suicidal ideation is rare in the absence of a diagnosable mental disorder (5), this chapter is based on the assumption that suicidal distress is an appropriate target for intervention, even in the absence of a major mental disorder.

Practicing clinicians have had far more experience with patients who have *attempted* suicide than those who have gone on to take their lives. Yet the desire to draw conclusions about completed suicide from research on attempted suicide, or clinical experience with patients who have attempted suicide, must be resisted. The demographic risk factors for attempted and completed suicide differ. Rates of attempted suicide are highest in young women (6), whereas suicide rates are highest in older men (7–9). A majority of suicides have never previously engaged in suicidal behavior (10). Men are nearly 70% more likely than women to have their first attempt be their last; people who have never made a prior suicide attempt account for approximately 75% of the suicides in older age (11,12). A prior history of suicide attempts amplifies risk in older adults (11,13,14), but it should not be assumed that risk factors for suicide attempts and completed suicide in seniors are similar, let alone identical. Unfortunately, suicidal ideation, attempted suicide, and completed suicide are conflated in discussions of suicidal behavior, leading to an inaccurate understanding of risk, and perhaps misguided and potentially iatrogenic treatments and prevention efforts. This chapter focuses principally on completed suicide.

EPIDEMIOLOGICAL DATA—TEN FACTS ABOUT SUICIDE

Scope of the Problem

Approximately 31,000 Americans take their own lives every year, leaving over 200,000 bereaved family members wondering if they could have done something to prevent the death. In 2000 there were over 5,300 suicides among senior citizens, an overall rate of 15.3 per 100,000 (8). There is no systematic surveillance mechanism in the United States to track attempted suicide, but it appears that attempted suicide is far less frequent in later life than among younger age groups (15).

Age and Gender Differences in Suicide Rates

Figure 27-1 depicts the significant age and gender differences in suicide rates. Rates increase with age and are greatest in older adults. The rate among white males 85 and older is almost six times the nation's age-adjusted rate; rates are even higher among those who are widowed or single. As shown in Fig. 27-1, rates for males in the United States increase with age, but rates for women peak in midlife and remain stable or decline slightly thereafter. Among individuals 65 and older in the United States, the ratio of male to female suicides approaches 7:1, but in most other countries

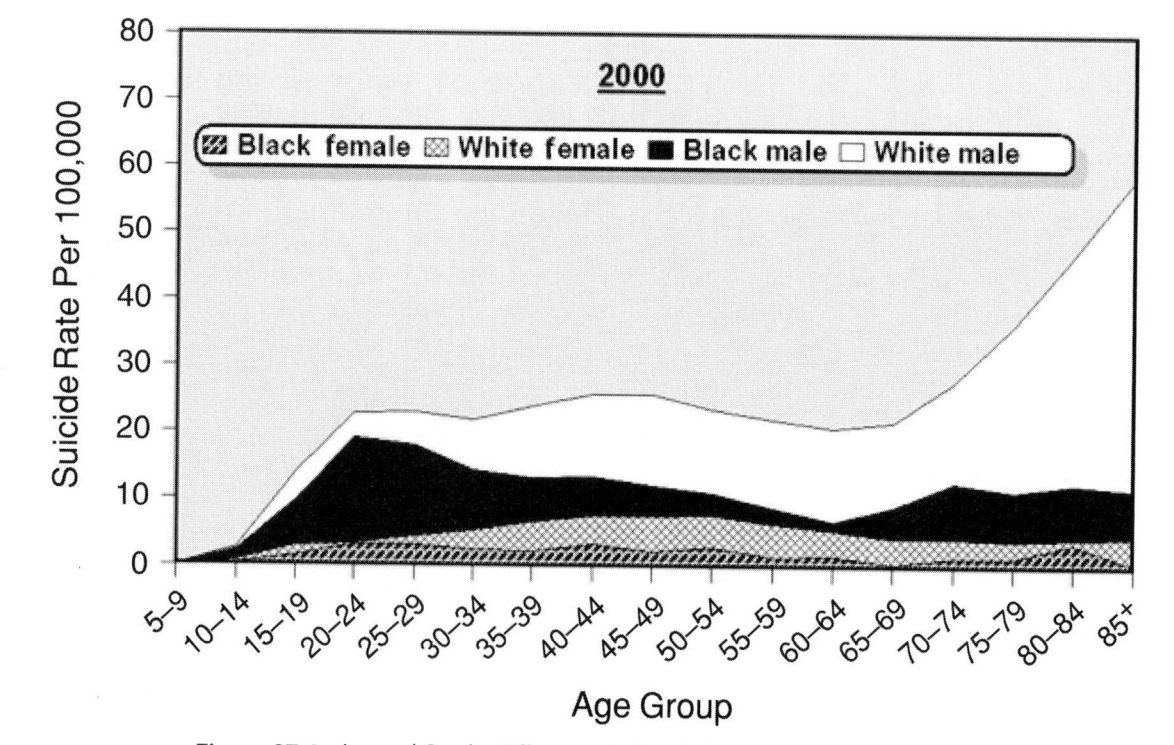

Figure 27-1 Age and Gender Differences in Suicide Rates
Source: National Institute of Mental Health
Data: Center for Disease Control and Prevention, National Center for Health Statistics

the ratio is closer to 3:1. Indeed, in many countries later life is the time of highest risk for both men and women, according to statistics reported by the World Health Organization (16).

Race Differences

In the United States, men have higher suicide rates than women, and Whites of both sexes have higher rates than Blacks (Fig. 27-1). Analyses of the 1993 National Mortality Follow-Back Survey showed that antisocial behaviors and problem-drinking history conferred suicide risk in Whites but not Blacks (17). The relevance of these findings to older adults is not clear, since the analyses were conducted on a mixed-aged sample. Still, the data suggest it is unwise to assume that risk factors for suicide are identical across demographic groups. Unfortunately, research on culturally sensitive markers of suicide risk (e.g., perceived discrimination, racism) has rarely been conducted in any age group.

Marital Status

It has been scientifically established since the 19th century that suicide rates for people who are single or widowed are higher than for married people (18). One study showed that suicide risk is elevated during the first 4 years of widowhood and decreases thereafter (19). Those who take their lives within a year or so of widowhood may be acting in the midst of complicated grief (20), but the symptoms of mental disorders in people who die by suicide after a longer period may be less severe and more difficult to detect (21). The problem for widowed people in accessing mental health services is compounded by the fact that they have fewer social contacts than married people, and thus fewer people in their social networks to encourage them to seek and adhere to treatment.

Living Arrangements

The data on this topic are mixed. Several studies have shown that living alone confers suicide risk (22–24), but others have not (13,25,26). The mixed findings may simply reflect the fact that residential choice, more so than marital status, is determined by local and not by universal conditions. Relevant local conditions include cultural and subcultural norms, housing prices, economic conditions, and population density. Given the variability in findings, the clinical significance of living arrangements remains unclear. On one hand, living alone may confer risk in some societies because it increases loneliness and compromises adherence to mental health treatments; the fewer people in the residence, the less likely that one will be encouraged to seek or adhere to treatment. On the other hand, living with others may not be protective in some societies or cultures because it increases the likelihood of family tension and discord.

Socioeconomic Status

There are well-established socioeconomic differences in all-cause mortality (27), but until recently there were no firm data on the question of socioeconomic status and suicide, particularly in older adults. Three studies of mixed-aged samples have shown that people with blue-collar occupations were more likely than white-collar employees to take their lives (28–30), but a fourth did not (31). Our own data suggest that older adults with less education may be at increased risk (14). In another study, adults 50 years of age and older who died by suicide had lower incomes and were more likely to have been unemployed or disabled (32). Age-stratified analyses revealed that people 50 to 64 years old who committed suicide were more likely than demographically matched controls to have experienced financial trouble or employment change in the prior year; these effects were not observed in those 65 years of age or older, perhaps due to insufficient statistical power. Alternatively, people born in later cohorts may be less accepting of financial and other challenges. Elevated suicide rates in groups with lower levels of income or education may reflect poorer access to quality mental health care, lower levels of mental health literacy, more stigmatized attitudes toward the receipt of mental health care, or the effects of job-related injuries on physical function and health.

Regional and National Differences

Regional differences in suicide rates have been observed since the early 19th century (18). Countries in Northern Europe (Sweden, Finland, Denmark, Norway, Iceland) have higher rates than those in Southern Europe (Italy, Spain). In the United States, the more densely populated states in the Mid-Atlantic region (New York, New Jersey) and New England (Massachusetts, Rhode Island, Connecticut) have lower rates than the Mountain states (Nevada, Wyoming, Montana, Arizona). Acknowledging minor annual variations, the crude rates in the Mountain states are nearly twice that of the Mid-Atlantic region. Possible explanations include firearm availability, population density, religious differences, ethnic variations across regions, and the availability of mental health services. These influences are not independent; for example, firearms are more plentiful and mental health services less accessible in the sparsely populated Mountain regions.

Temporal Fluctuations: Periodicity

The term periodicity refers to differences in rates as a function of time, defined as day-of-the-week, day-of-the-month, month-of-the-year, or season. In the early 19th century, Quetelet documented a spring peak in suicide rates (33). Durkheim later concluded that rates were highest in the summer months (18). Both agreed that rates in the northern hemisphere were higher, particularly when the weather was relatively warm. Goodwin and Jamison noted a spring peak, and ascribed it to rapid changes in the brightness and duration of light (34). Social and socioeconomic explanations have also been offered. In one study, suicide rates among men 60 and older were elevated from late spring through the summer, but teenage boys had higher rates in the autumn and winter (35). Month-of-the-year effects were not observed in females. Day-of-the-week effects were seen almost exclusively in individuals between the ages of 41 and 55, with a peak on Mondays. That peak may be attributable in part to the social, economic, and symbolic significance of Mondays for the middle aged.

Temporal Fluctuations: Historical Trends

Suicide rates have remained relatively stable in the general population throughout the second half of this century, but they have declined by up to 50% in seniors between 1930 and 1980 (36). That trend may have reversed, however. Data from the Centers for Disease Control and Prevention indicate that the suicide rate for the population 65 years and older rose 9% between 1980 and 1992, with increases of 35% among those aged 80 to 84 (37). More recent data indicate that suicide rates for seniors continued to rise until reaching a peak in the mid-to-late 1980s, with slight annual declines ever since (38). The significance and cause of these fluctuations is unknown. Changes in rates over time may be ascribed to birth cohort effects or historical influences. Due to shared early exposures to life-defining events (e.g., economic depressions, wars, political turmoil) or child-rearing practices, some birth cohorts may have an increased or decreased vulnerability to suicide. As birth cohorts age, they share exposures in adulthood life-defining events, technological developments (medications), and policy changes (e.g., insurance coverage) that may affect the suicide rate. The baby boom cohort has had substantially higher suicide rates than preceding generations (39).

Lethal Methods

Firearms account for more than 60% of the suicides in the United States annually, and close to 70% of the suicides among those 70 and older (8). Men are far more likely to use firearms than women. This gender difference appears to increase with age in the United States. In 1997, 2,857 men and only 237 women 70 and older used a firearm for suicide (40). In a study of 86 suicides in people 50 and older, and 86 community-control subjects individually matched on age, sex, race, and county of residence, the presence of a firearm in the home amplified the risk for suicide, even after statistically accounting for the effects of mental disorder (41). Education programs for older people, their families, and health care providers concerning the risks of having a gun in the home, and reinforcement

of rules for safe storage, may contribute to reducing the rate of suicide.

IDENTIFYING CLINICAL RISK FACTORS: TOWARD AN INTEGRATED CLINICAL AND PUBLIC HEALTH APPROACH TO SUICIDE PREVENTION

Psychiatric education about suicide is based on the premise that suicide risk is diminished by the development, implementation, and dissemination of treatments for the mental disorders that confer risk. It is expected that improved methods of treating depression will lead to a lowering of the suicide rate, especially if these treatments decrease the desire for suicide among individuals who are at high risk by virtue, for example, of a history of suicide attempts.

This idea has much commonsense, intuitive appeal; however, the majority of older people who take their lives have never made a prior suicide attempt (11,12) and have never received mental health treatment (12). These two facts have significant implications for how psychiatrists and other mental health providers are taught to conceptualize and formulate risk. Reflecting an interest in the suicidal mind, psychiatric education has historically (if implicitly) conceived of clinical risk factors in motivational terms: "Mr. X is suicidal because he is depressed". While it is true that clinical risk factors operate by providing a motive for the act, they may also amplify risk by undermining the receipt of timely and effective mental health treatment: "Mr. X took his own life because his depressive symptoms were not recognized as severe enough by his health care providers to indicate the need for aggressive intervention". An alternative explanation assigns a central role to the clinician's subjective discomfort: "Mr. X took his own life because he stopped discussing his depressive symptoms, after having noticed that those discussions made his clinician uncomfortable". Developing an understanding of the suicidal mind is a vital goal in the education of mental health practitioners. Gaining insight into the factors that undermine the delivery of effective interventions is just as vital.

As shown in Table 27-1, clinically important risk factors confer suicide risk by providing motive and undermining risk recognition and preventive efforts. All of these problems are compounded by sociocultural, economic, and structural barriers, as outlined in Table 27-2. Our culture has erected or inherited numerous barriers to the provision of mental health care, many of which are attitudinal and rooted in centuries of superstition (42). Somebody who is not particularly psychologically minded and is reluctant to seek mental health treatment under the best of circumstances is even less likely to do so in the face of cultural and economic barriers to treatment.

The clinical risk factors for suicide will be reviewed in four domains: mental disorders, personality traits and

TABLE 27-1

FACTORS AFFECTING THE RECOGNITION OF DEPRESSION IN OLDER ADULTS: CHARACTERISTICS OF ELDERS AND MEMBERS OF THEIR SOCIAL NETWORK

Characteristics	Domain	Potentially Pathogenic Process
Characteristics of at-risk elders	Psychopathology	■ Affective symptoms are mild and therefore difficult to detect. ■ The absence of a prior psychiatric history may make health professionals and family members less vigilant about looking for signs or symptoms of distress.
	Personality and social support	■ Low openness to experience and low extraversion are associated with smaller social networks and lower levels of perceived support, impeding detection.
	Physical parameters	■ Family members and physicians may be too preoccupied managing the elder's multiple medical problems to think about the elder's mental health. ■ Some symptoms of affective disorder (e.g., fatigue, insomnia) are also symptoms of physical disease, which can confound diagnosticians and confuse family members.
	Demographics	■ Older people are less likely to report psychiatric symptoms than younger people. ■ Men are less likely to report symptoms than women. ■ Unmarried people spend less time with others than married people, and are therefore less likely to have their symptoms recognized.
Characteristics of members of the elder's social network	Psychopathology	■ Friends and family members who themselves have not been treated for a depressive disorder will be less likely to detect depressive symptoms in the at-risk elder.
	Physical health	■ Friends and family members who are preoccupied with their own physical problems may be less likely to recognize specific psychiatric symptoms in the at-risk elder, despite being sensitive to the elder's overall level of distress.

disorders, physical illnesses and functional impairment, and stressful life circumstances.

Mental Disorders

Retrospective studies of later-life suicides have shown that from 71% to over 90% had a major mental disorder at the time of death (1). Mood disorders, in particular, amplify suicide risk (11–14,43,44). Recurrent major depressive disorder, single-episode major depression, dysthymia, and minor depression all increase the likelihood of suicide (44). Alcohol and substance-use disorders also confer risk (13,14,44,45). People with histories of remitted alcoholism and substance abuse may represent a population of special concern (46).

The contribution of the retrospective case-control design to the understanding of suicide risk is undeniable (47,48), but it is vulnerable to numerous biases, chief of which is hindsight and the inability of researchers to collect data directly from those who died by suicide. Prospective cohort studies of high-risk samples overcome both of these limitations but are themselves severely limited. They can provide data on only a tiny fraction of people who die by suicide in a given community, and these samples are unrepresentative (48). Still, it is reassuring that findings from prospective

studies of older samples reinforce data collected retrospectively. For example, using data from the Established Populations for Epidemiologic Studies of the Elderly, researchers compared 20 completed suicides with 420 controls randomly selected from a sample of 14,456 participants 65 and older (49). Higher self-rated depression scores were significantly associated with suicide risk.

Implications for Risk Detection and Health Services Utilization

The phenomenology of mood disorders in older adults has important implications for risk detection. Older people are less likely to report depressed or sad moods than younger people. This is true of psychiatric inpatients (50) and of community dwellers (51,52). In addition, older inpatients (53) and community dwellers (51) are less likely to report suicidal ideation than younger people. These age effects would drive depressive diagnoses toward the apparently less-severe end of a diagnostic continuum, perhaps without decreasing risk for suicide or other causes of death. Our motive-missed opportunity framework suggests that mild-to-moderate depressive symptoms in people with histories of adequate adjustment may amplify risk because health care providers, friends, relatives, and others in their social network are not cued in to the possibility of imminent danger.

TABLE 27-2

CULTURAL, FINANCIAL, AND INFRASTRUCTURE BARRIERS TO THE DETECTION AND EFFECTIVE TREATMENT OF DEPRESSION AND OTHER MENTAL DISORDERS IN OLDER ADULTS

Level of Analysis	Barrier to Effective Treatment	Comment
Cultural attitudes and values	Ageism	▪ People may not label their abnormally low mood as sadness unless they are motivated to return to normal, but the media shapes their concept of normal; media depictions of aging show a distinct negative bias. ▪ Myth that depression is a normal aspect of aging could discourage people from seeking mental health treatment, while also making physicians less likely to diagnose and treat depression in older adults. ▪ Public education is needed to combat the myth that depression is normal and expected.
	Pathological self-reliance	▪ In the United States, the belief that people are supposed to "pick themselves up by the bootstraps" and not rely on others discourages treatment-seeking. ▪ Pathological self-reliance also associated with mistrust of government and the belief that government is too intrusive. ▪ This belief may be more pernicious in some regions of the United States (Mountain States) than others (e.g., New England, Middle Atlantic).
	Stigmatization of the mentally ill	▪ Physicians may refrain from diagnosing depression if they are concerned about stigmatizing their patients. ▪ Patients are less likely to seek treatment for disorders that have historically been viewed as marks of shame. ▪ Individuals with negative attitudes towards mental illness are less likely to appreciate the need for treatment, reveal their distress, and seek help from a medical or mental health provider. ▪ Public education is needed to de-stigmatize the diagnosis and treatment of mental disorders.
Health services: access and financing	Poor access to palliative care	▪ Severely ill patients may be more likely to take matters into their own hands by killing themselves out of fear of burdening family members. ▪ Better access to affordable palliative care may lead to a lower suicide rate. ▪ Earlier referral to hospice care may lead to a lower suicide rate.
	Poor mental health reimbursement	▪ Limited Medicare reimbursement for mental health services (50% co-pay) may discourage their use. ▪ Patients are less likely to seek costly mental health treatment as a means of saving money; primary care physicians are less likely to make referrals for the same reason. ▪ Mental health parity may lead to more appropriate use of primary care, enhanced use of mental health services, and a decreased suicide rate.
Health services: "bricks and mortar" infrastructure	Design of health care delivery settings	▪ Seniors are much less likely to see a mental health provider than they are a primary care provider. ▪ Most primary care (and specialty medical care) settings do not have an on-site or co-localized mental health provider. ▪ Co-localized practices have been shown to enhance the uptake of mental health services, and may also diminish suicide risk. ▪ Financially disadvantaged seniors may not be able to afford mental health fees or co-pays.
	Transportation	▪ As they become increasingly frail, seniors are less likely to drive and less able to drive safely. ▪ Safety concerns diminish the appeal of public transportation, particularly in high-crime areas. ▪ Transportation problems are also particularly severe in rural and outlying areas. ▪ Seniors may be reluctant to seek needed treatment, for fear of having their driving privileges revoked.

Personality Disorders and Traits

Approximately 30% to 40% of suicides in mixed-aged samples had personality disorders. Elevated rates in these mixed-aged studies have been observed in patients with antisocial, borderline, schizoid, and avoidant personality disorders. Only one controlled study of suicide in older adults has yielded data on both personality disorders and traits (43). Levels of anankastic (obsessional) and anxious traits significantly distinguished suicides from those who died of natural causes, but rates of personality disorder did not. Duberstein and colleagues (54) administered an informant-report version of the NEO Personality Inventory (55) to friends and relatives of suicides and controls 50 years of age or older. The NEO yields scores on domains of personality identified in the Five Factor Model—Neuroticism, Extraversion, Openness to Experience, Agreeableness, and Conscientiousness (55). Higher levels of neuroticism and lower levels of openness to experience distinguished suicides; the latter trait describes muted affective and hedonic responses, a constricted range of interests, and a strong preference for the familiar over the novel. Other research points to the role of introversion in attempted suicide in older adults (56).

Implications for Risk Detection and Services Utilization

Undoubtedly, younger patients with Cluster B disorders who have histories of mental health treatment are at elevated risk; however, people who are less outspoken about their suicidal thoughts and intent also kill themselves. Our motive-missed opportunity framework suggests that some people are at increased risk because they do not seek help, either from health care providers or members of their social network. This might be particularly true of patients who have avoidant or schizoid tendencies, and those who are introverted and low in openness (57).

CASE EXAMPLE

Mr. Y was a retired security guard and 78-year-old separated father of two adult sons. He shot himself in the head with a shotgun that belonged to one of his sons. His single-sentence suicide note, addressed to "all the loved ones I leave," stated, "I cannot stand the pain any longer." He had suffered from severe arthritis and required a walker. As a consequence of his sexual liaisons as an adolescent and young adult, Mr. Y had contracted gonorrhea, and a permanent catheter had been inserted years earlier. Mr. Y had been unfaithful to his wife throughout their 50-year marriage. When she died, he married a much younger woman, Ms. X, with whom he had been having an affair. When Ms. X moved out of the house following a dispute with Mr. Y's adult son, Mr. Y grew depressed. His affective illness, however, was not

particularly severe, a phenomenon that might be related to his longstanding personality traits—low neuroticism, low extraversion, and low openness. He spoke of wanting to die, but he did not speak of suicide. Believing he was being punished for his infidelity and alcohol dependence, he had a bleak outlook and displayed a general sense of worthlessness. Despite these symptoms, he did maintain some of his activities. He still had an interest in sex, and enjoyed watching pornographic videos and calling sex hotlines. But he had no higher order defenses (intellectualization, sublimation) to fall back on (reflected in his low openness) and a very small social circle (a result of low extraversion and low openness). He never received any mental health treatment.

Physical Illness

In a review of 235 prospective studies with at least 2 years of follow-up and no more than 10% attrition, Harris and Barraclough calculated standardized mortality ratios for suicide in over 60 medical disorders and treatments (58). HIV/AIDS, head and neck cancers, Huntington disease, multiple sclerosis, peptic ulcer, renal disease, spinal cord injury, and systemic lupus erythematosus conferred increased suicide risk. The data could not be adjusted for the effects of comorbid affective disorders, and the authors made no mention of age effects. In a record-linkage study of 2,323 suicides among 1,978,527 persons 50 years or older in Denmark, Erlangsen and Jeune showed that neoplasms and circulatory, respiratory, and digestive diseases all conferred risk; infections and nutritional and metabolic disorders were associated with suicide in hospitalized men, but not hospitalized women (59). Again the findings were not adjusted for the effects of mental disorders.

Conwell and colleagues (14) demonstrated that greater physical illness burden and functional impairment significantly distinguished elderly primary care patients who took their own lives from aged-matched primary care controls. However, after controlling for mood disorders, physical health and functional measures no longer distinguished the groups. Other data suggest that objective indicators of illness could amplify suicide risk in older adults, even after controlling for mental disorders (60–62). For example, in a study of 822 suicides and 944 controls 55 years of age and older, cancer was a significant predictor of suicide risk, even after adjusting for depression (62). Chronic pulmonary disease also amplified risk; interestingly, this effect was confined to those who were married. Waern and colleagues showed that cancer, visual impairment, and neurological disorder conferred risk, after adjusting for the effects of depression history and interpersonal conflicts (61). In that study, the association between objectively measured physical illness and suicide was stronger in men than women.

Other findings suggest that the relationship between physical illness and suicide depends in part on sampling characteristics. For example, in a comparison of suicides and accidental deaths, cancer amplified suicide risk even after controlling for depression, but when the authors compared suicides and natural death, physical illness did not confer risk (60). A record-linkage study showed that cancer decreases suicide risk among older adults with a history of mental services utilization (63).

Subjective indicators of health are also important considerations. Poor subjective health exerts independent effects on suicidal ideation (64) and suicide (32,49), although there has been at least one negative study (25). Physical illness could generate stress in caregivers, create family discord, and drain financial resources (65). Our data suggested that perceived physical illness drives suicide risk independent of the financial and family problems often associated with physical illness (32).

There are several possible explanations for the association between physical illness and suicide. Biological interpretations posit that there are pathophysiological pathways by which a particular disorder affects brain function, and thereby increases suicide risk (66,67). Some tumors could have specific effects on the central nervous system (67), increasing risk for depression and subsequent suicide (68). From a social-constructionist perspective, the symbolic meaning of the disease, as derived from societal norms as well as one's personal experiences, is potentially lethal, as in the case example. Growing infirm in a body that robs one's independence is unappealing, especially in societies that place a high premium on autonomy (69). On a positive note, those discovering sources of meaning despite their physical suffering may be less likely to report suicidal ideation (70).

Implications for Risk Detection and Services Utilization

Our motive-missed opportunity framework suggests a third possible explanation for the relationship between physical illness and suicide. Overburdened primary care physicians, striving to manage and treat patients with several comorbid chronic illnesses, may underappreciate their patients' mental health needs and refrain from diagnosing depression (71,72). This may be particularly true when the patients themselves attribute mental symptoms to medical causes (73).

Life-Event Stressors and Social Circumstances

Recent meta-analyses have documented significant associations of depression in older adults with severe physical illness, financial strain, relationship difficulties (74) and caregiver burden (75). Controlled data on life events and suicide in older adults first became available in 2002 (12,13,25,32). Beautrais reported bivariate analyses of data collected on 31 older adults who died by suicide and 269 controls 55 years of age and older in Christchurch, New Zealand (13). Suicides were more likely to have experienced serious relationship and financial problems during the past year, but were not more likely to have suffered physical illness. Rubenowitz et al. compared 85 seniors who took their own lives and 153 demographically matched controls 65 years of age and older in Göteborg, Sweden (25). Multivariate analyses showed that suicides were more likely to have had family discord and financial trouble in the previous 24 months. Family discord, but not financial trouble, was associated with suicide after controlling for mental disorders. Duberstein and colleagues showed that family discord and employment change distinguished from controls those 50 years and older who died by suicide, after adjusting for sociodemographic covariates and mental disorders that developed prior to the last year (32).

Implications for Risk Detection and Services Utilization

The motive-missed opportunity framework suggests that life events and chronic strains can deflect attention away from treatable mental disorders. For example, families may rally to provide financial assistance to a senior in need, but remain silent about his or her mental disorder. Similarly, the involvement of at-risk seniors in arguments and conflicts may lead family members and friends to distance themselves from the senior and view him or her as difficult, combative, or irritable. The need for mental health intervention is not perceived.

CASE EXAMPLE

Mr. W was a married, White, college-educated, practicing Catholic and father of seven children. He died of a self-inflicted gunshot wound to the right thigh a week prior to his 61st birthday. The victim had prepared for his death, leaving a suit and shirt hanging on a door, and two suicide notes, one of which contained detailed directions about the maintenance of the lawnmower. While Mr. W had been mildly and intermittently depressed for more than 2 years, his mood grew notably worse about 6 months prior to death, when he was laid off from the company that had employed him for more than 30 years. Symptoms included depressed mood, psychomotor restlessness, diminished self-esteem, and fitful sleep. The latter symptom was particularly disturbing to his wife, since he had been urgently crying out in his sleep, "Why me?" The atmosphere at home had been unpleasant for quite some time. Hopelessness about financial affairs was a prominent theme in the family's conversations. Mr. W would remark that there appeared to be no end to the country's economic miseries, and he could not foresee getting a job.

Three days prior to his death, Mr. W gave his wife a rose and took her to dinner. When they returned, his daughter helped him polish his resume in preparation for yet another job application. After looking through the paper the next morning, he sighed, "There is not one single job." That evening the family ate dinner together. Before his son left for school the next morning, Mr. W hugged him goodbye. It was unusual for Mr. W to hug his son. By the time his wife came downstairs an hour later, he had already left for church, where he went to confession. Mrs. W left the home to take care of some errands shortly before noon, and discovered her husband's body when she returned several hours later.

RELEVANT TREATMENTS AND PREVENTION STRATEGIES

Treatment

Treating the disorders that confer suicide risk is expected to lower the suicide rate, but this assumption has not been adequately tested. Lithium has been proven effective in the reduction of suicide risk among individuals with bipolar affective disorder (76), but it is not known whether these effects persist into older adulthood. This question could be addressed via meta-analysis. For treatment of individual disorders, readers should refer to those specific chapters in this textbook.

Prevention

Older people who take their lives rarely receive any mental health treatment. No matter how well they are designed, randomized controlled trials conducted on treatment-seeking, or even treatment-referred populations cannot address this problem. Developing mechanisms to get at-risk elders into some form of effective treatment is as pressing a public health need as developing more potent treatments. More effective treatment referral mechanisms can lead to a cascade of other benefits, such as decreased depression-related morbidity and all-cause mortality. Two theoretical approaches to suicide prevention have been identified: population-based strategies (also called universal prevention) and high-risk models (77).

Population-Based Strategies

Population-based strategies involve interventions or initiatives that decrease mortality risk by affecting large segments of a society, rather than targeting at-risk individuals. Examples include restricting access to lethal means, crafting economic policies that lead to the creation of new jobs, improving access to palliative care, and developing policy initiatives designed to decrease ageism. Many population-based strategies are unpopular because they are perceived as restricting a freedom rather than conferring a benefit.

Population-based strategies have not received strong empirical support. For example, with respect to firearm access, there is some evidence that decreasing access to one method only serves to increase the rate at which another is used, while having no impact on the overall suicide rate

(78). Other studies find no evidence of method substitution (79). Of course, decreasing firearm access is desirable, even if it does not lead to a lower suicide rate, because it could lower the accident rate. With respect to self-poisonings, Hawton (80) reported that the initial year following a legislated reduction in maximum package size of analgesics in the United Kingdom saw a decrease in nonfatal overdoses, treatment of liver toxicity, and deaths due to analgesic self-poisoning. Given that suicide prevention resources are finite and scarce, they may best be used for developing and implementing strategies that are both potent and politically palatable.

Strategies for High-Risk Groups

High-risk approaches to suicide prevention can be offered in both primary care settings and community service agencies. They are less controversial because they typically involve providing a service, not placing limits on autonomy (e.g., to own a gun).

Primary care

Primary care offices are suitable contexts for the implementation of suicide-prevention initiatives, as many older adults visit a primary care physician (81). Educating overburdened primary care physicians about treating depression does not confer significant benefits (82), nor does screening (83) or providing treatment recommendations based on computer algorithms (84). Active collaborations between mental health and primary care practitioners are more effective for the treatment of depression (85).

Many studies of collaborative-care models in younger and mixed-aged populations excluded patients with suicidal ideation. Still, their findings are instructive. Treatments tend to be effective in the short term for major depression, but ineffective in the long term and for people with milder forms of depression (86–90).

Several recent studies have evaluated collaborative-care models for the treatment of depressed older adults (91–94). Early results are encouraging, but the treatment responses are relatively modest and not as robust as those observed in specialty treatment settings. The Improving Mood-Promoting Access to Collaborative Treatment Study examined the effectiveness of a primary-care-based collaborative model that included a depression clinical specialist, patient education, case management, antidepressants, and problem-solving therapy according to a stepped care protocol (92). The study found that only half of intervention patients experienced a 50% reduction in depressive symptoms, and only 25% to 30% became asymptomatic. Similar data were reported from the Prevention of Suicide in Primary Care Elderly—Collaborative Trial (PROSPECT). Intervention patients compared to those in usual care had a more favorable course of their depression, as measured by severity of symptoms and depression remission (93). Decreases in depressive symptoms were greater in the intervention group at 4 months, 8 months, and 1 year. Four-month remission rates were significantly higher in the intervention group (48.2% versus 34.2%), but this difference narrowed and was not statistically significant at 8 months or 1 year. The PROSPECT study was the first to show that collaborative care may decrease rates of suicidal ideation. Whether collaborative treatments reduce the risk of completed suicide or attempted suicide remains unknown.

The rather lackluster findings in these trials of collaborative and stepped care suggest that further refinement of these approaches is warranted. Treatment effects could be enhanced by conducting moderator analyses to identify subgroups (defined demographically or otherwise) of responders, and offering tailored treatments to those with a greater likelihood of responding. On the other hand, treatment effects are often influenced by sample characteristics. For example, inpatients may improve more with treatment than outpatients, perhaps because treatment staff administer medication and control the treatment milieu. No matter how potent treatments may be in theory, they are only effective in practice if patients actively partner with the clinician and engage in the treatment. Developing novel approaches to increasing treatment adherence in outpatient collaborative care is as important as creating mechanisms and incentives to get patients into treatment in the first place.

Community Service Agencies

Although primary-care-based approaches show promise, they do not reach all elders with mental illness, and their effectiveness is limited. Outreach programs are required, particularly for those with mobility and transportation problems, which may prevent access to care, inadequate insurance coverage, and high Medicare co-pays. The Spokane Mental Health Center, Elder Services Division, has developed a program with the capability to mount acute, multi-disciplinary in-home assessments, combined with the *Gatekeeper model*, a method for reaching at-risk elders living in the community (95). The Gatekeeper model relies on nontraditional community referral sources to identify older individuals at risk for self-harm. Meter readers, utility workers, bank personnel, apartment and mobile-home managers, postal carriers, and others likely to observe older people in their homes or community during the course of their routine business serve as gatekeepers. With a small amount of education and training, they refer elders judged to be at risk to a program equipped to respond with clinical referrals; in-home medical, psychiatric, family, and nutritional assessments; medication management and respite services; and crisis intervention. The impact of the Gatekeeper model on suicide risk has not been rigorously examined.

The Baltimore-based Psychogeriatric Assessment and Treatment in City Housing (PATCH) study was another attempt to overcome barriers to care (96). Researchers screened 945 residents of six urban public-housing sites for disadvantaged older adults; 342 individuals (36%) screened positive for mental illness. The intervention combined gatekeeper training in the identification of older adults at risk of mental disorder, and referral by gatekeepers to a nurse-clinician who provided in-home psychiatric evaluation and treatment. Mental health treatment consisted of interventions ranging from monitoring vital signs to provision of counseling, significantly improving psychological functioning (96). Findings suggest the PATCH intervention was effective for public-housing residents who were depressed at baseline. Improvements were not observed for residents who were not depressed at baseline. Psychotic and demented residents also did not benefit. The impact of PATCH on suicide risk has not yet been examined, although descriptive statistics on suicidal ideation have been published for the six housing facilities studied (97).

Enthusiasm for community models must be weighed against the sobering findings from a recent meta-analysis of the effects of preventive home visits to community-dwelling elders. No clear evidence of the effectiveness of home visits was observed (98). For example, a rigorously conducted British study sought to decrease social isolation among seniors 75 or older that lived alone (99). Half of the experimental group declined repeated offers of help, perhaps reflecting longstanding personality traits and a desire to "go it alone". Other studies (100) and meta-analyses (101) have reached more optimistic conclusions. Studies yielding more promising findings are those that identify a circumscribed problem, seek out a well-defined and motivated target population, and implement a treatment tailored to the needs of that population.

CONCLUSIONS

Older adults at risk for suicide pose specific public health challenges, because health care professionals and members of their social network may not recognize their risk. A public health approach to suicide prevention requires intensive research on how symptoms of mental disorders are reported, recognized, and treated—or not treated—in a variety of contexts. Interventions are also needed to increase the ability of all health care providers to treat depression, and to decrease the likelihood that they will miss opportunities for intervention. Health care providers, including experienced psychiatrists, must remain vigilant about seeking and seizing such opportunities. Patients may be at risk even if they do not have a prior history of suicide attempt, and even if they do not report dysphoria. They may steadfastly deny feeling sad, but may admit to feeling blue, irritable, disgusted, and so on. Some patients will work hard to avoid reporting sadness even when they are experiencing it; clinicians need to explore a range of negative emotions, and use the language of the patient's sub-culture. This may be facilitated by involving the patient's friends and family members in treatment. Even if patients deny sadness or other negative emotions, clinicians must still inquire about thoughts and plans for suicide. Excellent books on the art of eliciting suicidal ideation are available (102). Other missed opportunities stem from the clinician's own biases, ageist or otherwise. As a consequence of misplaced empathy, some clinicians may believe that suicide is expected under certain circumstances, and may be less likely to offer vigorous treatments. In this scenario, peer consultation and referral to another provider may be advisable.

Advertising campaigns are needed to educate the public and medical professionals, to dispel the myths that depression and suicidal ideation are normal aspects of aging. These initiatives should also target seniors and their families and friends. When depression and suicide are no longer seen as normal or expected, people will be more likely to seek treatment. Policy initiatives designed in part to mitigate the stigmatization of mental illness will improve quality of life, and increase the likelihood that people will seek mental health treatment. While individuals' attitudes cannot be legislated, treatment parity can. Mental health parity, long overdue in the United States, may decrease the available opportunities for suicide by removing financial barriers, shifting cultural attitudes toward mental illness, and encouraging people to seek and adhere to life-saving treatments.

REFERENCES

1. Conwell Y, Duberstein PR, Caine ED. Risk factors for suicide in later life. *Biol Psychiatry.* 2002;52:193–204.
2. Erlangsen A, Bille-Brahe U, Jeune B. Differences in suicide between the old and the oldest old. *J Gerontol B Psychol Sci Soc Sci.* 2003;58B:S314–S322.
3. Waern M, Rubenowitz E, Wilhelmson K. Predictors of suicide in the old elderly. *Gerontology.* 2003;49:328–334.
4. Werth JL Jr, ed. *Contemporary Perspectives on Rational Suicide.* Philadelphia, PA: Brunner/Mazel, Inc.; 1999.
5. Chochinov HM, Wilson KG, Enns M, et al. Desire for death in the terminally ill. *Am J Psychiatry.* 1995;152:1185–1191.
6. Kessler RC, Borges G, Walters EE. Prevalence of and risk factors for lifetime suicide attempts in the National Comorbidity Survey. *Arch Gen Psychiatry.* 1999;56:617–626.
7. Office of the U.S. Surgeon General. *The Surgeon General's Call to Action to Prevent Suicide.* 1999. Available at: http://www.surgeon-general.gov/osg/calltoaction/default.htm. accessed March 30, 2004.
8. Minino AM, Arias E, Kochanek KD, Murphy SL, Smith BL. Deaths: final data for 2000. *National Vital Statistics Reports.* 2002;50(15). Hyattsville, MD. National Center for Health Statistics. DHHS Publication No. (PHS) 2002;1120.
9. Centers for Disease Control. Suicide among older persons—United States. *MMWR Surveill Summ.* 1996;45:3–6.
10. Isometsä ET, Lönnqvist JK. Suicide attempts preceding completed suicide in personality disorders. *Br J Psychiatry.* 1998;173:531–535.
11. Conwell Y, Duberstein PR, Conner KR, Eberly S, Wadkins H, Caine ED. Suicide in the second half of life—a psychological autopsy study. Paper presented at the 11th International Congress of the International Psychogeriatrics Association. 2003; Chicago.
12. Phillips M, Yanping Z, Gonghuan Y. Elderly suicides in China: a controlled psychological autopsy study. Paper presented at the

11th International Congress of the International Psychogeriatrics Association. 2003; Chicago.
13. Beautrais, AL. A case control study of suicide and attempted suicide in older adults. *Suicide Life Threat Behav.* 2002;32:1–9.
14. Conwell Y, Lyness JM, Duberstein PR, et al. Suicide among older patients in primary care practices. *J Am Geriatr Soc.* 2000;48:23–29.
15. Mooecicki EK. Identification of suicide risk factors using epidemiologic studies. *Psychiatr Clin North Am.* 1997;20(3):499–517.
16. Pearson JL, Conwell Y. Suicide in late life: challenges and opportunities for research. *Int Psychogeriatr.* 1995;7:131–136.
17. Castle K, Duberstein PR, Meldrum S, Conner KR, Conwell Y. Risk factors for suicide in blacks, with an examination of race differences. *Am J Psychiatry.* 2004;161:452–458.
18. Durkheim E. *Suicide: A Study in Sociology.* New York: Free Press; 1951.
19. MacMahon B, Pugh TF. Suicide in the widowed. *Am J Epidemiol.* 1965;81:23–31.
20. Prigerson HG, Frank E, Kasl SV, et al. Complicated grief and bereavement-related depression as distinct disorders: preliminary empirical validation in elderly bereaved spouses. *Am J Psychiatry.* 1995;152:22–30.
21. Duberstein PR, Conwell Y, Cox C. Suicide in widowed persons: a psychological autopsy comparison of recently and remotely bereaved older subjects. *Am J Geriatr Psychiatry.* 1998;6(4):328–334.
22. Barraclough BM, Pallis DJ. Depression followed by suicide: a comparison of depressed suicides with living depressives. *Psychol Med.* 1975;5:55–61.
23. Boardman AP, Grimbaldeston AH, Handley C, Jones PW, Willmott S. The North Staffordshire Suicide Study: a case-control study of suicide in one health district. *Psychol Med.* 1999;29:27–33.
24. Cheng AT, Chen TH, Chen CC, Jenkins R. Psychosocial and psychiatric risk factors for suicide: case-control psychological autopsy study. *Br J Psychiatry.* 2000;177:360–365.
25. Rubenowitz E, Waern M, Wilhelmsson K, Allebeck P. Life events and psychosocial factors in elderly suicides: a case control study. *Psychol Med.* 2001;31:1193–1202.
26. Phillips MR, Yang G, Zhang Y, Wang L, Ji H, Zhou M. Risk factors for suicide in China: a national case-control psychological autopsy study. *Lancet.* 2002;360(9347):1728–1736.
27. Adler NE, Boyce T, Chesney M, et al. Socioeconomic status and health: the challenge of the gradient. *Am Psychol.* 1994;49(1):15–24.
28. Kung HC, Liu X, Juon HS. Risk factors for suicide in Caucasians and in African-Americans: a matched case-control study. *Soc Psychiatry Psychiatr Epidemiol.* 1998;33:155–161.
29. Drever F, Whitehead M, Roden M. Current patterns and trends in male mortality by social class (based on occupation). *Popul Trends.* 1996;86:15–20.
30. Kagamimori S, Matsubara I, Sokejima S, et al. The comparative study on occupational mortality, 1980 between Japan and Great Britain. *Ind Health.* 1998;36:252–257.
31. Brown GK, Beck AT, Steer RA, Grisham JR. Risk factors for suicide in psychiatric outpatients: a 20-year prospective study. *J Consult Clin Psychol.* 2000;68:371–377.
32. Duberstein PR, Conwell Y, Conner KR, Eberly S, Caine ED. Suicide at 50 years of age and older: perceived physical illness, family discord, and financial strain. *Psychol Med.* 2004;44:137–146.
33. Quetelet MA. *A Treatise on Man and the Development of His Faculties.* Farnborough, UK: Gregg International Publishers; 1973.
34. Goodwin FK, Jamison K. *Manic Depressive Illness.* New York: Oxford University Press; 1990.
35. McCleary R, Chew KS, Hellsten JJ, Flynn-Bransford M. Age- and sex-specific cycles in United States suicides, 1973 to 1985. *Am J Public Health.* 1991;81:494–497.
36. McIntosh JL, Santos JF, Hubbard RW, Overholser, JC. *Elder Suicide: Research, Theory, and Treatment.* Washington, DC: American Psychological Association; 1994.
37. Centers for Disease Control. Suicide among older persons—United States. *MMWR Surveill Summ.* 1996;45:3–6.

38. Centers for Disease Control and Prevention. Web-based injury statistics query and reporting system (WISQARS) [online]. 2002. National Center for Injury Prevention and Control, Centers for Disease Control and Prevention (producer). Available at: http://www.cdc.gov/ncipc.wisqars. Accessed November 3, 2003.

39. McIntosh JL. Older adults: the next suicide epidemic? *Suicide Life Threat Behav.* 1992;22:322–332.

40. Centers for Disease Control and Prevention. US injury mortality statistics. Firearm suicide deaths and rates per 100,000. Available at: http://www.cdc.gov.ncipc.osp.usmort.htm. Accessed October 9, 1999.

41. Conwell Y, Duberstein PR, Conner K, Eberly S, Cox C, Caine ED. Access to firearms and risk for suicide in middle-aged and older adults. *Am J Geriatr Psychiatry.* 2002;10:407–416.

42. Hinshaw SP, Cicchetti DL. Stigma and mental disorder: conceptions of illness, public attitudes, personal disclosure and social policy. *Dev Psychopathol.* 2000;12:555–598.

43. Harwood D, Hawton K, Hope T, Jacoby R. Psychiatric disorder and personality factors associated with suicide in older people: a descriptive and case-control study. *Int J Geriatr Psychiatry.* 2001; 16:155–165.

44. Waern M, Runeson B, Allebeck P, et al. Mental disorder in elderly suicides: a case-control study. *Am J Psychiatry.* 2002;159(a):450–455.

45. Waern M. Alcohol dependence and misuse in elderly suicides. *Alcohol.* 2003;38:249–254.

46. Conner KR, Duberstein PR, Conwell Y, et al. After the drinking stops: completed suicide in individuals with remitted alcohol use disorders. *J Psychoactive Drugs.* 2000;32:33–37.

47. Cavanagh JTO, Carson AJ, Sharpe M, Lawrie SM. Psychological autopsy studies of suicide: a systematic review. *Psychol Med.* 2003;33:395–405.

48. Duberstein PR, Conwell Y. Personality disorders and completed suicide: a methodological and conceptual review. *Clin Psychol: Science and Practice.* 1997;4:359–376.

49. Turvey CL, Conwell Y, Jones MP, et al. Risk factors for late-life suicide: a prospective community-based study. *Am J Geriatr Psychiatry.* 2002;10:398–406.

50. Lyness JM, Cox C, Curry J, Conwell Y, King DA, Caine ED. Older age and the underreporting of depressive symptoms. *J Amer Geriatr Soc.* 1995;43:216–221.

51. Gallo JJ, Anthony JC, Muthen B. Age differences in the symptoms of depression: a latent trait analysis. *J Gerontol B Sci Soc Sci.* 1994;49:251–264.

52. Allen-Burge R, Storandt M, Kinscerf DA, Rubin EH. Sex differences in the sensitivity of two self-reported depression scales in older depressed inpatients. *Psychol Aging.* 1994;9:443–445.

53. Duberstein PR, Conwell Y, Seidlitz L, Lyness JM, Cox C, Caine ED. Age and suicidal ideation in older depressed inpatients. *Am J Geriatric Psychiatry.* 1999;7:289–296.

54. Duberstein PR, Conwell Y, Caine ED. Age differences in the personality characteristics of suicide completers: preliminary findings from a psychological autopsy study. *Psychiatry.* 1994;57:213–224.

55. Costa PT Jr, McCrae RR. *Revised NEO Personality Inventory and NEO Five Factor Inventory: Professional Manual.* Odessa, FL: Psychological Assessment Resources; 1992.

56. Duberstein PR, Conwell Y, Seidlitz L, Denning D, Cox C, Caine ED. Personality traits and suicidal behavior and ideation in depressed inpatients 50 years of age and older. *J Gerontol B Psych Sci Soc Sci.* 2000;55B:P18–P26.

57. Duberstein, PR. Shneidman Award Address: are closed-minded people more open to the idea of killing themselves? *Suicide Life Threat Behav.* 2001;31:9–15.

58. Harris EC, Barraclough BM. Suicide as an outcome for medical disorder: a meta-analysis. *Medicine.* 1994;73:281–296.

59. Erlangsen A, Vach W, Jeune B. The effect of hospitalization with medical illnesses on the suicide risk in the oldest old: a population-based register study. *J Am Geriatr Soc.* 2005;53(5):771–776.

60. Grabbe L, Demi A, Camann MA, Potter L. The health status of elderly persons in the last year of life: a comparison of deaths by suicide, injury, and natural causes. *Am J Public Health.* 1997;87:434–437.

61. Waern M, Rubenowitz E, Runeson B, Skoog I, Wilhelmsson K, Allebeck P. Burden of illness and suicide in elderly people: a case-control study. *BMJ.* 2002;324:1355–1358.

62. Quan H, Arboleda-Florez J, Fick GH, Stuart HL, Love EL. Association between physical illness and suicide among the elderly. *Soc Psychiatry Psychiatr Epidemiol.* 2002;37:190–197.

63. Lawrence D, Almeida OP, Hulse GK, Jablensky AV, Holman CDJ. Suicide and attempted suicide among older adults in Western Australia. *Psychol Med.* 2000;30:813–821.

64. Goodwin R, Olfson M. Self-perception of poor health and suicidal ideation in medical patients. *Psychol Med.* 2002;32:1293–1299.

65. Emanuel EJ, Fairclough DL, Slutsman J, Emanuel LL. Understanding economic and other burdens of terminal illness: the experience of patients and their caregivers. *Ann Intern Med.* 2000;132:451–456.

66. McDaniel JS, Musselman DL, Porter MR, Reed DA, Nemeroff CB. Depression in patients with cancer. Diagnosis, biology, and treatment. *Arch Gen Psychiatry.* 1995;52(2):89–99.

67. Musselman DL, Evans DL, Nemeroff CB. The relationship of depression to cardiovascular disease: epidemiology, biology, and treatment. *Arch Gen Psychiatry.* 1998;55(7):580–592.

68. Szigethy E, Conwell Y, Forbes NT, Cox C, Caine ED. Adrenal weight and morphology in victims of completed suicide. *Biological Psychiatry.* 1994;36:374–380.

69. Bellah RN, Madsen R, Sullivan WM, Swidler A, Tipton SM. *The Good Society.* New York: Random House; 1991.

70. Heisel MJ, Flett GL. Meaning in life and the prevention of elderly suicidality. In: Wong PTP, McDonald M, Klaassen D, eds. *Advances in the Positive Psychology of Meaning and Spirituality.* Abbotsford, BC: INPM Press. In press.

71. Rost K, Smith G, Matthews D, Guise B. The deliberate misdiagnosis of major depression in primary care. *Arch Fam Med.* 1994;3:333–337.

72. Klinkman MS. Competing demands in psychosocial care: a model for the identification and treatment of depressive disorders in primary care. *Gen Hosp Psych.* 1997;19:98–111.

73. Kessler D, Lloyd K, Lewis G, Gray DP. Cross sectional study of symptom attribution and recognition of depression and anxiety in primary care. *BMJ.* 1999;318:436–440.

74. Kraaij V, Arensman E, Spinhoven P. Negative life events and depression in elderly persons: a meta-analysis. *J Gerontol Psych Sci Soc Sci.* 2002;57B:P87–P94.

75. Pinquart M, Sörensen S. Differences between caregivers and non-caregivers in psychological health and physical health: a meta-analysis. *Psychol Aging.* 2003;18:250–267.

76. Tondo L, Hennen J, Baldessarini RJ. Lower suicide risk with long-term lithium treatment in major affective illness: a meta-analysis. *Acta Psychiatr Scand.* 2001;104(3):163–172.

77. Lewis G, Hawton K, Jones P. Strategies for preventing suicide. *Br J Psychiatry.* 1997;171:351–354.

78. Rich CL, Young D, Fowler RC, Wagner J, Black NA. Guns and suicide: possible effects of some specific legislation. *Am J Psychiatry.* 1990;147(3):342–346.

79. Ludwig J, Cook PJ. Homicide and suicide rates associated with implementation of the Brady Handgun Violence Prevention Act. *JAMA.* 2000;284(5):585–591.

80. Hawton K. United Kingdom legislation on pack sizes of analgesics: background, rationale, and effects on suicide and deliberate self-harm. *Suicide Life Threat Behav.* 2002;32(3):223–229.

81. Luoma JB, Martin CE, Pearson JL. Contact with mental health and primary care providers before suicide: a review of the evidence. *Am J Psychiatry.* 2002;159:909–916.

82. Lin EH, Katon WJ, Simon GE, et al. Achieving guidelines for the treatment of depression in primary care: is physician education enough? *Med Care.* 1997;35(8):831–842.

83. Gilbody SM, House AO, Sheldon TA. Routinely administered questionnaires for depression and anxiety systematic review. *BMJ.* 2001;322:406–409.

84. Simon GE, VonKorff M, Rutter C, Wagner E. Randomised trial of monitoring, feedback, and management of care by telephone to improve treatment of depression in primary care. *BMJ.* 2000;320:550–554.

85. Oxman TE, Dietrich AJ, Schulberg HC. The depression care manager and mental health specialist as collaborators within primary care. *Am J Geriatr Psychiatry.* 2003;11:507–516.

86. Schulberg HC, Pilkonis PA, Houck P. The severity of major depression and choice of treatment in primary care practice. *J Consult Clin Psychol.* 1998;66(6):932–938.

87. Katon W, Robinson P, Von Korff M, et al. A multifaceted intervention to improve treatment of depression in primary care. *Arch Gen Psychiatry.* 1996;53:924–932.

88. Von Korff M, Katon W, Bush T, et al. Treatment costs, cost offset, and cost-effectiveness of collaborative management of depression. *Psychosom Med.* 1998;60(2):143–149.

89. Lin EH, Katon WJ, Von Korff M, et al. Relapse of depression in primary care: rate and clinical predictors. *Arch Fam Med.* 1998;7:443–449.

90. Lin EH, Simon GE, Katon WJ, et al. Can enhanced acute-phase treatment of depression improve long-term outcomes? A report of randomized trials in primary care. *Am J Psychiatry.* 1999;156(4):643–645.

91. Bartels SJ, Coakley E, Zubritsky C, et al. Improving engagement in mental health services for older adults in primary care: a randomized trial comparing integrated and enhanced referral care for depression, anxiety disorders, and at-risk alcohol use. *JAMA.* In press.

92. Unutzer J, Katon W, Callahan CM, et al. Improving mood-promoting access to collaborative treatment. Collaborative care management of late-life depression in the primary care setting: a randomized controlled trial. *JAMA.* 2002;288:2836–2845.

93. Bruce ML, Ten Have TR, Reynolds CF III, et al. Reducing suicidal ideation and depressive symptoms in depressed older primary care patients: a randomized controlled trial. *JAMA.* 2004;291:1081–1091.

94. Dietrich AJ, Oxman TE, Burns MR, Winchell CW, Chin T. Application of a depression management office system in community practice: a demonstration. *J Am Board Fam Pract.* 2003;16:107–114.

95. Florio ER, Rockwood TH, Hendryx MS, Jensen JE, Raschko R, Dyck DG. A model gatekeeper program to find the at-risk elderly. *J Case Manag.* 1996;5:106–114.

96. Roca RP, Storer DJ, Robbins BM, Tlasek ME, Rabins PV. Psychogeriatric assessment and treatment in urban public housing. *Hospital and Community Psychiatry.* 1990;41(8):916–920.

97. Cook JM, Pearson JL, Thompson, R, Black BS, Rabins PV. Suicidality in older African Americans: findings from the EPOCH study. *Am J Geriatr Psychiatry.* 2002;10(4):437–446.

98. Van Haastregt JC, Diederiks JP, Rossum EV, de Witte LP, Crebolder HF. Effects of preventive home visits to elderly people living in the community: systematic review. *BMJ.* 2000;320:754–758.

99. Clarke M, Clarke SJ, Jagger C. Social intervention and the elderly: a randomized control trial. *Am J Epidemiol.* 1992;136:1517–1523.

100. Rabins PV, Black BS, Roca R, et al. Effectiveness of a nurse-based outreach program for identifying and treating psychiatric illness in the elderly. *JAMA.* 2000;283:2802–2809.

101. Elkan R, Kendrick D, Dewey M, et al. Effectiveness of home-based support for older people: systematic review and meta-analysis. *BMJ.* 2001;323(7315):719–725.

102. Shea SC. *The Practical Art of Suicide Assessment: A Guide for Mental Health Professionals and Substance Abuse Counselors.* New York: John Wiley & Sons; 1999.

Psychosis in the Elderly 28

Salman Karim   Alistair Burns

The notion that mental disorders could occur in particular periods of life appeared only in the second half of the nineteenth century (1). During the present time, there has been much discussion regarding the nosology and classification of late-life mental disorders, particularly in the area of psychotic disorders (2).

WHAT IS PSYCHOSIS?

In his seminal work on clinical psychopathology, Fish opined that there were no specific criteria that would allow a clear distinction to be made between psychotic phenomena and neurotic symptoms. He described a person suffering from psychotic symptoms as "an individual who lacks insight, has the whole of his personality distorted by illness and constructs a false environment out of his or her subjective experiences" (3). Medical dictionaries define psychosis as a mental disorder characterized by gross impairment in *reality testing*, as evidenced by delusions, hallucinations, marked incoherent speech, or disorganized and agitated behavior, without apparent awareness on the part of the patient on the incomprehensibility of his or her behavior. In clinical practice, most psychiatrists are accustomed to using the word psychosis to describe a severe mental illness in which delusions and hallucinations are prominent.

This chapter will focus on the psychotic illnesses in the elderly, traditionally called functional psychoses, which include late-onset schizophrenia, chronic schizophrenia, and delusional disorders. Psychosis associated with dementia is covered elsewhere in this textbook.

CASE EXAMPLE

Mr. W, a 71-year-old widower, presented himself at the doctor's office saying that his neighbors had been planning to kill him for the last year. On further enquiry, Mr. W said he had seen them standing outside his house dis-

---

cussing ways of murdering him, and was sure one of them had decided to stab him if he returned home. He had tried calling the police a number of times, but they did not believe him. He also claimed he was the last descendent of a royal family that had ruled the world, and his neighbors were jealous of him.

On mental state examination, Mr. W appeared disheveled and pale and had not eaten for days for fear of being poisoned. He muttered to himself while sitting alone in the waiting room, and during the interview his speech was interrupted by pauses when he would simply stare into space and mutter abuse. He was having persistent auditory hallucinations, which he described as two voices of his neighbors constantly ridiculing him and talking to each other about plans to kill him. He expressed delusions of reference, persecution, and grandiosity, and had no insight into his problem.

Mr. W was previously known as a retired teacher who was pleasant and courteous, but did not socialize with the neighbors. Neighbors had noticed he was becoming more reclusive, avoiding the milk man and neglecting his garden for the last 6 to 8 months. There was no history of a medical or psychiatric illness, apart from hypertension.

When seen, Mr. W got agitated, started shouting, and threatened to sue his doctor. After discussions with the psychiatric emergency services, he was admitted on the acute psychiatry ward for assessment.

On the ward, he was prescribed 0.5 mg of risperidone, which he refused to take orally. He had to be given 1 mg of lorazepam intramuscularly twice a day for his agitation. His physical examination and investigation was normal. On the fourth day of admission his agitation began to settle, and he started taking risperidone orally, at which point it was increased to 1 mg twice a day over 3 weeks. He was noted to be suspicious of the food and members of the staff, and was often seen muttering to himself. After 4 weeks, his auditory hallucinations began to subside, he started looking after his hygiene, and became more interested in the ward activities. He gradually developed a positive relationship with some of the staff members. He remained convinced about his royal descent and the plot to kill him for 8 to 12 weeks, but was less concerned about them. Through discussions with the doctors, he gradually became more aware of the nature of his illness and the role of medication. On discharge from hospital, he was free of psychotic features and was willing to take medication regularly. It was arranged that Mr. W have weekly home visits by a community psychiatric nurse, and regular follow-up appointments in the outpatient clinic.

LATE-ONSET SCHIZOPHRENIA

Historical Development

In 1893, Kraepelin used the term *dementia praecox* to describe an endogenous psychotic illness starting at an early age and progressing to dementia in late life (4). He later conceded that dementia praecox did not always begin in youth, and that two-thirds of patients experienced onset between the ages of 15 and 30. The number of first episodes of illness dwindled as age progressed, although in a small number of cases the illness developed in the fourth, fifth, or even the sixth decade of life (5). In 1908, Bleuler suggested the term *schizophrenia* instead of Kraepelin's dementia praecox (6), and later Bleuler's son coined the term *late-onset schizophrenia* to describe a group of psychoses fulfilling the following criteria (7):

■ The psychosis must begin after age 40.
■ Symptomatology does not differ from that of schizophrenia, which develops in early life.
■ There is neither an amnestic syndrome nor accompanying physical findings linking the symptoms to brain disease.

Bleuler reported that 15% of all schizophrenic disorders began after the age of 40, and that they could be divided into two groups according to their symptomatology (7). In somewhat more than half of the late-onset schizophrenics, the range of symptoms may include paraphrenia-like states on the one hand, and depressive, anxious, and catatonic states on the other. They may also exhibit confusion and agitation that can easily be mistaken for dementia. In the second, smaller subset of late-onset schizophrenics, symptomatology does not show anything differing from early-onset schizophrenics.

In the early 1950s, Roth and Morrissey described a group of patients who developed an illness after the age of 60, characterized by primary delusions associated with volitional disturbances, and hallucinations in clear consciousness (8). These symptoms were similar to a subgroup of dementia praecox, as described by Kraepelin. He had characterized this group as having a minimal disturbance of affect and will, and having a very insidious development of delusions and hallucinations, with relative preservation of personality and no progression to dementia. Kraepelin described the symptoms as beginning mostly between the ages of 30 and 50, and called them *paraphrenia*. Roth coined the term *late paraphrenia* to describe elderly patients with paraphrenia-like symptoms (9). In 1960, Fish criticized the term late paraphrenia on the grounds that, firstly, the studies conducted in Germany showed that the diagnosis of paraphrenia merged into that of paranoid schizophrenia and, secondly, that late paraphrenia could also be confused with Bleuler's late-onset schizophrenia (10). The term late paraphrenia has also been criticized as being over-inclusive and ill-defined, described by Howard as a British concept with no international counterpart (11). However, it did have an impact on international research and literature, and can serve a useful purpose by embracing conditions whose boundaries and relationship to schizophrenia are yet unclear (12).

In summary, there has been much debate on the nomenclature of psychosis in old age over the last 50 years. Until the 1980s, these nomenclature debates caused widespread disputes among the psychiatrists in Europe and the United States with regard to the diagnosis of psychosis (13). Howard and Rabins attempted to resolve these differences in 1997 by suggesting the term of *late-onset schizophrenia* for psychotic illnesses developing between the ages of 45 to 59, and *late life onset schizophrenia-like psychosis* for psychotic illnesses with an onset after 60 years of age (14). Andreasen criticized the use of the term late-onset schizophrenia for psychotic illnesses in old age by arguing that schizophrenia, according to current evidence, is a neurodevelopmental disorder, in contrast to the psychosis developing in old age, which occurs after the full development of the brain and is therefore likely to be a degenerative process (15). Andreasen further argued that although both these conditions have common symptoms, they should be treated as separate conditions to avoid the risk of pooling heterogenous disorders that have different etiologies. The recent versions of the Diagnostic and Statistical Manual of American Psychiatric Association, 4th Edition, Text Revision (DSM-IV-TR), and the International Classification of Diseases (ICD-10) have no special categories for late-onset psychosis, although schizophrenia can be diagnosed at any age (16,17).

Clinical Features

Psychopathology

Delusions are the most common presenting symptom in late-onset schizophrenia. Persecutory delusions are most frequent, although grandiose, erotic, or somatic delusions are not uncommon. In a series of 101 patients, Howard et al.

reported delusions of reference in 76% of patients, delusions of control in 25%, grandiosity in 12%, and hypochondriasis in 11% (18). Hallucinations, in all sensory modalities, are also common, with auditory hallucinations most common. Schneiderian first-rank symptoms are less common, and formal thought disorder and negative symptoms are rare (19,20). Depressive symptoms are known to be associated with late-onset schizophrenia and are reported by a number of patients (21).

Neuropsychology

The development of neurocognitive deficits in schizophrenia has been widely reported and will be discussed in detail under chronic schizophrenia, but very few studies have looked at development of neurocognitive deficits in late-onset schizophrenia. Late-onset schizophrenia patients show a generalized pattern of cognitive deficits that is similar to younger schizophrenics but is different, both quantitatively and qualitatively, from those observed in patients with dementia of the Alzheimer's disease or Lewy-body type. The schizophrenia deficits seem to spare the patients' learning capacity (22). Almeida et al. studied a group of 40 patients with late paraphrenia and 33 age-matched controls on a number of cognitive tasks (23). Patients with paraphrenia showed worse performance than that of the controls in all tasks, even though the groups were matched for premorbid IQ and educational attainment. When these results were compared with a similar study done on younger-onset schizophrenia patients, it was noted that, regardless of the age of onset, people with schizophrenia displayed a similar pattern of generalized cognitive impairment.

In a recent study, Brodaty et al. studied groups of early onset, late onset, and healthy controls, after excluding dementia, for 5 years (24). All groups were assessed on measures of psychopathology, cognition, and general functioning, and compared on rates of decline and incidence of dementia at the start, at 1 year, and at 5 years of the study. No differences were observed between the early-onset and late-onset schizophrenia groups in cognitive decline at the start and year one of the study, but at 5 years the differences in cognitive decline became more marked, as a number of patients from the late-onset schizophrenia group developed dementia, and about half of the sample of the early-onset schizophrenia group remained cognitively stable. This suggested that late-onset schizophrenia is a heterogeneous syndrome, and relatively little is known about the interaction between cognitive deficits associated with schizophrenia, dementia, and ageing.

Diagnostic Criteria

There is no separate category for late-onset schizophrenia in DSM-IV-TR or ICD-10. The diagnosis will be based on the general criteria for schizophrenia using DSM-IV-TR

TABLE 28-1
DIAGNOSTIC CRITERIA FOR SCHIZOPHRENIA

Characteristic Symptoms: Two (or more) of the following, each present for a significant portion of time during a 1-month period (or less if successfully treated):
- Delusions
- Hallucinations
- Disorganized speech (e.g., frequent derailment or incoherence)
- Grossly disorganized or catatonic behavior
- Negative symptoms (e.g., affective flattening, alogia, or avolition)
- Social/occupational dysfunction

Duration: Continuous signs of the disturbance persist for at least 6 months
Exclusion of schizoaffective and mood disorder
Exclusion of substance abuse/general medical condition

Adapted from Reference 25.

(25); however, it is important to realize that the symptoms may be milder in elderly people (Table 28-1).

Epidemiology

There have been a few studies detailing the prevalence of schizophrenia and related disorders in late life. The Epidemiological Catchment Area study reported a 1-year prevalence rate of schizophrenia of 0.6% for people between 45 and 64 years old, and 0.2% for people older than 65 (26). Copeland et al. reported the prevalence of schizophrenia as 0.12% and of delusional disorder as 0.04% in a sample of 5,222 individuals 65 and older in Liverpool, England (27). The same study reported the incidence rates of schizophrenia and delusional disorder as three per 100,000 per year.

Studies conducted on the frequency of late-onset schizophrenia amongst patients in psychiatric facilities have reported a range from 3% to 4% (28) to as high as 8% to 10% (29,30). In a review of early studies, Harris and Jeste estimated that 13% of the hospitalized patients with schizophrenia were reported to have had onset of psychosis in their 40s, 7% had onset in their 50s, and only 3% first presented after the age of 60 (31). These percentages cannot be considered definitive, since studies were conducted on samples of patients treated for their illnesses and not on the general population, thus missing undiagnosed patients living in the community who are known to be reluctant to seek help from the mental health services (32).

Assessment

Since paranoid symptoms are not uncommon in elderly people (33) and late-onset schizophrenia is relatively uncommon, the schizophrenia diagnosis should be made by ruling out other possible causes of psychotic symptoms.

It is important to rule out organic brain pathology by carrying out the following:

- Neurological examination.
- Laboratory investigations (blood counts, liver function tests, and renal function tests). These investigations are intended to rule out underlying metabolic or inflammatory conditions that could present with psychosis in elderly patients.
- Brain scan or imaging studies may be done if organic brain pathology is suspected.

Typical late-onset schizophrenia patients present with delusions (most commonly persecutory delusions) and hallucinations. They have no history of such problems and have functioned moderately well in the past.

Differential Diagnosis

The three important conditions in the differential diagnosis of late-onset schizophrenia are as follows:

Dementia

It is important clinically to rule out dementias of all three common types, which include Alzheimer's disease, vascular dementia, and dementia with Lewy bodies. They can all present with psychotic symptoms. In most cases, a detailed psychiatric history and careful mental state examination, supported by a brain scan, should be sufficient to reach the diagnosis. In some cases there might be an overlap between the psychotic symptoms and the onset of cognitive problems, and a detailed neuropsychological assessment may be required.

Mood Disorders with Psychotic Features

The overlap between late-onset schizophrenia and affective features is commonly seen clinically. In a 10-year follow-up study of 24 late paraphrenia patients, Holden reported that 10 of the group had affective or schizoaffective illnesses, and that these patients had a better outcome as compared to the purely psychotic patients (34). Mood disorders with psychotic features can present for the first time after the age of 45 and can be confused with late-onset schizophrenia. Predominance of affective symptoms and a periodical course of illness can be helpful in differentiating mood disorders from late-onset schizophrenia patients, whose psychotic symptoms start earlier and persist for a longer time as compared to affective symptoms.

Delusional Disorders

Delusional disorders can be differentiated from late-onset schizophrenia since they present with delusions with a single, often encapsulated, theme. Hallucinations are not prominent with delusional disorders, and the overall psychosocial functioning is not markedly impaired.

In late-onset schizophrenia the common presentation is of delusions that may have multiple themes, hallucinations, and generalized deterioration of psychosocial functioning (25). It may be difficult at times to differentiate between the two conditions, and the diagnosis is reached after considering the course of illness and response to medication.

Etiology

Genetics

Family studies have shown the overall risk of schizophrenia in relatives of an affected person to be about 10%, compared with the risk of about 1% for the general population (35). Few studies have looked at the familiarity in late-onset schizophrenia due to the difficulties inherent in conducting such studies, like tracing first degree relatives due to untimely deaths and geographic relocation. The overall prevalence and risk of schizophrenia in first degree relatives of late-onset schizophrenia patients is lower than that in families of early-onset schizophrenia (36,37). The prevalence of schizophrenia amongst relatives of late-onset cases is no higher than the general population (38,39).

An association of HLA-A9 genotype has been reported for early-onset schizophrenia, but this finding could not be replicated in late-onset schizophrenia patients. It has been postulated that the syndrome of late-onset schizophrenia is genetically different from early-onset schizophrenia. The mode of inheritance is postulated to be polygenic and influenced by nongenetic factors (40,41).

Gender Differences

Many studies on late-onset psychosis have described a majority of women as compared to men (42). In a magnetic resonance imaging (MRI) study of gender differences in age-related brain changes in the elderly population, Murphy et al. found increased brain volume loss in parietal lobes of females as compared to males (43). The antidopaminergic action of estrogen may have a protective function at delaying the onset of schizophrenia (44). However, the incidence of schizophrenia does not rise around menopause, when there is the biggest drop in estrogen levels, and schizophrenia can manifest for the first time at a very advanced age.

Brain Imaging

Computed tomography (CT) and MRI studies looking at ventricular enlargements and cerebral atrophy in late-onset schizophrenia, compared to age and sex-matched healthy controls, have not revealed any significant differences. In 1989, Burns et al. (45) found no significant differences in lateral and third ventricular changes compared to healthy control subjects, and suggested that in late-onset schizophrenia an uncoupling of the normal association between ventricular and cortical size occurs, which could be responsible for the onset of psychotic symptoms (46). These findings were replicated in 1992 (47), although Pearlson and colleagues found insignificant lateral but significant third ventricular enlargements in late-onset schizophrenia (48).

The regional cerebral blood flow studies using single positron emission computed tomography (SPECT) have suggested the contribution of vascular structural brain abnormalities in the etiology of late-onset schizophrenia. Miller et al. (49) studied 18 late-onset schizophrenia patients compared with 30 healthy controls, using SPECT. Thirteen patients out of the 18 late-onset schizophrenia patients showed unilateral or bilateral temporal hypoperfusion, as compared to seven out of 30 healthy controls. In addition to the blood perfusion changes, some studies have also reported an increased number of vascular lesions (50,51), and others have documented large areas of white matter hyperintensities in patients with late-onset schizophrenia as compared to age-matched controls (52).

Sensory Deficits

Several studies have reported an association between hearing impairment and late-onset schizophrenia. Deafness has been clinically associated with paranoid symptoms, since it can reinforce the pre-existing tendency to social isolation, withdrawal, and suspiciousness (53,54). Keshavan et al. (55) noted that auditory hallucinations, of all the psychopathological phenomena, were most consistently associated with deafness, and Almeida and colleagues reported improvement in psychotic symptoms after the fitting of a hearing aid (56).

Visual impairments, such as cataracts, have also been associated with paranoid psychosis and visual hallucinations (57,58). In a case control study, Prager and Jeste assessed visual and hearing impairments in 87 middle-aged and elderly subjects, including 16 with late-onset schizophrenia, 25 with early-onset schizophrenia, 20 with mood disorder, and 26 normal comparison subjects, uncorrected and corrected (with eye glasses and hearing aids) (59). They concluded that late-onset schizophrenia, early-onset schizophrenia, and mood disorder patients may all have equivalent sensory deficits, but inadequate correction of their sensory impairments compared to normal comparison subjects. Therefore, a specific contribution of sensory deficits to the etiology of late-onset schizophrenia remains uncertain.

Causation of Late-Onset Schizophrenia

Two possible hypotheses have been suggested for the causation of late-onset schizophrenia. The first suggests a genetic susceptibility to the illness, with the onset of illness in late life brought about by neuronal loss due to aging and vascular or other age-related functional changes, particularly those affecting women with post-menopausal estrogen loss and consequent alteration in the relative balance of basal ganglia dopamine D2 receptors (60). The second hypothesis suggests no genetic etiology, but rather that a single event occurring in late life precipitates the onset of illness. This event could be an age-associated pathology such as a microvascular disease, or the early manifestations of a primary dementia. Pearlson concluded that late-onset psychosis represents the end result of diverse etiopathologies, perhaps a mixture of delayed classical early onset and organic secondary causes (61).

Management

Antipsychotics

Antipsychotic medications are the most effective symptomatic treatment for both early-onset and late-onset schizophrenia, because they improve the acute symptoms and prevent relapses (62). Elderly people are known to show variable responses and increased sensitivity to medications (63). Age-related bodily changes are known to affect the pharmacokinetics and pharmacodynamics of neuroleptics in the elderly. It is important to avoid doing more harm than good, and to follow the principle of "start low and go slow" when initiating antipsychotic medication in the elderly (64).

Conventional Antipsychotics

Conventional antipsychotics are known to be effective for the positive symptoms of schizophrenia, but have little impact on the negative symptoms. The research literature on the use of conventional antipsychotics in late-onset schizophrenia is sparse, and their use should be weighed against the potential side-effect risks. Significant improvements in psychotic symptoms with the use of haloperidol, trifluoperazine (10 to 30 mg/day), and thioridazine (50 to 400 mg/day) have been reported (65,66). However, thioridazine has been reported to cause prolongation of QT interval, and its use in the elderly is not recommended. More recent studies, conducted from the 1980s onwards, have reported modest response to conventional antipsychotic medication. Pearlson et al. reported no improvement or only partial improvement in 54% of their patients, and found poor response to be associated with the presence of thought disorder and with schizoid premorbid personality traits, but not with presence of first-rank symptoms, a family history of schizophrenia, or gender (67).

Howard and Levy reported that the use of depot antipsychotic medication (either 14.4 mg of flupenthixol decanoate or 9 mg of fluphenazine decanoate every 2 weeks) was associated with better compliance and treatment outcome at a reduced amount of neuroleptic medication, as compared to patients receiving oral medication (68).

Conventional antipsychotics are known to have a wide variety of side effects related to their affinity for dopamine, cholinergic, and alpha adrenergic receptors. Table 28-2 gives a list of commonly seen side effects of conventional antipsychotics, which need to be considered when prescribing these

TABLE 28-2
POTENTIAL SIDE EFFECTS OF ANTIPSYCHOTICS IN THE ELDERLY

Extrapyramidal
- Pseudoparkinsonism
- Akathisia
- Acute dystonia
- Tardive dyskinesia

Anticholinergic
- Urinary hesitancy
- Constipation
- Blurred vision
- Dry mouth
- Delirium

Postural Hypotension
Sedation
Hypersalivation
Gastrointestinal
- Nausea
- Constipation
- Diarrhea

Liver
- Cholestatic jaundice
- Raised transaminase enzyme activities

Cardiovascular
- Electrocardiogram abnormalities: QTc prolongation

Endocrine
- Weight gain
- Diabetes mellitus

Epilepsy

medications to elderly patients. Conventional antipsychotics can also affect cognitive performance in the elderly, cause significant functional impairment, and increase the incidence of falls and hip fractures. A greater susceptibility to cardiac side effects and the risk of tardive dyskinesia should be given special consideration. Jeste et al. reported the cumulative incidence of dyskinetic movements in elderly patients to be 29% following 12 months of typical neuroleptic use (69). Higher dosage and longer duration of neuroleptic treatment is known to increase the risk of tardive dyskinesia.

Atypical Antipsychotics

The newer antipsychotics have been found more effective in treating negative symptoms and patients who are treatment resistant. They also have the advantage of having fewer side effects, although some of these medications can cause sedation and postural hypertension (70). Clozapine has been widely used in young-onset cases of schizophrenia, and has been found effective in managing treatment-resistant cases and cases of severe tardive dyskinesia. It is known to cause agranulocytosis in 1% of the adult population, but the rates may be higher in the elderly population. Other potentially problematic side effects in the elderly are sedation and postural hypotension (71). Keeping in mind

the side-effect profile and potential difficulties in monitoring blood white-cell count, clozapine is not a first-line antipsychotic for elderly patients, and should only be used in cases of treatment resistance and severe dyskinesia (72).

Risperidone is the most extensively studied atypical antipsychotic in the elderly population. Jeste and colleagues reported that risperidone is effective as a first-line antipsychotic agent. It is well tolerated if prescribed in low doses, and produces significant clinical improvement in elderly patients with schizophrenia (73). It is available in depot form and has also been shown to improve cognitive functions (69,74). Also, it has a reduced risk of causing tardive dyskinesia as compared to haloperidol. In a few recent studies, risperidone use was associated with an increased risk of cerebrovascular events (CAE) in demented patients with psychosis and agitation. This is thought to be a class effect for all atypicals; thus, their use in people with a history of or high risk for cerebrovascular events should be based on a thorough assessment of the potential risks and benefits.

Olanzapine has also been shown to reduce positive and negative symptoms in elderly patients with schizophrenia; however, there have been concerns of olanzapine causing weight gain, worsened diabetes mellitus, and adverse effects on lipid metabolism.

Quetiapine has also been shown effective in treating elderly patients with schizophrenia. Dizziness and postural hypotension are the commonly reported side effects, which may be avoided by gradual titration of dose (75).

Other atypical antipsychotics like ziprasidone and aripiprazole have been shown effective in young-onset cases, but there are little data available on their use in the elderly. Aripiprazole, with its unique mode of action as a partial agonist at D2 receptors, and reduced likelihood of causing extrapyramidal side effects, cardiovascular problems, sedation, and weight gain, holds promise for the elderly population (76). In a recently published open-label study of aripiprazole use on 10 elderly patients, Madhusoondanan et al. found it was safe and improved both positive and negative symptoms (77). The suggested daily doses of atypical antipsychotics are given in Table 28-3, but should be taken as a guide only. For more information on use of atypicals in the elderly, see the chapter on agitation and psychosis associated with dementia, and Appendix A in this textbook.

Psychosocial Therapies

Psychosocial interventions are important in improving the treatment outcome of late-onset schizophrenia, due to the chronic nature of the illness. Moreover, a significant number of patients fail to show a complete response to antipsychotic medication (72). A number of psychosocial interventions, like social skills training, cognitive retraining, and family counseling, have been shown to have positive effects in the treatment of young adults with schizophrenia. Jeste and Winnett stressed the importance of addressing cognitive and sensory impairments through individual or group therapy sessions (78).

TABLE 28-3
RECOMMENDED DOSES OF ATYPICAL ANTIPSYCHOTICS IN THE ELDERLY

Name	Starting Dose	Typical Dose Range
Clozapine	6.25–12.5 mg/day	12.5–100 mg/day
Risperidone	0.25–0.5 mg/day	0.5–4 mg/day
Olanzapine	2.5–5 mg/day	5–20 mg/day
Quetiapine	12.5–50 mg/day	50–450 mg/day
Ziprasidone	20–40 mg/day	20–160 mg/day
Aripiprazole	5 mg/day	20–30 mg/day

Cognitive Behavioral Therapy

The efficacy of cognitive behavioral techniques has been widely reported in early-onset schizophrenia, and these techniques have been found useful in treatment-resistant patients (79). Techniques aimed at modification of delusional beliefs and control over hallucinations (80), and reinforcement of coping strategies have also been reported effective. There is a dearth of research on the use of psychotherapeutic interventions in elderly patients with schizophrenia, but perhaps these interventions can be used to address coping strategies and to help patients gain insight into their illness and live a meaningful life (81).

Electroconvulsive Therapy (ECT)

Most of the research work on the efficacy of ECT for elderly patients with schizophrenia comes from the 1950s and 1960s. Kay and Roth reported temporary remissions occurring with the use of ECT in about 25% of their patients (82), and Frost reported a positive response to ECT in patients of late paraphrenia presenting with dominant mood symptoms (83). With the introduction of a variety of typical and atypical antipsychotic medications, the use of ECT in elderly patients with schizophrenia has become rare in clinical practice. See figure 28.1 for a protocol of managing schizophrenia in the elderly.

Course and Outcome

Little is known about the long-term course of late-onset schizophrenia, and there have been few studies on the topic in recent years. Earlier studies found that late-onset schizophrenia runs a chronic course, and the causes of death are similar to the general population (82,84). In a 3-year follow-up study of elderly patients with schizophrenia, Hoffman et al. reported the prevalence of moderately severe negative symptoms that tend to remain stable over time (85). The outcome studies on schizophrenia in general have reported either a general decline in the severity of positive symptoms, or remission over the long term. The long-term outcome of chronic schizophrenia will be discussed in detail in the following section.

CHRONIC SCHIZOPHRENIA

This section deals with schizophrenic patients who had an onset of illness at a younger age, ran a chronic course, and have now joined the elderly age group. This group of patients has also been called *graduates*, a term coined by Arie and Jolley in 1982 (86). Unfortunately, the literature and research work on this population has been sparse; Bridge et al. called schizophrenia in old age "the stepchild of psychiatric research" (87).

Clinical Features

Bleuler (88) described the reduction of delusions, hallucinations, and dysfunctional effects of schizophrenia in elderly patients, phenomena described as *burning out* by Bridge et al. (87). Recent studies have reported a gradual decline of positive symptoms and an increase of negative symptoms over time (89,90), correlating with cognitive deficits (91). Depressive symptoms are not uncommon and are linked to positive symptoms, poor physical health, low income, and diminished network support (92).

Neuropsychological Deficits

Cognitive impairment associated with schizophrenia has been widely reported (93), and severe cognitive impairment is the most important single predictor of poor outcome (94). Specific cognitive deficits, such as in executive functioning (95), use of language (96), and memory functions (97) have been reported. Whether these cognitive impairments are progressive is controversial. One school of thought believes that cognitive deficits occur at an early stage of the illness and remain more or less stable over the rest of the lifespan, and cross-sectional studies have suggested that cognitive functions do not decline over time (93,98). The other school of thought suggests that cognitive impairments are progressive over time. Harvey et al. studied at least 26 elderly patients with schizophrenia over 13 months and found that 30% of the patients showed cognitive decline (99). Low education, older age, and severe positive symptoms were the major predicting factors of the cognitive decline.

These neurocognitive deficits are more or less permanent and do not improve with antipsychotic medication. They have a negative effect on community functioning and social adaptation (100,101), and are responsible for the failure of the patient's social rehabilitation (93). It is important to consider the possibility of the comorbid onset of dementia in elderly patients with schizophrenia, which can act as a confounder in the studies done on neurocognitive deficits in this population.

Medical Comorbidity

Medical problems are known to increase with age (102), and some medical illnesses, like cardiovascular disorders, diabetes mellitus, Parkinson's disease, peptic ulcers, epilepsy, asthma, cancer, and rheumatoid arthritis, have been associated with schizophrenia (103,104). Koranyi reported that nonpsychiatric physicians missed one-third and psychiatrists missed one-half of their psychiatric patients' comorbid medical conditions (105), and Koran et al. reported that half of the public psychiatric patients' physical illnesses went unrecognized (106). Jeste and colleagues reported that schizophrenic patients received less adequate health care compared to the general population, and the elderly population of schizophrenics can be at risk of being undiagnosed or inadequately cared for regarding their comorbid physical problems (107). It is important to be aware of the possibility of concomitant physical illness, since patients with schizophrenia may under-report symptoms because of increased pain tolerance. Furthermore, lack of knowledge can cause noncompliance with treatment, and comorbid conditions can adversely affect the clinical course and treatment of schizophrenia (108).

Social Disabilities

Most elderly patients with schizophrenia suffer from varying degrees of social disabilities, due to the chronic nature of their symptoms and neurocognitive deficits (105). In a study of long-term hospitalized patients, Wing and Furlong found that a majority of patients were unmarried and had lost contact with their relatives and the outside community (109). The major factors that contributed to their social disabilities were risk of harm, unpredictability of behavior, poor motivation, lack of insight, and low public acceptability.

Elderly patients with schizophrenia are known to develop relatively better coping skills for their illness (110), but they continue to have problems in their daily functioning while living in the community. Klaplow et al. studied a group of 55 patients between the ages of 45 and 86, and compared them with normal controls (111). Although the schizophrenic patients were similar to the controls in the more basic living skills, like time, orientation, and eating, they were significantly impaired on higher-order functioning skills, like communication, transportation, finance, shopping, and grooming.

Epidemiology

The epidemiologic catchment area study reported the prevalence rate of schizophrenia in the elderly population to be 0.3%, but was criticized for under-reporting the prevalence in the elderly population (112). In North America, the prevalence of schizophrenia in the elderly population is believed to be about 1% (113), and various studies have reported the prevalence in Europe as 0% to 2.22% (114).

Cunningham and Johnstone (115) reported an equal sex distribution in long-stay hospitalized elderly patients with schizophrenia, but later studies reported a predominance of males, with a male to female ratio of 2:1. These results could be biased, as male elderly patients are more likely to be hospitalized for a longer time due to the difficulties of housing them in the community (89).

Since the shift of the psychiatric services from hospital-based to community-based care, and the closure of the majority of mental hospitals in the U.K. and North America, the majority of elderly patients with schizophrenia are living in the community. In 1987, Goldman et al. reported that about 200,000 elderly people with schizophrenia had been discharged to nursing homes in the United States (116). The population of elderly patients with schizophrenia living in the community has been gradually rising since then, and Cohen and colleagues reported that approximately 85% of elderly patients with schizophrenia were living in the community in the United States in the year 2000 (108).

Management

Antipsychotics

Several studies done on young patients with schizophrenia have indicated the favorable long-term effects of the use of antipsychotic medication (117). Fewer studies have looked at the use of neuroleptics in elderly patients, but antipsychotics are reportedly the most commonly used medication for patients living in institutions (118). Older patients are known to be at greater risk of developing extrapyramidal symptoms and tardive dyskinesia. These symptoms can affect functional performance to a greater extent than positive or negative symptoms for the duration of psychosis (119). The use of atypical antipsychotics, which have fewer side effects and a better effect on negative symptoms than the typicals, along with psychosocial therapies, seems to produce the most favorable results (Table 28-3).

Psychological Therapies

The role of cognitive behavioral therapy (CBT) in alleviating symptoms and improving the quality of life in younger patients with schizophrenia has been widely reported (120). McQuaid and colleagues suggested the usefulness of an integrated treatment combining CBT and social skills training (SST) for elderly schizophrenic patients (121). This treatment approach suits the needs of elderly patients, and is aimed at reducing their cognitive vulnerabilities, improving abilities to cope with stress, and adherence to other forms of treatment. The use of SST alone, in order to facilitate the rehabilitation of elderly patients with schizophrenia in the community, by improving their social skills (122) and interpersonal skills (123), has also been reported.

Rehabilitation

The rehabilitation of elderly patients with schizophrenia is aimed at enabling them to make the best use of their residual abilities to function at an optimal level in as normal a social context as possible (124). It is important to look at the range of disabilities of this group of patients in order to plan their rehabilitation. The disabilities can be divided into the following classifications (125):

- Primary disabilities: emotional, cognitive, motivational, and behavioral dysfunction.
- Secondary disabilities: loss of self-esteem, social withdrawal, and loss of social network.
- Tertiary disabilities: unemployment, stigma, homelessness, and poverty.

A comprehensive rehabilitation plan would include medication and compliance, housing and financial support, support for daily activities and social contacts, education, and treatment of physical illness. This rehabilitation plan can be achieved by adopting a multi-disciplinary approach, with the involvement of the psychiatrist, physician, psychiatric nurse, occupational therapist, social worker, and the patient's relatives.

Course and Outcome

Kraepelin (126) described a bleak outcome of schizophrenia, but more recent studies have reported a heterogeneous outcome. Abrahamson et al. studied a population of elderly patients with schizophrenia and found improvement in 25% and deterioration in only 10%, indicating a trend towards improvement in late age (127). But McGlashan noted that the improvement in late age was highly variable and impossible to predict (128). Many patients developed multiple exacerbations of their illness throughout their lives, requiring hospitalization and continued long-term treatment (129). The most common indicators of a poor outcome are unmarried status, social isolation, long duration of episode, a history of psychiatric treatment, and a history of behavioral disturbance in childhood (130).

DELUSIONAL DISORDERS

Delusional disorders are characterized by nonbizarre and circumscribed delusions, less frequent hallucinations (if at all), and relatively better-preserved psychosocial functioning. Delusions are deemed nonbizarre if they can conceivably occur in real life (e.g., being poisoned, plotted against, or deceived).

TABLE 28-4
DIAGNOSTIC CRITERIA FOR DELUSIONAL DISORDER

Characteristic Symptoms
- Nonbizarre delusions (i.e., involving situations that can occur in real life, such as being followed, poisoned, infected, loved at a distance, deceived by spouse or lover, giving a disease) of at least 1 month's duration
- Not meeting the criteria for schizophrenia
- No marked social or occupational dysfunction
- Exclusion of mood disorder
- Exclusion of substance abuse

Subtypes
- Erotomanic: delusions that another person, usually of higher status, is in love with the individual
- Grandiose: delusions of inflated worth, power, knowledge, identity, or special relationship to a deity or famous person
- Jealous: delusions that the individual's sexual partner is unfaithful
- Persecutory: delusions that the person (or someone to whom the person is close) is being malevolently treated in some way
- Somatic: delusions that the person has some physical defect or general medical condition
- Mixed: delusions characteristic of more than one of the above types, but no one theme predominates

Adapted from Reference 25.

Clinical Features

The symptomatology of delusional disorders in the elderly has not been studied in detail. While looking at its presentation in general, the delusions are nonbizarre and can have different themes like persecution, infection, love, or infidelity. Persecutory delusions are most commonly seen. Auditory and visual hallucinations, if present, are not prominent. Hallucinations in other modalities, like olfaction and touch, can be present in relation to the delusional theme, e.g., tactile hallucinations along with delusions of infestation (131).

Diagnostic Criteria

There are no separate diagnostic criteria for delusional disorders in the elderly in DSM-IV-TR. The criteria for delusional disorder for adults are used for the elderly population, but the symptoms can be milder (Table 28-4).

Epidemiology

The prevalence of delusional disorder in the elderly was reported by Copeland and colleagues to be 0.04% in a randomly selected sample of 5,222 people (27). The minimum incidence for delusional disorder estimated in this study was 15.6 per 100,000 per year. In a case register study of 440 patients with DSM-IV delusional disorder in Spain, 122 (27%) were older than 65 (131). In hospital-based studies, delusional disorder accounts for 1% to 2% of the admissions (adults and elderly combined) to inpatient mental health facilities (16).

Assessment and Diagnosis

The typical patient is an elderly man, with no psychiatric history, presenting with a strong conviction that one of his ex-colleagues is plotting to kill him. Social functioning is relatively preserved, and there might not be any other associated symptom.

It is important to exclude delirium, dementia, drug abuse, psychotic depression, and schizophrenia before making the diagnosis. It may be difficult to establish whether a delusion is bizarre or not, particularly if the patient comes from a different culture. The diagnosis can be further divided into various sub-types according to the predominant delusional theme, such as erotomanic, grandiose, jealous, persecutory, somatic, and mixed types (Table 28-4).

Management

Very few studies have looked at the treatment of delusional disorder in the elderly. Antipsychotics are the most commonly used medication. Brietner and Anderson reported that the delusions tended to be chronic and did not respond well to antipsychotic medication (132). However, these medications did tend to decrease agitation and the intensity of delusions (133).

Considering the current evidence, it would be sensible to suggest the use of antipsychotics (preferably atypical) as

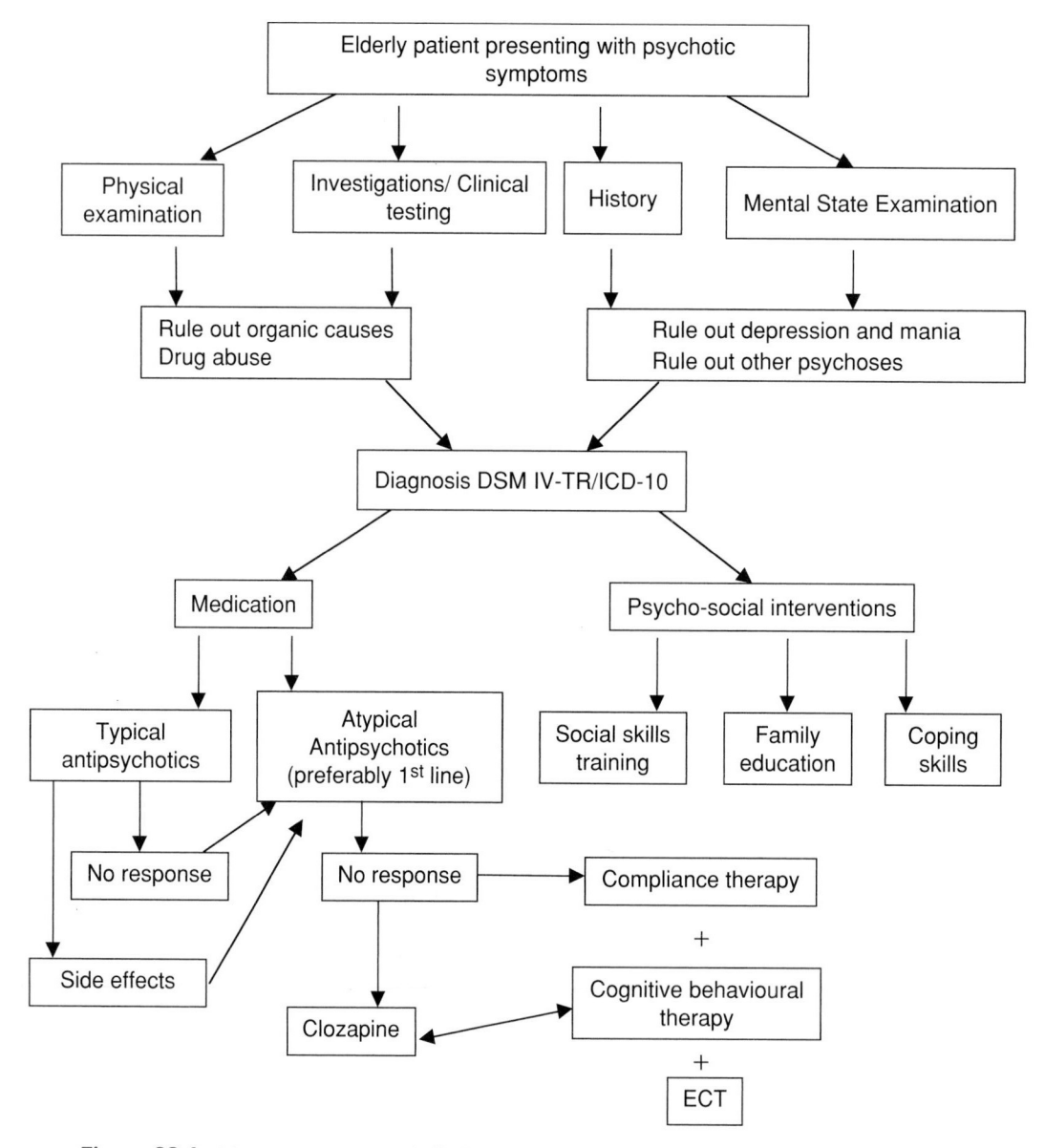

Figure 28-1   Management protocol of schizophrenia in the elderly.
DSM-IV-TR, Diagnostic and Statistical Manual of Mental Disorders, 4th Edition, Text Revision; ECT, electroconvulsive therapy; ICD-10, International Classification of Mental and Behavioral Disorders, 10th Edition.

first-line treatment, starting from a smaller dose and titrating according to the response and side effects experienced by the individual patient.

Course and Outcome

Little is known about the course and outcome of delusional disorder in the elderly. In a follow-up study of 23 patients with somatic delusions, Opjordsmoen reported that delusional disorder had the worst outcome (134). The course is variable in the adult population, with some showing full periods of remission and relapses, while others run a chronic course. In some patients, remission occurs in a few months without subsequent relapses.

REFERENCES

 1. Berrios BE. Late-onset mental disorders: a conceptual history. In: *Late-Onset Mental Disorders: The Postdam Conference*. Glasgow, UK: Bell & Bain; 1999:1–23.
 2. Lisa T, Zorrilla E, Jeste D. Late-life psychotic disorders: nosology and classification. In: Copeland JRM, Abou-Saleh MT, Blazer D, eds. *Principles and Practices of Geriatric Psychiatry*. 2nd ed. Chichester, UK: John Wiley; 2002:493–496.
 3. Hamilton M, ed. *Fish's Clinical Psychopathology: Signs and Symptoms in Psychiatry*. 2nd ed. Bristol, UK: Wright; 1985.
 4. Kraepelin E. *Psychiatrie, Ein Lehrbuch Für Studierende Und Ärzte*. Vol. 4. Barth: Leipzig; 1893.
 5. Kraepelin E. Fragestellungen der klinischen psychiatrie. *Zentralblatt Nervenheilkunde Psychiatrie*. 1905;28:573–590.
 6. Bleuler E. Due Prognose der dementia praecox (schizophreniegruppe). *Allg Z Psychiatr*. 1908;65:436–464.
 7. Bleuler M. Die spätschizophrenen krankheitsbilder. *Fortschr Neurol Psychiatr*. 1943;15:259–290.
 8. Roth M, Morrissey JD. Problems in the diagnosis and classification of mental disorders in old age. *J Mental Sci*. 1952;98: 66–80.
 9. Roth M. The natural history of mental disorders in old age. *J Mental Sci*. 1955;101:281–301.
10. Fish F. Senile schizophrenia. *J Mental Sci*. 1960;106:938–946.
11. Howard R. Late paraphrenia: an update. *J Roy Soc Med*. 1992;3:63–65.
12. Kay WK. The English-language literature on late-paraphrenia from the 1950s. In: Howard R, Rabins PV, Castle DJ, eds. *Late Onset Schizophrenia*. Stroud, UK: Wrightson Biomedical Publishing Ltd; 1999:17–43.
13. Rabins PV, Pauker S, Thomas J. Can schizophrenia begin after age 44? *Compr Psychiatry*. 1984;25:290–293.
14. Howard R, Rabins PV. Late-paraphrenia revisited. *Br J Psychiatry*. 1997;171:406–408.
15. Andreasen NC. I don't believe in late-onset schizophrenia. In: Howard R, Rabins PV, Castle DJ, eds. *Late Onset Schizophrenia*. Stroud, UK: Wrightson Biomedical Publishing Ltd; 1999: 111–123.
16. American Psychiatric Association. *Diagnostic and Statistical Manual of Mental Disorders*. 4th ed. Washington, DC: American Psychiatric Association; 1995.
17. World Health Organization. *The Tenth Revision of the International Classification of Diseases (ICD10)*. Geneva: World Health Organization; 1992.
18. Howard R, Almeida O, Levy R. Phenomenology, demography and diagnosis in late paraphrenia. *Psychol Med*. 1994;24(a): 397–410.
19. Pearlson GD, Kreger L, Rabins, et al. A chart-review study of late-onset and early-onset schizophrenia. *Am J Psychiatry*. 1989;146: 1568–1574.
20. Almeida O, Howard R, Levy R, David A. Psychotic states arising in late life (late paraphrenia). Psychopathology and nosology. *Br J Psychiatry*. 1995;166(a):205–215.
21. Jeste DV, Harris MJ, Pearlson GD, et al. Late-onset schizophrenia: studying clinical validity. *Psychiatr Clin North Am*. 1988;11:1–14.
22. Almeida OP. The neuropsychology of schizophrenia in late life. In: Howard R, Rabins PV, Castle DJ, eds. *Late Onset Schizophrenia*. Stroud, UK: Wrightson Biomedical Publishing Ltd; 1999: 181–189.
23. Almeida OP, Howard RJ, Levy R, David AS, Morris RG, Sahakian B. Cognitive features of psychotic states arising in late life (late paraphrenia). *Psychol Med*. 1995;25:685–698.
24. Brodaty H, Sachdev P, Koschera A, Monk D, Cullen B. Long-term outcome of late-onset schizophrenia: 5-year follow-up study. *Br J Psychiatry*. 2003;183:213–219.
25. American Psychiatric Association. Diagnostic and Statistical Manual of Mental Disorders (DSM-IV-TR). 4th ed. Text Revision. Washington, DC: American Psychiatric Association; 2000.
26. Keith SJ, Regier DA, Rae DS. Schizophrenic disorders. In: Robins LN, Regier DA, eds. *Psychiatric Disorders in America*. New York: Free Press; 1991.
27. Copeland JRM, Dewey ME, Scott A, et al. Schizophrenia and delusional disorder in older age: community prevalence, incidence, comorbidity and outcome. *Schizophr Bull*. 1998;24:153–161.
28. Yassa R, Dastoor D, Nastase C, Camille Y, Belzile L. The prevalence of late-onset schizophrenia in a psychogeriatric population. *J Geriatr Psychiatry Neurol*. 1993;6:120–125.
29. Leuchter AF, Spar JE. The late-onset psychoses. *J Nerv Ment Dis*. 1985;173:488–494.
30. Roth M. The natural history of mental disorder in old age. *J Ment Sci*. 1955;101:281–301.
31. Harris MJ, Jeste DV. Late-onset schizophrenia: an overview. *Schizophr Bull*. 1988;14:39–55.
32. Castle DJ. Epidemiology of late-onset schizophrenia. In: Howard R, Rabins PV, Castle DJ, eds. *Late Onset Schizophrenia*. Stroud, UK: Wrightson Biomedical Publishing Ltd; 1999:139–146.
33. Grief C, Eastwood RM. Paranoid disorders in the elderly. *Int J Geriatr Psychiatry*. 1993;8:681–684.
34. Holden N. Late paraphrenia or the paraphrenias: a descriptive study with a 10-year follow-up. *Br J Psychiatry*. 1987;150:635–639.
35. Gottesman II, Shields J. Schizophrenia, the epigenetic puzzle. Cambridge, UK: Cambridge University Press; 1982.
36. Rokhlina ML. A comparative clinico-genetic study of attack-like schizophrenia with late and early manifestations with regard to age [in Russian]. *Zh Nevropatol Psikhiatr*. 1975;75:417–424.
37. Castle DJ, Howard R. What do we know about the aetiology of late-onset schizophrenia? *European Psychiatry*. 1992;7:99–108.
38. Brodaty H, Sachdev P, Rose N, Rylands K, Prenter L. Schizophrenia with onset after age 50 years. 1. Phenomenology and risk factors. *Br J Psychiatry*. 1999;175:410–415.
39. Howard R, Graham C, Sham P, et al. A controlled family study of late-onset non-affective psychosis (late paraphrenia). *Br J Psychiatry*. 1997;170:511–514.
40. Naguib M, McGuffin R, Levy R, Festenstein H, Alonso A. Genetic markers in late paraphrenia: a study of HLA antigens. *Br J Psychiatry*. 1987;150:124–127.
41. Funding T. Genetics of paranoid psychosis of later life. *Acta Psychiatr Scand*. 1961;37:267–282.
42. Robbins TW, Sahakian B. Computer methods of assessment of cognitive function. In: Copeland JRM, Abou-Saleh MT, Blazer D, eds. *Principles and Practice of Geriatric Psychiatry*. 2nd ed. Chichester, UK: John Wiley; 2002:147–151.
43. Murphy DGM, DeCarli C, McIntosh AR. Sex differences in human brain morphometry and metabolism: as in-vivo quantitative magnetic resonance imaging and positron emission tomography study on the effect of aging. *Arch Gen Psychiatry*. 1996;53:585–594.
44. Seeman MV. Gender differences in schizophrenia. *Can J Psychiatry*. 1982;27:107–111.
45. Burns A, Carrick J, Ames D, Naguib M, Levy R. The cerebral cortical appearance in late paraphrenia. *Int J Geriatr Psychiatry*. 1989; 4:31–34.
46. Burns A, Carrick J, Ames D, et al. The cerebral cortical appearance in late paraphrenia. *Int J Geriatr Psychiatry*. 1988;12:712–717.
47. Howard RJ, Forstl H, Almeida O, et al. Computer-assisted CT measurements in late paraphrenia with and without Schneiderian first-rank symptoms: a preliminary report. *Int J Geriatr Psychiatry*. 1992;7:35–38.

48. Pearlson G, Tune L, Wong D, et al. Quantitative D2 dopamine receptor PET and structural MRI changes in late-onset schizophrenia. *Schizophr Bull.* 1993;19:783–795.

49. Miller BL, Lesser IM, Boone KB, Hill E, Mehringer CM, Wong K. Brain lesions and cognitive function in late-life psychosis. *Br J Psychiatry.* 1991;158:76–82.

50. Breitner J, Husain M, Figiel G, Krishnan K, Boyko O. Cerebral white matter disease in late-onset psychosis. *Biol Psychiatry.* 1990;28:266–274.

51. Flint AJ, Rifat SI, Eastwood MR. Late-onset paranoia: distinct from paraphrenia? *Int J Geriatr Psychiatry.* 1991;6:103–109.

52. Lesser IM, Jeste DV, Boone KB, et al. Late-onset psychotic disorder, not otherwise specified: clinical and neuroimaging findings. *Biol Psychiatry.* 1992;31:419–423.

53. Moore NC. Is paranoid illness associated with sensory deficits in the elderly? *J Psychosom Res.* 1981;25:69–74.

54. Corbin S, Eastwood MR. Sensory deficits and mental disorders of old age: causal or coincidental associations? *Psychol Med.* 1976;16:251–256.

55. Keshavan MS, David AS, Steingard S, Lishman WA. Musical hallucinations: a review and synthesis. *Neuropsychiatry Neuropsychol Behav Neurol.* 1992;5:211–223.

56. Almeida O, Forstl H, Howard R, David AS. Unilateral auditory hallucinations. *Br J Psychiatry.* 1993;162:262–264.

57. Cooper AF, Porter R. Visual acuity and ocular pathology in the paranoid and affective psychoses of later life. *J Psychosom Res.* 1976;20:107–114.

58. Howard R, Levy R. Charles Bonnet syndrome plus: complex visual hallucinations of Charles Bonnet type in late paraphrenia. *Int J Geriatr Psychiatry.* 1994;9:399–404.

59. Prager S, Jeste DV. Sensory impairment in late-life schizophrenia. *Schizophr Bull.* 1993;19(4):755–772.

60. Pearlson GD, Petty R. Late life onset schizophrenia. In: Cummings J, Coffey CE, eds. *Textbook of Geriatric Neuropsychiatry.* Washington, DC: APA Press; 1994.

61. Pearlson G. Brain imaging studies in late-onset schizophrenia. In: Howard R, Rabins PV, Castle DJ, eds. *Late Onset Schizophrenia.* Petersfield, UK: Wrightson Biomedical Publishing Ltd; 1999:50–65.

62. Jeste DV, Lacro JP, Gilbert PL, Kline J, Kline N. Treatment of late-life schizophrenia with neuroleptics. *Schizophr Bull.* 1993;19: 817–830.

63. Avorn J, Gurwitz J. Principles of pharmacology. In: Cassel K, Riesenberg D, Sorenson L, Walsh J, eds. *Geriatric Medicine.* 2nd ed. New York: Springer-Verlag; 1990:66–77.

64. Zayas EM, Grossberg GT. Treatment of late-onset psychotic disorders. In: Copeland JRM, Abou-Saleh MT, Blazer DG, eds. *Principles and Practice of Geriatric Psychiatry.* 2nd ed. Chichester, UK: Wiley; 2002:511–525.

65. Tsuang MM, Lu LM, Stotsky BA, Cole JO. Haloperidol versus thioridazine for hospitalized psychogeriatric patients: double-blind study. *J Am Geriatr Soc.* 1971;19:593–600.

66. Post F. Persistent persecutory states of the elderly. Oxford, New York: Pergamon Press; 1966.

67. Pearlson GD, Kreger L, Rabins RV, et al. A chart review study of late-onset and early-onset schizophrenia. *Am J Psychiatry.* 1989;146:1568–1574.

68. Howard R, Levy R. Which factors affect treatment response in late paraphrenia? *Int J Geriatr Psychiatry.* 1992;7:667–672.

69. Jeste DV, Lacro JP, Palmer B, Rockwell E, Harris MJ, Caligiuri MP. Incidence of tardive dyskinesia in early stages of neuroleptic treatment for older patients. *Am J Psychiatry.* 1999;156(a): 309–311.

70. McClure FS, Jeste DV. Treatment of late-onset schizophrenia and related disorders. In: Howard R, Rabins PV, Castle DJ, eds. *Late Onset Schizophrenia.* Petersfield, UK: Wrightson Biomedical Publishing Ltd; 1999:217–232.

71. Salzman C, Vaccaro B, Lieff J, et al. Clozapine in older patients with psychosis and behavioural disruption. *Am J Psychiatry.* 1995;3:26–33.

72. Howard R. Late onset schizophrenia and very late-onset schizophrenia-like psychosis. In: Jacoby R, Oppenheimer C, eds. *Psychiatry in the Elderly.* Oxford, UK: Oxford University Press; 2002:744–761.

73. Jeste DV, Eastham JH, Lacro JP, Gierz M, Field MG, Harris MJ. Management of late-life psychosis. *J Clin Psychiatry.* 1996;57 (suppl 3):39–45.

74. Berman I, Merson A, Allen E, Alexis C, Sison C, Losonczy M. Poster No. 93: Effect of risperidone on cognitive performance in elderly schizophrenic patients: a double blind comparison with haloperidol. NCDEU 35th Annual Meeting. Orlando, Florida.

75. Jaskiw GE, Thyrum PT, Fuller MA, Arvanitis LA, Yeh C. Pharmacokinetics of quetiapine in elderly patients with select psychotic disorders. *Clinical Pharmacokinet.* 2004;43(14): 1025–1035.

76. Hirose T, Uwahodo Y, Yamada S, et al. Mechanism of action of Aripiprazole predicts clinical efficacy favourable side-effect profile. *J Psychopharmacology.* 2004;18(3):375–383.

77. Madhusoodanan S, Brenner R, Gupta S, Reddy J, Bogunovic O. Clinical experience with aripiprazole treatment in ten elderly with schizophrenia or schizoaffective disorder: retrospective studies. *CNS Spectr.* 2004;9(11):862–827.

78. Jeste CCB, Winnett RL. Late-onset paranoid disorder. *Am J Orthopsychiatry.* 1987;57:485–493.

79. Garety P, Kuipers E, Fowler D, Chamberlain F, Dunn G. Cognitive-behavioural therapy for drug resistant psychosis. *Br J Med Psychol.* 1994;67:259–271.

80. Fowler D, Garety P, Kuipers E. Cognitive behaviour therapy for psychosis: theory and practice. Chichester, UK: Wiley; 1995.

81. Agüera-Ortiz L, Reneses-Prieto B. The place of non-biological treatments. In: Howard R, Rabins PV, Castle DJ, eds. *Late onset schizophrenia.* Winchester, UK: Wrightson Biomedical Publishing Ltd; 1999:50–65.

82. Kay DWK, Roth M. Environmental and hereditary factors in the schizophrenias of old age ("late paraphrenia") and their bearing on the general problem of causation in schizophrenia. *J Ment Sci.* 1961;107:649–686.

83. Frost JB. Paraphrenia and paranoid schizophrenia. *Psychiatr Clinica.* 1969;3:129–138.

84. Herbert ME, Jacobson S. Late paraphrenia. *Br J Psychiatry.* 1967; 113:461–469.

85. Hoffman WF, Ballard L, Turner EH, Casey DE. Three-year follow-up of older schizophrenics: extrapyramidal syndromes, psychiatric symptoms, and ventricular brain ratio. *Biol Psychiatry.* 1991;30:913–926.

86. Arie T, Jolly DJ. Making services work: organization and style of psychogeriatric services. In: R Levy, F Post, eds. *The Psychiatry of Late Life.* Oxford: Blackwell; 1982:222–251.

87. Bridge TP, Cannon HE, Wyatt RJ. Burned-out schizophrenia: evidence for age effects on schizophrenic symptomatology. *J Gerontol A Biol Sci Med Sci.* 1978;33:835–839.

88. Bleuler M. *The Schizophrenic Disorders.* Yale University Press: New Haven and London; 1978.

89. Soni SD, Mallik A. The elderly chronic schizophrenic inpatient: a study of psychiatric morbidity in 'elderly graduates.' *Int J Geriatr Psychiatry.* 1993;8:665–673.

90. Davidson M, Harvey PD, Powchik P, et al. Severity of symptoms in chronically institutionalized geriatric schizophrenic patients. *Am J Psychiatry.* 1995;152:197–207.

91. Lindenmayer JP, Negron AE, Shah S, et al. Cognitive deficits and psychopathology in elderly schizophrenic patients. *Am J Psychiatry.* 1997;5:31–42.

92. Cohen CI, Talavera N, Hartung R. Predictors of subjective well-being among older, community-dwelling persons with schizophrenia. *Am J Psychiatry.* 1997;5:145–155.

93. Goldberg TE, Hyde TM, Kleinman JE, et al. Course of schizophrenia: neuropsychological evidence for a static encephalopathy. *Schizophr Bull.* 1993;19:797–804.

94. Perlick D, Mattis S, Stastny P, et al. Neuropsychological discriminators of long-term inpatient or outpatient status in chronic schizophrenia. *J Neuropsychiatry Clin Neurosci.* 1992;4:428–434.

95. Shallice T, Burgess PW, Frith CD. Can the neuropsychological case-study approach be applied to schizophrenia? *Psychol Med.* 1991;21:661–673.

96. Faber R, Abrams R, Taylor MA, et al. Comparison of schizophrenic patients with formal thought disorder and neurologically impaired patients with aphasia. *Am J Psychiatry.* 1983;140: 1348–1351.

97. Saykin AJ, Shtasel DL, Gur RE, et al. Neuropsychological deficits in neuroleptic naive patients with first-episode schizophrenia. *Arch Gen Psychiatry.* 1994;51:124–131.

98. Russell AJ, Munro JC, Jones PB, et al. Schizophrenia and the myth of intellectual decline. *Am J Psychiatry.* 1997;154: 635–639.

99. Harvey PD, Silverman JM, Mohs RC, et al. Cognitive decline in late-life schizophrenia: a longitudinal study of geriatric chronically hospitalized patients. *Biol Psychiatry.* 1999;45:32–40.

100. Green MF. What are the functional consequences of neurocognitive deficits in schizophrenia? *Am J Psychiatry.* 1996;153:321–330.

101. Harvey PD, Howanitz E, Parrella M, et al. Symptoms, cognitive functioning, and adaptive skills in geriatric patients with lifelong schizophrenia: a comparison across treatment sites. *Am J Psychiatry.* 1998;155:1080–1086.

102. Kovar MG. Health of the elderly and use of health services. *Public Health Reports.* 1977;92:9–19.

103. Harris AE. Physical disease and schizophrenia. *Schizophr Bull.* 1988;14:85–96.

104. Jeste DV, Gladsjo JA, Lindamer LA, et al. Medical comorbidity in schizophrenia. *Schizophr Bull.* 1996;22:413–430.

105. Koranyi EA. Morbidity and rate of undiagnosed physical illnesses in a psychiatric clinic population. *Arch Gen Psychiatry.* 1979;36: 414–419.

106. Koran LM, Sox HC, Marion I, et al. Medical evaluation of psychiatric patients. *Arch Gen Psychiatry.* 1989;46:733–740.

107. Jeste DV, Patterson TL, Zorrilla LE, et al. Schizophrenia and aging: myths and reality. Presented at the American Psychiatric Association, 152nd Annual Meeting. May 15–20, 1999; Washington DC.

108. Cohen CI, Cohen, GD, Blank K, et al. Schizophrenia and older adults. An overview: directions for research and policy. *Am J Geriatr Psychiatry.* 2000;8:19–28.

109. Wing JK, Furlong RA. A haven for the severely disabled within the context of a comprehensive psychiatric community service. *Br J Psychiatry.* 1986;149:449–457.

110. Cohen, CI. Age-related correlations in patient symptom management strategies in schizophrenia: an exploratory study. *International Journal of Geriatric Psychiatry.* 1993;8:211–213.

111. Klaplow JC, Evans J, Patterson TL, et al. Direct assessment of functional status in older patients with schizophrenia. *Am J Psychiatry.* 1997;154:1022–1024.

112. Rabins PV, Black B, German P, et al. The prevalence of psychiatric disorders in elderly residents of public housing. *J Gerontol A Bio Sci Med Sci.* 1996;51:M319–M324.

113. Gurland B J, Cross PS. Epidemiology of psychopathology in old age: some implications for clinical services. *The Psychiatr Clin North Am.* 1982;5:11–26.

114. Dale MC, Burns A. Graduates. *Rev Clin Gerontol.* 1997;7:273–285.

115. Cunningham Owens DG, Johnstone EC. The disabilities of chronic schizophrenia—their nature and the factors contributing to their development. *Br J Psychiatry.* 1980;136:384–395.

116. Goldman HH, Manderscheid RW. Epidemiology of chronic mental disorder. In: WH Menninger, GT Hannah, eds. *The Chronic Mental Patient.* Vol II. Washington, DC: American Psychiatric Press; 1987:41–63.

117. Hegarty JD, Baldessarini RJ, Tohen M, et al. One hundred years of schizophrenia: a meta-analysis of the outcome literature. *Am J Psychiatry.* 1994;151:1409–1416.

118. Ray WA, Federspiel CF, Schaffner W. A study of antipsychotic drug use in homes: epidemiological evidence suggesting misuse. *Am J Public Health.* 1980;70:485–491.

119. Eastham JH, Patterson TL, Rockwell E, et al. Movement disorders and functional impairment in middle-aged and elderly schizophrenic patients. Presented at the American Psychiatric Association 150th Annual Meeting. May 17–22, 1997; San Diego, CA.

120. Sensky T, Turkington D, Kingdon D, et al. A randomized controlled trial of cognitive-behavioural therapy for persistent symptoms in schizophrenia resistant to medication. *Arch Gen Psychiatry.* 2000;57:165–172.

121. McQuaid JR, Granholm E, McClure FS, et al. Development of an integrated cognitive-behavioural and social skills training intervention for older people with schizophrenia. *J Psychother Prac Res.* July 2000;149–156.

122. Liberman RP, et al. *Social Skills for Psychiatric Patients.* New York: Pergamon Press; 1989.

123. Bartels S. Community service needs of severe and persistent mentally ill elderly. Presented at the American Psychiatric Association, 150th Meeting. May 17–22, 1997; San Diego, CA.

124. Bennett DH. The historical development of rehabilitation services. In: Watts FN, Bennett DH, eds. *The Theory and Practice of Rehabilitation.* Chichester, UK: Wiley; 1983.

125. Royal College of Psychiatrists. *Rehabilitation in the 1980s.* London: Royal College of Psychiatrists; 1981.

126. Kraepelin E. *Psychiatrie ein Lehrbuch fur Studierende and Artze (Psychiatry, a text for students and practitioners).* 8th ed. Leipzig: Barth; 1913.

127. Abrahamson D, Swatton J, Wills W. Do long-stay patients want to leave hospital? *Health Trends.* 1989;21:17–19.

128. McGlashan TH. A selective review of recent North American long-term follow-up studies of schizophrenia. *Schizophr Bull.* 1988;14:515–542.

129. Davidson M, Harvey PD, Powchik P, et al. Severity of symptoms in chronically institutionalized geriatric schizophrenic patients. *Am J Psychiatry.* 1995;152:197–207.

130. Cutting J. Outcome of schizophrenia: overview. In: Kerr A, Snaith P, eds. *Contemporary Issues in Schizophrenia.* London: Gaskell; 1986.

131. Cervilla JA. PC-009. A delusional disorder case register study. *Int Psychogeriatr* 2003;15(2):300.

132. Breitner JCS, Anderson DN. The organic and psychological antecedents of delusional jealousy in old age. *Int J Geriatr Psychiatry.* 1994;9:703–707.

133. Schneider LS, Olin JT, Pawluczyc S. A double-blind crossover pilot study of 1-deprenyl selegiline combined with cholinesterase inhibitor in Alzheimer's disease. *Am J Psychiatry.* 1993;150: 321–323.

134. Opjordsmoen J. Hypochondriacal psychoses: a long-term follow-up. *Acta Psychiatr Scand.* 1985;77:587–597.

Adjustment Disorders in Late Life

29

Melinda Lantz

Older adults face numerous stressors from medical problems, disability, loss of roles, and death of friends and loved ones. They must constantly cope and adjust to the ongoing changes in their lives. An adjustment disorder is a time-limited maladaptive response to a life stress that results in significant distress, or impairment of social or occupational functioning (1). The clinical presentation of an adjustment disorder may include a variety of emotional and behavioral features (Table 29-1). These features are typically short-term in nature; improvement is expected after the stress resolves. In cases where the stressor is chronic (e.g., diagnosis of cancer, amputation of a limb due to complications of diabetes, economic deprivation due to loss of a job), a new pattern of coping and adaptation develops (2). The management of these disorders in late life must address the multifactorial nature of the stress of old age (3–5).

It is believed that the diagnosis of adjustment disorder is underutilized, in part due to a lack of recognition by clinicians, combined with the reluctance of older adults to seek help for emotional distress (6). This group of disorders has received very little attention in both research and clinical literature (7).

PHENOMENOLOGY

DSM-IV-TR criteria for the diagnosis of an adjustment disorder require the presence of an identifiable stressor. The symptoms must develop within 3 months of the onset of the stressor. Resolution is expected within 6 months following termination of the stressor, but may last longer if the stress is chronic in nature (1–5). There are six types of adjustment disorders described in DSM-IV-TR (1):

- With depressed mood.
- With anxiety.
- With mixed anxiety and depressed mood.
- With disturbance of conduct.
- With mixed disturbance of emotions and conduct.
- Unspecified.

The duration of the symptoms is described with a modifier of *acute* (less than 6 months) or *chronic* (the stressor is ongoing).

The degree of morbidity associated with adjustment disorders is believed to be significant (7). Patients diagnosed with adjustment disorder with depressed mood are more likely to report poor health status and impaired physical functioning than those with other mood disorders (8). Unfortunately, very little research has focused on long-term outcome.

EPIDEMIOLOGY

In the general population, adjustment disorders have a prevalence rate ranging from 2% to 8% (7), and vary widely among the populations studied. Older adults are particularly vulnerable to develop an adjustment disorder, due to the numerous medical, psychosocial, and economic stressors that elderly persons are subject to. Adjustment disorders account for 7% of admissions to acute psychiatric inpatient units (9). Jones et al. reported that while readmission rates for these patients were lower than for those with major depressive disorder, schizophrenia, or bipolar disorder, one-third required hospitalization again within 3 years (10).

TABLE 29-1

COMMON SYMPTOMS IN ADJUSTMENT DISORDERS

Acting-out behavior
Anxiety
Depression
Destructive behavior
Fearfulness
Irritability
Neglect of roles or activities
Recklessness

Medical inpatients have some of the highest reported prevalence of adjustment disorders—up to 20% of those referred for psychiatric consultation—in part due to the clear stressor of the need for hospitalization and treatment (11–13). Among patients evaluated in the period following onset of an acute stroke, 27% of older adults were diagnosed as having an adjustment disorder (14). Participants in adult day health centers who did not display dementia were often diagnosed with an adjustment disorder (15), and residents of long-term care facilities commonly display symptoms of adjustment disorder following admission (16). However, the recognition and treatment of the disorder is unfortunately low in many settings (6).

The most common type among elderly patients is adjustment disorder with depressed mood, followed by those with anxious mood, mixed anxiety and depressed mood, and disturbance of conduct (17). These disorders are time-intensive for clinicians, and may prolong hospital length of stay (11–13).

ASSESSMENT AND DIAGNOSIS

Unlike mood and anxiety disorders, there are no readily available screening tools for the diagnosis of an adjustment disorder. The identification of a recent or chronic source of stress is a necessary feature of the disorder (1). Since older adults are often reluctant to seek help, and face many stresses associated with aging, there is often a significant delay in identifying the disorder and providing treatment and support (6). Furthermore, the diagnosis is based on the individual patient's response to the identified stressor, not the stress itself. The factors involved in making a diagnosis of an adjustment disorder include the determination of whether the response to the stressor is in excess of what is typical or expected, and if significant functioning impairment occurs (1,7).

Adjustment disorders are often difficult to diagnose, because the nature and severity of the stressor is not specified. Many older adults have acquired significant coping skills and react with resilience to a variety of stressful events. Others may suffer significant distress and functional decline in response to stressors that appear minor (18). Utilizing the patient's response to a stressor provides a means to identify emotional and behavioral symptoms that require further evaluation and treatment.

Differential Diagnosis

Clinical evaluation, including an adequate psychiatric history and assessment of the current stressors, is vital to diagnosis. The type and nature of reaction to the stressor must also be evaluated. Symptoms within the range considered normal and attributable to the stress do not meet criteria for a psychiatric disorder (1,6). The other DSM-IV-TR disorders that often present with symptoms similar to adjustment disorders include acute stress disorder, post-traumatic stress disorder, and the mood disorders. Patients with a prior psychiatric history of major depressive disorder, bipolar disorder, or an anxiety disorder may suffer an exacerbation of this condition when faced with a stressful event. Patients suffering from personality disorders are by definition likely to suffer a maladaptive response related to poor coping skills, and are at high risk for developing comorbid adjustment disorders (1).

When evaluating an older adult with psychiatric symptoms, it is always important to consider cognitive impairment as a related or pre-existing condition. It is also a time when screening for substance abuse should be performed. Elder abuse and neglect must be considered, as the stressor may be related in part to unrecognized physical, emotional, or financial exploitation. Sleep disorders, such as nocturnal myoclonus and sleep apnea, must be considered, since these conditions are highly prevalent yet often unrecognized in older adults. It is obviously important to have contact with the patient's primary care physician and to coordinate care as much as possible (19). Grief and bereavement are common in late life, and are discussed later in this chapter.

ETIOLOGY

By definition, adjustment disorders are associated with an identifiable stressor. As noted, the nature and severity of the stressor is not specified in DSM-IV-TR (1). Among medically ill patients diagnosed with an adjustment disorder, 69% of patients suffered from a stressor directly related to their medical illness (12). Cancer, diabetes, and a prolonged hospital stay were commonly cited stressors. In the 32% of patients who cited stressors other than their medical illness, many suffered from pre-existing psychiatric disorders and had problems related to personal relationships and financial hardship (13). This illustrates the clinical importance of identifying the stressor for each individual through their history and a clinical interview.

PSYCHOSOCIAL ISSUES

The diagnosis of adjustment disorder is made often in late life, in part due to the number and magnitude of losses that older adults encounter. Normal or adaptive adjustment to a stressor occurs in patients who are able to remain active in their life role, find outlets for emotional distress, and continue to engage in activities that are meaningful and important. The ability to successfully cope with a stressor is related to the patient's personality, psychosocial supports, and ability to adapt to change (20).

Suicide attempts occur in the context of adjustment disorders, particularly among women with stressors related to problems with their primary support system (21). Asking about suicidal thoughts is always prudent.

TREATMENT APPROACHES

Psychotherapy is the treatment of choice for older patients suffering from adjustment disorders. Unfortunately, it is an underutilized modality in this population. Studies examining preference for mental health services among older medical patients find high levels of interest in psychosocial treatments, but very low rates of physician referral of older patients to psychotherapy (22,23).

Psychotherapy for adjustment disorders should focus on minimizing the impact of the identified stressor, improving the patient's coping skills, and promoting the use of support systems to enhance adaptation and accommodation (24). Brief, goal-directed psychotherapy has been successfully utilized for the treatment of adjustment disorders, but many other therapies may be helpful (25,26). Several forms of psychotherapy have been found effective for older patients with depression, and may be adapted for the treatment of an adjustment disorder. These include problem-solving therapy, cognitive behavioral therapy (CBT), interpersonal therapy (IPT), brief focused psychodynamic psychotherapy, family therapy, and group therapy. All of these approaches employ strategies aimed at changing information processing and building skills in problem-solving, communication, and mood regulation. CBT has the greatest amount of empirical data supporting its use, and has been found to be a viable treatment option for mild-to-moderate major depressive disorder in late life (23). The use of CBT for adjustment disorders offers significant advantages, but formal clinical trials are lacking.

IPT has been less studied in older adults than CBT, but includes more longitudinal data. IPT plus the antidepressant nortriptyline was superior to medication or psychotherapy alone in a randomized, double-blind, placebo-controlled trial to maintain recovery over 3 years (26,27). Patients suffering from bereavement-related depression displayed the greatest rate of treatment compliance when treated with a combination of nortriptyline and IPT (28).

Clinicians vary greatly in their recommendation of when to treat an adjustment disorder with medications. The only consensus appears to be that medications should be considered when patients are significantly impaired by their symptoms, have suicidal ideation, or have not responded to psychotherapy after a 3-month period (5,17). Antidepressants are often used in clinical practice to treat adjustment disorders, regardless of age, in a manner similar to that for other Axis I and II disorders (12,29). The need for such medications, however, begs the question of whether symptom severity indicates a different diagnosis, such as a major depressive episode or an anxiety disorder. Short-term symptomatic relief for adjustment disorders is likely to involve the use of benzodiazepine anxiolytics such as alprazolam or lorazepam, or sedative-hypnotic medications such as zolpidem and zaleplon, or even the antidepressant trazodone.

COURSE

Adjustment disorders are one of the few DSM-IV-TR disorders that have a specified time limit of 6 months beyond the resolution of the stressor. The prognosis for most adjustment disorders is positive, with some improvement or resolution of symptoms noted within the first 3 months. Poor prognostic features include multiple chronic stressors, multiple medical problems, financial hardship, and limited psychosocial support (1,17). Suicide attempts among patients with adjustment disorders have been documented. Suicidal behavior is more common among patients with pre-existing personality disorders and substance use disorders, and among those with a history of suicide attempts (10,21).

CASE EXAMPLE

ADJUSTMENT DISORDER WITH MIXED DISTURBANCE OF EMOTIONS AND CONDUCT

Mrs. P is a 72-year-old woman who was referred for a court-ordered evaluation of her mental status and capacity to assist her court-appointed attorney. She was arrested after being found shoplifting multiple items of men's clothing from a well-known designer store. Mrs. P has no prior criminal record, and had several hundred dollars in cash as well as credit cards with her when she was arrested. She refused to cooperate with her attorney, and at her arraignment told the judge that she wanted to stay in jail. Her attorney was able to contact her daughter, who arranged for bail and agreed to supervise her. The judge ordered a psychiatric evaluation to determine Mrs. P's capacity to understand the legal proceedings.

Mrs. P arrived at the psychiatrist's office with her daughter. She was alert and very neatly dressed and groomed, wearing designer clothes and a great deal of jewelry. Her daughter explained that Mrs. P was in an unhappy marriage for 61 years, and was widowed 1 year ago. Mrs. P came from a wealthy family, and her husband became part of a successful import/export business. He traveled frequently and was often away from home for long periods of time. The family recently found out that their father had six other children from relationships with three other women. He married two of the women while still married to Mrs. P. There was a complex legal situation currently being managed by the family's many attorneys due to claims by the other wives and children on Mr. P's estate. The daughter explained that following the emergence of these new "family members" and the many lawsuits filed over the past 3 months, Mrs. P had been irritable and angry and engaging in strange behavior, such as packing up all of her late-husband's underwear and sending it to one of the other women. She continued to perform many of her civic and charity activities, but would come home and often scream and cry. The daughter was overwhelmed by the whole situation, especially the thought that she had six half-bothers and half-sisters who were suing her. After going to the county jail to arrange bail for her mother, she felt that things had hit rock bottom.

On examination, Mrs. P appeared angry but was cooperative. She related the details of the recent events in a careful, deliberate manner. She reported that for years she always thought her husband was having an affair, but she never thought he would "sink this low." Since finding out about the other wives and the six children, and having to deal with multiple lawsuits against an estate that was built from her family business, Mrs. P felt angry and outraged, and admitted to doing "stupid things." Her mood was somewhat labile, but she stopped herself at times during the interview, stating that she did not wish to lose control. She reported significant insomnia, often sleeping only 2 hours per night and feeling constantly tired. She denied weight loss. Her affect was reactive and angry, but appropriate given her situation. She had no signs of psychotic symptoms, and admitted that while getting arrested was "a stupid thing to do," she really wanted some help for herself. Her cognitive functioning was intact. Her score on a Mini Mental State Examination was 30/30, and her clock drawing had no errors. She was willing to cooperate with her lawyer, who arranged a plea bargain that would require a fine and community service.

Mrs. P presented with significant disturbance of conduct and emotional changes following a prominent psychosocial stressor. While acting out through criminal behavior more commonly occurs in adolescents and young adults, it is not unheard of in the elderly. Mrs. P agreed to see a social worker for individual psychotherapy, using an interpersonal model. She performed her community service at a shelter for homeless adolescents. The psychotherapy helped Mrs. P examine her grief, role transitions, unresolved conflicts, and personal relationships that were disrupted both before and after her husband's death. Due to the severity of her insomnia, she was treated with an intermittent course of zolpidem 5 mg as needed. Mrs. P still faced many issues over finances and her husband's estate, but after 6 months of treatment she felt stronger and more able to cope.

RELATED LIFE EVENTS AND CONDITIONS

Grief and Bereavement

Mourning is a process involving the social and emotional expression of a loss. This includes feelings or sensations of grief, and the global process of loss that is referred to as bereavement. The word bereavement literally means *to be deprived by death*. As the definition implies, it is associated with a range of reactions including denial, disbelief, sadness, anger, despair, guilt, and a sense of yearning for the deceased (30).

The acute phase of grief typically lasts for 2 months, but ongoing mild symptoms may persist (30). Normal bereavement, with an ongoing sense of loss, may last for years. For instance, it is common for widows to talk to a deceased spouse and gain comfort from the sense of their presence. A sense of loneliness may persist, but older adults will gradually learn to function, perform routine tasks, and adapt to life roles after the loss. Anniversary reactions are common. Holidays, birthdays, and family events may trigger a return of more acute grief symptoms that typically resolve over time. The range of physical and emotional responses to grief is quite varied, and the physician must be prepared to provide support and empathy while monitoring for more pathological signs of depression or anxiety requiring further treatment (2).

The loss of a spouse or significant other is not only a time of grief and bereavement, but also puts an older adult at risk of increased medical and psychiatric morbidity (31,32). One year following the loss of a spouse, 15% to 25% of the elderly meet criteria for major depression (32). The majority of these older adults do not receive any treatment for their symptoms. This is due, in part, to the incorrect assumption that all symptoms related to bereavement will resolve in time. It appears that patients who develop symptoms of major depression following a loss will remain symptomatic and suffer additional morbidity due to decline in health and functional status, unless treatment is provided (31). Differences between normal bereavement and major depression are outlined in Table 29-2.

An older adult who experiences the loss of a spouse may develop multiple somatic complaints and visit his or her physician often (31). This offers an opportunity to screen the patient for depression and anxiety, and to offer treatment when significant symptoms are present. Patients at risk for developing significant depression following a loss include those with a psychiatric history of depression or anxiety. Patients who have substance abuse problems, suffer from personality disorders, or who have a history of significant trauma are also at risk for developing major depression in the bereavement period. Medication treat-

TABLE 29-2
SYMPTOMS OF NORMAL BEREAVEMENT VERSUS MAJOR DEPRESSION

Common in Bereavement

Anger	Disbelief	Sadness
Denial	Guilt	Shock
Despair	Humiliation	Yearning

Indicative of Major Depression

Symptom persistence for at least 2 months following the loss
Worthlessness
Psychomotor retardation
Poor grooming and self-care
Apathy
Suicidal ideation
Psychotic symptoms (Note: talking to or hearing the deceased is not considered a psychotic symptom)
Marked functional impairment
Weight loss
Persistent sense of guilt or inadequacy

Source: References 1, 30, and 31.

ment and counseling should be considered when patients display significant symptoms more than 2 months following the loss (28,31,32).

Antidepressants have been useful in treating symptoms of major depression and anxiety disorders that develop during grief and bereavement. Many types of antidepressants, including selective serotonin re-uptake inhibitors, tricyclic agents, and bupropion have been utilized successfully. Short courses of benzodiazepines have been utilized for anxiety and insomnia, typically while awaiting response to antidepressant medications (31). In addition, supportive psychotherapy, bereavement counseling, and psychosocial support is vital to help the older adult develop coping skills and new sources of social support. Social service agencies and senior centers may be valuable sources of assistance for an older adult who needs help with finances, housing, and legal issues following a loss (3).

Most older adults have experienced multiple losses throughout their lives, and are often quite resilient at coping with grief and bereavement. Mourning rituals are extremely important, and may help the elderly prepare for and cope with a significant loss. Religious, social, and cultural factors also play an important role in how an older adult copes with loss. Grief responses will vary depending on the circumstances associated with the death. An accidental, unexpected, or violent death may lead to a greater sense of shock, loss, and denial, while the loss of a loved one from a chronic illness is often associated with some degree of anticipatory grief (33).

Women greatly outnumber men by the 8th and 9th decades of life, and often have additional sources of

activity and social support following the loss of a spouse. Women are more likely than men to attend support groups, seek help from a physician, or visit a senior center. In contrast, older men often have great difficulty coping with the loss of a spouse and are at significant risk for pathological grief, depression, and suicide if they remain isolated and are unable to access assistance (34,35).

It is important to recognize that other losses, although less obvious, may be traumatic, such as the loss of a companion animal. The grief an older adult suffers following the loss of a companion animal is often trivialized and minimized, because society views these companions as replaceable. It is important to acknowledge such a loss and offer an opportunity for the expression of grief and mourning rituals.

In general, older adults have learned to live with periods of economic hardship, deprivation, disappointment, and loss. We can often learn valuable lessons from their ability to cope with grief and bereavement. When symptoms of worthlessness, hopelessness, guilt, apathy, or expressions of depressed mood persist beyond 2 months, further evaluation of depression is indicated. If complicating factors such as alcohol or drug use, severe anxiety, suicidal ideation, or poor self-care emerge, immediate psychiatric evaluation is warranted.

CASE EXAMPLE

NORMAL BEREAVEMENT

A 78-year-old woman came to a psychiatrist for evaluation, accompanied by her two daughters, who had scheduled the appointment. The daughters appeared anxious and restless, and insisted on speaking with the psychiatrist before their mother's evaluation. The daughters reported that their father had died 6 months earlier of colon cancer, following a lengthy course of surgery and chemotherapy. Their mother had cared for her husband throughout his illness, and he died at home with his wife beside him in bed. The daughters reported that their mother had been withdrawn and isolative since his death. She had worn black clothing every day and sat in a chair by the bed where her husband died.

Despite their many requests for her to move in with them, the patient chose to remain in her own apartment, stating that she planned to live there until her own death. The daughters became worried when they visited and heard their mother talking to her husband as if he were still present. They thought she must be having "some kind of nervous breakdown." They requested that medication be prescribed for their mother, and wanted the psychiatrist to "tell her to get on with her life." It became apparent during the interview that the daughters were having difficulty coping with the loss of their father. They were tearful and expressed feelings of guilt over not being with him more at the end of his life. The daughters had to be asked to leave the office several times, so their mother could be interviewed.

The patient appeared very calm and cooperative. She was neatly dressed and groomed, wearing a black dress, hat, and gloves. She explained that her father died when she was 8 years old, and all of the female relatives in her family wore black for 1 year afterwards as part of a mourning ritual. She reported feeling lonely since the death of her husband, whom she described as her best friend. The patient reported that she married at the age of 17, and celebrated her 60th wedding anniversary with her husband a few weeks before his death. She fondly described their life together, and stated that she would one day join her husband in heaven. Her affect was reactive. She had no psychotic symptoms and no suicidal ideation. The patient reported that she liked to keep to her usual routine, and felt that her husband was still with her and was helping her.

The patient had suffered many losses in her life. In addition to the death of her father, she lost two infants shortly after birth due to heart defects, and two of her brothers died while serving in World War II. She reported that she attended church and did the shopping, but otherwise preferred to be alone. The patient periodically attended a senior center near her apartment and a widow's support group at her church. The patient was aware of her daughters' concerns, but felt that *they* needed help. She expressed a sense of frustration at being unable to comfort them.

The "patient" in this case was displaying many of the features associated with normal grief and bereavement. She was drawing on her prior experiences of mourning, and was following family rituals to cope with her loss. Her daughters, however, were having far greater difficulty dealing with the death of their father. The psychiatrist encouraged the mother to share her life experiences with her daughters, and referred them to a bereavement group offered by a local hospice. The patient continued to function in the community and was doing well one year following the death of her husband. Her daughters attended the bereavement group, and started researching their family history as part of their recovery.

REFERENCES

1. American Psychiatric Association. *Diagnostic and Statistical Manual of Mental Disorders. 4th ed. Text Revision.* Washington, DC: American Psychiatric Association; 2000.
2. Andreasen NC, Hoenk PR. The predictive value of adjustment disorders: a follow-up study. *Am J Psychiatry.* 1982;139:584–590.
3. Cobb S. Social support as a moderator of life stress. *Psychosom Med.* 1976;3:300–314.
4. Lazarus RS, DeLongis A. Psychological stress and coping in aging. *Am Pschol.* 1983;38:245–254.
5. American Psychiatric Association. *Practice Guideline for the Treatment of Patients With Major Depressive Disorder.* 2nd ed. Washington, DC: American Psychiatric Association; 2000.
6. Blazer DG. Depression in late life: review and commentary. *J Gerontol A Biol Sci Med Sci.* 2003;58A(3):249–265.
7. Casey P, Dowrick C, Wilkenson G. Adjustment disorders: fault line in the psychiatric glossary. *Br J Psychiatry.* 2001;179: 479–481.
8. Jones R, Yates WR, Williams S, Zhou M, Hardman L. Outcome for adjustment disorder with depressed mood: comparison with other mood disorders. *J Affect Disord.* 1999;55:55–61.
9. Greenberg WM, Rosenfeld DN, Ortega EA. Adjustment disorder as an admission diagnosis. *Am J Psychiatry.* 1995;152:459–461.
10. Jones R, Yates WR, Zhou MH. Readmission rates for adjustment disorders: comparison with other mood disorders. *J Affect Disord.* 2002;71:199–203.
11. Popkin MK, Callies AL, Colon EA, Steibel V. Adjustment disorders in medically ill inpatients referred for consultation in a university hospital. *Psychosomatics.* 1990;31:410–414.
12. Strain JJ, Smith GC, Hammer JS, et al. Adjustment disorder: a multisite study of its utilization and interventions in the consultation-liaison psychiatry setting. *Gen Hosp Psychiatry.* 1998;20: 139–149.
13. Snyder S, Strain JJ, Wolf D. Differentiating major depression from adjustment disorder with depressed mood in the medical setting. *Gen Hosp Psychiatry.* 1990;12:159–165.
14. Kellermann M, Fekete I, Gesztelyi R, et al. Screening for depressive symptoms in the acute phase of stroke. *Gen Hosp Psychiatry.* 1999;21:116–121.
15. Cohen-Mansfield J, Lipson S, Brenneman KS, Pawlson LG. Health status of participants of adult day care centers. *J Health Soc Policy.* 2001;14:71–89.
16. Loebel JP, Borson S, Hyde T, et al. Relationships between requests for psychiatric consultations and psychiatric diagnoses in long-term care facilities. *Am J Psychiatry.* 1991;148(7): 898–903.
17. Sampang JA. Adjustment disorder with depressed mood. A review of diagnosis and treatment. *Adv Nurse Pract.* 2003;11:51–54.
18. Cole MG, Dendukuri N. Risk factors for depression among elderly community subjects: a systematic review and meta-analysis. *Am J Psychiatry.* 2003;160:1147–1156.
19. Lynes JM, Caine ED, King DA. Psychiatric disorders in older primary care patients. *J Gen Intern Med.* 1999;14(4):249–254.
20. Wortman CB, Silver RC. The myths of coping with loss. *J Consult Clin Psychol.* 1989;57:349–357.
21. Kryzhanovskaya L, Canterbury R. Suicidal behavior in patients with adjustment disorders. *Crisis.* 2001;22:125–131.
22. Alvidrez J, Arean PA. Physician willingness to refer older depressed patients for psychotherapy. *Int J Psychiatry Med.* 2002; 32(1):21–35.
23. Arean PA, Cook BL. Psychotherapy and combined psychotherapy/pharmacotherapy for late life depression. *Biol Psychiatry.* 2002;52: 293–303.
24. Nierderehe GT. Psychosocial therapies with depressed older adults. In: Schneider LS, Reynolds CF, Lebowitz BD, Friedhoff AJ, eds. *Diagnosis and Treatment of Depression in Late Life: Results of the NIH Consensus Development Conference.* Washington DC: American Psychiatric Association; 1994.
25. Mossey JM, Knott KA, Higgins M, Talerico K. Effectiveness of a psychosocial intervention, interpersonal counseling, for subdysthymic depression in medically ill elderly. *J Gerontol A Biol Sci Med Sci.* 1996;51A(4):M172–M178.
26. Gonzalez-Jaimes EI, Turnbill-Plaza B. Selection of psychotherapeutic treatment for adjustment disorder with depressive mood due to acute myocardial infarction. *Arch Med Res.* 2003;34(4): 298–304.
27. Reynolds CF, Frank E, Perel J, et al. Nortriptyline and interpersonal psychotherapy as maintenance therapies for recurrent major depression: a randomized controlled trial in patients older than 59 years. *JAMA.* 1999;2381(1):39–45.
28. Reynolds CF, Miller MD, Pasternak RE, et al. Treatment of bereavement-related major depressive episodes in later life: a controlled study of acute and continuation treatment with nortriptyline and interpersonal psychotherapy. *Am J Psychiatry.* 1999;156(2): 202–208.
29. Schatzberg AF. Anxiety and adjustment disorder: a treatment approach. *J Clin Psychiatry.* 1990;51(suppl):20–24.
30. Zisook S, Shuchter SR. Uncomplicated bereavement. *J Clin Psychiatry.* 1993;54:365–372.
31. Rosenzweig A, Prigerson H, Miller MD, Reynolds CF III. Bereavement and late-life depression: grief and its complications in the elderly. *Annu Rev Med.* 1997;48:421–428.

32. Turvey CL, Carney C, Arndt S, Wallace RB, Herzog R. Conjugal loss and syndromal depression in a sample of elders aged 70 years or older. *Am J Psychiatry*. 1999;156(10):1596–1601.

33. Prigerson HG, Bierhals AJ, Kasl SV, et al. Traumatic grief as a risk factor for mental and physical morbidity. *Am J Psychiatry*. 1997; 154(5):616–623.

34. Chen JH, Bierhals AJ, Prigerson HG, Kasl SV, Mazure CM, Jacobs S. Gender differences in the effects of bereavement-related psychological distress in health outcomes. *Psychol Med*. 1999;29(2): 367–380.

35. Byrne GJ, Raphael B. The psychological symptoms of conjugal bereavement in elderly men over the first 13 months. *Int J Geriatr Psychiatry*. 1997;12(2):241–251.

Anxiety Disorders in the Elderly

30

Sean A. Lauderdale   Kacie Kelly   Javaid I. Sheikh

Anxiety symptoms have a dramatic and pervasive impact on older adults' lives, radiating beyond the affective domain and producing changes across the biopsychosocial spectrum. Anxious older adults are more likely to report that their activities are limited by their health, and more physical activity limitations compared to nonanxious elderly. Anxious elderly also experience greater loneliness, are less satisfied with their life, and rate their perceived health as lower compared to nonanxious elderly. These findings are not limited to older adults with diagnosable anxiety disorders. Elders with subsyndromal anxiety symptoms report more days in bed and more activity limitations due to their health compared to nonanxious elders. Additionally, elderly with subsyndromal anxiety symptoms describe loneliness and more limitations in their physical activities, as well as decreased perceived health and life satisfaction compared to nonanxious elders (1).

Although anxious older adults use health services at an increased rate compared to a nonanxious reference group, many are treated only by their primary care providers, and few receive treatment from mental health care professionals. These elders are often dissatisfied with the treatment they receive, and a substantial proportion are treated with benzodiazepines (1), potentially increasing their risk for adverse side effects such as cognitive impairment and falls. Despite the obvious need, very few prospectively designed pharmacological treatment studies of older patients with anxiety disorders have been implemented (2).

Knowledge regarding anxiety disorders experienced by older adults has steadily, albeit slowly, accumulated over the past decade. Although we have entered the new century with greater knowledge, there is still much to learn. Questions remain regarding symptom presentation, course,

assessment, and age-appropriate treatment of anxious elderly. In this chapter, we will review the current state of knowledge regarding prevalence rates, assessment, phenomenology, and treatment of anxiety syndromes experienced by older adults. We conclude by reviewing contemporary assessment and treatment models implemented in primary care.

CASE EXAMPLE

Mr. S was an 85-year-old White male admitted to a short-stay inpatient psychiatric unit for difficulties with severe anxiety. He was widowed twice but had been married to his third wife for approximately 10 years. Mr. S and his wife lived in their own home in a large metropolitan community.

When admitted to the psychiatric inpatient unit, Mr. S reported recurrent panic attacks entailing severe shortness of breath, dizziness, headaches, diaphoresis, and trembling. He also reported decreasing appetite, fatigue, nausea, nocturnal sweating, muscle tension, restlessness, and difficulty sleeping over the past couple of years, and increased dysphoria regarding his symptoms. Cognitively, Mr. S stated that he could not "think straight," specifically reporting difficulties understanding what he had heard and read, trouble concentrating, and decreased memory efficiency. He also described a range of worries regarding his finances, his wife's health, his personal health, and his safety at home.

In a separate interview, Mrs. S described her husband as always wanting to have control and being a "worrier." He had become increasingly socially withdrawn, anxious, dysphoric, and rigid (e.g., insistent on the same daily routine) over the last 6 months, while she received treatment for cancer. She described his current hospitalization as a respite from his constant worrying, and expressed concern that his discharge would elevate her stress. Mr. S reported that he had been discharged from military service due to anxiety symptoms, and described himself as a "worrier" since adolescence.

Mr. S had been prescribed a variety of psychotropic medications during his past psychiatric treatment, although he had principally taken alprazolam for the last 20 years. Multiple efforts to discontinue alprazolam were unsuccessful due to exacerbation of anxiety symptoms. On admission, Mr. S reported taking regularly scheduled doses as prescribed by his psychiatrist (0.5 mg TID), but also indicated taking extra doses to manage exacerbation of anxiety symptoms.

Mr. S's medical history was noncontributory to his anxiety symptoms. A computerized tomography (CT) scan of the brain revealed age-appropriate generalized atrophy, and a carotid Doppler revealed no significant lesions. Mr. S denied a history significant for head injuries, substance abuse (except for prolonged use of alprazolam), cerebrovascular accidents, or other neurological disorders. There was no evidence of any potential underlying medical reason for his anxiety, such as hyperthyroidism, chronic obstructive lung disease, or congestive cardiac failure. Based on the information provided, it was determined that Mr. S met DSM-IV-TR criteria for generalized anxiety disorder (GAD) and dysthymic disorder.

Pharmacologically, Mr. S's treatment goals included stabilizing his daily intake of alprazolam and slowly initiating (starting at 25 mg/day) and titrating sertraline to therapeutic levels (50 to 100 mg/day). From a psychotherapeutic standpoint, the goals of Mr. S's treatment were to:

- Teach him basic relaxation strategies for effective management of physiological anxiety symptoms.
- Teach him basic components of the cognitive-behavioral model and how these are related to the experience of anxiety symptoms.
- Teach him to recognize common maladaptive thoughts associated with anxiety symptoms, particularly probability overestimation and catastrophic thinking, and help him develop problem-solving strategies for coping with worry-provoking situations.
- Teach him basic cognitive strategies for recognizing and countering maladaptive beliefs generating anxiety.

During the course of treatment, Mr. S learned and implemented relaxation exercises combining deep breathing and muscle relaxation. He reported using these exercises frequently and independently during his stay on the ward. He also reported these exercises were useful in decreasing his physiological symptoms for a short period of time, but that his worries "kept pushing in." During sessions, Mr. S readily appreciated the cognitive model and identified thoughts contributing to his anxiety. He was able to apply cognitive strategies, countering catastrophic thinking and identifying helping resources and

problem-solving for potentially difficult situations, when in sessions with a significant amount of structure. His ability to counter overestimation of negative events was frequently derailed, however, by anxiety provoking thoughts, making it difficult for him to consistently use introduced cognitive strategies. To help maintain his concentration, frequent breaks were taken, information was repeated frequently, and skills were practiced in session. Recurrent review of intrasession goals, tasks, and negative cognitions was also implemented. Mr. S was provided with written summaries of cognitive strategies learned during the session, and concrete, step-by-step guides to prompt use of these strategies outside of session.

Over the course of treatment, Mr. S was best able to apply a strategy in which he used past events and experiences to accurately gauge the likelihood of future feared events (e.g., falling outside or being abandoned by a transportation service). He had the greatest difficulty identifying potential coping resources, possibly due to his belief that he should not ask for assistance. As Mr. S's symptoms stabilized, he was discharged to his home. He was scheduled for continued outpatient psychotherapy and medication management with his psychiatrist. His discharge medications included alprazolam 0.5 mg three times a day and sertraline 75 mg/day with breakfast. It was also recommended that he and his wife participate in couples therapy and that Mr. S participate in activities outside of his home to provide his wife regular respite. Finally, Mrs. S was strongly encouraged to closely monitor Mr. S's use of alprazolam, and to notify his psychiatrist if his anxiety symptoms resulted in misuse.

PREVALENCE OF ANXIETY DISORDERS IN OLDER ADULTS

Over the years, it has been assumed that young and middle-aged adults experience a higher prevalence rate of anxiety disorders compared to older adults. This assumption, possibly stemming from dated epidemiological surveys, is difficult to assess because of the myriad of methodological differences characterizing national epidemiological surveys of young and older adults. For instance, substantial differences emerge across surveys in the timeframe used to assess prevalence rates (e.g., 1 month, 6 months, 12 months), the types of assessment instruments (e.g., checklist versus structured interviews), and the use of diagnostic hierarchical rules. Differences also exist in recruitment, sampling strategies, and age groupings used (e.g., groups of participants ≥65 years old versus ≥55 years old). Compounding these difficulties are potential age-related changes in anxiety symptoms, frequent comorbidity of anxiety and medical conditions, potential increased mortality of anxious individuals (compared to nonanxious), and cohort biases

TABLE 30-1
PREVALENCE RATES OF ANXIETY DISORDERS IN OLDER ADULTS

	1 Month	6 Month	12 Month
Generalized Anxiety Disorder			
Lindesay et al. 1989[5]	3.7%		
Manela et al. 1996[6]	4.7%		
Blazer et al. 1991[7]		1.9%	
Beekman et al. 1998[8]			
65–74 years		11.5%	
75–85 years		6.9%	
Uhlenhuth et al. 1983[9]			7.1%
Simple/Specific Phobias			
Lindesay et al. 1989[5]	2.1%		
Manela et al. 1996[6]	5.9%		
Weissman et al. 1985[19]		3.1%	
Uhlenhuth et al. 1983[9]			1.4%
Phobic Disorders			
Regier et al. 1988[20]	4.8%		
Beekman et al. 1998[8]			
65–74 years		2.9%	
75–85 years		3.5%	
Bland et al. 1988[21]		3.0%	
Panic Disorder			
Lindesay et al. 1989[5]	0%		
Manela et al. 1996[6]	.1%		
Weissman et al. 1985[19]		.1%	
Bland et al. 1988[21]		.3%	
Beekman et al. 1998[8]			
65–74 years		1.7%	
75–85 years		.5%	
Uhlenhuth et al. 1983[9]			1.7%
Social Phobia			
Lindesay et al. 1989[5]	1.3%		
Manela et al. 1996[6]	.6%		
Myers et al. 1984[22]			
Men		.1–1.5%	
Women		.3–1.9%	
Obsessive Compulsive Disorder			
Regier et al. 1988[20]	.8%		
Beekman et al. 1998[8]			
65–74 years		1.6%	
75–85 years		.4%	
Bland et al. 1988[21]		1.5%	

in symptom reports (3). For these reasons, it is more informative to examine prevalence rate ranges across investigations of younger and older adults to identify possible age-related trends in anxiety disorder prevalence. Accordingly, we will review and compare prevalence rate data for adults 65 and older to young and middle-aged adults (18 to 64 years old). For comparison, results from epidemiological surveys of older adults are compared to recently revised prevalence rates identified for young and middle-aged respondents from the Epidemiological Catchment Area Survey (ECA) and the National Comorbidity Survey (NCS) (4). Following the prevalence rates review, we summarize age-associated symptom differences identified between young and old anxious adults to draw attention to unique symptom presentations that may be seen clinically.

GENERALIZED ANXIETY DISORDER

Prevalence

Prevalence rates of GAD for 1, 6, and 12 months are shown in Table 30-1. The lower 6-month rate reported by Blazer and associates may have resulted from their use of the hierarchical diagnostic rule excluding comorbid diagnoses of major depressive disorder (MDD) and GAD (7).

Summing across surveys, prevalence rates of GAD for older adults exceeds the 12-month revised prevalence rate of 2.8% identified for young and middle-aged adults from the ECA and NCS (4). Age-related trends indicate that GAD symptom onset occurs most commonly in early adulthood and late middle age (9,10), persists into old age, and shows a slight decline in the middle and oldest old (≥75 years of age) (5,6,8). Amongst older adults with GAD, approximately 52% reported a 5-year history of symptoms, 9% reported a 10-year history, while 39% reported a 21-year or more symptom history (7), indicating that GAD is highly prevalent in the elderly and characterized by a chronic and pervasive course.

Phenomenology

Beck et al. characterized GAD in older adults by comparing a sample of older adults who met DSM-III-R criteria for GAD (mean age 67.6 years) to a sample without GAD symptoms (mean age 66.7 years) using self-report measures of anxiety symptoms, fears, and worries, as well as a clinician-rated measure of anxiety and depression (11). As expected, elderly patients with GAD reported more transient and trait-like anxiety symptoms, worry, and social fears compared to the nonclinical sample. Furthermore, patients with GAD were rated by clinicians as having more severe anxiety symptoms than the nonclinical group. More recently, Wetherell and colleagues found that older adults with GAD reported greater worry, worry more days than not, worry about a greater range of topics (e.g., family, finances, personal health, social/interpersonal matters), and had more difficulty controlling their worry compared to a group of elders with subsyndromal anxiety and asymptomatic elderly controls (12). Older adults with GAD also reported more restlessness, irritability, fatigue, and muscle tension relative to the two non-GAD groups. Having some but not all symptoms of GAD can also negatively affect older adults. Elders with subsyndromal symptoms of GAD (excessive worry for at least 6 months, but without experiencing uncontrollable worry at clinically significant levels) experience intermediate symptoms of worry, trait anxiety, and depression relative to elderly GAD patients and normal elderly controls. Older adults with subsyndromal symptoms of GAD are also likely to be misidentified as having GAD (13).

Further research is needed to quantify anxiety symptom differences between younger and older adults. In nonclinical samples, the findings are equivocal. Surveys of nonclinical community samples suggest older adults report less intense worry (14,15), anxiety, avoidance, and obsessive-compulsive symptoms (15) relative to nonclinical young adult samples, but these findings are not consistently replicated (16). Findings from clinical samples are clearer, although limited to a single study. Results indicate that older GAD patients are comparable to younger GAD patients on measures of trait anxiety and fear-associated avoidance (15). Caution in interpreting such findings is warranted, though, given evidence that measures developed with young and middle-aged adult samples may require modification when used with older adults to improve psychometric characteristics (17,18).

PHOBIC DISORDERS

Prevalence

Prevalence rates of phobic disorders are presented in two sections in this chapter. The first section presents prevalence rates of simple and specific phobias (SSP), which entails intense and unreasonable fear of objects, animals, or situations. The second section presents combined prevalence rates for phobic disorders, which include agoraphobia, SSP, and social phobia. Social phobia will be discussed later in the chapter due to the lack of studies examining prevalence rates and phenomenology in older adults. Organizing the discussion this way allows for comprehensive coverage of available epidemiologic surveys, which includes those parsing SSP from other phobic disorders as well as surveys collapsing prevalence rates data across phobic disorders (agoraphobia, SSP, and social phobia).

Phobic disorders are common in the elderly, although slightly less prevalent compared to young and middle-aged adults. One-month, 6-month, and 12-month prevalence rates for SSP are shown in Table 30-1. The 12-month prevalence rate for SSP was from an investigation employing hierarchical diagnostic rules, possibly explaining the reduced prevalence rate compared to the 1-month and 6-month rates. Summing across surveys, the prevalence rate range for older adults was slightly lower than the revised 12-month prevalence rate (4.4%) identified for young and middle-aged adults from the ECA and NCS (4).

Surveys combining prevalence rates for phobic disorders (i.e., agoraphobia, SSP, and social phobia) reported slightly elevated prevalence rates compared to the rates reported for SSP (Table 30-1). The range of rates for phobic disorders among older adults is consistent with the 6-month prevalence rates for men less than 65 years old from the New Haven and St. Louis sites of the ECA (2.5% to 4.8%), but below the rates identified for women less than 65 (5.3% to 11.3%) (22).

Phenomenology

In a recent community-based survey, Fredrikson and associates found older respondents (50 years of age and older) were more likely to report situational phobias (e.g., intense fear and avoidance of lightning and heights), while younger respondents reported more fears of animals and injections (23). Fears and phobias of older adults were speculated to develop from learning experiences over the lifespan.

Although not specifically focusing on older adults, Anthony et al. found similar results with patients meeting DSM-IV criteria for specific phobias (24). Patients reporting fears of heights and driving were older (mean 50.9 years) compared to patients with animal and blood/injection phobias or with agoraphobia (42.5 years). Finally, older adults with specific phobias have higher psychiatric and medical morbidity as well as more primary care physician visits relative to normal elderly controls. Unfortunately, successful treatment rates are extremely low (25).

PANIC DISORDER (PD)

Prevalence

PD prevalence rates for the elderly vary widely across surveys (Table 30-1). One-month prevalence estimates for older adults fall below rates (ranging from 0.4% to 0.6%) identified for young and middle-aged respondents to the ECA (20). Six-month prevalence rates demonstrated wide variation, but a potential age-related trend was observed given the lower prevalence rates among adults 75 to 85 years old (8). The lower estimate for adults 75 to 85 years old is consistent with estimates from surveys combining elderly samples without parsing rates for younger, middle, and older participants (19,21). Thus, combining young-old with middle-old and old-old respondents may result in lower overall prevalence estimates of PD. Consistent with this possibility, Weissman and colleagues observed that rates of DSM-III disorders remain constant for adults 65 to 79 years old, and subsequently decline thereafter for both men and women (19). Dovetailing with these findings, Uhlenhuth and associates found a 12-month prevalence estimate of 1.7% in adults 65 to 79 years old, which was only slightly decreased from the 1.8% estimate for adults between 50 and 64 (9). The 12-month prevalence rate identified by Uhlenhuth and associates is comparable to the 12-month 1.4% revised prevalence estimate identified for young and middle-aged adults from the ECA and NCS (4).

Phenomenology

With a goal of investigating the impact of aging on the symptoms and clinical characteristics of PD, we recently reported a study of 167 outpatients with PD (26). Dividing patients into a younger group (less than 60 years, N = 93) and older group (60 years and older, N = 74), we found that the older patients reported higher levels of functioning, fewer panic symptoms during attacks, less anxiety and arousal, less severe PD, and lower levels of depression. Additionally, older patients with onset after 35 years of age reported less distress during panic attacks in relation to body sensations, as well as less panic-related cognitions and negative emotions. Multiple regression analysis of the entire sample showed that chronological age and age of onset of PD predicted distinct domains of panic phenomenology. Although fulfilling DSM-IV criteria, PD was consistently less severe in older patients.

POSTTRAUMATIC STRESS DISORDER (PTSD)

Prevalence

In the third cycle of the Longitudinal Study of Aging Amsterdam (LASA), measures were included to assess PTSD in a community-dwelling sample of older adults, whose ages ranged from 61 to 95 (27). Using strict diagnostic criteria for establishing diagnosis, the 6-month population prevalence was estimated to be 0.9%, which is greater than the 0.44% 6-month prevalence rate reported for a community sample of adults between the ages of 18 and 95 (28). The PTSD LASA estimate falls below the 12-month 3.6% revised prevalence estimate identified for young and middle-aged adults from the ECA and NCS (4).

Prior to the findings reported from LASA, rates of PTSD in the elderly have been difficult to estimate because this disorder has not been regularly assessed in large epidemiological surveys. Nonetheless, PTSD rates have been reported for discrete groups of older adults, such as natural disaster survivors, veterans groups (combat and former prisoners of war), and Holocaust survivors.

In a large community survey with the goal of assessing the impact of Hurricane Hugo, Norris examined past and current rates of PTSD and traumatic event exposure in Black and White, community-dwelling men and women across several broad age categories (young, middle-aged, and older adults) (29). Summing across nine traumatic events such as robbery, physical assault, sexual assault, and combat, the percentage of older adults (≥60 years of age) reporting lifetime exposure did not differ relative to young (18 to 39 years) and middle-aged (40 to 59 years) adults. When examining lifetime exposure to discrete traumatic events, older men were more likely to have experienced combat compared to young and middle-aged adults. In contrast, older adults were less likely to report a lifetime history of physical assault or sexual assault, or injury or damage due to natural or manmade disasters. When evaluating trauma exposure the year prior to the survey, older adults experienced fewer traumatic events (14.2%) compared to young (27%) and middle-aged adults (21%). With regard to current rates of PTSD, the overall percentage was lower for older adults (3.1%) compared to rates found for young (9.0%) and middle-aged (9.9%) adults.

Evidence from older adults exposed to other natural disasters, such as earthquakes, indicates that severe trauma exposure is associated with PTSD symptoms for up to 2 years following exposure (30,31). Available evidence also indicates similarity in rates of PTSD symptoms following natural disasters for young and older adults (30), although prior exposure to a similar traumatic event may act as a buffer, diminishing reactions to future similar traumatic events (32).

Rates of PTSD in elderly war veterans vary substantially depending on a number of issues, such as sample composition, recruitment site, and severity of traumatic exposure. Spiro et al. (33) found that 1.15% of World War II (WWII) survey respondents, rigorously screened and selected to represent a healthy sample of men, exceeded the recommended cutoff for PTSD on the Mississippi Scale for Combat Related PTSD (M-PTSD) (34) 45 to 50 years after combat exposure. The prevalence was higher (3.45%) for WWII veterans who reported moderate-to-heavy combat exposure. Within elderly veteran samples, severe trauma exposure is associated with higher rates of PTSD. Current (70%) and lifetime (78%) prevalence rates of PTSD amongst elderly former prisoners of war (POWs) exceed percentages found for elderly combat veterans (current: 18%, lifetime: 29%) (35). Rates of PTSD in clinical settings are also substantial. Blake and colleagues found approximately 19% of WWII and 30% of Korean War (KW) combat veterans in a Veterans Affairs (VA) hospital medical ward exceeded the M-PTSD cutoff (36). Within a VA skilled nursing home, 23% of cognitively intact veterans met lifetime diagnostic criteria for PTSD, with 57% of veterans reporting chronic PTSD symptoms (37). Rates of PTSD are higher among older veterans seeking psychiatric treatment (38).

Finally, Holocaust survivors have also been found to report significant symptoms of PTSD. Yehuda and associates found approximately 56% of nontreatment-seeking Holocaust survivors met clinician-rated criteria for PTSD (39).

Comparative Prevalence Rates

Across several investigations, Vietnam veterans report more severe PTSD symptoms compared to WWII and KW veterans (36,40,41). Although few differences were found across Symptom Checklist 90-Revised scales (42) when comparing Vietnam and WWII veterans diagnosed with PTSD, Vietnam veterans reported more severe PTSD symptoms (e.g., survivor guilt, trauma avoidance, startle reaction), as well as frequent suicidal ideation/attempts and a higher prevalence of PD (40). In contrast, Fontana and Rosenheck reported that KW veterans experienced more general psychiatric symptoms than WWII and Vietnam veterans (41). KW veterans also exhibited more suicidal severity (i.e., required hospitalization for physical consequences of suicide attempts) relative to WWII veterans, but had less severity than Vietnam veterans. Vietnam veterans reported more survivor guilt than either WWII or KW veterans.

The mechanisms explaining decreased PTSD symptom severity amongst older adults are not well understood and may be related to several variables, such as increased mortality among older PTSD survivors, age-related changes in coping strategies, cohort biases in symptom reports, and public support received by WWII veterans upon return from war (41,43). Nonetheless, it should not be overlooked that prevalence rates of PTSD are substantial amongst older combat veterans and POWs, despite the passage of four to five (or more) decades since trauma exposure. Furthermore, a small but emerging literature suggests that these individuals may be vulnerable to symptom reactivation in late life. Relevant identified triggers include media reminders on anniversary dates (44), compromised health, death of loved ones, retirement (45,46), dementia (47,48), and institutionalization in skilled-nursing settings (49).

Despite recognition that PTSD symptoms are present in older trauma survivors, the symptom course of PTSD has only recently received empirical attention. In their investigation, Port et al. found an increase of participants reporting substantial PTSD symptoms (from 27% to 34%) over 4 years among WWII and KW POWs 50 years after discharge from military service (50). Increases in PTSD symptomology dovetailed with the POWs' retrospective accounts of being "seriously troubled" by PTSD symptoms since discharge. Retrospective judgment of serious trouble with PTSD symptoms by POWs was highest immediately following repatriation and discharge from the military. The initially high percentage of POWs' symptom troubles slowly declined over three decades, but was followed by an increased percentage of symptom troubles over the two decades just prior to the investigation (1980–1999). The percentage of POWs reporting serious trouble with symptoms later in life was smaller than the percentage reporting concerns about symptoms immediately following discharge from service. These findings are consistent with previous observations (43,51), suggesting that PTSD symptoms are better characterized as ebbing and flowing rather than as a constant flood over the life span.

CASE EXAMPLE

Mr. C was a 73-year-old White male admitted to a short-stay inpatient psychiatric unit. He was an honorably discharged Marine veteran (infantry) who reported experiencing extensive ground combat during the Korean War. His first marriage following his discharge from the service ended in divorce. He was married to his second wife for approximately 40 years. At the time of his admission, his second wife had been deceased for close to 7 years. He blamed himself for her death, noting that he was unable to get her to the hospital in time after she suffered a major cardiac infarct during the night.

Mr. C was admitted to the unit after eviction from a local residential care home, where he had lived since his last psychiatric hospitalization. The eviction was served because of increasing agitation and aggression, including shouting and threatening staff and others (e.g., a bank teller), refusing to take his medications as prescribed, not completing basic self-care activities (e.g., bathing, eating regular meals), and refusing to keep his medical appointments. He specifically reported not liking the food in the residential care home and believing his prescribed medications were unnecessary because he was not experiencing symptoms of depression. He also described them as "poison" to his psychiatrist. His predominant affect expressed during his stay on the unit was intense anger.

Mr. C's previous psychiatric hospitalization followed his removal from his home by Adult Protective Services because of severe depression, suicidality, weight loss (40 to 50 pounds), and failure to complete basic and instrumental activities of daily living (e.g., buying and preparing food, paying his bills, cleaning his apartment). During this hospitalization he reported an adequate premorbid work history as a self-employed construction contractor. His psychiatric history since military discharge was notable for heavy daily alcohol use and intense anger. He had previously been prescribed diazepam for anger management. Following the death of his wife, he described an evolving pattern of persistent and intrusive recollections about her death, accompanied by increasing rumination about friends lost in combat during the Korean War. In fact, he reported difficulty sleeping because he was unable to "quiet his mind" or "shut out" intrusive and painful recollections. His sleep was also unsatisfying and he reported waking early and daytime fatigue. Additionally, he described not having a desire to interact with others and diminished interest and energy needed to prepare his meals, bathe, clean his home, or visit with friends from church, his main social outlet. He also expressed beliefs that he should not have outlived his wife or his friends lost in the war. When discussing his emotional experiences, he described cycling between intense anger and intense emotional pain. Interviews with him were kept abbreviated because of his fatigue, difficulty concentrating, and intense headaches. Early interviews were punctuated by silence, because he was reluctant to answer questions regarding his psychiatric symptoms and potential eliciting stressors.

Mr. C had at least two psychiatric hospitalizations for benzodiazepine abuse (reportedly taking two to three times the amount prescribed for emotional pain), suicidal ideation, and depression. He had also experienced other intermittent episodes of decompensation following the death of his wife, and had been diagnosed with MDD, recurrent (without full inter-episode recovery) and chronic PTSD with delayed onset.

Phenomenology

Older adults who suffered trauma early in life report specific symptoms that span the PTSD spectrum. Kuch and Cox reported that Holocaust survivors describe high rates of sleep disturbance (96%), recurrent nightmares (83%), intense distress when confronted with trauma cues (75%), difficulty concentrating (67%), diminished interest in activities (65%), and physiological reactivity (61%) (52). Other symptoms reported by over half their sample included intrusive trauma recollections, hypervigilance, irritability/ anger, and avoidance of activities or situations

reminiscent of trauma experiences. Approximately one-third of participants reported avoidance of thoughts and feelings associated with traumatic experiences, detachment from others, restricted affect, and expectations of a short future. Least frequently reported was exaggerated startle response, flashbacks, and psychogenic amnesia. Holocaust survivors suffering the most-severe traumatic experiences reported a greater frequency of intrusive recollections, avoidance of activities and situations consistent with traumatic events, hypervigilance, and greater diagnosis of PTSD relative to those with exposure to less-severe traumas, similar to findings reported by Yehuda and associates (39). Additionally, Holocaust survivors with PTSD were more likely to report dissociative experiences, psychogenic amnesia (53), depression (54), and alexethymia (55) compared to a control group of Holocaust survivors without PTSD.

Similar symptom reports have been observed in combat veterans. In their chart review of WWII veterans referred for mental health services, Kaup et al. reported that 80% of veterans reported sleep disturbance, 75% experienced nightmares, 65% experienced irritability, and 50% reported social isolation and detachment from others (45). Other symptoms frequently reported were flashbacks (45%), intrusive thoughts (35%), distress at trauma reminders (35%), and increased startle response (30%). Far fewer WWII veterans reported avoidance, restricted affect, or decreased interest in activities. To clarify the most relevant PTSD symptoms in older combat veterans, Hyer and colleagues assessed the association between PTSD symptoms and a blind clinician-assigned diagnosis of PTSD (43). Although all PTSD symptoms were predictive of PTSD diagnosis, emotional distress when exposed to reminders, diminished interest in activities, and inability to recall aspects of the trauma accounted for substantial unique variance. In a sample of WWII veterans seeking compensation for exacerbation of traumatic symptoms in late life, Macleod described intrusive recollections, nightmares, insomnia, irritability, and hypervigilance as frequently reported (46).

As with Holocaust survivors, severity of trauma exposure affects symptom reports. Zeiss and Dickman found former WWII POWs reported excessive startle responses and persistent painful memories more frequently than other PTSD symptoms (51). Survivor guilt and flashbacks were reported less frequently in their sample. Similarly, in their investigation of former WWII POWs, Goldstein and associates found sleep disturbance, nightmares, and intrusive recollections were the most frequently reported symptoms (56). Detachment from others was also frequently reported, as were concentration/memory difficulties and physiological reactivity to trauma cues. Less frequently reported were hyperarousal, flashbacks, avoidance of activities, survivor guilt, restricted affect, and diminished interest in activities. Common comorbid conditions associated with the PTSD syndrome in combat veterans include depression, alcohol abuse, and other anxiety disorders (37,57). Some evidence also suggests increased physical health vulnerability and mortality in older combat veterans and POWs (58–61), although these findings are not consistently replicated (57).

Symptom differences between young and older adult survivors of natural disasters have emerged and are useful for highlighting phenomenology of PTSD in older adults. In a report assessing the development of PTSD for the first time in older adults, older survivors of the 1988 Armenian earthquake reported less re-experiencing but more symptoms of hyperarousal compared to younger survivors, although the overall severity of PTSD was similar among both age groups (30). Not all studies of natural disasters have replicated these findings, and extensive methodological limitations have been cited (62).

Posttraumatic sequela experienced by older crime victims is also substantial. In their assessment of older adults seeking treatment for past and recent trauma exposure, Gray and Acierno reported that 44% of participants experienced intrusive thoughts (63). Thirty-six percent reported sleep disturbance, psychological distress when exposed to trauma cues, and diminished interest in daily activities. Approximately 33% reported experiencing nightmares; avoidance of trauma-related thoughts, feelings, and conversations; and difficulty concentrating. A quarter of participants reported experiencing physiological reactivity to traumatic events; avoidance of trauma-related places, people, and activities; and hypervigilance and exaggerated startle. Remaining symptoms (e.g., flashbacks, restricted affect, irritability/anger outbursts) were experienced less frequently. Additionally, depression (e.g., sadness, fatigue, weight changes, feelings of worthlessness) and panic symptoms (e.g., panic attacks, particularly rapid heart rate, shortness of breath, trembling, worrying about future attacks) were frequently reported by study participants.

Although potential differential symptom presentations across traumatic events (e.g., Holocaust, combat/POW, natural disasters, crime victims) have been observed, the available research is insufficient to assess the validity of these findings independent of methodological limitation (38).

SOCIAL PHOBIA

The 1-month, 6-month, and 12-month prevalence rates of social phobia in older adults is shown in Table 30-1. The overall social phobia prevalence in the elderly falls below the revised 12-month prevalence (3.7%) identified for young and middle-aged participants in the ECA and NCS (4), and social phobia appears to be a relatively rare syndrome amongst the elderly. No studies comparing symptoms of young and older adults were found in the literature.

OBSESSIVE-COMPULSIVE DISORDER (OCD)

OCD exhibits less age-related variation than the other anxiety disorders previously discussed. Prevalence rates for OCD in older adults are shown in Table 30-1. The 1-month prevalence rate of OCD in older adults from the ECA and as reported by Regier and associates (20) is consistent with the 0.9% rate identified for adults between 45 and 64, but lower than the range of rates (1.3% to 1.8%) identified for adults 18 to 44 years old. The 6-month prevalence rates of OCD suggest a possible diminishment with advanced age. The 6-month prevalence estimates of OCD from the ECA revealed a relatively even age distribution, although estimates varied across sites and gender (22). No studies comparing symptoms of young and older adults were found in the literature.

MIXED ANXIETY AND DEPRESSION

Less commonly discussed are findings regarding the comorbid prevalence rate of anxiety and mood disorders. Estimates from the NCS indicate that 58% of young and middle-aged adults (15 to 54 years old) with a lifetime history of MDD had a comorbid anxiety disorder. The 12-month prevalence rate of MDD and any anxiety disorder was similar in magnitude (51.2%) (64). Amongst older adults, Beekman et al. (65) reported the comorbid prevalence rate of primary MDD and any anxiety disorder as 47.5%, while the prevalence rates of any primary anxiety disorder and MDD were 26.1% in the LASA survey. Significant comorbidity of depressive and anxious symptoms has also been reported in elderly primary care patients, psychiatric outpatients, psychiatric inpatients (66), elderly residents of residential care facilities (67), and in geriatric primary care centers (68).

ANXIETY AND DEMENTIA

Several recent investigations suggest patients with dementia frequently experience comorbid anxiety symptoms and disorders. Using caregiver ratings from the anxiety subscale of the Neuropsychiatric Inventory (NPI), patients with dementia had higher anxiety levels compared to normal elderly controls (69). After controlling for age, education level, severity of cognitive impairment, and age of dementia onset, patients with Alzheimer's disease (AD) exhibited less anxiety relative to patients with vascular dementia (VaD) and frontotemporal dementia (FTD) (70). Approximately 30% of AD, 39% of FTD, and 46% of VaD patients were rated as having clinically relevant levels of anxiety symptoms on the NPI. After controlling for the level of cognitive impairment, anxiety was associated with depression/dysphoria for patients with AD, FTD, and VaD. For patients with AD and FTD, anxiety was associated with delusions, while for patients with FTD and VaD, anxiety was associated with agitation and irritability/lability. For patients with AD, anxiety was also correlated with symptoms of elation/euphoria, hallucinations, aberrant motor behaviors, and behavioral disinhibition. Follow-up analyses of anxious patients with AD revealed they had a younger age of dementia onset, greater severity of cognitive impairment, and more severe impairment in instrumental activities of daily living. Small sample size of the VaD and FTD patients prohibited follow-up analyses. Amongst the anxious AD patients, only four of 30 were receiving antidepressant treatment, leading the authors to suggest the need for aggressive treatment of these patients.

In an investigation of 398 consecutive patients with AD seeking neurological services, approximately 5% met DSM-III-R criteria for GAD, 2% met diagnostic criteria for PD, and one patient (<1%) met diagnostic criteria for social phobia (71). Compared to AD patients without GAD, the AD-GAD patients were more likely to have a psychiatric history. Patients with AD-GAD also had higher clinician-rated levels of depression and anxiety, as well as irritability, pathological crying, and delusions.

The evidence summarized above suggests that a sizeable number of patients with dementia experiences anxiety symptoms and disorders. Prevalence of anxiety symptoms varies across dementias, and is more prominent in FTD and VaD than AD. It was suggested that comorbid anxiety and dementia was not being aggressively treated despite its association with prominent cognitive, affective, and behavioral symptoms.

Summary

Overall, the assumption that anxiety disorders are quite uncommon in the elderly is an unfortunate overgeneralization, masking a rather complex pattern of prevalence rates. GAD is as prevalent in older adults as it is in young and middle-aged adults, while the prevalence rates of PD for older adults varied, with 6-month and 12-month rates consistent with young and middle-aged adults. Prevalence rates of OCD among older adults were consistent with rates for adults 45 to 64 years old, but lower relative to adults between 18 and 44. Rates of phobic disorders, PTSD, and mixed anxiety and depression amongst older adults are lower than rates for young and middle-aged adults. Finally, the prevalence of anxiety symptoms in older patients with dementia is substantial.

Some conclusions regarding the phenomenology of late-life anxiety disorders can be drawn from the limited available data. First, PD begins earlier in life and runs a chronic course continuing into old age, although symptom severity seems to lessen with age. New onset of PD in late life is rare; however, when it does occur, symptoms are

milder in severity. Second, some epidemiological data indicates approximately 39% of elderly patients with GAD report a chronic course of 21 or more years, while the remaining patients report a course of less than 10 years. More data are required to replicate findings suggesting few differences between early onset and late-onset GAD. Third, specific phobias of older adults seem more likely to encompass situational fears (e.g., heights, driving, flying) while those of younger adults focus on animals, blood, and injections. Fourth, PTSD symptoms follow a chronic, waxing and waning course, and anecdotal evidence suggests that symptoms may be exacerbated in old age. Empirical data on phenomenological manifestations of other anxiety disorders in late life are virtually nonexistent.

EVALUATION OF ANXIETY IN THE ELDERLY

Assessment of anxiety in elders is complicated by a number of variables, including a confounding of the symptom picture by medical comorbidity, polypharmacy (including over-the-counter and prescribed medications), frequent use of alcohol or substance use, difficulty of differentiation from depression, and resistance to psychiatric evaluation in older cohorts. Despite these substantial challenges, evaluation of anxiety in the elderly can be accomplished through several routes: clinical evaluation, rating scales, and laboratory evaluations.

Clinical Evaluation

A clinical evaluation should incorporate a recent history of presenting symptoms, characteristics of past symptoms (e.g., PD can be characterized by relapses), a detailed accounting of current prescribed and over-the-counter medications (including analgesics, cold medications, anticholinergic medications, and herbal and vitamin supplements), a history of substance use (alcohol, drug), and a medical history. Family history of anxiety symptoms may also be informative. Cognitively, evidence of worry, apprehension, fearfulness, and distractibility may be present in addition to common behavioral symptoms of hyperkinesis and exaggerated startle response. Physiological signs may include increased pulse rate, rapid breathing, sweating, and trembling.

Assessing Anxiety with Rating Scales

Anxiety rating scales can be used as adjuncts to the clinical evaluation of anxiety. These measures are quickly administered and useful for initial screening of symptoms, assessing symptom severity, and for documenting effectiveness of various psychological and pharmacological interventions. These scales are primarily of two kinds: observer-rated and self-rated. The most commonly used observer-rated scale is the Hamilton Anxiety Rating Scale (HARS) (72). This 14-item scale requires clinicians to rate the severity of each anxiety symptom from none (0) to very severe (4). A total rating of 18 or above is generally considered suggestive of clinically significant anxiety. A recent study suggests that the HARS has adequate inter-rater reliability, high specificity, and high sensitivity, and it successfully differentiates older patients with GAD from normal elderly controls (11).

Commonly used self-rated scales are the State-Trait Anxiety Inventory (STAI) (73) and the Beck Anxiety Inventory (BAI) (74). The STAI is a 40-item measure that assesses both transient (STAI-State) and enduring (STAI-Trait) symptoms of anxiety. The psychometric properties (i.e., adequate reliability and validity) of the STAI-State and STAI-Trait have been found adequate in a normal elderly sample (11) and an elderly sample with GAD (15,17). The BAI, which is a quick and easy-to-understand scale, is a 21-item symptom inventory in which patients rate the severity of anxiety symptoms. Recent studies suggest the BAI has good internal consistency and evidence of validity in a diverse and socially disadvantaged sample of older medical patients (75,76). In fact, in a sample of elderly psychiatric outpatients, the BAI sub-scales significantly correlated with the STAI-State and STAI-Trait. Elderly psychiatric outpatients diagnosed with anxiety disorders also had significantly higher scores on BAI sub-scales compared to elderly psychiatric outpatients without anxiety disorders (76). The BAI has also been found to differentiate elderly psychiatric outpatients from elderly medical outpatients (77).

Other self-report measures used to assess anxiety symptoms, such as the Penn State Worry Questionnaire (78), the Worry Scale (79), the Fear Questionnaire (80), and the Padua Inventory (81), have been extensively evaluated in older adults with GAD in several investigations (11,15,17, 18). Both self-report and structured clinician-rating scales of PTSD symptoms, such as the Mississippi Scale for Combat Related PTSD (34), the Impact of Events Scale (82), and the Clinician Administered PTSD Scale (83) have also been evaluated in a series of investigations with older combat veterans with PTSD (84–86). Many of these measures have adequate psychometric properties with anxious older adults.

Finally, efforts have been made to combine brief self-report measures screenings with clinical diagnostic interviews for use by primary care physicians (87,88). The Primary Care Evaluation of Mental Disorders (PRIME-MD) (88) allows diagnosis of 18 specific disorders (grouped into anxiety, mood, alcohol, somatoform, and eating disorder categories) using DSM-IV diagnostic criteria. This measure has been found to have adequate evidence of brevity, sensitivity, specificity, inter-rater agreement, and construct validity (88). Valenstein and associates found that use of the PRIME-MD increased recognition of psychiatric symptoms for older adults (≥65 years of age) attending a veterans' primary care clinic (89). Older adults were as likely to complete the PRIME-MD as younger adults (≤65 years of age),

but were less likely to be diagnosed with a psychiatric disorder or receive an intervention from physicians relative to adults younger than 65. Post-hoc analyses revealed older adults were less likely to be diagnosed with a mood disorder and probable alcohol abuse relative to younger adults; however, no differences in anxiety or somatoform disorder diagnoses were found. Lower rates of psychiatric diagnoses amongst older adults were speculated to reflect several processes, such as decreased rates of psychiatric disorders in older adults and increased endorsement of somatic symptoms in lieu of affective symptoms (e.g., feeling down or depressed) by older adults. Other issues complicating psychiatric diagnoses in older adults may include primary care physicians' focus on emergent medical issues as well as hesitancy to raise concerns of psychiatric diagnoses for fear that older patients will have a negative emotional reaction and resist acknowledgment and treatment of psychiatric symptoms.

Laboratory Investigations

Laboratory evaluations can help diagnose underlying medical conditions that produce symptoms of anxiety. A complete blood count, electrocardiogram, thyroid function tests, blood sugar, blood gases, and drug/alcohol screening are helpful to exclude more common medical conditions associated with anxiety, such as anemia, endocrine disorders, arrhythmias, and substance abuse.

Summary

Assessing anxiety disorders experienced by older adults can be accomplished through the use of clinical evaluation, self-report measures, clinician-rated measures, and laboratory evaluations. Given the potentially complex interaction amongst diverse causal mechanisms (e.g., medical comorbidity, polypharmacy, cohort bias in symptom reports) and lack of clear-cut empirically validated guidelines demonstrating the superiority of one assessment strategy over others, clinicians are urged to use a multi-method strategy, combining assessment techniques to adequately identify the range of anxiety disorder symptoms experienced by older adults.

GERIATRIC ANXIETY DISORDER MANAGEMENT

Effective management of geriatric anxiety is accomplished through both pharmacological and psychological treatments. Collaborative care models addressing physician, patient, and health care delivery system barriers show promise for treating anxiety disorders experienced by older adults.

Pharmacologic Treatments

Several factors may complicate psychopharmacologic management of the anxious older patient, most notably the physiological changes of aging that may affect pharmacokinetics and pharmacodynamics of drugs, the presence of comorbid medical conditions, and polypharmacy. Prior treatment response, the nature of the targeted symptoms, and the most tolerable side-effect profile should also be taken into account. To reach the optimal dose for an older patient without causing intolerable side effects, the old adage "start low and go slow" should be followed.

Over the years, numerous compounds have been used as anxiolytics. These have included benzodiazepines, azapirones, tricyclic antidepressants, monoamine oxidase inhibitors, neuroleptics, beta-adrenergic receptor antagonists, barbiturates, anticonvulsants, and antihistamines. More recently, newer antidepressants such as selective serotonin-reuptake inhibitors (SSRIs), serotonin/norepinephrine reuptake inhibitors (SNRIs), other dual-action antidepressants, and 5-HT2 antagonists have emerged as the first-line treatment for several anxiety disorders and mixed anxiety-depression syndromes in younger patients. While the data from controlled trials of newer compounds in the elderly will accumulate slowly, clinical experience of geriatric psychiatrists suggests similar efficacy of these compounds in late-life anxiety syndromes. Furthermore, newer antidepressants seem to be much better tolerated by older people than many of the anxiolytic medications used in the past, particularly over longer periods of time. Some of these compounds (e.g., venlafaxine—an SNRI, and sertraline—an SSRI) have also been recently studied for late-life anxiety syndromes (90,91).

Selective Serotonin Reuptake Inhibitors
Several investigations have documented the efficacy of SSRIs for anxiety disorders in younger patients. SSRIs have been shown in several randomized and controlled clinical trials to demonstrate superior efficacy to placebo, and at least equal efficacy to tricyclic antidepressants for PD, generally in younger patients (92–95). There is also preliminary evidence of efficacy of sertraline in older patients with PD (91). SSRIs such as fluoxetine, sertraline, fluvoxamine, and paroxetine, have all been found to be superior to control groups for OCD in younger patients (96–100). Sertraline has also shown promise as a long-term treatment for patients with OCD (101), and is efficacious in treating comorbid symptoms of OCD and MDD (102). There is also evidence of the efficacy of SSRIs in GAD, as demonstrated by a randomized, placebo-controlled trial with paroxetine (103). Finally, several randomized, controlled trials of SSRIs indicate their efficacy in addressing PTSD symptoms (104–107). Given the propensity for antidepressants to worsen anxiety in the beginning of the therapeutic regimen, it is recommended that starting doses be very small (e.g., sertraline 12.5 mg once daily, to be increased gradually to 50 mg once daily over a period of 2 to 4 weeks).

SNRIs and Other Newer Antidepressants
There is emerging evidence that newer antidepressants, such as SNRIs like venlafaxine, are efficacious in PD (108) and GAD (109). More importantly, a recent retrospective, pooled

analysis of five randomized, placebo-controlled trials of extended-release venlafaxine, in doses of 37.5 to 225 mg/day, demonstrated efficacy compared to placebo in participants older than 60 (110). We recommend a starting dose of venlafaxine at 37.5 mg/day with breakfast, to be increased to 75 mg/day after 1 week. The dose can then be further increased by 37.5 mg on a weekly basis, depending upon the patient's response. Considering the variation in individual responses, patients with GAD or mixed anxiety-depression may require doses varying from 75 to 225 mg/day. Several recent randomized, placebo-controlled trials support the prolonged (6 months) use of extended-release venlafaxine as an effective, safe, and tolerable treatment for GAD symptoms (111,112). There is some preliminary evidence of efficacy of mirtazapine, which enhances both noradrenergic and serotonergic neurotransmission, in PTSD (113). We recommend a starting dose of 7.5 mg at bedtime, which can be increased to 15 mg/day in a week, depending upon tolerance to sedation. Dose range is 15 to 45 mg/day, with most elderly patients responding well at or near the 15 to 30 mg/day range. Similarly, there is some evidence of the efficacy of the 5-HT2 antagonist nefazodone in PTSD (114) and mixed anxiety-depression (115), although it should be used with extreme caution due to the Food and Drug Administration's boxed warning regarding potential hepatotoxicity.

As is apparent from this brief review, SSRIs and SNRIs are considered the drugs of choice for anxiety in older patients. Noncompliance associated with delayed onset of action and initial transient jitters can be minimized by patient education, the addition of a benzodiazepine in the first few weeks of treatment, and using small doses at the beginning of treatment, which can then be gradually increased for therapeutic effect.

Benzodiazepines
After being the mainstay of anxiolytic therapy for more than three decades, benzodiazepines have recently been supplanted by SSRIs and SNRIs as the most frequently prescribed anxiolytic agents for both young and older patients. Benzodiazepines, however, remain the mainstay of pharmacological therapy for acute management of anxiety, and as initial short-term adjuncts to therapy with SSRIs and SNRIs. Benzodiazepines are beneficial because they have a rapid onset and little effect on cardiovascular status. However, potential complications of long-term benzodiazepine use in older patients include excessive daytime drowsiness, cognitive impairment and confusion, psychomotor impairment and risk of falls, depression, paradoxical reactions, amnestic syndromes, respiratory problems, abuse and dependence potential, and breakthrough withdrawal reactions. Because of these complications, use of benzodiazepines for more than a few weeks is generally not recommended.

For older patients, short half-life benzodiazepines (e.g., lorazepam or oxazepam) are preferred because they require only phase II metabolism and are inactivated by direct conjugation in the liver, mechanisms minimally impacted by normal aging. A typical starting dose of lorazepam would be 0.25 mg twice a day, which can be increased over the next several days to a total daily dose ranging from 1 to 3 mg, divided into two or three doses.

Azapirones

Buspirone has demonstrated efficacy comparable to diazepam in double-blind studies in patients with GAD (116,117). A decreased probability of dependence, absence of withdrawal symptoms upon discontinuation (118), and lack of psychomotor impairment even with long-term usage (119) seems to be an advantage over benzodiazepines. Studies in geriatric samples indicate that buspirone is well tolerated, does not cause adverse interactions when coprescribed with other medications (including antihypertensives, cardiac glycosides, and bronchodilators), and is effective for remediation of chronic anxiety symptoms in this population (10 to 30 mg/day in BID or TID regimen) (120, 121). Despite efficacy in clinical trials, however, experience with this medication in clinical settings suggests an inconsistent therapeutic response. Because buspirone may require 4 weeks to manifest therapeutic effects, it may at times be prudent to initially combine buspirone with a short-acting benzodiazepine as an adjunct that can be withdrawn once the therapeutic effects of buspirone begin.

Atypical Neuroleptics and Miscellaneous Others

Evidence from meta-analyses of controlled trials of traditional neuroleptics suggests a moderate effect for management of agitation and behavioral symptoms associated with dementia (122). Because of data suggesting reduced rates of adverse side effects (e.g., extrapyramidal symptoms) and comparable efficacy to the traditional neuroleptics, the atypical antipsychotic agents (e.g., risperidone, olanzapine) have been recommended for treating agitation and behavioral symptoms associated with dementia (123). In a post-hoc analysis, the efficacy of olanzapine for anxiety symptoms experienced by Alzheimer's patients was demonstrated relative to patients receiving placebo (124). We recommend a typical starting dose for olanzapine of 2.5 mg/day, with an eventual range of 2.5 to 7.5 mg/day. Similarly, risperidone can be started at 0.25 mg twice a day with an upper limit of therapeutic dose at 0.75 mg twice a day, and quetiapine starting at 25 mg at bedtime to be increased to 25 mg twice a day in a few days, with an eventual dose range of 100 to 200 mg/day divided into two doses in agitated patients with dementia.

Antihistamines like hydroxyzine and diphenhydramine are used sometimes to manage mild anxiety with varying degree of success, though empirical data are in general lacking regarding their efficacy, and hence we prefer not to use them in our practice. Further, if used, antihistamines should only be considered for the short term (2 to 4 weeks) in the elderly, due to their anticholinergic and antihistaminic actions.

Recommendations for pharmacological treatments are summarized in Table 30-2.

Psychological Treatments

Psychopharmacological interventions are the first-line intervention for older adults with anxiety disorders in psychiatric settings; however, older patients' vulnerability to

---

TABLE 30-2

MANAGEMENT STRATEGIES FOR ANXIETY DISORDERS IN LATE LIFE

Disorder	First-Line Treatment(s)	Second-Line Treatment(s)
Panic disorder with or without agoraphobia	SSRIs, SNRIs, and/or CBT	Newer antidepressants and TCAs
Generalized anxiety disorder	SNRIs, SSRIs, Buspirone, and/or CBT	Newer antidepressants, TCAs
Obsessive compulsive disorder	SSRIs plus CBT	Clomipramine, combination pharmacotherapy
Social phobia		
Generalized	SSRIs plus CBT	Benzodiazepines
Specific	Buspirone and/or CBT	Benzodiazepines
Simple (specific) phobia	CBT	Benzodiazepines
Posttraumatic stress disorder	SSRIs or SNRIs	CBT, newer antidepressants
Mixed anxiety-depression	SSRIs or SNRIs	Buspirone, CBT
Anxiety and agitation in dementia	Atypical antipsychotics	Benzodiazepines, Anticonvulsants
Anxiety and medical disorders	Identify and treat underlying cause, use SSRIs or SNRIs in primary anxiety disorder	Benzodiazepines

SSRIs, selective serotonin reuptake inhibitors; SNRIs, serotonin/norepinephrine reuptake inhibitors; CBT, cognitive behavioral therapy; TCA, tricyclic antidepressants.

adverse medication side effects, polypharmacy, and lack of prospectively designed, placebo-controlled clinical trials of pharmacological interventions suggests that other strategies for managing anxiety disorder symptoms, such as psychotherapy, should be considered. Skills learned in psychotherapy can also be applied beyond the course of treatment, a benefit not typically expected or associated with psychopharmacological interventions (125).

A recent meta-analysis of 15 studies encompassing 20 interventions that included 495 adults with a mean age of 69.5 years indicated that psychotherapeutic interventions for older adults with late-life anxiety symptoms and/or disorders were reliably more effective than no treatment and treatment-control conditions (126). Unfortunately, many of the investigations evaluated interventions for general anxiety symptoms rather than specific syndromes, such as GAD or PD. Investigations reporting intervention efficacy for specific anxiety syndromes evaluated cognitive behavioral therapy (CBT). CBT, which integrates cognitive (e.g., monitoring and reformulating inaccurate and/or maladaptive beliefs) and behavioral (e.g., exposure, relaxation training) strategies, has proven to be a highly successful intervention choice for the treatment of depression experienced by older adults (127). Substantial empirical evidence documenting the efficacy of CBT for anxiety disorders among younger populations exists (129,129), but only recently have well-controlled studies evaluating interventions for anxious older adults been published.

Panic Disorder

Preliminary evidence supports the use of CBT for PD experienced by older adults. We found significant improvement among older adults with PD using CBT at posttreatment and 3-month follow-up on all measured domains (cognitive, behavioral, physiological, depression) (130). Greater reductions in anxiety and depressive symptoms were also found in a randomized trial of CBT for anxious older adults, most of whom were diagnosed with PD, receiving individual in-home CBT compared to patients receiving individual in-home supportive therapy (131).

Conceptualizing PD as stemming from catastrophic interpretations of physiological symptoms, such as rapid heart rate and breathing, the investigations described above implemented multicomponent treatment packages addressing cognitive, physiological, and behavioral (e.g., avoidance) symptoms of PD modified from a protocol developed by Barlow and Cerny (132). A detailed overview of the rationale, risks, benefits, and evidence of efficacy of a similar protocol are provided by Craske and Barlow (133). A summary of interventions from these protocols follows.

In the initial phase of treatment, clinicians primarily play a psychoeducational role. Patients receive extensive education regarding the dynamic interplay of cognitions and PD symptoms, with the primary goal of emphasizing the connections between thoughts, anxiety, and the non-pathological nature of autonomic arousal. By providing accurate information about autonomic arousal, patients

learn to re-conceptualize panic symptoms as normal physiological arousal.

After learning about the development of maladaptive cognitions and developing skills to recognize and monitor these thoughts, patients learn specific cognitive strategies for countering maladaptive misinterpretations of physiological symptoms in anxiety-provoking situations. Crucial to treatment is encouraging patients to conceptualize maladaptive thoughts as hypotheses to be logically evaluated. This opens thoughts for critical evaluation through strategies such as accurately estimating the probabilities of negative events occurring based on past experiences ("Although I believe I may have a panic attack and pass out in public, I have never passed out in public before when I have had a panic attack, so the probability that I will pass out this time is unlikely."), and de-catastrophizing or realistically examining how feared events can be coped with and managed ("If I had a panic attack in public, others may help me rather than think I am crazy."). Other strategies used may include *thought stopping*, in which patients interrupt misinterpretations through simultaneous use of visual imagery (e.g., vividly imagining a bright red stop sign) and refocusing their attention to current ongoing activities, such as becoming more aware of activities going on around them. Helping patients develop cognitive coping statements ("Although I am starting to breath quickly, I can do this if I just stick with it.") and re-conceptualizing feared situations ("Going to the store gives me a chance to test my belief that I will have a panic attack.") may also be crucial cognitive strategies.

To manage physiological arousal, patients learn a number of breathing and relaxation strategies. As with cognitive restructuring, these interventions are introduced following a detailed explanation of the rationale for the procedures in relation to the presumed etiology of PD. For breathing control, patients are taught slowed diaphragmatic breathing for use during episodes of intense arousal. Saying a calming word, such as "relax," on exhale is also encouraged. Initially, therapists model breathing retraining in the session, and patients are encouraged to practice in the session so they may receive corrective feedback. Patients are also urged to use breathing retraining at home and eventually in stressful situations, once they are proficient.

Additionally, early in treatment, patients are taught the use of progressive muscle relaxation (PMR), in which eight specific muscle groups are tensed and relaxed in succession, affording patients the opportunity to discriminate muscular tension from relaxation. Assisting patients to recognize building muscular tension enables them to rapidly deploy easily implemented relaxation interventions learned later in treatment. Once eight-muscle PMR is mastered through repeated practise in and out of session, patients learn relaxation by recall, in which they are instructed to recall the experience of relaxation in four major muscle groups (such as the stomach, chest, shoulders, and forehead, although these can be tailored to problematic areas specific to individual patients), rendering

PMR portable and not requiring muscular tensing. Achieving the greatest portability of PMR comes from cue-controlled relaxation, in which patients take slow breaths while instructing themselves to relax on each exhale and release tension from their muscles. Over the course of treatment, therapists help patients troubleshoot difficulties and increasingly encourage practise of relaxation and breathing strategies in stressful situations, providing opportunities for patients to manage and master intense physiological arousal.

Interoceptive exposure is used to decrease fearful reactions to specific symptoms of physiological arousal, while agoraphobic avoidance is addressed through imaginal and in vivo exposure. Through interoceptive exposure, patients are exposed to panicogenic interoceptive cues through purposeful shallow breathing, spinning in a chair, breathing through a straw, or effortful exercises (to name but a few strategies) to induce sensations such as hyperventilation, light-headedness, dizziness, or cardiovascular reactions. Patients are required to perform these exercises for a specified amount of time to decrease use of avoidance strategies and induce habituation to physiological arousal. Exercises that produce sensations similar to the patients' panic symptoms are ranked according to the amount of anxiety produced, and patients are asked to induce these sensations in sessions and at home in a graduated fashion, starting with those that produce less anxiety and working up a hierarchy to those that produce the greatest arousal. After induction, cognitive restructuring and breathing control are used in-session and at home to manage symptoms and re-conceptualize maladaptive beliefs elicited before or during the exposure.

Interoceptive exposure is extended to naturally occurring situations (e.g., exercising) that patients have avoided due to physiological arousal. As with the interoceptive induction exercises, naturally occurring situations are ranked in terms of the amount of anxiety generated in a hierarchical fashion, and patients gradually expose themselves to these situations for specified periods of time to induce panic-like physiological arousal. Again, cognitive restructuring and breathing strategies can be used after exposure to decrease the strength of maladaptive beliefs and help patients manage physiological symptoms. Over the course of exposure work, it is critical that therapists help patients engage in exposure while gradually phasing out the use of objects (e.g., lucky charms, cellular phones), people (e.g., significant others), behaviors (e.g., lying down to reduce dizziness, or avoidance), or places (e.g., near hospitals) that provide a sense of safety and reinforce misattributions and maladaptive beliefs regarding the meaning of physiological arousal. Similar strategies (constructing a hierarchy, requiring exposure for a specified amount of time in a clearly defined fashion, implementation of cognitive restructuring, and breathing control) are used for imaginal and in vivo exposure to agoraphobic situations as well.

Generalized Anxiety Disorder

GAD has received substantial research attention, although findings have been equivocal. In a controlled study comparing group CBT and nondirective supportive psychotherapy for older adults with GAD, participants in both conditions manifested significantly lower worry, anxiety, and depression scores posttreatment and at 6-month follow-up. No statistically significant differences were found between the groups in responder status and high end-state functioning (134).

Similarly, Wetherell and associates found few differences between older adults with GAD randomly assigned to either a CBT group or a discussion group (DG) that focused on worry-provoking events (135). Relative to a wait-list control group, both the CBT and DG groups improved on measures of GAD severity and pathological worry at posttreatment. The CBT group also improved in depression symptom severity and select quality-of-life subscales at posttreatment relative to the wait-list control condition. Both the CBT and the DG group improved across a range of measures from pretreatment to posttreatment (GAD severity, clinician-rated and self-rated anxiety, self-rated depression), while the wait-list control condition did not. However, no statistically significant differences were found between the CBT group and DG across self-report and clinician-rated measures, treatment responder status, and high-end state functioning immediately following treatment or at 6-month follow-up, with the exception of decreased time spent worrying by the CBT group immediately following treatment.

Addressing methodological limitations of these previous investigations, Stanley and associates found that older adults with GAD randomly assigned to a group CBT intervention improved on measures of anxiety, worry, depression, and fears relative to a minimal contact group immediately following treatment (136). At posttreatment, more patients in the CBT group were rated as responders relative to the minimal contact group (45% versus 8%). Likewise, only 55% of CBT participants met diagnostic criteria for GAD relative to 81% of patients in the minimal contact group. Only one participant in the CBT and none in the minimal contact group met criteria for high-end state functioning, highlighting the pervasive, entrenched quality of GAD in the elderly. For the most part, the CBT group patients maintained improvements across measured domains (worry, anxiety, depression, fears, and quality of life) at 3-month, 6-month, and 12-month assessments.

Treatments used in these investigations were adapted for older adults from multicomponent protocols addressing the cognitive, physiological, and behavioral symptoms of GAD (137,138). A brief overview of interventions used in these protocols is discussed next.

In the initial session, patients receive information regarding the nature of cognitive, behavioral, and physiological symptoms of anxiety. Specifically, patients receive a description of the role maladaptive thoughts, such as catastrophizing and probability overestimation, play in generating and maintaining anxiety symptoms. Behavioral consequences of these thoughts, such as seeking excessive reassurance, worry, and avoidance, are also discussed as contributing issues in the maintenance of symptoms. Patients also receive information regarding the adaptive and maladaptive nature of physiological anxiety reactions. Time in the initial session is also devoted to providing an overview of the treatment and the rationale for specific strategies used over the course of treatment, such as self-monitoring of thoughts, relaxation training, cognitive restructuring, and exposure strategies.

Following the educational discussion of the first session, sessions two through five focus on helping patients learn to practise and implement breathing training and PMR to manage physiological symptoms of anxiety. As with the PD protocols discussed above, patients learn to implement diaphragmatic breathing. The PMR training incorporates discrimination, recall, and cue-controlled procedures similar to those discussed previously.

In sessions six through 10, patients are taught specific strategies for addressing maladaptive thoughts associated with GAD. As a starting point, patients are encouraged to conceptualize maladaptive thoughts as hypotheses that can be examined logically and critically through scrutiny of available evidence, past or present. Maladaptive thinking patterns identified for patients with GAD include probability overestimation and catastrophic thinking. Probability overestimation results when patients overestimate the possibility of negative events occurring, such as assuming they have a major medical illness when experiencing physiological arousal. Catastrophic thinking results when patients believe they will be unable to manage or cope with a feared event. For example, in the first case study, Mr. S believed he would be unable to find a way of returning home if he and his wife were not picked up by the transportation service they used to get to his medical appointments. Catastrophic thoughts may also involve patients assuming extremely negative consequences will result from the occurrence of minor events (e.g., they will be fired for being 5 minutes late), or assuming personal responsibility for the occurrence of minor events (e.g., poor investment of a small sum of money will ruin the family's finances).

Specific strategies are used to address these cognitions. For example, for probability overestimation patients are asked to examine past and present experiences to evaluate the actual likelihood of feared negative events occurring. In initial stages therapists play an active role, helping patients to identify evidence suggesting that feared negative events are unlikely and represent maladaptive thinking. Generating evidence to counter probability overestimation is done in therapy session and outside of therapy. In the case study, Mr. S was asked to critically examine evidence that he would not be picked up by the transportation service. The fact that Mr. S and his wife had never been left behind by the transportation service countered

his belief that he and his wife would be abandoned. For catastrophic thoughts, patients are asked to generate plausible but less-negative outcomes using past or present experience. Patients may also be asked to imagine the worst possible outcomes of feared events, and realistically evaluate the duration of these events and their ability to cope based on past experiences. For example, Mr. S was asked to imagine the worst possible outcome if he fell on the sidewalk outside of his home. Noting that his street saw a moderate amount of traffic, he acknowledged that someone would probably stop to help him, call an ambulance, or notify his wife that he needed help, weakening the belief that he would die of exposure. To weaken maladaptive beliefs regarding being abandoned by the transportation company, Mr. S was encouraged to think of all possible ways he and his wife could cope with this situation, such as calling the transportation dispatch or arranging for alternative transportation by calling a taxi service or friends. Through these procedures, completed both in and out of session, patients learn that their feared events are unlikely, that if they did occur the consequences would probably be time-limited, and that they have some abilities to cope with these events.

In implementing these strategies, therapists should avoid conveying that maladaptive thoughts are replaced with more positive ones. Rather, therapists emphasize that the connection between negative thoughts and excessive anxiety can be addressed through repeated practice of critically evaluating maladaptive thoughts and reformulating those thoughts so they are less negative, more adaptive, and more realistic. Critically important to this process is that elicitation and challenging of maladaptive beliefs be thorough. If patients continue to experience maladaptive beliefs and act accordingly, any reformulation of thoughts will be weakened.

Exposure strategies are used in sessions 10 through 15 to help patients practice and implement relaxation and cognitive skills through graduated practise. Patients and therapists develop a fear hierarchy of worry-producing situations. Exposure to worrisome situations is accomplished imaginally and in vivo, both of which are paired with cognitive restructuring and relaxation strategies. Patients implement exposure both in and out of session.

Finally, other interventions included in GAD treatment protocol are worry exposure, time management, and problem solving.

Modifying Cognitive-Behavioral Therapy for Older Adults

As with psychopharmacological interventions, psychotherapeutic strategies found effective with younger adults are generally implemented with older adults (139). Modifying CBT for the needs of older adults (e.g., age-associated memory changes) has been suggested but not widely or systematically investigated (140); however, a recent study investigated the use of a modified CBT treatment package for older patients. Using strategies to enhance compliance with cognitive-behavioral procedures (e.g., weekly readings, graphing symptom changes, reminder/troubleshooting phone calls) resulted in lower anxiety and worry symptoms, as well as fewer symptoms of GAD or comorbid disorders for a small group of older adults with GAD (N = 8) randomly assigned to receive enhanced individual CBT relative to those assigned to a wait-list condition (141). Only a small difference in GAD symptom severity was found comparing older adults randomly assigned to receive either standard individual CBT or wait-list control, highlighting the potential usefulness of the enhanced CBT package. These conclusions are tentative, however, because a direct comparison between the standard and enhanced CBT conditions was not made. Further research investigating modifications for CBT is required.

COLLABORATIVE CARE

As with young and middle-aged adults, many elderly patients first seek psychiatric treatment from their primary care physician. Thus, increased recognition of psychiatric symptoms by primary care physicians may be necessary for appropriate treatment implementation and cost-savings associated with treating anxiety disorders. However, acknowledging that physicians' recognition of symptoms is but one piece of an interdependent system, which includes both patient and physician variables that unfold against the backdrop of complex health-delivery systems, Roy-Byrne and Katon recommend a model of collaborative care targeting each major variable in the healthcare delivery system (e.g., patient, physician, health care system) (142). This model includes:

- Intensive patient education about psychiatric symptoms and encouraging active participation in treatment.
- Preliminary and ongoing primary care physician education and consultation regarding psychiatric symptoms and interventions.
- More frequent and extended contact with patients emphasizing symptom education, symptom prevention, social support, trouble-shooting barriers to treatment compliance, and continued follow-up.

Patient education and skill-building components are commonly emphasized in cognitive CBT, suggesting that such interventions could easily be incorporated into collaborative care models (143).

Collaborative models integrating these components have been found effective (e.g., reduced depressive symptom severity, increased treatment adherence with antidepressant medication, increased satisfaction with treatment for depression) in several randomized, controlled trials for young and middle-aged adults (143) as well as older patients with MDD (144). Similar findings have been found for young and middle-aged adults with PD (145). A small pilot study that screened and provided individual CBT for older adults meeting diagnostic criteria for GAD in the primary care setting reported statistically and clinically significant declines in self-reported worry, depression, and GAD symptom severity relative to patients receiving care as usual (146). Combined, these investigations provide promising models of intervention for the treatment of anxiety symptoms experienced by older adults, but have yet to be empirically evaluated.

Overall, CBT holds promise as an effective therapeutic approach for anxiety disorders, particularly PD and GAD, in older adults. For the treatment of PD, further efforts are needed to replicate the reviewed results using appropriately controlled investigations. The tenacity of GAD symptoms is evident from the investigations reviewed above, and highlights the need for continued efforts to address anxiety and worry in older adults through the use of innovative interventions. No other well-controlled studies have evaluated the efficacy of CBT for older adults with other anxiety disorders such as PTSD and OCD, and recommendations for treatment cannot be made. Overall, psychotherapeutic approaches to treating anxiety disorders in older adults are in need of vigorous research efforts to identify and evaluate efficacious interventions in the context of well-controlled investigations.

CONCLUSIONS

Recent epidemiological surveys indicate that anxiety disorders in older adults are characterized by a complex pattern of prevalence rates that challenges the view that these disorders are rare relative to young and middle-aged adults. Knowledge regarding the clinical characteristics of anxiety disorders in older adults is slowly emerging, but suggests potential age-related symptom differences compared to young and middle-aged adults. Detection of anxiety symptoms in elders is complicated by several factors, including a confounding of the symptom picture by high medical comorbidity, frequent use of multiple prescribed and over-the-counter medications, difficulty in differentiating anxiety from depression, and the tendency of some older adults to resist psychiatric evaluation. Nonetheless, a comprehensive evaluation including a clinical interview, self-report measures, and laboratory results, can improve detection and accurate assessment of anxiety in the elderly. Empirically validated knowledge regarding appropriate pharmacological interventions in the elderly is still sparse, and inferences from data in young and middle-aged populations form the basis of clinical practice in the elderly. SSRIs and SNRIs are considered first-line interventions because of their efficacy and relative tolerability in the elderly. Psychotherapy, particularly CBT, has also been found efficacious for older adults with anxiety disorders. Collaborative care models, which address physician, patient, and health care service-delivery barriers, hold promise for assessing and treating anxiety disorders experienced by older adults in the primary care setting.

REFERENCES

1. de Beurs E, Beekman ATF, van Balkom AJL, Deeg DJH, van Dyck R, van Tilburg W. Consequences of anxiety in older persons: its effect on disability, well-being, and use of health services. *Psychol Med.* 1999;29:583–593.
2. Sheikh JI, Cassidy EL. Treatment of anxiety disorders in the elderly: issues and strategies. *J Anxiety Disord.* 2000;14: 173–190.
3. Krasucki C, Howard R, Mann A. The relationship between anxiety disorders and age. *Int J Geriatr Psychiatry.* 1998;13:79–99.
4. Narrow WE, Rae DS, Robins LN, Regier DA. Revised prevalence estimates of mental disorders in the United States: using a clinical significance criterion to reconcile two surveys' estimates. *Arch Gen Psychiatry.* 2002;59:115–123.
5. Lindesay J, Briggs K, Murphey E. The Guy's/Age Concern Survey: prevalence rates of cognitive impairment, depression, and anxiety in an urban elderly community. *Br J Psychiatry.* 1989;155:317–329.
6. Manela M, Katona C, Livingston G. How common are the anxiety disorders in old age? *Int J Geriatr Psychiatry.* 1996;11: 65–70.
7. Blazer D, George LK, Hughes D. The epidemiology of anxiety disorders: an age comparison. In: Salzman C, Lebowitz BD, eds. *Anxiety in the Elderly: Treatment and Research.* New York: Springer; 1991:17–30.
8. Beekman ATF, Bremmer MA, Deeg DJH, et al. Anxiety disorders in later life: a report from the Longitudinal Aging Study, Amsterdam. *Int J Geriatr Psychiatry.* 1998;13:717–726.
9. Uhlenhuth EH, Balter MB, Mellinger GD, Cisin IH, Clinthorne J. Symptom checklist syndromes in the general population: correlations with psychotherapeutic drug use. *Arch Gen Psychiatry.* 1983;40:1167–1173.
10. Wittchen HU, Zhao S, Kessler RC, Eaton WW. DSM-III-R Generalized Anxiety Disorder in the National Comorbidity Survey. *Arch Gen Psychiatry.* 1994;51:355–364.
11. Beck JG, Stanley MA, Zebb BJ. Characteristics of generalized anxiety disorder in older adults: a descriptive study. *Behav Res Ther.* 1996;34:225–234.
12. Wetherell JL, Le Roux H, Gatz M. DSM-IV criteria for generalized anxiety disorder in older adults: distinguishing the worried from the well. *Psychol Aging.* 2003;18:622–627.
13. Diefenbach GJ, Hopko DR, Feigon S, et al. Minor GAD: characteristics of subsyndromal GAD in older adults. *Behav Res Ther.* 2003;41:481–487.
14. Babcock RL, Laguna LB, Laguna KD, Urusky DA. Age differences in the experience of worry. *J Mental Health Aging.* 2000;6: 227–235.
15. Stanley MA, Beck JG, Zebb BJ. Psychometric properties of four anxiety measures in older adults. *Behav Res Ther.* 1996;34: 827–838.
16. Fuentes K, Cox B. Assessment of anxiety in older adults: a community-based survey and comparison with younger adults. *Behav Res Ther.* 2000;38:297–309.
17. Stanley MA, Novy DM, Bourland SL, Beck JG, Averill PM. Assessing older adults with generalized anxiety: a replication and extension. *Behav Res Ther.* 2001;39:221–235.
18. Hopko DA, Stanley MA, Reas DL, et al. Assessing worry in older adults: confirmatory factor analysis of the Penn State Worry Questionnaire and psychometric properties of an abbreviated model. *Psychol Assess.* 2003;15:173–183.
19. Weissman MM, Myers JK, Tischler GL, et al. Psychiatric disorders (DSM-III) and cognitive impairment among the elderly in a US urban community. *Acta Psychiatr Scand.* 1985;71:366–379.
20. Regier DA, Boyd JH, Burke JD, et al. One-month prevalence of mental disorders in the United States. *Arch Gen Psychiatry.* 1988;45:977–986.
21. Bland RC, Newman SC, Orn H. Prevalence of psychiatric disorders in Edmonton. *Acta Psychiatr Scand.* 1988;77:57–63.
22. Myers JK, Weissman MM, Tischler GL, et al. Six-month prevalence of psychiatric disorders in three communities. *Arch Gen Psychiatry.* 1984;41:959–967.
23. Fredrikson M, Annas P, Fischer H, Wik G. Gender and age differences in the prevalence of specific fears and phobias. *Behav Res Ther.* 1996;34:33–39.
24. Anthony MM, Brown TA, Barlow DH. Heterogeneity among specific phobia types in DSM-IV. *Behav Res Ther.* 1997;35: 1089–1100.
25. Lindesay J. Phobic disorders in the elderly. *Br J Psychiatry.* 1991;159:531–541.
26. Sheikh JI, Swales PJ, Carlson EB, Lindley SE. Aging and panic disorder: phenomenology, comorbidity, and risk factors. *Am J Geriatr Psychiatry.* 2004;12:102–109.
27. van Zelst WH, de Beurs E, Beekman ATF, Deeg DJH, van Dyck R. Prevalence and risk factors of posttraumatic stress disorder in older adults. *Psychother Psychosom.* 2003;72: 333–342.
28. Davidson JR, Hughes D, Blazer DG, George LK. Post-traumatic stress disorder in the community: an epidemiological study. *Psychol Med.* 1991;21:713–721.
29. Norris FH. Epidemiology of trauma: frequency and impact of different potentially traumatic events on different demographic groups. *J Consult Clin Psychol.* 1992;60:409–418.
30. Goenjian AK, Najarian LM, Pynoos RS, et al. Posttraumatic stress disorder in elderly and younger adults after the 1988 earthquake in Armenia. *Am J Psychiatry.* 1994;151:895–901.
31. Ticehurst S, Webster RA, Carr VJ, Lewin TJ. The psychosocial impact of an earthquake on the elderly. *Int J Geriatr Psychiatry.* 1996;11:943–951.
32. Norris F, Murrell SA. Prior experiences as a moderator of disaster impact on anxiety symptoms in older adults. *Am J Community Psychol.* 1988;16:665–683.
33. Spiro A, Schnurr PP, Aldwin CM. Combat-related posttraumatic stress disorder symptoms in older men. *Psychol Aging.* 1994;9: 17–26.
34. Keane TM, Caddell JM, Taylor KL. Mississippi scale for combat-related posttraumatic stress disorder: three studies in reliability and validity. *J Consult Clin Psychol.* 1988;56:85–90.
35. Sutker PB, Allain AN, Winstead DK. Psychopathology and psychiatric diagnoses of World War II Pacific Theater prisoner of war survivors and combat veterans. *Am J Psychiatry.* 1993;150: 240–245.
36. Blake DD, Keane TM, Wine PR, Mora C, Taylor KL, Lyons JA. Prevalence of PTSD symptoms in combat veterans seeking medical treatment. *J Trauma Stress.* 1990;3:15–27.
37. Hermann N, Eryavec G. Posttraumatic stress disorder in institutionalized World War II veterans. *Am J Geriatr Psychiatry.* 1994;2:324–331.
38. Averill PM, Beck JG. Posttraumatic stress disorder in older adults: a conceptual review. *J Anxiety Disord.* 2000;14:133–156.
39. Yehuda R, Kahana B, Schmeidler J, Southwick SM, Wilson S, Giller EL. Impact of cumulative lifetime trauma and recent stress on current posttraumatic stress disorder symptoms in Holocaust survivors. *Am J Psychiatry.* 1995;152:1815–1818.
40. Davidson JRT, Kudler HS, Saunders WB, Smith RD. Symptom and comorbidity patterns in World War II and Vietnam veterans with posttraumatic stress disorder. *Compr Psychiatry.* 1990;31: 162–170.
41. Fontana A, Rosenheck R. Traumatic war stressors and psychiatric symptoms among World War II, Korean, and Vietnam War veterans. *Psychol Aging.* 1994;9:27–33.
42. Derogatic LR, Lipman RS, Covi L. SCL 90: an outpatient psychiatric rating scale—preliminary report. Psychopharmacol Bull 1973;9:13–27.
43. Hyer L, Summers MN, Braswell L, Boyd S. Posttraumatic stress disorder: silent problem among older combat veterans. *Psychotherapy.* 1995;32:348–364.
44. Hilton C. Media triggers of post-traumatic stress disorder 50 years after the Second World War. *Int J Geriatr Psychiatry.* 1997;12:862–867.
45. Kaup BA, Ruskin PE, Nyman G. Significant life events and PTSD in elderly World War II veterans. *Am J Geriatr Psychiatry.* 1994;2:239–243.

46. Macleod AD. The reactivation of post-traumatic stress disorder in later life. *Aust NZ J Psychiatry.* 1994;28:625–634.

47. Hamilton JD, Workman RH. Persistence of combat-related post-traumatic stress symptoms for 75 years. *J Trauma Stress.* 1998;11: 763–768.

48. Johnson D. A series of cases of dementia presenting with PTSD symptoms in World War II combat veterans. *J Am Geriatr Soc.* 2000;48:70–72.

49. Cook JM, Cassidy EL, Ruzek JI. Aging combat veterans in long-term care. *NC-PTSD Clinical Quarterly.* 2001;10:26–30.

50. Port CL, Engdahl B, Frazier P. A longitudinal and retrospective study of PTSD among older prisoners of war. *Am J Psychiatry.* 2001;158:1474–1479.

51. Zeiss RA, Dickman HR. PTSD 40 years later: incidence and person-situation correlates in former POWs. *J Clin Psychol.* 1989;45:80–87.

52. Kuch K, Cox BJ. Symptoms of PTSD in 124 survivors of the Holocaust. *Am J Psychiatry.* 1992;149:337–340.

53. Yehuda R, Elkin A, Binder-Brynes K, et al. Dissociation in aging Holocaust survivors. *Am J Psychiatry.* 1996;153:935–940.

54. Yehuda R, Kahana B, Southwick SM, Giller EL Jr. Depressive features in Holocaust survivors with post-traumatic stress disorder. *J Trauma Stress.* 1994;7:699–704.

55. Yehuda R, Steiner A, Kahana B, et al. Alexithymia in Holocaust survivors with and without PTSD. *J Trauma Stress.* 1997;10:93–100.

56. Goldstein G, van Kammen W, Shelly C, Miller DJ, van Kammen DP. Survivors of imprisonment in the Pacific theater during World War II. *Am J Psychiatry.* 1987;144:1210–1213.

57. Eberly RE, Engdahl BE. Prevalence of somatic and psychiatric disorders among former prisoners of war. *Hosp Community Psychiatry.* 1991;42:807–813.

58. Elder GH Jr, Shanahan MJ, Clipp EC. Linking combat and physical health: the legacy of World War II in men's lives. *Am J Psychiatry.* 1997;154:330–336.

59. Lee KA, Vaillant GE, Torrey WC, Elder GH. A 50-year prospective study of the psychological sequelae of World War II combat. *Am J Psychiatry.* 1995;152:516–522.

60. Lipton MI, Schaffer WR. Physical symptoms related to post-traumatic stress disorder (PTSD) in an aging population. *Mil Med.* 1988;153:316–318.

61. Schnurr PP, Spiro A III. Combat exposure, posttraumatic stress disorder symptoms, and health behaviors as predictors of self-reported physical health in older veterans. *J Nerv Ment Dis.* 1999;187:353–359.

62. Falk B, Hersen M, van Hasselt VB. Assessment of post-traumatic stress disorder in older adults: a critical review. *Clin Psychol Rev.* 1994;14:383–415.

63. Gray MJ, Acierno R. Symptom presentations of older adult crime victims: description of a clinical sample. *J Anxiety Disord.* 2002;16:299–309.

64. Kessler RC, Nelson CB, McGonagle KA, Lie J, Swartz M, Blazer DG. Comorbidity of DSM-III-R major depressive disorder in the general population: results from the US National Comorbidity Survey. *Br J Psychiatry.* 1996;168:17–30.

65. Beekman ATF, de Beurs E, van Balkom AJLM, Deeg DJH, van Dyck R, van Tilburg W. Anxiety and depression in later life: co-occurrence and communality of risk factors. *Am J Psychiatry.* 2000;157:89–95.

66. Lenze EJ, Mulsant BH, Shear MK, et al. Comorbid anxiety disorders in depressed elderly patients. *Am J Psychiatry.* 2000;157: 722–728.

67. Casten RJ, Parmelee PA, Kleban MH, Lawton MP, Katz IR. The relationships among anxiety, depression, and pain in a geriatric institutionalized sample. *Pain.* 1995;61:271–276.

68. Smith SL, Colenda CC, Espeland MA. Factors determining the level of anxiety state in geriatric primary care patients in a community dwelling. *Psychosomatics.* 1994;35:50–58.

69. Cummings JL, Mega M, Gray K, et al. The neuropsychiatric inventory: comprehensive assessment of psychopathology in dementia. *Neurology.* 1994;44:2308–2314.

70. Porter VR, Buxton WG, Fairbanks LA, et al. Frequency and characteristics of anxiety among patients with Alzheimer's disease and related dementias. *J Neuropsychiatry Clin Neurosci.* 2003;15:180–186.

71. Chemerinski E, Petracca G, Manes F, Leiguarda R, Starkstein SE. Prevalence and correlates of anxiety in Alzheimer's disease. *Depress Anxiety.* 1998;7:166–170.

72. Hamilton M. The assessment of anxiety states by rating. *Br J Med Psychol.* 1959;32:50–55.

73. Spielberger C, Gorsuch R, Lushene R. *STAI Manual for the State-Trait Anxiety Inventory.* Palo Alto, CA: Consulting Psychologists Press; 1970.

74. Beck AT, Epstein N, Brown G, Steer A. An inventory for measuring clinical anxiety: psychometric properties. *J Consult Clin Psychol.* 1988;56:893–897.

75. Wetherell JL, Arean PA. Psychometric evaluation of the Beck Anxiety Inventory with older medical patients. *Psychol Assess.* 1997;9:136–144.

76. Kabacoff RI, Segal DL, Hersen M, van Hasselt VB. Psychometric properties and diagnostic utility of the Beck Anxiety Inventory and State-Trait Anxiety Inventory with older adult psychiatric outpatients. *J Anxiety Disord.* 1997;11:33–47.

77. Steer RA, Willman M, Kay PAJ, Beck AT. Differentiating elderly medical and psychiatric outpatients with the Beck Anxiety Inventory. *Assessment.* 1994;1:345–351.

78. Myer TJ, Miller ML, Metzger RL, Borkovec TD. Development and validation of the Penn State Worry Questionnaire. *Behav Res Ther.* 1990;28:487–495.

79. Wisocki PA, Handen B, Morse CK. The Worry Scale as a measure of anxiety among homebound and community active elderly. *The Behavior Therapist.* 1986;5:91–95.

80. Marks IM, Mathews AM. Brief standardization self-rating for phobic patients. *Beh Res Ther.* 1979;17:263–267.

81. Sanavio E. Obsessions and compulsions: the Padua inventory. *Behav Res Ther.* 1988;26:169–177.

82. Horowitz M, Wilner N, Alvarez W. Impact of Events Scale: a measure of subjective distress. *Psychosom Med.* 1979;41:209–218.

83. Blake DD, Weathers F, Nagy LM, et al. A clinician rating scale for assessing clinical and lifetime PTSD: the CAPS-1. *The Behavior Therapist.* 1990;13:187–188.

84. Engdahl BE, Eberly RE, Blake JD. Assessment of posttraumatic stress disorder in World War II veterans. *Psychol Assess.* 1996;8:445–459.

85. Hyer L, Summers MN, Boyd S, Litaker M, Boudewyns P. Assessment of older combat veterans with the Clinician-Administered PTSD Scale. *J Trauma Stress.* 1996;9:587–593.

86. Summers MN, Hyer L, Boyd S, Boudewyns PA. Diagnosis of late-life PTSD among elderly combat veterans. *J Clin Geropsych.* 1996;2:103–115.

87. Broadhead WE, Leon AC, Weissman MM, et al. Development and validation of the SDDS-PC screen for multiple mental disorders in primary care. *Arch Fam Med.* 1995;4:211–219.

88. Spitzer RL, Williams JBW, Kroenke K, et al. Utility of a new procedure for diagnosing mental disorders in primary care: the PRIME-MD 1000 study. *JAMA.* 1994;272:1749–1756.

89. Valenstein M, Kales H, Mellow A, et al. Psychiatric diagnosis and intervention in older and younger patients in a primary care clinic: effect of a screening and diagnostic instrument. *J Am Geriatr Soc.* 1998;46:1499–1505.

90. Katz IR, Reynolds CF, Alexopoulos GS, Hackett D. Venlafaxine ER as a treatment for generalized anxiety disorder in older adults: pooled analysis of five randomized placebo-controlled clinical trials. *J Am Geriatr Soc.* 2002;50:18–25.

91. Sheikh JI, Lauderdale SA, Cassidy EL. Efficacy of sertraline for panic disorder in older adults: a preliminary open-label trial. *Am J Geriatr Psychiatry.* 2004;12:230.

92. Boyer W. Serotonin uptake inhibitors are superior to imipramine and alprazolam in alleviating panic attacks: a meta-analysis. *Int Clin Psychopharmacol.* 1995;10:45–49.

93. Coplan JD, Pine DS, Papp LA, Gorman JM. An algorithm-oriented treatment approach for panic disorder. *Psychiatr Ann.* 1996;26:192–201.

94. Oehrberg S, Christiansen PE, Behnke K, et al. Paroxetine in the treatment of panic disorder: a randomized, double-blind, placebo-controlled study. *Br J Psychiatry.* 1995;167:374–379.

95. Otto MW, Tuby KS, Gould RA, McLean RYS, Pollack MH. An effect size-analysis of the relative efficacy and tolerability of

serontonin selective reuptake inhibitors for panic disorder. *Am J Psychiatry.* 2001;158:1989–1992.

96. Greist J, Chouinard G, DuBoff E, et al. Double-blind parallel comparison of three doses of sertraline and placebo in outpatients with obsessive-compulsive disorder. *Arch Gen Psychiatry.* 1996;52:289–295.

97. Jenike MA, Baer L, Minichiello WE, Rausch SL, Buttolph ML. Placebo-controlled trial of fluoxetine and phenelzine for obsessive-compulsive disorder. *Am J Psychiatry.* 1997;154:1261–1264.

98. McDougle CJ, Goodman WK, Leckman JF, Barr LC, Heninger GR, Price LH. The efficacy of fluvoxamine in obsessive compulsive disorder: effects of comorbid chronic tic disorder. *J Clin Psychopharmacol.* 1993;13:354–358.

99. Tollefson GD, Rampey AH, Potvin JH, et al. A multicenter investigation of fixed-dose fluoxetine in the treatment of obsessive-compulsive disorder. *Arch Gen Psychiatry.* 1994;51:559–567.

100. Zohar J, Judge R. Paroxetine versus clomipramine in the treatment of obsessive-compulsive disorder. *Br J Psychiatry.* 1996;169:468–474.

101. Koran LM, Hackett E, Rubin A, Wolkow R, Robinson D. Efficacy of sertraline in the long-term treatment of obsessive-compulsive disorder. *Am J Psychiatry.* 2002;159:88–95.

102. Hoehn-Saric R, Ninan P, Black DW, et al. Multicenter double-blind comparison of sertraline and desipramine for concurrent obsessive-compulsive and major depressive disorders. *Arch Gen Psychiatry.* 2000;57:76–82.

103. Pollack MH, Zainelli R, Goddard A, et al. Paroxetine in the treatment generalized anxiety disorder: results of a placebo-controlled, flexible dosage trial. *J Clin Psychiatry.* 2001;62:350–357.

104. Brady K, Pearlstein T, Asnis GM, et al. Efficacy and safety of sertraline treatment of posttraumatic stress disorder: a randomized controlled trial. *JAMA.* 2000;283:1837–1844.

105. Davidson J, Pearlstein T, Longborg P, et al. Efficacy of sertraline in preventing relapse of posttraumatic stress disorder: results of a 28-week double-blind, placebo-controlled study. *Am J Psychiatry.* 2001;158:1974–1981.

106. Marshall RD, Beebe KL, Oldham M, Zaninelli R. Efficacy and safety of paroxetine treatment for chronic PTSD: a fixed-dose, placebo-controlled study. *Am J Psychiatry.* 2001;158:1982–1988.

107. Connor KM, Sutherland SM, Tupler LA, Malik ML, Davidson JRT. Fluoxetine in post-traumatic stress disorder: randomised, double-blind study. *Br J Psychiatry.* 1999;175:17–22.

108. Geracioti TD. Venlafaxine treatment of panic disorder: a case series. *J Clin Psychiatry.* 1995;56:408–410.

109. Rickels K, Pollack MH, Sheehan DV, Haskins JT. Efficacy of extended-release venlafaxine in nondepressed outpatients with generalized anxiety disorder. *Am J Psychiatry.* 2000;157:968–974.

110. Katz IR, Reynolds CF, Alexopoulos GS, Hackett D. Venlafaxine ER as a treatment for generalized anxiety disorder in older adults: pooled analysis of five randomized placebo-controlled clinical trials. *J Am Geriatr Soc.* 2002;50:18–25.

111. Allgulander C, Hackett D, Salinas E. Venlafaxine extended release (ER) in the treatment of generalised anxiety disorder: twenty-four week placebo-controlled dose-ranging study. *Br J Psychiatry.* 2001;179:15–22.

112. Gelenberg AJ, Lydiard RB, Rudolph RL, Aguiar L, Haskins JT, Salinas E. Efficacy of venlafaxine extended-release capsules in non-depressed outpatients with generalized anxiety disorder: a 6-month randomized controlled trial. *JAMA.* 2000;283:3082–3088.

113. Conner KM, Davidson JRT, Weisler RH. A pilot study of mirtazepine in posttraumatic stress disorder. In: *Scientific Abstracts of the 37th Annual Meeting of the American College of Neuropsychopharmacology.* December 14–18, 1998; Las Croabas, Puerto Rico.

114. Davis LL, Nugent AL, Murray J, Kramer GL, Petty F. Nefazodone treatment for chronic posttraumatic stress disorder: an open trial. *J Clin Psychopharmacol.* 2000;20:159–164.

115. Fawcett J, Marcus RN, Anton SF, O'Brien K, Schwiderski U. Response of anxiety and agitation symptoms during nefazodone treatment of major depression. *J Clin Psychiatry.* 1995;56(suppl 6):37–42.

116. Rickels K, Weisman K, Norstad N, et al. Buspirone and diazepam in anxiety: a controlled study. *J Clin Psychiatry.* 1982;43:81–86.

117. Rickels K, Schweizer EE. Current pharmacotherapy of anxiety and panic. In: Meltzer HA, ed. *Psychopharmacology: The Third Generation of Progress.* New York: Raven Press; 1987:1–14.

118. Rickels K, Schweizer EE, Csanalosi I, Case WG, Chung H. Long-term treatment of anxiety and risk of withdrawal: prospective comparison of clorazepate and buspirone. *Arch Gen Psychiatry.* 1988;45:444–450.

119. Smiley A, Moskowitz H. Effects of long-term administration of buspirone and diazepam on driver steering control. *Am J Med.* 1986;80:22–29.

120. Boehm C, Robinson DS, Gammens RE. Buspirone therapy for elderly patients with anxiety or depressive neurosis. *J Clin Psychiatry.* 1990;51:309.

121. Napoliello MJ. An interim multicenter report on 677 anxious geriatric outpatients treated with buspirone. *Brit J Clin Prac.* 1986;40:71–73.

122. Hemels ME, Lanctot KL, Iskedjian M, Einarson TT. Clinical and economic factors in the treatment of behavioural and psychological symptoms of dementia. *Drugs Aging.* 2001;18:527–550.

123. Kindermann SS, Dolder CR, Bailey A, Katz IR, Jeste DV. Pharmacological treatment of psychosis and agitation in elderly patients with dementia: four decades of experience. *Drugs Aging.* 2002;19:257–276.

124. Mintzer J, Faison W, Street JS, Sutton VK, Breier A. Olanzapine in the treatment of anxiety symptoms due to Alzheimer's disease: a post hoc analysis. *Int J Geriatr Psychiatry.* 2001;16:S71–S77.

125. Gould RA, Otto MW, Pollack MH, Yap L. Cognitive behavioral and pharmacological treatment of generalized anxiety disorder: a preliminary meta-analysis. *Behavior Therapy.* 1997;28:285–305.

126. Nordhus IH, Pallesen S. Psychological treatment of late-life anxiety: an empirical review. *J Consult Clin Psychol.* 2003;71:643–651.

127. Scogin F, McElreath L. Efficacy of psychosocial treatments for geriatric depression: a quantitative review. *J Consult Clin Psychol.* 1994;62:69–74.

128. Barlow DH, Lehman CL. Advances in the psychosocial treatment of anxiety disorders: implications for national health care. *Arch Gen Psychiatry.* 1996;53:727–735.

129. DeRubeis RJ, Crits-Christoph P. Empirically supported individual and group psychological treatments for adult mental disorders. *J Consult Clin Psychol.* 1998;66:37–52.

130. Swales PJ, Solfvin JF, Sheikh JI. Cognitive-behavioral therapy in older panic disorder patients. *Am J Geriatr Psychiatry.* 1996;4:46–60.

131. Barrowclough C, King P, Colville J, Russell E, Burns A, Tarrier N. A randomized trial of the effectiveness of cognitive-behavioral therapy and supportive counseling for anxiety symptoms in older adults. *J Consult Clin Psychol.* 2001;69:756–762.

132. Barlow DH, Cerny JA. *Psychological Treatment of Panic.* New York: Guilford; 1988.

133. Craske MG, Barlow, DH. Panic disorder and agoraphobia. In: Barlow DH, ed. *Clinical Handbook of Psychological Disorders.* 3rd ed. New York: Guilford; 2001:1–59.

134. Stanley MA, Beck JG, Glassco JD. Treatment of generalized anxiety in older adults: a preliminary comparison of cognitive-behavioral and supportive approaches. *Behavior Therapy.* 1996;27:565–581.

135. Wetherell JL, Gatz M, Craske MG. Treatment of generalized anxiety disorder in older adults. *J Consult Clin Psychol.* 2003;71:31–40.

136. Stanley MA, Beck JG, Novy DM, et al. Cognitive-behavioral treatment of late-life generalized anxiety disorder. *J Consult Clin Psychol.* 2003;71:309–319.

137. Borkovec TD, Costello E. Efficacy of applied relaxation and cognitive-behavioral therapy in the treatment of generalized anxiety disorder. *J Consult Clin Psychol.* 1993;61:611–619.

138. Craske MG, Barlow DH, O'Leary TA. *Mastery of Your Anxiety and Worry.* New York: Graywind; 1992.

139. Sheikh J, Salzman C. Anxiety in the elderly: course and treatment. *Psychiatr Clin North Am.* 1995;18:871–883.

140. Beck JG, Stanley MA. Anxiety disorders in the elderly: the emerging role of behavior therapy. *Behavior Therapy.* 1997;28:83–100.

141. Mohlman J, Gorenstein EE, Kleber M, de Jesus M, Gorman JM, Papp L. Standard and enhanced cognitive-behavioral therapy for

late-life generalized anxiety disorder: two pilot investigations. *Am J Geriatr Psychiatry.* 2003;11:24–32.

142. Roy-Byrne PP, Katon W. Anxiety management in the medical setting: rationale, barriers to diagnosis and treatment, and proposed solutions. In: Mostofsky DI, Barlow DH, eds. *The Management of Stress and Anxiety in Medical Disorders.* Boston: Allyn and Bacon; 2000:1–14.

143. Katon W, von Korff M, Lin E, et al. Collaborative management to achieve treatment guideline: impact on depression in primary care. *JAMA.* 1995;273:1026–1031.

144. Unutzer J, Katon W, Callahan CM, et al. Collaborative care management of late-life depression in primary care setting: a randomized control trial. *JAMA.* 2002;288:2836–2845.

145. Roy-Byrne PP, Katon W, Cowley DS, Russo J. A randomized effectiveness trial of collaborative care for patients with panic disorder in primary care. *Arch Gen Psychiatry.* 2001;58:869–876.

146. Stanley MA, Hopko DR, Diefenbach GJ, Bourland SL, Rodriguez H, Wagener P. Cognitive-behavior therapy for late-life generalized anxiety disorder in primary care. *Am J Geriatr Psychiatry.* 2003;11:92–96.

Personality Disorders in Late Life

31

Richard A. Zweig   Marc E. Agronin

Despite decades of clinical and empirical inquiry, consensus regarding the core manifestations, etiology, clinical course, and treatment of personality disorders (PDs) remains elusive. Yet clinicians are aware that this group of patients, to which we attach our most pejorative labels (e.g., *hateful, manipulative, help-rejecting, toxic*) remain among our most difficult to diagnose and treat. Because of the complexity of PDs and the rudimentary state of our diagnostic and intervention methods, clinicians vaguely speak of a patient's axis II problem or render the diagnosis invisible (1) through indefinite deferral of diagnosis. Persisting recognition of the continued relevance of PDs to clinical practice as well as trends toward evidence-based treatment have led to the development of a PD-specific practice guideline (2). While inherently flawed by an insufficient database and a lack of clinical consensus regarding borderline PD, such guidelines represent an effort to provide recommendations to practitioners when evidence is slim (3).

For older adults suffering from PD, clinical guidelines regarding assessment, management, and intervention are no less needed or compelling (4). Personality disordered older adults often present with a bewildering array of problems including polymorphous psychiatric symptoms, vague physical complaints, ill-managed medical problems, cognitive "soft-signs," and interpersonal/familial conflict, all of which may be superimposed upon personality pathology. Geriatric mental health clinicians face the usual challenge of sorting out various components of the presenting problem (5), and the added challenge of using assessment and treatment technologies with uncertain applicability for older adults. Given the nascent state of the literature in this area, this chapter will draw upon empirical studies of PDs in

adults and older adults, provide a descriptive phenomenology of PDs in late life, and use diverse theoretical perspectives to propose diagnostic and treatment guidelines for intervention.

ASSESSMENT AND DIAGNOSIS

Definition

Efforts to define criteria for PDs are complicated by the heterogeneity, conceptual fuzziness, and sociocultural relativity of the construct. Recent iterations of the *Diagnostic and Statistical Manual of Mental Disorders* (DSM) improve conceptual clarity by differentiating personality traits from disorders (6,7). Personality traits are defined as "enduring patterns of perceiving, relating to, and thinking about the environment and oneself . . . exhibited in a wide range of social and personal contexts. It is only when personality traits are inflexible and maladaptive and cause either significant functional impairment or subjective distress that they constitute personality disorders" (6).

A more recent general definition of PD in the DSM emphasizes both core criteria and the sociocultural relativity of the construct, defining a PD as "an enduring pattern of inner experience and behavior that deviates markedly from the expectations of an individual's culture" (8). General diagnostic criteria for PD propose that these deviant experiences and behaviors are evident in at least two of four putative domains (cognition, affectivity, interpersonal functioning, and impulse control) (8). In accord with earlier definitions, PD experiences and behaviors must be demonstrated to be inflexible, maladaptive, and pervasive, and not as a result of Axis I or physical disorders.

The DSM-IV-TR provides prototypal criteria sets for 10 PD types, and groups them into three higher-order clusters:

- Cluster A: Odd/eccentric (schizoid, schizotypal, and paranoid)
- Cluster B: Dramatic/emotional (histrionic, borderline, narcissistic, and antisocial)
- Cluster C: Anxious/fearful (dependent, avoidant, and obsessive-compulsive)
- NOS: A category of PD, *not otherwise specified* (NOS) may also be employed to describe individuals who meet criteria for a provisional PDs type (e.g., passive-aggressive PD, depressive PD) or who meet general diagnostic criteria for PDs but do not meet criteria for a specific PD.

Application of General Diagnostic Criteria

The general diagnostic criteria for PD require that maladaptive behaviors and experiences be differentiated from those attributable to clinical state, situational context, or cultural role. These usual suspects invalidate or confound a diagnosis of PD, but may be difficult to fully evaluate in clinical practice. Acute states such as mood disorder can mimic PD features (9), and this is no less true for personality disordered elderly (10). Clinicians are advised to avoid a definitive Axis II diagnosis until comorbid Axis I disorders are maximally treated (11). Similarly, clinicians must ascertain that a patient's purported maladaptive behavior or experience is inflexibly displayed across varied settings and is truly deviant within the patient's cultural/ethnic or other reference group. For example, suspiciousness regarding the motives of authority figures may be normative in some cultures. Ruling out potential confounds thus requires culturally informed careful assessments of mood as well as personality, evaluation of the patient's temporal relationship, use of professional and familial informants regarding historically dysfunctional behaviors, and longitudinal assessment during treatment to provide a definitive PD diagnosis (12). Such guidelines reduce the likelihood of false-positive errors in detecting PDs, support aggressive treatment efforts for PD patients with comorbid axis I conditions, and are necessary given the cultural relativity of PDs. However, in a health care environment that is rapidly paced, resource thin, and reimbursement driven, clinicians have formidable obstacles to overcome when diagnosing PDs.

Assessment technologies ranging from self-report measures to semistructured interviews provide increasingly sophisticated methods to assist clinicians in the diagnosis of adults with PDs; to date, however, no clear gold standard exists (13). Structured interviews for PDs are more reliable than unstructured clinical interviews (14), and self-report measures assist in differentiating personality traits from mood states (12). However, measures of PDs remain limited by several factors related to the complexity of the phenomenon:

- Self-report data are hampered by patient nonrecognition of ego dystonic behaviors and traits.

- Interview-based data remain vulnerable to clinician judgments regarding traits/behaviors that fluctuate in the context of acute mood states.
- Most measures do not fully capture the longitudinal history of deviant experiences/behaviors or current dysfunctional interpersonal patterns (15).

On a broader level, results of interview-based and self-report methods of PDs are often discordant (16), a fact partly attributable to the diverging conceptual models (categorical versus dimensional) upon which each is based.

In regard to practice implications, it may be helpful for clinicians to think categorically and dimensionally to reach an empirically based diagnosis of a PD. Livesley proposes a two-step diagnostic process, based on current DSM nosology, which attempts to combine categorical and dimensional assessment (17). As a first step, the general diagnostic criteria for PD provide a categorical method to differentiate PDs from other mental disorders and from normal variations in personality manifested in various roles and contexts. In the second diagnostic step, specific PD criteria sets are assessed dimensionally, using the techniques outlined above, to describe individual differences in personality.

In the context of geriatric diagnostic assessment, how is a clinician to differentiate normal from dysfunctional traits and behaviors? Are DSM-IV-TR PD criteria sets valid for the elderly (7)? Does what is known of the natural history of PDs shed light on these questions? Perhaps due to the scarcity of empirical data, the DSM-IV-TR is less than clear in describing the longitudinal course of PD. By definition, PDs are enduring and pervasive maladaptive and deviant experiences and behaviors. Although the pervasiveness criterion requires that maladaptive personality features and patterns of functioning be evident by early adulthood, the current definition allows for the possibility of exacerbation of PDs in later life "following the loss of significant supportive persons (e.g., a spouse) or previously stabilizing social situations (e.g., a job)" (7). Furthermore, because "some types of personality disorder (notably antisocial and borderline PDs) tend to become less evident or to remit with age," the possibility of PD attenuation is suggested (7). Current definitions thus endeavor to describe PD as both a static and dynamic construct that may present in stable or emergent/residual forms over the life course (7,18). A geriatric clinician might reasonably conclude that pervasiveness is a relevant but insufficient criterion upon which to base a PD diagnosis for older adults. To assess for personality dysfunction in older adults, consideration must first be given to empirical findings regarding the relationship of personality and aging.

Obstacles to Diagnosis

The paucity of research regarding PDs and aging, and an underappreciation of the relevance of studies of normal personality and aging, has resulted in a trend among some geriatric mental health clinicians to be guided more by opinion and myth rather than science (Table 31-1). These

TABLE 31-1

MYTHS AND OBSTACLES TO PERSONALITY DISORDER DIAGNOSIS IN OLDER ADULTS

Myths regarding normal personality and aging:
- *Downward drift* stereotypes
- *Brittle adaptation* viewed as normative
- *Developmental stagnation* viewed as normative

Clinician-related factors that may impede detection of PD in elderly:
- Assumption that PD is rare in late life
- Difficulty distinguishing Axis II disorders from other medical/psychiatric disorders, especially if Axis I disorder is chronic

Challenges related to DSM criteria and assessment methods:
- DSM criteria fail to capture age-related manifestations of PD
- Unclear applicability of impaired social/occupational functioning criterion
- Uncertain reliability, validity, and utility of assessment instruments designed for younger adults
- Uncertain reliability of longitudinal histories provided by patient/informant

DSM, *Diagnostic and Statistical Manual of Mental Disorders*. PD, personality disorder.
Adapted from References 19 and 27.

myths then negatively affect diagnostic decision making and treatment planning, with particularly adverse consequences for personality disordered elderly.

What is the effect of aging on individuals with normal or adaptive personality traits? Some clinicians mistakenly endorse a *downward drift* theory of personality and aging, believing that most older adults become more dependent, stubborn, hypochondriacal, or regressive and child-like in their behavior. Hence, personality features are presumed to become more maladaptive with age. Such ageist stereotypes are sharply refuted by empirical evidence (19). Several longitudinal studies have found substantive stability of basic personality traits with age (20), and found no evidence of age-related increases in specific maladaptive traits such as hypochondriasis (21).

Other clinicians mistakenly endorse a *brittle adaptation* theory, in which age-associated physical frailty is believed to coincide with increased frailty of the personality, resulting in a marginal adaptation to life circumstances. Gutmann has similarly described the *camel's back* theory in which clinicians presume that the volume of psychosocial stressors common in late life overwhelms the frail older patient and results in psychopathology (22). Again, empirical evidence suggests otherwise; for example, in reaction to natural disasters and trauma, older adults exhibit comparable or lower rates of subsequent posttraumatic stress disorder (PTSD) than younger adults, and premorbid functioning clearly appears more predictive than age (23). One might speculate that a subgroup of older adults who are marginally adaptive always "walked with a limp" as a result

of long-standing PD, and may be more prone to develop pathology, even in response to objectively mild stressors.

Finally, some view the personality-related behaviors and coping styles of older adults as increasingly rigid and inflexible, as if endorsing a *developmental stagnation* theory of aging. The elderly are perceived as too old to change (a phrase sometimes echoed by pessimistic older adults themselves), unable to harness any positive developmental trends, and devoid of any inclination toward modifying coping styles or personal development. However, empirical research suggests normative positive developmental changes in late life, including improved cognitive complexity and self-regulation of affect (24,25), and finds that modifiable traits such as perceived self-efficacy exert a salutary effect on maintaining functioning in late life (26).

Why do these myths persist? Myths that associate age with maladaptive personality changes may persist due to the well-known tendency of clinicians to attribute an illusory correlation (in this case, between age and maladaptive personality) to unrelated characteristics present in select populations. In addition, myths regarding older adults' brittle adaptation or developmental stagnation may arise from clinicians' well-known tendency to confuse age with disease (in this case, PD) and draw spurious conclusions about all older adults.

In addition to clinicians' persisting myths, other clinician-related factors may affect detection of PDs in older adults. Perhaps due to beliefs that PDs burn out with age (27), or biases based on institutionalized samples with disproportionate rates of dementia (28), some clinicians assume that PDs are rare in older adults, despite growing evidence to the contrary (29–31). Furthermore, as mentioned earlier, PD detection in the elderly is often obfuscated by multiple comorbid Axis I conditions and amplified functional impairment (32), complicating the process of differential diagnosis. These and other clinician-related factors, including concerns regarding stigmatizing the patient, counter-transferential avoidance, and the uncertain heuristic value of the diagnosis (19) all likely result in underdetection of PDs in older adult clinical samples.

Other obstacles and challenges to diagnosis arise from the uncertain applicability of DSM criteria and assessment methods for personality disordered elderly. First, many have raised concerns about the possible age bias of DSM criteria for selected PDs, arguing that the behavioral manifestations of PD change in later life (19,27,33,34). Sadavoy and Fogel cogently describe that "as the changes that accompany old age begin to impinge, the individual's behavioral responses become less reliable measures of personality (i.e., internal) processes or disorder" (18). This represents a formidable obstacle for clinicians, because diagnostic reliability often hinges on observable behavioral manifestations of PD rather than inferences about internal processes. It is therefore unclear whether DSM criteria accurately capture the phenomenology of PDs in older adults or, for that matter, whether manifestations of PDs in the elderly are affected by cohort (35). Second, Segal et al. note that normative age-related changes in occupational and social roles require clinicians to recalibrate estimations of impaired role functioning before diagnosing elders with PDs (27). Third, as mentioned earlier, assessing for the pervasiveness of PDs in older adults requires clinicians to gather longitudinal histories of uncertain veracity, whether obtained from patients or ancillary sources (19,36). Finally, while technologies for assessing PDs in younger adults have become more varied (categorical or dimensional, self-report or interviewer-rated) and rigorous (37,38), many have not been normalized or validated for use with older adult samples (27), and their clinical utility remains untested.

In clinical practice, the persistence of myths regarding personality and aging may skew clinicians' understanding of what is normative, resulting in providers' underestimation of older adults' personality resiliency and a spurious view of aberrant traits as normative in late life. This mistaken understanding likely results in underdetection of PDs in the elderly, or a misattribution of the relationship between Axis I and Axis II disorders. Furthermore, conceptual challenges and limitations of our diagnostic technologies may leave even the most experienced clinicians frustrated and uncertain of their findings. While these obstacles appear daunting, they call for an empirically informed approach, using extant data regarding prevalence rates and the natural history of PDs to guide the application of criteria sets for use with the elderly.

EPIDEMIOLOGY

Clinical diagnostic assessment begins with an understanding of a disorder's epidemiology, characteristic features, and natural history. What is known regarding the overall prevalence rate of PDs in older adults? Are PDs more or less common in the elderly than in younger adults? A recent meta-analysis and a review of prevalence studies of both nonclinical and clinical populations (30,39) suggests an overall PD prevalence rate of 10% in adults over age 50, which does not differ significantly from younger adults. The authors caution that definitive conclusions are precluded by differences in methodology across various studies. Studies of nonclinical elderly samples find prevalence rates of any PD ranging from 6% to 13% (29,39,40), an estimate that appears comparable to the 9% to 13.5% rate found in studies of mixed-age samples (15,41). The National Epidemiologic Survey, which assessed seven PD types in a mixed-age nonclinical sample, found lower prevalence rates for specific PDs in elderly compared to younger groups, and an overall prevalence rate of 15% for "any PD" in the sample (31). Rates for specific PDs among the elderly ranged from 0.3% to 5.2%, whereas rates for younger adults ranged from 0.4% to 9%. Of note, age differences in prevalence rates seem to vary by PD type, in that age differences in prevalence rates are most marked for borderline, antisocial, and schizotypal PDs when evaluated in cross-sectional studies (17).

Not surprisingly, clinical samples of depressed elderly have notably higher rates (24–67%) of PDs (28,42,43) especially when assessed with self-report diagnostic techniques, in the context of depression, or in outpatient psychiatric settings (30). These rates again appear comparable to those obtained (36–65%) in younger-adult depressed samples (44). In depressed or anxious elderly samples, cluster C PDs or mixed/NOS types appear prevalent (29).

What clinical implications may be drawn regarding PD prevalence rates in late life? First, since extant epidemiologic data suggest relatively high rates of PDs in the elderly (possibly comparable to that in younger adults), routine screening of depressed elderly for PDs is warranted. Second, because sizable proportions of treatment-seeking older adults appear to manifest comorbid PDs, clinicians should consider listing "rule-out" Axis II diagnoses more frequently. Third, existing base rates of PD, while preliminary, can inform diagnostic decision making and treatment planning.

WHAT IS THE NATURAL HISTORY OF PERSONALITY DISORDERS?

While this issue is critical in order to evaluate the longitudinal stability of patients' PD traits, the definitive answer to this basic question is currently unknown, owing to differing definitions of *personality* and *personality disorder* and the rarity of longitudinal studies. Over the lifecycle, the course of PD could follow multiple potential trajectories for different individuals (19,29). This complex question might best be addressed by posing several related questions for which there are data:

- Do individuals with early manifestations of maladjusted personality improve with age?
- Might fluctuations or quantitative changes in PD severity (attenuated or exacerbated forms) occur over the life span, as suggested by DSM-IV-TR?
- Is age associated with qualitative changes in the phenotypic expression of PD?

With respect to the question of age-associated improvement in PD, clinical observational studies suggest a maturation effect, particularly for cluster B PDs (45,46). However, empirical studies present mixed findings. Longitudinal studies using self-report personality measures find that people with high neuroticism (a trait purportedly related to PD) tend to remain maladjusted throughout their lives (47,48). Long-term follow-up studies using categorical PD diagnoses find general consistency of traits and diagnoses over time (49). Yet, cross-sectional retrospective chart review studies often find fewer cluster B PD diagnoses (50) but possibly more cluster C PD diagnoses (51) in older compared to younger patient groups, and epidemiologic studies note lower prevalence rates of antisocial PD with advancing age (52). Longitudinal follow-up studies (ranging 2–16 years) of young adults with borderline or antisocial PD find fewer patients meeting criteria for a categorical diagnosis over time, but all patients manifesting persisting impairments in social functioning (53). These seemingly contradictory findings may be partly because of age at index evaluation, since normal maturational changes in personality often occur through the third decade of life (54).

If maturational changes in personality (and PD) are possible, might they be manifested quantitatively (PD severity), qualitatively (PD trait expression), or in both ways? Some clinicians propose that older adults experience a quantitative attenuation or exacerbation of PD manifestations (residual or emergent subtypes) mediated by age-associated changes in neurotransmitter functioning (29) or psychosocial and life circumstances (18,22). Again, in the absence of longitudinal studies following personality disordered adults into late life, no conclusions can be drawn. Cross-sectional studies, for example, of dimensional scores of histrionic and antisocial PD traits, find lower trait scores for middle-aged than for younger groups (55). Furthermore, cross-sectional studies of dimensional personality traits find trends toward age-related decreases in impulsivity and activity and increased conscientiousness (18,36,40) in both nonclinical (56) and clinical samples (57). Overall, studies of quantitative changes in PD-related traits suggest that attenuation or exacerbation is possible, but whether this represents a true age effect or a cohort effect (58) remains unknown.

With regard to age-associated qualitative changes in the expression of PD traits, some clinicians have proposed that the manifestations of PD may shift in late life, while underlying dispositions persist (18,19,36,40). Such heterotypic continuity (59) occurs frequently in complex psychological phenomena. Several clinicians have noted that DSM Axis II criteria sets fail to capture problem behaviors manifested in late life (18,19,36) and may result in disproportionate diagnoses of PD NOS (60). With regard to borderline PD, for example, case series reports and cross-sectional studies find less impulsivity, but possibly more somatization, when comparing older and younger patients with borderline PD (61–63). This is congruent with subjective reports of older adults with cluster B PDs, who often acknowledge that their levels of impulsivity and affective dyscontrol have diminished over their lifetime.

Hence, while the natural history of PDs throughout the lifecycle is unknown, preliminary evidence suggests the potential for maturational, quantitative, and qualitative changes. Most likely, taxonomies of PD related to temperament (64), basic tendencies (65), or underlying personality structure display substantial stability, whereas characteristic adaptations or the behavioral expressions of PD are less consistent over the lifespan (10).

DIFFERENTIAL DIAGNOSIS

By definition, a diagnosis of PD requires that long-standing maladaptive experiences and behaviors do not represent aspects of an Axis I disorder. However, given the frequent comorbidity of Axis I and Axis II disorders, their complex and uncertain etiologic relationship, and practical difficulties differentiating personality traits from persisting mood states, distinguishing between the two can present a formidable challenge. Furthermore, the behavioral features of some neurocognitive syndromes (e.g., impulse dyscontrol) and other medical disorders can mimic manifestations of PD. Since psychiatric, medical, and cognitive disorders are relatively prevalent in treatment-seeking older adults with Axis II disorders, a strategy of sorting out rather than ruling out (5) seems warranted.

Several diagnostic challenges seem particularly common in efforts to differentiate PD pathology from other psychiatric or physical disorders (Table 31-2). Some older adults present with chronic unremitting Axis I disorders (e.g., mood and anxiety disorders) and severe functional impairment. Clinicians may confuse a chronic treatment-refractory Axis I disorder, and the hopelessness and exhaustion this engenders in patients, families, and care providers, with an "untreatable" Axis II disorder. In elderly patients with persisting severe depression and comorbid Axis II pathology, manifestations of the PD may overshadow Axis I symptoms.

CASE EXAMPLE

Mrs. P is an 83-year-old woman recently admitted to a nursing home and referred for psychiatric evaluation due to her irritable mood, demanding and verbally abusive behavior toward staff, and poor motivation for rehabilitative activities. She acknowledges feeling depressed and anxious throughout much of her life, but received some symptom relief from combined pharmacotherapy and psychotherapy in the past. Recent physical impairment prompted her nursing home placement and forced reliance on others, which she experienced as deeply humiliating, and frayed her already estranged relations with her children.

She currently presents with symptoms of recurrent major depression and panic disorder, for which she receives subtherapeutic doses of a selective serotonin-reuptake inhibitor (SSRI), and with evidence of a narcissistic PD. When it was suggested that she suffers from a treatable mood and anxiety disorder, staff members disagreed. Angered by her verbally abusive behavior, they viewed her long-standing mood symptoms as yet another form of manipulation due to her personality, and expressed a fear that more aggressive pharmacotherapy and psychotherapy would only make things worse.

TABLE 31-2

DIFFERENTIAL DIAGNOSIS OF PERSONALITY DISORDER: CHALLENGES AND STRATEGIES

Diagnostic Challenge	Diagnostic Strategy
Detecting Axis II disorders in elderly with complex array of medical, psychiatric, psychosocial, and behavioral problems	General strategies: Use multimethod approach including structured interview, self-report assessment, and longitudinal data from multiple informants. Begin with DSM-IV-TR general diagnostic criteria for PD. Use specific PD criteria sets flexibly to allow for age-associated changes. Avoid use of Axis II as a diagnosis of exclusion.
Distinguishing Axis II from persisting axis I condition (e.g., depressive PD versus unremitting dysthymia)	Evaluate historical temporal relationship of objective/behavioral manifestations of each disorder. Maximize treatment of Axis I condition and reevaluate.
Distinguishing Axis II from personality change due to a medical condition or behavioral sequelae of a mild neuropsychiatric syndrome (e.g., borderline PD versus early frontal-temporal dementia)	Identify cognitive manifestations of neurocognitive syndrome using neuropsychological techniques. Evaluate temporal relationship of behavioral manifestations of each potential disorder.
Distinguishing Axis II from moderate-severe neurocognitive impairment with nonvolitional disturbed behavior (e.g., antisocial PD versus moderate dementia with impulse dyscontrol)	Evaluate medical or environmental etiologies for problem behavior. Evaluate capacity for volitional maladaptive behavior.
Distinguishing Axis II from chronic regressive behavior arising in the context of persisting physical illness or changes in the psychosocial environment (e.g., dependent PD versus "sick role" behavior following physical illness onset)	Evaluate historical temporal relationship of persisting physical illness or psychosocial environment changes and onset of regressive behavior. Evaluate functional significance of "sick role" behavior.

DSM-IV-TR, *Diagnostic and Statistical Manual of Mental Disorders*. 4th Ed. Text Revision; PD, personality disorder.
Adapted from References 19 and 36.

Some older adults present with the behavioral features of early neurocognitive syndromes, whose manifestations can mimic symptoms of PD. Symptoms that seem to represent an amplification of premorbid behaviors can be particularly confusing to family members.

CASE EXAMPLE

Mrs. S is a 79-year-old married woman and mother of three sons seen in a psychiatric outpatient clinic. She suffered from recurrent depressive episodes since her 30s, some severe enough to warrant hospitalization and treatment with electroconvulsive therapy (ECT). She experienced chronic depression and increasingly frequent hospitalization over the past 10 years, with only modest benefit from antidepressants or ECT. She exhibited no focal neurological signs, and achieved a Mini-Mental State Examination score of 26/30.

In the past 8 years Mrs. S had become notorious among various treatment providers for her increasingly attention-seeking, frustration-intolerant, and rejection-sensitive behavior. For example, she would speak in a plaintive tone, moan at regular intervals, request help with simple tasks, become enraged in response to perceived rejection by others, and express vague suspicious that others were lying to her. Her relationship with her husband had recently become stormy, characterized by her anger at his need for time away during the day. Her husband endorsed the treatment team's provisional diagnosis of recurrent depression and mixed PD with borderline and dependent features.

However, closer inquiry revealed that other relevant information had been overlooked. She had been college educated and enjoyed a brief but successful work career. She had been married for over 55 years and had stable and supportive relations with her husband and adult children prior to the last 10 years. With the help of old medical records, it was learned that she had been diagnosed with a "frontal lobe blood clot" at about that time. A subsequent magnetic resonance image found "focal atrophy in the right frontal region of unclear etiology," and a neuropsychological evaluation found significant impairments of verbal and visual memory, initiation, and executive functioning. The revision of Mrs. S's working diagnoses led to more realistic treatment goals and modified interventions for her and her family.

Behavioral sequelae of this type are appropriately diagnosed as personality change due to a medical disorder, rather than as PD. When presenting at a severity level of mild cognitive impairment, or with a static or slowly progressing course, the persisting behavioral symptoms of these disorders may appear prominent and the underlying neurocognitive disorder may go undetected. Sadavoy and Fogel (18) suggest that dysfunction in three neuroanatomical areas can result in behavioral syndromes that amplify underlying personality traits:

- Orbital frontal lobe dysfunction, associated with Alzheimer's disease (AD) and frontotemporal dementia, resulting in reduced empathy and disinhibition
- Dorsolateral frontal lobe dysfunction, associated with AD and frontotemporal dementias as well as Parkinson's disease and long-term neuroleptic use, producing impaired initiation, planning, and social awareness
- Parietal and temporal lobe dysfunction, associated with AD and vascular dementias, producing misperception of sensory stimuli and of the emotional content of speech

A third diagnostic challenge arises when some health care providers encounter maladaptive behavior in elderly with moderate-severe dementia, and spuriously attribute behaviors of uncertain etiology to personality, as if PD were a diagnosis of exclusion.

CASE EXAMPLE

Mrs. W, an 89-year-old female nursing home resident with moderate-severe dementia, is rarely communicative but described by nursing staff as having recently become agitated and bulimic. When staff approach her to assist with dressing, she repeatedly yells, "Help me!" and tries to strike them. Following staff assistance with feeding, she often vomits her food, and on several occasions has been observed to place her finger in her mouth prior to vomiting.

A medical record review revealed a history of gastric reflux and esophageal strictures, but no recent gastrointestinal consultation or treatment. Staff view her agitation and vomiting as volitional and due to her personality, and attribute it to Mrs. W's anger at her sister, who has been expressing concerns to the staff about the patient's disheveled appearance and recent weight loss.

In noncommunicative elderly with severe dementia, the extent to which personality governs behavior is ambiguous. Observed inconsistencies in behavior and functioning, even in the context of objectively reduced competence, provide fertile ground for care providers to view maladaptive behaviors as volitional and ascribe them to the patient's personality. This may represent another manifestation of the fundamental attribution error well known to social psychologists, in which ambiguous interpersonal events are ascribed to dispositional rather than environmental (or biological) factors.

A fourth diagnostic challenge arises when an older patient displays regressive behavior that emerges in the context of persisting physical disability or other marked changes in the individual's psychosocial environment. While such maladaptive behavior could be a manifestation

of an underlying PD that has become exacerbated, it may also represent a situational adaptation that arose in the context of a less-than-optimal environment. For example, passive and dependent behaviors in elderly with disabling physical illness are often unintentionally reinforced by caregivers in institutional settings (66).

Recommendations for Assessment and Diagnosis

Based on available evidence regarding the prevalence and natural history of PDs, and the specific challenges of evaluating PDs in the elderly, the following diagnostic assessment strategies are recommended:

- Given estimates of the base rate for PDs in late life, screening for PDs in clinical samples is warranted.
- Given possible age and cohort effects affecting the validity of criteria for PD types and the uncertain reliability of PD categorical thresholds (67), diagnostic screening for PDs in older adults should use general criteria for PDs (DSM-IV-TR) as an initial step.
- Manifestations of PDs may be sorted out from the effects of persisting Axis I mood disorders through careful historical assessment of both, using validated assessment methods and maximal treatment of the Axis I disorder.
- Manifestations of PDs in late life may be differentiated from personality change due to a medical condition through comprehensive neurocognitive evaluation, historical assessment of the temporal relationship between cognitive symptoms and personality manifestations, and a review of medical antecedents to problem behaviors.
- PDs may be differentiated from behaviors arising in specific contexts, situations, or roles through a careful evaluation of the temporal relationship between the niche-changing situational context and PD-related behaviors, as well as assessment of the functional significance of role behavior within the individuals' cohort, culture, and environment.

In general, definitive diagnosis of specific PD types requires a multimethod approach that ideally includes:

- Dimensional ratings of personality and functional impairment, based on self-report measures
- Categorical ratings based on structured interviews
- Longitudinal data based on informant reports, clinical records, or serial assessments by multidisciplinary staff

PD should not be employed as a diagnosis of exclusion. However, to maximize diagnostic sensitivity and specificity in older clinical populations, dimensional and categorical measures that adhere closely to DSM-IV-TR PD criteria may need to be interpreted more flexibly to account for the possible age/cohort bias of DSM criteria. Hence, diagnostic assessment of PDs must be informed by an understanding of both age-normative and of maladaptive age-deviant experiences and behaviors that characterize PDs in late life (19).

PERSONALITY DISORDERS IN LATE LIFE: A DESCRIPTIVE PHENOMENOLOGY

The core features of PDs may be described as "the failure to solve life tasks related to the establishment of stable and integrated representations of self and others; the capacity for intimacy, attachment, and affiliation; and the capacity for prosocial behavior and cooperative relationships. In essence, it involves chronic interpersonal problems and self pathology" (17). How might these features manifest in the context of the developmental tasks of late life? Knight (35) has proposed that psychological problems of older adults be evaluated by considering the individual's cohort, environmental context, and maturational or developmental stage, as well as current situational challenges. Similarly, an understanding of the normative challenges and developmental processes of late life informs an evaluation of PDs in this age group.

Aging is associated with a myriad of normative stressors and developmental transitions (10,68,69). Older adults normatively experience numerous direct challenges to the self-system, including age-associated physical changes (e.g., in appearance, perception, strength, and sexual functioning) and cognitive changes (e.g., in short-term memory, processing speed, and novel problem solving). Such challenges threaten the self-system with a sense of reduced competence and self-efficacy, activate existential concerns, and may narrow coping options and prompt an increased reliance on a cocreated sustaining environment (or psychosocial niche [22]) to maintain a sense of identity and self-continuity. Yet the psychosocial niche of the elderly also undergoes change; psychosocial challenges common to late life (e.g., retirement, familial and spousal loss, debilitating illness in self or others) force a series of role losses or transitions to new roles within work, family, and social environments. For most elderly, such stressful events are variably experienced as a threat/loss or a challenge/ opportunity for personal development. Most elderly adapt well to these age-normative developmental challenges (70), and modify their characteristic adaptation (e.g., by developing more interdependent relationships within their families, or by recognizing the new potentials that accompany loss and transition) to account for changes in their self-system and psychosocial niche. Yet for older adults with PDs, whose chronic interpersonal problems and self pathology are often accompanied by more narrow or inflexible coping styles (71), such normative developmental stressors are the psychosocial equivalent of infectious disease in an immunocompromised individual (22), and thus may prompt psychopathology.

In addition to the normative stressors described above, older adults experience normative developmental changes in how they manage their social and emotional well being. One such normative developmental change is *socioemotional selectivity*, a process that describes older adults' tendencies toward more selective engagement in familiar, close, interpersonal relationships in order to optimize energy expenditure and maximize positive emotional experiences. A growing body of literature supports the universality of this adaptive developmental process in older adulthood (72). How might such a process affect elders with PDs? Due to their long-standing difficulties managing close interpersonal relationships and rigid coping styles, older adults with PDs would likely experience developmental trends toward socioemotional selectivity as a double-edged sword; some may experience an unwanted sense of forced intimacy and come to experience relationships as emotional traps rather than as potential sources of support (68).

Emotion and aging research suggests a second normative developmental trend that may ameliorate features of PD in late life. In cross-sectional studies, older adults show greater cognitive complexity and self-regulation of affect, and more flexible reasoning when faced with emotion-laden dilemmas when compared with younger adults (24,25,73). A growing body of research finds that older adults "exercise greater control of affective arousal by acting proactively to avoid conflict or the escalation of conflict ... show greater affective control, greater avoidance of stressors, engage in less negative start-up with partners, and de-emphasize the negative in interpersonal relations" (25). For personality disordered elderly, such trends would be consistent with aforementioned findings of positive maturational effects and beneficial changes in traits such as impulsivity and conscientiousness. In sum, normative stressors and developmental processes may modify differential aspects of personality functioning, possibly contributing to changes in the expression of PD traits in later life. While these developmental processes may color the phenomenology of PD in late life, we are not aware of empirical studies seeking to investigate this question.

Findings from the clinical and developmental gerontology research described earlier may inform and broaden our notions of domains of functional impairment commonly observed in individuals with PDs, and assist in deriving a descriptive phenomenology of PDs in late life (19,29,68). Any such phenomenology presumes more continuity than change in core features of PDs over the lifecycle, but broadens functional impairment indicators to underscore differences in the behavioral manifestations of PD in older adults. Congruent with the DSM-IV-TR general diagnostic criteria for a PD (7), this phenomenology may be broadly described in terms of dysfunction in cognitive, affective, interpersonal, and impulse-control domains (Table 31-3; more detailed descriptions of individual PDs appear in Table 31-6).

This phenomenology largely reflects cross-sectional research findings and clinical observations of PDs in treatment-seeking depressed older adults. As such, its susceptibility to cohort effects and clinician and selection biases is unknown, and must await further empirical confirmation. In routine clinical practice, evaluation of the psychosocial

TABLE 31-3

PERSONALITY DISORDERS IN LATE LIFE: MANIFESTATIONS OF DYSFUNCTION IN VARIOUS DOMAINS

Domain of Dysfunction	Phenomenology in Adults	Phenomenology in Elderly
Cognitive	■ Unstable or distorted representations of self, others, or environment ■ Impaired relationship to reality (depersonalization, body image distortion, idealization/devaluation, mini-psychoses) ■ Distorted representations of self resulting in identity disturbance in select PD types (e.g., borderline)	■ Distorted representations/schemas exacerbated by age-associated changes in executive functioning, memory/learning, processing speed ■ Difficulties in self-monitoring of affect and behavior, linking past and present or cause and effect, accurate recall of emotion-laden experiences, organizing experience to plan action ■ Failure of self-cohesion rather than identity; difficulty integrating disparate self experiences results in heightened interpersonal sensitivity, denial of areas of reduced competence, pseudo self-sufficiency
Affective	■ Difficulty modulating affect, manifesting as tendencies toward mood dysregulation (e.g., anxiety proneness, rage, panic, suspiciousness, emptiness) or affective inhibition ■ Marked affective constriction, or transient intense affective experience, often following personal or interpersonal stressors	■ Developmental improvement in affect modulation manifested in reduced affective intensity and lability (e.g., rage, panic) but continued difficulty modulating anxiety, suspiciousness, anger ■ Less extreme affective experience in response to personal and interpersonal stressors ■ Increased somatic expression of affective distress
Interpersonal	■ Difficulty forming and maintaining close relationships, regulating intimacy, resolving interpersonal conflict; deficient social skills ■ In cluster B PDs: Behaviors that push others' limits (controlling/inflexible, manipulative/exploitive, critical/argumentative) ■ In cluster B PDs: Behaviors that push therapist/system limits (e.g., nonattentive, noncollaborative, noncompliant behaviors)	■ Developmental trend toward socioemotional selectivity results in fewer, but more emotionally salient relationships, and further challenges marginal interpersonal functioning ■ Continued manifestation of behaviors that push limits of significant others and health care providers ■ Interpersonal dysfunction most manifest in maladaptive response to normative stressors such as loss, role transition, familial conflict, interpersonal context of physical illness/disability, and reduced competence
Impulse control	■ Maladaptive impulse dyscontrol manifesting in self-injurious behavior (e.g., self-mutilation), self-damaging behavior (e.g., sexual promiscuity, reckless sensation-seeking, substance abuse), and behaviors harmful to others (e.g., violent, unethical, or criminal acts)	■ Developmental trend toward reduced impulse dyscontrol, change in manifestations of self-injurious behavior (e.g., medical noncompliance, refusal of nutrition/hydration or self-care activities), self-damaging behavior (e.g., excessive or inappropriate use of health services, medication misuse/abuse, financial recklessness), and behavior harmful to others (e.g., noncompliance with local regulations/norms, abusive speech, domestic violence, abuse, or neglect)

PD, personality disorder.
Sources: References 10, 18, 19, 25, 36, 38, 40, 68, 72, and 88.

history may best be supplemented by empirical findings regarding demographic and clinical features associated with PDs across the lifespan.

A growing body of evidence suggests specific demographic and clinical features associated with PD in adults, in some cases replicated in older samples, which may represent the beginnings of an epidemiology of the disorder. For example, psychosocial histories of adults and older adults with PDs often reveal a higher preva-

lence of single/unmarried or separated/divorced marital status (74), several marriages but few children (40), and downward occupational change (47). The clinical histories of adults with PDs evidence a higher prevalence of sexual trauma or PTSD (75,76), early-onset Axis I disorders, comorbid substance abuse, suicide attempts (44,74), and mental health treatment (77). Related studies in older adults find PDs associated with a higher prevalence of early-onset depression (40,60), recurrent depression, comorbid anxiety disorder, past suicide attempts (28), and negative life events (43). While the association of lifetime trauma and PDs in older adults is not known, it has been tied to impaired health and functional status in older samples (78), suggesting its potential relevance. These empirical findings, when used in tandem with the descriptive phenomenology described earlier, may further assist in the detection and diagnosis of personality-disordered elderly.

TREATMENT STRATEGIES

While there is limited consensus as to the best treatment approaches for individuals with PDs, clinical and empirical research in the past three decades has provided a compelling rationale for treatment. The prevalence of PDs in the general population and its adverse impact on daily functioning has led some to suggest that PDs "constitute one of the most important sources of long-term impairment in both treated and untreated populations" (15). Standardized short-term treatments for Axis I disorders, whether using somatic or psychotherapeutic modalities, are generally weakened or impeded when applied to adults with Axis II disorders. For example, several studies find that depressed adults with PDs present with higher depression severity and experience poorer outcomes than those without PDs (44,79–82). Similarly, while depressed elderly without PDs respond well to standardized psychotherapeutic and/or somatic approaches (83,84), those with PDs experience increased depressive symptom severity, greater residual symptoms following standardized psychotherapeutic treatment (42,43,85), and persisting decreases in functioning and quality of life, even following remission of most depressive symptoms (32,86).

Growing awareness of the significance of PDs in adults has prompted the development and evaluation of more targeted treatment strategies. Evaluation of these treatments is complicated, however, by the multifaceted nature of PDs, which may be manifest in subjective symptoms, functional impairment, maladaptive behavioral and interpersonal patterns, and distressing inner experiences. Because most treatments cannot target all levels at once, and treatment difficulty varies across different levels, "conclusions about the effectiveness of treatment can vary considerably depending on the objective" (87). Yet, initial findings from recent treatment studies are encouraging. For example, aspects of borderline PD show sustained improvement following dialectical behavior therapy (88) or interpersonal group psychotherapy (89). Cluster C PD symptoms and social functioning improve following brief adaptational therapy (90) or cognitive-behavioral therapy (91). In general, the strongest treatment effects are achieved by studies using powerful combinations of modalities, such as psychotherapeutic and somatic treatments, individual and group therapy, and milieu or day-treatment approaches (87). Given preliminary empirical evidence of the targeted beneficial effects of diverse treatments, a growing consensus of clinicians believe the treatment of PDs merits a *common factors integrative approach* (17). Such an approach may provide broad guidelines for the management and treatment of personality-disordered elderly as well.

A Common Factors Approach to Treatment

A common factors integrative treatment approach begins with several general premises, based on extant empirical research, which provide a rationale for management and treatment strategies (3,17,87). First, given the wide range of potential treatment targets for individuals with PDs (e.g., symptoms, functional impairment, behavior patterns, internal personality structure), effective treatment strives to employ a combination of modalities tailored to individualized treatment goals. Hence, a common factors approach combines psychotherapeutic modalities (e.g., individual plus group therapy) and psychotherapeutic treatment techniques (e.g., psychodynamic and cognitive-behavioral) for maximal benefit. Second, as PDs are understood to have both genetic and psychosocial etiologies, a common factors approach uses both somatic and psychotherapeutic interventions and sets realistic treatment goals focused on maximizing adaptation and psychosocial competence. Hence, suitable treatment objectives may include promoting the adaptive expression of basic personality traits, promoting a cohesive self-system and integrated mental representations of others, and modifying maladaptive self-schema and dysfunctional interpersonal patterns. Third, as PD is understood to be tied to earlier experiences of psychosocial adversity that interact with a personality trait diathesis, the overall treatment approach strives to acknowledge and address the consequences of trauma for the patient (17).

A common factors approach provides a premise for management strategies in the elderly, for which there is substantial clinical consensus. The following section outlines strategies developed to treat PDs in adults that may be readily adapted for use with older adults.

Managing Crises and Ensuring Safety

Because patients with PDs are prone to experience impulsive behaviors involving harm to self and others, as well as overwhelming symptoms and psychosocial crises, ensuring patient safety and affect containment are foremost management goals. This may include therapist monitoring of suicidal or violent ideations/behaviors, therapist availability during periods of crisis, medication interventions, involvement of significant others to ensure a safe environment, and the application of therapeutic techniques directed toward crisis management and containment (17,92). Since depressed older adults' interpersonal context has been tied to subsequent suicidal behavior (93), and personality disordered elders exhibit high rates of past suicide attempts (28), ensuring patient safety also requires careful evaluation of the clinical history and the quality of the older adult's current interpersonal environment.

Establishing and Maintaining a Consistent Therapeutic Process

Adults with PDs are prone to experience distorted perceptions of self and others, and to engage in maladaptive interpersonal interactions and behaviors that may thwart the therapeutic process. Subsequently, appropriate management requires that all treatment team members vigilantly maintain a consistent therapeutic process. Elements of a consistent therapeutic process include:

- Clearly defined treatment goals and roles and responsibilities of patient and treatment team members
- Close coordination of treatment modalities (and team members)
- Clear identification of and adherence to treatment parameters (e.g., frequency and duration of treatment, and policies regarding confidentiality, consent, treatment attendance, and availability of treatment team or other resources during nontreatment hours)
- Provision of a consistently supportive and validating therapeutic stance (17,92)

Individuals with PDs tend to push the boundaries of the therapeutic process, and thus management of this tendency requires vigilance and consistent but nonpunitive limit setting by treating clinicians.

In older adults with PD, and especially those with mild cognitive impairment, a written behavioral contract may assist in this process (68). If formulated with a realistic appreciation of the patient's functional level and the treatment team's resources, this contract may specify the mutual expectations of the patient and team in regard to treatment goals and patient behavior, and the consequences of behavioral success or failure. In addition, personality-disordered elderly tend to be sensitive to the comings and goings of treatment personnel, and benefit from efforts to maximize staff continuity or to provide predictable notification of changes. Both of these approaches may also assist in coordinating the efforts of a treatment team represented by several disciplines in disparate settings.

Establishing and Maintaining a Collaborative Therapeutic Relationship

Given that dysfunctional interpersonal functioning is a hallmark of PDs, establishing and maintaining a collaborative relationship is arduous; when such an alliance is achieved, it is often tenuous and subject to ruptures. Yet consensus opinion suggests that the clinician's ability to manage the therapeutic alliance may be integral to the treatment's effectiveness. Livesley describes that a collaborative therapeutic relationship is achieved by interventions that establish and maintain therapist credibility, and that provide an experience of collaboration (17). For example, therapist credibility and optimism is conveyed through respect and acceptance, exploration of doubts and fears regarding treatment, summarizing and educating, collaborative goal-setting, and highlighting of all signs of progress in achieving goals. The experience of collaboration is fostered by a joint search for therapeutic understanding, references to a shared therapeutic history, and recognition of evidence of learning. Most importantly, it is fostered by a sensitive and nondefensive approach to detecting and repairing inevitable ruptures of the alliance (94). Clinicians from varied orientations agree that therapist empathy and validation, balanced with recognition of the patient's capacity and responsibility for change, are key ingredients in building a collaborative relationship (92).

Therapeutic Encirclement by the Treatment Team

Personality disordered adults are best treated by an interdisciplinary team of mental health professionals, rather than an individual clinician. Managing older adults with PDs often requires broadening the definition of the treatment team to include significant family members, primary care physicians, and other health care providers. Additionally, many personality-disordered elderly present with a fractured psychosocial niche, in that social and professional supports are limited or fragmented. Effective treatment of personality disordered elderly often requires *environmental splinting* (10) or the augmenting of traditional services with approaches to modify the psychosocial environment. Community social programs may be arranged to provide structured activity and social interaction; family and health care providers can be enlisted to ensure appropriate maintenance of physical health and safety; and home health aides or supported living environments may be required to improve the well being of low-functioning elders with PDs.

Effective management of older adults with PDs thus requires a primary mental health clinician to coordinate the efforts of an expanded treatment team and to assist the team in developing and maintaining a collaborative relationship with the patient. Of course, this strategy of direct involvement in the patient's interpersonal world must respect therapeutic boundaries of confidentiality, and must proceed with the awareness and consent of the patient (36). Achieving a cohesive team approach may require repeated contacts with family, health care, and social agency personnel, and the use of education and reframing to achieve a consensual working model of the patient's disorder, needs, and realistic capacities. This strategy of *therapeutic encirclement* (68) assists in containing affective instability and limiting maladaptive behavior patterns. However, given the propensity of personality-disordered patients to burn bridges in their relationships and leave a trail of angry and depleted caregivers behind, establishing a team of personnel who are willing to join together in pursuing treatment goals and strategies may itself be a gradual and effortful process.

Psychopharmacologic Strategies

As with any treatment modality for late-life PDs, the use of pharmacologic agents must be incorporated into a broader psychotherapeutic strategy based upon the best possible diagnostic formulation. This formulation will help the clinician avoid the pitfall of trying to cure the PD, but instead focus on three primary goals of pharmacotherapy:

1. Reduce the intensity and frequency of maladaptive behaviors
2. Avoid behavioral crises
3. Treat comorbid psychiatric disorders

Target symptoms vary based upon the PD or PD cluster, but typically include depressed or anxious moods, transient psychosis, and agitated or impulsive behaviors. In older individuals, there are unique considerations that must be factored into therapy, including the presence of comorbid medical illnesses, the role of cognitive impairment, the use of multiple medications, the effects of aging on drug metabolism, and late-life psychosocial issues that influence medication adherence. In all cases, it is important to obtain and document informed consent for the use of psychotropic medications, especially when there is a history of dementia, recent delirium, paranoia, or conflictual doctor–patient relationships.

The theoretical basis for the use of psychopharmacologic agents to treat PDs stems in part from two psychobiologic models that describe a relationship between certain personality traits and underlying neurotransmitter systems. Cloninger and colleagues (95,96) have described four dimensions of personality: novelty-seeking, harm avoidance, reward dependence, and persistence. They believe that empirical evidence points to the first three traits being mediated by respective neurotransmitter pathways containing dopamine, serotonin, and norepinephrine. A second model, proposed by Siever and Davis (97), is based upon four behavioral dimensions that they believe are mediated by monoamine pathways:

1. Cognitive-perceptual organization (impairment leads to symptoms of paranoia, transient psychosis, and perceptual distortions)
2. Affective regulation (accounts for symptoms of depression and anger)
3. Impulse control (underlies self-injurious and reckless behaviors)
4. Anxiety modulation

Each dimension is anchored in specific Axis I syndromes, with PDs representing less extreme forms of disturbance. At the other side of each dimension lie healthier defensive mechanisms and adaptive behaviors.

In terms of empirical support for the link between neurotransmitter pathways and personality traits, there is strong evidence linking serotonergic dysfunction to compulsive behaviors, impulsive aggression, and suicidality (98,99). Pharmacologic strategies that modulate monoamine activity would be expected, then, to alter corresponding trait vulnerabilities. In fact, the models just described are based, in part, on observations of how certain pharmacologic agents affect behavior. Soloff argues, however, that pharmacologic treatment cannot be reduced to a one-to-one correspondence between a specific medication with its target neurotransmitter and a single behavior or personality trait (100). Rather, it is the complex interaction among multiple neurotransmitters that gives rise to certain behaviors and traits, and pharmacologic strategies that fail to modulate these complex interactions are only modestly effective, at best. Soloff further notes that the use of pharmacologic agents with PDs is usually targeted at acute symptoms rather than long-standing traits.

There has been limited research of pharmacotherapy for PDs in adults, and no studies looking specifically at older individuals. Most studies in the literature have focused on three PDs: borderline, schizotypal, and antisocial (100–102). The majority of these studies looked at treatment for comorbid symptoms of anxiety, depression, or psychosis instead of treatment for specific maladaptive traits. Basic psychopharmacologic strategies are outlined in Table 31-4.

The problematic and disruptive behaviors seen with each PD often extend into the use of pharmacologic agent (112). Consider the following case examples.

TABLE 31-4
PHARMACOLOGIC STRATEGIES FOR LATE-LIFE PERSONALITY DISORDERS

Personality Disorder	Pharmacologic Strategies
Paranoid	Atypical antipsychotics may reduce transient psychosis and agitation. Antidepressants may target recurrent rage and aggression.
Schizoid	Anxiolytics and/or antidepressants may reduce excess avoidance or anxiety.
Schizotypal	Studies have shown both conventional and atypical antipsychotics to be useful in treating schizotypal PD, particularly psychotic symptom clusters (103–106). Antidepressants may play a beneficial role in reducing anxiety and depression seen in schizotypal PD (107,108).
Antisocial	Psychotropic medications shown to reduce aggressive, impulsive, and disinhibited behaviors seen in antisocial PD include antipsychotic agents (109), antidepressants (110), and mood stabilizers (lithium, divalproex, and carbamazepine). Comorbid substance abuse can interfere with psychotropic medications or increase the chances of medication-seeking behaviors, polypharmacy, or medication abuse (111).
Borderline	Psychopharmacologic treatment should be considered early on for symptom clusters of BPD such as depression, anxiety or panic, and impulsivity (112). Despite numerous studies, there is no single medication of choice, and little research to support the long-term efficacy of any agent (101,102,113). A variety of antidepressants have demonstrated efficacy in treating impulsive, aggressive, self-injurious, and depressive behaviors (113–118). SSRIs are usually first-line agents (119).
	Antipsychotic medications have been shown helpful for transient paranoia, impulsive aggression, agitation, and self-injurious behaviors (103), including clozapine (120,121), risperidone (122,123), olanzapine (124), quetiapine (125), and the combination of olanzapine and fluoxetine (126).
	Mood stabilizers such as divalproex sodium (127–129), carbamazepine (130), and lithium carbonate have reduced symptoms of anxiety and agitation.
Histrionic	There have been virtually no studies of pharmacologic treatment of HPD. One study found that patients with HPD had an increased number of hypochondriacal complaints, and that these complaints decreased after treatment with fluoxetine (131). It is not clear whether this decrease represented a true change in a personality trait (in this case a decreased tendency to focus on bodily symptoms) versus an improvement in more acute depressive symptoms, which in turn resulted in fewer somatic complaints. The study does suggest a role for SSRIs and perhaps other antidepressants for HPD.
Narcissistic	Consider the use of antidepressants or anxiolytics to reduce anger and depression.
Avoidant	Several antidepressants have been found to decrease avoidant behaviors (132). Antidepressants can also be used to treat comorbid major depression or anxiety disorders, in particular social phobia, which has shown significant overlap with avoidant PD (133,134).
Dependent	Consider anxiolytics or antidepressants to attenuate symptoms of anxiety and depression.
Obsessive-Compulsive	OC individuals might insist upon precise routines for scheduling, ingesting, and managing medication regimens. Clinicians need to provide sufficient detail without losing the focus of treatment. Antidepressants may reduce associated anger and depression, and possibly improve OC symptoms. However, SSRI antidepressants used to treat OCD have not been studied in OCPD.
Depressive	Antidepressants are the treatment of choice. Engaging depressive individuals in pharmacologic treatment might be challenged by their pessimistic and critical attitudes towards their prognosis and the efficacy of medications.
Passive-Aggressive	Avoid medications if patient is not fully compliant. No specific pharmacologic strategies have been developed.

BPD, borderline personality disorder; HPD, histrionic personality disorder; OC, obsessive-compulsive; OCD, obsessive-compulsive disorder; OCPD, obsessive-compulsive personality disorder; PD, personality disorder; SSRIs, selective serotonin-reuptake inhibitors.

CASE EXAMPLE

Side Effects and Noncompliance as an Expression of the Underlying PD

Mr. P had been treated sporadically by clinic psychiatrists for 20 years, and carried a diagnosis of PD with passive-aggressive and narcissistic traits. He always demonstrated the same pattern: he would demand a medication, and then return in several days or weeks complaining that the medication was "killing" him by causing terrible pain in the back of his head. He refused to continue taking the medication after several doses. Mr. P would then become fed up with his psychiatrist's failed attempts to treat him and request transfer to a new physician, who also tried and failed to find a satisfactory medication. On a regular basis, Mr P. complained to the clinic's director that the psychiatry staff was incompetent.

CASE EXAMPLE

Hazardous Use of Medications

Mr. M had a history of alcohol abuse, major depression, and PD with antisocial and narcissistic traits. Over the years he had managed to get himself on an antidepressant, two benzodiazepines (lorazepam for anxiety and temazepam for sleep), a narcotic analgesic for arthritic pain, and a muscle relaxant. Despite warnings from his psychiatrist, Mr. M continued to drink alcohol intermittently while on this medication regimen.

CASE EXAMPLE

Medications Used to Perpetuate PD Traits

Mrs. Y had a history of PD with obsessive-compulsive and dependent traits. She had been on a benzodiazepine for many years, but for unclear reasons. Her current psychiatrist had not prescribed the benzodiazepine initially, but was reluctant to discontinue it given Mrs. Y's protestations at every attempt of a taper. Mrs. Y spent most of the time during sessions with her psychiatrist discussing in great detail ways to alter the medication's dose and schedule to maximize several vaguely described benefits.

At the heart of each of these cases lie characteristic personality disturbances being expressed through maladaptive responses to pharmacotherapy. Mr. P never took any medication long enough to experience benefit, and his incessant complaints regarding side effects shielded him from talking about more substantive issues. Mr. M was clearly dependent on several psychotropics, and demonstrated an abusive and frankly hazardous pattern of medication use. Mrs. Y did not have a clearly established clinical need for her medication, but she relied on it to maintain a sense of dependency and control within the therapeutic relationship.

Some of the most common complications and forms of resistance to psychopharmacologic treatment are listed in Table 31-5. The table divides these problems into three areas: noncompliance, poor treatment relationships, and abuse of medications (112). On the basis of these issues, it may be prudent not to use medications as part of treatment. When concerns about medication use arise, the treating clinician must be prepared to discuss them with the patient and modulate treatment appropriately. Treatment failure is likely if the clinician does not recognize and intervene with these maladaptive behavioral patterns.

Psychotherapeutic Techniques

To evaluate and treat older adults with specific PDs, the generic management strategies described earlier must be aug-

---

TABLE 31-5

COMMON COMPLICATIONS AND FORMS OF RESISTANCE IN THE PHARMACOLOGIC TREATMENT OF PERSONALITY DISORDERS

Noncompliance with Medications
- Refusing to take medications
- Frequent forgetting of doses
- Experiences of repetitive, suspect, idiosyncratic, and/or inconsistent side effects that derail treatment
- Excessive or unrealistic fears of side effects
- Angry, belligerent responses to side effects

Poor Relationship with Prescribing Clinician
- Difficulty forming stable working relationship
- Distrust of clinician's intentions or recommendations
- Repetitive questions, complaints, or demands

Abuse of Medications
- Polypharmacy/abusive patterns of use
- Self-injurious or suicidal use of medications
- Unsupervised and/or unwarranted use of medications

---

mented by specific diagnostic approaches informed by the biopsychosocial factors influencing PD phenomena in late life. This may then form the basis for targeted psychotherapeutic techniques and pharmacologic treatment approaches for specific PD types. General descriptions of each PD along with management strategies are summarized in Table 31-6.

While there is substantial consensus regarding common factors management strategies, there is less consensus regarding specific techniques for modifying dysfunctional interpersonal patterns, promoting the adaptive expression of basic personality traits, or assisting patients to develop a cohesive self-system. Treatment models have been proposed for personality disordered elderly based on psychodynamic or cognitive-behavioral approaches used with younger adults (10,68,135–137).

An integrative approach to treating personality disordered elders builds upon psychodynamic and cognitive-behavioral techniques used in individual psychotherapy, and incorporates the necessary augmenting roles of pharmacotherapy, milieu and community programs, and a cohesive treatment team. The following case example illustrates some practical strategies based on an integrative approach employed in a hospital-based outpatient geriatric psychiatry setting.

CASE EXAMPLE

The Case of Mrs. L: Introduction

Mrs. L, a 72-year-old married woman and mother of two adult children, came to the psychiatric clinic seeking help for her cognitively impaired husband and her own attendant depression and anxiety. In her initial interview, she described that their 27-year marriage (her second) had been tumultuous and was characterized by marital infidelity, arguments escalating to bilateral domestic violence, and a mutually condoned flamboyant lifestyle that resulted in financial strain. She acknowledged a proneness to abandonment fears and depression since childhood, a sporadic academic and work history, an impulsive suicide attempt during young adulthood, and episodic substance abuse in the past, but she had never sought treatment. As a result of her husband's cognitive changes in the past 2 years, she stated that she no longer knew who he was. While acknowledging being informed that her husband's stroke had affected his memory and behavior, she was nonetheless unable to comprehend or tolerate his inability to recall their conversations, his dependent behavior and lack of initiative, and his emotional unresponsiveness to her. Overwhelmed with caregiving for her husband and frustrated by his unawareness of his behavioral changes or gratitude for her assistance, she perceived his neediness as volitional and manipulative and responded to his dependent behaviors by yelling, "You have dementia!" and threatening him with nursing home placement.

Mrs. L presented herself to clinic staff as acutely depressed, angry, and anxious, at once demanding of treatment for her husband and assistance for her, only to be suspicious or rejecting of recommendations. Her personality characteristics appeared consistent with a late-life manifestation of borderline PD. In a later conjoint session with her husband, when staff did not accede to her demand that her husband be told to stop behaving this way and instead recommended that Mrs. L alter her own approach, she became enraged, impulsively left the clinic, and threatened to seek treatment at another facility that would be more responsive to her needs.

Psychotherapeutic treatment with personality disordered older adults is initiated following a careful diagnostic evaluation of Axis I and Axis II disorders, and often occurs in combination with pharmacotherapy for Axis I symptoms (Table 31-6). The common factors management strategies outlined earlier serve as a general framework for organizing and coordinating the early stage of treatment. Hence, the initial phase begins with a focus on crisis management, ensuring patient safety, establishing a collaborative relationship, and therapeutic encirclement.

From an integrative perspective, the clinician's primary task during the initial phase is to carefully balance psychotherapeutic techniques that establish a collaborative relationship with those that treat symptoms and limit maladaptive behaviors (68). Older adults with PDs often present in the context of an Axis I disorder, and can benefit from empirically supported techniques to assist in regulating mood and managing symptoms. Cognitive behavioral techniques, such as pleasant-events scheduling, monitoring of automatic thoughts and mood, cognitive restructuring, relaxation training, and week-to-week goal setting may be particularly effective in containing depressive and anxiety symptoms. Psychodynamic techniques, such as labeling of affects, linking affects to maladaptive coping techniques or defenses, identifying focal interpersonal patterns, and facilitating self-observation are equally critical during this phase. Many personality-disordered older adults benefit from clinicians who provide an auxiliary source of executive functioning in assisting them to distinguish experiences of self versus others and past versus present, to recognize cause and effect relationships, and to organize experience to guide planned action. Pharmacologic approaches may assist in managing target symptoms and reducing the frequency of behavioral crises during this phase.

To foster a collaborative relationship, clinicians must initially validate the patient's subjective explanatory model of his or her problem, while independently assessing the objective realities of the patient's situation. To align with the patient's vantage point, particularly with patients who express distress somatically or through entitled behavior, clinicians must avoid directly challenging the patient's explanatory model during this initial phase. Concurrently, however, nonpunitive confrontation and limit setting is required for patients who evidence maladaptive coping styles or defenses that may be self-damaging or undermine treatment (e.g., acting on impulses rather than understanding uncomfortable affects). These maladaptive defenses are manifest in behaviors that typically seek to push the limits of the clinician or system, and understandably evoke strong counter-transference feelings (140). Hence, nonpunitive confrontation and limit setting requires clinicians to be aware of normative counter-transference feelings, avoid reflexively responding to provocative patient behavior, and to identify the maladaptive behavior and its consequences for the patient and the treatment enterprise (141).

CASE EXAMPLE

The Case of Mrs. L: Follow-Up

Mrs. L was contacted by phone and invited to discuss her concerns regarding her husband's care prior to finalizing her treatment decision. In a subsequent session, as she and the clinician reviewed and validated her experience of caregiving, difficulty comprehending her husband's behavior changes, and limited social supports and coping resources, Mrs. L's anger and anxiety began to diminish. She responded well to an initial treatment contract in which the treatment team assumed responsibility for evaluating and managing her husband's depression, cognitive impairment, and dependent behavior, in exchange for Mrs. L's agreement to maintain a safe environment, bring her husband for scheduled appointments, and initiate her own treatment to help alleviate her stress. Her initial treatment modalities included weekly individual psychotherapy (using psychodynamic and cognitive-behavioral techniques) and biweekly to monthly pharmacotherapy (SSRI and mood-stabilizing medications) visits.

TABLE 31-6

PERSONALITY DISORDER TYPES: DESCRIPTION, LIFECYCLE COURSE, AND MANAGEMENT APPROACHES

Type/Description	Lifecycle Course	Management in Elderly
Paranoid PD Pattern in which others are viewed with suspicion and distrust, prompting querulous, hyper-sensitive, hostile, accusatory, or guarded behavior.	Frequent occupational and marital/familial problems in middle age. Clinical reports suggest insidious decline in social functioning over lifecycle, proneness to transient agitation and psychosis, possible exacerbation in late life due to forced reliance on others.	Screen for psychosis, dementia. Psychotherapeutic interventions include empathizing with distressing affects, straightforward explanations, reframing anger due to situational factors as misdirected at others. Reframe antipsychotic medication as means to alleviate stress.
Schizoid/Schizotypal PD Pattern of social detachment and restricted range of emotions in interpersonal situations. Schizotypal PD characterized by discomfort and diminished capacity for intimate relationships as well as by cognitive/perceptual distortion and behavioral eccentricity.	Schizoid and schizotypal PD may persist with age. Possible decline in social functioning over lifecycle. Clinical reports suggest problems in late-life relationships with caregivers, increased risk for late-onset schizophrenia.	Screen for psychosis, dementia; respect need for interpersonal distance. Psychotherapeutic intervention to assist in compensating for interpersonal deficits. Consider antipsychotic medications.
Antisocial PD Pattern of disregard for social norms, manifested in unremorseful, reckless/aggressive, irresponsible, and deceitful behavior.	Cross-sectional and longitudinal data suggest decreasing prevalence over lifecycle but persisting social impairment and suicide risk. Clinical reports suggest less aggressive, impulsive, and criminal behavior, but persisting risk for depression and substance abuse.	Screen for substance abuse, mania/psychosis, impulse-control disorder, neurological impairment. Psychotherapeutic interventions focus on firm, nonpunitive limit setting, behavioral contracting. Monitor for suicide risk. Consider mood-stabilizing, antipsychotic, or antidepressant medications.
Borderline PD Pattern of unstable interpersonal relationships, self-image and affects, and significant impulsivity. Frequent states of crisis.	Longitudinal data suggest decreasing prevalence of major traits and improved occupational functioning over lifecycle, but persisting social impairment and suicide risk. Clinical reports suggest decreased impulsivity and self-injurious behavior, but persisting emotional lability and possible exacerbation in late life due to forced reliance on others.	Screen for neurological impairment, substance abuse, mania/psychosis. Psychotherapeutic interventions include consistent, cohesive team approach; firm limit setting regarding behavior harmful to others or self-damaging behavior; techniques to reduce mood dysregulation. Consider use of antidepressant, antipsychotic, and mood-stabilizing medications.
Histrionic PD Pattern of attention-seeking and excessive emotionality, manifested in transient but dramatic emotional displays, seductive and provocative behavior, naïve suggestibility, and impressionistic speech.	Clinical reports suggest cluster B PD types may "mature" with age. Clinical reports suggest age-associated changes in physical attributes may exert adverse impact, trends toward disinhibited or hypochondriacal behavior.	Screen for mania, intoxication, disinhibition associated with neurocognitive impairment. Psychotherapeutic interventions include appreciation of preserved physical attributes despite age, clarification of fears, warm support but firm limits on excessive neediness.
Narcissistic PD Pattern of excessive need for admiration, grandiose self-perception, and reduced empathy, manifested in self-important beliefs, arrogant or entitled behavior, and interpersonal exploitation.	Clinical reports suggest cluster B PD types may mature with age. Clinical reports suggest age-associated changes in physical or social/occupational status may exert adverse impact and prompt rage, suspiciousness, or depression, but also increase malleability of personality defenses and coping styles.	Screen for mania, personality change due to a medical illness or medication (e.g., steroid use) or neurocognitive impairment. Psychotherapeutic interventions include making patient an independent and equal partner in treatment. Assist in restoring aspects of former social/occupational status in new roles; validation regarding emotional needs but firm limit setting regarding unrealistic expectations for care.

(continued)

TABLE 31-6
(continued)

Type/Description	Lifecycle Course	Management in Elderly
Avoidant/Dependent PD Avoidant PD characterized by pattern of social inhibition, feelings of inadequacy, and hypersensitivity to negative evaluation. Dependent PD characterized by excessive need to be taken care of, with associated significant reliance on others for advice and decision-making, submissive behavior, and separation fears.	Cluster C often associated with comorbid mood or anxiety disorder in elderly. Clinical reports suggest cluster C PD types may persist through life course, may have special vulnerability to loss of significant others. Changes in functional or physical status (e.g., ambulation, early dementia) may exert adverse impact or give rise to avoidant or dependent behaviors.	Screen for persisting anxiety or mood disorder, situational "sick role" behavior due to perceived disability, or personality change due to a medical condition. Psychotherapeutic interventions include identifying reversible and irreversible areas of functional impairment, recommending rehabilitative or compensatory strategies, providing support for gradual exposure to feared situations, and pairing limit-setting regarding needy behavior with regular scheduling of brief clinical contacts. Consider use of antidepressant medications.
Obsessive-Compulsive PD Pattern of excessive need for orderliness and perfectionism at the expense of flexibility, openness, and efficiency.	Cluster C associated with comorbid depressive disorder in elderly. Clinical reports suggest cluster C PD types may persist through life course. Age-associated changes in role, environment, and cognitive or physical performance may be particularly stressful and increase vulnerability to mood/anxiety disorder and resistant and belligerent behavior.	Screen for persisting anxiety or mood disorder or neurocognitive impairment. Psychotherapeutic interventions include providing detailed explanations of treatment rationale, yielding control regarding treatment planning when feasible, but limit-setting regarding excessive demands on clinician time. Consider use of antidepressant and antianxiety medications.
Passive-Aggressive PD Pattern of negative attitudes and passive resistance to demands.	May be relatively common in late life, suggesting persistence of symptoms.	Screen for persisting anxiety or mood disorder. Psychotherapeutic interventions include validation of underlying anger and disappointment. Consider pharmacotherapy for comorbid anxiety or depression.
Depressive PD Pattern of depressive cognitions and behaviors.	Underreported in late life because typical presentation is submerged within comorbid Axis I depressive disorders.	Screen for persisting mood disorder. Psychotherapeutic interventions include cognitive behavioral schema-focused techniques. Consider antidepressants for acute symptoms.

PD, personality disorder.
Adapted from References 8, 29, 38, 45, 62, 68, 137, 138, and 139.

As symptoms and maladaptive behaviors are more contained and a collaborative relationship develops, personality disordered elders may benefit from therapeutic efforts to clarify and examine focal interpersonal patterns evidenced in their current relationships. Weissman and colleagues' (142) interpersonal psychotherapy model, adapted to address problems of personality-disordered adults and applicable to older adults, describes five areas of interpersonal difficulty:

- Managing familial interpersonal conflict
- Managing loss
- Managing role transition
- Managing interpersonal skills deficits
- Managing self-image disturbance, which in the elderly may manifest as difficulty adapting to functional deficits

and dependency needs in the context of physical or emotional illness/disability

Interpersonal and psychodynamic techniques, such as clarifying central patterns in interpersonal relationships, linking distressing affects to these patterns, and exploring ties between current interpersonal patterns and those evidenced in past relationships (as well as the doctor–patient relationship) may be of particular benefit during this phase. Interpersonal techniques that focus on addressing dysfunctional communication patterns, interpersonal conflicts, and difficulty engaging in role transitions because of unresolved prior experiences may help patients begin to contemplate more adaptive interpersonal patterns.

CASE EXAMPLE

The Case of Mrs. L: Treatment Course

Over the next several months, Mrs. L responded well to symptom-focused cognitive-behavioral techniques, such as activity scheduling, relaxation training, and modeling of communication skills, as well as symptom-focused psychodynamic techniques including clarifying recurrent interpersonal patterns in her relationships, identifying and linking current affects to maladaptive coping strategies, and facilitating self-observation. While she experienced episodic behavioral crises, at which time she would contemplate impulsively altering treatment parameters for herself or her husband, these became less frequent and responded to limit setting so as not to derail the treatment.

Initial treatment modalities were augmented by involving Mrs. L in a caregiver support group and in conjoint meetings with her adult children, and by frequently consulting (with mutual consent) with her husband's treatment team. Her children, with whom she previously had only limited contact, were enlisted to provide occasional caregiver respite when she became overwhelmed. The caregiver support group assisted Mrs. L to extend her resources for coping with her husband's behaviors. Her husband's treatment team collaborated by providing a neuropsychological evaluation of her husband that served to clarify his cognitive deficits, objectify the functional and behavioral changes that were expected given his mild vascular dementia, and initiate his referral to a structured day program that proved beneficial for them both.

After one year of treatment, while still manifesting social functioning impairments common to individuals with PDs, Mrs. L reported feeling less distressed by anxious and depressive symptoms and more accepting of her husband's illness.

In later phases of treatment, as gains with regard to containing symptoms and maladaptive behaviors are consolidated and dysfunctional interpersonal patterns are acknowledged, personality-disordered older adults may benefit most from interventions that directly address the self-system. Cognitive-behavioral techniques that identify and modify self-schema, address social skills deficits, and reinforce the adaptive expression of basic personality traits may be employed. Psychodynamic techniques that address fears and wishes that underlie dysfunctional interpersonal patterns, link these to historical experiences (e.g., trauma, family of origin issues), and promote integrated representations of self and others (e.g., through life review and facilitated mourning) may further augment this process. It is often during this phase, having achieved a greater sense of mastery over their symptoms and behaviors and broader options for interpersonal functioning, that patients may experience a greater sense of self-efficacy or psychosocial competence.

REFERENCES

1. Zimmerman M, Mattia J. Differences between clinical and research practices in diagnosing borderline personality disorder. *Am J Psychiatry*. 1999;156:1570–1574.
2. Oldham JM, Gabbard GO, Goin MK. Practice guideline for the treatment of patients with borderline personality disorder. *Am J Psychiatry*. 2001;158:1–52.
3. Paris J. Commentary on the American Psychiatric Association Guidelines for the treatment of borderline personality disorder: evidence-based psychiatry and the quality of the evidence. *J Personal Disord*. 2002;16(2):130–134.
4. Rosowsky E, Abrams RC, Zweig RA. *Personality Disorders in Older Adults: Emerging Issues in Diagnosis and Treatment*. Mahwah: Lawrence Erlbaum Assoc; 1999.
5. Kennedy G. *Geriatric Mental Health Care: A Treatment Guide for Health Professionals*. New York: Guilford Press; 2000.
6. American Psychiatric Association. *Diagnostic and Statistical Manual of Mental Disorders*. 3rd Ed. Revised. Washington: American Psychiatric Association; 1987.
7. American Psychiatric Association. *Diagnostic and Statistical Manual of Mental Disorders*. 4th Ed. Washington: American Psychiatric Association; 1994.
8. American Psychiatric Association. *Diagnostic and Statistical Manual of Mental Disorders*. 4th Ed. Text Revision. Washington: American Psychiatric Association; 2000.
9. Hirshfeld RM, Cross CK. The measurement of personality in depression. In: Marsella AJ, Hirshfeld R, Katz M, eds. *The Measurement of Depression*. New York: Guilford Press; 1987.
10. Sadavoy J. The effect of personality disorder on axis I disorders in the elderly. In: Duffy M, ed. *Handbook of Counseling and Psychotherapy with Older Adults*. New York: Wiley; 1999; 397–412.
11. Jacobsberg L, Goldsmith S, Widiger T, et al. Assessment of DSM-III personality disorders. In: Wetzler S, ed. *Measuring Mental Illness: Psychometric Assessment for Clinicians*. Washington: American Psychiatric Association; 1989;141–159.
12. Klein MH. Issues in the assessment of personality disorders. *J Personal Disord*. 1993;7(Suppl):18–33.
13. Pilkonis PA. Measurement issues relevant to personality disorders. In: Strupp HH, Horowitz LM, Lambert MJ, eds. *Measuring Patient Changes in Mood, Anxiety, and Personality Disorders*. Washington: American Psychological Association; 1997.
14. Frances AJ, Widiger TA. Personality disorders. In: Skodol AE, Spitzer RL, eds. *An Annotated Bibliography of DSM-III*. Washington: American Psychiatric Association; 1987;125–133.
15. Weissman M. The epidemiology of personality disorders: a 1990 update. *J Personal Disord*. 1993;7(Suppl):44–62.
16. Perry JC. Problems and considerations in the valid assessment of personality disorders. *Am J Psychiatry*. 1992;149(12): 1645–1653.
17. Livesley WJ. *Handbook of Personality Disorders: Theory, Research, and Treatment*. New York: Guilford; 2001.
18. Sadavoy J, Fogel B. Personality disorder in old age. In: Birren JE, Sloane B, Cohen GD, eds. *Handbook of Mental Health and Aging*. 2nd Ed. San Diego: Academic Press; 1992.
19. Agronin M, Maletta G. Personality disorders in late life: understanding and overcoming the gap in research. *Am J Geriatr Psychiatry*. 2000;8(1):4–18.
20. Costa PT, McCrae RR. Personality in adulthood: a six-year longitudinal study of self-reports and spouse ratings on the NEO Personality Inventory. *J Pers Soc Psychol*. 1988;54:853–863.
21. Costa PT, McCrae RR. Hypochondriasis, neuroticism, and aging: when are somatic complaints unfounded? *Am Psychologist*. 1985;40:19–28.
22. Gutmann D. Late onset pathogenesis: dynamic models. *Topics in Geriatric Rehabilitation*. 1988;3:1–8.
23. Averill PM, Beck JG. Post-traumatic stress disorder in older adults: a conceptual review. *J Anxiety Disord*. 2000;14(2): 133–156.
24. LaBouvie-Vief G, DeVoe M, Bulka D. Speaking about feelings: conceptions of emotion across the life span. *Psychol Aging*. 1989;4:425–437.

25. Magai C, Passman V. The interpersonal basis of emotional behavior and emotion regulation in adulthood. In: Lawton MP, Schaie K, eds. *Annual Review of Geriatrics and Gerontology.* 1997;17:104–137.
26. Rowe JW, Kahn RL. *Successful Aging: The MacArthur Foundation Study.* New York: Pantheon Books; 1998.
27. Segal DS, Hersen M, Van Hasselt VB, et al. Diagnosis and assessment of personality disorders in older adults: a critical review. *J Personal Disord.* 1996;10:384–399.
28. Kunik ME, Mulsant BH, Rifai AH, et al. Personality disorders in elderly inpatients with major depression. *Am J Geriatr Psychiatry.* 1993;1(1):38–45.
29. Agronin M. Personality disorders in the elderly: an overview. *J Geriatr Psychiatry.* 1994;27(2):151–191.
30. Abrams RC, Horowitz SV. Personality disorders after age 50: a meta-analytic review of the literature. In: Rosowsky E, Abrams R, Zweig R, eds. *Personality Disorders in Older Adults: Emerging Issues in Diagnosis and Treatment.* Mahwah: Lawrence Erlbaum; 1999; 31–53.
31. Grant BF, Hasin DS, Stinson FS, et al. Prevalence, correlates, and disability of personality disorders in the United States: results from the National Epidemiologic Survey on Alcohol and Related Conditions. *J Clin Psychiatry.* 2004;65:948–958.
32. Abrams RC, Alexopoulos GS, Spielman LA, et al. Personality disorder symptoms predict declines in global functioning and quality of life in elderly depressed patients. *Am J Geriatr Psychiatry.* 2001;9(1):67–71.
33. Fogel BS, Westlake R. Personality disorder diagnoses and age in inpatients with major depression. *J Clin Psychiatry.* 1990;51: 232–235.
34. Krossler D. Personality disorders in the elderly. *Hosp Community Psychiatry.* 1990;41:1325–1329.
35. Knight BG. Personality disorders in late life and public policy: implications of the contextual, cohort-based, maturity, specific challenge model. In: Rosowsky E, Abrams R, Zweig R, eds. *Personality Disorders in Older Adults: Emerging Issues in Diagnosis and Treatment.* Mahwah: Erlbaum; 1999;289–294.
36. Abrams R. Personality disorders in the elderly. In: Binenfeld D, ed. *Verwoerdt's Clinical Geropsychiatry.* Baltimore: Williams & Wilkins; 1990;151–163.
37. Clark LA, Harrison JA. Assessment instruments. In: Livesley WJ, ed. *Handbook of Personality Disorders: Theory, Research, and Treatment.* New York: Guilford; 2001;277–306.
38. Zweig RA, Hillman J. Personality disorders in adults: a review. In: Rosowsky E, Abrams R, Zweig R, eds. *Personality Disorders in Older Adults: Emerging Issues in Diagnosis and Treatment.* Mahwah: Erlbaum; 1999;31–53.
39. Abrams RC, Horowitz SV. Personality disorders after age 50: a meta-analysis. *J Personal Disord.* 1996;10(3):271–281.
40. Ames A, Molinari V. Prevalence of personality disorders in community-living elderly. *J Geriatr Psychiatry Neurol.* 1994;7:189–194.
41. Samuels J, Eaton WW, Bienvenu OJ, et al. Prevalence and correlates of personality disorders in a community sample. *Brit J Psychiatry.* 2002;180:536–542.
42. Thompson L, Gallagher D, Czirr R. Personality disorder and outcome in the treatment of late-life depression. *J Geriatr Psychiatry.* 1998;21:133–146.
43. Vine R, Steingart A. Personality disorder in the elderly depressed. *Can J Psychiatry.* 1994;39(7):392–398.
44. Farmer R, Nelson-Gray RO. Personality disorders and depression: hypothetical relations, empirical findings, and methodological considerations. *Clin Psychol Rev.* 1990;10:453–476.
45. Kernberg O. *Severe Personality Disorders: Psychotherapeutic Strategies.* New Haven: Yale University Press; 1984.
46. Vaillant GE, Perry JC. Personality disorders. In: Kaplan HI, Sadock BJ, eds. *Comprehensive Textbook of Psychiatry.* 5th Ed. Vol 2. Baltimore: Williams & Wilkins; 1990;1352–1387.
47. Costa PT, McCrae RR. Influence of extraversion and neuroticism on subjective well-being: happy and unhappy people. *J Pers Soc Psychol.* 1980;38(4):668–678.
48. McCrae RR, Costa PT. Personality, coping, and coping effectiveness in an adult sample. *J Pers.* 1986;54(2):385–405.
49. Drake RE, Vaillant GE. A validity study of axis II of DSM-III. *Am J Psychiatry.* 1985;142:553–558.
50. Kenan MM, Kendjelic EM, Molinari VA, et al. Age-related differences in frequency of personality disorders among inpatient veterans. *Int J Geriatr Psychiatry.* 2000;15:831–837.
51. Agbayewa MO. Occurrence and effects of personality disorders in depression: are they the same in the old and young? *Can J Psychiatry.* 1996;41:223–226.
52. Robins L, Regier D. *Psychiatric Disorders in America: The Epidemiologic Catchment Area Study.* New York: The Free Press; 1991.
53. Perry JC. Longitudinal studies of personality disorders. *J Personal Disord.* 1993;7(Suppl):63–85.
54. Costa P, McCrae R. Trait psychology comes of age. In: Sonderegger T, ed. *Nebraska Symposium on Motivation 1991.* Lincoln: University of Nebraska Press; 1992;169–204.
55. Tyrer P, Sieverwright H. Studies of outcome. In: Tyrer P, ed. *Personality Disorders: Diagnosis, Management, and Course.* London: Wright; 1988;119–136.
56. Butcher JN, Aldwin CM, Levenson MR, et al. Personality and aging: a study of the MMPI-2 among older men. *Psychol Aging.* 1991;6:361–370.
57. Molinari V, Kunik ME, Snow-Turek AL, et al. Age-related personality differences in inpatients with personality disorder: a cross-sectional study. *J Clin Geropsychology.* 1999;5:191–202.
58. Botwinick J. *Aging and Behavior.* New York: Springer; 1984.
59. Mroczek DK, Hurt SW, Berman WH. Conceptual and methodological issues in the assessment of personality disorders in older adults. In: Rosowsky E, Abrams R, Zweig R, eds. *Personality Disorders in Older Adults: Emerging Issues in Diagnosis and Treatment.* Mahwah: Erlbaum; 1999;135–152.
60. Abrams RC, Rosendahl E, Card C, et al. Personality disorder correlates of late and early onset depression. *J Am Geriatr Soc.* 1994;42:727–731.
61. Stevenson J, Meares R, Comerford A. Diminished impulsivity in older patients with borderline personality disorder. *Am J Psychiatry.* 2003;160:165–166.
62. Rosowsky E, Gurian B. Borderline personality disorder in late life. *Int Psychogeriatr.* 1991;3:39–52.
63. Trappler B, Backfield J. Clinical characteristics of older psychiatric inpatients with borderline personality disorder. *Psychiatr Q.* 2001;72:29–40.
64. Bengtson V, Reedy M, Gordon C. Aging and self-conceptions: personality processes and social contexts. In: Birren JE, Schaie KW, eds. *Handbook of the Psychology of Aging.* New York: Van Nostrand Reinhold; 1985;544–593.
65. Costa PT, McCrae RR. Set like plaster? Evidence for the stability of adult personality. In: Heatherton TF, Weinberger JL, eds. *Can Personality Change?* Washington: American Psychological Association; 1994;21–40.
66. Baltes MM, Honn S, Barton EM, et al. On the social ecology of dependence and independence in elderly nursing home residents. *J Gerontol.* 1973;38:760–774.
67. Shea MT, Stout R, Gunderson JG, et al. Short-term diagnostic stability of schizotypal, borderline, avoidant, and obsessive-compulsive personality disorders. *Am J Psychiatry.* 2002;159: 2036–2041.
68. Sadavoy, J. Character disorders in the elderly: an overview. In: Sadavoy J, Leszcz M, eds. *Treating the Elderly with Psychotherapy: The Scope for Change in Later Life.* Madison: International Universities Press; 1987;175–229.
69. Nemiroff RA, Colarusso CA. *New Dimensions in Adult Development.* New York: Basic Books; 1990.
70. Neugarten B. Time, age, and the life cycle. *Am J Psychiatry.* 1979;136:887–894.
71. Jacobowitz J, Newton N. Time, context, and character: a lifespan view of psychopathology during the second half of life. In: Nemiroff RA, Colarusso CA, eds. *New Dimensions in Adult Development.* New York: Basic Books; 1990;306–329.
72. Carstensen LL. Social and emotional patterns in adulthood: support for socio-emotional selectivity theory. *Psychol Aging.* 1992;7:331–338.
73. Isaacowitz DM, Charles ST, Carstensen LL. Emotion and cognition. In: Craik FIM, Salthouse TA, eds. *Handbook of Aging and Cognition.* 2nd Ed. Mahwah: Erbaum; 2000;593–631.
74. Zimmerman M, Coryell W. DSM-III personality disorder diagnoses in a nonpatient sample: demographic correlates and comorbidity. *Arch Gen Psychiatry.* 1989;46:682–689.

75. Shea MT, Zlotnick C, Dolan R, et al. Personality disorders, history of trauma, and posttraumatic stress disorder in subjects with anxiety disorders. *Compr Psychiatry.* 2000;41(5):315–325.

76. Yen S, Shea MT, Battle C, et al. Traumatic exposure and posttraumatic stress disorder in borderline, schizotypal, avoidant, and obsessive-compulsive personality disorders: findings from the collaborative longitudinal personality disorders study. *J Nerv Ment Dis.* 2002;190(8):510–518.

77. Bender DS, Dolan RT, Skodol AE, et al. Treatment utilization by patients with personality disorders. *Am J Psychiatry.* 2001;158(2):295–302.

78. Krause N, Shaw BA, Cairney J. A descriptive epidemiology of lifetime trauma and the physical health status of older adults. *Psychol Aging.* 2004;19:637–648.

79. Shea MT, Glass DR, Pilkonis P, et al. Frequency and implications of personality disorders in a sample of depressed outpatients. *J Personal Disord.* 1987;1:27–42.

80. Pfohl B, Coryell W, Zimmerman M, et al. Prognostic validity of self-report and interview measures of personality disorder in depressed inpatients. *J Clin Psychiatry.* 1987;48:468–472.

81. Frank E, Kupfer DJ, Jacob M, et al. Personality features and response to acute treatment in recurrent depression. *J Personal Disord.* 1987;1:14–26.

82. Beardon C, Lavelle N, Buysse D, et al. Personality pathology and time to remission in depressed outpatients treated with interpersonal psychotherapy. *J Personal Disord.* 1996;10:164–173.

83. Scogin F, McElreath L. Efficacy of psychosocial treatments for geriatric depression: a quantitative review. *J Consult Clin Psychol.* 1994;62:69–74.

84. Niederehe G, Schneider LS. Treatments for depression and anxiety in the aged. In: Nathan PE, Gorman JM, eds. *A Guide to Treatments That Work.* New York: Oxford; 1998;270–287.

85. Gradman T, Thompson L, Gallagher-Thompson D. Personality disorders and treatment outcome. In: Rosowsky E, Abrams R, Zweig R, eds. *Personality Disorders in Older Adults: Emerging Issues in Diagnosis and Treatment.* Mahwah: Erlbaum; 1999; 69–94.

86. Abrams RC, Spielman LA, Alexopoulos GE, et al. Personality disorder symptoms and functioning in elderly depressed patients. *Am J Geriatr Psychiatry.* 1998;6(1):24–30.

87. Piper WE, Joyce AS. Psychosocial treatment outcome. In: Livesley WJ, ed. *Handbook of Personality Disorders: Theory, Research, and Treatment.* New York: Guilford; 2001;323–343.

88. Linehan MM, Heard HL, Armstrong HE. Naturalistic followup of a behavioral treatment for chronically parasuicidal borderline patients. *Arch Gen Psychiatry.* 1993;50:971–974.

89. Munroe-Blum H, Marziali E. A controlled trial of short-term group treatment for borderline personality disorder. *J Personal Disord.* 1995;9:190–198.

90. Winston A, Laikin M, Pollack J, et al. Short-term psychotherapy of personality disorders. *Am J Psychiatry.* 1994;151:190–194.

91. Hardy GE, Barkham M, Shapiro DA, et al. Impact of cluster C personality disorders on outcomes of contrasting brief psychotherapies for depression. *J Consult Clin Psychol.* 1995;63:997–1004.

92. Sanderson C, Swensen C, Bohus M. A critique of the American Psychiatric Practice Guideline for the treatment of patients with borderline personality disorder. *J Personal Disord.* 2002;16(2): 122–129.

93. Zweig RA, Hinrichsen GA. Factors associated with suicide attempts in depressed older adults: a prospective study. *Am J Psychiatry.* 1993;150:1687–1692.

94. Safran JD, Crocker P, McMain S, et al. Therapeutic alliance rupture as a therapy event for empirical investigation. *Psychotherapy.* 1990;27:154–165.

95. Cloninger CR. A systematic method for clinical description and classification of personality variants. *Arch Gen Psychiatry.* 1987;44:573–588.

96. Cloninger CR, Svrakic DM, Przybeck TR. A psychobiologic model of temperament and character. *Arch Gen Psychiatry.* 1993;50:975–990.

97. Siever LJ, Davis KL. A psychobiological perspective on the personality disorders. *Am J Psychiatry.* 1991;148:1647–1658.

98. Coccaro EF, Siever LJ, Kla HM, et al. Serotonergic studies in patients with affective and persoanlity disorders: correlates with suicidal and impulsive aggressive behavior. *Arch Gen Psychiatry.* 1989;46:587–599.

99. Stein DJ, Trestman RL, Mitropoulou V, et al. Impulsivity and serotonergic function in compulsive personality disorder. *J Neuropsychiatry Clin Neurosci.* 1996;8:393–398.

100. Soloff PH. Psychobiologic perspectives on treatment of personality disorders. *J Personal Disord.* 1997;11(4):336–344.

101. Markovitz PJ. Pharmacotherapy. In: Lively WJ, ed. *Handbook of Personality Disorders.* New York: Guilford Press; 2001;475–493.

102. Markovitz PJ. Recent trends in the pharmacotherapy of personality disorders. *J Personal Disord.* 2004;18(1):90–101.

103. Goldberg SC, Schulz SC, Schulz PM, et al. Borderline and schizotypal personality disorders treated with low-dose thiothixene vs placebo. *Arch Gen Psychiatry.* 1986;43:680–686.

104. Hymowitz P, Frances A, Jacobsberg LB, et al. Neuroleptic treatment of schizotypal personality disorder. *Compr Psychiatry.* 1986;27:267–271.

105. Schulz SC. The use of low-dose neuroleptics in the treatment of "schizo-obsessive" patients. *Am J Psychiatry.* 1986;143: 1318–1319.

106. Koenigsberg HW, Reynolds D, Goodman M, et al. Risperidone in the treatment of schizotypal personality disorder. *J Clin Psychiatry.* 2003;64:628–634.

107. Jensen HV, Anderson J. An open, comparative study of amoxapine in borderline disorders. *Acta Psychiatr Scand.* 1989;79:89–93.

108. Markowitz PJ, Calabrese JR, Schulz SC, et al. Fluoxetine treatment of borderline and schizotypal personality disorders. *Am J Psychiatry.* 1991;148,1064–1067.

109. Hirose S. Effective treatment of aggression and impulsivity in antisocial personality disorder with risperidone. *Psychiatry Clin Neurosci.* 2001;55:161–162.

110. Penick EC, Powell BJ, Campbell J, et al. Pharmacological treatment for antisocial personality disorder in alcoholics: a preliminary study. *Alcoholism Clin Exp Res.* 1996;20(3):477–484.

111. Arndt IO, McLellan AT, Dorozynsky L, et al. Desipramine treatment for cocaine dependence. Role of antisocial personality disorder. *J Nerv Ment Dis.* 1994;182(3):151–156.

112. Agronin M. Pharmacologic treatment of personality disorders in late life. In: Rosowsky E, Abrams RC, Zweig RA, eds. *Personality Disorders in Older Adults.* Mahwah: Lawrence Erlbaum Associates, Publishers; 1999;229–254.

113. Cowdry RW, Gardner DL. Pharmacotherapy of borderline personality disorder. Alprazolam, carbamazepine, trifluoperazine, and tranylcypromine. *Arch Gen Psychiatry.* 1988;45: 111–119.

114. Coccaro EF, Astill JL, Herbert JA, et al. Fluoxetine treatment of impulsive aggression in DSM-III-R personality disorder patients. *J Clin Psychopharmacol.* 1990;10:373–375.

115. Links PS, Steine M, Boiageo BA, et al. Lithium therapy for borderline patients: preliminary findings. *J Personal Disord.* 1990;4: 173–181.

116. Kavoussi RJ, Liv J, Cocarro EF. An open trial of sertraline in personality disorder patients with impulsive aggression. *J Clin Psychiatry.* 1994;55:137–141.

117. Salzman C, Wolfson AN, Schatzberg A, et al. Effect of fluoxetine on anger in symptomatic volunteers with borderline personality disorder. *J Clin Psychopharm.* 1995;15(1):23–29.

118. Markovitz PJ, Wagner SC. Venlafaxine in the treatment of borderline personality disorder. *Psychopharm Bull.* 1995;31(4): 773–777.

119. Rinne T, Van den Brink W, Wouters I, et al. SSRI treatment of borderline personality disorder: a randomized, placebo-controlled clinical trial for females with BPD. *Am J Psychiatry.* 2002;159: 2048–2054.

120. Frankenburg FR, Zanarini MC. Clozapine treatment of borderline patients: a preliminary study. *Compr Psychiatry.* 1993;34(6): 402–405.

121. Chengappa KNR, Ebeling T, Kang JS, et al. Clozapine reduces severe self-mutilation and aggression in psychotic patients with borderline personality disorder. *J Clin Psychiatry.* 1999;60: 477–484.

122. Khouzam HR, Donnelly NJ. Remission of self-mutilation in a patient with borderline personality during risperidone therapy. *J Nerv Ment Dis.* 1997;185(5):348–349.

123. Rocca P, Marchiaro L, Cocuzza E, et al. Treatment of borderline personality disorder with risperidone. *J Clin Psychiatry.* 2002;63: 241–244.

124. Zanarini MC, Frankenberg FR. Olanzapine treatment of female borderline patients: a double-blind, placebo-controlled pilot study. *J Clin Psychiatry*. 2001;62:849–854.

125. Adityanjee, Schulz SC. Clinical uses of quetiapine in disease states other than schizophrenia. *J Clin Psychiatry*. 2002;63: 32–38.

126. Zanarini M, Frankenberg F, Parachini EA. A preliminary, randomized trial of fluoxetine, olanzapine, and the olanzapine-fluoxetine combination in women with borderline personality disorder. *J Clin Psychiatry*. 2004;65(7):903–907.

127. Stein DJ, Simeon D, Frenkel M, et al. An open trial of valproate in borderline personality disorder. *J Clin Psychiatry*. 1995;56(11): 506–510.

128. Frankenberg FR, Zanarini MC. Divalproex sodium treatment of women with borderline personality disorder and bipolar II disorder: a double-blind, placebo-controlled pilot study. *J Clin Psychiatry*. 2002;63:442–446.

129. Wilcox JA. Divalproex sodium as a treatment for borderline personality disorder. *Ann Clin Psychiatry*. 1995;7(1):33–37.

130. Gardner DL, Cowdry RW. Positive effects of carbamazepine on behavioral dyscontrol in borderline personality disorder. *Am J Psychiatry*. 1986;143:519–522.

131. Demopulos C, Fava M, McLean NE, et al. Hypochondriacal concerns in depressed outpatients. *Psychosom Med*. 1996;58(4): 314–320.

132. Deltito JA, Stam M. Psychopharmacological treatment of avoidant personality disorder. *Compr Psychiatry*. 1989;30:498–504.

133. Schneier FR, Chin SJ, Hollander E, et al. Fluoxetine in social phobia. *J Clin Psychopharmacol*. 1992;12:62–64.

134. Fahlén T. Personality traits in social phobia, II: changes during drug treatment. *J Clin Psychiatry*. 1995;56(12):569–573.

135. Jacobowitz J, Newton N. Dynamics and treatment of narcissism in late life. In: Duffy M, ed. *Handbook of Counseling and Psychotherapy with Older Adults*. New York: Wiley; 1999; 453–469.

136. Lynch TR. Treatment of elderly depression with personality disorder co-morbidity using dialectical behavior therapy. *Cognitive and Behavioral Practice*. 2000;7:447–456.

137. Agronin M. Personality disorders. In: DV Jeste, JH Friedman, eds. *Psychiatry for Neurologists*. Totowa, NJ: Humana Press; 2005; 105–121.

138. Agronin ME, Orr WB. Personality disorders in a geriatric psychiatry outpatient clinic. Poster/abstract presented at: Annual Meeting of the American Association for Geriatric Psychiatry; March 8–11, 1998; San Diego, CA.

139. Agronin ME. Depressive personality disorder in late life: a descriptive study of 11 cases. Poster/abstract presented at: Annual Meeting of the American Association for Geriatric Psychiatry; March 16, 1999; New Orleans, LA.

140. Groves JE. Taking care of the hateful patient. *N Engl J Med*. 1978;298(16):883–887.

141. Zweig RA. Personality disorders in older adults: managing the difficult patient. *Clin Geriatr*. 2003;11(5):22–25.

142. Weissman MM, Markowitz JC, Klerman GL. *Comprehensive Guide to Interpersonal Psychotherapy*. New York: Basic Books; 2000.

Substance Use Disorders in the Elderly

32

Maria D. Llorente   *David W. Oslin*   *Julie Malphurs*

Substance use disorders in older adults are a significant public health problem that has only recently begun to receive attention, particularly among women. As our nation ages, this problem is likely to increase because the current cohort of baby boomers grew up during a time when the use of substances, such as alcohol, marijuana, cocaine, and narcotics, became more widespread. In the current group of older adults, these disorders are often underrecognized and untreated (1). Older adults are highly heterogeneous when it comes to the impact of substances of abuse, and can present with substantial variability in physical and social functioning. This chapter will review the four most commonly encountered problematic substances in older adults: alcohol, tobacco, benzodiazepines, and opioids.

ALCOHOL

While diagnostic criteria from the Diagnostic and Statistical Manual of Mental Disorders, 4th edition, Text Revision (DSM-IV-TR) exist for both alcohol abuse and dependence, these criteria are often inconsistently applied or difficult to interpret in older adults (2). Alcohol abuse is defined as the recurrent use of alcohol that results in failure to fulfill roles and responsibilities. Similarly, dependence criteria include alcohol-related problems in occupational or social activities. This would be very difficult to assess in an older person who drinks alone at home and is thus less likely to become involved in fights, get arrested, or drive while intoxicated. Care providers may easily overlook the effects of alcohol use, attributing them instead to common disorders of late life. This is likely to be the main reason for the consistent finding that older problem drinkers are identified less often by clinicians and are less

often referred for treatment than their younger counterparts (1).

Due to the difficulties in assessing older adults for alcohol use, several guidelines now recommend that older primary care patients be screened on an annual basis for alcohol consumption (1,3). Further, the Center for Substance Abuse Treatment (CSAT) Treatment Improvement Protocol Panel has proposed the use of the terms *at-risk* and *problem drinkers* to better address alcohol-related issues in older adults. At-risk drinking is defined as alcohol use that does not yet cause problems, but may lead to adverse consequences for the drinker or others. Problem drinking is the consumption of any amount of alcohol with at least one problem related to this use.

The National Institute on Alcohol Abuse and Alcoholism and the CSAT panel further recommend that the upper limit of alcohol consumption for persons older than 65 be no more than one *standard drink* per day (see Figure 32-1), with a maximum of two drinks on a single occasion (1,4). These drinking limits are consistent with data regarding the relationship between consumption and alcohol-related problems within this age group, while keeping in mind the current evidence on the beneficial health effects of drinking (5–7).

Epidemiology

The prevalence of alcohol use disorders declines with age, and men are far more likely to be diagnosed than women. The prevalence is also higher in health care settings. Prevalence rates are summarized in Table 32-1. Unlike younger adults, most older persons (60–70%) are abstainers from alcohol (defined as no alcohol use at all in the past year). Reasons for abstention can vary, and include continued life-long patterns, recent medical illness, desire to avoid

TABLE 32-1
PREVALENCE OF ALCOHOL USE DISORDERS IN OLDER SAMPLES

Study	Age	Population	Diagnostic Criteria	12-Month Prevalence
Helzer et al. (8)	65+	Community dwelling	DSM-III alcohol abuse/dependence	M: 3.1% F: 0.46%
Barry et al. (9)	65+	Primary care	At-risk/problem drinking	15%
Callahan et al. (10)	60+	Primary care	Problem drinking	10.6%
Holroyd et al. (11)	65+	Mental health outpatient clinic	DSM-IV alcohol dependence	8.6%
Joseph et al. (12)	65+	VA nursing home	Alcohol dependence	18%
Oslin et al. (13)	65+	Nursing home	Alcohol dependence	10%
Speer et al. (14)	65+	Acute geropsychiatry inpatient	Alcohol dependence	23%

DSM-III, Diagnostic and Statistical Manual of Mental Disorders 3rd Ed; DSM-IV, Diagnostic and Statistical Manual of Mental Disorders 4th Ed; F, female; M, male; VA, Veterans Administration.

medication–alcohol or disease–alcohol interactions, lower income due to retirement, religious beliefs, and previous history of alcohol abuse/dependence. This last group may benefit from further inquiry about prior triggers for drinking, current life stressors, and screening for depression and cognitive impairment. Problems related to past history of heavy or problematic drinking are also important to ascertain since this is a known risk factor for developing difficult-to-treat late-life depression and dementia (15,16).

Assessment and Diagnosis

Few older adults seek help for alcohol-related problems. As a result, and given the increased prevalence of these disorders in clinical settings, the health care provider must have a high index of suspicion and inquire about the quantity and frequency of alcohol intake. This is best done as part of a routine visit, embedding alcohol use questions in the context of other health behaviors (such as diet, exercise, and smoking). In order to improve assessment, clinicians should clarify that alcohol includes beer, wine, sherry, and hard liquor and explain the amount of these drinks that contain similar amounts of alcohol, known as a *standard drink* (see Figure 32-1).

Additionally, several screening instruments have been developed to probe for alcohol-related problems. The CAGE is the most widely used and is easy to administer because it has only four items regarding an individual's alcohol use: felt they should *Cut down*, felt *Annoyed* that people criticized their drinking, felt *Guilty* about their drinking, and had a drink upon waking in the morning—an *Eye opener* (17). In older adults, one positive response is an indicator of problems. The Short Michigan Alcoholism Screening Instrument—Geriatric Version was developed specifically for use among older persons in a variety of settings and its psychometric properties are superior to other

available instruments for the identification of alcohol abuse/dependence in the elderly (18).

Positive screens should be further assessed for abuse and dependence with additional questions regarding alcohol-related problems, such as accidents and falls; a history of failed attempts to stop or to cut back; withdrawal symptoms; insomnia; alcohol–medication interactions, particularly with warfarin or digoxin (19); and alcohol-related medical illness, such as out-of-control diabetes, poor nutrition, and peripheral neuropathy. Physical findings are frequently absent but can help to confirm the diagnosis when present; they include an enlarged, tender liver, peripheral neuropathy, cerebellar ataxia, and cognitive impairment. Several abnormal laboratory values have been found to occur more often in older alcoholics than in younger ones and include increases in mean corpuscular hemoglobin and mean corpuscular volume, elevated aspartate aminotransferase and serum uric acid levels, and decreases in serum albumin (20).

1 Standard Drink =

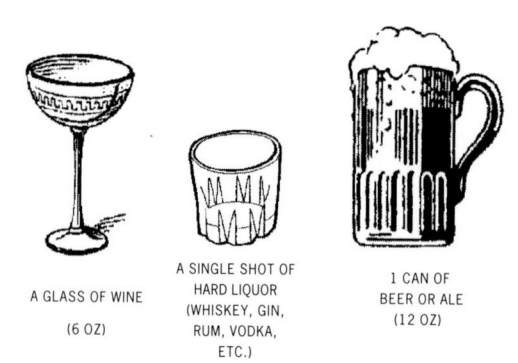

A GLASS OF WINE (6 OZ)

A SINGLE SHOT OF HARD LIQUOR (WHISKEY, GIN, RUM, VODKA, ETC.) (1.5 OZ)

1 CAN OF BEER OR ALE (12 OZ)

A SMALL GLASS OF LIQUEUR, OR APERITIF (4 OZ)

Figure 32-1   What is a standard drink?

Differential Diagnosis

Intoxication and withdrawal states, as well as alcohol-related cognitive disorders, can cause symptoms that mimic other psychiatric illnesses, such as anxiety, depression, psychosis, or dementia. Home visits can occasionally identify an alcohol problem, particularly when part of the nutritional evaluation includes asking the patient for permission to look in his/her refrigerator or pantry: food items are often absent, but beer, wine, or liquor are present. When patients are asked about this, they frequently admit that they have a problem with alcohol.

Depression and Anxiety

Reports have consistently found that depression and alcohol dependence frequently co-occur (21). Mood disorders were found to be the most common comorbid condition among 22,463 veterans presenting for alcohol treatment (22). Additionally, an age-related increase in comorbid major depression occurred across the life span, such that comorbidity of depression and alcoholism was a more significant issue for older than younger adults. The effect of past heavy alcohol use is highlighted in the Liverpool Longitudinal Study, which demonstrated a five-fold increase in psychiatric illness among elderly men who had a lifetime history of 5 or more years of heavy drinking (15). Current and past history of heavy consumption is also related to suicide in late life.

The relationship between alcohol use disorders and depression is complex. Depressive symptoms can precede alcohol use (*primary depression*), with alcohol often functioning to self-medicate these symptoms. Depressive symptoms can also develop as a consequence of alcohol use (*reactive* or *secondary depression*). For example, while 42% of subjects presenting to alcohol detoxification had significant depressive symptoms, only 6% continued to have these symptoms 4 weeks later (23). Lastly, depressive symptoms can occur simultaneously with (*indeterminate*) alcohol use. Clinically, making the distinction is critical to the development of the treatment plan. Primary depression would be treated concurrently with the alcohol use disorder, whereas secondary depression would likely resolve with treatment of the addiction. A reliable method for categorizing depression is to examine the temporal relationship of depressive symptoms and abstinence periods. Similarly, anxiety symptoms that precede the alcohol use or occur during abstinence are likely to indicate a primary anxiety disorder. Anxiety symptoms can occur during detoxification due to withdrawal, which will resolve once detoxification is complete.

Cognitive Disorders

Rates of alcohol-related dementia vary based on diagnostic criteria used and populations studied. The prevalence of lifetime alcohol abuse/dependence among subjects age 55 and older in the Epidemiologic Catchment Area study was 1.5 times greater among persons with mild and severe cognitive impairment than those with no cognitive impairment (24). Unlike Alzheimer's disease, however, patients with alcohol-related dementia who become and remain abstinent do not show progressive cognitive decline, and occasionally demonstrate improved cognitive functioning with sobriety (25). Alcohol-related dementia can be further distinguished from Alzheimer's disease in that ataxia and peripheral neuropathy occur frequently in the former, while naming deficits are uncommon.

Etiology

For many individuals, drinking patterns are stable over many years, (26), such that the risk factors for alcohol abuse and dependence are similar for older and younger adults. As in younger patients, psychological distress increases alcohol consumption or relapse risk in older adults being treated for alcoholism (27). A number of older adults will increase drinking in late life due to boredom, unstructured or excess free time, available disposable income, and psychiatric disorders, particularly depression.

A second group of older adults may develop alcohol-related problems in the absence of increased consumption due to the physical and physiologic changes that occur with aging. For example, as we age, lean body mass and total body water are reduced, leading to higher peak blood alcohol levels. An individual who typically consumed two to three standard drinks per day for most of his/her life without difficulties may experience falls or mental confusion in later life.

Some of the neuropsychological changes associated with chronic alcoholism stem from direct effects of thiamine-deficient diets. The primary lesion occurs in the mammillary bodies, where petechial hemorrhages can be seen and, microscopically, capillary dilatation and hemorrhage occur (28). In Korsakoff's psychosis, the mammillary bodies show severe neuronal loss and reactive astrocytosis. Atrophy of the frontal and parietal lobes can occur, with ventricular dilatation (28). Older adults with current or lifetime histories of alcohol abuse should therefore be screened for cognitive impairment.

CASE EXAMPLE: AT-RISK ALCOHOL INTAKE

Mr. T is a 72-year-old Hispanic man who came in for his annual physical exam in a veteran's primary care clinic. A brief interview inquired about health habits, including exercise, nutrition, and tobacco use. The concept of a standard drink was explained using Figure 32-1. Inquiry regarding alcohol use was made as follows: "During the past week, on how many days did you drink alcohol [frequency], and on these days, how many standard drinks did you have [quantity]? Were there any days during the past month on which you drank four or more standard drinks [binge drinking]?"

He responded that he drank daily, usually having two beers with lunch, and a mixed drink with dinner, for a total of 21 standard drinks per week (three times more than the recommended daily limits). He was then given education regarding alcohol consumption patterns among older adults in the United States and saw that his level of drinking placed him in the at-risk group. Mr. T remarked that he had just realized how much alcohol he was consuming each week. Both positive and negative consequences of alcohol use were discussed, as well as possible reasons for cutting back on his alcohol use. He stated that he now was concerned about an alcohol–medication interaction because he was taking an antihypertensive and digoxin for his heart. Spontaneously, he stated that he wanted to cut back on his alcohol intake for his health. A drinking agreement was drawn up to establish daily limits on alcohol intake. He was given a drinking diary card to monitor his alcohol use until his next appointment 2 weeks later.

At his follow-up visit his wife came. He had successfully cut down his alcohol use so that he was choosing to have either a beer with lunch or a drink with dinner. There were several days that he chose not to drink at all. He noticed that his thinking was clearer and he reported that his memory and concentration had improved, as had his balance. His wife noted that his personality had changed and he was less moody and irritable.

CASE EXAMPLE: COMORBIDITY OF ALCOHOL USE AND DEPRESSION

Mr. J is an 84-year-old White man who was referred to mental health for increased alcohol consumption, anorexia with a 20-pound weight loss, and fatigue. The primary care provider was specifically referring him for alcohol treatment. Upon initial evaluation, Mr. J reported that he never drank very much alcohol until he retired the year before. He reported feelings of worthlessness now that he was not working. He reported insomnia with early-morning awakening that preceded his alcohol intake, and the main reason he had started to drink alcohol was "to help me sleep better." He also reported sad mood and loss of interest in things he used to enjoy. It was determined that Mr. J met criteria for a primary major depressive episode with secondary alcohol abuse. He was started on an antidepressant and given recommendations to taper his alcohol intake. At 3 months, he was able to discontinue his alcohol intake and his depressive symptoms had resolved.

Treatment

Recommended strategies to identify, evaluate, and treat alcohol use disorders in older adults are summarized in Figure 32-2. Experts recommend making every reasonable effort to ensure that older adults with at-risk or problem drinking enter treatment. Intervention strategies need to be nonconfrontational and supportive because older adults, particularly older women, experience a significantly greater amount of stigma associated with alcohol use than do

younger adults. The goals of treatment vary depending on the severity of the problem, and range from reduction of alcohol consumption to sobriety. Brief intervention is the recommended first step, supplemented by motivational interviewing. Patients should also be evaluated for potential withdrawal symptoms and a determination made as to whether detoxification is indicated and can be done on an outpatient basis.

Detoxification

Alcohol withdrawal symptoms are more likely to occur in patients who dramatically reduce or stop their drinking after regular consumption. Because the severity of withdrawal symptoms typically peak around 72 hours after cessation of drinking, the clinician must know the time of the last drink. The patient is the best source of information regarding past withdrawal symptoms during periods when he or she tried to cut down or stop. It is likely that if withdrawal occurred in the past, it will occur again in the future. Patients who have previously been hospitalized for detoxification or who report seizures or delirium tremens should be monitored carefully when trying to reduce alcohol intake. Patients currently drinking more than 28 drinks per week who want to reduce or eliminate alcohol intake should be assessed with an objective measure of alcohol withdrawal such as the Clinical Institute Withdrawal Assessment for Alcohol Scale (CIWA-Ar) (29). If the total score is less than 8, patients can be followed-up in 2 to 3 days and the CIWA-Ar repeated. If the score is again less than 8, the patient can be given a routine follow-up appointment following the brief intervention (typically within 2 weeks). If the total CIWA-Ar score is between 8 and 20, patients should be started on a benzodiazepine. Benzodiazepines can reduce severity of withdrawal symptoms, and decrease the incidence of seizures and delirium. The preferred agent to use in older adults is oxazepam, since it has no active metabolites and a short half-life. If the total CIWA-Ar score is greater than 20, hospitalization should be considered.

Brief Alcohol Interventions

Two studies have been conducted among older adults to determine the efficacy of this type of intervention (30,31). Patients receiving the intervention significantly reduced alcohol use, particularly episodes of binge drinking. The intervention in this study utilizes motivational interviewing and includes the FRAMES model developed by Miller and Rollnick (32). Table 32-2 describes the elements of this particularly effective model for older adults. It emphasizes personal choice and responsibility for change, focuses on the patient's own concerns, and uses negotiation rather than prescription.

Pharmacotherapy

Some of the general principles used in treating younger patients also should be applied to older drinkers. The use of medications to support abstinence may be of benefit, but

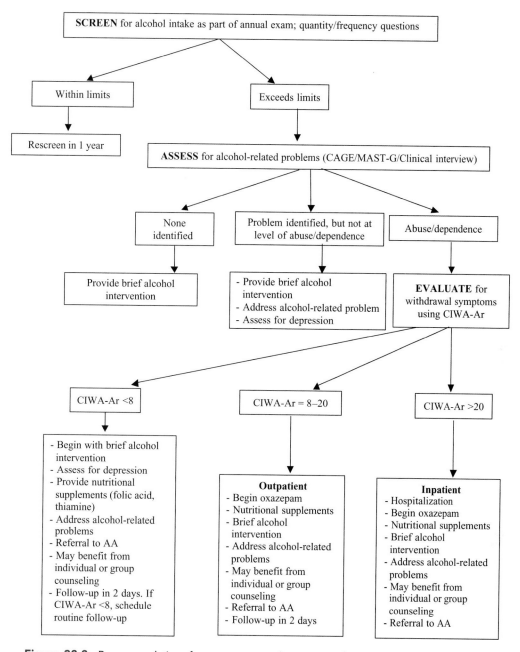

Figure 32-2 Recommendations for assessment and treatment of alcohol use disorders in older adults. AA, Alcoholics Anonymous; CAGE, cut down-annoyed-guilty-eye opener alcohol screening questionnaire; CIWA-Ar, Clinical Institute Withdrawal Assessment for Alcohol Scale; MAST-G, Michigan Alcoholism Screening Test—Geriatric Version.

is not well studied in older adults. Naltrexone has been demonstrated to be safe and helpful in older adults and should be considered in the treatment of alcohol dependence (33). The use of serotonin selective reuptake inhibitors is currently being studied and should be used with caution among patients without primary depression. Disulfiram may benefit some well-motivated patients, but cardiac and hepatic disease limit its use in geriatric patients. Acamprosate is a promising drug whose mechanism of action is unknown, although it is thought to modulate glutamate response. In a clinical trial in younger adults, twice as many acamprosate users maintained abstinence throughout the trial as compared to the placebo group. This drug, however, has not yet been studied in the elderly. Acamprosate has been used widely in Europe for several years and was approved by the Food and Drug Administration (FDA) for the US market in early 2005.

Psychosocial Treatments
For older adults, peer-specific group activities are superior to mixed-age group activities, and include supportive group psychotherapy and regular attendance at self-help

TABLE 32-2

ELEMENTS OF FRAMES MODEL FOR APPROACHING OLDER DRINKERS

Element	What the Provider Does	Example
Feedback	Provide educational information based on screening	Comparing patient's intake to recommended limits and other older alcohol consumption patterns
Responsibility	Focus on change as the personal responsibility of the patient, not the clinician	Negotiating change behaviors, such as reduction rather than abstinence
Advice	Provide specific recommendations for change	Drink below weekly recommended limits
Menu	Offer options so that change is more likely to occur	Reduction in drinking vs. abstinence
Empathy	Demonstrate understanding of the patient's personal goals and the role alcohol plays in his/her life	"I understand that alcohol is part of your social group. Maybe you could order nonalcoholic beer when you go out with them."
Self-efficacy	Validate the patient's ability to accomplish his/her goals	"I think you can do this too."

Adapted from Reference 32.

group meetings such as Alcoholics Anonymous (AA). Use of resources such as day programs and senior centers can be especially beneficial, and may effectively address time management issues.

Course and Prognosis

Most patients treated for alcohol dependence are able to successfully abstain from alcohol, or experience brief relapses that do not progress to abuse or dependence (34). For older adults who do seek treatment, success is far greater than that seen in younger adults (35). Nearly 90% of patients who remain abstinent for 2 years are alcohol free at 10 years. Of those who remain alcohol free for 10 years, more than 90% are alcohol free at 20 years (36,37). Very little is known about the long-term course of alcohol abuse/dependence with late-life onset.

Until recently, few studies examined whether negative consequences associated with alcohol could be reversed in older adults. Residents of nursing homes with recent histories of alcohol-related problems who were able to discontinue drinking were more likely to be discharged back to the community (38). Similarly, older adults with alcohol-related problems who were able to initiate abstinence from alcohol experienced an associated improvement in functioning as measured by activities of daily living (13). These reports of improved physical functioning associated with alcohol reduction provide the best argument for initiating treatment in older adults.

Cultural Factors

Ethnic minority elderly are a rapidly expanding demographic group. Most epidemiologic studies that have included African-American, Hispanic, and Asian elderly have found similar or lower rates of alcohol abuse and dependence compared to Caucasian elderly and greater prevalence among men than women (8,39,40,41). As foreign-born individuals become more acculturated, the prevalence of drinking problems increases and rates approach that of the United States in general. Alcohol-related problems are thus likely to increase in the next generation of ethnic minority elderly.

Among Hispanics, the fastest growing minority group, treatment interventions are effective. Hispanic men use alcohol treatment out of proportion to their numbers in the population (41). Outpatient services are the most common form of treatment, but Hispanics are less likely than non-Hispanic Whites to attend AA. Family involvement is of critical importance in engaging Hispanics in treatment. Because they are more than twice as likely to seek mental health care from primary care, the brief alcohol intervention strategy may be particularly useful.

Women and Alcohol

Women are more vulnerable to the effects of alcohol and develop alcohol-related diseases more quickly than men (42). More older female alcoholics (50%) begin their problem drinking in late life than do older male alcoholics (25%). As with men, both benefits and negative consequences have been associated with alcohol use. Moderate alcohol intake has been associated with higher bone mineral density in postmenopausal elderly women (43). Alcohol abuse/dependence, however, leads to osteopenia and increased incidence of skeletal fractures. Research has indicated that the risk of breast cancer increases by approximately 50% in women who consume three to nine drinks per week, compared to women who drink fewer than three drinks per week (44). The risk of cardiovascular disease and ischemic strokes is reduced with moderate drinking. Women alcoholics are four times more likely than alcoholic men to suffer from depression and twice as likely as nonalcoholic females to be depressed (42).

Functional Loss

Among otherwise-healthy, primarily middle-aged adults, a substantial amount of evidence suggests that moderate (defined as no more than one standard drink per day) alcohol use has beneficial effects, including reduction of cardiovascular disease and vascular dementias, and may reduce cancer risk (44–46). Much less is known about the effects of low-risk use in the elderly, or moderate alcohol use in the context of comorbid medical and/or psychiatric disorders.

The negative health-related consequences of at-risk and problem drinking are well described and include hepatic cirrhosis, alcohol-related cardiomyopathy, hypertension, fractures and subdural hematomas associated with falls and motor vehicle accidents, impaired driving-related skills, memory problems, and sleep disturbances (47). Of particular concern in the elderly are the interactions between alcohol and medications, both prescribed and over-the-counter.

TOBACCO

Cigarette smoking is the leading cause of premature and preventable morbidity and death in the United States (48). Approximately, 23% of the population smokes, with one out of every five smokers age 50 years or older (49). About 70% of smokers see their physician each year, yet only half report ever being advised to quit smoking by this physician. Among older adults, 15.2% of community-dwelling individuals age 65 to 74 and 8.4% of those age 75 and older are smokers, with higher rates among African-American men (22.1% between the ages of 65–74, and 12% for age 75 or older) (50). The prevalence of smoking is two-to-three-times higher, however, for individuals with chemical dependency or mental illness, such that almost half of all cigarettes consumed in the United States are smoked by individuals who have suffered from a psychiatric disorder within the past 30 days (51). Because older smokers have typically consumed large amounts of tobacco in their lifetimes, they are disproportionately affected by tobacco-related disease.

Assessment

The degree of physical dependence on tobacco is an important predictor of the likelihood and severity of withdrawal symptoms. Greater dependency is associated with increased difficulty in quitting. Several biochemical markers of nicotine dependence exist but are not readily available in routine clinical practice: serum nicotine levels; cotinine (the main metabolite of nicotine) levels in serum, saliva, or urine; and carbon monoxide levels (expired breath or serum carboxyhemoglobin). Clinicians can assess dependence through interview questions. The Fagerstrom Test for Nicotine Dependence (FTND) is a six-item questionnaire that is useful in predicting severity of nicotine craving and withdrawal and is the most widely used measure (52); however, the two-item Heaviness of Smoking Index performs as well as the FTND and correlates with biochemical indices of nicotine intake (53). There is general consensus that persons who smoke at least 10 cigarettes per day or within 60 minutes of waking up are moderately nicotine dependent. Individuals who smoke at least 20 cigarettes per day or within 30 minutes of waking are highly dependent.

CASE EXAMPLE: TOBACCO DEPENDENCY

Mr. C is a 68-year-old White divorced man who has a history of peripheral vascular disease, coronary artery disease, diabetes, and past history of alcohol dependence who was admitted to the hospital for congestive heart failure and his fourth myocardial infarction. Mr. C reported that he had been smoking cigarettes his entire life, starting at the age of 14, and currently smoked one-to-two packs per day. He typically smoked his first cigarette shortly after waking up. He had tried to quit on several occasions, including one time when he remained abstinent for 2 years. He reported that he usually resumed smoking when under stress, and that smoking relaxed him and alleviated his anxiety.

While in the intensive care unit, he was asked whether he might be interested in quitting. He stated that he realized he was going to have to quit because of his heart, but was not sure if he would be able to do so. The clinician asked a few questions to enhance her understanding of the patient's desires. He explained that on admission he had felt as if "there was an elephant sitting on my chest, making it impossible to breathe." The clinician suggested that whenever he began to experience cravings for tobacco, he visualize an elephant sitting on his chest and recall how uncomfortable he felt. Mr. C agreed that this would be useful. During this admission, he was also evaluated by psychiatry and found to meet criteria for major depressive disorder and generalized anxiety disorder. He expressed a desire to quit smoking, and was started on bupropion, gradually titrated to 300 mg daily.

He was seen in follow-up 4 days after his discharge. The clinicians emphasized their belief in the patient's ability to remain smoke free. At subsequent follow-ups, Mr. C was encouraged to discuss social cues that led to

> desires to smoke and positive reinforcement was utilized to reward his ability to abstain from smoking. His depressive and anxiety symptoms responded well to bupropion and he has remained smoke free 3 years later. Importantly, he has had no further hospital admissions.

Treatment

Current recommendations are similar to those for younger adults with a few exceptions. For example, aversion therapy (a type of behavioral therapy in which a smoker is placed in a confined smoke-filled room for a specified period of time) is potentially hazardous for older adults, particularly those with underlying medical conditions. A complete treatment plan for tobacco cessation provides a reduction in withdrawal symptoms together with the development of coping skills and alternative behaviors to remain smoke free. A very brief intervention—usually lasting less than 5 minutes—in which the patient is firmly and nonjudgmentally advised to quit smoking, is sometimes effective in increasing the proportion of patients who quit smoking in primary care settings and can be adapted for use in other settings (54). However, most patients will require an approach that combines behavioral and pharmacotherapies.

Behavioral Modalities

Table 32-3 describes the U.S. Public Health Service Clinical Practice Guideline on Treating Tobacco Use and Dependence. The five A's provide a road map for facilitating a patient's desire to quit smoking and use the principles of *motivational interviewing* (55). Motivational interviewing is a counseling approach with empirical support in a wide range of addictive behaviors including alcohol and tobacco. Essential to this approach is a respectful, empathic, patient-centered attitude. The patient is an active collaborator in the treatment planning process, rather than a passive recipient of information. There are four general strategies: *roll with resistance, express empathy, develop discrepancy,* and *support self-efficacy.*

In rolling with resistance, the clinician avoids direct confrontations or arguments. Rather, the focus is on responding empathically, reflective listening, and redirecting the conversation. A smoker may express irritation at "being nagged" about smoking or resentment over many failed attempts. Responses such as, "this must be very frustrating for you," are likely to help the patient become receptive to cessation interventions.

The expression of empathy allows the clinician to demonstrate that he or she understands how difficult the task of quitting tobacco is for the patient. Many smokers describe sadness and fear at the idea of giving up tobacco, which has often become an integral part of their lives. Clinicians can also help patients recognize the discrepancy

TABLE 32-3

THE FIVE A'S FOR FACILITATING TOBACCO CESSATION

	Suggested Interventions
Ask about smoking	1. How many cigarettes do you smoke each day? 2. How soon after you wake up do you smoke your first cigarette?
Advise to quit	1. Educate about specific effects of tobacco on this person's health. 2. Express your personal concern about his/her well-being 3. Provide a firm, nonjudgmental and personal recommendation to quit
Assess willingness to quit	1. Assess interest in quitting 2. Provide motivational counseling
Assist in quit attempt	1. Emphasize that successful cessation is associated with multiple failed attempts 2. Explain potential withdrawal symptoms 3. Review pharmacologic and NRT options 4. Develop coping strategies to deal with cravings and smoking cues 5. Teach smoking refusal skills 6. Select a quit date
Arrange follow-up contact	1. First contact ideally within 4–7 days of quit date 2. Reinforce self-efficacy 3. Review coping strategies 4. Practice smoking refusal skills

NRT, nicotine replacement therapy.
Adapted from Reference 55.

between their desired behavior (to be smoke free) and current behavior. Strategies include identifying immediate and certain consequences, such as those on health (chronic cough, shortness of breath, heart problems), finances (costs of cigarettes), or social interactions (friend/significant others' attitudes, no smoking policies in public areas).

Lastly, the clinician must believe in and openly discuss the patient's ability to change, or self-efficacy. The majority of smokers have tried to quit and have failed several times. They are often afraid of failing again. This is an ideal time to discuss with the patient the various treatment options that are available.

Nicotine Replacement Therapy

Nicotine replacement therapy (NRT), summarized in Table 32-4, is the cornerstone of nicotine addiction treatment. The success of NRT is due to its ability to prevent and treat the signs and symptoms of nicotine withdrawal. These include irritability, anxiety, depression, fatigue, decreased alertness, lightheadedness, headache, body aches, hunger, urges to smoke, weight gain, insomnia, constipation, sweating, and decreased heart rate. The choice of agent is based on several factors that include the severity of withdrawal and cravings, adherence, and cost. A typical approach, however, is to use a patch to achieve steady-state levels of nicotine to prevent withdrawal, and then use the other modalities for treatment of acute cravings, especially in social-cue situations such as restaurants or bars.

Regardless of modality, all have been shown to be effective and safe, such that at 3 months, 40% of individuals using one of these modalities are abstinent. These abstinence rates typically decline to 15% to 30% at 12 months. NRT is not associated with increased cardiovascular risks, even in patients with chronic obstructive pulmonary disease (COPD) or those who have pre-existing cardiac disease (56–58). NRT is intended for time-limited treatment, and there are currently no data available on the use of any of these modalities for long-term treatment.

Pharmacotherapy

The only FDA-approved nonnicotine treatment is the antidepressant bupropion SR. In addition to its unique antidepressant properties, bupropion also acts as a noncompetitive nicotinic receptor antagonist. It is most effective at doses of 300 mg per day. Treatment should begin 1 week before the quit date, usually at a dose of 150 mg per day. The effect of bupropion on tobacco dependence is independent of its effect on depression. It is effective in smokers, even if they are not depressed, and its effects are independent of gender or race (59–61), or prior history of alcoholism (62).

Because of the relationship between smoking and depression, other antidepressant drugs have been tested. The tricyclic antidepressant nortriptyline (10 mg per day) in combination with cognitive behavioral counseling, was found to be effective for smoking cessation (63). Doxepin has also been shown to effective in a small sample of patients.

Course and Prognosis

Even after 30 or more years of regular smoking, there are significant benefits to cessation (64). Older smokers actually have a higher probability of success on any quit-attempt than do younger ones (65). In fact, positive predictors of sustained abstinence (12–24 months) include previous attempts to stop smoking and greater age (for each 10 years, the adjusted odds ratio was found to be 1.3) (66). Combining behavioral treatments with medical treatments doubles the chances of successfully quitting smoking. Older smokers should be educated on the health benefits of quitting. A recent study reviewed 20 prospective cohort studies of smokers who were diagnosed with coronary heart disease (CHD) that included reports of all-cause mortality and had at least 2 years of follow-up (67). Results showed a 36% reduction in relative risk of mortality for patients with CHD who quit compared with those who continued smoking. This risk reduction was consistent regardless of age, gender, or index cardiac event.

Further, unlike alcohol, reducing tobacco use is not associated with health benefits. A recently pooled analysis of 19,732 persons, followed at 5-year to 10-year intervals, found that heavy smokers (15 or more cigarettes per day) who reduced their daily tobacco intake without quitting, had the same risk of tobacco-related mortality as persons who continued to smoke heavily (68). For subjects who quit smoking, however, the estimates were significantly lower than that of the smokers. Similarly, quitting smoking was associated with a significant reduction in the risk of hospital admission for patients with COPD (69). Those who reduced but did not quit did not achieve a similar advantage. These results demonstrate that smoking reduction is not associated with decreased mortality or morbidity from tobacco-related diseases and confirm that smoking cessation is effective. Every effort should be made to encourage smokers to quit.

Patients with tobacco dependence should be evaluated for depression during the early phases of a quit-attempt, and then again at regular intervals during abstinence. Smokers with a history of depression are at increased risk of a depressive episode in the 6 months after they quit smoking (70). The presence of depressive symptoms during tobacco abstinence is associated with resumption of tobacco use, failed quit-attempts, and a higher number of quit attempts (71). Depressive episodes should, therefore, be treated.

Women and Tobacco

The vast majority of American women are nonsmokers (72). Women with less than a high school education are about three times more likely to be smokers than are women with a college education. Native American or Alaskan women are much more likely to smoke than are Hispanic women and Asian or Pacific Islander women.

TABLE 32-4

FEATURES OF NICOTINE REPLACEMENT THERAPY MODALITIES

Modality	Route of Administration	Dosing	Adverse Events	Advantages	Disadvantages

Gum	■ "Bite and park"
	■ Absorption through buccal mucosa
		■ >25 cigs/day: 4 mg
		■ <24 cigs/day: 2 mg
		■ USE:
		  ■ Weeks 1–6: one piece every 1–2 hours
		  ■ Weeks 7–9: one piece every 2–4 hours
		  ■ Weeks 10–12: one piece every 4–8 hours
		  ■ Maximum dose: 24 pieces/day
			■ Tingling sensation
			■ Hiccups
			■ Upset stomach
			■ Sore jaws
				■ Immediate relief	■ Improper use or underdosing frequently occur

Patch	■ Dermal absorption
	■ Daily administration
	■ Two durations:
	  ■ 16 hour: Nicotrol
	  ■ 24 hour: Nicoderm
	■ Patch is taken off at night if sleep disturbance occurs
		■ Nicotrol: 15, 10, and 5 mg/day
		■ USE: Start with 15 mg patch for 6 weeks, then go to10 mg patch for 2 weeks, then go to 5 mg patch for 2 more weeks, then discontinue
		■ Nicoderm: 21, 14, and 7 mg/day
		■ USE:
		  ■ >10 cigs/day start with 21mg, otherwise, begin with 14 mg dose.
		  ■ Start 21 mg/day dose for 6 weeks, then go to 14 mg/day for 2 weeks, then go to 7 mg/day for 2 weeks, then discontinue
			■ Insomnia
			■ Skin irritation
			■ Skin itching
			■ Skin redness
				■ Adherence is more likely than other modalities	■ Not effective for immediate relief
					■ Frequently must be used with another agent

Inhaler	■ Oral puffer with cartridges ■ Absorption through buccal mucosa	■ Cartridge used for 20–60 min ■ Maximum dose is 16 cartridges/day	■ Irritation of throat/ mouth ■ Cough	■ Simulates sensory/ ritual aspects of smoking	■ Considerable puffing is needed for absorption
Nasal spray	■ Absorption through nasal mucosa	■ 1 mg/dose ■ 1–2 sprays per hour for 1st 8 weeks; then reduce dose by 1/2 for next 2 weeks, then discontinue	■ Nasal irritation ■ Sneezing ■ Lacrimation ■ Rhinorrhea ■ Nosebleeds ■ Headaches	■ Most rapid delivery ■ May be especially useful in severely dependent smokers ■ Highest peak serum levels	■ AEs common (80%) ■ Discontinuation due to AEs ■ Available via prescription only

Lozenge	■ Absorption through buccal mucosa	■ Maximum of 32 doses/day
		■ If time to 1st cig is <30 minutes: 4 mg
		■ If time to 1st cig is >30 min: 2 mg
		■ USE:
		  ■ Weeks 1–6: one piece every 1–2 hours
		  ■ Weeks 7–9: one piece every 2–4 hours
		  ■ Weeks 10–12: one piece every 4–8 hours
			■ Heartburn
			■ Indigestion
			■ Insomnia
			■ Nausea
			■ Hiccups
			■ Coughing
				■ Immediate relief	■ If chewed or swallowed, dosing is incorrect and can lead to AEs

Sublingual tablet	■ Placed under tongue, buccal absorption
	■ Lasts up to 15–20 minutes
		■ 2 mg/tablet
		■ USE:
		  ■ <20 cigs/day: one tablet per hour
		  ■ >20 cigs/day: two tablets per hour
		  ■ Full dose for first 3 months, then taper
			■ Mouth irritation
			■ Coughing
			■ Hiccups
			■ Dizziness
				■ Immediate relief
				■ Easier to use than other modalities
					■ Not available in United States

AEs, adverse events; cig, cigarette.

In 1987, lung cancer surpassed breast cancer as the leading cause of cancer deaths in American women. Two years earlier, the tobacco industry specifically targeted women by linking cigarette use with women's rights and progress in society. Interestingly, the women most empowered in our society, as measured by educational attainment, are the least likely to be smokers. This recognition can be an important tool in helping women quit smoking.

Among women, tobacco has also been associated with greater risk of cancers of the oropharynx, bladder, kidney, larynx, cervix, colon, rectum, liver, and esophagus. Smoking is a major cause of CHD, ischemic stroke, and peripheral vascular disease among women. Similarly, cigarette smoking is the primary cause of COPD in women, and mortality rates for COPD have increased among women for the past 20 to 30 years. The risk for these disorders increases with the amount and duration of cigarette use. Women smokers have natural menopause at a younger age than do nonsmokers, may experience more severe menopausal symptoms, and postmenopausal women who smoke have lower bone density than women who never smoked. As a result, women who smoke have an increased risk for hip fracture. Women smokers have an increased risk for cataracts, and may have an increased risk for age-related macular degeneration.

Women who stop smoking greatly reduce their risk of dying prematurely. Smoking cessation reduces the excess risk of CHD, no matter at what age women stop smoking. The risk is substantially reduced within 1 or 2 years after they stop smoking. The increased risk of stroke associated with smoking begins to reverse after women stop smoking, and approaches that of a woman who never smoked about 10 to 15 years after stopping.

Functional Loss

Smoking is a major risk factor for a number of chronic illnesses, including cardiovascular disease, COPD, hypertension, cancer, diabetic complications, and osteoporosis. Women smokers who die of a smoking-related disease, on average, lose 14 years of potential life. Approximately 10% of all current and former adult smokers have a smoking-attributable chronic disease, which often leads to a poorer quality of life (73). Among current smokers, chronic bronchitis was the most prevalent (49%) condition, followed by emphysema (24%). For former smokers, the three most prevalent conditions were chronic bronchitis (26%), emphysema (24%), and previous heart attack (24%).

Legal and Ethical Issues

The Centers for Medicare and Medicaid Services is conducting a demonstration to test smoking cessation as a Medicare benefit. The demonstration will compare the impact on quit rates from offering three different types of benefits for smoking cessation services: 1) reimbursement for provider counseling only; 2) reimbursement for provider counseling and NRT; 3) a telephone counseling quit line and reimbursement for NRT. The study was completed in 2004. A smoking cessation benefit could be legislated pending the results of this demonstration and Congressional approval.

PRESCRIPTION DRUG ABUSE

The misuse of prescribed medications is commonly problematic for the elderly. Older people are prescribed medications about three times more frequently than the general population, and have poorer compliance with directions for use. The two classes most commonly misused by the elderly are benzodiazepines and narcotics.

Benzodiazepines

Benzodiazepine (BZD) use in older adults can be categorized as *acute, intermittent* (either short or long term), or *continuous* (74). Acute use lasts 7 days or less, frequently consists of a single dose, and typically occurs in a health care setting. Examples are preoperative or premedication for uncomfortable or painful procedures, or the treatment of insomnia or agitation in the hospital. Acute use has not been historically associated with BZD use disorders, but 3% to 6% of older adults begin taking BZDs while in the hospital (2,3). Unfortunately, indications for new BZD prescriptions in hospitalized elderly are poorly documented in a third of cases. As many as 12% of older adults, supplied with a BZD prescription at hospital discharge, were prescribed the BZD "routinely" at the time of admission, without a specific indication (75). As many as 38% of older adults will refill these BZD discharge prescriptions for an additional 3 or more months following discharge (76). Medical hospitalization is thus a significant risk factor for initiation and continuation of BZD use for some elderly, even where there may be no medical indication.

Short-term intermittent use occurs when a BZD is taken sporadically, generally less than two to three times per week or for periods not exceeding 60 to 90 days. Long-term intermittent use is the same pattern of use but occurring for 4 months or longer. Intermittent use was the predominant pattern of prescription hypnotic use in a national study of more than 3,000 community-dwelling American adults older than 18. Among the elderly, reports of intermittent use vary from 36% to 70%, and community studies have found that 6% to 50% continue this usage pattern for 5 or more years (74).

Continuous use is defined as daily administration of at least one dose of BZD for 4 months or longer. Among BZD users, 21% and 17%, are continuous users for anxiety and insomnia, respectively (77). This is equal to a prevalence rate of 3% continuous use in the general population between the ages of 18 and 79. Compared to nonusers, *continuous* anxiolytic users are elderly, female, more likely to take other psychotropic medications, and have significantly more chronic medical problems, particularly cardiovascular and rheumatologic conditions (77). These patients are high utilizers of medical services, with 39% visiting their physician seven or more times per year.

One study reported that most, but not all, patients exposed to long-term, continuous, use of BZDs will develop physiological dependence (78). BZD dependence was defined in the study as having at least three of the following: physiological tolerance; withdrawal symptoms; impaired control; preoccupation with acquisition and/or use; persistent desire or unsuccessful efforts to quit; sustained social, occupational or recreational disability; or use continued despite adverse consequences (78). Many older adults, however, do not meet these criteria for BZD dependence. Some experts use withdrawal symptoms alone to define BZD dependence. However, older adults may not experience withdrawal symptoms, and, as a result, consensus has not yet been reached on the definition of BZD dependence as a disorder. Dose escalation is rare in the elderly, with only 1.8% using higher daily doses than originally prescribed (79).

Epidemiology

While older adults represent about 13% of the population, they receive 27% of all prescriptions for anxiolytic BZDs and 38% of hypnotic BZDs (77). Current and 1-year exposure to BZD use for the elderly average 15.2% (range 10.7–42%) and 32% (range 9–54%), respectively (74). As many as one in four elderly BZD users currently take a long half-life BZD.

Among older community-dwelling adults referred for prescription drug abuse, a 1990 study reported that most were abusing BZDs (80). The majority of these individuals were women who took three or more prescription drugs of abuse simultaneously. Almost one in three had histories of prior psychiatric hospitalizations, 36% started abusing prescription drugs after age 65, 92% had abused prescription drugs longer than 5 years, and 24%, longer than 21 years. The long-acting BZDs diazepam and flurazepam accounted for 76% of BZD prescriptions. A 60% correlation between prescription drug abuse and alcoholism was found.

Among geriatric psychiatry outpatients, prevalence of BZD dependence was reported to be 11.4% (81). These patients were again mostly women, taking 5.5 medications for 4.3 medical diagnoses and 62.5% and 43.8% experienced comorbid depression and dementia, respectively. Among psychiatrically hospitalized elderly, 18% met criteria for BZD dependence (82), with 89% having comorbid depression and 89% having histories of drug abuse.

Assessment and Diagnosis

Despite consistent recommendations to prescribe BZDs for short-term intermittent periods, a small but significant group of mostly elderly women use BZDs daily for extended time periods, often years. The clinician must therefore determine whether BZD use is appropriate and should continue, whether an attempt should be made to discontinue BZD use, or whether there is evidence of abuse and/or dependence.

DuPont has developed a checklist to assist the clinician in the assessment of BZD treatment (83). The four areas of assessment are:

- Indication: What is the indication for BZD use and is it appropriate? Are the quality of life and functioning improved for the patient through this use?
- Drug use: Is the dose escalating or stable? Is there evidence or history of abuse of other substances, particularly alcohol or prescription narcotics?
- Toxic behavior: Is the patient experiencing adverse events as a result of the BZD use, and to what extent do they interfere with the patient's daily functioning? Could these adverse events result in serious injury to the patient or others?
- Family monitor: What impact, positive or negative, do family members ascribe to the BZD, and how do they feel about continued use?

If there is no indication for the use of a BZD, a patient's daily functioning is impaired, the dose of medication is escalating, or use is in conjunction with alcohol or other psychotropics, discontinuation should be strongly recommended. The Severity of Dependence Scale has been validated as a sensitive (97.9%) and specific (94.2%) instrument to screen for BZD dependence (84). It is a brief self-report questionnaire asking the following questions: 1) Did you think your use of tranquilizers was out of control? 2) Did the prospect of missing a dose make you anxious or worried? 3) Did you worry about your use of tranquilizers? 4) Did you wish you could stop? 5) How difficult would you find it to stop or go without your tranquilizers?

Differential Diagnosis

Among 153 adult patients with BZD dependence, (15% of sample older than 65), comorbid disorders were as follows: 31% anxiety disorders, 20% affective disorders, 53% personality disorders (59% anxious cluster disorders) (85). Depressed elderly often receive prescriptions for BZDs to treat the anxiety symptoms associated with unrecognized depression. This may explain the high association of BZD dependence and depression. Of great concern is that BZDs have no demonstrated efficacy for depression. Older depressed adults inappropriately treated with BZDs may experience worsening of their depression, further feelings of despondency due to their perceived lack of response to treatment and, as a result, may attempt or commit suicide. Conversely, BZDs may act like alcohol in disinhibiting individuals, particularly older men, who are contemplating suicide. BZDs were found in the serum of 30% and 47% of a sample of older Hispanic men and women, respectively, who committed suicide (86), and 15% of all elderly perpetrators of homicide-suicide events (87). None of those individuals committed suicide via overdose. Thus, patients taking BZDs should always be screened for depression and suicidality.

Pharmacology of Benzodiazepine Use

Changes that occur with aging (e.g., increases in body fat, decreases in lean body mass, and decreases in body water) increase the volume of distribution of BZDs, particularly in women. Serum albumin levels may decrease by 15% to 20% in some older patients, without a change in total protein levels, leading to an increase in the pharmacologically active free drug fraction, and in some cases potentiation of the medication effect. Therefore, geriatric patients are more sensitive to the clinical effects of BZDs, and often require a lower dose of a BZD to achieve sedation.

Metabolism of many drugs decreases with age, such that after 70 years of age it may be reduced by up to 30% (88). Age-related reductions in the clearance of BZDs that are metabolized by phase I oxidation (such as diazepam, desalkylflurazepam, alprazolam, and triazolam) are known to occur. BZDs metabolized mainly by glucuronide (phase II) conjugation (e.g., oxazepam, lorazepam, and temazepam), have minimal age-related decreases in active drug clearance. Therefore, BZDs metabolized through phase II pathways are considered safer and more appropriate for older patients.

Treatment

A strategy of periodic discontinuation to identify the subgroup of patients whose anxiety is truly persistent and may require long-term BZD treatment is often helpful (89). These patients may also be candidates for trials of antidepressants to manage anxiety symptoms. Additionally, this strategy will identify people who no longer need medication. Often, an older female patient may not realize this class of medications may be habit-forming. Once educated about this, many older patients will spontaneously request discontinuation.

A brief intervention strategy, similar to the brief alcohol intervention, may prove useful in the prevention and management of continuous BZD use, as well as abuse and dependence in the elderly. To facilitate the decision to discontinue a BZD, a review of the negative and positive aspects of BZD use, including potential for physiological dependence, drug-drug interactions, and adverse effects, helps the patient set personal goals based on a logical rationale. A review of withdrawal symptoms that are common is helpful and reassurance that symptoms will abate within 4 to 5 weeks is provided. Behavioral treatments, including sleep hygiene techniques and exercise plans, can be discussed and should be implemented prior to discontinuation. Written instructions detailing the tapering schedule should be given to the patient. It is advisable to administer increasingly smaller doses at several times throughout the day, until the end of the taper period when the last dose is given at bedtime. Doses can be reduced by 12.5% to 25%

of the total daily dose each week. Some patients will require slowing of this taper to a reduction every 2 weeks.

Withdrawal

About one-third of patients who attempt to discontinue a BZD will do so easily, another one-third will experience some difficulty, and the final third will have significant or prolonged problems. Elderly patients, when compared to younger adults, experience less severe withdrawal, with fewer symptoms and less anxiety, and fewer require slowing of the taper rate (90). In older adults, BZD plasma levels decline more slowly, possibly explaining this attenuation of withdrawal symptoms.

Factors associated with increased risk for withdrawal symptoms include abrupt discontinuation (particularly with short–half-life agents), rapid rate of decline of plasma BZD levels, higher daily BZD dosage, and longer duration of treatment (91,92). Insomnia is the most troubling symptom that leads to resumption of BZD use (92). Withdrawal that leads to delirium or psychotic symptoms should trigger immediate replacement of 50% to 75% of the total daily dose taken by the patient, followed by a gradual taper of 10% to 20% (93). With the exception of alprazolam, which is a high-potency drug, short–half-life BZDs can be replaced with longer half-life agents for purposes of detoxification. Clonazepam, a high-potency BZD with a long half-life, may be used to detoxify patients from alprazolam. The dose of the longer-acting agent is then tapered over 6 to 8 weeks. These guidelines, however, have been developed for younger patients, and treatment considerations always need to be individualized for older patients. A small number of patients may require inpatient detoxification.

Course and Prognosis

Older adults can be successfully detoxified from BZDs. In fact, at 6 weeks, more than 60% remain BZD free and remain off these medications at 12 months (94,95). Importantly, elderly nursing home residents who discontinue BZDs often demonstrate improved cognitive functioning.

Psychosocial Issues

Older adults who initiate treatment with a long-acting BZD exhibited a 50% increased rate of involvement in injurious motor vehicle accidents within the first week of treatment, and this risk remains elevated for up to 1 year of continuous use (96). No increased risk was associated with continuous use of short–half-life BZDs. The increasing number of older drivers, combined with the high prevalence of BZD prescriptions, make this a significant public health problem and an important consideration prior to starting a BZD in older drivers. Moreover, older drivers should never be prescribed long-acting BZDs.

Special Populations

BZDs have been prescribed to treat behavioral disturbances associated with dementia (97). The Omnibus Budget

Reconciliation Act of 1987 mandated that all residents of skilled nursing facilities have the right to be free of psychotropic drugs, unless indicated to treat a specific condition. A review of the literature found that sedative–hypnotics were the second most commonly prescribed class of psychotropics in the nursing home setting, with a range of 7% to 40% of residents (98).

Beers and colleagues developed explicit criteria for the determination of appropriate use of 26 medication categories including BZDs (99). According to these criteria, BZD use in frail elderly is inappropriate, as follows: 1) any use of flurazepam, diazepam, or chlordiazepoxide; 2) if daily recommended dosing limits are exceeded (3 mg of lorazepam; 60 mg of oxazepam; 2 mg of alprazolam; 15 mg of temazepam; and 0.25 mg of triazolam. Utilizing these criteria, almost 2 million physician office visits in 1992 involved an inappropriate prescription of flurazepam, diazepam, or chlordiazepoxide (100).

Narcotics

As with BZDs, older patients are more likely to be prescribed narcotics for longer periods of time than younger patients (101). Compared with younger patients, older adults who misuse and abuse these drugs are more likely to have other primary psychiatric diagnoses (particularly depression), have cognitive impairment, and report sleep disturbances, irritability, delusions, violent behavior, and have a diminished ability to perform activities of daily living (102). Distinguishing among normal use, misuse, abuse, and dependence in an older population is a major challenge to clinicians, and the presence of multiple medical disorders can add to the difficulty (103).

Misuse
Most problems with drug dependency in an older population involve misuse of prescription drugs. Misuse is often unintentional due to such factors as an older adult's inability to manage the schedule and number of prescribed medications, failure to follow instructions, cognitive impairment, and interaction of multiple medications (104). Specifically, older adults can misuse opioid analgesics for a variety of reasons including: 1) a lack of judgment or misconceptions about the drugs; 2) an inability to manage the medication regimen due to complexity or cognitive impairment; 3) insufficient resources for purchasing or storing medications; and 4) intentional misuse to obtain results other than for those prescribed (e.g., to sleep, relax, or self-medicate depression or anxiety) (1).

Abuse and Dependence
There is little available information about narcotics abuse and dependence in the older population, but they are generally thought to be underdiagnosed (105). Criteria for abuse/

dependence are generally similar to those for younger adults. Older patients who abuse opioids are more likely than younger patients to underreport the extent of their use, be socially isolated, and are less likely to engage in criminal behavior. Consequently, older adults typically have suffered fewer social consequences of their addictive behavior, and this makes it difficult for a clinician to identify the problem. Additionally, other negative consequences of opioid abuse and dependence can be confused with problems that frequently occur with aging including constipation, falls, and impaired cognition (106).

Epidemiology
It is generally believed that older adults who abuse narcotics in late life are simply younger addicts grown old because very few older adults initiate opioid drug use in their later years. When opioid dependence does develop late in life it may be the result of a failure to cope with late-life stressors, including retirement, loss of spouse or other loved ones, and loss of function due to illness (102).

An estimated 2% of community-dwelling older adults receive prescriptions for opioid analgesics (107). Propoxyphene, a synthetic narcotic, is among the most frequently misused drugs by community-based older adults (108). The mean annual admission rate for prescription drug substance use disorders among all older patients in one study was 16%, and of these, half reported addiction to opioid analgesics (103).

Alarmingly, while only 3.6% of emergency room visits for heroin or morphine abuse are in persons older than 55 (109), this figure has doubled in the past 10 years. Of equal concern are reports that some older adults are obtaining prescription narcotics, in particular oxycodone, and then selling the medications for financial gain (104).

Assessment and Diagnosis
Older adults should be asked on an annual basis about their use of prescription narcotics including codeine, morphine, oxycodone, propoxyphene, hydrocodone, and hydromorphone, as well as meperidine. There are some elderly who may not realize that these are narcotics. In other cases, they may be taking the medication inappropriately. The health care provider must often have a high index of suspicion and actively inquire about usage patterns. Table 32-5 summarizes signs that should prompt a more in-depth assessment for narcotics abuse/dependence. The Dupont checklist previously described can be adapted to narcotics use and is helpful in determining when an attempt at discontinuing a narcotic is in the patient's best interests.

It is often helpful to track refills once it is known that a patient is taking a narcotic, for two reasons. First, abuse and misuse is more easily identified. Second, undermed-

TABLE 32-5

WARNING SIGNS THAT SHOULD PROMPT A MORE IN-DEPTH ASSESSMENT FOR NARCOTIC ABUSE

- Excessively worrying about whether opioid analgesics are "really working" to alleviate numerous physical complaints; complaints that the drug prescribed has lost its effectiveness over time (evidence of tolerance)
- Displaying detailed knowledge about a specific opioid drug and attaching great significance to its efficacy and personal impact
- Worrying about having enough pills or whether it is time to take them, to the extent that other activities revolve around the dosage schedule
- Continuing to use and to request refills when the physical or psychological condition for which the drug was originally prescribed has or should have improved; resisting cessation or decreasing doses of a prescribed opioid analgesic
- Complaining about doctors who refuse to write prescriptions for preferred drugs, who taper dosages, or who do not take symptoms seriously
- Self-medicating by increasing doses of opioids that are not "helping anymore" or supplementing prescribed drugs with over-the-counter medications of a similar type

icating may be a reason for uncontrolled pain, and this is a useful way to make this determination clinically.

Additionally, if a provider becomes aware that a patient is receiving narcotics from several providers, he/she should contact those providers to make them aware of the potential abuse. They can then agree as to which provider will manage the narcotics. It is important to recognize that older patients may not accept a diagnosis of addiction because they are taking medications that have been prescribed to them by their physician (102).

Pharmacology of Narcotics

Narcotic dose requirements can decrease with age, while the duration of action increases. Older persons develop tolerance and physical dependence more rapidly, and are more likely than younger persons to experience respiratory depression and other side effects of opioid use including sedation, constipation and fecal impaction, substantial vision impairment, decrease in attention and motor coordination, and falls with hip fractures (1,110).

Treatment

An important aspect of initiating treatment is to provide education regarding the habit-forming potential of these medications, and the use of phrases such as "the body becomes used to having the medication," rather than the term "addiction." Older patients with addiction to prescription narcotics should be referred early for appropriate psychiatric, addiction, and pain management services; and age-specific treatment is preferable to mixed-age groups (104).

Biopsychosocial Treatments

Psychotherapeutic approaches are similar to those that have been previously described for other addictive disorders.

Pharmacotherapy

Pharmacologic treatment has historically consisted of drug cocktails that treat withdrawal symptoms. An example would be a combination of a BZD (for symptoms of anxiety, tremors, insomnia), an antihistamine (for symptoms of rhinorrhea, watery eyes, pruritis), and a belladonna alkaloid antispasmodic (for diarrhea and cramping). A possible regimen would be: 1 mg lorazepam twice a day, plus 25 mg diphenhydramine twice or three times a day, plus one to two tablets of Donnatal twice or three times a day. This regimen is given to the patient for the first 3 to 5 days, and then gradually tapered during the next 5–9 days. Dosages may have to be adjusted either up or down, depending on the severity of withdrawal symptoms, adverse effects of the medications, duration and dosage of narcotic use, age, and comorbid medical disorders of the patient. There is little empirical evidence either in favor of or against this method of detoxification in the elderly, although for individuals with mild-to-moderate narcotic dependence this may be a useful regimen.

For significant opioid addiction, methadone treatment has been used for more than 30 years. The medication is taken orally and has a duration of action of about 24 hours, four to six times longer than heroin. Methadone relieves the craving associated with heroin addiction, a major reason for relapse. Levo-alpha-acetyl-methadol (LAAM), like methadone, is a synthetic opiate that can be used to treat heroin addiction and was approved by the FDA for this indication in 1993. LAAM can block the effects of heroin for up to 72 hours with minimal side effects when taken orally. Its long duration of action permits dosing just three times per week, thereby eliminating the need for daily dosing and take-home doses for weekends. Naloxone and naltrexone are opiate antagonists, which are especially useful as antidotes. The efficacy and safety of these agents have not been specifically evaluated in the elderly.

Buprenorphine is a partial opioid agonist. At low doses, it enables opioid-addicted individuals to discontinue the opioid use without experiencing withdrawal symptoms. It has the potential of causing respiratory depression in higher doses, and should be used cautiously in patients with hepatic or gall bladder disease and in the elderly in general. There are three phases of buprenorphine maintenance therapy: induction, stabilization, and maintenance. Buprenorphine is unlikely to be as effective as optimal-dose methadone, and therefore may not be the treatment of choice for patients with higher levels of physical dependence. Few studies have been reported on the efficacy of buprenorphine for completely withdrawing patients from opioids. Buprenorphine, however, is known to cause a milder withdrawal syndrome compared to methadone and thus may be the better choice if opioid withdrawal is the goal.

Women and Narcotics

Older women are more likely to have problems with prescription drug abuse and dependence. This is due to their being more likely than older men to visit physicians and to be given prescriptions (42,103,111). A study of consecutive admissions to a substance abuse treatment program noted that 70% admitted for prescription drug abuse were women, and of those, 50% were admitted for dependence on opioids (111). Physicians may not recognize or suspect prescription drug abuse in older women even when faced with multiple symptoms and signs. Only 2% of physicians, for example, presented with a hypothetical case of an older woman with signs of prescription drug abuse considered substance abuse as a leading diagnosis (112).

Chronic Pain

Opioids are essential for the medical management of moderate-to-severe acute pain, pain due to cancer, and certain types of chronic pain. There is little evidence that addictive problems are more prevalent in older patients with chronic pain than any other groups (42,111,112). Many health care providers underprescribe narcotics because they overestimate the potential for addiction. Although these drugs carry a heightened risk, research has shown that providers' concerns that patients will become addicted to pain medication are largely unfounded. Most patients who are prescribed opioids for pain, even long-term therapy, do not develop addiction. Those who do develop rapid and marked tolerance for opioids usually have a history of psychological problems or prior substance abuse. One study found that only four out of about 12,000 patients who were given opioids for acute pain became addicted. In a study of 38 chronic pain patients, most of whom received opioids for 4 to 7 years, only two patients became addicted, and both had a history of drug abuse (111).

REFERENCES

1. Blow F. Substance abuse among older adults. Treatment Improvement Protocol (TIP) series 26. Rockville, MD: U.S. Dept. Health and Human Services, Public Health Service, Substance Abuse and Mental Health Services, Center for Substance Abuse Treatment, 1998.
2. American Psychiatric Association. *Diagnostic and Statistical Manual of Mental Disorders, Fourth Edition, Text Revision.* Washington, DC: American Psychiatric Press, 2000.
3. Department of Defense and Veterans Health Administration. VHA/DoD Clinical practice guideline for the management of substance use disorders. http://www.guideline.gov/summary/summary.aspx?ss=15&doc_id=3169. Accessed September 6, 2003.
4. National Institute on Alcohol Abuse and Alcoholism. Diagnostic criteria for alcohol abuse. *Alcohol Alert.* 1995;30(PH 359):1–6.
5. Chermack ST, Blow FC, Hill EM, Mudd SA. The relationship between alcohol symptoms and consumption among older drinkers. *Alcohol Clin Exp Res.* 1996;20:1153–1158.
6. Klatsky AL, Armstrong MA. Alcohol use, other traits, and risk of unnatural death: a prospective study. *Alcohol Clin Exp Res.* 1993;17:1156–1162.
7. Poikolainen K. Epidemiologic assessment of population risks and benefits of alcohol use. *Alcohol Alcohol Suppl.* 1991;1:27–34.
8. Helzer JE, Burnam A, McEvoy LT. Alcohol abuse and dependence. In Robins LN, Regier DA, eds. *Psychiatric Disorder in America: The Epidemiologic Catchment Area Study.* New York: Free Press; 1991:81–115.
9. Barry KL, Blow FC, Walton MA, et al. Elder-specific brief alcohol intervention: 3-month outcomes. *Alcohol Clin Exp Res.* 1998;22:32A.
10. Callahan CM, Tierney WM. Health services use and mortality among older primary care patients with alcoholism. *J Am Geriatr Soc.* 1995;43:1378–1383.
11. Holroyd S, Duryee JJ. Substance use disorders in a geriatric psychiatry outpatient clinic: prevalence and epidemiologic characteristics. *J Nerv Ment Dis.* 1997;185:627–632.
12. Joseph CL, Ganzini L, Atkinson R. Screening for alcohol use disorders in the nursing home. *J Am Geriatr Soc.* 1995;43: 368–373.
13. Oslin DW, Streim JE, Parmelee P, Boyce AA, Katz IR. Alcohol abuse: a source of reversible functional disability among residents of a VA nursing home. *Int J Geriatr Psychiatry.* 1997;12: 825–832.
14. Speer DC, Bates K. Comorbid mental and substance disorders among older psychiatric patients. *J Am Geriatr Soc.* 1992;40: 886–890.
15. Saunders PA, Copeland JR, Dewey ME, et al. Heavy drinking as a risk factor for depression and dementia in elderly men. Findings from the Liverpool longitudinal community study. *Br J Psychiatry .*1991;159:213–216.
16. Cook BG, Winokur G, Garvey MJ, Beach V. Depression and previous alcoholism in the elderly. *Br J Psychiatry.* 1991;158:72–75.
17. Ewing JA. Detecting alcoholism. The CAGE questionnaire. *JAMA.* 1984;252:1905–1907.
18. Blow FC, Brower KJ, Schulenberg JE, Demo-Dananberg LM, Young KJ, Beresford, TP. The Michigan Alcoholism Screening Test—Geriatric Version (MAST-G): A new elderly-specific screening instrument [Abstract]. *Alcohol Clin Exp Res.* 1992;16:372.
19. Fraser AG. Pharmacokinetic interactions between alcohol and other drugs. *Clin Pharmacokinet.* 1997;33:79–90.
20. Hurt RD, Finlayson RE, Morse RM, Davis LJ Jr. Alcoholism in elderly persons: medical aspects and prognosis of 216 inpatients. *Mayo Clin Proc.* 1988;63:753–760.
21. Kessler RC, Berglund P, Demler O, et al. The epidemiology of major depressive disorder: results from the National Comorbidity Survey Replication (NCS-R). *JAMA.* 2003; 3095–3105.
22. Blow FC, Cook CA, Booth BM, Falcon SP, Friedman MJ. Age-related psychiatric comorbidities and level of functioning in alcoholic veterans seeking outpatient treatment. *Hosp Community Psychiatry.* 1992;43:990–995.
23. Brown SA, Schuckit MA. Changes in depression among abstinent alcoholics. *Journal J Stud Alcohol.* 1988;49:412–417.
24. George LK, Landerman R, Blazer DG, et al. Cognitive impairment. In Robins LN, Regier DA, eds. *Psychiatric Disorders in America: The Epidemiologic Catchment Area Study.* New York: Free Press; 1991:291–327.
25. Oslin DW, Cary MS. Alcohol-related dementia: validation of diagnostic criteria. *Am J Geriatr Psychiatry.* 2003;11:441–447.
26. Kerr WC, Fillmore KM, Bostrom A. Stability of alcohol consumption over time: evidence from three longitudinal surveys from the United States. *J Stud Alcohol.* 2002;63:325–333.
27. Schutte KK, Brennan PL, Moos RH. Predicting the development of late-life late-onset drinking problems: a 7-year prospective study. *Alcohol Clin Exp Res.* 1998;22:1349–1358.
28. Mann DMA, Neary D, Testa H. *Color Atlas and Text of Adult Dementias.* New York: Mosby-Wolfe; 1994:95–96.
29. Stuppaeck CH, Barnas C, Falk M, et al. Assessment of the alcohol withdrawal syndrome: validity and reliability for the translated and modified Clinical Institute Withdrawal Assessment for Alcohol Scale (CIWA-A). *Addiction.* 1994;89:1287–1292.
30. Fleming MF, Manwell LB, Barry KL, Adams W, Stauffacher EA. Brief physician advice for alcohol problems in older adults: a randomized community-based trial. *J Fam Pract.* 1999;48: 378–384.
31. Barry KL, Oslin DW, Blow FC. *Prevention and Management of Alcohol Problems in Older Adults.* New York: Springer Publishing, 2001.
32. Miller W, Rollnick S. *Motivational Interviewing: Preparing People to Change Addictive Behavior.* New York: Guilford Press; 1991.
33. Oslin D, Liberto JG, O'Brien J, Krois S, Norbeck J. Naltrexone as an adjunctive treatment for older patients with alcohol dependence. *Am J Geriatr Psychiatry.* 1997;5:324–332.

34. American Psychiatric Association. Practice guideline for the treatment of patients with substance use disorders: alcohol, cocaine, opioids. *Am J Psychiatry* 1995; 152(Nov Suppl): 1–59.

35. Oslin DW, Pettinati H, Volpicelli JR. Alcoholism treatment adherence: older age predicts better adherence and drinking outcomes. *Am J Geriatr Psychiatry*. 2002;10:740–747.

36. Vaillant GE. What can long-term follow-up teach us about relapse and prevention of relapse in addiction? *Br J Addict*. 1988;83:1147–1157.

37. Vaillant GE. A 20-year follow-up of New York narcotic addicts. *Arch Gen Psychiatry*. 1973;29:237–241.

38. Joseph C, Rasmussen J, Ganzini L, Atkinson RM. Outcome of nursing home care for residents with alcohol use disorders. *Int J Geriatr Psy*. 1997;12:767–772.

39. Alderete E, Vega WA, Kolody B, Aguilar-Gaxiola S. Lifetime prevalence of and risk factors for psychiatric disorders among Mexican migrant farmworkers in California. *Am J Public Health*. 2000;90:608–614.

40. Yamamoto J, Yamamoto M, Steinberg A, et al. Alcohol abuse among elderly Asians in Los Angeles: a pilot study. *Pacific/Asian American Mental Health Research Center Research Review*. 1988;6:26–27.

41. Arroyo JA, Westerberg VS, Tonigan JS. Comparison of treatment utilization and outcome for Hispanics and non-Hispanic Whites. *J Stud Alcohol*. 1998;59:286–291.

42. The National Center on Addiction and Substance Abuse at Columbia University. Under the rug: substance abuse and the mature woman. http://www.casacolumbia.org/publications 1456/publications. Accessed September 6, 2003.

43. Rapuri PB, Gallagher JC, Balhorn KE, Ryschon KL. Alcohol intake and bone metabolism in elderly women. *Am J Clin Nu*. 2000;72:1206–1213.

44. Thun MJ, Peto R, Lopez AD, et al. Alcohol consumption and mortality among middle-aged and elderly US adults. *N Engl J Med*. 1997; 337:1705–1714.

45. de Labry LO, Glynn RJ, Levenson MR, Hermos JA, LoCastro JS, Vokonas PS. Alcohol consumption and mortality in an American male population: recovering the U-shaped curve—findings from the normative Aging Study. *J Stud Alcohol*. 1992;53:25–32.

46. Stampfer MJ, Colditz GA, Willett WC, Speizer FE, Hennekens CH. A prospective study of moderate alcohol consumption and the risk of coronary disease and stroke in women. *N Engl J Med*. 1988;319:267–273.

47. Liberto JG, Oslin DW, Ruskin PE. Alcoholism in older persons: a review of the literature. *Hosp Community Psychiatry*. 1992;43:975–984.

48. US Department of Health and Human Services. The Health Consequences of Smoking. Nicotine addiction: a report of the Surgeon General (Publication No. CDC 88-8406). Washington DC: US Department of Health and Human Services, 1988.

49. US Department of Health and Human Services. Psychological and behavioral consequences and correlates of smoking cessation. In: Health Benefits of Smoking Cessation: a report of the US Surgeon General. Washington, DC, US Government Printing Office, 1990;517–578.

50. Centers for Disease Control and Prevention. Surveillance for five health risks among older adults—United States, 1993–1997. *Morbidity and Mortality Weekly Report*. 1999;48:89–130.

51. Lasser K, Boyd JW, Woolhandler S, Himmelstein DU, McCormick D, Bor DH. Smoking and mental illness: a population-based prevalence study. *JAMA*. 2000;284:2606–2610.

52. Payne TJ, Smith PO, McCracken LM, McSherry WC, Antony MM. Assessing nicotine dependence: a comparison of the Fagerstrom Tolerance Questionnaire (FTQ) with the Fagerstrom Test for Nicotine Dependence (FTND) in a clinical sample. *Addict Behav*. 1994;19:307–317.

53. Kozlowski LT, Porter CQ, Orleans CT, Pope MA, Heatherton T. Predicting smoking cessation with self-reported measures of nicotine dependence: FTQ, FTND, and HIS. *Drug Alcohol Depend*. 1994;34:211–216.

54. Katz DA, Muehlenbruch DR, Brown RB, Fiore MC, Baker TB; AHRQ Smoking Cessation Guideline Study Group. Effectiveness of a clinic-based strategy for implementing the AHRQ Smoking Cessation Guideline in primary care. *Prev Med*. 2002;35:293–301.

55. Fiore MC, Bailey WC, Cohen SJ, et al. *Treating Tobacco Use and Dependence. Clinical Practice Guideline*. Rockville, MD: US Department of Health and Human Services; 2000.

56. Murray RP, Bailey WC, Daniels K, et al. Safety of nicotine polacrilex gum used by 3,094 participants in the Lung Health Study. Lung Health Study Research Group. *Chest*. 1996;109: 438–445.

57. Benowitz NL, Gourlay SG. Cardiovascular toxicity of nicotine: implications for nicotine replacement therapy. *J Am Coll Cardiol*. 1997;29:1422–1431.

58. Joseph AM, Norman SM, Ferry LH, et al. The safety of transdermal nicotine as an aid to smoking cessation in patients with cardiac disease. *New England Journal of Medicine*. 1996;335:1792–1798.

59. Jorenby DE, Leischow SJ, Nides MA, et al. A controlled trial of sustained-release bupropion, a nicotine patch, or both for smoking cessation. *N Engl J Med*. 1999;340:685–691.

60. Ahluwalia JS, Harris KJ, Catley D, Okuyemi KS, Mayo MS. Sustained-release bupropion for smoking cessation in African-Americans: a randomized controlled trial. *JAMA*. 2002;288:468–474.

61. Gonzales D, Bjornson W, Durcan MJ, et al. Effects of gender on relapse prevention in smokers treated with bupropion SR. *Am J Prev Med*. 2002;22:234–239.

62. Evins AE, Mays VK, Rigotti NA, Tisdale T, Cather C, Goff DC. A pilot trial of bupropion added to cognitive behavioral therapy for smoking cessation in schizophrenia. *Nicotine Tob Res*. 2001;3:397–403.

63. Hall SM, Reus VI, Muñoz F, et al. Nortriptyline and cognitive-behavioral treatment of cigarette smoking. *Arch Gen Psychiatry*. 1998;55:683–690.

64. Morgan GD, Noll EL, Orleans CT, Rimer BK, Amfoh K, Bonney G. Reaching midlife and older smokers: tailored interventions for routine Medicare care. *Prev Med*. 1996;26:346–354.

65. Stapleton JA, Russell MA, Feyerabend C, et al. Dose effects and predictors of outcome in a randomized trial of transdermal nicotine patches in general practice. *Addiction*. 1995;90:31–42.

66. Grandes G, Cortada JM, Arrazola A, Laka JP. Predictors of long-term outcome of a smoking cessation programme in primary care. *Br J Gen Pract*. 2003;53:101–107.

67. Critchley JA, Capewell S. Mortality risk reduction associated with smoking cessation in patients with coronary heart disease: a systematic review. *JAMA*. 2003;290:86–97.

68. Godtfredsen NS, Holst C, Prescott E, Vestbo J, Osler M. Smoking reduction, smoking cessation, and mortality: a 16-year follow-up of 19,732 men and women from the Copenhagen Centre for Prospective Population Studies. *Am J Epidemiol*. 2002;156:994–1001.

69. Godtfredsen NS, Vestbo J, Osler M, Prescott E. Risk of hospital admission for COPD following smoking cessation and reduction: a Danish population study. *Thorax*. 2002;57:967–972.

70. Glassman AH, Covey LS, Stetner F, Rivelli S. Smoking cessation and the course of major depression: a follow-up study. *Lancet*. 2001;357:1929–1932.

71. Glassman AH, Helzer JE, Covey LS, et al. Smoking, smoking cessation and major depression. *JAMA*. 1990;64:1546–1549.

72. US Department of Health and Human Services. Women and smoking: a report of the Surgeon General 2001. http://www.cdc.gov/tobacco. Accessed September 21, 2003.

73. Centers for Disease Control and Prevention. Surveillance for five health risks among older adults—United States, 1993–1997. *Morbidity and Mortality Weekly Report*. 2003;52:842–844.

74. Llorente MD, David D, Golden A, Silverman MA. Defining patterns of benzodiazepine use in older adults. *J Geriatr Psychiatry Neurol*. 2000;13:150–160.

75. Surendrakumar D, Dunn M, Roberts CJ. Hospital admission and the start of benzodiazepine use. *BMJ*. 1992;304:881.

76. Grad R, Tamblyn R, Holbrook AM, Hurley J, Feightner J, Gayton D. Risk of a new benzodiazepine prescription in relation to recent hospitalization. *J Am Geriatr Soc*. 1999;47:184–188.

77. Pincus HA, Tanielian TL, Marcus SC, et al. Prescribing trends in psychotropic medications: primary care, psychiatry and other medical specialties. *JAMA*. 1998;279:526–531.

78. Linsen SM, Breteler MH, Zitman FG. Defining benzodiazepine dependence: the confusion persists. *European Psychiatry*. 1995;10:306–311.

79. Woods JH, Katz JL, Winger G. Benzodiazepines: use, abuse, and consequences. *Pharmacol Rev*. 1992;44:151–347.

80. Jinks MJ, Raschko RR. A profile of alcohol and prescription drug abuse in a high-risk community-based elderly population. *DICP*. 1990;24:971–975.

81. Holroyd S, Duryee JJ. Substance use disorders in a geriatric psychiatry outpatient clinic: prevalence and epidemiologic characteristics. *J Nerv Ment Dis*. 1997;185:627–632.

82. Whitcup SM, Miller F. Unrecognized drug dependence in psychiatrically hospitalized elderly patients. *J Am Geriatr Soc*. 1987;35:297–301.

83. DuPont RL. A practical approach to benzodiazepine discontinuation. *J Psychiatr Res*. 1990;24:81–90.

84. de las Cuevas C, Sanz EJ, de la Fuente JA, Padilla J, Berenguer JC. The Severity of Dependence Scale (SDS) as screening test for benzodiazepine dependence: SDS validation study. *Addiction*. 2000;95:245–250.

85. Martinez-Cano H, de Iceta Ibanez de Gauna M, Vela-Bueno A, Wittchen HU. DSM-III-R co-morbidity in benzodiazepine dependence. *Addiction*. 1999;94:97–107.

86. Llorente MD, Eisdorfer C, Zarate Y, Lowenstein D. Suicide among Hispanic elderly: Cuban-Americans in Dade County, Florida, 1990–93. *J Ment Health Aging*. 1996;2:79–87.

87. Cohen D, Llorente MD, Eisdorfer C. Homicide-suicide in older persons. *American Journal of Psychiatry*. 1998;155:390–396.

88. Sotaniemi EA, Arranto AJ, Pelkonen O, Pasanen M. Age and cytochrome P450-linked drug metabolism in humans: an analysis of 226 subjects with equal histopathologic conditions. *Clin Pharmacol Ther*. 1997;61:331–339.

89. Shader RI, Greenblatt DJ. Use of benzodiazepines in anxiety disorders. *N Engl J Med*. 1993;328:1398–1405.

90. Schweizer E, Case WG, Rickels K. Benzodiazepine dependence and withdrawal in elderly patients. *Am J Psychiatry*. 1989;146: 529–531.

91. Rickels K, Schweizer E, Case WG, Greenblatt DJ. Long-term therapeutic use of benzodiazepines: I. Effects of abrupt discontinuation. *Arch Gen Psychiatry*. 1990;47:899–907.

92. Schweizer E, Rickels K, Case WG, Greenblatt DJ. Long-term therapeutic use of benzodiazepines: II. Effects of gradual taper. *Arch Gen Psychiatry*. 1990;47:908–915.

93. Moss JH, Lanctot KL. Iatrogenic benzodiazepine withdrawal delirium in hospitalized older patients. *J Am Geriatr Soc*. 1995; 46:1020–1022.

94. Habraken H, Soenen K, Blondeel L, et al. Gradual withdrawal from benzodiazepines in residents of homes for the elderly: experience and suggestions for future research. *Eur J Clin Pharmacol*. 1997;51:355–358.

95. Salzman C, Fisher J, Nobel K, Glassman R, Wolfson A, Kelley M. Cognitive improvement following benzodiazepine discontinuation in elderly nursing home residents. *Int J Geriatr Psychiatry*. 1992;7:89–93.

96. Hemmelgarn B, Suissa S, Huang A, Boivin JF, Pinard G. Benzodiazepine use and the risk of motor vehicle crash in the elderly. *JAMA*. 1997;278:27–31.

97. Small GW, Rabins PV, Barry PP, et al. Diagnosis and treatment of Alzheimer disease and related disorders: consensus statement of the American Association for Geriatric Psychiatry, the Alzheimer's Association, and the American Geriatrics Society. *JAMA*. 1997;278:1363–1371.

98. Harrington C, Tompkins C, Curtis M, Grant L. Psychotropic drug us in long-term care facilities: a review of the literature. *Gerontologist*. 1992;32:822–833.

99. Beers MH. Explicit criteria determining potentially inappropriate medication use by the elderly. *Arch Intern Med*. 1997;157: 1531–1536.

100. Aparasu RR, Fliginger SE. Inappropriate medication prescribing for the elderly by office-based physicians. *Ann Pharmacother*. 1997;31:823–829.

101. Patterson TL, Jeste DV. The potential impact of the baby-boom generation on substance abuse among elderly persons. *Psychiatr Serv*. 1999;50:1184–1188.

102. Juergens SM. Prescription drug dependence among elderly persons. *Mayo Clinic Proc*. 1994;69:1215–1217.

103. Finlayson RE, Davis LJ Jr. Prescription drug dependence in the elderly population: demographic and clinical features of 100 inpatients. *Mayo Clinic Proc*. 1994;69:1137–1145.

104. Substance abuse among aging adults: a literature review. Fairfax, VA: Substance Abuse and Mental Health Services Administration (SAMHSA), 2002.

105. Miller NS, Belkin BM, Gold MS. Alcohol and drug dependence among the elderly: epidemiology, diagnosis, and treatment. *Compr Psychiatry*. 1991;32:153–165.

106. Ozdemir V, Fourie J, Busto U, Naranjo CA. Pharmacokinetic changes in the elderly: do they contribute to drug abuse and dependence? *Clin Pharmacokinet*. 1996;31:372–385.

107. Chrischilles EA, Lemke JH, Wallace RB, Drube GA. Prevalence and characteristics of multiple analgesic use in an elderly study group. *J Am Geriatr Soc*. 1990;38:979–984.

108. Willcox SM, Himmelstein DU, Woolhandler S. Inappropriate drug prescribing for the community-dwelling elderly. *JAMA*. 1994;272:292–296.

109. National Institute of Drug Abuse. Annual medical examiner data 2002: data from the Drug Abuse Warning Network. http://www.samhsa.gov. Accessed September 26, 2003.

110. Cepeda MS, Farrar JT, Baumgarten M, Boston R, Carr DB, Strom BL. Side effects of opioids during short-term administration: effect of age, gender, and race. *Clin Pharmacol Ther*. 2003;74: 102–112.

111. National Institute of Drug Abuse. Prescription drugs: misuse, abuse and addiction: a research update. 2001. http://www.drugabuse.gov. Accessed September 4, 2003.

112. Fishbain DA, Rosomoff HL, Rosomoff RS. Drug abuse, dependence, and addiction in chronic pain patients. *Clin J Pain*. 1992;8:77–85.

Somatoform Disorders in Late Life

33

Terry Rabinowitz *John P. Hirdes* *Isabelle Desjardins*

The somatoform disorders comprise a collection of ailments that share as their common feature the presence of bodily symptoms suggestive of a physical disorder, but for which no physical cause or causes can be found. The term *somatoform* has its roots in Greek and Latin: *somat* (body) + *form* (having the shape of). Thus, someone with a somatoform disorder has symptoms that appear related to the body as opposed to the mind. The symptoms suggest that a general medical condition is present, must cause significant distress or impairment in one or more important domains (e.g., social, occupational), and are not intentionally produced. The *Diagnostic and Statistical Manual of Mental Disorders*, 4th Edition, Text Revision (DSM-IV-TR) separates the somatoform disorders into seven categories:

- Somatization disorder
- Undifferentiated somatoform disorder
- Conversion disorder
- Pain disorder
- Hypochondriasis
- Body dysmorphic disorder
- Somatoform disorder not otherwise specified

Clinical features of these disorders in adult and elderly individuals are described in Table 33-1.

Somatoform disorders have received increased attention over the last decade. These disorders are common in primary care and general hospital settings, and manifest with equal frequency among different cultures. They produce significant physical, psychological, and occupational disability, and considerable economic burden (1). Somatization is recognized as a major worldwide public health problem, and is a common way that psychiatric disorders present in primary care (2,3).

Before these disorders are discussed, it must be strongly advised that physical symptoms in elders are common and are often signals that a true pathological condition is present,

even if relatively benign. Moreover, the presence of nearly all physical illnesses increases with age (4). Therefore, when considering a diagnosis of a somatoform disorder in the elderly population, it is of vital importance that the clinician thoroughly rules out possible physiological causes of the symptoms before the diagnosis of somatoform disorder is proffered. A premature incorrect diagnosis of a somatoform disorder may not only be wrong, but may be particularly harmful if it prevents identification and treatment of true disease, thus leading to increased morbidity and mortality (5).

On the other hand, we caution that it is equally important to diagnose a somatoform disorder when it *is* present. For example, Mouradian et al. examined the medical records of 85 patients who received intravenous recombinant tissue plasminogen activator for symptoms of acute stroke (6). They reported that two patients (2.4%) who received this drug had never sustained a stroke, but instead had symptoms of a somatoform disorder. Thus, these patients were unnecessarily exposed to a potent thrombolytic agent. Ferrante et al. described a patient who presented with signs and symptoms of a thalamic stroke following spinal cord stimulator implantation (7). Prior to implantation, psychological evaluation detected no pathology. Eleven days after implantation, the patient complained of right-sided numbness and burning dysesthesia. A diagnosis of thalamic stroke was given and symptoms waxed and waned over the next several weeks. On subsequent admission to a psychiatric unit, conversion disorder was suspected, the stimulator was removed, and within 6 months all sensory and motor symptoms completely resolved.

BACKGROUND

Because the age of onset of the individual somatoform disorders is often in early adulthood, data concerning these

TABLE 33-1
SOMATOFORM DISORDERS AT A GLANCE

Condition	Features	Epidemiology/ Family History	Comorbid Conditions	Treatment	Course	Elders
Somatization disorder	Chronic multiple physical complaints that began before age 30. Must include: four or more pain symptoms, two or more gastrointestinal symptoms, one or more sexual symptoms, and one or more pseudoneurological symptoms. Symptoms often described in a dramatic manner.	Female, 2–3%; male, 0.2%. Prevalence rates much higher (~50%) when less restrictive criteria used. Ten to 20% of first-degree female relatives have the disorder. Male relatives of affected women have higher rates of antisocial personality disorder and substance-related disorders. Affected women often with history of parental dysfunction and sexual or physical abuse.	Major depression, dysthymia, substance abuse, panic disorder, personality disorder (prevalence rates for any co-occurring psychiatric condition may be as high as 75%), any physical illness.	CBT or other psychotherapy. Very few studies to support use of medication for primary disorder.	Chronic. Complete remissions very rare.	History may be difficult or impossible to obtain. Use extreme caution when making this diagnosis—make sure you rule out true pathology.
Undifferentiated somatoform disorder	Somatoform symptoms that do not meet full criteria for somatization disorder. Requires presence of only one or more unexplained physical complaint that lasts for 6 months or longer.	Widely variable prevalence depending on patient population, study site, comorbid conditions.	Not available.	Not available. Treat as for somatization disorder.	Erratic. A final diagnosis of a general medical condition or another mental disorder is common.	Treat as for somatization disorder.
Pain disorder	Chronic pain causes significant disruption, impairment, or distress, and psychological factors must be significant contributors to the onset, severity, exacerbation, or maintenance of the pain. Three subtypes: 1. Associated with psychological factors 2. Associated with both psychological factors and a general medical condition 3. Associated with a general medical condition (this last subtype is not considered a mental disorder and is coded on axis III)	Prevalence among nursing home residents is 50–85%, and about 40% have moderate or excruciating daily pain. In community, prevalence rates of any pain about 70%, higher in women. In general, prevalence is extensive. Depressive disorders, alcohol dependence, and chronic pain more common among first-degree relatives.	Mood disorders (most often depression), posttraumatic stress disorder, anxiety, substance abuse, panic disorder, sleep disturbance and fatigue, decreased appetite, functional limitation. Common general medical conditions associated with chronic pain include musculoskeletal conditions, neuropathies, and malignancies.	Antidepressants may be effective primary treatment. CBT or other psychotherapy.	Variable. Many cases resolve quickly, others may last for decades.	Pain is common in the elderly—often a way of life—disabling pain is not uncommon. Before giving this diagnosis, make sure all causes of pain have been identified and treated, if possible. Overtreatment may also cause morbidity (confusion, constipation, urinary

Disorder	Description	Epidemiology	Associated features/comorbidity	Treatment	Course	Elders
Conversion disorder	A loss of or deficit in sensory or motor function suggestive of a neurological or other general medical condition that occurs in relation to psychological stress. *La belle indifference*. Symptoms do not conform to known anatomical pathways or physiological mechanisms.	Often begins in childhood but rarely before the age of 10. Prevalence 0.3% in general population, 1–3% in medical outpatient settings, 1–4.5% among medical inpatients. Female:male ratio from 2:1–10:1. More common among those of lower socioeconomic status, with less education, less psychological sophistication, and from rural settings. Risk factors: history of physical or sexual abuse, maternal parent dysfunction, personality disorder, neurological illness.	Depression, anxiety, schizophrenia, histrionic and dependent personality disorder. Dissociative phenomena reported.	CBT or other psychotherapy, hypnosis.	Single episodes of short duration, but reoccurrence is common.	In elders, it may not always be possible to discover the link between symptoms and the preceding stressor. First onset in old age is unlikely and should raise suspicion of a real medical condition.
Hypochondriasis	Preoccupation with the fear or belief that one has a serious, undiagnosed disease.	Men and women affected equally. Prevalence of 1–5% in general population, but approaches 40% in inpatient settings. Prevalence may increase with age.	Major depression (in approximately 40% of cases), panic disorder, OCD, generalized anxiety disorder.	Important to treat comorbid psychiatric conditions. Insufficient medication trials to support their use for primary condition. CBT or other psychotherapy, hypnosis.	Chronic. Complete remissions rare.	Strong association with depression makes evaluation for and treatment of this comorbid disorder essential.
Body dysmorphic disorder	Preoccupation with an imagined or real defect in appearance—if real, the concern is markedly out of proportion to the magnitude of the defect. Most often concern about face, breasts, genitals. Often leads to seeking and receiving medical or surgical treatment.	Usually begins in adolescence. Prevalence estimated at about 5% for general population—higher among adolescents, young adults, and those seeking cosmetic medical treatment. Some studies report higher prevalence among females, others do not.	Major depression, social phobia, OCD, substance use disorders, personality impairment. Impairment in functioning, poor quality of life, high suicide attempt rates.	Antidepressants and antipsychotics useful. Psychotherapy perhaps less useful than for other somatoform disorders.	Few symptom-free intervals. Referenced body part may change over time.	No prevalence data in elders. An unlikely diagnosis in the absence of history of body dysmorphic disorder symptoms.

CBT, cognitive-behavioral therapy; OCD, obsessive-compulsive disorder.

disorders in the elderly population are sparse. Prevalence rates for somatoform disorders vary by diagnosis (8), and recent investigations suggest that somatization is common among elders (2), with prevalence rates as high as about 5% for some somatoform disorders (9). Somatization is more prevalent among depressed elders (10) and may occur with greater frequency in the context of physical illness (11). Thus, its presence may confound not only its own diagnosis but also the diagnosis of comorbid nonpsychiatric illnesses. In fact, it may be the most common way for depression to present in older adults (12). A recent study of 140 primary care patients with a mean age of 76.8 years found that somatic symptom scores were significantly higher among depressed than nondepressed subjects (13). Individual symptoms that occurred at higher frequency among the depressed cohort were weakness/dizziness, numbness, a feeling of a lump in the throat, heaviness of the limbs, and muscle soreness.

Some researchers assert that somatoform disorders have been ignored by geriatric psychiatry (1,14,15), and propose several reasons why:

- Conceptual, diagnostic, and classification problems, which are particularly prevalent in the elderly population
- The belief that somatoform disorders occur infrequently among elders and are of little consequence
- The perception that somatoform disorders have not been validated as independent clinical disorders
- General difficulties in the assessment of psychiatric disorders in primary care
- Barriers to the provision of adequate management

Somatoform disorders in elders with cognitive impairment have received virtually no attention, perhaps because the presenting symptoms were incorrectly attributed to a dementing illness. Sheehan and Banerjee attribute this oversight partly to the traditional view that somatization in the elderly is a masked presentation of depression (11).

Sheehan et al. reported that general practitioners thought almost three-quarters of their elderly patients had some psychological component associated with their physical complaints, and believed 13% had complaints that were primarily or entirely psychological (16). Female gender, frequent attendance at medical clinics, and taking antidepressant medication were associated with higher somatization ratings. Another study (2) found that somatic symptoms were persistent and associated with depression, physical illness and perceived poor social support, and Gureje and Simon (17) reported that individuals with depression at baseline and those with a poor view of their health were more likely to develop new episodes of somatic complaints following an index episode of somatization.

A provocative study by Rief and colleagues, with a total of 150 patients with somatization versus controls, examined the possible role of serotonergic and noradrenergic systems in this disorder (18). They found decreased levels of l-tryptophan, a branched-chain heterocyclic amino acid, and other serotonergic amino acids in patients with somatoform symptoms, even when depression was not present, and concluded that serotonergic amino acids might be biological correlates of unexplained physical symptoms. Given that the aged brain may be deficient in one or more of these components, a higher prevalence of somatoform symptoms in older patients would not be surprising.

Each somatoform disorder from DSM-IV-TR will be discussed in this chapter, addressing each one's diagnostic criteria and epidemiology. Following that, somatoform disorder symptom correlative data collected on a large cohort of older psychiatric inpatients will be presented. Lastly, treatment of these disorders will be addressed.

SOMATIZATION DISORDER

Diagnostic criteria for somatization disorder vary depending on the particular reference used, which may cause confusion when interpreting the findings and conclusions from various studies. For example, somatization disorder became an official diagnosis in the *Diagnostic and Statistical Manual of Mental Disorders*, 3rd edition (DSM-III) in 1980, and diagnostic criteria included "a history of physical symptoms of several years' duration beginning before the age of 30" (19). In addition, women were required to have at least 14 of 37 listed physical symptoms, and men had to have at least 12 symptoms. Seven years later, the revised third edition (DSM-III-R) criteria included the presence of 13 physical symptoms with no distinction made between men and women (20). In DSM-IV-TR, the required total number of physical symptoms was decreased to eight, from four separate categories (described below) (15). In addition, some studies of somatization used *International Classification of Mental and Behavioral Disorders* (ICD) classification schemata that, at times, were not concordant with DSM. Therefore, there is a risk of comparing apples to oranges when reviewing studies of somatization, and this is true for the other somatoform disorders. For this chapter, diagnostic criteria for each somatoform disorder come from DSM-IV-TR.

Originally termed *Briquet's syndrome* (21,22), somatization disorder is a chronic syndrome of reoccurring multiple somatic complaints that are not explainable medically, and are associated with significant psychosocial distress, impairment, and medical help-seeking. Of particular importance for the geriatric psychiatrist is the requirement that the complaints began before the age of 30, and that they occurred over a period of several years. Thus, it may be very difficult to apply this diagnosis to an older patient whose medical history is unknown or uncertain.

In addition to a history of many physical complaints that began before the age of 30, there must be a history of:

- *Four* or more pain symptoms related to at least four different sites or functions (e.g., head, chest, rectum, genitals, sexual intercourse, defecation, urination, walking, using a wheelchair, brushing teeth)

- *Two* or more gastrointestinal symptoms (e.g., diarrhea, flatulence, constipation, nausea, food intolerance, cramps)
- *One* or more sexual symptoms other than pain (e.g., erectile dysfunction, orgasmic dysfunction, sexual indifference)
- *One* or more pseudoneurological symptoms (e.g., blindness, hallucinations, deafness, difficulty swallowing, paralysis, or localized weakness)

In addition to the criteria above, another requirement *for all somatoform disorders* is that each of the above symptoms:

- Cannot be fully explained by a known general medical condition or the direct effects of a substance (e.g., illicit drugs, prescribed or over-the-counter medications), *or*
- The intensity of symptoms or degree of impairment is far in excess of what would be expected, and
- The symptoms are not intentionally produced or feigned

Prevalence rates are variable, but the disorder is more common in women, with prevalence rates as high as about 2% to 3% versus 0.2% in men, when very strict diagnostic criteria are used. However, when diagnostic criteria are not as stringent, prevalence rates may be as high as 50% (17) and vary with respect to patient type (e.g., primary care, psychiatric, geriatric), setting (e.g., hospital, outpatient primary care clinic, outpatient specialty clinic), and comorbid diagnoses (e.g., depression, anxiety).

About 10% to 20% of first-degree female relatives of affected individuals also have the disorder, and male relatives of women with somatization disorder have higher rates of antisocial personality disorder and substance-related disorders. Females with the disorder often have a history of missing, disturbed, or defective parents, and of sexual or physical abuse (5). Symptoms often fluctuate over time and there are rarely complete remissions. Flare-ups may occur during times of increased psychosocial stress that reactivate maladaptive coping strategies.

Many patients with somatization disorder describe their symptoms in a dramatic and exaggerated way. Thus, in an elder whose personality style has always been histrionic or flamboyant, one must be careful not to automatically attribute new symptoms to personality style or somatization, thereby missing real illness. Clues to diagnoses include early onset and chronic course without development of physical signs of structural abnormalities, lack of characteristic laboratory values or diagnostic findings of the suggested physical disorder, and the simultaneous involvement of multiple systems (5,8).

As part of their DSM-IV field trial of somatization disorder performed in five states at family practice, general medicine, and psychiatry clinics, Pribor and colleagues found no difference in prevalence rates or in the number of somatic complaints between younger (<55 years) and older (≥55 years) women (22). In addition, no differences were found in younger versus older somatizers with respect to race, education, or marital history, and similar results were obtained when the cohort was separated into <65 years versus ≥65 years groups. In their study of somatic complaints in men, Costa and McCrae found no association between age and rate of reporting of physical symptoms in a large community sample of men between 17 to 97 years old (23). Two studies reported a slight increase in somatization symptoms with age, but one (24) did not include subjects 65 years or older, and the other (3), a large cross-national study performed at 15 separate sites, had significant between-site variation, with the strongest age association occurring at European sites.

Using reliable and validated instrumentation to assess psychiatric patients (25), we analyzed a large cohort of older inpatients for the presence of somatization and associated symptoms, and describe our instrument and findings below. The *Resident Assessment Instrument-Mental Health* is a comprehensive assessment system designed to support care planning, outcome measurement, quality indicators, and case mix-based resource allocation in inpatient psychiatry (26,27). Psychometric properties of the instrument are the focus of ongoing research, including studies of inter-rater agreement and convergent validity.

A sample of 6,282 adult psychiatric inpatients was constrained to include only people 65 and older who had no medical diagnoses recorded in a list of 28 possible health conditions (N = 229). About 75% of the original sample of elderly patients had one or more medical diagnoses.

We defined people with potential somatization as those who self-rated as having poor health, or who made repetitive health complaints over a 7-day observation period, despite the absence of co-occurring medical conditions. This broad definition captured 34.4% of the sample, and a narrower definition based on both poor self-rated health *and* repetitive health complaints included 10.9% of the elderly patients. About half the sample (55%) was female, with an average age of 74.6 years.

The most common comorbid psychiatric diagnoses were mood disorders (36.5%), organic disorders (23%), substance use disorders (22.2%), schizophrenia (14.4%), and anxiety disorders (9.6%), and 54.9% of the sample had no previous psychiatric admissions, while 23.5% had been admitted seven times or more in their lifetimes.

Figure 33-1 shows the most common physical symptoms among elderly patients with no medical diagnosis by the broad definition of potential somatization. The five most common health complaints in the group with indicators of somatization were pain, constipation, fatigue/weakness, headache, and impaired balance. Rates for all of these complaints were significantly higher than rates in the group without somatization indicators.

Figure 33-2 shows the rates of provisional psychiatric diagnoses at the time of assessment by the presence of indicators of somatization. Mood and anxiety disorders were significantly more likely to be present among those with somatic complaints, whereas substance use and organic disorders were significantly less common.

There were also a number of important social differences in those with indicators of somatization compared to those without indicators. Somatizers were significantly more likely to report feeling lonely (50.6% versus 35.1%), having no confidante (15.2% versus 7.3%), and dissatisfaction with the support received from others (22.8% versus 8.2%) than those with no indicators of somatization. Similarly, their families were more likely to report feeling overwhelmed by the patient's illness (27.9% versus 15.9%). A particularly striking difference is the higher rates of death of a family member or close friend in patients with indicators of somatization compared to those with no such indicators (25.3% versus 6%).

These results raise some interesting issues regarding somatization in the aged that deserve further exploration:

■ Only about one-quarter of elderly patients can be expected to have no medical diagnoses evident. Among those with known medical problems, it will be particularly difficult to differentiate nonpsychiatric from psychiatric causes of somatic complaints.
■ Despite the absence of corresponding medical diagnoses, patients with indicators of somatization experienced a number of important health problems that might have an adverse impact on their quality of life.
■ There appears to be an overlap with indicators of mood disorders, suggesting it may also be difficult to disentangle somatization from depression among the elderly.

■ Patients with indicators of somatization had a number of social concerns, suggesting the problems were having an important negative impact on both the individual and family.
■ The finding of a higher rate of death of family members or close friends of those with somatization indicators suggests that additional research should focus on the potential relationship between somatization and bereavement.

Although we found no specific studies of somatization in elders with cognitive impairment, Riello et al. conducted a study that examined differential associations of head and body symptoms with depression and physical comorbidity in 129 patients with cognitive impairment (28). They found that physical symptoms of the head reported by patients with mild-to-moderate cognitive impairment were associated with depressive symptoms but not with physical illness. In contrast, physical symptoms of other body regions were associated with physical illness but not with depressive symptoms. They concluded that "head symptoms" are suggestive of depressive illness while "body symptoms" are suggestive of true physical illness in those with cognitive impairment, and that somatization in demented patients may be specific to some (the head) but not to other (the body) physical symptoms.

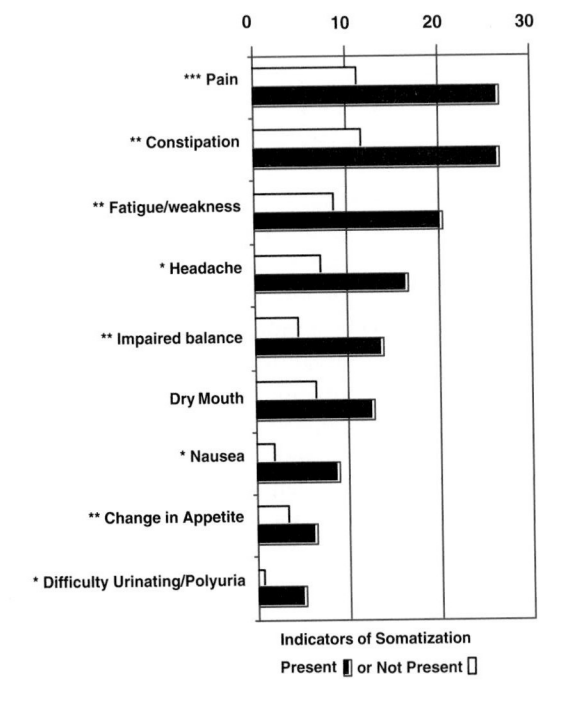

+ -p<.10; * -p<.05; **<.01; *** -p<.001;

Figure 33-1   Rates (%) of selected physical symptoms in elderly psychiatric inpatients with no medical diagnoses recorded, by indicators of somatization.

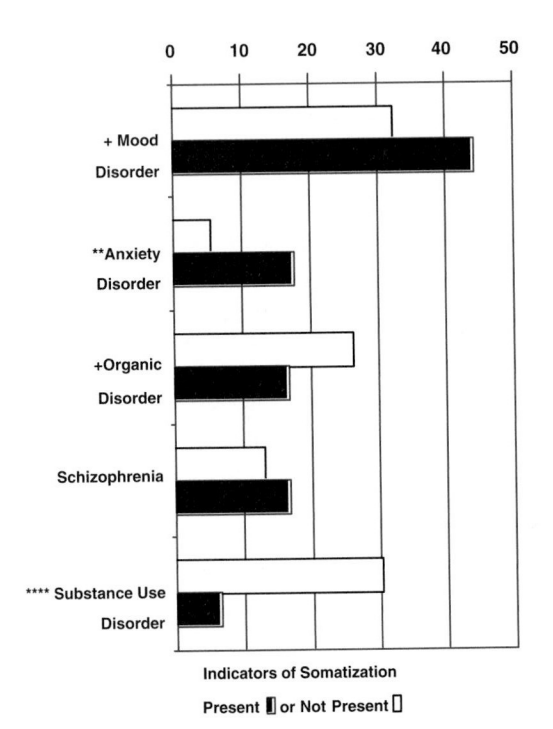

+ -p<.10; * -p<.05; **-p<.01; *** -p<.001; **** -p<.0001

Figure 33-2   Rates (%) of selected provisional psychiatric diagnoses among elderly psychiatric inpatients with no medical diagnoses recorded, by indicators of somatization.

UNDIFFERENTIATED SOMATOFORM DISORDER

This is a residual category comprising somatoform symptoms that do not meet full criteria for somatization disorder, requiring the presence of only *one* or more unexplained physical complaints that lasts for 6 months.

Given that diagnostic criteria are much less restrictive than those for somatization disorder, this diagnosis is much more likely, and perhaps much more applicable, for many elders. However, in our opinion, physicians run a greater risk of misdiagnosis and of incurring the wrath of patient and family if he or she implies this diagnosis, given that many elders have one or more comorbid medical conditions and may misattribute their somatoform symptoms to those of a real medical condition. Moreover, because only one physical complaint is necessary for diagnosis, the chances that a few symptoms, even though not characteristic of a comorbid medical condition, are *not* related to *that* condition are much lower than the possibility that multiple, simultaneous, medically unexplainable symptoms are associated with true disease.

As is true for all somatoform disorders, prevalence rates vary significantly with respect to the population studied, study site, and presence or absence of comorbid medical or psychiatric illness. A recent study by Grabe et al. of specific somatoform disorders in a general population of 4,075 subjects reported a prevalence rate of 19.7% for undifferentiated somatoform disorder compared to the 1.3% prevalence rate of a specific somatoform disorder (29). Of 4,401 consecutive inpatients seen by a consultation-liaison psychiatry service, 0.6% were diagnosed with hypochondriasis or undifferentiated somatoform disorder versus 0.2% with somatization disorder (30). A primary care prevalence study of somatoform disorders performed on 191 consecutive patients (31) found that 27.3% had undifferentiated somatoform disorder, and Altamura et al. (32), who evaluated 2,620 community or hospital psychiatric patients from 50 centers throughout Italy, reported a prevalence rate of 1.6%. These data lead us to conclude that, because prevalence rates are so variable and study conditions and subjects so heterogeneous, neither a single prevalence rate nor a range of rates can be assigned to this disorder.

CONVERSION DISORDER

The patient with conversion disorder has a loss of or deficit in sensory or motor function, suggestive of a neurological or other general medical condition that occurs in relation to psychological stress. Thus, the psychological suffering is unconsciously "converted" into physical or neurological symptoms. Because it may be difficult or impossible to elicit an accurate history from an elder, it is not always possible to discover the link between the symptoms and the preceding stressor, making the diagnosis difficult. Furthermore, conversion symptoms often co-occur with real disease and may be overlooked (33).

Ford and Folks describe conversion disorder symptoms as "nonverbal communications facilitated by nonspecific factors that inhibit a more articulate verbal expression of ideas and emotions" (34). This description is particularly applicable to elders, because many of them lack sufficient communication skills because of cognitive dysfunction or comorbid medical conditions, and must express their suffering in ways other than finding the right words to say how they feel.

Common symptoms in conversion disorder include paralysis, aphonia, seizures, gait or coordination disturbances, blindness or tunnel vision, or anesthesia. However, any sensory or motor complaint is possible. Per DSM-IV-TR, complaints of pain or sexual dysfunction alone cannot be considered symptoms of conversion disorder.

Prevalence rates vary according to the setting and population studied. The prevalence in the general population is about 0.3%, 1% to 3% in general medical outpatient settings, and 1% to 4.5% among medical inpatients. The female-to-male ratio ranges from 2:1 to 10:1, and conversion disorder is found more frequently among those of lower socioeconomic status, with less education and psychological sophistication, and from rural settings (5).

In one study comparing somatization and conversion disorder (35), age of onset occurred throughout the life span in conversion disorder patients, but mostly before the age of 21 for somatization disorder. Another study found symptoms of conversion disorder begin in young adulthood and, as the duration of the disorder increases, anxiety level and prevalence of depression also increase (36). A common subtype of conversion disorder is *psychogenic nonepileptic seizures,* also called *nonconvulsive seizures* and frequently but incorrectly (and often pejoratively) called *pseudoseizures.* Risk factors for conversion disorder include a history of physical or sexual abuse and maternal parent dysfunction (37), personality disorder, and neurological illness (8).

In a sample of 85 patients originally diagnosed with conversion disorder, 11.8% had a true neurological condition. Variables associated with the neurological condition included prior suspicion of a neurological disorder, older age at onset of symptoms, and longer duration of symptoms. Therefore, it is imperative that a thorough examination be performed for every patient to rule out organic pathology before a diagnosis of conversion disorder is considered (38).

In a prospective study of 30 patients with motor symptom conversion disorder (39), 19 had completely recovered and eight had improved at reassessment 2 to 5 years later. Worse outcomes were associated with the presence of a personality disorder or comorbid medical illness.

As is true for all somatoform disorders, symptom presentation and interpretation as well as treatment may be influenced by the ethnicity and culture of both the patient and clinician (5), and clinical presentations may vary from culture to culture depending on what symptoms are considered acceptable among that population. For example, Pineros et al. (40) reported a collective episode of psychogenic illness in response to psychosocial stress in an indigenous group of Colombians that affected nine people simultaneously. The condition, called *ataques de locura* (madness attacks) by those affected, was diagnosed by psychiatrists as a conversion disorder with dissociative features. Standard therapies, including antipsychotic medication, were ineffective in treating symptoms, which resolved after exposure to shamans of similar ethnic background.

Conversion symptoms may also have genuine physiological correlates, as suggested by studies by Yazici and colleagues. In one study, cerebral blood flow was measured in five patients with conversion disorder (41). The investigators found decreased cerebral perfusion in four of five subjects. In another study, two subjects with severe gait disturbance, with almost complete absence of somatosensory-evoked potentials (SEPs) and motor-evoked potentials during their unexplained symptoms, showed complete normalization of SEPs with resolution of the gait disturbance (42). Thus, there may be true physiologic disruption when conversion symptoms appear.

Associated psychiatric conditions include depression, anxiety, schizophrenia, and histrionic and dependent personality disorder (5). In addition, dissociative phenomena have been reported in patients with conversion disorder (43).

PAIN DISORDER

Chronic pain is a frequent symptom among older ambulatory and hospital patients as well as those in nursing homes (44), with prevalence rates that vary depending on complex characteristics and interrelationships among the patient, caregiver, assessor, and study site. Despite published guidelines for its assessment and management (45–47), pain in elders is often ignored, misdiagnosed, underdiagnosed, or poorly treated. For example, as part of a care quality indicator study, Chodosh et al. (48) found that fewer than 40% of vulnerable patients reported having been screened for the presence of pain over a 2-year period. They also found about 60% of patients treated with opioids were not placed on an appropriate bowel regimen, and approximately 10% of patients placed on noncyclooxygenase-selective nonsteroidal anti-inflammatory medications were monitored properly for gastrointestinal toxicity.

Prevalence rates of chronic pain among nursing home residents vary from about 50% to 85%, with approximately one-quarter of residents reporting daily pain and about 40% suffering moderate or excruciating daily pain at 6-month follow-up assessments (49,50). Among community-dwelling elders, prevalence rates of chronic pain also vary widely. Thomas et al. report a 4-week prevalence rate of any pain of about 72% among 11,230 adults 50 years and older,

with no differences across 10-year groups but with higher prevalence among women (51). In this study, the median number of painful areas was six (out of a possible 14) and 12.5% of the subjects were felt to have widespread pain. Weiner and colleagues (52) reported very poor agreement between resident and caregiver with respect to interpretation of pain-related behaviors and pain intensity, and Chibnall and Tait (53), who compared pain assessment of cognitively impaired and unimpaired adults using four different pain scales, stated, "Pain is a serious and undertreated health problem among older adults, both in the community and institutions." Bernabei and colleagues reported that age, gender, race, marital status, physical function, depression, and cognitive status were all independently associated with the presence of pain in elderly nursing home residents with cancer, and independent risk factors predictive of failure to receive *any* analgesic agents were minority race, low cognitive performance, and the number of other medications received (54).

Chronic pain is associated with significant comorbidity. Sleep disturbance and fatigue (55), substance abuse (56), decreased appetite (57), functional limitation (55), gait impairment (48), low levels of self-care (58), increased use of health services, and poorer overall quality of life (55,59) are all associated with chronic pain.

Psychiatric conditions associated with or that may exacerbate chronic pain symptoms include mood disorders (most often depression) (60–65), posttraumatic stress disorder (66,67), anxiety (62), and panic disorder (68,69). The detection and treatment of pain may be complicated in elders because of poor pain assessment (70), impaired pain perception (71), or both.

In pain disorder (PD), the chief symptom and predominant focus of the affected person is pain. However, what differentiates the typical geriatric patient with pain from one with PD is the effect the chronic pain has on that patient. Those with PD must experience significant disruption, impairment, or distress, and psychological factors must be significant contributors to the onset, severity, exacerbation, or maintenance of the pain.

DSM-IV-TR divides PD into three subtypes:

1. PD associated with psychological factors
2. PD associated with both psychological factors and a general medical condition.
3. PD associated with a general medical condition

For subtypes 1 and 2, either one or both factors has been determined to play a major role in the onset, severity, exacerbation, or maintenance of the pain. Subtype 3 is not considered a mental disorder and is coded on axis III.

Because pain symptoms are the rule rather than the exception among the elderly (8), and comorbid conditions are so common, PD is likely the most common somatoform disorder in this group, although prevalence rates are not clear. However, assigning this diagnosis may lead to prejudice among those who care for the affected patient, given that the patient has now received a psychiatric diagnosis that is often interpreted as an explanation for presenting symptoms rather than as a pathological response to pain symptoms that may have received no or suboptimal treatment. Therefore, we strongly advise the clinician to keep a high threshold when considering this diagnosis. Be certain that all appropriate diagnostic and treatment interventions have been considered and tried before making this diagnosis. For more information, see the chapter on pain in this textbook.

HYPOCHONDRIASIS

Author and humorist Erma Bombeck (1927–1996) has engraved on her tombstone the declaration, "I told you I was sick," and composer, musician, and actor, Oscar Levant (1906–1972), well known for his frequent somatic complaints, said, "I have given up reading books; I find it takes my mind off myself." Together, these statements capture the essence of the hypochondriac, a person certain that he or she has a serious medical condition based on their misreading of and constant preoccupation with benign bodily sensations or signs. However, the hypochondriac's beliefs never reach delusional proportions. Thus, reality testing remains intact and those with the disorder are able to acknowledge that there may indeed be significant hyperbole associated with their symptom reports, or that no real disease is present.

Descriptions of hypochondriasis date back to 350 B.C., but it was not until many centuries later that the disorder was viewed as an indicator of psychological dysfunction (72). Charatan (73) states that hypochondriasis in elders may serve a number of psychological functions.

- "Withdrawal of psychic interest from other persons and objects and a centering of this interest on oneself, one's own body, and its functioning
- Shift of anxiety from a specific psychic area to a less threatening concern with bodily pain or discomfort
- Use of physical symptoms as a means of self-punishment and atonement for unacceptable hostile or vengeful feelings towards individuals close to the person; in the case of the elderly patient, this usually means a spouse or children
- Use of physical symptoms to excuse the patient from all social responsibilities, the so-called secondary gain"

These observations provide a stable base from which to consider the psychodynamic underpinnings of this distressing disorder, and should be borne in mind when providing care.

Somatic symptoms are experienced by 60% to 80% of healthy persons in any given week, and about 10% to 20% of people worry intermittently about illness (74). Therefore, the hypochondriac presents as an outlier among these individuals because of his or her inability to appreciate

the nonthreatening quality of their symptoms, viewing them instead as indicators of real pathology. These unfortunate people chronically seek attention and treatment for their imagined maladies and, as Barsky states (75), "Patients with hypochondriasis have a characteristically paradoxical history of medical care—extensive, yet unsatisfactory."

Positive predictors of the disorder include disease or significant stressors at an early age, and the first onset of the disorder may occur in the context of real disease (5). Therefore, it may be very difficult or impossible to rule in this diagnosis in an elderly patient. Common comorbid psychiatric conditions, seen in about two-thirds of affected patients, include major depression (in approximately 40% of cases), PD, obsessive-compulsive disorder (OCD), and generalized anxiety disorder (76).

Studies not restricted to elders report a prevalence of about 1% in the general population (77,78), and studies of the disorder in primary care patients (75,79–82) report prevalence rates of between 1% and 9%. Inpatient prevalence rates approach 40%, and men and women are affected equally (5).

Prevalence rates among elders are sparse, with one study by Blazer and Houpt (83) reporting that 15% of community-dwelling elders felt their physical health was poorer than their actual health state, and another study by Ghubash et al. (9) reporting a prevalence rate of 4.4% among a cohort of community-dwelling persons aged 60 and older. Ruegg et al. reported that depressed elders are at greater risk for both hypochondriasis and somatization (84). Kramer-Ginsberg and colleagues examined the extent of hypochondriacal complaints in elderly inpatients with depression, and found that 60% had symptoms of the disorder on admission and that hypochondriasis was associated with anxiety and somatic concerns (85). Barsky et al. found that elderly patients with hypochondriasis did not differ significantly from their younger counterparts with respect to attitudes about their symptoms or assessment of their overall health (86). For about one-third of elders, symptoms spontaneously remit (87), and the disorder may be preventable if potential environmental stressors are identified early (88).

BODY DYSMORPHIC DISORDER

The main feature of body dysmorphic disorder (previously called dysmorphophobia) is preoccupation with an imagined or real physical defect, most often of the face, breasts, or genitals. If the defect is real, the preoccupation and worry is far out of proportion to the extent of the defect. The disorder is associated with many time-consuming behaviors, such as mirror-gazing, constant comparing, scrutinizing of the defect, and excessive grooming (89,90). Age of onset is usually adolescence (91), and there are no prevalence data specific to elders. Some experts feel that body dysmorphic disorder may have a delusional subtype (92–94); however, DSM-IV-TR recommends an additional diagnosis of delusional disorder, somatic type in people with body dysmorphic disorder if the belief of a physical defect is held with delusional intensity.

There are few studies of prevalence rates in the general population, but it appears the disorder is common among certain cohorts. A recent investigation by Cansever et al. of 420 Turkish female college students found a prevalence rate of 4.8%, with the head, face, and hips as most common areas of concern (95). Similarly, Bohne et al. found a prevalence rate of 5.3% among 133 male and female German college students, and of 4% among 101 American college students (96). A point prevalence of 0.7% was reported by Otto and colleagues when they examined a cohort of 976 women between the ages of 36 and 44 (97).

Body dysmorphic disorder is more common among people seeking cosmetic treatments for their physical defect (98). For instance, Uzun et al. (99) evaluated its prevalence among 159 patients with mild acne who presented to a dermatology clinic and found a prevalence of 8.8%, and Phillips and colleagues (100) report a prevalence of 11.9%, with similar rates for those seen in a community dermatology setting or a university cosmetic surgery setting. Body dysmorphic disorder occurs in about 5% to 15% of patients seeking cosmetic surgery or dermatological care (101).

Comorbid psychiatric conditions are common and include major depression, social phobia, OCD, substance use disorders, and personality impairment (97,102–104). Body dysmorphic disorder is associated with marked impairment in functioning, poor quality of life, and high suicide attempt rates (105,106). One prevalence study of adolescent and adult psychiatric inpatients reported a rate of 13.1%, suggesting that body dysmorphic disorder is a common condition in this group (107).

SOMATOFORM DISORDER NOT OTHERWISE SPECIFIED (NOS)

Included here are disorders with somatoform symptoms that do not meet criteria for any specific somatoform disorder. DSM-IV-TR includes pseudocyesis—the false belief that one is pregnant, with accompanying objective signs of pregnancy (abdominal enlargement, decreased menstrual flow, nausea, etc.)—in this category. Also included would be somatoform symptoms that have not persisted long enough to qualify as a somatoform disorder.

This NOS category of somatoform disorders seems at first not to capture much that might be relevant to elders. However, pseudocyesis is reported in both elderly men (108) and women (109). In Harland and Warner's case report, five women (aged 71 to 86 years old, three with dementia and two with a mood disorder) all presented with at least one physical symptom mimicking pregnancy (109). Two of the three patients with dementia and the two with

mood disorders responded to antipsychotic or antidepressant medication, all with resolution of their symptoms.

ETIOLOGY

Sheehan and Banerjee suggest that traditional views of somatization in elders have focused on the concept of *masked depression*, in which the depressed elder turns his or her unbearable feelings into physical complaints that may be more easily expressed or accepted, or both (11). This is an interesting idea and makes intuitive sense; however, it does not completely explain the often chronic course of most somatoform disorders, or their tendency to occur first in adolescence or young adulthood.

Therefore, it is likely that even the very old patient who shows *new* signs and symptoms of a somatoform disorder may have had the condition for many years before the diagnosis was made. We hypothesize that for many such elders, somatoform symptoms were present at a younger age, either when sufficient stress was occurring or when psychopathology was present; but these symptoms were not reported, misdiagnosed as a true medical condition, ignored, or indirectly treated with one or more psychotropic medications in the absence of a somatoform disorder diagnosis.

This hypothesis is supported by the many referenced studies throughout this chapter showing that the stage is set for developing one or more somatoform disorders by childhood or young adulthood. However, the disorder may never manifest if stress does not reach sufficient magnitude to disrupt psychological homeostasis.

There is a strong association of the somatoform disorders with one or more other psychiatric disorders, with anxiety, substance use, personality, and major depressive disorders as the most common. Conditions in childhood conducive for the development of somatoform disorders include adversity or trauma (110–112), serious illness in early life (113), and parental dysfunction (37).

Thus, a somatoform disorder is much less likely to be a new condition in an elderly patient. Instead, the condition may have been present for many years but not diagnosed because it was not considered or symptoms were not reported. As the patient aged and defenses—both physical and psychological—deteriorated, somatoform symptoms and complaints reached a crescendo that then received appropriate attention.

A somatoform disorder in an elderly patient may represent the outcome of a failed attempt of a depressed or anxious individual to deal with significant and accumulating losses. These might include losses of independence or loved ones and stresses such as deteriorating health, chronic pain, cognitive deficits, and approaching death. In a society where beauty, youth, and health are revered and where psychological distress is often considered a sign of weakness, an affected elder may have no choice but to develop physical symbols of mental anguish in hopes that these will be more acceptable not only to the elder, but to others as well.

MANAGEMENT

The somatoform disorders are generally chronic conditions. Therefore, the term *management* is preferred to *treatment* when considering options. Management of these disorders in elders poses significant challenges for the geriatric psychiatrist who struggles to help a patient, perhaps with disintegrating cognitive abilities, cope with a disorder for which explanation and empathy do little to soothe symptoms. Likewise, the patient, family and others may cause even the most talented physicians to doubt their diagnostic and treatment skills when confronted by anger, helplessness, and the threat to seek yet another opinion.

It is important to emphasize again that a somatoform disorder should be diagnosed only after exhaustively ruling out a general medical condition that may be responsible for symptoms. Likewise, because the somatoform disorders are so closely associated with mood, anxiety, and personality disorders, searching for these comorbid conditions and treating them when found may lead to significant attenuation of somatoform symptoms. Finally, it is unfortunate that many older patients with or without a somatoform disorder receive one or more medications that are given:

- At inappropriate dosages or intervals
- For too long
- In the absence of convincing pathology
- For the wrong symptoms
- Because it is the newest medication in its class

In elders, where polypharmacy is rampant (114), significant morbidity and death can occur when symptoms are indiscriminately chased with multiple medications (115,116).

In developing a management schema, the following interventions for hypochondriasis adapted from Barsky et al. (75) will serve equally well for any of the somatoform disorders in an older patient.

Schedule Regular Primary Care Visits
Keep visits brief and focused. Discourage visits at patient's discretion. In many cases, having the older patient come with a family member or other interested person may be helpful, especially if this person appreciates and understands the condition and its challenges.

Practice Diagnostic and Therapeutic Conservatism
Avoid diagnostic or laboratory studies or surgical procedures except when indicated by clinical presentation. Try

to keep the number of consultations and treaters to a minimum. The primary care physician (ideally, a geriatrician) should take charge and be the sole prescriber to avoid polypharmacy, untoward drug interactions, and drug duplication (whether intentional or accidental).

Validate the Patient's Symptoms, and Provide an Explanatory Model
Never suggest that symptoms are not real. Reassure the patient that what they are experiencing is not just happening in their head, but also make it clear that symptoms are not life threatening and may be explained by the patient's unique response to stress, depression, anxiety, etc.

Aim to Care Rather than Cure
Most somatoform disorders are chronic, which should be communicated in such a way so the patient can appreciate the disorder's chronicity and thus, its benignity. Here is an example of a clinician making this point to the patient:

You know, Mrs. P, these feelings you have that you are critically ill will sometimes get better and sometimes worsen, as they have in the past, but I do not think they will ever entirely go away. The good news is that your symptoms do not indicate a serious health problem. But I know they are distressing, so I will do everything I can to help you cope. I think it is a very good idea to make sure we take care of your anxiety and depression, so that you can be as emotionally strong as possible.

Psychotherapy

In one study, cognitive-behavioral therapy (CBT) was implemented in cognitively intact older patients with chronic low back pain, and led to significant reductions in reports of pain intensity and pain-related disability (117). Other studies of CBT in somatoform disorders found it was effective in reducing symptoms as well as health costs (118,119). Other forms of psychotherapy including brief dynamic psychotherapy (120), brief family therapy (121), exposure plus response prevention (122), and behavioral stress management (123) have also shown efficacy. Hypnosis also has documented efficacy in treating some somatoform disorders (124,125). Some older patient characteristics that could adversely affect the success of psychotherapy or hypnosis include the presence of cognitive disorders, hearing or speech impairment, and poor insight.

Psychopharmacologic Treatments

From our review of the literature, we found that the somatoform disorders have not received sufficient clinical attention with respect to medication management, especially in elders. Therefore, we cannot endorse pharmacotherapy as a first-line approach to management, except in the case of body dysmorphic disorder and PD, for which adequate clinical studies have documented the efficacy of pharmacological interventions. However, pharmacotherapy may be very helpful in any of the somatoform disorders when aimed at treatment of coexisting depression, anxiety, and delusional symptoms.

For body dysmorphic disorder, including the delusional variant, symptom improvement was achieved after treatment with standard selective serotonin-reuptake inhibitor antidepressants (126–131), clomipramine (132), and antipsychotics (131,133). Fishbain et al. performed a meta-analysis of 11 studies of PD or psychogenic pain, and found that antidepressant treatment significantly reduced pain intensity in treated subjects versus controls (134). Pirildar and colleagues reported the beneficial effects of the antidepressant moclobemide, a reversible inhibitor of monoamine oxidase-A, in an open-label study of PD (135). Turkington et al. found fluvoxamine helpful in treating symptoms of prostatodynia, a male somatoform PD, in a randomized double-blind trial (136). A case report by Maurer et al. describes a woman with continuous whole-body pain following herniorrhaphy who was refractory to antidepressant and carbamazepine treatment, but who responded to gabapentin (137). However, we found no other reports of the usefulness of anticonvulsants in PD.

There are a few small studies and case reports of the pharmacological treatment of somatization disorder with antidepressants (138,139) and anticonvulsants (140). However, given the small number of patients treated so far, we cannot endorse medications as first-line treatment for this disorder.

SUMMARY

Some somatoform disorders are common among elders (PD, hypochondriasis), while others are uncommon or so rare that prevalence, correlative, and management data are not available. Therefore, management recommendations rely extensively on studies performed on younger (and likely healthier) populations, guided by clinical experience with elders. These approaches are grounded in good clinical medicine, but elders, especially those who are frail, may be exquisitely sensitive to *any* intervention, pharmacological or otherwise, sometimes with unexpected or exaggerated responses. Therefore, whatever the intervention, start low and go slow!

If these disorders were more aggressively sought out in elders, there would be a higher capture rate that would provide a more accurate reflection of rates of occurrence and correlative conditions of these disorders. Moreover, better treatment would ensue, increasing the chances that a suffering elder would receive appropriate care for a potentially disabling condition.

REFERENCES

1. Wijeratne C, Brodaty H, Hickie I. The neglect of somatoform disorders by old age psychiatry: some explanations and suggestions for future research. *Int J Geriatr Psychiatry.* 2003;18(9):812–819.
2. Sheehan B, Bass C, Briggs R, Jacoby R. Somatization among older primary care attenders. *Psychol Med.* 2003;33(5):867–877.
3. Gureje O, Ustun TB, Simon GE. The syndrome of hypochondriasis: a cross-national study in primary care. *Psychol Med.* 1997;27 (5):1001–1010.
4. Bienenfeld D. Nosology and classification of neurotic disorders. In: Copeland JRM, Abou-Saleh MT, Blazer DG, eds. *Principles and Practice of Geriatric Psychiatry.* London: John Wiley & Sons, Ltd.; 2002.
5. Rabinowitz T, Lasek J. An approach to the patient with physical complaints or irrational anxiety about an illness or their appearance. In: Stern TA, ed. *The 10-Minute Guide to Psychiatric Diagnosis and Treatment.* New York, NY: Professional Publishing Group, Ltd.; 2005,225–238.
6. Mouradian MS, Rodgers J, Kashmere J, et al. Can rt-PA be administered to the wrong patient? Two patients with somatoform disorder. *Can J Neurol Sci.* 2004;31(1):99–101.
7. Ferrante FM, Rana MV, Ferrante MA. Conversion disorder mimicking Dejerine-Roussy syndrome (thalamic stroke) after spinal cord stimulation. *Reg Anesth Pain Med.* 2004;29(2):164–167.
8. Agronin ME. Somatoform disorders. In: Blazer DG, Steffens DC, Busse EW, eds. *American Psychiatric Publishing Textbook of Geriatric Psychiatry.* Washington, D.C.: American Psychiatric Press, Inc.; 2004.
9. Ghubash R, El-Rufaie O, Zoubeidi T, Al-Shboul QM, Sabri SM. Profile of mental disorders among the elderly United Arab Emirates population: sociodemographic correlates. *Int J Geriatr Psychiatry.* 2004;19(4):344–351.
10. Waxman HM, McCreary G, Weinrit RM, Carner EA. A comparison of somatic complaints among depressed and non-depressed older persons. *Gerontologist.* 1985;25(5):501–507.
11. Sheehan B, Banerjee S. Review: somatization in the elderly. *Int J Geriatr Psychiatry.* 1999;14(12):1044–1049.
12. Bridges KW, Goldberg DP. Somatic presentation of DSM III psychiatric disorders in primary care. *J Psychosom Res.* 1985;29(6):563–569.
13. Sheehan B, Bass C, Briggs R, Jacoby R. Somatic symptoms among older depressed primary care patients. *Int J Geriatr Psychiatry.* 2003;18(6):547–548.
14. Wijeratne C, Hickie I. Somatic distress syndromes in later life: the need for paradigm change. *Psychol Med.* 2001;31(4):571–576.
15. American Psychiatric Association. *Diagnostic and Statistical Manual of Mental Disorders.* 4th Ed. Text Revision. Washington, D.C.: American Psychiatric Association; 2000.
16. Sheehan B, Bass C, Briggs R, Jacoby R. Do general practitioners believe that their older patients' physical symptoms are somatized? *J Psychosom Res.* 2004;56(3):313–316.
17. Gureje O, Simon GE. The natural history of somatization in primary care. *Psychol Med.* 1999;29(3):669–676.
18. Rief W, Pilger F, Ihle D, Verkerk R, Scharpe S, Maes M. Psychobiological aspects of somatoform disorders: contributions of monoaminergic transmitter systems. *Neuropsychobiology.* 2004;49(1):24–29.
19. American Psychiatric Association. *Diagnostic and Statistical Manual of Mental Disorders.* 3rd ed. Washington, D.C.: American Psychiatric Association; 1980.
20. American Psychiatric Association. *Diagnostic and Statistical Manual of Mental Disorders.* 3rd Ed. Revised. Washington, D.C.: American Psychiatric Association; 1987.
21. Pribor EF, Yutzy SH, Dean J, Wetzel RD. Briquet's syndrome, dissociation, and abuse. *Am J Psychiatry.* 1993;150(10):1507–1511.
22. Pribor EF, Smith DS, Yutzy SH. Somatization disorder in elderly patients. *Am J Geriatr Psychiatry.* 1994;2(2):109–117.
23. Costa PT Jr, McCrae RR. Somatic complaints in males as a function of age and neuroticism: a longitudinal analysis. *J Behav Med.* 1980;3(3):245–257.
24. Wittchen HU, Essau CA, von Zerssen D, Krieg JC, Zaudig M. Lifetime and six-month prevalence of mental disorders in the

Munich Follow-Up Study. *Eur Arch Psychiatry Clin Neurosci.* 1992;241(4):247–258.

25. Hirdes JP, Smith TF, Rabinowitz T, et al. The resident assessment instrument-Mental Health (RAI-MH): inter-rater reliability and convergent validity. *J Behav Health Serv and Res.* 2002;29(4): 419–432.

26. Hirdes JP, Marhaba M, Smith TF, et al. Development of the Resident Assessment Instrument-Mental Health (RAI-MH). *H Q.* 2001;4(2):44–51.

27. Hirdes JP, Perez E, Curtin-Telegdi N, et al. *Resident Assessment Instrument-Mental Health for In-Patient Adult Psychiatry—RAI-MH Training Manual and Resource Guide Version 2.0.* Toronto: Queen's Printer for Ontario; 2003.

28. Riello R, Geroldi C, Zanetti O, Vergani C, Frisoni GB. Differential associations of head and body symptoms with depression and physical comorbidity in patients with cognitive impairment. *Int J Geriatr Psychiatry.* 2004;19(3):209–215.

29. Grabe HJ, Meyer C, Hapke U, et al. Specific somatoform disorder in the general population. *Psychosomatics.* 2003;44(4):304–311.

30. Smith GC, Clarke DM, Handrinos D, Dunsis A, McKenzie DP. Consultation-liaison psychiatrists' management of somatoform disorders. *Psychosomatics.* 2000;41(6):481–489.

31. Fink P, Sorensen L, Engberg M, Holm M, Munk-Jorgensen P. Somatization in primary care. Prevalence, health care utilization, and general practitioner recognition. *Psychosomatics.* 1999;40(4): 330–338.

32. Altamura AC, Carta MG, Tacchini G, Musazzi A, Pioli MR. Prevalence of somatoform disorders in a psychiatric population: an Italian nationwide survey. Italian Collaborative Group on Somatoform Disorders. *Eur Arch Psychiatry Clin Neurosci.* 1998; 248(6):267–271.

33. Silver FW. Management of conversion disorder. *Am J Phys Med Rehabil.* 1996;75(2):134–140.

34. Ford CV, Folks DG. Conversion disorders: an overview. *Psychosomatics.* 1985;26(5):371–374.

35. Tomasson K, Kent D, Coryell W. Somatization and conversion disorders: comorbidity and demographics at presentation. *Acta Psychiatr Scand.* 1991;84(3):288–293.

36. Uguz S, Toros F. Sociodemographic and clinical characteristics of patients with conversion disorder. *Turk Psikiyatri Derg.* 2003; 14(1):51–58.

37. Roelofs K, Keijsers GP, Hoogduin KA, Naring GW, Moene FC. Childhood abuse in patients with conversion disorder. *Am J Psychiatry.* 2002;159(11):1908–1913.

38. Martin RL. Diagnostic issues for conversion disorder. *Hosp Community Psychiatry.* 1992;43(8):771–773.

39. Binzer M, Kullgren G. Motor conversion disorder. A prospective 2- to 5-year follow-up study. *Psychosomatics.* 1998;39(6): 519–527.

40. Pineros M, Rosselli D, Calderon C. An epidemic of collective conversion and dissociation disorder in an indigenous group of Colombia: its relation to cultural change. *Soc Sci Med.* 1998; 46(11):1425–1428.

41. Yazici KM, Kostakoglu L. Cerebral blood flow changes in patients with conversion disorder. *Psychiatry Res.* 1998;83(3): 163–168.

42. Yazici KM, Demirci M, Demir B, Ertugrul A. Abnormal somatosensory evoked potentials in two patients with conversion disorder. *Psychiatry Clin Neurosci.* 2004;58(2):222–225.

43. Tezcan E, Atmaca M, Kuloglu M, Gecici O, Buyukbayram A, Tutkun H. Dissociative disorders in Turkish inpatients with conversion disorder. *Compr Psychiatry.* 2003;44(4):324–330.

44. Won AB, Lapane KL, Vallow S, Schein J, Morris JN, Lipsitz LA. Persistent nonmalignant pain and analgesic prescribing patterns in elderly nursing home residents. *J Am Geriatr Soc.* 2004; 52(6):867–874.

45. Stjernsward J. WHO cancer pain relief programme. *Cancer Surv.* 1988;7(1):195–208.

46. Stjernsward J. Cancer pain relief—an urgent public health problem. *J Palliat Care.* 1986;1(2):29–30.

47. Feldt KS. The complexity of managing pain for frail elders. *J Am Geriatr Soc.* 2004;52(5):840–841.

48. Chodosh J, Solomon DH, Roth CP, et al. The quality of medical care provided to vulnerable older patients with chronic pain. *J Am Geriatr Soc.* 2004;52(5):756–761.

49. Won A, Lapane K, Gambassi G, et al. Correlates and management of nonmalignant pain in the nursing home. SAGE Study Group. Systematic Assessment of Geriatric Drug Use via Epidemiology. *J Am Geriatr Soc.* 1999;47(8): 936–942.

50. Teno JM, Weitzen S, Wetle T, Mor V. Persistent pain in nursing home residents. *JAMA.* 2001;285(16):2081.

51. Thomas E, Peat G, Harris L, Wilkie R, Croft PR. The prevalence of pain and pain interference in a general population of older adults: cross-sectional findings from the North Staffordshire Osteoarthritis Project (NorStOP). *Pain.* 2004;110(1–2): 361–368.

52. Weiner D, Peterson B, Keefe F. Chronic pain-associated behaviors in the nursing home: resident versus caregiver perceptions. *Pain.* 1999;80(3):577–588.

53. Chibnall JT, Tait RC. Pain assessment in cognitively impaired and unimpaired older adults: a comparison of four scales. *Pain* 2001;92(1–2):173–186.

54. Bernabei R, Gambassi G, Lapane K, et al. For the SAGE Study Group. Management of pain in elderly patients with cancer. *JAMA* 1998;279(23):1877–1882.

55. Jakobsson U, Hallberg IR, Westergren A. Overall and health related quality of life among the oldest old in pain. *Qual Life Res.* 2004;13(1):125–136.

56. Trafton JA, Oliva EM, Horst DA, Minkel JD, Humphreys K. Treatment needs associated with pain in substance use disorder patients: implications for concurrent treatment. *Drug Alcohol Depend.* 2004;73(1):23–31.

57. Bosley BN, Weiner DK, Rudy TE, Granieri E. Is chronic nonmalignant pain associated with decreased appetite in older adults? Preliminary evidence. *J Am Geriatr Soc.* 2004;52(2): 247–251.

58. Hunt IM, Silman AJ, Benjamin S, McBeth J, Macfarlane GJ. The prevalence and associated features of chronic widespread pain in the community using the 'Manchester' definition of chronic widespread pain. *Rheumatology.* 1999;38(3):275–279.

59. Petrak F, Hardt J, Kappis B, Nickel R, Tiber Egle U. Determinants of health-related quality of life in patients with persistent somatoform pain disorder. *Eur J Pain.* 2003;7(5):463–471.

60. Rethelyi JM, Berghammer R, Ittzes A, Szumska I, Purebl G, Csoboth C. Comorbidity of pain problems and depressive symptoms in young women: results from a cross-sectional survey among women aged 15–24 in Hungary. *Eur J Pain.* 2004;8(1): 63–69.

61. Smith GR. The epidemiology and treatment of depression when it coexists with somatoform disorders, somatization, or pain. *Gen Hosp Psychiatry.* 1992;14(4):265–272.

62. Slocumb JC, Kellner R, Rosenfeld RC, Pathak D. Anxiety and depression in patients with the abdominal pelvic pain syndrome. *Gen Hosp Psychiatry.* 1989;11(1):48–53.

63. Ciaramella A, Grosso S, Poli P, et al. When pain is not fully explained by organic lesion: a psychiatric perspective on chronic pain patients. *Eur J Pain.* 2004;8(1):13–22.

64. Dworkin SF, Von Korff M, LeResche L. Multiple pains and psychiatric disturbance. An epidemiologic investigation. *Arch Gen Psychiatry.* 1990;47(3):239–244.

65. Carrington Reid M, Williams CS, Concato J, Tinetti ME, Gill TM. Depressive symptoms as a risk factor for disabling back pain in community-dwelling older persons. *J Am Geriatr Soc.* 2003; 51(12):1710–1717.

66. Geisser ME, Roth RS, Bachman JE, Eckert TA. The relationship between symptoms of post-traumatic stress disorder and pain, affective disturbance and disability among patients with accident and non-accident related pain. *Pain.* 1996;66(2–3):207–214.

67. Kulich RJ, Mencher P, Bertrand C, Maciewicz R. Comorbidity of post-traumatic stress disorder and chronic pain: implications for clinical and forensic assessment. *Curr Rev Pain.* 2000;4(1): 36–48.

68. McWilliams LA, Cox BJ, Enns MW. Mood and anxiety disorders associated with chronic pain: an examination in a nationally representative sample. *Pain.* 2003;106(1–2):127–133.

69. Fleet RP, Dupuis G, Marchand A, Burelle D, Arsenault A, Beitman BD. Panic disorder in emergency department chest pain patients: prevalence, comorbidity, suicidal ideation, and physician recognition. *Am J Med.* 1996;101(4):371–380.

70. Teno JM, Kabumoto G, Wetle T, Roy J, Mor V. Daily pain that was excruciating at some time in the previous week: prevalence,

characteristics, and outcomes in nursing home residents. *J Am Geriatr Soc.* 2004;52(5):762–767.

71. Moore AR, Clinch D. Underlying mechanisms of impaired visceral pain perception in older people. *J Am Geriatr Soc.* 2004; 52(1):132–136.

72. Dorfman W. Hypochondriasis—revisited: a dilemma and challenge to medicine and psychiatry. *Psychosomatics.* 1975;16(1): 14–16.

73. Charatan FB. Hypochondriasis in the elderly. *Psychosomatics.* 1980;21(11):880–883.

74. Kellner R. Hypochondriasis and somatization. *JAMA.* 1987;258 (19):2718–2722.

75. Barsky AJ. Clinical practice. The patient with hypochondriasis. *N Engl J Med.* 2001;345(19):1395–1399.

76. Barsky AJ, Wyshak G, Klerman GL. Psychiatric comorbidity in DSM-III-R hypochondriasis. *Arch Gen Psychiatry.* 1992;49(2): 101–108.

77. Wilhelmsen I. Hypochondriasis and cognitive therapy. *Tidsskr Nor Laegeforen.* 2002;122(11):1126–1129.

78. Magarinos M, Zafar U, Nissenson K, Blanco C. Epidemiology and treatment of hypochondriasis. *CNS Drugs.* 2002;16(1):9–22.

79. Hardy RE, Warmbrodt L, Chrisman SK. Recognizing hypochondriasis in primary care. *Nurse Pract.* 2001;26(6):26, 29, 33, 34, 36, 38, 41.

80. Faravelli C, Salvatori S, Galassi F, Aiazzi L, Drei C, Cabras P. Epidemiology of somatoform disorders: a community survey in Florence. *Soc Psychiatry Psychiatr Epidemiol.* 1997;32(1):24–29.

81. Barsky AJ, Wyshak G, Klerman GL, Latham KS. The prevalence of hypochondriasis in medical outpatients. *Soc Psychiatry Psychiatr Epidemiol.* 1990;25(2):89–94.

82. Escobar JI, Gara M, Waitzkin H, Silver RC, Holman A, Compton W. DSM-IV hypochondriasis in primary care. *Gen Hosp Psychiatry.* 1998;20(3):155–159.

83. Blazer D, Houpt JL. Perception of poor health in the healthy older adult. *J Am Geriatr Soc.* 1979;27(4):330–334.

84. Ruegg RG, Zisook S, Swerdlow NR. Depression in the aged. An overview. *Psychiatr Clin North Am.* 1988;11(1):83–99.

85. Kramer-Ginsberg E, Greenwald BS, Aisen PS, Brod-Miller C. Hypochondriasis in the elderly depressed. *J Am Geriatr Soc.* 1989;37(6):507–510.

86. Barsky AJ, Frank CB, Cleary PD, Wyshak G, Klerman GL. The relation between hypochondriasis and age. *Am J Psychiatry.* 1991;148(7):923–928.

87. Busse EW. Hypochondriasis in the elderly. *Am Fam Physician.* 1982;25(2):199–202.

88. Busse EW. Hypochondriasis in the elderly: a reaction to social stress. *J Am Geriatr Soc.* 1976;24(4):145–149.

89. Veale D. Body dysmorphic disorder. *Postgrad Med J.* 2004; 80 (940):67–71.

90. Allen A, Hollander E. Body dysmorphic disorder. *Psychiatr Clin North Am.* 2000;23(3):617–628.

91. Phillips KA, McElroy SL, Keck PE Jr, Pope HG Jr, Hudson JI. Body dysmorphic disorder: 30 cases of imagined ugliness. *Am J Psychiatry.* 1993;150(2):302–308.

92. Phillips KA, McElroy SL, Keck PE Jr, Hudson JI, Pope HG Jr. A comparison of delusional and nondelusional body dysmorphic disorder in 100 cases. *Psychopharmacol Bull.* 1994;30(2):179–186.

93. Phillips KA. Psychosis in body dysmorphic disorder. *J Psychiatr Res.* 2004;38(1):63–72.

94. O'Sullivan RL, Phillips KA, Keuthen NJ, Wilhelm S. Near-fatal skin picking from delusional body dysmorphic disorder responsive to fluvoxamine. *Psychosomatics.* 1999;40(1):79–81.

95. Cansever A, Uzun O, Donmez E, Ozsahin A. The prevalence and clinical features of body dysmorphic disorder in college students: a study in a Turkish sample. *Compr Psychiatry.* 2003;44(1): 60–64.

96. Bohne A, Keuthen NJ, Wilhelm S, Deckersbach T, Jenike MA. Prevalence of symptoms of body dysmorphic disorder and its correlates: a cross-cultural comparison. *Psychosomatics.* 2002; 43(6):486–490.

97. Otto MW, Wilhelm S, Cohen LS, Harlow BL. Prevalence of body dysmorphic disorder in a community sample of women. *Am J Psychiatry.* 2001;158(12):2061–2063.

98. Sarwer DB, Crerand CE, Didie ER. Body dysmorphic disorder in cosmetic surgery patients. *Facial Plast Surg.* 2003;19(1) 7–18.

99. Uzun O, Basoglu C, Akar A, et al. Body dysmorphic disorder in patients with acne. *Compr Psychiatry.* 2003;44(5):415–419.

100. Phillips KA, Dufresne RG Jr, Wilkel CS, Vittorio CC. Rate of body dysmorphic disorder in dermatology patients. *J Am Acad Dermato* 2000;42(3):436–441.

101. Veale D, De Haro L, Lambrou C. Cosmetic rhinoplasty in body dysmorphic disorder. *Br J Plast Surg.* 2003;56(6):546–551.

102. Gunstad J, Phillips KA. Axis I comorbidity in body dysmorph disorder. *Compr Psychiatry.* 2003;44(4):270–276.

103. Nierenberg AA, Phillips KA, Petersen TJ, et al. Body dysmorph disorder in outpatients with major depression. *J Affect Disord* 2002;69(1–3):141–148.

104. Cohen LJ, Kingston P, Bell A, Kwon J, Aronowitz B, Hollander E Comorbid personality impairment in body dysmorphic disorder. *Compr Psychiatry.* 2000;41(1):4–12.

105. Phillips KA, Dufresne RG Jr. Body dysmorphic disorder: a guide fc primary care physicians. *Prim Care.* 2002;29(1):99–111.

106. Phillips KA. Quality of life for patients with body dysmorphi disorder. *J Nerv Ment Dis.* 2000;188(3):170–175.

107. Grant JE, Kim SW, Crow SJ. Prevalence and clinical features o body dysmorphic disorder in adolescent and adult psychiatri inpatients. *J Clin Psychiatry.* 2001;62(7):517–522.

108. Novotny V, Mayer A. A case of male pseudopregnancy. *Cesko slovenska Psychiatrie.* 1989;85(6):398–401.

109. Harland RF, Warner NJ. Delusions of pregnancy in the elderly *Int J Geriatr Psychiatry.* 1997;12(1):115–117.

110. Imbierowicz K, Egle UT. Childhood adversities in patients wit fibromyalgia and somatoform pain disorder. *Eur J Pain.* 2003; (2):113–119.

111. Nijenhuis ER, Spinhoven P, van Dyck R, van der Hart C Vanderlinden J. Degree of somatoform and psychological disso ciation in dissociative disorder is correlated with reporte trauma. *J Trauma Stress.* 1998;11(4):711–730.

112. Maaranen P, Tanskanen A, Haatainen K, Koivumaa-Honkaner H, Hintikka J, Viinamaki H. Somatoform dissociation and adverse childhood experiences in the general population. *J Nerv Ment Dis.* 2004;192(5):337–342.

113. Smith C, Steiner H. Respiratory stridor and repressive defense style in adolescent somatoform disorders. *Acta Paedopsychiatr* 1992;55(4):199–202.

114. Gray SL, Lai KV, Larson EB. Drug-induced cognition disorders in the elderly: incidence, prevention and management. *Drug Safety* 1999;21(2):101–122.

115. Rabinowitz T, Murphy KM, Nagle KJ, Bodor CI, Kennedy SM Hirdes JP. Delirium: pathophysiology, recognition, preventior and treatment. *Expert Rev Neurotherapeutics.* 2003;3(3):89–101.

116. Rabinowitz T. Delirium: an important (but often unrecog nized) clinical syndrome. *Curr Psychiatry Rep.* 2002;4(3) 202–208.

117. Reid MC, Otis J, Barry LC, Kerns RD. Cognitive-behavioral therapy for chronic low back pain in older persons: a preliminary study. *Pain Med.* 2003;4(3):223–230.

118. Hiller W, Kroymann R, Leibbrand R, et al. Effects and cost-effectiveness analysis of inpatient treatment for somatoform disorders. *Fortschr Neurol Psychiatr.* 2004;72(3):136–146.

119. Hiller W, Leibbrand R, Rief W, Fichter MM. Predictors of course and outcome in hypochondriasis after cognitive-behavioral treatment. *Psychother Psychosom.* 2002;71(6):318–325.

120. Treatment outlines for the management of the somatoform disorders. The Quality Assurance Project. *Aust NZ J Psychiatry* 1985;19(4):397–407.

121. Real Perez M, Rodriguez-Arias Palomo JL, Cagigas Viadero J, Aparicio Sanz MM, Real Perez MA. Brief family therapy: an option for the treatment of somatoform disorders in primary care. *Aten Primaria.* 1996;17(4):241–246.

122. Visser S, Bouman TK. The treatment of hypochondriasis: exposure plus response prevention vs cognitive therapy. *Behav Res Ther.* 2001;39(4):423–442.

123. Clark DM, Salkovskis PM, Hackmann A, et al. Two psychological treatments for hypochondriasis. A randomised controlled trial. *Br J Psychiatry.* 1998;173:218–225.

124. Moene FC, Spinhoven P, Hoogduin KA, van Dyck R. A randomized controlled clinical trial of a hypnosis-based treatment for patients with conversion disorder, motor type. *Int J Clin Exp Hypn.* 2003;51(1):29–50.

125. Moene FC, Spinhoven P, Hoogduin KA, van Dyck R. A randomised controlled clinical trial on the additional effect of hypnosis in a comprehensive treatment programme for in-patients with conversion disorder of the motor type. *Psychother Psychosom.* 2002;71(2):66–76.

126. Phillips KA, Najjar F. An open-label study of citalopram in body dysmorphic disorder. *J Clin Psychiatry.* 2003;64(6): 715–720.

127. Phillips KA, Albertini RS, Rasmussen SA. A randomized placebo-controlled trial of fluoxetine in body dysmorphic disorder. *Arch Gen Psychiatry.* 2002;59(4):381–388.

128. Phillips KA, McElroy SL, Dwight MM, Eisen JL, Rasmussen SA. Delusionality and response to open-label fluvoxamine in body dysmorphic disorder. *J Clin Psychiatry.* 2001;62(2): 87–91.

129. Rao S. Fluoxetine was safe and effective for body dysmorphic disorder. *Evid Based Ment Health.* 2002;5(4):119.

130. Phillips KA. Body dysmorphic disorder: clinical aspects and treatment strategies. *Bull Menninger Clin.* 1998;62(4, Suppl A): A33–A48.

131. Phillips KA. Body dysmorphic disorder: diagnosis and treatment of imagined ugliness. *J Clin Psychiatry.* 1996;57(Suppl 8):61–65.

132. Hollander E, Allen A, Kwon J, et al. Clomipramine vs desipramine crossover trial in body dysmorphic disorder: selective efficacy of a serotonin reuptake inhibitor in imagined ugliness. *Arch Gen Psychiatry.* 1999;56(11):1033–1039.

133. Grant JE. Successful treatment of nondelusional body dysmorphic disorder with olanzapine: a case report. *J Clin Psychiatry.* 2001;62(4):297–298.

134. Fishbain DA, Cutler RB, Rosomoff HL, Rosomoff RS. Do antidepressants have an analgesic effect in psychogenic pain and somatoform pain disorder? A meta-analysis. *Psychosom Med.* 1998;60(4):503–509.

135. Pirildar S, Sezgin U, Elbi H, Uyar M, Zileli B. A preliminary open-label study of moclobemide treatment of pain disorder. *Psychopharmacol Bull.* 2003;37(3):127–134.

136. Turkington D, Grant JB, Ferrier IN, Rao NS, Linsley KR, Young AH. A randomized controlled trial of fluvoxamine in prostatodynia, a male somatoform pain disorder. *J Clin Psychiatry.* 2002;63 (9):778–781.

137. Maurer I, Volz HP, Sauer H. Gabapentin leads to remission of somatoform pain disorder with major depression. *Pharmacopsychiatry.* 1999;32(6):255–257.

138. Menza M, Lauritano M, Allen L, et al. Treatment of somatization disorder with nefazodone: a prospective, open-label study. *Ann Clin Psychiatry.* 2001;13(3):153–158.

139. Okugawa G, Yagi A, Kusaka H, Kinoshita T. Paroxetine for treatment of somatization disorder. *J Neuropsychiatry Clin Neurosci.* 2002;14(4):464–465.

140. Garcia-Campayo J, Sanz-Carrillo C. Gabapentin for the treatment of patients with somatization disorder. *J Clin Psychiatry.* 2001;62(6):474.

Sleep Disorders in the Elderly

34

Yohannes Endeshaw   *Donald L. Bliwise*

Sleep, referred to as the "brother of death" in Greek mythology, has been mostly considered a passive state where the individual disengages from his or her surroundings and becomes unresponsive (1). With the discovery of *electroencephalography* (EEG), which made possible the recording of brain waves during sleep in the early 1920s and the discovery of *rapid eye movement* (REM) sleep in the early 1950s, the perception of sleep as a passive process started to change (2–4). Although great progress has been made in the field of sleep medicine to date, the function of sleep is still not completely understood. Various theories have been offered for explanation, including the restorative theory (body and brain tissue restoration occurs during non-REM [NREM] and REM sleep respectively), energy conservation theory, adaptive theory, memory reinforcement, and consolidation theory, to name but a few (4–6). It is possible that the functions of sleep may encompass all the elements stated in these different theories. Studies in animals and humans have revealed that sleep deprivation results in physical, social, and emotional consequences that include loss of physical and cognitive performance, mood changes with increased irritability, difficulty concentrating, disorientation, decrease in immune function, and metabolic abnormalities (7–14).

Sleep problems are described as prevalent among older adults (15–17). In this chapter, we will describe the changes in sleep that are reported to occur with aging, and to discuss the common sleep disorders seen in older adults. We will also outline the approach to diagnosis and management of these sleep disorders.

CHANGES IN SLEEP ASSOCIATED WITH AGING

Sleep Architecture

The normal sleep architecture consists of five stages of sleep: stage 1 through stage 4 of NREM, and REM sleep. Human adults enter sleep through NREM sleep and progress from stage 1 (light sleep) to stages 3 and 4 (deep sleep), and then enter REM sleep. This cycle repeats itself about every 90 to 110 minutes throughout the sleep period. Stage 1 sleep is considered a transitory stage and constitutes only 2% to 5% of the total sleep time (TST). Stage 2 consists of 45% to 55%, while stages 3 and 4 comprise 15% to 20% of TST. REM sleep, also known as *paradoxical sleep*, consists of 20% to 25% of TST. Stages 3 and 4, also referred to as *slow wave sleep*, occur more during the first third of the night, while REM sleep occurs more during the last third of the night (18). Dreaming mostly occurs during REM sleep. Atonia of most of the major skeletal muscles occurs during REM sleep, to keep the person from acting out his or her dreams. This important phenomenon, absent in a disorder called *REM sleep behavior disorder*, is discussed later in the chapter.

Changes in sleep stage distribution occur with aging. Although older adults spend more time in bed, their TST is decreased, resulting in decreased sleep efficiency (sleep efficiency is equal to TST divided by total time in bed). Other reported changes in sleep architecture of older adults include decreases in stages 3 and 4 sleep, and increases in stages 1 and 2 sleep, with this change more marked in men than in women (19–24). Transient arousals, awakenings,

TABLE 34-1

SLEEP ARCHITECTURE AMONG HEALTHY YOUNG AND OLDER ADULTS

	30–39 years Mean ± SD (N = 11; Female = 6)	>60 years Mean ± SD (N = 12; Female = 6)
Total recording time (mins)	404 ± 46	422 ± 58
Total sleep time (mins)	386 ± 40	364 ± 47
Sleep efficiency (%)	95.5	86.4
Stage 1 (%)	5.7 ± 2.7	11.3 ± 4.8
Stage 2 (%)	45.5 ± 3.3	42.6 ± 6.8
Stages 3 and 4 (%)	27.1 ± 3.4	18.7 ± 8.7
REM sleep (%)	21.1 ± 3.5	14.9 ± 4.6
Wake after sleep onset (mins)	10.7 ± 11	46.1 ± 34.8

Adapted from Reference 28.

and difficulty going back to sleep are also increased among older adults (25). The reports on the changes in REM sleep are not as remarkable, although REM density (the number of actual eye movements during REM sleep) is reported to be decreased, once again more in men than in women (26,27). Table 34-1 shows the results of a study reported by Naifeh and colleagues comparing sleep architecture in healthy young and older adults (28).

Circadian Rhythm

In humans, as in most living things, most functions of the different organ systems follow a circadian rhythm (about 24 hours). For example, the sleep-wake cycle, body temperature, autonomic nervous system activity, cardiovascular system activity, and hormone secretion all show a regular pattern of change during a 24-hour period. The circadian rhythm is controlled and coordinated by the suprachiasmatic nucleus (SCN) in the hypothalamus. Common environmental factors that influence the SCN include light and physical and social activities. These environmental cues (also known as *zeitgebers*) are essential in synchronizing the activities of the different organ systems with the environment, such that the activities coincide with the appropriate environmental condition in a 24-hour period. Activities that disrupt the established harmony between the circadian rhythm and the environment (for example, shift work, travel across time zones) result in sleep problems (29). The SCN has been reported to show age-dependent changes, and the circadian rhythm is believed to become *phase advanced* (shifted to earlier period) and less robust as a result (30–32). Furthermore, insufficient exposure to light and decreased physical and social activities can result in inadequate stimulation of the SCN, contributing to disruption of the circadian rhythm in old age.

Although changes in sleep architecture associated with aging have been reported, there are mixed reports about their role in the sleep complaints of older adults. Recent epidemiologic studies have shown that older adults with no significant primary sleep problems or other medical, neurological, or psychiatric problems do not have increased sleep complaints (16,33), suggesting that the previously reported increased sleep complaints may be predominantly due to accompanying health problems(16,33–35). This underscores the importance of a comprehensive approach while addressing sleep complaints in the elderly.

Sleep in Nursing Home Residents

Sleep problems are even more prevalent among nursing home residents (NHRs) than among community-dwelling older adults (36,37). In fact, sleep problems may be one of the factors that influence families to place their loved ones in nursing homes (38,39). In addition to primary sleep problems, factors that contribute to sleep problems in NHRs include:

- Most NHRs have multiple medical problems that may affect their sleep.
- Most NHRs take multiple medications that may have sleep-related side effects.
- The nursing home environment may not be conducive to sleep because of increased noise and other disruptions (40,41).
- Some nursing home practices (e.g., medication administration, incontinence care) may disrupt sleep (40,41).
- NHRs may not get enough light exposure and physical activity during the day.

Steps to improve sleep in NHRs should take these factors into consideration.

APPROACH FOR PATIENTS WITH SLEEP PROBLEMS

Sleep History

A detailed history is crucial to reaching a working diagnosis when evaluating an older patient with sleep problems. The history should establish both the pattern of nocturnal sleep and daytime activities. Whenever possible, the history should be corroborated by a bed partner or roommate.

Nighttime Sleep

Information about the nighttime sleep habits of the patient helps to determine the presence of problems related to sleep schedules, sleep hygiene, initiating sleep (sleep latency ≥30 minutes), maintaining sleep, and early-morning awakenings.

Useful information in assessing nighttime sleep pattern includes:

- Time the person goes to bed
- How long it takes the person to fall asleep (sleep latency)
- Number of awakenings during the night, and reasons for the awakenings, if known (e.g., nocturia, pain, shortness of breath, etc.)
- Difficulty falling back to sleep after awakenings
- Unintended early-morning awakenings
- Time out of bed in the morning
- Whether the person feels well rested upon awakening in the morning
- Different activities performed while in bed (e.g., reading, watching TV, etc.)
- Time and amount of caffeine intake, alcohol intake, physical exercise
- Time and dose of medications taken
- Any drugs or supplements taken to promote sleep

Daytime Sleep-Wake Pattern

The objective is to determine the presence of excessive daytime sleepiness (EDS) and associated consequences, if any. Helpful information includes:

- Whether the individual:
  - Feels sleepy during the day
  - Takes naps; if so, the time and duration of naps
  - Dozes off during different activities (unintended sleep)
- Whether unintended sleepiness (EDS) occurs at rest or during activities that may put the person or other people in danger (e.g., while driving, operating machinery, etc.). If so, the person should be advised not to perform these activities until the sleep disorder is successfully treated. Common causes of EDS are described below.
- Epworth Sleepiness Scale is a questionnaire-based assessment of sleepiness during different daytime activities that helps to quantify the degree of sleepiness. It is used in sleep clinics for this purpose (42).

Excessive Daytime Sleepiness

The sleep-wake cycle is organized in such a way that the individual is awake and alert during the day and sleepy during the night. Some degree of sleepiness may be observed between the hours of 1:00 PM and 3:00 PM in the 24-hour cycle in normal individuals, but this sleepiness usually lasts less than 30 minutes and does not signifi-

cantly disrupt daytime activities (29). Sleepiness, like hunger and thirst, is considered a physiological need state and typically has an inverse relationship with the quantity and quality of nocturnal sleep. In addition to negatively affecting the quality of life, EDS is associated with serious consequences like motor vehicle accidents and mistakes and accidents at work. The most common causes of EDS include (43):

- *Sleep disorders:* Disruption of nocturnal sleep by primary or secondary sleep disorders (e.g., *sleep apnea, periodic limb movement disorder* (PLMD), uncontrolled pain, depression) may result in increased daytime sleepiness. In these situations, successful treatment of the nocturnal sleep disorder usually improves the daytime sleepiness. Other primary sleep disorders like *narcolepsy* should also be considered in the differential diagnosis.
- *Medications:* Sedative-hypnotics taken at night may have prolonged effects into the next day. This is particularly true in older adults where age-related changes in drug metabolism and/or drug-drug interactions might lead to prolonged drug effect. On the other hand, some medications (e.g., theophylline) may have wake-promoting effects, and if taken in the evening hours may interfere with nocturnal sleep and result in daytime sleepiness. This calls for a detailed scrutiny of medications (prescribed or over-the-counter [OTC], both conventional and herbal) during the history-taking process.
- *Neurodegenerative disorders:* In patients with neurodegenerative diseases like Alzheimer's disease, degenerative changes may occur in brain structures involved in the control of circadian rhythms and/or wakefulness. This can result in daytime sleepiness, regardless of the quality and quantity of nocturnal sleep.
- *Insufficient nighttime sleep:* Although this may not be relevant for older adults, it is a common cause of daytime sleepiness in younger people who intentionally decrease the duration of their nocturnal sleep time to accommodate ever-increasing work demands and leisure activities. The individual may not be aware of the relationship between daytime sleepiness and insufficient nighttime sleep. Therefore, a careful history of the quantity and quality of nocturnal sleep and an explanation of the relationship between nocturnal sleep and daytime sleepiness is important in the management of these patients.

Sleep Diary

In addition to the history taken in the clinic, it is essential to ask patients to keep a sleep diary for a period of 1 to 2 weeks, where they record their bedtime, sleep time, wake-up time, nighttime awakenings, daytime naps, and time of consumption and amount of caffeine-containing drinks, alcohol, etc. The information obtained from the diary is used in conjunction with the patients' complaints to better understand their sleep patterns (44).

Physical Examination

During physical examination, the physician should observe if the patient is sleepy or dozing off during the clinic visit (while in the waiting room, during interview, etc.). A complete physical examination is required to make sure there are no medical or neurological problems that may be responsible for the sleep complaints. Abnormal physical findings specific to the different sleep disorders are described later.

Laboratory Investigations

Laboratory-based investigations used in the diagnosis of sleep disorders include polysomnography (PSG), multiple sleep latency test (MSLT), actigraphy, ambulatory sleep study, and monitoring of leg movements.

Polysomnography

This is a procedure by which several physiological characteristics are monitored during sleep. These include: sleep-wake activity using EEG, eye movements using electro-oculogram, muscle activity using electromyogram, breathing (air flow, respiratory effort, and pulse oximetry), and heart rate and rhythm. The procedure is usually done in a sleep laboratory and requires technician supervision. Information obtained through PSG includes sleep latency, sleep efficiency, the proportion of the different stages of sleep, the pattern of breathing, the presence of leg movements, and cardiac arrhythmia. It is considered the gold standard for the evaluation of sleep disorders such as sleep-disordered breathing (SDB). Medicare and most insurance companies cover the cost of the procedure when ordered with appropriate indications. Figure 34-1 shows a normal PSG tracing of a person in REM sleep.

Multiple Sleep Latency Test

The MSLT is used to confirm the complaint of daytime sleepiness in subjects with no obvious etiology, or when narcolepsy is suspected. The MSLT measures the amount of time it takes a person to fall asleep at different times of day. In an environment conducive to sleep (dark, quiet, comfortable), the person is asked to lie down and try to go to sleep for 30 minutes. This procedure is repeated every 2 hours for a total of four to five naps. It starts about 2 hours after an overnight PSG and continues throughout the day. In between the naps, the person stays out of bed and engages in different activities such as reading. Mean sleep latency less than 10 minutes is considered abnormal. MSLT is performed on the day after an overnight PSG to make certain that primary sleep disorders, such as SDB or PLMD, are excluded as possible causes of daytime sleepiness.

Actigraphy

Actigraphy is the recording of movement (wrist movement) using actigraphs, small devices with movement detectors that are placed on the wrist like a watch. The procedure is based on the assumption that movement is minimal during sleep and increased during wake periods. The actigraph has sufficient memory to record up to a week of information and can thereby give the pattern of wake and sleep over a longer period of time (45). It is a simple and noninvasive method that can be used even in patients with dementia and abnormal behavior. But because sleep and wake are assessed indirectly (absence or presence of activity), the information may not be as accurate as the results obtained by PSG.

GENERAL PRINCIPLES OF TREATMENT OF SLEEP DISORDERS

Both pharmacologic and nonpharmacologic treatments are important in the management of sleep disorders. The mainstay of nonpharmacologic treatment is sleep hygiene. Sleep hygiene refers to performance of activities that are consistent with maintenance of good quality nocturnal sleep and daytime alertness, and is considered the cornerstone in the management of sleep disorders in general. Sleep hygiene instructions that help to initiate and maintain good quality of sleep are listed below (46).

- Keep a regular bedtime and wake time.
- Go to bed only when sleepy and get out of bed when you are unable to fall asleep after trying for 20 minutes. Engage in activities until you feel sleepy (avoid excessively stimulating activities).
- Use the bedroom only for sleep and sex. Avoid doing other activities (e.g., reading, watching TV, talking on the phone) while in bed.
- Avoid naps during the day if possible, or limit daytime naps to 10 to 15 minutes in duration 8 hours after rising (unless specifically advised to take longer or more frequent naps by a physician).
- Get regular exercise during the day but avoid vigorous physical exercise in the evening hours (at least 4 hours before bedtime).
- Limit caffeine intake in general and avoid caffeine intake in the afternoon and evenings.
- Avoid smoking in the evening and while awake at night.
- Avoid heavy meals within 3 to 4 hours before bedtime.
- Avoid alcohol intake within 3 to 4 hours before bedtime.
- Develop relaxing bedtime routines (warm bath within 2 hours of sleep, relaxing activities, etc.).

Pharmacologic treatment includes the use of both prescription and nonprescription drugs. The use of nonprescription sleep-promoting agents is not uncommon among older adults (47,48), and these medications may be used without the advice of a physician. This pattern of use of OTC sleep-promoting agents may expose patients to side effects that they are not aware of. For this reason, the physician should enquire about the use of these medications and determine whether their use is appropriate.

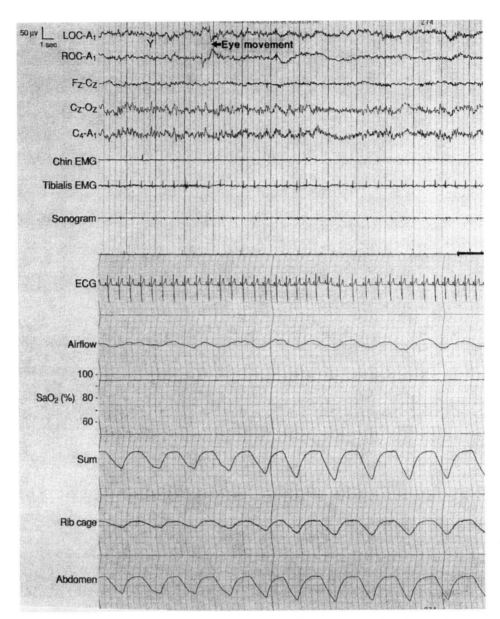

Figure 34-1   Normal polysomnography tracing. (Adapted with permission from Sheppard JW, ed. *Atlas of Sleep Medicine*. Mount Kisco, New York: Futura Pub Co; 1991.)

Referral to a sleep specialist is indicated for appropriate diagnosis and management of sleep problems that cannot be managed by the nonsleep specialist. In the United States, the American Academy of Sleep Medicine gives accreditation to individual specialists and sleep centers, and can be accessed at its Web site at www.aasmnet.org.

COMMON SLEEP PROBLEMS AMONG OLDER ADULTS

Nocturnal sleep problems and EDS can be caused by primary sleep disorders or secondary to medical, neurological, or psychiatric conditions. Table 34-2 shows the common causes of primary and secondary sleep disorders.

DISORDERS OF INITIATION AND MAINTENANCE OF SLEEP

Disorders of initiation and maintenance of sleep (DIMS), commonly referred to as *primary insomnia*, is characterized by increased sleep latency, increased awakenings after sleep onset with difficulty going back to sleep, and early-morning awakenings, in the absence of other primary sleep disorders, medical, neurological, or psychiatric conditions known to disrupt sleep.

Primary insomnia is subclassifed into psychophysiological insomnia, inadequate sleep hygiene, and idiopathic insomnia. Psychophysiological insomnia is characterized by physical tension and learned sleep-preventing behaviors.

TABLE 34-2

COMMON PRIMARY AND SECONDARY SLEEP DISORDERS AMONG OLDER ADULTS

Primary Sleep Disorders	Secondary Sleep Disorders (causes)
Primary insomnia	Medical disorders
Sleep-disordered breathing (sleep apnea)	Neurological disorders
Restless legs syndrome	Psychiatric disorders
Periodic limb movement disorder	Medication side effects
REM sleep behavior disorder	Alcohol dependent problems
Disorders of circadian rhythm	
■ Advanced sleep phase syndrome	
■ Delayed sleep phase syndrome	

REM, rapid eye movement.

The problem usually starts with an acute stressful event that renders the patient unable to fall asleep. The inability to fall asleep makes the person anxious and frustrated, and this results in worsening of the insomnia. In addition, the patient may develop maladaptive behaviors (drinking alcohol to initiate sleep, performing different activities while in bed) to overcome the insomnia. These behaviors may make the insomnia worse in the short term and also perpetuate the insomnia, even after the actual stressful event is over (49). Subjects with a hyperarousal state are reported to be predisposed to develop insomnia (50). Figure 34-2 depicts the relationship between insomnia and the factors involved in its initiation and maintenance. These patients usually sleep better when they spend the night at a different location (e.g., in a hotel or sleep laboratory).

Inadequate sleep hygiene refers to practices that interfere with initiation or maintenance of sleep. Idiopathic insomnia occurs when difficulty with initiating and maintaining sleep has occurred since childhood with no factors identified as causing the problem. These conditions are well described in the *International Classification of Sleep Disorders: Diagnostic and Coding Manual* (51). The diagnosis is based on suggestive history in a patient with normal physical examination after excluding other primary or secondary sleep disorders. Treatment includes both nonpharmacologic and pharmacologic approaches.

Nonpharmacologic Treatment

This is commonly known as cognitive-behavioral therapy (CBT) and includes stimulus control, sleep restriction, cognitive therapy, sleep hygiene education, and relaxation therapy. Nonpharmacologic treatments have been shown to work effectively for treatment of primary insomnia in older adults (52,53). This method of treatment is preferred whenever possible because it prevents the chronic use of pharmacologic agents for insomnia. Treatment with CBT usually requires referral to a sleep specialist who provides this form of therapy.

Pharmacologic Treatment

The use of sleep-promoting medications is recommended for initiation and maintenance of sleep in conjunction with nonpharmacologic approaches during the first few weeks of treatment (54–57). The two common groups of medications used in the treatment of insomnia are short-acting benzodiazepines and the nonbenzodiazepine hypnotics (Table 34-3). These drugs are preferred to other medications like barbiturates and benzodiazepines, that have a longer duration of action (e.g., estazolam), because of their wider margin of safety and less residual sedation the next day. This is particularly important in older adults for whom the half-life of most medications is prolonged due to age-related changes in drug metabolism.

The duration of most of the studies that examine the effect of sleep-promoting agents in patients with insomnia is less than 4 to 6 weeks. For this reason, there is no clear consensus on the beneficial effects of the chronic use of sleep-promoting agents in patients with insomnia. Furthermore, chronic use of sleep-promoting agents may be associated with side effects that include dependence, tolerance, rebound insomnia, daytime fatigue, impaired memory, and falls (55–57). These side effects are reported to be less with the use of nonbenzodiazepine hypnotics such as zolpidem or zaleplon, as compared to short-acting

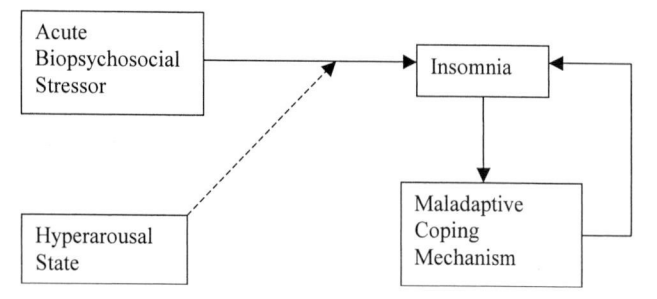

Figure 34-2 Relationship among insomnia and related factors.

TABLE 34-3

COMMONLY PRESCRIBED SLEEP PROMOTING MEDICATIONS

Drug	Half-Life[a]	Dose
Benzodiazepine hypnotics		
▪ Triazolam	1.5–5.5 hours	0.125–0.25 mg
▪ Temazepam	3.5 to >10 hours	7.5–30 mg
Nonbenzodiazepine hypnotics		
▪ Zolpidem	2.6 hours	5–10 mg
▪ Zaleplon	1 hour	5–10 mg
▪ Eszopiclone	5.8 hours	1–3 mg

[a]The half-life may be longer in older adults.

benzodiazepines (55). The use of these agents in combination with other drugs like alcohol or other sedative-hypnotic agents may increase their sedating potential and predispose subjects to more side effects. For these reasons, the chronic use of sleep-promoting agents is not recommended.

The practice of prescribing antidepressants with sedating properties (e.g., trazodone, mirtazapine, amitriptyline) for promoting sleep is common, and has increased over the last decade (58). These medications have been shown to increase sleep latency and decrease awakening from sleep in healthy subjects (59). In patients with depression, trazodone has been shown to improve the quality and quantity of sleep as compared to placebo (60), but there are no studies to show that the use of these antidepressant agents for sleep promotion is superior to or safer than the use of standard sedative-hypnotics. In addition, clinicians must be aware of the potentially hazardous side effects of tricyclic antidepressants (e.g., amitriptyline, imipramine) such as anticholinergic activity, orthostasis, excess sedation, and slowing of cardiac conduction (61). Trazodone has infrequently been associated with priapism, ventricular arrhythmias at high doses, and hyponatremia and seizures in overdose (62). This situation calls for studies that would examine the efficacy and safety of these antidepressant medications in comparison to the short-acting hypnotics that are widely used for sleep problems.

As mentioned earlier, the use of OTC drugs is common among older adults. Some of the major ones are described below.

Diphenhydramine, sold in generic form and under the brand name Benadryl, is also a common ingredient in many brand name OTC sleep-promoting agents like Tylenol PM, Unisom, and others. It is a first-generation antihistamine with anticholinergic and antiadrenergic properties. In older adults, its actions may persist into the next day and cause daytime sedation. Diphenhydramine's anticholinergic effects may result in other unwanted side effects such as dry mouth, worsening of bladder outlet obstruction in men with prostate problems, blurred vision, and constipation. An association between serum anticholinergic levels and decreased cognitive function among older adults has also been reported (63). For these reasons, the use of this medication for sleep promotion in the elderly is not recommended.

Melatonin is another widely used OTC supplement in older adults. Melatonin is a hormone produced by the pineal gland and regulated by the SCN. Physiological levels of melatonin increase at night and decrease during the day. Melatonin has sleep-promoting properties and is used in the treatment of specific conditions such as jet lag and delayed sleep phase syndrome. But because of its availability, melatonin is also used by many older adults for nonspecific sleep problems. Although melatonin levels have been shown to be reduced in older adults with insomnia, replacement of melatonin has not been shown to consistently improve the insomnia (64). Furthermore, the side effects of chronic use of melatonin have not been clearly established. For these reasons, the random use of melatonin is not advised.

Alcohol is one of the common "drugs" used by many as a sleep-promoting agent. Mild-to-moderate alcohol intake decreases sleep latency due to its sedative effect, but also leads to awakenings in the second half of the night (rebound effect). The awakenings in the second part of the night are believed to be a result of the effect of the body's adjustment to the increased alcohol level, which results in sleep disruption when the alcohol is metabolized and eliminated from the body. Because of inadequate sleep in the second part of the night, daytime fatigue and sleepiness may be a problem the next day. In addition, when taken on a daily basis tolerance to the sleep-inducing effects develops, which may result in the individual drinking more and more alcohol to get the sedating effect, resulting in worsening of sleep disruption later in the night (65). Alcohol use may be one of the more common causes of sleep problems among older adults.

There is an increasing trend among older individuals to use herbal supplements or alternative medications to treat sleep problems (66). Valerian is one such popular herbal medicine. However, its effectiveness in promoting sleep has not been well established (67), and as a result it is not recommended for older adults.

SLEEP-DISORDERED BREATHING

SDB comprises three conditions, namely *obstructive sleep apnea and hypopnea* (OSAH), *central sleep apnea* (CSA), and *upper airway resistance syndrome*. In this chapter we will limit the discussion to OSAH and CSA.

Obstructive Sleep Apnea and Hypopnea

OSAH is characterized by cessation of or decrease in airflow (apnea and hypopnea respectively) for a period of 10 seconds or more during sleep, and mostly associated with a decrease in oxygen saturation and/or arousal from sleep (51,68). The apnea and hypopnea is accompanied by continuing activity of the muscles of respiration (the intercostals, abdominal muscles, and the diaphragm) and occurs as a result of complete or partial obstruction of the upper airway.

Epidemiology

The prevalence of OSAH is reported to be high among older adults. In a recent population-based survey, the prevalence of OSAH with an apnea-hypopnea index (AHI) ≥5 episodes per hour of sleep was 52.8% among participants ≥60 years old. Of these, 32.8% had an AHI between 5 and 14, while 19.9% had an AHI of 15 or more per hour of sleep (69). This was significantly higher than the rate for subjects less than 60 years old in the same study. The male-to-female ratio is reported to be 2–3:1 (70,71), even though a higher ratio has been reported among sleep-clinic populations (72).

Risk factors for OSAH include snoring, increased body mass index (BMI), increased neck circumference (>17 inches in males and >16 inches in females), and craniofacial abnormalities (e.g., micrognathia). However, these risk factors may not be as important in older adults as they are in middle-aged adults (69). Among older adults, a common condition associated with OSAH is edentulism (73). Edentulism leads to a decrease in the vertical dimension of occlusion, which may result in a reduction of upper airway size and altered upper-airway-dilating muscle activity, probably predisposing these subjects to partial or complete obstruction of the upper airway during sleep.

Clinical Manifestation

The symptoms of OSAH include snoring, which may be loud enough to waken the bed partner or roommate, breathing pauses associated with snoring, unexplained awakenings, nonrefreshing sleep in the morning, and daytime sleepiness. The patient may admit to recent weight gain. Depending on the severity of OSAH, the daytime

sleepiness may occur while at rest or during different activities. OSAH is a common cause of sleeping while driving and consequent motor vehicle accidents (74,75). Abnormal findings on physical examination include increased BMI, increased neck circumference, micrognathia, and retrognathia. Blood pressure may be elevated, but low blood pressure and orthostatic hypotension have also been described in subjects with OSAH (76).

The manifestations of OSAH among older adults, however, may be more subtle or nonspecific. Snoring may not be as commonly reported in older adults; snoring may be less loud, the subject may not have a bed partner or roommate, or the hearing ability of the roommate or bed partner may be decreased. Obesity may not be as common as it is among middle-aged adults; therefore, the BMI may not be a useful indicator of risk. On the other hand, two other important symptoms of OSAH among older adults are increased frequency of nocturia and decline in mental function (77–79). Nocturia is a significant problem among older adults because it is associated with sleep disruption, falls, and possible fractures (80,81). Decline in mental function may interfere with day-to-day activities. Furthermore, both nocturia and decline in mental function may be considered normal with aging and not given the appropriate attention. Thus, physicians taking care of older adults should be cognizant of the atypical presentations of OSAH.

Complications

Daytime sleepiness as a result of OSAH has been reported in association with motor vehicle accidents. Furthermore, several studies have reported significant association between OSAH and acute and chronic cardiovascular and cerebrovascular diseases (82–85), making the prompt diagnosis and management of SDB a priority.

Laboratory Investigation

Clinical suspicion of SDB is confirmed by monitoring of breathing during sleep. PSG is the diagnostic method of choice to confirm the diagnosis of OSAH (86), because it monitors both brain activity and respiration during sleep. The results of the test include the number of apneas and hypopneas per hour of sleep (i.e., the AHI), the degree of desaturation associated with these events, and the number of arousals caused by the apneas or hypopneas. The AHI is used to determine the OSAH severity, categorized as follows (87):

- Mild OSAH: AHI 5 to 14/hour of sleep
- Moderate OSAH: AHI 15 to 29/hour of sleep
- Severe OSAH: AHI ≥30/hour of sleep

Other respiratory monitoring systems are also available. These instruments monitor several respiratory parameters during sleep, including airflow, chest and abdominal movements, and pulse oximetry, and they determine the AHI and degree of O_2 desaturation associated with these events. The

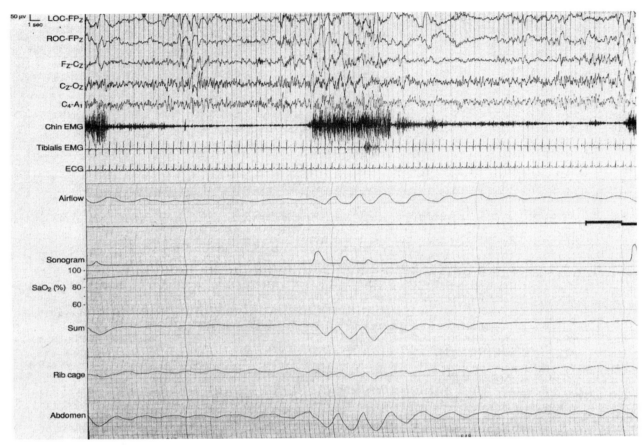

Figure 34-3   Polysomnographic tracing showing an obstructive sleep apnea event. (Adapted with permission from Sheppard JW, ed. *Atlas of Sleep Medicine*. Mount Kisco, New York: Futura Pub Co; 1991.)

advantage of these systems is that they can be used in a person's home, and do not require the presence of a technician during the procedure. A disadvantage, however, is that the information obtained is limited to the respiratory system, and provides no information about the quality and quantity of sleep. As a result, the total sleep time used to calculate the AHI may not be accurate. Such home monitoring is recommended as an acceptable method for the diagnosis of OSAH in situations where PSG is not possible (87).

Another system used to screen for OSAH is overnight pulse oximetry. This system measures O_2 saturation during sleep. The information obtained using this system is limited to the frequency and severity of desaturation only, with no information about an individual's breathing pattern. For this reason, it is not considered an acceptable method for the diagnosis of OSAH (87). Figure 34-3 shows a PSG tracing in a patient with OSAH. Note the flat line in the airflow tracing accompanied with some activity in the rib cage and abdominal tracings.

Treatment of Sleep-Disordered Breathing

Conservative Management

This includes measures like weight loss and avoiding the supine position during sleep, especially if the apnea and hypopnea are supine-position dependent. Most PSG and ambulatory sleep recordings record the position of the subject during sleep. Drugs that worsen SDB (alcohol, sedative-hypnotics) should be avoided.

Continuous Positive Pressure Ventilation

Continuous positive pressure ventilation (CPAP) is the treatment of choice for SDB. The CPAP equipment consists of a face mask attached by tubing to an air pump. The CPAP machine blows air into the mask, and the air pressure keeps the airway patent during breathing. The minimum CPAP pressure required to successfully eliminate both apneas and hypopneas during sleep will vary across individuals, and is determined during an overnight CPAP titration study in a sleep laboratory.

Although CPAP treatment is effective, tolerance has been a problem, with noncompliance rates ranging from 25% to 50% (88,89). There are many biological and psychological factors that may predict compliance with CPAP treatment, but in most studies age was not found to be a factor. Information on long-term CPAP use in older adults is limited. A small preliminary study with nine subjects reported encouraging results about CPAP use in patients with Alzheimer's disease (90), suggesting that CPAP use

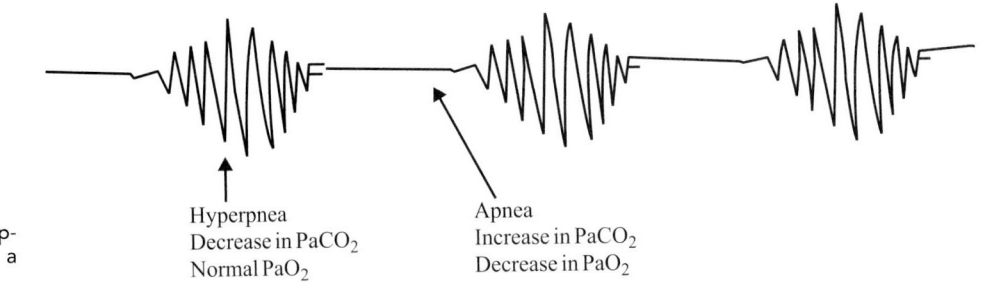

Figure 34-4 Periods of hyperpnea alternating with apnea in a patient with CSA.

Hyperpnea
Decrease in $PaCO_2$
Normal PaO_2

Apnea
Increase in $PaCO_2$
Decrease in PaO_2

should not be ruled out as possible treatment for older adults with dementia and OSAH.

Oral Appliances

Oral appliances are used to increase the upper airway caliber by advancing the mandible forward. Oral appliance therapy is performed by dentists who have a special interest and expertise in sleep disorders. Oral appliances are indicated for treatment of snoring and mild sleep apnea (91).

Surgical Treatment

Surgical treatment may be indicated for individuals with anatomic abnormalities that are felt to be causing the problem, and that are amenable to correction (92). Tracheostomy was the first treatment used for SDB, even before the advent of CPAP. Current techniques include nasal reconstruction, uvulopalatopharyngoplasty (removal of redundant tissue in the oropharynx), and a mandibular osteotomy and genioglossus advancement with hyoid myotomy and suspension in order to prevent both the posterior displacement of the tongue during sleep and the narrowing of the airway at the level of the hypopharynx. The success of surgical treatments is variable (93), and depends on the correct identification and correction of the actual cause.

Drug Treatment

Drugs that have been attempted in the treatment of SDB include protriptyline, medroxyprogesterone, acetazolamide, clonidine, and aminophylline. None have been found to be effective (94).

Central Sleep Apnea

CSA is characterized by cessation of breathing with no accompanying respiratory effort (i.e., no activity of the respiratory muscles) and may be associated with nighttime O_2 desaturation, arousals, and awakenings. It is due to malfunction in the control of breathing by the respiratory center. CSA is seen in different medical conditions, including congestive heart failure (CHF), chronic obstructive pulmonary disease, uremic encephalopathy, and cerebrovascular accidents involving the respiratory center in the ventrolateral medulla. In CHF, the patient is observed to have a repeating pattern of hyperventilation followed by hypoventilation and apnea, also known as Cheyne-Stokes breathing. It is believed that CSA in CHF occurs as

a result of increased sensitivity to arterial carbon dioxide tension, or $PaCO_2$, such that CHF patients may develop hyperventilation at a normal $PaCO_2$ level. This hyperventilation results in a decline in the $PaCO_2$ levels, and when the level decreases below a certain level (known as the apnea threshold), the patient develops apnea and an increase in $PaCO_2$ (95,96). This cycle continues during the period of Cheyne-Stokes breathing. Figure 34-4 shows the relationship between ventilation and the $PaCO_2$ level.

PSG is indicated to confirm the diagnosis and determine the severity of CSA. Treatment of CSA should be directed at the primary medical problem whenever possible. In a situation where that is not adequate, treatment with CPAP or bilevel positive airway pressure may be considered.

RESTLESS LEGS SYNDROME AND PERIODIC LIMB MOVEMENT DISORDER

Restless Legs Syndrome

Restless legs syndrome (RLS) is a condition characterized by a constellation of symptoms without obvious abnormal physical findings. The diagnosis is based on diagnostic criteria established by the International Restless Legs Syndrome Study Group (97), presented in Table 34-4.

Epidemiology

RLS is a common condition with a prevalence rate of about 5% among the general population. Its prevalence increases with age, with a prevalence of up to 35% reported in the elderly (98–101). RLS symptoms are referred to by different names in different populations, such as the *heebie-jeebies* in the Southern United States and *growing pains* in children.

RLS occurs in two forms: the familial form, which is transmitted as an autosomal dominant trait with variable penetrance, and the idiopathic form. In the familial form the symptoms mostly start before age 40, while in the idiopathic form symptoms usually occur after the age of 50 (102–104). Risk factors associated with RLS include increasing age, family history, pregnancy, iron deficiency anemia (serum ferritin <50 µg/L), and uremia. Drugs reported to precipitate or exacerbate the symptoms of RLS include selective serotonin-reuptake inhibitors (SSRIs), tricyclic antidepressants, lithium carbonate, dopamine antagonists,

TABLE 34-4
ESSENTIAL DIAGNOSTIC CRITERIA FOR RESTLESS LEGS SYNDROME

1. An urge to move the legs, usually accompanied or caused by uncomfortable and unpleasant sensations in the legs. Sometimes the urge to move is present without the uncomfortable sensations, and sometimes the arms or other body parts are involved in addition to the legs.
2. The urge to move or unpleasant sensations begin to worsen during periods of rest or inactivity, such as when lying or sitting.
3. The urge to move or unpleasant sensations are partially or totally relieved by movement, such as walking or stretching, as long as the activity continues.
4. The urge to move or unpleasant sensations are worse in the evening or night than during the day, or only occur in the evening or night. When symptoms are very severe, the worsening at night may not be noticeable, but must have been present previously.

Adapted from Reference 97.

and withdrawal of benzodiazepines, barbiturates, and anticonvulsants (105). Spinal cord lesions with impairment of sensory pathways (which interrupts the descending inhibitory spinal pathway) have been reported to result in RLS symptoms (106,107). PLMD is reported to occur in up to 80% of subjects with RLS (99–102).

The exact nature of the disorder that leads to symptoms of RLS is not clearly understood. There are suggestions that it may represent dopamine dysfunction in the central nervous system. Decreased cerebrospinal fluid ferritin and decreased iron in nigrostriatal areas of the brain have also been reported in association with RLS. It is postulated that cerebral iron insufficiency may lead to dopamine abnormalities in the central nervous system, resulting in RLS. Iron is a required metal for the function of tyrosine hydroxylase, the enzyme that catalyzes the conversion of tyrosine to L-hydroxyphenylalanine, the rate-limiting step in the synthesis of dopamine (108–111).

Clinical Manifestations
The clinical features of RLS are described in Table 34-4. The unbearable discomfort in the legs may be described as creepy, crawly, and achy sensations. The symptoms are typically limited to the lower extremities, but may involve the upper extremities in severe cases. Symptoms mostly occur during the evening hours and at bedtime, and may result in problems falling asleep. Some patients may come to see the doctor with a primary complaint of insomnia, not realizing a potential association with RLS. The differential diagnosis includes peripheral polyneuropathy, nocturnal leg cramps, and akathisia. Detailed history and neurological examination helps to exclude these condi-

tions. Once the diagnosis is made, treatable secondary causes of RLS should be excluded. The diagnosis of RLS remains a challenge in subjects with impaired cognitive function. It is not known how much of the restlessness and agitation that occurs in the evening hours in subjects with dementia could be due to discomfort caused by RLS symptoms.

Periodic Limb Movement Disorder

PLMD is a condition characterized by repetitive movements of the lower extremities (big toe extension, ankle dorsiflexion, with or without knee and hip flexion) that occur during sleep or relaxed wakefulness. These movements may be associated with arousals from sleep, resulting in nocturnal sleep disruption and daytime sleepiness. The diagnosis is based on the number of leg movements found during an overnight PSG, although leg monitors designed to detect movements can also be used. The movement occurs intermittently, lasting for 0.5 to 10 seconds, at intervals of 5 to 90 seconds (112). A PLM index of five or more movements per hour of sleep is considered abnormal. The PLM arousal index is used to determine the severity of sleep disruption. Most people with PLMD complain of daytime fatigue or sleepiness and are not aware of the problem. PLMs mostly occur during the NREM sleep cycle. The prevalence of PLMD increases with age, with a reported prevalence of 5% between the ages of 30 and 50, and 44% in individuals older than 65 (113,114).

Pharmacologic Treatment

The pharmacologic treatment of RLS and PLMD is the same. Although the Food and Drug Administration has not approved pharmacologic agents for either disorder, several drugs have been used successfully. Dopaminergic agents are considered the drugs of choice (113,114) and are listed in Table 34-5. Opioids have also been proven beneficial in the treatment of RLS, but they carry the risk of abuse and addiction. Gabapentin has been found effective in the treatment of RLS in a double-blind cross-over study, although the mean dose of the drug used to control symptoms was about 1,800 mg/day (115). Benzodiazepines such as clonazepam, temazepam, nitrazepam (sold only in Canada), and lorazepam have been used for the treatment of RLS and PLMD, but they are not drugs of choice. This may be because they do not eliminate the PLM, although they may improve nighttime sleep by allowing the subject to sleep through the events (i.e., causing a decrease in the PLM arousal index but not the PLM index itself). Benzodiazepines with longer half-lives may be associated with daytime sleepiness in older individuals, and can potentially worsen apnea and hypopnea events in subjects with SLB.

TABLE 34-5
COMMONLY USED DOPAMINERGIC DRUGS FOR RESTLESS LEGS SYNDROME

Drug	Dose	Half-Life[a]	Comment
Levodopa/carbidopa (Sinemet) 25/100	25/100 mg	1.5 hours	Greater risk for augmentation of RLS symptoms compared to other dopamine agonists
Pramipexole (Mirapex)	0.125 mg	8–12 hours	Somnolence reported as a side effect
Ropinirole HCl (Requip)	0.25 mg	6 hours	Somnolence reported as a side effect

[a]Half-life may be longer in the elderly.
RLS, restless legs syndrome.

Of concern regarding the use of dopaminergic agents is the occurrence of symptom rebound or augmentation (105). Rebound of symptoms of RLS may begin to occur 2 to 6 hours after a dose, following a period of initial improvement. A greater risk for rebound symptoms is found with levodopa/carbidopa preparations (116). Appropriate scheduling of the drug usually takes care of this problem. Augmentation of symptoms is characterized by RLS symptoms that appear weeks to months after an initial improvement and may be even more severe than the first symptoms (e.g., occurring at earlier times, or in the upper extremities). This may respond to changing to another dopaminergic agent. The mechanism for this phenomenon is not clearly understood (116).

Drug Dosing and Scheduling

In general, it is advised to start low and go slow with drug scheduling, based on the frequency and timing of symptoms and the half-life. Since most RLS symptoms start in the evening, it is recommended to take the first dose about 45 minutes before the start of symptoms. To prevent rebound and treat accompanying PLMs, another dose may be taken at bedtime. In situations where the symptoms start in the afternoon, appropriate dosing modifications may be made.

RAPID EYE MOVEMENT SLEEP BEHAVIOR DISORDER

Rapid eye movement sleep behavior disorder (RBD) is a condition characterized by abnormal sleep behaviors in association with vivid dream enactment. In this condition, there is loss of the normal skeletal muscle atonia that accompanies REM sleep, resulting in enactment of dreams. Dream enactment activities range from simple movements of the extremities while in bed, to jumping out of bed while dreaming about playing games, or punching the bed partner while trying to protect oneself from an attack. The patient usually remembers these dreams but does not remember the dream enactment behavior (117–119). RBD is more commonly seen in older individuals and in males, with a reported mean age of onset of about 60 years (117–119).

Clinical Features

RBD may present in an acute or chronic form. The acute form of the disease is associated with withdrawal states, most commonly from alcohol. It is also described as a side effect of excessive caffeine intake and medications such as tricyclic antidepressants, monoamine oxidase inhibitors, SSRIs such as fluoxetine, and venlafaxine (117–119).

The chronic form of the disease may be idiopathic and appear in apparently healthy individuals, or may occur in association with neurodegenerative diseases such as Parkinson's disease and dementia (120–123). RBD has sometimes been reported to precede these conditions by a few years. The disease usually has an insidious onset, starting with sleep talking, yelling, and jerking movements of the extremities for years before the violent behavior is manifested. The dreams are reported to become more vivid and violent as the disease progresses. Patients may present to physicians with signs of injury (e.g., ecchymoses, fractures, lacerations) to themselves or their bed partner.

Diagnosis is based on history and confirmed by overnight PSG with video recording, where increased electromyographic activity and abnormal movements are observed during REM periods. Although the history is typical, PSG is essential to rule out other possible causes like a seizure disorder, sleep terrors, or nightmares.

Treatment

Clonazepam has been used successfully in the treatment of RBD with a reported response rate of up to 90% (118,119). Clonazepam is taken at bedtime, or 30 to 45 minutes before bedtime if sleep initiation is a problem. Response is reported as early as the first night, but mostly in the first week. Tolerance is not a reported problem. Successful treatment has also been reported in small samples of patients on donepezil (124), melatonin (125), and pramipexole (126). It is also important to make sure the patient is not taking any medications that may aggravate the symptoms of RBD.

DISORDERS OF SLEEP-WAKE CYCLE

The sleep-wake cycle is influenced by the *homeostatic factor* and the circadian rhythm. The homeostatic factor refers to the amount of sleep the person had during the previous night, and how this influences the sleep-wake cycle. The circadian rhythm refers to a 24-hour pattern of physiological functions of the different organ systems in the body. All physiological functions follow a pattern of activity during the 24-hour cycle that is synchronized with the environment. The sleep-wake cycle follows a similar pattern. This pattern of activity is coordinated by the SCN of the hypothalamus. Disruption of this pattern results in sleep-wake problems. Common circadian rhythm disorders seen in older individuals include *advanced sleep phase syndrome* and *irregular sleep pattern*.

Advanced Sleep Phase Syndrome

Advanced sleep phase syndrome is a condition in which the subjects are unable to stay awake until the desired bedtime, and remain asleep until the desired wake time. These individuals go to sleep early (e.g., 7:00 PM) and wake up early (e.g., 3:00 AM). Although they get an adequate amount of sleep each night, their sleep-wake schedule does not conform to sleep schedules of their families and friends, which may present a problem. Treatment strategies include:

- Chronotherapy, where bedtime is progressively delayed until the desired bedtime is reached
- Bright light therapy during the early evening period to help delay bedtime.

Delayed Sleep Phase Syndrome

Delayed sleep phase syndrome is a condition in which the subject is unable to sleep and wake up at the desired or conventional time. Sleep time and wake-up time are delayed by 3 to 6 hours as compared to the conventional time. If left uninterrupted, the person gets an adequate amount of sleep. But the sleep schedule may interfere with social activities and work schedules. This condition is more common among younger individuals. Treatment strategies include:

- Chronotherapy, where bedtime is progressively advanced until the desired bedtime is reached
- Bright light therapy during the early morning hours to help advance bedtime
- Melatonin given in the early evening hours to help advance bedtime.

Irregular 24-Hour Sleep-Wake Cycle

This occurs when the sleep-wake cycle is disorganized, with a variable amount of sleep or wake behavior occurring

TABLE 34-6
COMMON MEDICAL CONDITIONS AND ASSOCIATED SLEEP DISTURBANCES

Condition	Associated Symptoms	Sleep Disturbance
Congestive heart failure	Orthopnea Paroxysmal nocturnal dyspnea: (sudden awakening from sleep with shortness of breath ± cough, wheezing) Nocturia	Sleep-onset insomnia Sleep-maintenance insomnia
Osteoarthritis	Pain	Sleep-onset insomnia Sleep-maintenance insomnia
Chronic obstructive pulmonary disease	Hypoventilation and hypoxemia during sleep (especially REM sleep) Sleep fragmentation	Sleep-maintenance insomnia
Gastroesophageal reflux disease	Epigastric burning, reflux Sleep disruption	Sleep-maintenance insomnia Sleep-onset insomnia
Parkinson's disease	Stiffness, pain (motor symptoms) Associated PLMs, RBDs	Sleep-maintenance insomnia Excessive daytime sleepiness
Dementia	Degenerative CNS changes	Irregular sleep-wake pattern Excessive daytime sleepiness
Seizure disorders	Sleep disruption	Sleep-maintenance insomnia
Depression	Physiological arousal Emotional arousal Cognitive arousal Faulty conditioning	Sleep-onset insomnia Sleep-maintenance insomnia Early-morning awakenings Sleep-onset insomnia
Anxiety disorder	Worrying at bedtime Nocturnal panic	Sleep-maintenance insomnia

CNS, central nervous system; PLMs, periodic limb movements; RBDs, rapid eye movement sleep behavior disorders; REM, rapid eye movement.

at different times during a 24-hour period. Individuals with this disorder nap multiple times during the day, and their nocturnal sleep is poorly consolidated. This may be seen in patients with neurodegenerative diseases such as dementia. It can also be seen in individuals with poor sleep hygiene, or institutionalized individuals with inadequate exposure to light and activity (127). Treatment depends on the specific etiology, but practice of good sleep hygiene, adequate exposure to light, and participation in activities have all been shown to benefit most individuals.

Sundowning/Nocturnal Agitation

Sundowning is a term used to refer to abnormal behavior, manifested mostly by patients with dementia, in the late afternoon and evening hours. The abnormal behavior may range from inappropriate vocalizations to aggression. The condition may be seen more commonly in hospitalized and institutionalized dementia patients. Sundowning poses a significant management problem for family members and other caretakers at home, and may be a major reason for nursing home placement. The prevalence of sundowning has been reported to range from 12% to 24%, depending on the site of the study and the definition used (128,129). Factors that contribute to the occurrence of sundowning include:

- Cognitive dysfunction: Among NHRs, subjects with more severe dementia are more likely to show sundowning. Other factors associated with sundowning include a recent admission to a facility, a change of room, and other psychosocial stresses. It is postulated that neurode-

---

TABLE 34-7

SLEEP-RELATED EFFECTS OF COMMONLY PRESCRIBED MEDICATIONS

Medication	Sleep-Related Effects
Acetylcholinesterase Inhibitors	
Donepezil	nightmares, insomnia
Galantamine	Insomnia (9%), nightmares
Rivastigmine	Increased REM sleep and REM density
Antidepressants	
Selective serotonin-reuptake inhibitors	Insomnia about 20%; sleepiness 10–15%; some more sedating than others
	May increase symptoms of restless legs syndrome
	Decreased REM sleep
Tricyclic Antidepressants	Improved nocturnal sleep ± daytime sedation
	Decreased REM sleep
Venlafaxine	Insomnia
	Increased sleepiness also reported (not common)
	May increase symptoms of restless legs syndrome
Trazodone	Improved sleep ± daytime sedation
Mirtazapine	Improved nocturnal sleep ± daytime sedation. Lower doses may be more sedating compared to higher doses
Bupropion	Insomnia
Nefazodone	Daytime sedation
MAO inhibitors	Insomnia
Antihistamines	Daytime sedation
Antihypertensives	
β-blockers	Insomnia, nightmares (more common with lipophilic compounds)
Diuretics	Sleep disruption due to nocturia if taken later in the day
Angiotensin II receptor blockers	Insomnia (rare)
Clonidine	Decreased REM sleep
Terazosin	Somnolence
Doxazosin	Somnolence
Antipsychotics	Daytime sedation possible in all agents
Benzodiazepines	Daytime sedation
	May worsen sleep-disordered breathing
Dopaminergic Agents	
Levodopa-carbidopa	Sleep disruption in high dose
Other dopamine agonists	Sleepiness in low dose

MAO, monoamine oxidase; REM, rapid eye movement.

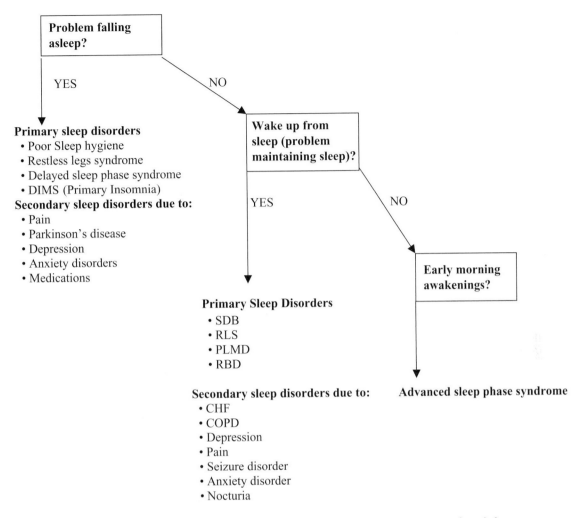

Primary sleep disorders
- Poor Sleep hygiene
- Restless legs syndrome
- Delayed sleep phase syndrome
- DIMS (Primary Insomnia)

Secondary sleep disorders due to:
- Pain
- Parkinson's disease
- Depression
- Anxiety disorders
- Medications

Primary Sleep Disorders
- SDB
- RLS
- PLMD
- RBD

Secondary sleep disorders due to:
- CHF
- COPD
- Depression
- Pain
- Seizure disorder
- Anxiety disorder
- Nocturia

Advanced sleep phase syndrome

Excessive daytime sleepiness may be the consequence of any of the sleep problems mentioned above. Conditions such as narcolepsy, idiopathic hypersomnia, and degenerative CNS diseases may also cause

Figure 34-5 An algorithm for the differential diagnosis of sleep disorders. CHF, congestive heart failure; CNS, central nervous system; COPD, chronic obstructive pulmonary disease; DIMS, disorders of initiating and maintaining sleep; PLMD, period limb movement disorder; RBD, rapid eye movement sleep behavior disorder; RLS, restless legs syndrome; SDB, sleep-disordered breathing.

generative changes in the SCN may explain why behavioral changes occur later in the day (130).

■ Unmet needs: Another factor that may contribute to sundowning is physical or mental stress (e.g., pain, anxiety) that may be aggravated during the late afternoon or evening hours. For example, pain due to osteoarthritis is reported to worsen towards the end of the day (131).

The treatment of sundowning involves first identifying and treating possible unmet needs, such as pain or excessive ambient commotion, or underlying medical conditions such as infection or metabolic alterations. The second step is to devise and implement a nonpharmacologic behavioral plan. The pharmacologic treatment of sundowning is

detailed in a separate chapter in this textbook on agitation and psychosis.

MEDICAL, NEUROLOGICAL, AND PSYCHIATRIC DISEASES

Many of the chronic medical, neurological, and psychiatric diseases that are common among older individuals could be associated with sleep problems. Conditions that can disrupt falling and/or staying asleep, or cause early-morning awakenings, include CHF, chronic pulmonary disease, osteoarthritis pain, depression, and Parkinson's disease, to name a few. A more complete list can be found in

Table 34-6. Advanced Parkinson's disease is also associated with daytime sleepiness, and disruption of the sleep-wake pattern is found in patients with Alzheimer's disease. Successful management of these conditions usually improves the nocturnal sleep of the patient as well.

MEDICATIONS

Older adults comprise only 12% of the population yet consume 25% of the medications prescribed each year. Some of these medications may directly and adversely affect the sleep-wake cycle. Others may alter the metabolism of sleep-promoting agents, thus prolonging their action. For this reason, a critical evaluation is required so that essential medications that are required for the management of the patients' medical problems are continued, and nonessential medications are discontinued. Table 34-7 lists commonly used drugs and their sleep-related effects.

An algorithm of the entire diagnostic process for sleep disorders in the elderly is presented in Figure 34-5.

REFERENCES

1. Borbely A. *Secrets of Sleep*. Library of Congress: New York: Basic Books; 1986.
2. Caton R. The electric currents of the brain. *BMJ*. 1875;2:278.
3. Asterinsky E, Kleitman N. Regularly occurring periods of eye motility and concomitant phenomena during sleep. *Science*. 1953;118:273.
4. Chokroverty S. An overview of sleep. In: Chokroverty S. *Sleep Disorders Medicine*. Woburn, MA: Butterworth-Hainemann; 1999;7–20.
5. Adam K, Oswald I. Sleep is for tissue restoration. *J Roy Coll Phys*. 1977;11:376.
6. Zepelin H, Rechtschaffen A. Mammalian sleep, longevity and energy metabolism. *Brain Behav Evol*. 1974;10:425.
7. Craskadon MA, Dement WX. Cumulative effects of sleep restriction on daytime sleepiness. *Psychophysiology*. 1981;18:107.
8. Koslowski M, Babkoff H. Meta-analysis of the relationship between total sleep deprivation and performance. *Chronobiol Int*. 1992;9:132–136.
9. Pilcher JJ, Huffcutt AI. Effects of sleep deprivation on performance: a meta-analysis. *Sleep*. 1996;19:318–326.
10. Van Dongen HA, Maislin G, Mullington J, Dinges DF. The cumulative cost of additional wakefulness: dose-response effects on neurobehavioral functions and sleep physiology from chronic sleep restriction and total sleep deprivation. *Sleep*. 2002;26: 117–126.
11. Irwin M, McClintick J, Costlow C, et al. Partial night sleep deprivation reduces natural killer and cellular immune responses in humans. *FASEB J*. 1996;10:643–653.
12. Dinges DF, Douglas SD, Zaugg L, et al. Leukocytosis and natural killer cell function parallel neurobehavioral fatigue induced by 64 hours of sleep deprivation. *J Clin Invest*. 1994;93:1930–1939.
13. Spiegel K, Leproult R, Van Cauter E. Impact of sleep debt on metabolic and endocrine function. *Lancet*. 1999;354:1435.
14. Mullington JM, Chan JL, Van Dongen HP, et al. Sleep loss reduces diurnal rhythm amplitude of leptin in healthy men. *J Neuroendocrinol*. 2003;15:851–854.
15. Schubert CR, Cruickshanks KJ, Dalton DS, et al. Prevalence of sleep problems and quality of life in an older population. *Sleep*. 2002;25:889–893.
16. Vitiello MV, Moe KE, Prinz PN. Sleep complaints congregate with illness in older adults: clinical research informed by and inform-

ing epidemiological studies of sleep. *J Psychosomatic Res*. 2002; 53:555–559.
17. National Institute of Health Conference Development Conference Statement: the treatment of sleep disorders of older people. *Sleep*. 1990;14:169–177.
18. Carskadon M, Dement W. Normal human sleep: an overview. In: Kryger MH, Roth T, Dement WC, eds. *Principles and Practice of Sleep Medicine*. Philadelphia: WB Saunders Company; 2000:15–25.
19. Hirshkowitz M, Moore CA, Hamilton CR, et al. Polysomnography of adults and elderly: sleep architecture, respiration, and leg movement. *J Clin Neurophysiol*. 1992;9:56–62.
20. Hoch CC, Dew MA, Reynolds CF III, et al. A longitudinal study of laboratory- and diary-based sleep measures in healthy "old old" and "young old" volunteers. *Sleep*. 1994;17:489–496.
21. Reynolds CF, Monk TH, Hoch CC, et al. Electroencephalographic sleep in the healthy "old old": a comparison with the "young old" in visually scored and automated measures. *J Gerontology*. 1991;4:M39–M46.
22. Webb WB, Dreblow LM. A modified method for scoring slow wave sleep of older subjects. *Sleep*. 1982;5:195–199.
23. Rediehs MH, Reis JS, Creason NS. Sleep in old age: focus on gender differences. *Sleep*. 1990;13:410–424.
24. Boselli M, Parrino L, Smerieri A, Terzano MG. Effect of age on EEG arousals in normal sleep. *Sleep*. 1998;21:351–357.
25. Webb WB, Campbell SS. Awakenings and the return to sleep in an older population. *Sleep*. 1980;3:41–46.
26. Bliwise D. Normal aging. In: Kryger MH, Roth T, Dement WC, eds. *Principles and Practice of Sleep Medicine*. Philadelphia: WB Saunders Company; 2000:26–42.
27. Wauquier A. Aging and changes in phasic events during sleep. *Physiol Behav*. 1993;54:803–806.
28. Naifeh K, Severinghaus J, Kamiya J. Effect of aging on sleep-related changes in respiratory variables. *Sleep*. 1987;10:160–171.
29. Turek F. Introduction to chronobiology: sleep and the circadian clock. In: Kryger MH, Roth T, Dement WC, eds. *Principles and Practice of Sleep Medicine*. Philadelphia: WB Saunders Company; 2000:315–333.
30. Hofman MA, Swaab DF. Influence of aging on the seasonal rhythm of the vasopressin-expressing neurons in the human suprachiasmatic nucleus. *Neurobiol Aging*. 1995;16:965–971.
31. Vitiello MV, Smallwood RG, Avery DH, et al. Circadian temperature rhythms in young adult and aged men. *Neurobiol Aging*. 1986;7:97–100.
32. Monk TH, Kupfer DJ. Circadian rhythms in healthy aging—effects downstream from the pacemaker. *Chronobiol Int*. 2000;17:355–368.
33. Foley DJ, Monjan AA, Brown SL, Simonsick EM, Wallace RB, Blazer DG. Sleep complaints among elderly persons: an epidemiologic study of three communities. *Sleep*. 1995;18(6):425–432.
34. Karacan I, Thomby J, Anch M, et al. Prevalence of sleep disturbance in a primary urban Florida County. *Soc Sci Med*. 1976;10: 239–244.
35. Bixler E, Kales A, Soldats C, Kales J, Hedley S. Prevalence of sleep disorders in the Los Angeles metropolitan area. *Am J Psychiatry*. 1979;136:1257–1261.
36. Fetveit A, Bjorvatn B. Sleep disturbances among nursing home residents. *Int J Geriatr Psych*. 2002;17:604–609.
37. Jacobs D, Ancoli-Israel S, Parker L, Kripke DF. Twenty-four-hour sleep-wake patterns in a nursing home population. *Psychol Aging*. 1989;4:352–356.
38. Sato R, Kanda K, Anan M, Watanuki S. Sleep EEG patterns and fatigue of middle-aged and older female family caregivers providing routine nighttime care for elderly persons at home. *Percept Mot Skills*. 2002;95(3 Pt 1):815–829.
39. Pollak CP, Perlick D. Sleep problems and institutionalization of the elderly. *J Geriatr Psych Neurol*. 1991;4:204–210.
40. Schnelle JF, Ouslander JG, Simmons SF, et al. The nighttime environment, incontinence care, and sleep disruption in nursing homes. *J Am Geriatr Soc*. 1993;41:910–914.
41. Schnelle JF, Cruise PA, Alessi CA, et al. Sleep hygiene in physically dependent nursing home residents: behavioral and environmental intervention implications. *Sleep*. 1998;21:515–523.
42. Johns W. A new method for measuring daytime sleepiness: the Epworth Sleepiness Index. *Sleep*. 1991;14:540–545.

43. Roehrs T, Carskadon M, Dement W, Roth T. Daytime sleepiness and alertness. In: Kryger MH, Roth T, Dement WC, eds. *Principles and Practice of Sleep Medicine*. Philadelphia: WB Saunders Company; 2000:43–52.

44. Monk TH, Reynolds CF III, Kupfer DJ, et al. The Pittsburgh Sleep Diary. *J Sleep Res*. 1994;3:111–120.

45. Ancoli-Israel S, Cole R, Alessi C, Chambers M, Moorcroft W, Pollak CP. The role of Actigraphy in the study of sleep and circadian rhythms. *Sleep*. 2003;26:342–392.

46. Zarcone V. Sleep hygiene. In: Kryger MH, Roth T, Dement WC, eds. *Principles and Practice of Sleep Medicine*. Philadelphia: WB Saunders Company; 2000:657–661.

47. Lasagna, L. Over-the-counter hypnotics and chronic insomnia in the elderly. *J Clin Psychopharmacol*. 1995;15:383–386.

48. Costa E, Silva JA, Chase M, Sartorius N, Roth T. Special report from a symposium held by the World Health Organization and the World Federation of Sleep Research Societies: an overview of insomnias and related disorders—recognition, epidemiology, and rational management. *Sleep*. 1996;19:412–416.

49. Morin CM, Hauri PJ, Espie CA, Spielman AJ, Buysse DJ, Bootzin RR. Nonpharmacologic treatment of chronic insomnia. An American Academy of Sleep Medicine review. *Sleep*. 1999;22(8):1134–1156.

50. Vgontzas AN, Bixler EO, Lin HM, et al. Chronic insomnia is associated with nyctohemeral activation of the hypothalamic-pituitary-adrenal axis: clinical implications. *J Clin Endocrinol Metab*. 2001;86:3787–3794.

51. American Academy of Sleep Medicine. International Classification of Sleep Disorders: Diagnostic and Coding Manual. Rochester, MN: American Academy of Sleep Medicine 1990.

52. Petit L, Azad N, Byszewski A, et al. Non-pharmacological management of primary and secondary insomnia among older people: review of assessment tools and treatments. *Age Ageing*. 2003;32:19–25.

53. Chesson L, Anderson W, Littner M, et al. Practice parameters for the non-pharmacologic treatment of chronic insomnia. *Sleep*. 1999;22:1128–1133.

54. Holbrook AM, Crowther R, Lotter A, et al. Meta-analysis of benzodiazepine use in the treatment of insomnia. *CMAJ*. 2000;162:225–233.

55. Montplaisir J, Hawa R, Moller H, et al. Zopiclone and zaleplon vs benzodiazepines in the treatment of insomnia: Canadian consensus statement. Consensus Development Conference. *Hum Psychopharmacol*. 2003;18:29–38.

56. Ray WA, Thapa PB, Gideon P. Benzodiazepines and the risk of falls in nursing home residents. *J Am Geriatr Soc*. 2000;48:682–685.

57. Herings RM, Stricker BH, de Boer A, Bakker A, Sturmans F. Benzodiazepines and the risk of falling leading to femur fractures. Dosage more important than elimination half-life. *Arch Int Med*. 1995;155:1801–1807.

58. Walsh JK, Schweitzer PK. Ten-year trends in the pharmacological treatment of insomnia. *Sleep*. 1999;22:371–375.

59. Schittecatte M, Dumont F, Machowski R, Cornil C, Lavergne F, Wilmotte J. Effects of mirtazapine on sleep polygraphic variables in major depression. *Neuropsychobiology*. 2002;46:197–201.

60. Kaynak H, Kaynak D, Gozukirmizi E, Guilleminault C. The effects of trazodone on sleep in patients treated with stimulant antidepressants. *Sleep Med*. 2004;5:15–20.

61. Godfrey RG. A guide to the understanding and use of tricyclic antidepressants in the overall management of fibromyalgia and other chronic pain syndromes. *Arch Int Med*. 1996;156:1047–1052.

62. Vanpee D, Laloyaux P, Gillet JB. Seizure and hyponatraemia after overdose of trazodone. *Am J Emerg Med*. 1999;17:430–443.

63. Mulsant BH, Pollock BG, Kirshner M, Shen C, Dodge H, Ganguli M. Serum anticholinergic activity in a community-based sample of older adults: relationship with cognitive performance. *Arch Gen Psychiatry*. 2000;57:1105–1114.

64. Hughes RJ, Sack RL, Lewy AJ. The role of melatonin and circadian phase in age-related sleep-maintenance insomnia: assessment in a clinical trial of melatonin replacement. *Sleep*. 1998;21:52–68.

65. Roehrs T, Roth T. Sleep, sleepiness and health. *Alcohol Res Health*. 2001;25:101–110.

66. Eisenberg DM, Davis RB, Ettner SL, et al. Trends in alternative medicine use in the United States, 1990–1997: results of a follow-up national survey. *JAMA*. 1998;280:1569–1575.

67. Glass JR, Sproule BA, Herrmann N, et al. Acute pharmacological effects of temazepam, diphenhydramine, and valerian in healthy elderly subjects. *J Clin Psychopharmacol*. 2003;23:260–268.

68. Bassiri AG, Guilleminault C. Clinical features and evaluation of obstructive sleep apnea-hypopnea syndrome. In: Kryger MH, Roth T, Dement WC, eds. Principles and practice of sleep medicine. Philadelphia: WB Saunders 2000;889–878.

69. Young T, Shahar E, Nieto FJ, et al. Sleep Heart Health Study Research Group. Predictors of sleep-disordered breathing in community-dwelling adults: the Sleep Heart Health Study. *Arch Int Med*. 2002;16:893–900.

70. Bixler EO, Vgontzas AN, Lin HM, et al. Prevalence of sleep-disordered breathing in women: effects of gender. *Am J Respir Crit Care Med*. 2001;163(3 Pt 1):608–613.

71. Redline S, Kump K, Tishler PV, et al. Gender differences in sleep disordered breathing in a community-based sample. *Am J Respir Crit Care Med*. 1994;149(3 Pt 1):722–726.

72. Guilleminault C, Quera-Salva MA, Partinen M, Jamieson A. Women and the obstructive sleep apnea syndrome. *Chest*. 1988;93:104–109.

73. Endeshaw Y, Katz S, Ouslander J, Bliwise D. Association between sleep-disordered breathing and denture use. *J Public Health Dent*. 2004;64:181–183.

74. Vorona RD, Ware JC. Sleep disordered breathing and driving. *Curr Opin Pulm Med*. 2002;8:506–510.

75. Teran-Santos J, Jimenez-Gomez A, Cordero-Guevara J. The association between sleep apnea and the risk of traffic accidents. *N Engl J Med*. 1999;340:847–851.

76. Guilleminault C, Faul JL, Stoohs R. Sleep-disordered breathing and hypotension. *Am J Respir Crit Care Med*. 2001;164: 1242–1247.

77. Foley DJ, Masaki KM, White L, et al. Sleep-disordered breathing and cognitive impairment in elderly Japanese-American men. *Sleep*. 2003;26:596–599.

78. Aloia MS, Ilniczky N, Di Dio P, Perlis ML, Greenblatt DW, Giles DE. Neuropsychological changes and treatment compliance in older adults with sleep apnea. *J Psychosom Res*. 2003;54:71–76.

79. Endeshaw Y, Johnson T, Kutner M, et al. Sleep-disordered breathing and nocturia among older adults. *J Am Geriatr Soc*. 2004;52:957–960.

80. Brown JS, Vittinghoff E, Wyman J, et al. Urinary incontinence: does it increase risk for falls and fractures? Study of Osteoporotic Fractures Research Group. *J Am Geriatr Soc*. 2000;48:721–725.

81. Stewart RB, Moore MT, May FE, et al. Nocturia: a risk factor for falls in the elderly. *J Am Geriatr Soc*. 1992;40:1217–1220.

82. Parish JM, Somers VK. Obstructive sleep apnea and cardiovascular disease. *Mayo Clin Proc*. 2004;79:1036–1046.

83. Quan SF, Gersh BJ, National Center on Sleep Disorders Research, National Heart, Lung, and Blood Institute. Cardiovascular consequences of sleep-disordered breathing: past, present and future: report of a workshop from the National Center on Sleep Disorders Research and the National Heart, Lung, and Blood Institute. *Circulation*. 2004;109:951–957.

84. Harding SM. Complications and consequences of obstructive sleep apnea. *Curr Opin Pulm Med*. 2000;6:485–489.

85. Fletcher EC. Cardiovascular consequences of obstructive sleep apnea: experimental hypoxia and sympathetic activity. *Sleep*. 2000;23(Suppl 4):S127–S131.

86. Standards of Practice Committee of the American Sleep Disorders Association. Practice parameters for the use of portable recording in the assessment of obstructive sleep apnea. *Sleep*. 1994;17:372–377.

87. American Academy of Sleep Medicine. Sleep-related breathing disorders in adults: recommendations for syndrome definition and measurement techniques in clinical research. *Sleep*. 2003;22:667–689.

88. Zozula R, Rosen R. Compliance with continuous positive airway pressure therapy: assessing and improving treatment outcomes. *Curr Opin Pulm Med*. 2001;7:391–398.

89. Mcardle N, Devereuxd G, Arnejad H, et al. Long-term use of CPAP therapy for sleep apnea/hypopnea syndrome. *Am J Respir Crit Care Med.* 1999;159:1108–1114.

90. Greenfield D, Gehrman P, Linn M, et al. CPAP compliance in mild-moderate Alzheimer's patients with SDB. *Sleep.* 2003; 26(Suppl):A154.

91. Standards of Practice Committee of the American Sleep Disorders Association. Practice parameters for the treatment of snoring and obstructive sleep apnea with oral appliances. *Sleep.* 1995;18:511–513.

92. Standards of Practice Committee of the American Sleep Disorders Association. Practice parameters for the treatment of obstructive sleep apnea in adults: the efficacy of surgical modifications of the upper airway. *Sleep.* 1996;19:152–155.

93. Riley R, Powell N, Li K, Guilleminault C. Surgical therapy for obstructive sleep apnea hypopnea syndrome. In: Kryger MH, Roth T, Dement WC, eds. *Principles and Practice of Sleep Medicine.* Philadelphia: WB Saunders Company; 2000: 913– 928.

94. Smith I, Lasserson T, Wright J. Drug treatments for obstructive sleep apnoea. *Cochrane Database Syst Rev.* 2002;(2):CD003002.

95. Wuyam B, Pepin JL, Tremel F, Levy P. Pathophysiology of central sleep apnea syndrome. *Sleep.* 2000;23(Suppl 4):S213–S219.

96. Javaheri S, Parker TJ, Wexler L, et al. Occult sleep-disordered breathing in stable congestive heart failure. *Ann Intern Med.* 1995;122:487–492.

97. Allen RP, Picchietti D, Hening WA, et al. Restless legs syndrome: diagnostic criteria, special considerations, and epidemiology: a report from the restless legs syndrome diagnosis and epidemiology workshop at the National Institutes of Health. *Sleep Med.* 2003;4:101–119.

98. Ohayon M, Roth T. Prevalence of restless legs syndrome and periodic limb movement disorder in the general population. *J Psychosom Res.* 2002;53:547–554.

99. Phillips B, Young T, Finn L, et al. Epidemiology of restless legs symptoms in adults. *Arch Intern Med.* 2000;160:2137–2141.

100. Nichols DA, Allen RP, Grauke JH, et al. Restless legs syndrome symptoms in primary care: a prevalence study. *Arch Intern Med.* 2003;163:2323–2329.

101. Milligan SA, Chesson AL. Restless legs syndrome in the older adult: diagnosis and management. *Drugs Aging.* 2002;19: 741–751.

102. Bonati MT, Ferini-Strambi L, Aridon P, et al. Autosomal dominant restless legs syndrome maps on chromosome 14q. *Brain.* 2003;126:1485–1492.

103. Winkelmann J, Muller-Myhsok B, Wittchen HU, et al. Complex segregation analysis of restless legs syndrome provides evidence for an autosomal dominant mode of inheritance in early age at onset families. *Annals Neurol.* 2002;52:297–302.

104. O'Keeffe ST. Restless legs syndrome. A review. *Arch Intern Med.* 1996;15:243–248.

105. Earley CJ. Clinical practice. Restless legs syndrome. *N Engl J Med.* 2003;348:2103–2109.

106. Hartmann M, Pfister R, Pfadenhauer K. Restless legs syndrome associated with spinal cord lesions. *J Neurol Neurosurg Psychiatry.* 1999;66:688–689.

107. Tings T, Baier PC, Paulus W, Trenkwalder C. Restless legs syndrome induced by impairment of sensory spinal pathways. *J Neurol.* 2003;250:499–500.

108. Michaud M, Soucy JP, Chabli A, Lavigne G, Montplaisir J. SPECT imaging of striatal pre- and postsynaptic dopaminergic status in restless legs syndrome with periodic leg movements in sleep. *J Neurol.* 2002;249:164–170.

109. Earley CJ, Allen RP, Beard JL, Connor JR. Insight into the pathophysiology of restless legs syndrome. *J Neurosci Res.* 2002;62: 623–628.

110. Allen RP, Barker PB, Wehrl F, Song HK, Earley CJ. MRI measurement of brain iron in patients with restless legs syndrome. *Neurology.* 2001;56:263–265.

111. Haavik J, Le Bourdelles B, Martinez A, et al. Recombinant human tyrosine hydroxylase isoenzymes. Recombination with iron inhibitory effect of other enzymes. *Eur J Biochem.* 1991;199: 371–378.

112. The Atlas Task Force. Recording and scoring periodic leg movements. *Sleep.* 1993;16:749–759.

113. Chesson AL Jr, Wise M, Davila D, et al. Practice parameters for the treatment of restless legs syndrome and periodic limb movement disorder. An American Academy of Sleep Medicine Report. Standards of Practice Committee of the American Academy of Sleep Medicine. *Sleep.* 1999;22:961–968.

114. Motplaisir J, Nicolas S, Godbout R, Walter A. Restless legs syndrome and periodic leg movement disorder. In: Kryger MH, Roth T, Dement WC, eds. *Principles and Practice of Sleep Medicine.* Philadelphia: WB Saunders Company; 2000:743.

115. Garcia-Borreguero D, Larrosa O, de la Llave Y, Verger K, Masramon X, Hernandez G. Treatment of restless legs syndrome with gabapentin: a double-blind, cross-over study. *Neurology.* 2002;59:1573–1579.

116. Comella CL. Restless legs syndrome: treatment with dopaminergic agents. *Neurology.* 2002;58(Suppl):S87–S92.

117. Ohayon MM, Caulet M, Priest RG. Violent behavior during sleep. *J Clin Psychiatry.* 1997;58(8):369–376.

118. Mahowald M, Schenck C. REM sleep parasomnias. In: Kryger MH, Roth T, Dement WC, eds. *Principles and Practice of Sleep Medicine.* Philadelphia: WB Saunders Company; 2000: 724– 733.

119. Olson EJ, Boeve BF, Silber MH. Rapid eye movement sleep behaviour disorder: demographic, clinical and laboratory findings in 93 cases. *Brain.* 2000;123:331–339.

120. Syed BH, Rye DB, Singh G. REM sleep behavior disorder and SCA-3 (Machado-Joseph disease). *Neurology.* 2003;60:148.

121. Turner RS. Idiopathic rapid eye movement sleep behavior disorder is a harbinger of dementia with Lewy bodies. *J Geriatr Psych Neurol.* 2002;15:195–199.

122. Friedman JH. Presumed rapid eye movement behavior disorder in Machado-Joseph disease (spinocerebellar ataxia type 3). *Mov Disord.* 2002;17:1350–1353.

123. Gagnon JF, Bedard MA, Fantini ML, et al. REM sleep behavior disorder and REM sleep without atonia in Parkinson's disease. *Neurology.* 2002;59:585–589.

124. Ringman JM, Simmons JH. Treatment of REM sleep behavior disorder with donezepil: a report of three cases. *Neurology.* 2000;55: 870–871.

125. Takeuchi N, Uchimura N, Hashizume Y, et al. Melatonin therapy for REM sleep behavior disorder. *Psychiatry Clin Neurosci.* 2001;55:267–269.

126. Fantini ML, Gagnon JF, Fillipini D, Montplaisir J. The effects of pramipexole in REM sleep behavior disorder. *Neurology.* 2003: 61:1418–1420.

127. Richardson G, Malin H. Circadian rhythm sleep disorders: pathophysiology and treatment. *Clin Neurophysiol.* 1996;13: 17–31.

128. Bliwise D. Dementia. In: Kryger MH, Roth T, Dement WC, eds. *Principles and Practice of Sleep Medicine.* Philadelphia: WB Saunders Company; 2000:1062–1067.

129. Bliwise D. What is Sundowning? *J Am Geriatr Soc.* 1994;42: 1009–1011.

130. Bliwise D. Circadian rhythms and agitation. *Int Psychogeriatr.* 2000;12(Suppl 1):143–146.

131. Labrecque G, Vanier MC. Biological rhythms in pain and in the effects of opioid analgesics. *Pharmacol Ther.* 1995;6:129–147.

Sexuality and Sexual Disorders in Late Life

35

Marc E. Agronin   Ruth K. Westheimer

The assessment and treatment of sexual disorders in late life has evolved considerably since the sexual revolution of the 1960s. Previous stereotypes of sexuality in late life as being inappropriate, unsafe, or even nonexistent have given way to more realistic and open perspectives that value the important role of sexuality throughout the adult lifecycle. This change has been fueled by demographic necessity: people are living longer and healthier lives, and as a result sexuality continues to play a vital role. Key factors that have influenced the role of clinicians in dealing with late-life sexuality include the successful treatment of menopause-induced sexual changes in women, the development and popularization of medications to treat erectile dysfunction (ED), and the increased recognition of sexual side effects due to many psychotropic medications. With a growing number of elderly individuals remaining sexually active, geriatric psychiatrists must be able to assess and treat sexual issues and disorders with understanding, empathy, comfort, and confidence.

I think that the main issue is one of attitude. Years ago, when anyone would say that sexuality exists in later life, people would say "You've got to be kidding." Attitudes are definitely changing, and the best example is that it is more acceptable even for an older woman to have a relationship with a younger man—unheard of several years ago. We have now come to a point where we can write and talk about sexuality in the older adult, and that has not been done before. This change has to do with sexual literacy, it has to do with television and the openness of discussing these issues, and it has to do with scientifically validated data about human sexual functioning that we now have available. Also—with a big exclamation mark—there is no question that the need for older people to be touched and caressed must be acknowledged. There are also several advantages for the older couple. One, she doesn't

have to worry about getting pregnant. Two, they have more time. There is no question that being able to remain sexually active will enhance an older individual's whole outlook on life.

■ *Dr. Ruth Westheimer*

THE ROLE OF THE GERIATRIC PSYCHIATRIST

There are several ways in which the geriatric psychiatrist might be involved in the assessment and treatment of sexual disorders. First, sexual dysfunction may be identified during a psychiatric evaluation for nonsexual symptoms, such as depression or anxiety. Second, patients may present with specific sexual concerns within the context of a relationship problem, a psychiatric disorder, or side effects of psychotropic medication. Finally, the geriatric psychiatrist may be consulted by another specialist to deal with psychiatric factors involved in a sexual problem (e.g., stress, anxiety, medication effects). In many cases, the most likely role for the geriatric psychiatrist will involve dealing with sexual side effects of medications; a section later in this chapter will present an algorithm for intervention. In terms of treatment for sexual disorders, the clinician should be prepared to listen in a supportive manner, offer suggestions on ways to enhance sexual function, and refer the patient for appropriate gynecologic or urologic consultation.

Treatment for ED with oral medications is usually done by internists, family practitioners, and urologists. Women with sexual complaints related to menopausal symptoms are best treated by gynecologists. More specific treatment for sexual disorders, such as premature ejaculation in men, or orgasmic dysfunction in women, is best managed by a clinician with training in sex therapy. That specialist may also be a geriatric psychiatrist who is able to combine expertise in both geriatrics and sexuality.

SEXUALITY IN LATE LIFE

The prevailing model of normal human sexual response describes five psychological and physiological stages that compose sexual activity (1–3):

1. Desire
2. Arousal or excitement
3. Plateau
4. Orgasm
5. Resolution

Sexual desire, or libido, is experienced as a psychological urge, and is centered in the hypothalamus and surrounding limbic structures. In both men and women, the hormone testosterone appears to play a key role in stimulating libido (4). Sexual response is also promoted by dopaminergic function and modulated by prolactin, serotonin, norepinephrine, and nitric oxide levels. Sexual arousal or excitement can be triggered by mental thoughts or fantasies, direct physical stimulation, or hormonal influences. In men, sexual arousal is manifested by a penile erection, while in women it involves swelling or vasocongestion of vaginal, clitoral, and breast tissue, along with vaginal lubrication.

In both sexes, physiological sexual arousal leads to increases in muscle tone, heart rate, respiration, and blood flow to the genitals. Sufficient genital stimulation during sexual arousal may lead to a brief sense of impending orgasm, called the plateau stage, followed by orgasm that is characterized by sensations of euphoria associated with rhythmic contractions of genital muscles. In men, orgasm is brief and accompanied by ejaculation, while in women orgasm tends to last longer and may involve multiple successive occurrences. During the resolution stage, individuals experience a state of mental and physical relaxation during which the genitals are refractory to further stimulation and orgasm. Intact and complimentary functioning of the sympathetic and parasympathetic branches of the autonomic nervous system is required for sexual response.

Normal aging is associated with a general decline in physiological sexual response, and more variable declines in sexual activity. For women, the experience of sexuality in late life is fundamentally shaped by the physiological and psychological changes that occur with *menopause*. This 2 to 10-year decline of ovarian function (termed *perimenopause*) typically begins in a woman's 40s and culminates in complete cessation of menses by the early 50s. For men, no comparable mid-life change in physiological function

occurs. With aging, however, many men can experience important changes in bodily function that are linked to declines in testosterone production. Some researchers have coined the term *andropause*, among others, to represent this change. Age-associated changes in sexual function are summarized in Table 35-1.

Menopause leads to important changes in female genital anatomy and function, including atrophy of urogenital tissue; decreased uterine and vaginal size; and decreases in vaginal lubrication, vasocongestion, and the erotic sensitivity of nipple, clitoral, and vulvar tissue during sexual activity (5). Accompanying changes in sexual function include declines in libido, sexual responsiveness, comfort level (sometimes resulting in uncomfortable intercourse, referred to as *dyspareunia*), and sexual frequency (6,7). During menopause up to 85% of women also experience symptoms such as hot flashes, head and neck aches, transient disruptions in mood (anxiety, irritability, and depression), sleep disturbances, and excess fatigue. Although these changes are primarily attributed to the loss of estrogen production, the role of age-related disruption in hypothalamic function has also been investigated for many menopausal symptoms, particularly hot flashes. Declines in testosterone production in premenopausal women may also lead to changes that affect sexual function, including loss of libido; decreased clitoral, vulvar, and nipple sensitivity; and fatigue (4).

As men age, there are gradual declines in sexual function that have variable impacts on sexual activity. There are no predictable changes in sexual desire, although it remains relatively stable in most men. Erections are less reliable and durable, and require more stimulation to achieve and sustain. Ejaculation during orgasm involves decreased amounts of seminal fluid, and the refractory period between orgasms can increase by hours to days. By middle age, testosterone levels begin to decrease by 1% to 2% per year, meaning that anywhere from 35% to 70% of men over the age of 70 suffer from hypogonadism, defined by a testosterone level less than 200 ng/dL (4,8). Terms such as andropause, *male climacteric*, and *androgen deficiency in aging men* have all been coined to refer to a symptom complex that results from age-related declines in testosterone levels (9). Clinical symptoms include decreased libido and sexual function; depression; decreased lean body mass, body hair, muscle power, and bone density; and increased visceral fat distribution. Some researchers also believe that andropause brings an increased risk for osteoporosis, bone fractures, obesity, insulin resistance, and cardiovascular disease (10,11).

For both men and women, the impact of age-related changes in sexual function has a variable effect on sexual attitudes and behaviors. In general, there is a decline in the frequency of sexual activity after the age of 65, but not as much as might be imagined. According to several major surveys, 50% to 80% of men and women over 60 continue

TABLE 35-1		
NORMAL AGE-ASSOCIATED CHANGES IN SEXUAL FUNCTION		
Function	**Changes in Men**	**Changes in Women**
Sex hormones	▪ Testosterone levels decline by 1–2% per year after age 40 ▪ Leydig cells become less sensitive to luteinizing hormone	▪ Menopause brings cessation of estrogen ▪ Testosterone levels decline gradually in premenopausal women
Genital anatomy	▪ Decreased penile blood flow	▪ Decreased pelvic blood supply ▪ Vaginal size shortens and narrows ▪ Urogenital tissue becomes atrophied and less lubricated
Fertility	▪ Fewer and less functional sperm ▪ Reduced rates of conception	▪ Ceases after menopause
Libido	▪ May decline relative to lower testosterone	▪ May decline with decreased testosterone and/or menopausal symptoms
Sexual arousal	▪ Erections require more tactile stimulation and take longer to achieve ▪ Erections are less rigid ▪ Erections are more difficult to sustain	▪ Requires more tactile stimulation ▪ Decreased vaginal swelling and lubrication ▪ Decreased erogenous sensitivity in clitoris
Orgasm	▪ Orgasm requires more tactile stimulation and takes longer to achieve ▪ Ejaculation is less forceful and has decreased volume	▪ Orgasm requires more tactile stimulation and takes longer to achieve ▪ Vaginal contractions are fewer and less forceful
Refractory period	▪ Lengthened by hours to days	▪ Lengthened

to be sexually active, usually defined as having sexual intercourse at least once a month (12–15). As illustrated in Table 35-2, older men tend to be more sexually active than older women, although sexual satisfaction remains relatively high in both sexes. The major predictors of both sexual interest and activity in late life include the previous level of sexual activity, an individual's physical and psychological health, and the availability, interest level, and health of a partner (16,17). These factors appear to be similar for both heterosexual and homosexual individuals.

Some individuals will react negatively to age-related changes, viewing them as harbingers of physical decline or sexual dysfunction. For men, declines in erectile function can symbolize a threat to their sense of masculinity, and lead to excessive worry, anger, or even depression. Some women grieve the loss of potential motherhood at menopause, particularly if they never had children. Negative reactions may reinforce stereotypes about late-life sexuality being inappropriate or dangerous, and may lead to less frequent and less enjoyable sexual relations (18). On the other hand, aging can bring increased emotional maturity and a heightened capacity for intimacy that can enhance sexual relationships. Older couples may also have greater privacy and more time for intimacy. Individuals who understand that certain changes in sexual function are normal are less

fearful and better able to adapt. For example, instead of dreading the effects of menopause, a woman may welcome the freedom from worry about contraception and unwanted pregnancy. Instead of focusing solely on sexual intercourse as the end-all and be-all of sexuality, a man may be able to shift his focus to the pleasurable sensual intimacy of sexual foreplay. Couples who communicate well can adjust sexual practices in order to maintain or even improve upon previous levels of enjoyment (18).

HOMOSEXUALITY

There are an estimated 1 to 3 million gay and lesbian people over the age of 60 in the United States, and this number is expected to double in the next 30 years. Gay and lesbian individuals and couples face similar issues to heterosexuals in terms of age-associated changes in sexual function and sexual relationships. Several studies indicate that older gay and lesbian people feel high levels of satisfaction with both their identity and lifestyle, and high levels of sexual satisfaction. For example, in one study of over 100 older gay men, 86% of respondents 60 years and older were sexually active, with two-thirds of them reporting sexual activity at least once a month (19).

TABLE 35-2	
SURVEYS OF SEXUAL ACTIVITY IN LATE LIFE	
Study	**Findings**
The Starr-Weiner Report on Sex and Sexuality (12)	▪ 80% of men and women aged 60 to 91 reported to have sex at least once a month
Marsiglio and Donnelly (13)	▪ 50% of married men and women aged 60 and older (N = 800) had sex at least monthly ▪ Mean frequency (age 60–75): 4.26 times/month ▪ Mean frequency (age >75): 2.75 times/month
National Council on the Aging (14)	▪ 80% of survey respondents aged 60–90 with sexual partners had sex at least once a month (N = 1292) ▪ 61% of men remained sexually active compared to 37% of women ▪ Men were twice as likely than women to want more sex than they were already having, and 79% of men sought partners who were interested in sex ▪ 61% of respondents with partners indicated that sex was as physically satisfying as it was in their 40s
American Association of Retired Persons (15)	▪ 75% of male and female survey respondents 45 or older (N = 1384) remained sexually active ▪ 84% of men and 78% of women aged 45–59 had steady sexual partners, compared to 58% of men and 21% of women older than 75 ▪ 50% of individuals aged 45–59 reported having sex at least once a week ▪ 30% of men and 24% of women aged 60–74 reported having sex at least once a week ▪ Of the respondents, the majority of men without partners said they masturbated, while over 77% of women did not ▪ Two-thirds of all respondents were extremely or somewhat satisfied with sex

SEXUALITY IN LONG-TERM CARE SETTINGS

Compared to elderly people living in the community, nursing home residents are significantly less likely to be sexually active (20,21). In one study of 250 nursing home residents, less than 10% reported being sexually active in the last month, although nearly 20% reported a desire for sexual activity but were limited by the lack of a partner or privacy (22). Barriers to sexuality in long-term care include loss of interest, poor health, sexual dysfunction, lack of partners, lack of privacy, and the negative attitudes of staff (23–25). Long-term care facilities have the responsibility, however, to educate both staff and residents about the residents' rights to privacy and to engage in intimate relationships. There are many accommodations that can be provided in a facility to appropriate individuals, such as beauty services, private rooms for conjugal visits, and medical and psychiatric consultation for sexual dysfunction (18).

SEXUALLY TRANSMITTED DISEASES

Sexually transmitted diseases (STDs) are at epidemic levels in the United States, affecting over 65 million people,

many with incurable viral infections (26). According to the Centers for Disease Control and Prevention (CDC), people under the age of 25 account for two-thirds of the 15 million new cases of STDs each year (27). CDC data indicate that individuals 65 and older, on the other hand, account for less than 1% of reported STDs including chlamydia, gonorrhea, and syphilis (28). A study from the State of Washington found that 1.3% of reported STDs were in individuals older than 50 years, with nongonococcal urethritis the most common STD in older men and genital herpes the most common STD in older women (29). Approximately 10% of AIDS patients in the United States are over 50 years old, with the age of diagnosis being greater than 60 in 3% of cases (30). Not all of these cases, however, resulted from sexual transmission.

Despite low prevalence rates, older people remain at risk for acquiring STDs, especially as they are increasingly sexually active. There are numerous reasons for this, including the fact that many older people never received the sex education provided to today's younger population. In addition, the knowledge that STDs are most prevalent in younger people may lead to a false sense of safety amongst older couples, causing them to neglect safe-sex practices. Older couples may also be less apt to use barrier contraceptives that protect against some STDs, because they do not have to worry about unwanted pregnancy. Given these potential lapses in safe-sex measures, education about sexuality, STDs, and safe-sex practices remains critical throughout the entire adult lifecycle.

SEXUAL DYSFUNCTION

The disorders of sexual dysfunction classified in DSM-IV-TR can be found in Table 35-3 (31). Recent statistics estimate that 20% to 30% of adult men and 40% to 45% of adult women suffer from at least one form of sexual dysfunction (32), with increased rates in later life. ED is the most common form of sexual dysfunction in older men, affecting 20% to 40% of men in their 60s, and 50% to 70% of men in their 70s and 80s (32–34). In older women, the most common forms of sexual dysfunction include hypoactive sexual desire, inhibited orgasm, and dyspareunia (35). The percentage of women with low sexual desire jumps from 10% of women under 50 to nearly 50% of women in their late 60s and 70s (32). Dyspareunia affects 8% to 30% of postmenopausal women not on hormone replacement therapy (HRT) (36).

The cause of sexual dysfunction in late life is typically multifactorial, involving the physical effects of medical

TABLE 35-3
SEXUAL DISORDERS

Sexual Desire Disorders
Hypoactive Sexual Desire Disorder
- Persistent or recurrent deficiency of sexual fantasies and desire for sex

Sexual Aversion Disorder
- Extreme aversion to and avoidance of genital sexual contact

Sexual Arousal Disorders
Female Sexual Arousal Disorder
- Persistent or recurrent difficulty to attain and/or maintain vaginal swelling and lubrication during sexual activity

Male Erectile Disorder (Impotence)
- Persistent or recurrent inability to attain and/or maintain an erection that is adequate for sexual activity

Orgasmic Disorders
Female/Male Orgasmic Disorder
- Persistent or recurrent delay in or absence of orgasm in response to sexual stimulation

Premature Ejaculation
- Persistent or recurrent, uncontrollable, rapid ejaculation that occurs just prior to or shortly after penetration

Sexual Pain Disorders
Dyspareunia
- Recurrent or persistent genital pain associated with sexual intercourse

Vaginismus
- Recurrent or persistent involuntary spasm of vaginal muscles that limits or prohibits vaginal penetration

illness and/or medications, comorbid psychiatric illness, and underlying maladaptive attitudes or dysfunctional relationships. Any medical illness that impairs the blood supply or nervous innervation of genital tissue can potentially serve as a primary cause of sexual dysfunction. Examples include impaired sexual arousal due to diabetic neuropathy, or impaired genital vasocongestion due to peripheral vascular disease. Secondary sexual dysfunction may result from fatigue, pain, physical disability, or some other effect of a medical illness. For example, a man with chronic obstructive pulmonary disease may become short of breath during sexual activity, causing him to become less aroused, with resultant ED. Or a woman with a history of cervical cancer who underwent surgery and radiation could have scarring and contractures of her vaginal tissue, resulting in pain during sex and subsequent loss of libido. Medical, psychiatric, medication-related, and psychosocial factors commonly associated with sexual dysfunction in late life are listed in Table 35-4.

Medications often play a role in precipitating sexual dysfunction, and can affect both sexes at any point in the sexual response cycle (37–39). Some of the most common culprits include antihypertensives (e.g., β-blockers, diuretics), antiandrogens, and many psychotropic medications, particularly antidepressants (39–41). One prospective study found that nearly 60% of individuals on selective serotonin-reuptake inhibitors (SSRIs) or venlafaxine suffered from sexual dysfunction, with higher rates in men (40). By contrast, up to 25% of those on mirtazapine and only 8% on nefazodone reported sexual dysfunction. Bupropion has also been associated with lower rates of sexual dysfunction, in the 5% to 15% range (42). The mechanism of action for some medication-induced sexual dysfunction can be found in Table 35-5.

Initial episodes of sexual dysfunction in the elderly are often precipitated by a major psychosocial stress, such as the loss of a job or loved one, a medical crisis or prolonged illness, or a hospitalization. Such major stresses may break sexual patterns and lead to uncertainty of how to resume sexual activity. The loss of a partner is particularly devastating, making the idea of sexuality moot in the short-term, and often suppressing sexual desire and the willingness to seek out a new partner in the long-term if grief or survivor guilt persists. In the face of an acute illness such as a recent heart attack or respiratory compromise, older individuals can suffer from performance anxiety if they anticipate pain, self-injury (or injury to a debilitated partner), or even death during sex. Some people may feel less sexual because they are embarrassed over changes in their personal appearance (e.g., due to a surgical scar or colostomy bag), or are fearful of body odors or incontinence during sex. Chronic illness can also sap one's energy and enthusiasm for sex.

Sexual dysfunction in late life is often comorbid with psychiatric illness, particularly mood and anxiety disorders

TABLE 35-4
FACTORS ASSOCIATED WITH SEXUAL DYSFUNCTION IN LATE LIFE

Medical Disorders

Cardiac disease (e.g., myocardial infarct, cardiomyopathy)
Chronic obstructive pulmonary disease
Degenerative joint disease/arthritis
Dementia (e.g., Alzheimer's disease and other types)
Diabetes mellitus
Genital and urological cancers and treatment effects (e.g., due to radiation or surgery)
Hyperlipidemia
Hypertension
Hypogonadism/low testosterone
Neurological disorders (e.g., multiple sclerosis, Parkinson's disease, spinal cord injury)
Organ failure (e.g., cardiac, hepatic, renal)
Peripheral vascular disease/atherosclerosis
Prostate surgery
Sexually transmitted diseases (e.g., urethritis, vaginitis, cervicitis, genital herpes)
Traumatic injury to genital or pelvic region
Urinary/fecal incontinence

Psychiatric Disorders

Anxiety disorders (e.g., panic disorder, generalized anxiety disorder, PTSD)
Mood disorders (e.g., major depression, bipolar disorder)
Schizophrenia and other psychotic disorders
Substance use disorders (e.g., alcohol, tobacco)

Medications

Antiandrogens (e.g., flutamide, leuprolide)
Antianxiety (e.g., benzodiazepines)
Anticholinergic medications (e.g., urinary antispasmodics)
Anticonvulsants (e.g., divalproex sodium, carbamazepine)
Antidepressants (SSRIs, TCAs, venlafaxine)
Antifungals (e.g., ketoconazole)
Antihistamines (e.g., diphenhydramine, hydroxyzine, H_2 blockers)
Antihypertensives (e.g., α-1 antagonists, α-2 agonists, β-blockers, diuretics)
Antipsychotic medications
Cardiac medications (e.g., amiodarone, digoxin)
Corticosteroids
Lipid-lowering agents (e.g., clofibrate, statins)
Lithium carbonate

Psychosocial Factors

Body image concerns (e.g., due to aging, bodily odors, disability, medical or prosthetic device, surgical scar)
Fear of injury or death due to physical exertion
Loss of partner (e.g., due to divorce or death)
Marital/relationship discord
Obesity
Persistent grief over major loss (e.g., financial setback, death of loved one)
Recent major illness, surgery, or hospitalization
Retirement
Sexual dysfunction in a partner

PTSD, post traumatic stress disorder; SSRIs, selective serotonin-reuptake inhibitors; TCAs, tricyclic antidepressants.

in which loss of libido is a frequent symptom (43). At baseline, 40% to 50% of individuals suffering from depression experience loss of sexual desire as a cardinal symp-tom, but up to 90% may experience any form of sexual dysfunction prior to the use of antidepressants (40). Individuals with sexual aversion or phobias often suffer from underlying panic disorder (44). Individuals with schizophrenia and other psychotic disorders may have fewer problems with sexual function per se, but more difficulty with managing sexual relationships. Specifically, they may experience difficulty relating to others in sexually comfortable or appropriate ways if they suffer from active positive symptoms such as delusions, hallucinations, and bizarre thought patterns, and/or negative symptoms including social withdrawal or discomfort in the presence of others, apathy, and blunted emotional affect.

SEXUAL DISORDERS IN MEN

As noted, ED is the most common sexual dysfunction in men. ED is a disorder of sexual arousal defined by the inability to achieve or sustain an erection that is adequate for sexual function. ED was previously called *impotence*, and thought to be largely due to psychological factors. In fact, the feelings of powerlessness and shame in front of one's partner connoted by the term impotence had a lot to do with ED often being a silent and hence untreated condition. Current research, however, indicates that up to 80% of ED cases are primarily caused by a physical problem with erectile physiology (33,34). The promotion of oral erectogenic agents to treat ED has helped educate the public that ED is a physical ailment that needs to be talked about openly with one's partner and physician. Psychological factors commonly associated with ED include discord in a relationship, performance anxiety, anger towards a partner, transient stress, anxiety, and depression.

Regardless of its cause, ED results from one of three physiological problems:

- Failure of initiation, due to psychological or neurological inhibition of neural stimulation
- Failure to attain penile arterial filling
- Failure to maintain penile veno-occlusion

The latter two causes are frequently associated with peripheral vascular disease. Erections occur when autonomic parasympathetic nervous innervation initiates relaxation of smooth muscle tissue in the two penile corpora cavernosa. These cylindrical bodies contain spongy erectile tissue, composed of vascular spaces or sinusoids. When the surrounding smooth muscle relaxes, blood flows into the vascular spaces and makes the penis erect. This muscle relaxation is mediated by the release of the neurotransmitter nitric oxide, with subsequent activation of cyclic guanosine monophosphate (GMP). As the vascular spaces in the spongy erectile tissue expand, the penile veins that drain them are compressed against the surrounding collagenous sheath or tunica albuginea, preventing outflow. The erection subsides when smooth muscles surrounding the vascular

TABLE 35-5
MECHANISM OF ACTION FOR MEDICATION-INDUCED SEXUAL DYSFUNCTION

Mechanism of Sexual Dysfunction	Potential Causative Agents
Suppression of testosterone levels leads to decline in libido and overall sexual response.	Antiandrogens
Dopamine blockade in the tuberoinfundibular pathway causes elevated prolactin levels, leading to decreased libido, sexual arousal, erectile function, and orgasm in some individuals.	Antipsychotics and other dopamine antagonists
Suppression of limbic system activation may decrease sexual drive.	Alcohol Anticholinergics Anticonvulsants Antihistamines Benzodiazepines CNS depressants
Peripheral noradrenergic inhibition can impair libido, sexual arousal, erectile function, and ejaculation (sometimes causing retrograde ejaculation).	α-1 antagonism (e.g., doxazosin, terazosin, antidepressants, antipsychotics) α-2 agonists (e.g., clonidine; potentially reversed by yohimbine, an α-2 antagonist) β-Blockers
Dopamine blockade can suppress sexual function, while dopamine agonists can enhance libido and sexual response.	Antipsychotics and other dopamine antagonists
Stimulation of the serotonin receptor 5-HT2A can inhibit sexual desire and overall response.	Antidepressants (except mirtazapine and nefazodone that selectively block 5-HT2A stimulation)
Anticholinergic effects on genitals can block sexual response.	Anticholinergic agents (e.g., urinary antispasmodics, digoxin, furosemide, prednisolone, H_2 blockers)

5-HT2A, 5-Hydroxytryptamine (or serotonin) 2A receptor; H_2, Histamine-2 receptor; CNS, central nervous system.

spaces contract, mediated by the breakdown of cyclic GMP back to GMP via the phosphodiesterase enzyme type 5 (PDE-5). Oral erectogenic agents, to be described later, work by inhibiting the action of PDE-5.

Premature ejaculation is more commonly seen in younger men. It is defined by the occurrence of persistent or recurrent, uncontrollable, rapid ejaculation that occurs just prior to or shortly after penetration. Such rapid ejaculation usually prohibits adequate sexual intercourse. In later life, premature ejaculation may be less common due to age-associated declines in penile sensitivity. Instead, delayed orgasm and ejaculation may be more of an issue, especially in the presence of medications such as antidepressants.

SEXUAL DISORDERS IN WOMEN

As noted, hypoactive sexual desire, defined by the persistent or recurrent deficiency of sexual fantasies and desire for sex, is likely the most common sexual disorder in older women, mediated in part by declines in testosterone levels

and changes in sexual function following menopause. Loss of libido frequently involves psychological factors, including poor body-image or self-image due to age-associated losses of physical beauty and strength, and internalized negative stereotypes of sexuality being inappropriate for older women. For many older women who are widowed, sex ceases to be a part of their life, although this does not necessarily indicate that they have a sexual dysfunction. Orgasmic disorder, defined by the persistent or recurrent delay in, or absence of, orgasm following normal sexual excitement is also common in late life, typically comorbid with low desire and associated with many of the same factors. Again, for many women who are not in active sexual relationships, or for whom orgasm was never a regular part of sex, a diagnosis of sexual dysfunction is not always appropriate.

The true prevalence of female sexual pain disorders in late life is not known, perhaps because they often go unreported. Dyspareunia consists of recurrent pain associated with sexual intercourse, and is common after menopause because vulvovaginal tissue is atrophied and becomes less engorged and lubricated during sexual arousal. Pain during intercourse is also associated with medical conditions that affect the genital region (e.g., vulvitis, vulvodynia, and vulvar vestibulitis) or pelvic organs (38). For example, scarring or atrophy due to surgery or radiation for gynecologic malignancies can also lead to pain during intercourse. The pain disorder *vaginismus,* characterized by recurrent or persistent involuntary spasm of vaginal muscles that limits or prohibits vaginal penetration, is typically seen in younger women after intercourse is first attempted. Without treatment, it can lead to an unconsummated marriage or a lifetime of avoidance or aversion to sexual relationships.

SEXUAL DYSFUNCTION AND DEMENTIA

The effect of dementia on sexual function poses a number of complex issues. On the one hand, sexual function and sexual needs continue throughout the course of most dementias, and can play an important role as a nonverbal form of communication and intimacy for couples. As dementia progresses, however, individuals become more prone to sexual dysfunction and to sexually disinhibited behaviors. Partners bear the brunt of these changes, as they struggle to maintain a relationship in the face of uncertainly about the appropriateness of sex with someone who is slowly losing the capacity to understand and consent to mutual sexual relations (45). Partners may lose the desire for sex from their partner, perhaps because they are "turned off" by the effects of the disease, or because they are frustrated by a partner who acts inappropriately, or repeatedly and perhaps uncharacteristically requests sexual gratification. Some partners may be torn by conflicting feelings of love and fidelity for their demented partner, and yet the desire for both emotional and physical intimacy from a nondemented individual.

In the early and middle stages of Alzheimer's disease (AD) there is no predictable change in sexual desire, with sexual desire declining in some individuals and increasing in others, perhaps due to cognitive disinhibition. Sexual activity does decline, however, with one study finding that only 27% of couples with a partner suffering from AD were sexually active, compared to 82% of couples without dementia (46). ED and female orgasmic disorder are the two most commonly reported forms of sexual dysfunction in demented men and women, respectively (46,47). Sexual dysfunction may result in part from the demented individual's impaired ability to maintain a coherent focus on physical or mental stimulation during sex, or to initiate and sequence components of lovemaking (48,49).

The ability to consent to sexual activity is a particularly sensitive issue for many partners, who fear that they may be coercing their loved one into something they can no longer fully understand (18). This is also an important issue in long-term care facilities, where an individual with dementia may be engaging in or attempting to engage in sexual activity with another demented individual. This behavior raises further ethical and clinical issues when it is being pursued by demented individuals, even when there are nondemented spouses or partners living outside of the facility. Both legally and ethically, the rights of an individual in a long-term care facility to engage in sexual activity depend on his or her ability to understand the nature of the relationship and provide reasonable consent. When there is concern about an individual's capacity to provide such consent, clinicians should attempt to determine how well the demented individual is able to understand the nature of the relationship, including its risks, and to what degree the demented individual can avoid coercion or exploitation (50).

Sexually disinhibited behaviors include inappropriate sexual comments or requests, public exposure or masturbation, and aggressive fondling, groping, or forced sexual activity. Not surprisingly, such behaviors generate a considerable amount of anxiety on the part of caregivers. They have been reported in 2% to 7% of demented individuals (51–53) and in 25% of residents on a dementia unit (54), and tend to be more common in men. Risk factors include frontal and temporal lobe impairment, mania, psychosis, substance abuse, stroke, head trauma, premorbid sexual aggression, and certain medications, such as dopaminergic agents used to treat Parkinson's disease (54–56).

The first step in the assessment of sexually aggressive or inappropriate behaviors is to make sure the problematic behavior is not actually an innocuous expression of confusion, delirium, or motor restlessness. For example, a demented man reported to be exposing himself in the hallway of a nursing home may have simply wandered out of a bathroom confused about how to dress himself. Similarly, a demented man accused of groping a nurse may have accidentally hit someone in the waist or chest while reaching out for attention from the level of a wheelchair. These examples illustrate the need to thoroughly investigate the context of the reported behaviors before making accusations that could be inaccurate. Staff can sometimes inadvertently and falsely label patients with loaded terms such as *pervert* or *molester,* causing the patients to be humiliated, ostracized, or even expelled from a facility. When behaviors are truly inappropriate, staff must assess and manage the situation in a sensitive and discrete manner, to preserve the dignity and privacy of both the offender and any victim, and of family members who may be horrified by the behaviors—even more so when the patient becomes the subject of inappropriate gossip, joking, and derision.

The most appropriate team to manage situations involving inappropriate sexual behaviors in institutional settings includes the geriatric psychiatrist; medical, nursing, and social work staff that work with the individual; members of the facility's abuse committee and the risk manager, when sexually aggressive behaviors are involved. In the latter situation, a safety assessment must be done; sexually assaultive patients may need 24-hour one-on-one monitoring or even emergent inpatient psychiatric hospitalization if staff cannot guarantee the safety of potential victims. It is important to avoid a situation in which staff ignore or tolerate episodic sexual fondling or groping behaviors that may represent more extensive or coercive behaviors that are not being seen. Consider the following case example.

CASE EXAMPLE

Mr. P, an 82-year-old man with a diagnosis of vascular dementia, had lived in a nursing home for 3 years. He had been labeled by staff as a "horny old man" who was frequently found in the rooms of demented female residents, fondling them sexually. His son would bring a "masseuse" by on a regular basis and stand outside the room while she "serviced" his father. Nursing staff assumed that the son was bringing in a prostitute, but when confronted by the social worker he denied this, and insisted that his father had the right to associate with whomever he wished. Mr. P was treated on and off for several years with various medications in an attempt to reduce his libido and extinguish his sexual behaviors, without success. Staff continued to tolerate his behaviors and redirect him when found in another resident's room.

A crisis developed when the mother of a young female resident in a persistent vegetative state discovered Mr. P in her daughter's room, forcing his penis into her mouth. The woman demanded an immediate investigation, and threatened to report the facility to the state if Mr. P was not immediately removed. The medical director hospitalized Mr. P involuntarily, over the objections of Mr. P's son.

Upon investigation, it was learned that Mr. P had a history of sexually aggressive behaviors for many years before becoming demented, and that while at the facility he had been seen on many different floors engaging in inappropriate and coercive sexual behaviors. Visits by the "masseuse" had actually seemed to reduce his behaviors, but the son had stopped bringing women by in the 3 months prior to Mr. P's hospitalization. A team meeting that included the medical director, risk manager, social worker, and director of nursing recommended that Mr. P not be allowed to return to the facility.

Unfortunately, the case example of Mr. P illustrates a situation in which a sexual predator was tolerated by staff without definitive intervention. It took a crisis and a near lawsuit against the facility to prompt action that might have been avoided by more intensive management. Although visits by prostitutes as provided by his son may have drawn off some of Mr. P's libido, their absence led to a rebound effect in which he sought out sexual gratification in a more aggressive manner. His disinhibited sexual behaviors were only partially attributed to his dementia, with another major risk factor being his previous sexual aggression.

Once the problematic behavior has been identified as involving true sexual disinhibition, treatment should begin with behavioral techniques to set limits on inappro-

priate verbalizations, redirect the individual to more appropriate behaviors, and eliminate inadvertent reinforcement of the behaviors by staff, such as laughing at obscene comments. In addition, clinicians must recognize when unmet needs for physical stimulation or intimacy are being expressed, and find appropriate ways for caregivers or partners to provide gratification. For example, the spouse of a demented individual who was attempting to fondle other residents in the special care unit agreed to provide increased physical stimulation through hugs, massages, and hand holding during visits.

When behavioral approaches are insufficient, psychopharmacologic intervention is often needed. Most of the psychotropic agents used to treat agitation and aggression in dementia can be used to treat sexually aggressive and inappropriate behaviors (57,58). For disinhibited and aggressive behaviors, the atypical antipsychotic medications are usually the quickest and most effective agents. Behaviors that are clearly associated with excessive libido may respond to antidepressants that have sexual side effects, such as the SSRIs (59,60). Disinhibited behaviors associated with hyperactivity or hypersexuality may respond to mood stabilizers such as divalproex sodium, carbamazepine, or lithium. Sexually aggressive behaviors in men that have not responded to more traditional psychotropic agents may sometimes respond to estrogen (61,62) or to an antiandrogen steroid hormone such as medroxyprogesterone (63,64). An algorithm for treating sexually disinhibited behaviors can be found in Figure 35-1.

ASSESSMENT OF SEXUAL DYSFUNCTION

The assessment of sexual dysfunction in an older individual depends, first and foremost, on an educated clinician who is comfortable and knowledgeable about late-life sexuality. If the clinician is embarrassed or uncomfortable asking questions about sexual function, it is unlikely that adequate assessment will occur. The clinician must be able to ask direct questions using common language, and to listen carefully and patiently, keeping in mind that older people will have many of the same sexual concerns as younger people (65). An indispensable source of information about a sexual problem is the partner. The partner's presence during an interview will help facilitate open communication with the affected partner that will prove key during the treatment phase.

Some clinicians are quite uncomfortable speaking with older individuals about sex. If the clinician in his own mind says, "I cannot ask that question, these people are the age of my parents, or grandparents," then there is a reluctance to ask those questions. But one can overcome that in two ways: one, by role playing an interview with someone taking the role of a patient; or two, by doing it in front of a mirror. If you

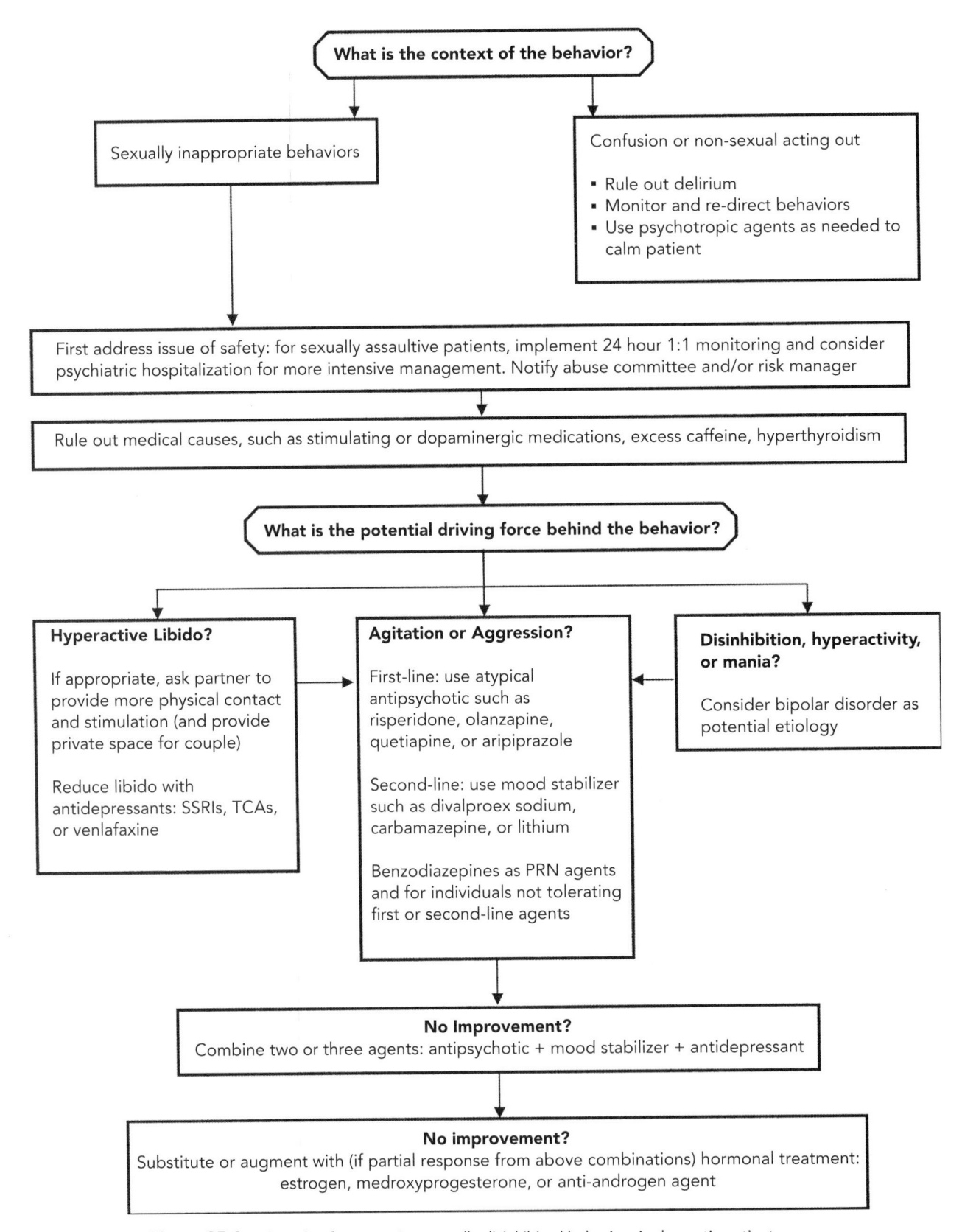

Figure 35-1 Algorithm for managing sexually disinhibited behaviors in dementia patients.

have asked the question, "Tell me, how firm is your erection?" 25 times in front of the mirror, the 26th time it will roll off your tongue easier. Do not feel that you are doing something wrong. For example, if a physician feels an erection coming on while interviewing or examining an older woman, he may naturally get quite upset, and think to himself, "This woman is the age of my mother! What's the matter with me that I get sexually aroused?" If it's a female physician, the same reaction may occur with an older man. It's very important to make sure that these kinds of happenings do not interfere with your ability to talk about sex. You have to say to yourself beforehand, "I am the physician, and this is a patient, and I have to get over this age barrier in terms of sexual questions."

The clinician needs to know how to take a sexual status examination in order to give some advice. They do not always have time to do the whole thing, but only to ask some specific questions as a matter of medical history: Do you have sex? How often? Any problems? For men: Do you have erections? For women: Do you lubricate enough? Can you have an orgasm? Are you angry with your partner? Any degree of anger—about anything—that gets taken into bed can be problematic. If you cannot clarify to the patient that he or she has to leave it outside the bedroom, you can be the best sex therapist and yet not be successful.

The older patient must also assume some responsibility here. They should come in with their questions in writing. They have to have a list, because otherwise they are not going to ask, or they are going to ask when they are on their way out—that is too late. They have to say to themselves, "Here is a person who knows about my body, whom I can ask a question about sex." We have to educate the patient to ask the physician.

■ *Dr. Ruth Westheimer*

One way to organize the assessment process and increase the comfort level of both the clinician and patient is to use a formal interview or *sexual status examination*. The goal of the sexual status examination is to identify the presence and degree of problematic changes in sexual function across the stages of the sexual response cycle. Inherent to this exam is a sex history that inquires about an individual's current sexual functioning, prior sexual experiences, attitudes towards sexuality, and the state of any current relationship. There are numerous standardized models that have been used clinically and in research, most of which take less than 10 minutes to administer. Several of these scales include the Sexual Function Questionnaire (66), the Changes in Sexual Functioning Questionnaire Clinical Version (67), the Derogatis Interview for Sexual Functioning (68), the Arizona Sexual Experience Scale (69), and the Sexual Function Questionnaire for Women (70). A sample sexual status examination that incorporates the above goals and many components of these scales can be found in Table 35-6.

The assessment process will also include a complete medical and psychiatric history, and a mental status examination to identify symptoms of anxiety or depression that may be blocking desire and performance, or certain thoughts (e.g., angry, obsessive, psychotic) that are interfering with

TABLE 35-6
SEXUAL STATUS EXAMINATION

Current History

1. Has there been a change in your sexual function?
2. Do you have any desire to be sexually active?
3. (For men): Can you still get an erection?
   Note: You can also clarify the question by asking if they get morning erections, erections while masturbating but not during sex, erections with one partner but not another, and whether the erection is sufficient for penetration.
4. (For women): Do you still lubricate when sexually aroused?
5. Does it take longer to get sexually aroused?
6. Can you have an orgasm?
7. Do you experience any pain during sexual activity?
8. Do you have any fears about being sexually active?
9. Do you use safe sex practices?

Relevant Medical and Psychiatric History

1. Are any medical or psychiatric problems (with you or a partner) interfering with your sexual function?
2. Do you have any genital rashes or irritations? New or unusual discharges?
3. Are any medications interfering with your sexual function?
4. Are you suffering from significant depression or anxiety?

Sexual History

1. Have you experienced sexual problems in the past?
2. Do you have a current partner? If so, are you having relationship problems?
3. Does your partner have sexual problems?
4. Do you have sufficient privacy for sexual intimacy?
5. How sexually active were you before your problem began? Currently?
6. Have you ever had a sexually transmitted disease?
7. Do you masturbate?
8. Do you feel that it is OK for you to be sexually active?

sexual arousal. A physical examination with a focus on urologic or gynecologic function done by a specialist will help rule out specific physical causes of sexual dysfunction. Select laboratory studies, including testosterone and prolactin levels, may also be necessary if a metabolic or hormonal etiology is suspected. Low testosterone and elevated prolactin levels (the latter sometimes resulting from the use of dopamine antagonists) have been associated with sexual dysfunction in both men and women. Finally, there are several diagnostic tests that can help identify relevant urologic or gynecologic pathology. Details of these tests can be found in Table 35-7. For men with ED, the introduction of oral erectogenic agents has greatly simplified the physical workup, since the medication may solve the issue without needing to search for an underlying cause.

TREATMENT

The role of the geriatric psychiatrist in the treatment of sexual dysfunction is to provide reassurance, education, and

TABLE 35-7

THE WORKUP FOR SEXUAL DYSFUNCTION

Diagnostic Test	Rationale
Sexual Status Examination (See Table 35-6)	Obtain basic information on presence and extent of sexual dysfunction, potential causes.
Physical examination (conducted by internist, gynecologist, or urologist, depending on the presentation)	Examine genital and pelvic anatomy for abnormalities or evidence of vascular or neurological compromise.
Basic laboratory studies: Including complete blood count, fasting glucose, lipid profile, thyroid function, and PSA (men)	Assess for presence of infection, anemia, diabetes, potential atherosclerosis, hypothyroidism, and prostate disease.
Hormone levels: Testosterone (both total and free), prolactin	Detect low testosterone or elevated prolactin levels.
Nocturnal penile tumescence and rigidity	Used in the workup of ED to determine whether natural erections occur during REM sleep.
Penile Doppler testing	Used in ED workup to assess penile arterial blood flow. A penile arteriogram can assess pelvic blood flow to the penis.
Penile cavernosography, cavernosometry	Used in ED workup to look for penile venous leakage.
Penile or vaginal cultures	Assess for the presence of suspected STDs.

ED, erectile dysfunction; PSA, prostate-specific antigen; REM, rapid eye movement; STDs, sexually transmitted diseases.

brief counseling. Sometimes this approach is sufficient; in other cases, a specialist is needed to treat physical causes or to implement sex therapy. All modalities will be described here. Reassurance of the patient depends on an enlightened clinician who understands that sexuality in general and sexual intercourse in particular remain important goals for many older patients. The clinician should listen empathically, and then emphasize in clear and nontechnical language the normality of sexuality in late life and the possibility of effective treatment for sexual problems. Keep in mind that many patients have internalized negative perspectives on late-life sexuality. The act of providing reassurance builds trust between patient and clinician, and this relationship will lay the basis for the patient feeling comfortable with being open about emotional reactions to the problem, and seeking follow-up treatment. Many treatments fail at this point—not because the treatment will not work, but because the patient and clinician never establish a solid working relationship, or the patient is overcome with pessimism or doubt and refuses to engage in treatment.

CASE EXAMPLE

Mr. J, a 78-year-old widower, was seen in a geriatric psychiatry clinic for symptoms of depression. He had been put on an SSRI antidepressant several months earlier by his internist, but with no improvement. In fact, he became quite upset with the physician, stating that the medication was worsening his situation. During the initial assessment,

the psychiatrist asked Mr. J about his sexual functioning, which prompted an outpouring of grief. Mr. J confided that he had suffered from ED ever since undergoing a prostatectomy 6 months prior to the appointment. When Mr. J asked the surgeon about changes in his sexual function, Mr. J paraphrased the response as, "Impotence is quite common after this surgery, but why would you worry about that anyway at your age?" Feeling humiliated and hopeless about regaining his sexual function, Mr. J broke up with his girlfriend and lapsed into a depression. The subsequent use of an SSRI antidepressant reduced his libido further, and felt like a double blow.

The psychiatrist spent a session reassuring Mr. J that treatment was available, and encouraged him to see a urologist who specialized in ED. He also educated Mr. J about erectile physiology, and discussed with him other potential causes of his ED, such as medication effects and unresolved grief over the death of his wife that manifested in anger directed towards his girlfriend. Even before treatment for his ED began, Mr. J reported feeling less depressed and more hopeful.

Educating patients about both normal and pathologic changes in sexual function in late life can reduce excessive fear and increase acceptance of these changes (71). For example, a man who does not understand the normal changes in erectile function may misinterpret them and believe he is suffering from a sexual problem. Similarly, a woman may misinterpret the experience of vaginal dryness to mean that she does not want to have sex. Such overreac-

TABLE 35-8

STRATEGIES TO ENHANCE SEXUAL FUNCTION IN LATE LIFE

Improve One's Health and Lifestyle
- Regular exercise
- Healthy diet
- Avoid tobacco products and excessive use of alcohol
- Identify and deal with excessive stress
- Identify and seek treatment for medical or psychiatric issues that may be affecting sexual function

Improve One's Relationship
- Open and honest communication about sexual preferences, changes, and problems
- Deal with anger directly and do not take it into the bedroom
- Plan for private, relaxed time together with and without sexual activity
- Seek counseling for long-standing, unresolved conflict or discord

Adapt Sexual Activity to the Realities of Aging
- Discuss sexual needs and desires and determine realistic expectations
- Address pain, discomfort, and physical mobility issues before sex
- Engage in relaxing activities prior to sex: mutual massage, taking a warm bath or shower together, listening to music
- Allow extra time and energy for sexual foreplay
- Use a water-based lubricant liberally to counteract vaginal dryness and sensitivity
- Select sexual positions that minimize exertion and maximize comfort, e.g., side-by-side

tions to normal changes can affect sexuality even more than actual physical changes, leading some individuals to engage in less frequent or more limited sexual activity (12). The clinician should review with the patient the normal changes in sexual function throughout each stage of the sexual response cycle, and discuss ways in which the patient's physical or mental state may be influencing these changes. For example, an older man with diabetes or atherosclerotic disease may have a more pronounced decline in erectile function or even ED, given possible compromise of penile blood flow. An older woman with a history of an arthritic hip might experience more limited pelvic movement or even pain during sex, in addition to potential discomfort due to decreased vaginal lubrication. A depressed patient may report significant reductions in libido. In each case, the patient can be reassured that his or her sexual changes have clearly identified causative factors, and treatment can improve or even alleviate these concerns.

Education should also focus on improving the quality of an individual's sexual relationship with his or her partner. Sometimes the clinician can provide a forum for the couple to discuss basic difficulties during sexual activity, and strategize on ways to improve them. When there is significant discord, a referral should be made to a couples or marital therapist. When one or both partners have suffered

from long-standing sexual dysfunction, a referral to a sex therapist should be strongly considered. The clinician should emphasize to the couple that sex can be more than just intercourse, and that physically pleasing each other can occur through massage and masturbation, and does not always have to be mutual. Couples often have to adapt sexual techniques and refocus more time on foreplay in order to preserve previous levels of sexual function and enjoyment. Several suggestions for older couples are described in Table 35-8.

When one or both partners suffer from chronic medical illness or disability, sexual practices may need to be adapted to account for physical limitations, fatigue, loss of muscle strength, and pain (72). Table 35-9 presents several useful strategies for these couples. A physician who treats the condition in question should be consulted on ways to minimize pain or discomfort and maximize function, perhaps by taking analgesics or other treatments (e.g., specific muscle stretches, nasal oxygen, inhalers) prior to sex. Sexual positions with the couple lying side-by-side, or rear entry braced by pillows, might minimize physical exertion or stress on certain parts of the body.

Helpful guides to sexuality in the setting of medical illness have been published by the American Cancer Society (74), the United Ostomy Organization, and the National Jewish Center for Immunology and Respiratory Medicine.

Sexuality in late life is massaging, it is touching, it is caressing, and it's certainly masturbating—or it is giving each other sexual pleasure so that she can masturbate him, and he can masturbate her without it being intercourse. For many couples sexual intercourse might be difficult, and the couple will need to engage in different positions. A crucial piece of advice that the clinician can offer is to recommend the use of a lubricant. Even if you think that you do not need it, use it so that the walls of the vagina—which become more brittle in late life—do not get hurt, because if there's pain she may say "it hurts" and "who needs it?" We need to teach them not to only be sexually active in the evening, when they are tired, but in the morning or early afternoon. I advise couples to get up in the morning, go to the bathroom, have a light breakfast, then go back to bed and take the phone off the hook. For older individuals who do not have partners, I suggest that they masturbate. And we have to tell them there's nothing to be ashamed of.

For many men it is important to know that the erection is not as firm as it once was. Such is a fact of life, and do not bemoan it, and do not mourn it, just say, "That's life. Thank God I still have erections, and that's my attitude." If a man's penis does not get fully erect, it is still possible for his partner to bring him to an orgasm. If intercourse is difficult but the woman wants the sensation of a penis in her vagina, then she should use a dildo, but always using a lubricant. Sex does not have to be a penis in a vagina—I think that's an important message—because in the olden days couples thought a penis had to be in a vagina or it's not sex—that's nonsense.

When one or both partners has a physical disability, or suffers from pain or some other medical condition, they should always discuss with their physician ways to adapt sex. For

TABLE 35-9
STRATEGIES TO IMPROVE SEXUALITY AFFECTED BY MEDICAL CONDITIONS

Medical Condition	Strategies
Cardiovascular disease/ recent myocardial infarct	▪ Discuss resumption of sexual activity with physician/cardiologist. ▪ Address underlying anxiety about sexual exertion. ▪ Sexual activity can be resumed when an individual can climb two flights of stair or elevate his or her heart rate to 120 beats per minute without chest pain or shortness of breath (73). ▪ Have nitroglycerin tabs on hand in the event of chest pain. ▪ For ED, consider the negative effects of cardiac medications.
Stroke	▪ Address potential ED due to use of antihypertensive medications. ▪ Suggest less strenuous positions or mutual masturbation for individuals with hemiparesis.
Prostate cancer/prostatectomy	▪ ED may result from nerve damage during surgery. An oral erectogenic agent may be used to reverse this. ▪ For men who received an orchiectomy, testosterone supplementation may be considered if the PSA has remained at 0 for 3 to 5 years (73).
Arthritis	▪ Painful or less mobile joints (especially hip or hands) can limit sexual activity and positioning. Analgesics/NSAIDS and/or a warm bath or shower prior to sex may help reduce pain and increase mobility. ▪ More accessible sexual positions include side-by-side and rear entry, with pillows for improved support. ▪ A vibrator may compensate for limited hand movement (73).
Diabetes mellitus	▪ ED is common due to both penile microvascular and neurologic damage, and can be treated with oral erectogenic agents or other modalities (See Table 35-10 and Table 35-11). ▪ For women with reduced lubrication, use a water-based vaginal lubricant.
Dry mouth/decreased saliva flow (due to medications, xerostomia, Sjögren's syndrome)	▪ If oral sex is limited, substitute sexual stimulation manually or with a vibrator. ▪ Edible lubricants or artificial saliva can also be used.
Pulmonary disease (COPD, asthma, etc.)	▪ Consider inhaler treatments prior to sex (and always have inhaler nearby) or supplemental oxygen if needed. ▪ Oxygen tanks can be hidden or creatively decorated in such a way as to enhance the sensuality of the setting. ▪ Consult a physician if shortness of breath during sex is a problem.
Colorectal disease with ileostomy or colostomy placement	▪ Ileostomy/colostomy bags should be changed before sexual activity. ▪ Couples who are distracted, anxious, or turned off by the presence of the bag can consider creatively covering it up with a colorful cloth wrap or item of clothing.
Urinary incontinence	▪ Treatment of urogenital atrophy with estrogen cream or ERT/HRT. ▪ Treat an associated cystocele, or other etiology. ▪ Void prior to sexual activity and use a water-based lubricant during sexual activity.
Urogenital pathology and treatment (e.g., hysterectomy, radiation for urogenital cancer, etc.)	▪ Liberal use of a water-based lubricant during sexual stimulation and intercourse ▪ Explore various positions to find one that will alleviate coital discomfort. ▪ For vaginal contractures, the use of graduated dilators can improve comfort during vaginal penetration (See treatment for vaginismus in Table 35-10).

COPD, chronic obstructive pulmonary disease; ED, erectile dysfunction; ERT/HRT, estrogen replacement therapy/hormone replacement therapy; PSA, prostate-specific antigen; NSAIDs, nonsteroidal anti-inflammatory drugs.
Adapted from References 38,72,73,74.

example, they can have sex right after they take a warm bath, or after they take painkillers. If one of them has a colostomy bag, they can find a way of putting a big bandage around it, or take the cummerbund of a tuxedo and put it around, something like this. Individuals have to force themselves to not think about upsetting issues during sex. I tell couples that it is OK to fantasize, even about other people, but just keep your mouth shut, and do not tell your partner now in bed that you are with the next door neighbor, or a movie star. It's perfectly all right to force your brain into some fantasy—that does not mean cheating. That's just putting your entire being into a mood that allows you to be sexually aroused and to have an orgasm.

■ *Dr. Ruth Westheimer*

HORMONE REPLACEMENT

HRT in women using oral or transdermal estrogen, or estrogen-progestin combinations, has three Food and Drug Administration-approved indications:

- Treatment of vasomotor symptoms of menopause
- Treatment of symptomatic vulvovaginal atrophy
- Prevention of postmenopausal osteoporosis

In the setting of female sexual dysfunction, HRT and/or the use of estrogen cream applied directly to genital tissues may help improve libido and reduce sexual pain by relieving vulvovaginal irritation and enhancing lubrication. Estrogen replacement therapy (ERT) alone has also been associated with a reduced risk of postmenopausal cardiovascular disease (75), but this effect appears to be reduced or even reversed in a certain subset of women by the addition of progestins, with an increased risk of cardiac events and stroke (75–77). ERT/HRT has also been reported to reduce the effects of osteoporosis, skin aging, and the risk of AD and colorectal cancer (75,77,78). At the same time, there is evidence to suggest a slightly increased risk of breast cancer in women on long-term HRT, likely due to the presence of progestin (75). All of these data can be quite confusing to interpret and explain to women, and the perception of increased risk has greatly reduced the use of ERT/HRT. It makes the most sense, then, for the geriatric psychiatrist to refer older female patients complaining of bothersome post-menopausal symptoms to their internist, family practitioner, or gynecologist to discuss the potential risks and benefits of ERT/HRT.

The use of testosterone replacement therapy depends on a number of factors for both men and women. It is reasonable to check a serum testosterone level in men with clinically significant symptoms of androgen deficiency, such as sexual dysfunction (loss of sexual desire, ED), lack of energy, decreased strength, and depression. Keep in mind, however, that these symptoms are common and usually not associated with hormonal changes. A low testosterone level (defined as total serum testosterone <200 ng/dL) or even a borderline level (200–400 ng/dL) should be confirmed with repeat testing and/or a free testosterone level (79). The timing of the level can be important in younger men, because they tend to have greater testosterone secretion in the morning; however, this rhythmic secretion may be attenuated in later life (80). Causes of symptomatic androgen deficiency should be ruled out and treated before testosterone supplementation is considered.

There are a number of testosterone preparations available, including an oral capsule, an intramuscular injection, a transdermal patch, and a skin gel, with the patch and gel being the easiest and hence most commonly used methods. With testosterone supplementation, clinicians should check for expected increases in testosterone levels, and monitor patients for improvements in libido, sexual responsiveness and activity, mood, energy, and sense of well-being (79,81,82). Potential side effects of testosterone supplementation in men include weight gain, increased lipid and hematocrit levels, and worsening of prostate disease. Contraindications to supplementation include the presence of prostate cancer, obstructive benign prostatic hypertrophy, polycythemia, and severely elevated lipid levels (79). All men on testosterone supplementation should have regular prostate examinations along with monitoring of prostate specific antigen, lipid, and hematocrit levels.

The use of supplemental testosterone (with or without estrogen) or the adrenal androgen dehydroepiandrosterone has been shown to increase libido and enhance sexual responsiveness in older women (83–85). Widespread use of androgen in women has been limited, however, by inconsistent data (86) and the risk of side effects, including weight gain, skin acne, virilization, and elevated lipid profiles (79).

DEALING WITH MEDICATION SIDE EFFECTS

There are a number of ways to deal with sexual side effects of medications other than stopping the offending agent, which is often not advisable. A treatment algorithm is outlined in Figure 35-2 (87,88). Before implementing any of these strategies, however, the clinician must first take a thorough sex history to make sure that the sexual dysfunction is not a pre-existing condition, or has causes other than the medication. In such circumstances, medication changes or the use of antidotes will not be helpful. For men with ED, however, oral erectogenic agents have quickly become the final common pathway of treatment, regardless of cause. Antidepressants tend to be the most common offending agents, and most of the suggested antidotes have been studied within this context.

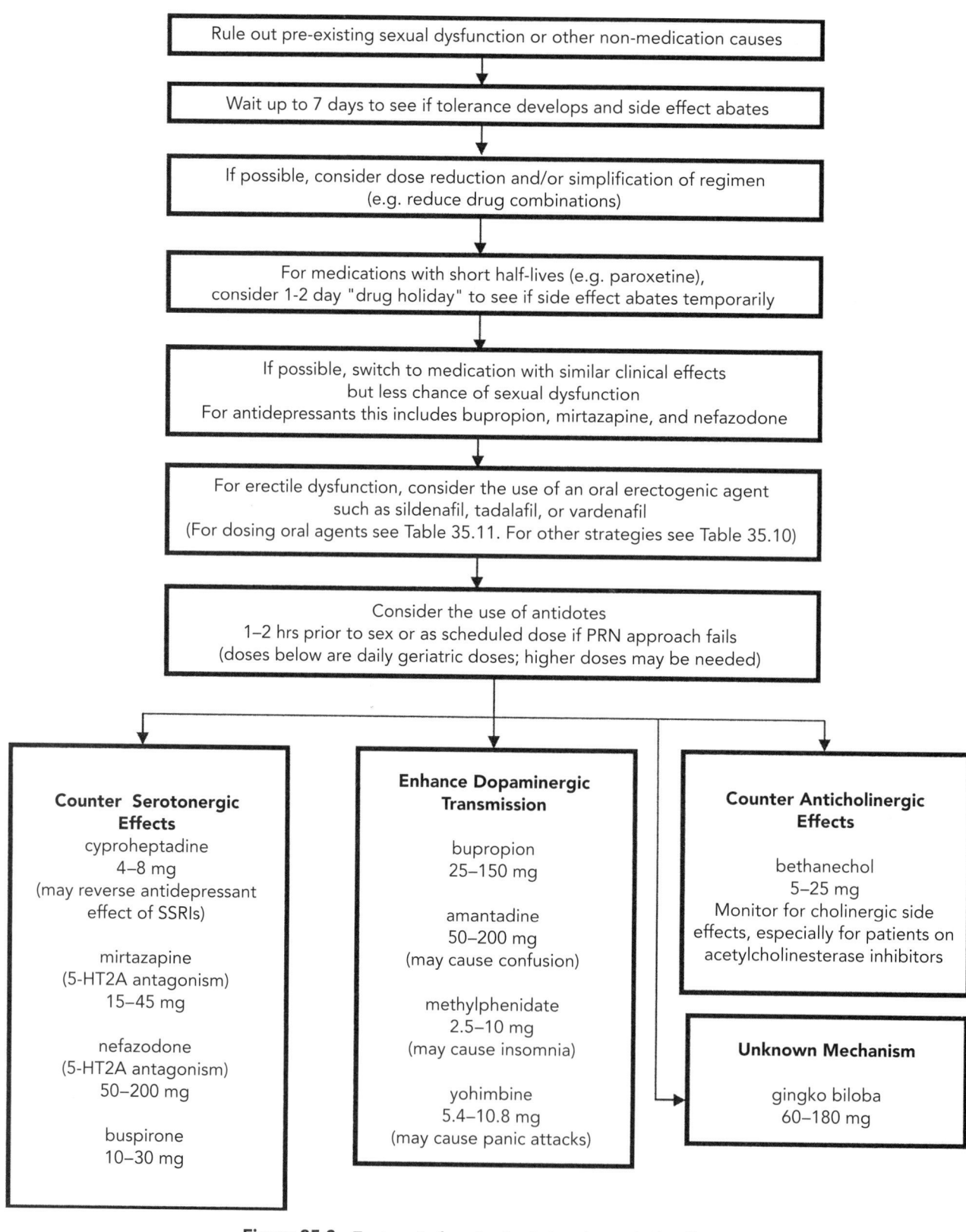

Figure 35-2   Treatment of medication-induced sexual side effects.

SEX THERAPY

Sex therapy is a psychotherapeutic process that combines supportive, insight-oriented, and cognitive-behavioral techniques to treat sexual dysfunction (89–91). The goal is to identify the psychological roots of the sexual dysfunction, if possible, and then help the individual or couple achieve normal, satisfying sexual function. Ideally, sex therapy is done conjointly, meaning that both partners are involved in the process. Conjoint therapy is a prerequisite when a dysfunctional relationship is at the root of the problem, and when expectations of sexual activity are discordant. The introduction of oral erectogenic agents has highlighted the issue of expectations, since many men have believed, incorrectly, that the simple correction of ED with a pill would resolve long-standing sexual and other relationship problems. In those situations and many others, enduring issues such as low desire, relationship discord, physical deconditioning, and medical problems must be dealt with at the outset of sex therapy. In order to accomplish this, a number of clinicians may be involved.

Sex therapy typically begins with a thorough sex history and discussion of the current problem. For the older individual or couple, an initial supportive and educational approach can build a crucial alliance with the therapist, and help to promote understanding of the problem and optimism towards improvement. Sometimes practical suggestions on sexual technique can bring immediate improvement; in other situations, the therapist needs to impose a moratorium on sex to reduce tension and eventually reintroduce a more relaxed and sensuous approach. In some cases, intensive couples therapy is necessary; in others, pharmacologic treatment of debilitating psychiatric symptoms (e.g., depression, panic attacks, psychosis) is needed, or the patient may need to be referred back to a specialist for further treatment of an enduring medical issue (e.g., joint or chest pain, or shortness of breath during exertion).

Once these barriers have been dealt with, the therapist can examine attitudes and responses to sexual stimulation and intimacy that are creating or exacerbating the dysfunction. Cognitive restructuring may be used to identify and alter cognitive distortions towards sexuality, such as a man believing that a failed erection means he is a failure *as a man*, or a woman viewing coital pain as a mental rejection of her partner. One common psychological barrier in ED is called *spectatoring*, in which a man is unable to remove his mind from the role of a spectator during sex, constantly monitoring the status of his erection rather than focusing on sexual arousal. The therapist may suggest that he adopt a self-indulgent focus on his own pleasure or on a fantasy in order to reduce the spectator mindset.

Lack of sexual arousal and inhibited orgasm may be perpetuated by the cognitive distortion termed *catastrophizing*, in which an individual thinks that if he does not achieve an erection or an orgasm during sex that he will be rejected not only by his partner, but by all future partners. Another common cognitive distortion is *all-or-nothing thinking*, in which an individual thinks that if he or she does not always achieve an erection or orgasm during sex, the whole thing is pointless. Although these cognitive distortions are quite unrealistic, the force of belief often leads to them becoming self-fulfilling prophecies. The sex therapist guides the patient to understanding the negative consequences of such thoughts, and then works on replacing them with more realistic and hopeful ones.

A special behavioral technique developed for couples in sex therapy is called *sensate focus*. The goal of sensate focus exercises is to create an association for the couple between sexual arousal and relaxed and sensuous time together, free of performance anxiety or other pressures. The couple is asked to not engage in sexual activity, but instead to practice relaxation techniques such as deep breathing and progressive muscle relaxation alone, and then together. Once they have achieved a state of relaxation, they apply this to nonpressured sensual touching. When the couple is able to feel relaxed and physically intimate together without sexual stimulation, they gradually progress to genital stimulation and then intercourse. Adjustments can be made in the exercises for older couples to account for any physical limitations (Tables 35-8 and 35-9).

It is quite common for sex therapy to become stalled at various points, often because of resistance on the part of one or both partners. This resistance, such as refusal to complete exercises, excuses, or procrastination, can reveal a lot about the underlying cause of the sexual dysfunction. Instead of becoming frustrated with each other, the couple is urged to use the resistance as an opportunity to understand their own sexuality better. It is quite common for the older couple in sex therapy to rediscover that they retain a considerable amount of sexual energy and ability, and this can lead to a newfound appreciation for their relationship and the life-affirming role of sexual intimacy.

CASE EXAMPLE

Mr. and Mrs. B, a couple in their late 70s, had been married for 45 years. They had previously experienced an enjoyable sexual relationship into their early 70s, but had stopped having sex several years ago, after Mrs. B was treated for breast cancer with a mastectomy and radiation. Afterwards she reported having no libido. Shortly after her surgery she fell and broke her hip, and thereafter resisted Mr. B's attempts at pleasuring her through oral sex, because she described it as uncomfortable to move her pelvis during arousal and orgasm. Mr. B subsequently began experiencing ED. Although the quality of their relationship was quite strong, they both missed the sexual intimacy of earlier years. Mrs. B began

TABLE 35-10

TREATMENT STRATEGIES FOR SPECIFIC SEXUAL DISORDERS

Sexual Disorder	Treatment Strategies
Medication-induced sexual dysfunction	See Figure 35-2
Hypoactive desire disorder	<ul><li>Rule out and treat underlying medical, medication-induced, or psychiatric causes, if identified.</li><li>Provide sex education and counseling to counter psychological barriers.</li><li>Estrogen replacement may help improve sexual arousal and comfort in women, which in turn may lead to increased desire.</li><li>Consider testosterone replacement in hypogonadal men and testosterone or DHEA in women.</li></ul>
Erectile dysfunction	<ul><li>Oral erectogenic medications (See Table 35-11)</li><li>Penile intracavernosal self-injection with alprostadil, a synthetic form of prostaglandin E1, into the base of the penis 10–20 minutes before sex leads to erections in 70–80% of men (34). Other injectable agents have included VIP, phentolamine, and papaverine HCl, sometimes in combination.</li><li>MUSE: Alprostadil given in the form of a urethral suppository (92).</li><li>Vacuum constriction devices (93)</li><li>Penile implants: Once a common treatment, now an option of last resort. Choice of devices includes semi-rigid or inflatable tubes with implantable pumps (94). Risks include infection and mechanical failure, which ranges from 5–20% (95). Prosthetic devices are permanent due to surgical destruction of erectile tissue; however, they can be repaired or reimplanted.</li><li>For hypogonadism: Testosterone supplementation</li><li>For anatomic curvature during erections (Peyronie's disease): Vacuum constriction devices may help break up scar tissue and restore normal shape</li></ul>
Premature ejaculation	<ul><li>Cognitive-behavioral techniques may help slow down the perception of sexual stimulation.</li><li>"Squeeze technique" during sex, in which the partner gently squeezes the man's penis prior to penetration to reduce sensation and stall ejaculation (96).</li><li>Use of antidepressant (SSRI or TCA) has been shown to significantly delay time to orgasm and ejaculation in some men (97,98).</li></ul>
Female arousal disorder	<ul><li>Identify and address both physical and psychological causes of impaired sexual arousal.</li><li>Use of ERT/HRT can improve arousal in postmenopausal women.</li><li>Use of lubricant to enhance erogenous sensitivity</li><li>Masturbation exercises using vibrator to stimulate arousal</li></ul>
Female orgasmic disorder	<ul><li>Cognitive-behavioral therapy to identify and address psychological inhibitions</li><li>Relaxation techniques that incorporate sensual self-stimulation and masturbation, usually with the aid of an electric vibrator to increase clitoral stimulation (99)</li><li>Short-term group therapy can also be helpful for women to provide education and support (100).</li><li>When orgasm is achieved, sensate focus exercises can help to incorporate orgasm into a couple's sexual relations.</li></ul>
Sexual pain disorder: Dyspareunia	<ul><li>Identification and management of underlying cause, especially pelvic pathology</li><li>Use of ERT/HRT for postmenopausal women</li><li>Topical estrogen creams may help alleviate vulvovaginal atrophy and irritation.</li><li>Liberal use of vaginal lubrication during sex</li><li>Sensate focus exercises can help maximize relaxation during sex.</li><li>Identification of sexual positions that minimize discomfort</li><li>Use of graduated vaginal cylinders to gradually stretch and desensitize vaginal tissue</li></ul>
Sexual pain disorder: Vaginismus	<ul><li>Gynecologic examination as first step to identify potential causes and gauge degree of vaginal spasm</li><li>Identify and treat underlying anxiety and/or panic disorder</li><li>Identify presence of sexual aversion or phobia</li><li>ERT/HRT; estrogen creams in women with spasm due to discomfort from vulvovaginal atrophy and irritation as a result of menopause; use of lubricants to decrease discomfort and friction during penetration</li><li>Relaxation techniques involving use of graduated vaginal cylinders to reduce fear reaction and desensitize vaginal musculature (38)</li><li>Sensate focus exercises with partner to build trust and decrease anxiety during sex</li></ul>

DHEA, dehydroepiandrosterone; ERT/HRT, estrogen replacement therapy/hormone replacement therapy; MUSE, Medicated Urethral Stimulation of Erection; SSRI, selective serotonin-reuptake inhibitor; TCA, tricyclic antidepressant; VIP, vasoactive intestinal polypeptide.

seeing a geriatric psychiatrist for treatment of depression. Mr. B accompanied her to one appointment, during which they were asked about their sexual relationship. Mrs. B became quite tearful when describing the impact of her experience with breast cancer, feeling that it had ruined her as a sexual being. Her hip fracture only made things worse for her, she believed. The psychiatrist referred the couple to a colleague trained in sex therapy.

After taking a careful sex history, the therapist felt that although Mrs. B's medical problems had disrupted the couple's sex life, they were not the insurmountable obstacles portrayed by the couple. In fact, Mr. B still retained erectile function (demonstrated by his having morning erections on a regular basis and occasionally masturbating to orgasm), but felt unable to get aroused with Mrs. B because he was both afraid to upset her and angry at her for resisting his attempts to be intimate. Mrs. B's loss of libido was traced to her loss of a breast being a blow to her body image and self-confidence. The therapist also learned that although Mrs. B experienced limited hip movement and pain after her surgery, this had largely resolved, whereas her fear of recurrent pain had not.

After discussing these issues with the couple, a series of sensate focus exercises were prescribed. The couple was amazed to find that just by gently massaging each other in bed without any expectation of sex, their libidos re-emerged. The therapist encouraged Mrs. B to wear loose-fitting lingerie that made her feel sexy and minimized the contour of her chest, helping lessen her focus on her surgery scar. The therapist also recommended a position for massage and then gentle genital fondling with plenty of lubrication that put minimal stress on Mrs. B's hip joint. Within several sessions Mr. and Mrs. B had progressed to sexual intercourse, which they both described as being comfortable and satisfying.

SPECIFIC TREATMENT MODALITIES

The treatment of specific forms of sexual dysfunction in older men and women will typically combine some form of sex therapy with many of the techniques described in Table 35-10. These approaches are similar for both younger and older patients. A list of oral erectogenic agents to treat ED is presented separately in Table 35-11. Until the introduction of the first oral erectogenic agent, sildenafil in 1998, there were many commonly used approaches for ED, including vacuum pumps, penile injections, a urethral suppository, and prosthetic devices. Now the overwhelming choice is to use an oral agent, sometimes even in lieu of a thorough workup and regardless of whether the cause is physical or psychological. For older men this trend has brought a revolution in terms of maintaining sexual potency and doing so in a discrete and uncomplicated way, assuming that there are not severe relationship issues.

An overall protocol to identifying, assessing, and treating sexual disorders is presented in Figure 35-3. It is important to recognize one's own clinical limitations in this area, and seek appropriate referrals where indicated. Given the growing role of sexuality in the geriatric patient, clinicians should also consider obtaining further training in sex therapy.

PARAPHILIAS

The focus of this chapter has been on sexual dysfunction that involves an interruption in the normal sexual response pathway. Paraphilias represent a very different type of sexual disorder, in which sexual function is intact but sexual excitement depends upon a particular stimulus

TABLE 35-11
USE OF ORAL ERECTOGENIC AGENTS/PDE-5 INHIBITORS[a]

Medication	Dosing Strategy	Time to Onset and Duration of Action
Sildenafil (Viagra)	25 mg or 50 mg initial dose and 100 mg if no response, 30 minutes to 4 hours prior to sex	Onset in 15 to 30 minutes Duration: 6 hours
Vardenafil (Levitra)	5 mg or 10 mg initial dose and 20 mg if no response, 30 minutes to 4 hours prior to sex	Onset in 15 to 30 minutes Duration: 6 hours
Tadalafil (Cialis)	10 mg initial dose and 20 mg if no response, 30 minutes to 30 hours prior to sex	Onset in 15 to 30 minutes Duration: 36 hours

[a]The advantages of PDE-5 inhibitors are ease of administration and high rates of success, regardless of cause, in up to 70% of users (101). Patients must be educated that erection requires physical stimulation—it is not automatic. If initial doses do not work, patients should be educated to take the higher dose, resulting in success in up to half of men not responding to the lower dose. Potential side effects include headache, flushing, gastrointestinal discomfort, blurred vision, and the potential for hazardous increases in blood pressure when taken concomitantly with nitrates (e.g., sublingual nitroglycerin, isosorbide, etc.). PDE-5, phosphodiesterase enzyme type 5.

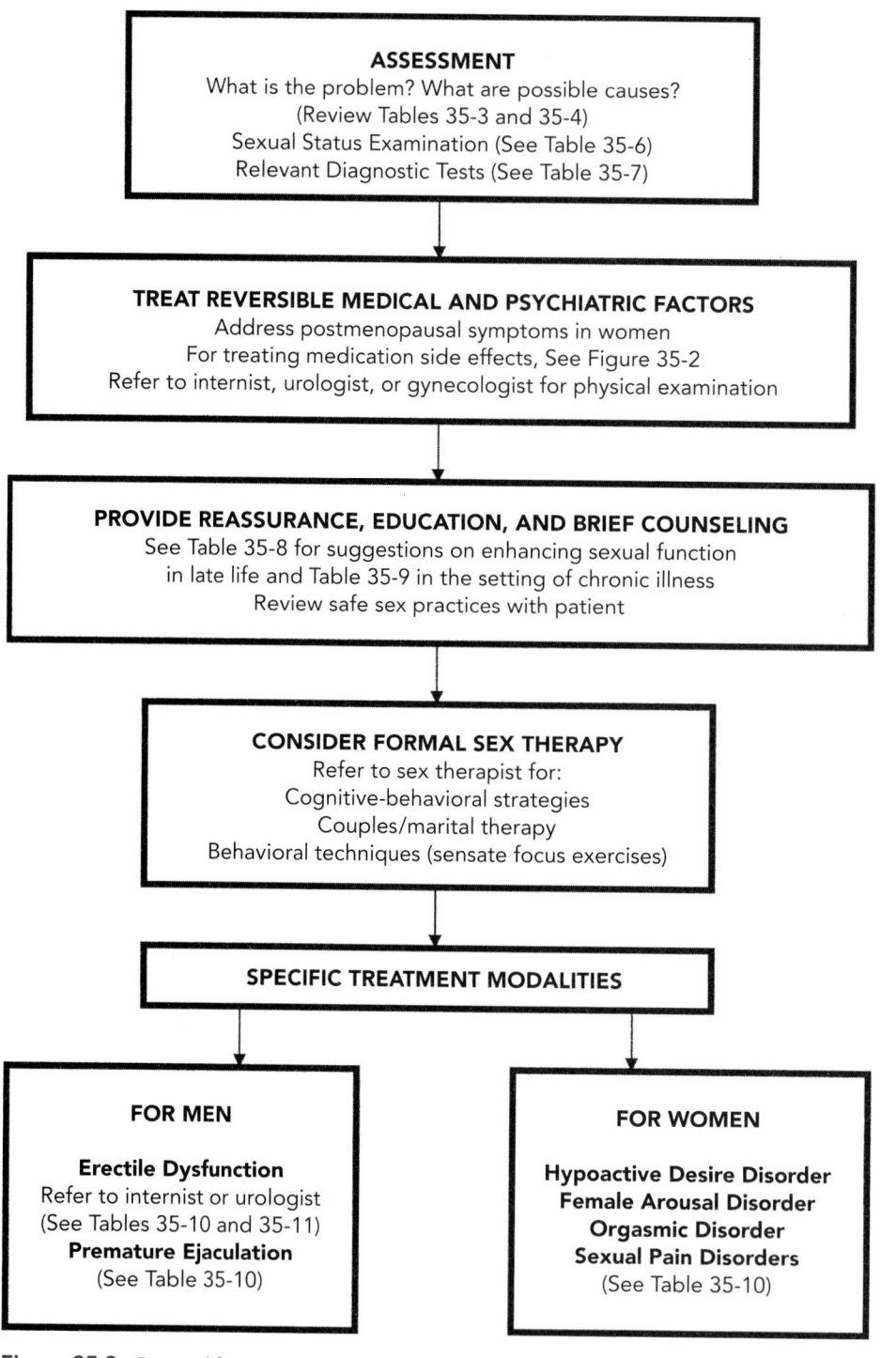

Figure 35-3 Protocol for assessment and treatment of sexual disorders in late life.

or activity that is often unusual or even bizarre (31,102). DSM-IV-TR defines paraphilias as involving "recurrent, intense sexually arousing fantasies, sexual urges, or behaviors generally involving nonhuman objects, the suffering or humiliation of oneself or one's partner, or children or other nonconsenting persons" (31). To make a DSM diagnosis, these behaviors have to persist for at least 6 months and be associated with distress or interpersonal difficulty.

Given this definition, paraphilias have historically been referred to as representing deviant or perverse sexual behaviors. Several forms of paraphilia cross into criminal behavior, such as exhibitionism, frotteurism, voyeurism, and pedophilia. Major forms of paraphilias are listed in Table 35-12.

Paraphilias are seen overwhelmingly in men. In older individuals they may represent long-standing behaviors,

TABLE 35-12
PARAPHILIAS

Paraphilia	Clinical Features
Paraphilia—recurrent, intense, sexually arousing urges, fantasies, or behaviors over a period of at least 6 months for the following:	
Exhibitionism	Exposure of one's genitals to unsuspecting stranger
Fetishism	Use of nonliving objects (e.g., woman's shoes or undergarments)
Frotteurism	Touching or rubbing against a nonconsenting person
Pedophilia	Sexual activity with children
Sexual masochism	Being humiliated or made to suffer, sometimes by being beaten or tied up
Sexual sadism	Causing mental or physical humiliation or suffering to another individual
Transvestic fetishism	Dressing in female clothing
Voyeurism	Watching an unsuspecting person naked or engaged in sexual activity

Sources: references 31 and 102.

or result from brain damage, particularly to frontotemporal regions (103,104). Research into paraphilias is sparse to begin with, and little is known about their presence in late life aside from several published case studies. They are believed to represent chronic conditions that are difficult to treat, because their very symptoms are a means of sexual gratification. For this reason, there may be limited incentive for treatment. Cognitive-behavioral, group, couples, and psychodynamic therapies may yield some success; in fact, rates of improvement are generally good and rates of relapse lower than typically reported (102,105). Both SSRI antidepressants and antiandrogens have been used to treat various forms of paraphilias (105,106). The geriatric psychiatrist should be aware of these conditions, because they can be major obstacles to treating comorbid relationship discord or sexual dysfunction, can be sources of inappropriate behaviors seen in long-term care settings, or can represent criminal behavior that must be reported to the proper authorities.

REFERENCES

1. Masters WH, Johnson VE. *Human Sexual Response*. Boston: Little, Brown & Company; 1966.
2. Kaplan HS. *The New Sex Therapy*. New York: Brunner/Mazel Inc.; 1974.
3. Snarch D. *Constructing the Sexual Crucible: An Integration of Sexual and Marital Therapy*. New York: W.W. Norton; 1991.
4. Morley JE. Testosterone and behavior. *Clin Geriatr Med*. 2003;19(3):605–661.
5. Wilson MG. Menopause. *Clin Geriatr Med*. 2003;19(3):483–506.
6. Hallstrom T, Samuelsson S. Changes in women's sexual desire in middle life: the longitudinal study of women in Gothenburg. *Arch Sex Behav*. 1990;19:259–268.
7. Dennerstein LL. The sexual impact of menopause. In: Levine SB, Risen CB, Althof SE, eds. *Handbook of Clinical Sexuality for Mental Health Professionals*. New York: Brunner-Routledge; 2003; 187–198.
8. Harman SM, Metter EJ, Tobin JD, et al. Longitudinal effects of aging on serum total and free testosterone levels in healthy men. Baltimore Longitudinal Study of Aging. *J Clin Endocrinol Metab*. 2001;86:724–731.
9. Hollander E, Samons DM. Male menopause: an unexplored area of men's health. *Psychiatr Ann*. 2003;33(8):497–500.
10. Shabsigh R. Urological perspectives on andropause. *Psychiatr Ann*. 2003;33(8):501–509.
11. Sternbach H. Psychiatric manifestations of low testosterone in men. *Psychiatr Ann*. 2003;33(8):517–524.
12. Starr BD, Weiner MB. *The Starr-Weiner Report on Sex and Sexuality in the Mature Years*. New York: McGraw-Hill; 1981.
13. Marsiglio W, Donnelly D. Sexual relations in later life: a national study of married persons. *J Gerontol*. 1991;46(6):S338–S344.
14. National Council on the Aging. *Healthy Sexuality and Vital Aging: Executive Summary*. Washington, DC: National Council on the Aging; 1998.
15. Jacoby S. Great sex. What's age got to do with it? *Modern Maturity*. 1999; Sept/Oct. Available at www.aarp.org/press/1998/nr100198.html. Accessed November 1, 2000.
16. Comfort A, Dial LK. Sexuality and aging: an overview. *Clin Geriatr Med*. 1991;7(1):1–7.
17. Kligman EW. Office evaluation of sexual function and complaints. *Clin Geriatr Med*. 1991;7(1):15–39.
18. Agronin ME. Geriatric psychiatry: sexuality and aging. In: Sadock BJ, Sadock VA, eds. *Kaplan & Sadock's Comprehensive Textbook of Psychiatry*. 8th Ed. Philadelphia: Lippincott Williams & Wilkins; 2005:3834–3838.
19. Adelman M. Stigma, gay lifestyles, and adjustment to aging: a study of late-life gay men and lesbians. *J Homosex*. 1991;20: 7–32.
20. Mulligan T, Palguta RF Jr. Sexual interest, activity, and satisfaction among male nursing home residents. *Arch Sex Behav*. 1987;20:199–204.
21. Spector IP, Fremeth SM. Sexual behavior and attitudes of geriatric residents in long-term care facilities. *J Sex Marital Ther*. 1996;22:235–246.
22. White CB. Sexual interests, attitudes, knowledge, and sexual history in relation to sexual behavior in the institutionalized aged. *Arch Sex Behav*. 1982;11:11–21.
23. Kaas MJ. Sexual expression of the elderly in nursing homes. *Gerontologist*. 1978;18:372–378.
24. Wasow M, Loeb MB. Sexuality in nursing homes. *J Am Geriatr Soc*. 1979;27:73–79.
25. Richardson JP, Lazur A. Sexuality in the nursing home patient. *Am Fam Physician*. 1995;51(1):121–124.
26. Wilson MG. Sexually transmitted diseases. *Clin Geriatr Med*. 2003;19(3):637–655.

27. Centers for Disease Control and Prevention. STDs Today. Available at: www.cdcnpin.org/scripts/std/std.asp#2a. Accessed March 26, 2005.

28. Centers for Disease Control and Prevention. STD Surveillance 2003. Available at: www.cdc.gov/std/stats/toc2003.htm. Accessed March 26, 2005.

29. Xu F, Schillinger JA, Aubin MR, et al. Sexually transmitted diseases of older persons in Washington State. *Sex Transm Dis.* 2001;28:287–291.

30. Centers for Disease Control and Prevention. *HIV/AIDS Surveillance Report.* 1998;10(2):1–43.

31. American Psychiatric Association. *Diagnostic and Statistical Manual of Mental Disorders.* 4th Ed. Text Revision. Washington, DC: American Psychiatric Association; 2000.

32. Lewis RW, Fugl-Meyer KS, Bosch R, et al. Epidemiology/risk factors of sexual dysfunction. *J Sexual Med.* 2004;1(1):35–39.

33. Feldman HA, Goldstein I, Hatzichristou DG, Krane RJ, McKinlay JB. Impotence and its medical and psychosocial correlates: results of the Massachusetts Male Aging Study. *J Urol.* 1994;151:54–61.

34. Althof SE, Seftel AD. The evaluation and management of erectile dysfunction. *Psychiatric Clin N Am.* 1995;18(1):171–192.

35. Bachmann GA, Leiblum SR. Sexuality in sexagenarian women. *Maturitas.* 1991;13:43–50.

36. Bachmann GA. Vulvovaginal complaints in treatment of the postmenopausal woman: basic and clinical aspects. In: Lobo RA, ed. *Treatment of the Postmenopausal Woman.* New York: Raven Press; 1994:137–142.

37. Crenshaw TL, Goldberg JP. *Sexual Pharmacology: Drugs that Affect Sexual Function.* New York: W.W. Norton; 1996.

38. Goodwin AJ, Agronin ME. *A Women's Guide to Overcoming Sexual Fear and Pain.* Oakland, CA: New Harbinger Press; 1997.

39. Gitlin MJ. Psychotropic medications and their effects on sexual function: diagnosis, biology, and treatment approaches. *J Clin Psychiatry.* 1994;55(9):406–413.

40. Montejo AL, Llorca G, Izquierdo JA. Incidence of sexual dysfunction associated with antidepressant agents: a prospective multicenter study of 1022 outpatients. *J Clin Psychiatry.* 2001;62 (Suppl 3):10–21.

41. Ferguson JM. The effects of antidepressants on sexual functioning in depressed patients: a review. *J Clin Psychiatry.* 2001;62(Suppl 3):22–34.

42. Kavoussi RJ, Segraves RT, Hughes AR, et al. Double-blind comparison of bupropion sustained release and sertraline in depressed outpatients. *J Clin Psychiatry.* 1997;58:532–537.

43. Clayton AH. Recognition and assessment of sexual dysfunction associated with depression. *J Clin Psychiatry.* 2001;62(Suppl 3):5–9.

44. Kaplan HS. *Sexual Aversion, Sexual Phobias, and Panic Disorder.* New York: Brunner/Mazel Inc.; 1987.

45. Haddad P, Benbow S. Sexual problems associated with dementia: part 2. Aetiology, assessment and treatment. *Int J Geriatr Psychiatry.* 1993;8:631–637.

46. Wright LK. The impact of Alzheimer's disease on the marital relationship. *Gerontologist.* 1991;31:224–237.

47. Zeiss AM, Davies HD, Wood M, Tinklenberg JR. The incidence and correlates of erectile problems in patients with Alzheimer's disease. *Arch Sex Behav.* 1990;19:325–332.

48. Duffy LM. Sexual behavior and marital intimacy in Alzheimer's couples: a family theory perspective. *Sexuality Disability.* 1995;13:239–254.

49. Redinbaugh EM, Zeiss AM, Davies HD, Tinklenberg JR. Sexual behavior in men with dementing illnesses. *Clin Geriatr.* 1997;5(13):45–50.

50. Lichtenberg PA, Strzepek DM. Assessments of institutionalized dementia patient's competencies to participate in intimate relationships. *Gerontologist.* 1990;30:117–120.

51. Rabins PV, Mace NL, Lucas MJ. The impact of dementia on the family. *JAMA.* 1982;248:333–335.

52. Kumar A, Koss E, Metzler D, et al. Behavioral symptomatology in dementia of the Alzheimer type. *Alzheimer's Disease Assoc Disord.* 1988;2:363–365.

53. Burns A, Jacoby R, Levy R. Psychiatric phenomena in Alzheimer's disease: IV. Disorders of behavior. *Br J Psychiatry.* 1990;157:86–94.

54. Hashmi FH, Krady AI, Qayum F, Grossberg GT. Sexually disinhibited behavior in the cognitively impaired elderly. *Clin Geriatr.* 2000;8(11):61–68.

55. Bowers MB, Woert MV, Davis L. Sexual behavior during L-dopa treatment for parkinsonism. *Am J Psychiatry.* 1971;127:1691–1693.

56. Uitti RJ, Tanner CM, Rajput AH, et al. Hypersexuality with antiparkinsonian therapy. *Clin Neuropharmacol.* 1989;12:375–383.

57. Kaiser FE, Morley JE. Sexuality and dementia. In: Morris JC, ed. *Handbook of Dementing Illnesses.* New York: Marcel Dekker, Inc.; 1994.

58. Levitsky AM, Owens NJ. Pharmacologic treatment of hypersexuality and paraphilias in nursing home residents. *J Am Geriatr Soc.* 1999;47:231–234.

59. Stewart JT, Shin KJ. Paroxetine treatment of sexual disinhibition in dementia. *Am J Psychiatry.* 1997;154:74.

60. Raji M, Liu D, Wallace D. Sexual aggressiveness in a patient with dementia: sustained clinical response to citalopram. *Ann Long-Term Care.* 2000;8(1):81–83.

61. Kyomen HH, Satlin A, Hennen J, Wei JY. Estrogen therapy and aggressive behavior in elderly patients with moderate-to-severe dementia. *Am J Geriatr Psychiatry.* 1991;7(4):339–348.

62. Lothstein LM, Fogg-Waberski J, Reynolds P. Risk management and treatment of sexual disinhibition in geriatric patients. *Conn Med.* 1997;61:609–618.

63. Cooper AJ. Medroxyprogesterone acetate (MPA) treatment of sexual acting out in men suffering from dementia. *J Clin Psychiatry.* 1987;48:368–370.

64. Weiner MF, Denke M, Williams K, et al. Intramuscular medroxyprogesterone acetate for sexual aggression in elderly men. *Lancet.* 1992;339:1121–1122.

65. Swabo PA. Counseling about sexuality in the older person. *Clin Geriatr Med.* 2003;19(3):595–604.

66. Burke MA, McEroy JP, Ritchie JC. A pilot study of a structured interview addressing sexual function in men with schizophrenia. *Biol Psychiatry.* 1994;35:32–35.

67. Clayton AH, McGarvey EL, Clavet GJ. The Changes in Sexual Functioning Questionnaire (CSFQ): development, reliability, and validity. *Psychopharmacol Bull.* 1997;33:731–745.

68. Derogatis LR. The Derogatis Interview for Sexual Functioning (DISF/DISF-SR): an introductory report. *J Sex Marital Ther.* 1997;23:291–304.

69. McGahuey CA, Gelenberg AJ, Laukes CA, et al. The Arizona Sexual Experience Scale (ASEX): reliability and validity. *J Sex Marital Ther.* 2000;26:25–40.

70. Quirk FH, Heiman JR, Rosen RC, et al. Development of a sexual function questionnaire for clinical trials of female sexual dysfunction. *J Womens Health Gend Based Med.* 2002;11(3):277–289.

71. Boyer G, Boyer J. Sexuality and aging. *Nurs Clin North Am.* 1982;17(3):421–427.

72. Schover LR, Jensen SB. *Sexuality and Chronic Illness.* New York: Guilford Press; 1988.

73. Morley JE, Tariq SH. Sexuality and disease. *Clin Geriatr Med.* 2003;19(3):563–573.

74. Schover LR. Sexuality and cancer. In: Randers-Pehrson M, ed. *Sexuality and Cancer.* Atlanta, GA: American Cancer Society; 1988.

75. Birge SJ. The use of estrogen in older women. *Clin Geriatr Med.* 2003;19(3):617–627.

76. Hulley S, Grady D, Busch T, et al. Randomized trial of estrogen plus progestin for secondary prevention of coronary heart disease in postmenopausal women. Heart and Estrogen/Progestin Replacement Study (HERS) Research Group. *JAMA.* 2002;288:321–333.

77. Writing Group for the Women's Health Initiative Investigators. Risks and benefits of estrogen plus progestin in healthy postmenopausal women. Principal results from the Women's Health Initiative Randomized Controlled Trial. *JAMA.* 2002;288(3):321–333.

78. Tang MX, Jacobs D, Stern Y, et al. Effect of oestrogen during menopause on risk and age at onset of Alzheimer's disease. *Lancet.* 1996;348:429–432.

79. Asnani S, Cefalu CA, Naval-Srinivas RM. Testosterone replacement in the elderly: a clinical approach. *Ann Long-Term Care.* 2003;11(12):44–50.

80. Bremner WJ, Vitiello MV, Prinz PN. Loss of circadian rhythmicity in blood testosterone levels with aging in normal men. *J Clin Endocrinol Metab*. 1983;56(6):1278–1281.
81. Morales A, Johnston B, Heaton JP, Lundie M. Testosterone supplementation for hypogonadal impotence: assessment of biochemical measures and therapeutic outcomes. *J Urol*. 1997;157:849–854.
82. Hajjar RR, Kaiser FE, Morley JE. Outcomes of long-term testosterone replacement in older hypogonadal males: a retrospective analysis. *J Clin Endocrinol Metab*. 1997;82(11):3793–3796.
83. Sherwin BN, Gelfand MM, Brender W. Androgen enhances sexual motivation in females: a prospective, crossover study of sex steroid administration in surgical menopause. *Psychosom Med*. 1991;49:45–50.
84. Shifren JL, Braunstein GD, Simon JA, et al. Transdermal testosterone treatment in women with impaired sexual function after oopherectomy. *N Engl J Med*. 2000;343:682–688.
85. Baulieu EE, Thomas G, Legruin S. Dehyoepiandrosterone, DHEA sulfate and aging: contributions of the DHEAge study to sociobiomedical issue. *Proc Natl Acad Sci USA*. 2000;97:4279–4284.
86. Dennerstein L, Dudley EC, Hopper JL, Burger H. Sexuality, hormones and the menopausal transition. *Maturitas*. 1997;26(2):83–93.
87. Zajecka J. Strategies for the treatment of antidepressant-related sexual dysfunction. *J Clin Psychiatry*. 2001;62(Suppl 3):35–43.
88. Labbate LA, Croft HA, Oleshansky MA. Antidepressant-related erectile dysfunction: management via avoidance, switching antidepressants, antidotes, and adaptation. *J Clin Psychiatry*. 2003;64(Suppl 10):11–19.
89. Kaplan HS. *The New Sex Therapy*. New York: Brunner/Mazel Inc.; 1974.
90. Kaplan HS. *The Evaluation of Sexual Disorders: Psychological and Medical Aspects*. New York: Brunner/Mazel; 1983.
91. Rosen RC, Leiblum SR. *Principles and Practice of Sex Therapy: Update for the 1990s*. New York: The Guilford Press; 1988.
92. Padma-Nathan H, Hellstrom WJG, Kaiser FE, et al. Treatment of men with erectile dysfunction with transurethral alprostadil. *New Engl J Med*. 1997;336(1):1–7.
93. Dutta TC, Eid JF. Vacuum constriction devices for erectile dysfunction: a long-term, prospective study of patients with mild, moderate, and severe dysfunction. *Urology*. 1999;54(5):891–893.
94. Evans C. The use of penile prostheses in the treatment of impotence. *Br J Urol*. 1998;81(4):591–598.
95. Lewis RW. Long-term results of penile prosthetic implants. *Urol Clin North Am*. 1995;22(4):847–856.
96. Kaplan HS. *Overcoming Premature Ejaculation*. New York: Bruner-Mazel; 1989.
97. Waldinger MD, Hengeveld MW, Zwinderman AH. Paroxetine treatment of premature ejaculation: a double-blind, randomized, placebo-controlled study. *Am J Psychiatry*. 1994;151(9):1377–1379.
98. Althof SE. Pharmacologic treatment of rapid ejaculation. *Psych Clin North Am*. 1995;18(1):85–94.
99. Heiman L, Lopiccolo J. *Becoming Orgasmic: A Sexual and Personal Growth Program for Women*. Revised Edition. New York: Prentice Hall; 1976.
100. Barbach L. *Women Discover Orgasm: A Therapist's Guide to a New Treatment Approach*. New York: The Free Press; 1980.
101. Boolell M, Gepi-Attee S, Gingell JC, Allen MJ. Sildenafil, a novel effective oral therapy for male erectile dysfunction. *Br J Urol*. 1996;78(2):257–261.
102. Person ES. Paraphilias. In: Sadock BJ, Sadock VA, eds. *Kaplan & Sadock's Comprehensive Textbook of Psychiatry*. 8th Ed. Philadelphia: Lippincott Williams & Wilkins; 2005:1965–1978.
103. Leo RJ, Kim KY. Clomipramine treatment of paraphilias in elderly demented patients. *J Geriatr Psychiatry Neurol*. 1995;8:123–124.
104. Philpot CD. Paraphilia and aging. *Clin Geriatr Med*. 2003;19(3):629–636.
105. Federoff JP. The paraphilic world. In: Levine SB, Risen CB, Althof SE, eds. *Handbook of Clinical Sexuality for Mental Health Professionals*. New York: Brunner-Routledge; 2003:333–356.
106. Bradford JM, Greenberg DM. Pharmacologic treatment of deviant sexual behavior. In: Rosen RC, Davis C, Rupple H Jr, eds. *Annual Review of Sex Research*. 1996;7:283–306.

NOTE: Selections from this chapter are based on excerpts from the following other chapters authored by Dr. Agronin:
Agronin ME. Sexuality and aging. In: Sadavoy J, Jarvik LF, Grossberg GT, Meyers BS, eds. *The Comprehensive Textbook of Geriatric Psychiatry*. 3rd Ed. New York: W.W. Norton and Company; 2004:789–816.
Agronin ME. Sexual disorders. In: Blazer DG, Steffens DC, Busse EW, eds. *Textbook of Geriatric Psychiatry*. 3rd Ed. Washington, DC: American Psychiatric Press; 2004:303–318.
Agronin ME. Geriatric psychiatry: sexuality and aging. In: Sadock BJ, Sadock VA, eds. *Kaplan & Sadock's Comprehensive Textbook of Psychiatry*. 8th Ed. Philadelphia: Lippincott Williams & Wilkins; 2005:3834–3838.
Agronin ME. Sexuality and aging: an introduction. *CNS Long-Term Care*. 2004;3(3):12–13.
Agronin ME. Sexuality and aging: the impact of menopause and andropause. *CNS Long-Term Care*. 2004;3(4):14–16.
Agronin ME. Sexuality and aging: an interview with Dr. Ruth Westheimer. *CNS Long-Term Care*. 2005;4 (1):7.

The Aging Patient with Intellectual Disabilities

36

John A. Tsiouris   Matthew P. Janicki
Kathryn Pekala Service

The number of adults with *intellectual disabilities* (ID)[a] surviving into middle and later age is increasing and so is the concern and awareness of clinicians about the coincident psychiatric problems presenting in this group. Studies suggest that, except for those individuals with Down syndrome (DS) or other specific syndromes limiting longevity (1), life expectancy of adults with ID is approaching that of the general population (2–5). Consequently, the mental health of this small but rapidly growing segment of the population of adults with lifelong disabilities has begun to attract the attention of professionals (6,7) and policymakers (8).

Although it is generally acknowledged that a high percentage of adults with ID have psychiatric or behavioral disorders, prevalence estimates have varied across studies (9–15) due in large part to diagnostic and sampling issues. However, there is evidence that at least some of these disorders may manifest themselves as often in older as in younger persons with ID (16). Prevalence studies show no overall differences based on gender (14); however, such studies do reveal prevalence differences for specific psychiatric or behavior disorders by level of ID (10).

For adults with ID, some parameters of aging may mirror those in the general population (4,7–19). In this regard,

Janicki et al. (4) reported that causes of death among New Yorkers were generally similar whether or not ID was present. van Schrojenstein Lantman-de Valk (19) found that frequencies of common medical morbidity in Dutch adults with ID were higher than might be expected in the Dutch population, while Kapell et al. (18) found that the frequency of common age-related disorders in American adults with ID was comparable to that in the general American population. Further, others report substantially increased risk of sensory disorders (18,20–24) and thyroid and heart disorders (18) among older adults with ID. Janicki et al. (25) reported that adults with ID over age 40 showed increases in the frequencies of most diseases of older adulthood that were comparable to expectations for the typical US population. Henderson and Davidson (26) reported the results of a geriatric assessment of a sample of adults with ID who were referred for functional decline. Of this group, about 14% had confirmed Alzheimer's-type dementia, while the rest had a wide variety of treatable medical conditions that were thought to cause alterations in function.

The aim of this chapter is to provide an overview of the epidemiology of psychopathology and behavioral disorders, a brief primer on assessment, differential diagnosis and treatment of aging adults with ID, and illustrations of some common situations and case studies to help provide a better understanding of variables that must be considered when making psychiatric diagnoses and treating aging persons with ID. Also covered will be reactive behaviors, stemming from life stressors, to help illustrate that not all problematic behaviors have a psychiatric etiology.

---

[a] The term *intellectual disabilities* is used in this chapter and supersedes the use of a variety of terms meaning the same condition, such as *mental retardation, mental handicap, learning disability* (as used in the United Kingdom)—see Fernald (27). *Developmental disability* is a broader term inclusive not only of intellectual but also of sensory, motor, and cognitive disabilities and when studies refer to this broader term it shall be so noted.

BEHAVIORAL ISSUES

Behavior disorders, which are often comorbid with functional decline in older persons with ID, may be related to medical morbidity to a greater degree than is presently appreciated. A number of reports have shown that presenting problems of age-associated conditions vary considerably across disease categories (18,28–31). Despite this, research on psychiatric issues in ID is often characterized by a benign neglect by the psychiatric establishment in most of the world. Geriatric psychiatry for the general population has been established as a discipline but its professionals have rarely applied their skills or undertaken research with populations of aging persons with ID. What is evident in the literature are attempts to modify or to develop new screening or diagnostic instruments, since the International Classification of Mental and Behavior Disorders (ICD-10) (32) and Diagnostic and Statistical Manual of Mental Disorders (DSM-IV-TR) (33) diagnostic criteria cannot be applied easily and reliably in clinical practice or in research to groups of people with ID. Few published studies have dealt with the rate of psychiatric disorders or *challenging behaviors*[b] in aging persons with ID and with the differences between groups with different etiologies (34,35). Most of the literature on aging and ID is associated with diagnosing dementia in persons with or without DS (36), and medical (20,21,25), nursing (37), rehabilitation, quality of life, ethical, and placement issues (38).

Chronic psychiatric disorders often follow adults with ID as they grow old, and at times, new age-associated psychiatric disorders emerge. With maturity, most challenging behaviors decrease, except in adults affected by dementia. Life stressors also produce changes in behavior, and these reactive behaviors often take on psychiatric overtones. When psychiatrists evaluate and treat older or elderly persons with ID, they have to apply their knowledge of geriatric psychiatry, but they also have to conduct the interview and think as child psychiatrists do when they evaluate children with ID.

MENTAL HEALTH ISSUES

Mental health and psychiatric impairments among older adults with ID have caught the eye of the world ID community and the World Health Organization (WHO). In the late 1990s, professionals in the field of ID and a variety of social and medical scientists addressing biobehavioral issues at the 1999 WHO Conference on "Healthy Aging: Adults with

Intellectual Disabilities" outlined 11 goals. Five of these goals were related to psychiatric issues in aging persons with ID and directed the world community to (39,40):

- Promote the detection of mental disorders such as depression, anxiety, and dementia
- Increase knowledge and skills in professionals, caregivers, and families on psychiatric and other mental health issues
- Develop living environments that are responsive to mental health needs
- Promote mental health and minimize negative outcomes secondary to mental health issues
- Increase mental health services and support in communities

In some developed nations, medical subspecialties have been established that provide focal assessment and treatment of mental health and psychiatric problems in people with ID. For example, recognition of the psychiatric subspecialty of *learning disability* in the United Kingdom and the Republic of Ireland has helped to advance research and offer optimal care to younger and older persons with ID, and has led to more focused guidelines on psychiatric assessment using established psychiatric assessment criteria. In general, medical practitioners and psychiatrists (both general and geriatric) are those usually called upon to diagnose and treat psychiatric and behavioral disorders in aging persons with ID.

Our hope is that practicing psychiatrists and researchers will become sensitized enough to approach the diagnosis, prevention, and treatment of psychiatric disorders in aging people with ID in the same manner that child and geriatric psychiatrists approach their patients. People with ID are unique. They were born with a specific temperament, were raised in different environments, and formed a certain personality and behavioral pattern as they have tried to survive with their limited cognitive abilities in a difficult world. At times, they are fixated on strategies that are maladaptive for the observer but are adaptive for themselves and have worked over the years. Noncompliance and aggressive, self-injurious, and destructive behaviors are their way of communicating their wishes, anger, protests, frustration, pain, anxiety, depression, psychosis, confusion, or disorganization.

The excessive use of neuroleptics in younger and older persons with ID for treatment of challenging behaviors (41), with their potential for negative side effects (42), reflects the current state of affairs in the psychiatric care of persons with ID. Except for emergencies, challenging behaviors should not simply be treated with neuroleptic drugs. If the behaviors are secondary to a psychiatric disorder, the acceptable and effective way of providing treatment in persons with ID is to investigate the reasons behind these behaviors, apply behavior modification and environmental changes, and prescribe the appropriate psychotropics when indicated (43).

---

[b] *Challenging behaviors* is a term in current usage in the ID community as a replacement for the term *maladaptive behaviors* (as many of these behaviors are adaptive for the person exhibiting them), or the common but nonspecific terms *behavioral problems* or *behavioral disorder,* used often as a diagnosis to justify interventions with psychotropics or behavior modification plans.

EPIDEMIOLOGY

Earlier studies found a much higher prevalence of psychiatric disorders in individuals with ID (44–46), but in a recent epidemiological study in which challenging behaviors were excluded, the prevalence of psychiatric disorders in persons with ID was found to be similar to the general population (47).

Prevalence studies of psychiatric disorders in older persons with ID are limited due to sampling bias, small number of subjects, use of case notes, different screening instruments, and rarely direct interviews, using different diagnostic schedules. The findings of these few studies are difficult to interpret, making it challenging to reach valid conclusions regarding prevalence of psychiatric disorders in older persons with ID (48). Between 1979 and 1987, five studies reported on the psychiatric disorders of 166 persons 60 years and older with ID, screened in different settings: schizophrenia was diagnosed in 27, mood disorder in 16, neuroses in 22, and dementia in 40.

A study using the Psychiatric Assessment Scale for Adults with Developmental Disabilities for 105 persons older than 50 years with ID reported a prevalence of dementia of 11.4%, mood disorder of 6.7%, and anxiety disorders of 5.8% (49). In a catchment area study of older people with ID, high rates of psychiatric disorders were reported in 134 adults older than 65 years of age (69.9%) and in 73 adults younger than 65 years of age (43.8%) (34). The Present Psychiatric State for Adults with Learning Disabilities, a novel screening tool, was used for this study. The rates of dementia and other psychiatric disorders were higher in this study than in others, and mood and anxiety disorders were diagnosed more often than schizophrenia or other psychotic disorders.

ASSESSMENT

Older people with ID are a heterogenous group. Their degree of disability ranges from mild to profound. Their ID is secondary to known or unknown underlying etiologies, and affected individuals have grown up in many different environments. Many are medically healthy, have not been diagnosed with any psychiatric disorder, and have not been on any psychotropic medication. Others have been on psychotropics for many years for challenging behaviors without any valid psychiatric assessment. Some individuals with chronic psychiatric disorders were diagnosed properly and responded well to psychotropics, with appropriate dose adjustment or replacement of older psychotropics with new ones. Thus, multiple factors must be considered during the assessment of challenging behaviors in a single older individual with ID (Table 36-1).

For a small percentage of individuals with refractory challenging behavior, many different psychiatric diagnoses

TABLE 36-1

THE ASSESSMENT OF CHALLENGING BEHAVIORS—CONSIDERATIONS

Characteristics

Adaptive from the person's point of view as he/she attempts to survive in his/her perceived world

Learned, and reinforced by others

Normal but exaggerated responses to environment or internal stimuli

Normal for the person's mental age

Due to side effects or in response to side effects of medication

Part of medical, neurological, or psychiatric syndromes

Preexisting but exacerbated because of medical, neurological, or psychiatric disorders

Secondary to caffeine intoxication or nicotine withdrawal

Function

Approach important subjects or objects

Avoid aversive stimuli or tasks

Communicate needs

Control the environment

Dominate others

Fulfill basic needs

Increase stimuli (internal–external)

Reduce stimuli (internal–external)

Soothe self

Baseline Variables

Diurnal variation

Frequency

Intensity

Persons around when exhibited

Place where exhibited

Response of others

Seasonal variation or cyclicity

Weekly variation

Precipitating Factors

Changes in room temperature

Dieting or overeating

Constipation

Hunger or thirst

Family visits

Hierarchy changes (dominance structure)

New clothing, tight shoes

New roommates

New classmates

Parents' illness or death

Problems among staff members

Program changes

Relocation of self/support network

Seasonal allergies

Seasonal changes

Adapted from Reference 180.

were made over the years, and most of the known psychotropics tried. Medical and neurological disorders of older age and sensory impairments (20,21) complicate the presentation of previously controlled psychiatric disorders and challenging behaviors, may precipitate new ones, or trigger past psychiatric disorders and behavioral patterns to re-emerge. In persons with ID and unique syndromes, older age has been associated with certain psychiatric disorders. Alzheimer's-type dementia has been known to occur in persons with Down Syndrome (DS) starting at around 45 years of age (36,50,51). Recently, psychotic illnesses were noted in older adults with velo-cardio-facial syndrome (52,53), and with Prader-Willi syndrome due to chromosome 15 maternal uniparental disomy (54). Persons with autism spectrum disorders and Asperger's disorder may present special diagnostic challenges in later life (55). Mood dysregulation, anxiety, impulse dyscontrol, and depressive disorders are the most common undiagnosed disorders in persons with autism spectrum disorders (43), fragile X syndrome (56), and DS (57,58), and a high prevalence of dementia and depression were found to be associated with older age and ID (59).

Aggressive, destructive, and self-injurious behaviors, hyperactivity, and screaming are the most common challenging behaviors for which help is often sought by caregivers and family members.

The challenging or maladaptive behaviors may be old, new, or old with an acute exacerbation. Baseline data and appropriate monitoring are essential for monitoring any intervention. The mental health clinicians who treat these behaviors often achieve less than optimal results if there is a lack of recognition that they might be the nonspecific expression of neurobiological, psychological, and socioenvironmental factors. The characteristics of challenging behaviors have to be assessed; their function analyzed; their precipitating factors investigated; their frequency, intensity, and variation measured; and the environment where they occured noted. Considerations are listed in Table 36-1 and 36-2.

CHALLENGING BEHAVIORS AND PSYCHIATRIC SIGNS/SYMPTOMS

It has been reported that the pattern of challenging behavior in people with ID generally remains the same across time (60,61). Most of the research in older adults with ID has been done on changes associated with significant regression in adaptive behaviors (60), and mental disorders or dementia in people with and without DS (16, 61–67).

The following challenging behaviors, psychiatric signs and symptoms, and factors contributing to psychiatric disorders have been reported to be associated with older age in people with ID:

1. **Challenging behaviors:**
   Disinhibition (e.g., impulsive acting out, overestimating own abilities)
   Lying, reacting poorly to frustration (obnoxious behavior)
   Noncompliance
   Overactivity–irritability

TABLE 36-2
PSYCHOSOCIAL LIFESPAN CONSIDERATIONS

Education: Very few have received any formal education, and those who have were either segregated from others or virtually ignored in the schoolroom.

Competency and Guardianship: Many are under guardianship, and competency is questioned much more frequently.

Locus of Control: Most reside with family or staff with whom control rests; however, the emphasis on personal choice is growing and becoming more accepted.

Income: Many are within a service network, with the provision of housing, food, and health through governmental benefits.

Activity Options: If connected with a formal system, these options are often dictated by an assessment, and are often limited.

Social Experience: In contrast to a lifetime of interactions with family, friends, and associates from work, church, clubs, and other social networks, for people with ID these experiences may be limited, particularly if institutionalized, due to staff turnover and relocation. Some families may have isolated their children from commonplace experiences, with most options being controlled by others.

Social Networks: They are frequently limited to paid staff and family, with occasional friends both with and without ID.

Family Experience: Marriage and/or children have been very rare.

Competitive Employment: For older people in the general population, most have had lifetime jobs and careers in competitive employment, particularly for men of this age cohort; while for older adults with ID, few have been competitively employed, although some have work histories.

Adapted from Reference 181.

Physical aggression
Self-injurious behavior
Stealing others' property, hoarding objects (lack of boundaries)
Tantrums and disruptive behavior
Verbal aggression
Wandering

2. **Psychiatric signs and symptoms:**
   Avoidance, fearful reactions (old, re-emerging, or new)
   Decreased communication
   Disorientation
   Drop in performance (e.g., not knowing how to dress)
   Forgetfulness (e.g., birth dates, names, what to do next)
   Willful incontinence
   Loss of interest, apathy, withdrawal
   Low self-esteem
   Low energy level
   Mood dysregulation (mood changes, affective lability)
   Ritualistic behavior
   Sleep disturbances
   Social isolation
   Weight loss

3. **Etiological factors contributing to psychiatric disorders:**
   Dementia
   Diminished physiological reserves associated with aging
   Emerging long-term side effects from the use of neuroleptics or other psychotropics
   Genetic factors
   Late-onset seizures
   Loss of support systems
   Loss of family members
   Medical problems
   Reduced mobility
   Relocations
   Sensory impairments
   Side effects from prescribed medications for medical illness and challenging behaviors

To document and monitor challenging behavior, different rating scales have been developed, but the Behavior Problems Inventory (68) is the basis for most of them. The Aberrant Behavior Checklist (69) is used to monitor treatment effects (70). The Overt Aggression Scale (71) has been used to study the treatment effects of medication on severe aggressive, destructive, and self-injurious behavior (43,72). Problems with the reliability and validity of behavior scales—self-report or informant-based—have been reported (73,74).

Medical illness associated with pain, reflux, nausea, dizziness, shortness of breath, fatigue, constipation, dysuria, depth perception, hearing impairment, and sensitivity to noise, heat, cold, or irritants (20,21) are often precipitants of challenging behavior. Psychiatric disorders are the most unrecognized persistent triggers and precipitants. Unfortunately, the psychiatric disorders are usually not in the differential diagnosis when parents, caretakers, behaviorists, or physicians of different specialties, including psychiatrists, are called upon to deal with challenging behaviors in persons with ID.

THE EVALUATION PROCESS

Psychiatrists, general practitioners, internists, neurologists, pediatricians, and nurse practitioners are the clinicians most often involved in the treatment of challenging behaviors and psychiatric disorders in persons with ID. These clinicians often are frustrated for the following reasons:

- Inability to make a clear psychiatric diagnosis in an uncooperative person with limited or impaired cognitive skills and often nonverbal
- Extensive time required in order to obtain information from others and analyze all the variables contributing to the behaviors
- Lack of biological markers or practical instruments that can be helpful in making a correct psychiatric diagnosis and prescribing the appropriate psychotropics

- In many instances, the cases are presented as an emergency situation, although the behaviors have been present for a long time and proper treatments were not implemented at the time that environmental variables initiated or sustained the challenging behaviors.

Researchers have also been frustrated when trying to develop research diagnostic criteria for psychiatric disorders in persons with ID. The many scales and questionnaires that have been developed reflect their frustration. The Psychopathology Inventory for Mentally Retarded Adults (75) is a self-report screening questionnaire, based on informants, for people with mild-to-moderate ID. The Reiss Screen for Maladaptive Behavior rating scale (76), another informant-based screening tool for people with mild-to-moderate ID only, detects eight psychiatric disorders. Another informant-based rating scale that taps into the symptoms of 13 psychiatric disorders, for people with severe and profound ID, is the Diagnostic Assessment Scale for the Severely Handicapped (DASH) (77).

The following scales, originally used to diagnose depression and anxiety disorders in people without ID, have been modified for people with ID, as these disorders are the most common disorders in both populations:

- Hamilton Depression Scale—Mental Handicap Version (78)
- Beck Depression Inventory (79)
- Zung Self-Rating Depression Inventory: Mental Handicap Version (80)
- Glasgow Anxiety Scale for People with an Intellectual Disability (81)
- Zung Anxiety Rating Scale: Adults Mental Handicap Version (82)
- Yale-Brown Obsessive Compulsive Scale in People with Prader-Willi Syndrome (83)

Others, specifically developed to diagnose depression in people with ID, are as follows:

- Self-Report Depression Questionnaire (84)
- Mental Retardation Depression Scale (85,86)
- Depression Subscale of DASH II (87)

Clinicians and researchers have added challenging behaviors as characteristics of depression in people with ID (88–93). This trend has been opposed by others (58,94,95), because the same behaviors can be exhibited by individuals without or with psychiatric disorders. Also, the same individual can exhibit self-injurious behavior during the depressive phase, but aggressive/assaultive and sexually inappropriate behavior during the hypomanic/manic phase of bipolar disorder (96).

According to a recent review (94), a consensus is emerging that the standard diagnostic criteria for depression are appropriate for those with mild-to-moderate degrees of ID. However, the assumption that certain challenging behaviors can be considered characteristic of depression has not been demonstrated effectively. Emerging behaviors or observed changes in their frequency and intensity can be considered red flags, which should alert caretakers and clinicians to search for adjustment reactions to changes in the environment and medical problems, or to investigate further for underlying psychopathology (43,58,95). The following instruments may be useful:

- The PAS-ADD (97) was developed and tested as an instrument for diagnosing psychiatric disorders in people with ID. It is based on ICD-10 criteria (32). Information is obtained from patient and informants by a trained interviewer.
- The mini-PAS-ADD was developed subsequently (98) as a screening tool.
- The Diagnostic Criteria for Psychiatric Disorders for use with Adults with Learning Disabilities/Mental Retardation (DC-LD) (99) represents a consensus of professional opinion in the United Kingdom and the Republic of Ireland. It is based on the ICD-10 (32) classification system with modification to facilitate the diagnosis of psychiatric disorders in adults with ID. DC-LD is not the *gold standard*, but its use in providing research diagnoses and enhancing clinical practice skills can be of value in the future (94).

The instruments above provide descriptive information across a broad range, but relatively little about specific psychiatric disorders (81).

Psychiatric diagnoses, although difficult to make, can be done using DSM IV-TR or ICD-10 diagnostic criteria (100). If the psychiatrist has experience with children or was trained in child psychiatry, he or she may be more comfortable with persons with ID and may reach a diagnosis through observing and interacting with the patient, e.g., asking simple questions in different ways, and validating the answers. Information regarding historical data and present problems obtained from family members, direct care staff, and nurses and psychologists who have been in contact with the patients are invaluable in deriving the final diagnosis. Response to treatment with certain categories of psychotropics can be a helpful, but not always accurate, indicator of the underlying diagnosis (92). Different psychotropics are used for symptomatic treatment of various psychiatric disorders. For example, selective serotonin reuptake inhibitors (SSRIs) may control symptoms of anxiety, including panic attacks, depressive disorders, and impulse control disorders, and atypical antipsychotics can be used for psychotic and mood disorders.

Depression

Most of the work regarding psychiatric diagnoses in adults with ID has been done on diagnosing depressive disorders (58,101,102), or Alzheimer's-type dementia in adults with

DS, and differentiating between depression and dementia in adults with DS at 35 to 60 years of age (57,103,104). In adults with DS, the prevalence of depressive disorders is high between 35 and 50 years of age. Alzheimer's disease (AD), although observed at age 40 in a few cases, increases in prevalence after age 50 in adults with DS (36). In many persons with DS, as with the rest of the population, depression can be independent of dementia, a prodromal stage to dementia, associated with dementia or secondary to dementia (57,104,105). Suicidal ideation, threats, and suicidal attempts have rarely been reported in people with ID (106,107), but the expressed wishes to join dead relatives "up in heaven" or crude suicidal attempts must be recognized as suicidal phenomena and be dealt with appropriately (101).

Anxiety

Tension, irritability, difficulty getting to sleep, obsessive fears, ritualistic behaviors, and somatic complaints have been reported as manifestations of an anxiety disorder (108,109). Avoidance of, or running away from, certain environments and engaging in self-injurious or aggressive behavior when escape is not an option suggests the diagnoses of claustrophobia, agoraphobia, or a specific fear of doctors or procedures. Nightmares and unexplained reactions to certain people or other stimuli suggest the presence of posttraumatic stress disorder, a common but unrecognized disorder in the ID population (110).

Mania

There are no specific studies regarding mania in older people with ID. Increased energy levels, hyperactivity, irritability, aggression, psychomotor excitation, increased rate and volume of speech or self-talk, noncompliance accompanied with grandiosity ("I am the manager;" "I am not retarded"), and other delusions or hallucinations, are the most common symptoms of mania in adults with ID (111–113). Mania was reported to be less common in people with DS than in others with ID or in the general population (114,115).

Schizophrenia

Studies to evaluate late-onset schizophrenia in people with ID do not exist, and the difficulty in diagnosing schizophrenia in adults with severe and profound ID is known (116,117). In a review article of 86 published cases of dementia in DS, only one case with a delusion and another with hallucinations were reported (118). It is important to re-evaluate an existing diagnosis of schizophrenia in older people with ID, as this was a common diagnosis given in the past to people with ID and behavior problems. In a tertiary clinic, where the most refractory cases were seen (a biased sample), psychotic disorders were diagnosed in only six of 102 adults with DS between 50 and 71 years of age, and in 10 of 91 adults without DS between 50 and 86 years of age (119). Many of the patients who already had the diagnosis of schizophrenia or psychotic disorder, not otherwise specified (NOS), were rediagnosed as having autistic disorder, intermittent explosive disorder, or bipolar disorder who developed psychotic features.

The symptoms of schizophrenia in adults with mild-to-moderate ID are similar to those in adults without ID (120). Deterioration in adaptive functioning, changes in behavior and affect, new fearful and avoidance responses with regard to others, aggressive behavior in the form of preemptory strikes when staff and others approach, insomnia, locking doors or windows, changes in self-talk or talking in a way that suggests hallucinatory experiences, are a few of the observable behaviors that suggest psychotic symptomatology. Reports of persons with ID talking to themselves when they exhibit challenging behaviors is considered by many clinicians a sign of underlying psychotic process. Talking to themselves actually may be part of an internal dialogue in persons with mild, moderate, and even severe ID without any psychopathology or challenging behaviors. Further, self-talk is prevalent in children with ID without any psychopathology (121, 122). Change in expressed emotions associated with self-talk is another flag that suggests emerging psychopathology.

Twenty-five percent of both a group of 206 adults with DS (20 to 71 years of age) and 142 without DS (40 to 86 years of age) seen in a tertiary clinic were noted to engage in self-talk without any evidence of psychosis (119). The presence of catatonic features is considered a symptom of psychosis in adults with autistic disorder (123); but in our experience, it was associated most often with major depression in adults with autistic disorder or with DS (67).

Dementia

The diagnosis of dementia in people with ID, and especially with DS, has attracted a lot of attention, and much has been written on the topic (124,125). Baseline cognitive evaluation after 40 years of age for people with DS and after 50 years of age for people with ID, but without DS, is recommended in order to assess future cognitive decline. In the absence of baseline evaluation, informant-based questionnaires are recommended with someone who has known the person for at least 6 months.

A review of research in the area of diagnosing dementia in people with ID suggested the following (124,126): a determination of dementia can be considered only if there is a decline from baseline and not from a level of functioning that is considered normal. Repeated testing over time is necessary, taking into account the level of functioning

prior to the decline. Moreover, there are unique problems among older individuals with DS. They are at higher risk than others for the development of thyroid abnormalities (127), superoxide dismutase abnormalities (128), immune system changes (129), auditory and visual problems (130), and arthritis and osteoporosis (131). At the same time, they appear to be less likely to develop other conditions such as delusions and hallucinations (62,118), high blood pressure, heart attacks, emphysema, chronic lung disease, and bone fractures (131) than persons of comparable age with ID of other etiologies. These are unique problems that require innovative and imaginative approaches to the evaluation of both preserved and deteriorating functions, as well as extra thought in the development of appropriate care plans and programs when dementia is also present. Many of these issues have been reviewed elsewhere (51,132).

There is a consensus among investigators (103,133–138) that the first signs of dementia in people with ID, and especially those with DS, include the observed non-cognitive aspects: irritability, emotional lability, noncompliance, loss of interest, apathy, and personality changes; the cognitive aspects, which include memory loss, difficulty in learning and retaining new information, disorientation to time and place, reduced verbal skills; and the loss of activities of daily living (ADLs) skills. The cognitive aspects can be detected before, at the same time as, or after the observation of non-cognitive changes, depending on the instruments used. Gradual deterioration in all aspects (cognitive, ADL skills, emotional, motoric) follows at different rates.

Dyspraxia, which is defined as a "partial loss of the ability to perform purposeful or skilled motor acts in the absence of paralysis, sensory loss, abnormal posture or tone, abnormal involuntary movements, incoordination, poor comprehension or inattention," (139) follows memory loss in people with DS and dementia. Challenging behaviors, with or without depressive or anxiety disorders, and at times psychotic symptoms, complicate the presentation. Late-onset seizures, seen in 75% of people with DS and dementia (140), bring further deterioration in overall functioning. It is not clear if late-onset seizures were responsible for a shortening of life expectancy to an average of 1.5 years after their onset (140), or whether treatment of the seizures with phenytoin, which may produce severe side effects at therapeutic levels and an overall decline in cognitive and ADL skills, affected the life expectancy of the reported cases (141).

The Dementia Scale for Down Syndrome (142) is the best informant-based instrument for monitoring changes, but it requires an informant who has known the person for at least 2 years. The Dementia Questionnaire for Mentally Retarded Persons (143) and the Multi-Dimensional Observation Scale for Elderly Subjects adapted for persons with DS (144) are informant-based questionnaires to evaluate memory, cognitive, and adaptive daily living skills in persons with ID.

Dalton/McMurray Visual Memory Tests (145) trace visual memory decline in persons with severe/profound ID. The Dyspraxia Test for Adults with Development Disabilities (146) is a valid test for the later stages of dementia. About 21 cases of misdiagnosed dementia in persons with DS have been reported in the literature. The correct diagnosis was depression in 17 cases (57,67,103, 142,147), hypothyroidism in two cases (134,142), or uncontrolled seizures and side effects due to neuroleptics in three cases (142). In our experience, many other such cases are not recognized, or recognized but not reported. Clinicians have been taught to consider first the diagnosis of dementia in persons with DS and a decline in ADL skills after 40 years of age. Unfortunately, further investigation into possible other reasons for the decline is not pursued in a vigorous manner.

CASE EXAMPLE

A mother of Mrs. W, an adult with DS and moderate ID who was diagnosed with and treated for depression told me, "Doctor, before, my daughter used to talk to herself when she was drying the plates in the kitchen, and I knew what was her mood and what was bothering her. Since she became sick (depressed), she does not to talk to herself anymore or talks so quietly that I cannot understand what she says."

Ms. W.'s elderly mother and older sister had taken her to a hospital one day when she was age 42. She had been getting up during the night screaming and crying, appearing scared, and behaving and talking in quiet, different ways than before. "She was not herself," her mother reported. Although her menses were irregular, her mother said that she had her period that night. Ms. W. was seen by a psychiatrist at the hospital's emergency room. The psychiatrist at the emergency room said that she did not know what Ms. W. was suffering from and suggested that she be seen by specialists in an Alzheimer clinic because "according to the textbooks, persons with DS develop early Alzheimer's after the age of 40."

Ms. W. was seen by a specialist in the dementia clinic for persons without ID, who diagnosed AD and psychotic disorder and prescribed haloperidol 1 mg twice a day. The mother and sister were devastated with the diagnosis of AD given to Ms. W. They stopped giving the haloperidol after 10 days because she "became worse" and "could not move." She had developed a dystonic reaction. [Personal observations suggest that older and younger people with DS are very sensitive to the side effects of high-potency neuroleptics. On the files of many older patients, we have seen a red tag with the note: "Allergic to haloperidol."]

Ms. W. was subsequently seen by a neurologist who did not find strong evidence for the diagnosis of demen-

tia and referred her for psychiatric evaluation. When she was seen, Ms. W. could not sleep alone, and her mother had to hold her hand so she could sleep for a few hours next to her. She lost weight, as her appetite had declined. She was constantly anxious and was crying and clinging to her mother.

Loss of ADL skills; reduction in social interaction, communication, and mobility; and decline in overall function were observed and reported by informants close to Ms. W. On mental status examination, she was alert, casually dressed, ambulated slowly, and was overall cooperative. She was wearing corrective glasses. Facial features of DS were evident. She was withdrawn. Head and shoulders were kept down and the corners of her mouth were down. Mood was depressed and anxious. Affect was constricted. Speech was sparse, not spontaneous, low in volume and dysarthric. She could not stay alone in the examining room without her mother or sister next to her. A few times she was observed talking to herself, but her self-talk would stop if she was asked questions. When questioned about the self-talk, she answered "nothing." No signs or symptoms of a psychosis (hallucinations, delusions, loosening of association) were reported, observed, or elicited. Her mother denied observing or hearing Ms. W. express suicidal or homicidal ideations. She was oriented to person and place, but not to time. Memory (immediate recall and after 10-minute intervals) was intact. It took 15 minutes for her to warm up to the examiner and there was a consistent wait for her answers after repeating questions. Insight was impaired and judgment was fair to poor.

The diagnosis of major depression was made, and Ms. W. was treated successfully with a tricyclic antidepressant: desipramine first and with fluoxetine and sertraline when they became available. She exhibited a few falling episodes from hypotension secondary to desipramine, experienced sedation when on fluoxetine, but tolerated and responded very well to sertraline. She was maintained on sertraline 50 mg/day for many years. She later developed hypothyroidism, which was treated successfully with Synthroid 50 µg/day.

Currently, at age 57, Ms. W. has not shown any signs of AD. She was able to mourn the death of her 95-year-old mother a year ago. Her communication skills and overall function, which had improved in the first months of treatment, increased further since she has been living with her sister and her sister's husband. It is of interest to note the precipitating factors in Ms. W.'s original onset of depression: her aunt died soon after Ms. W. and her mother had accompanied the aunt to a clinic where the aunt was examined. Three months after the death of the aunt, Ms. W. accompanied her mother to the same clinic, where Ms. W.'s mother had a checkup before they both went upstate to Ms. W.'s sister for a vacation, something they did every summer. According to the mother, Ms. W. became anxious and started clinging after the visit to the clinic. Questioning Ms. W., she revealed that she was afraid that her mother would die like her aunt did after the visit to the clinic and she would be left alone or would be "put away."

Psychosocial Issues

With increases in life expectancy, losses and changes are experienced by older people with and without ID. The interactions among the biological, psychological, and social aspects of aging are contributing factors to functional outcome (39). These age-related stressors not only impinge upon the quality of life, but also increase morbidity and mortality. Geriatric care providers know that even a relatively small change can have grave consequences; and, at the same time, even small or inexpensive interventions that improve one's functional status can have significant positive results (37). Likewise, clinical practice that considers a lifespan perspective can capitalize on the older person's repertoire of personal attributes and social supports. Historically, many of the present cohort of older individuals with ID have experienced psychosocial limitations during their lives (see Table 36-2). In spite of these limitations, many individuals have developed traits that demonstrate resilience and they should be used in building the plan of medical care.

Death, relocation, and illness may remove people upon whom the older person has depended for support, encouragement, and caring. Until the 1970's, it was widely believed that people with ID could not experience grief or recognize and understand loss. Paradoxically, people were even protected from death experiences because it was felt that they would not be able to "handle it" (148). Many have never been afforded the opportunity to face the reality of life and death, of "learning a language," (148) or the means with which to express their feelings.

Grief may be expressed through behaviors. Many professionals have been more likely to attribute behavioral symptoms to pathology or the ID itself (*diagnostic overshadowing*) and not to grief or bereavement (149). Symptoms of grief reactions can range from apathy or self-injurious behaviors to anorexia or incontinence. There has been increasing recognition and acknowledgment of end-of-life care needs of adults with ID to deal with these issues (148,150,151).

Palliative Care

Although there has been a lack of empirical data surrounding palliative care for needs of people with ID (38), a recent literature review noted some common potential issues. These include: the late presentation of illness and delays and difficulties around diagnosis; difficulties in assessing symptoms and in understanding the illness and its implications; and the ethical issues around decision making and consent to treatment. Other specific concerns include truth-telling, conflicts between the paid carers and family, and recognition of the need for professional support. These are unique issues that often confound the assessment for the clinician.

Death and Dying

Increasing resources are becoming available to support these older individuals and their carers about death and dying, whether their own or their loved ones (150). Basically, people with ID need to have concrete explanations of death in terms that are easily understood. The use of inclusive strategies like memorials and other rituals have been shown to be effective and meaningful (150).

While it is not possible for anyone to be fully prepared for death, it is vital to have an appreciation of such a loss. Preparation means inclusion, information, and detail. Detail includes such activities as a memory box or photograph albums (148). With the notion of a lifespan approach, which incorporates proactive planning (like the development of advanced directives), these older individuals may be more prepared for the idea of a loss and the intense feelings of grief. Through opportunities of inclusion, they may accumulate knowledge and experience that can be linked to their coping abilities. Historically, many elderly parents have been reluctant, when it comes to issues of death, to plan for and with their adult child with ID. Frequently, many assumptions are made about the role of the adult child's siblings. With all families, clinicians are advised to assess the history, characteristics, unique family dynamics, and negotiated commitments. This leads to an important activity for clinicians: the gentle exploration and negotiation of any plans with parents (including other children or sibling involvement), and the provision of support through referrals to social workers or nurses for follow-up with other community resources.

TREATMENT AND MANAGEMENT ISSUES

Immediate family members and care providers often find themselves confronted with agencies poorly equipped to provide practical guidance on management and care of adults with ID experiencing psychiatric disorders or dementia. Physicians with experience in the diagnosis and treatment of these older individuals are hard to find. Family practitioners, geriatricians, and many other health professionals who are accessible may not be aware of the special needs of individuals with ID and their impact on care providers. Many persons with ID are unable to provide verbal self-reports and often cannot follow verbal or spoken instructions readily. These problems hamper the introduction of effective care management strategies.

Without specific guidance, providers may offer inappropriate programs or services for this population or refer them to other care systems too soon. For example, persons with ID and dementia may be referred to long-term care settings, thereby exposing them to unnecessary and possibly inappropriate or overly restrictive conditions that may hasten or aggravate their functional decline. Janicki and Dalton (152) have reported that most referrals for diagnosis originally came about as a result of staff suspicions and that staff indicated a high need for training to help them deal more effectively with the complex problems they encounter in providing care for these persons. Agencies are now seeing greater numbers of older ID individuals in their care who are showing signs of dementia, and the staff needs much more support to cope with their own feelings as well as with the increasingly heavy demands of providing appropriate care (133,153–155).

Useful information regarding interventions for persons affected by dementia and ID is emerging (153,156,157). Specific practice guidelines have been promulgated jointly by the American Association on Mental Retardation (AAMR) and the International Association for the Scientific Study of Intellectual Disabilities (IASSID) (158). These AAMR/IASSID guidelines provide specific suggestions for assessment and service provision, as well as a rational basis for making clinical decisions and developing programs that are specifically responsive to the needs of individuals affected with dementia. The guidelines were developed with the following operating assumptions: 1) each person's needs must determine how care is provided; 2) age-associated changes are a normal part of life; 3) persons with DS are at greater risk for AD; 4) some behavioral changes may look like AD but may be due to other causes and be reversible; and, 5) the individual's own abilities and levels of function should be the basis for evaluating subsequent changes.

The AAMR/IASSID guidelines call for an initial screening for dementia, followed by periodic reviews combined with the implementation of care management practices that are tightly coupled to the expected sequence of functional changes as the individual progresses through the stages of AD. For example, a program for managing incontinence should be prepared and kept in reserve to be available when needed so that it can be implemented immediately at the time when it may be most effective and least embarrassing. The guidelines distinguish situations that require only a screening procedure from those that require a more comprehensive assessment. A three-step course of action is recommended: 1) recognize changes; 2) conduct assessments and evaluations; and 3) institute medical and care management.

Treatment of Challenging Behaviors

Treatment of challenging behaviors in persons with ID has similarities to treatment in persons without ID who developed difficult-to-manage behaviors after they sustained traumatic brain injury or developed dementia. In these three groups, multiple psychotropics have been tried, as well as β-blockers, opioid receptor blockers, acetylcholinesterase inhibitors, herbs, vitamins and, recently, the cannabinoid dronabinol.

Studies assessing the effectiveness and side effects of psychotropics prescribed for psychiatric disorders or chal-

lenging behaviors are very limited in older people with ID, although all the existing psychotropics are currently being used in this population. Clinical experiences suggest that these psychotropics are effective in older people with ID when prescribed for the same psychiatric disorders as in the general population, and the same side effects have been observed in both populations (159). As mentioned, older people with DS are more sensitive to the potential side effects of high-potency neuroleptics, (dystonic reactions), and to tricyclic antidepressants (orthostatic hypotension, constipation, urine retention). Amphetamine-like reactions have been observed with stimulants and tricyclic antidepressants; but fewer side effects overall were observed with SSRIs prescribed for various disorders (43). Paradoxical reactions or disinhibition were reported (160) or observed with benzodiazepines, especially the short-acting ones given to people with ID for control of anxiety, agitation, and aggression. It has been suggested that early, aggressive treatment of depressive disorders may relieve symptoms and improve function (161).

Tricyclic antidepressants in a few case reports appeared to have reversed the symptoms of depression in people with ID (57,101,162,163); but, since their introduction, SSRIs also have been effective in reversing symptoms of depression in younger and older adults with ID (164–166), or of depression associated with dementia (57,67,101). No serious side effects from the use of SSRIs were reported, although in certain cases, they could not be tolerated and had to be discontinued and replaced by other antidepressants because of increased irritability, aggressivity, sedation, insomnia, and gastrointestinal problems. Patience is recommended in the treatment of depression in people with DS, as it may take 3 to 6 months of treatment for full reversal of the symptoms.

Anxiolytics have been used for control of disruptive behaviors (167), with equivocal results (168). Clinical experience suggests anxiolytics can be used for the same indications and precautions as in the general aging population. For example, fluvoxamine was effective in the treatment of a 60-year-old man with ID who developed troublesome obsessive compulsive behaviors after the death of his mother, who was his main support (163).

CASE EXAMPLE

A 40-year-old male with DS and severe ID was treated with thioridazine for self-injurious behavior, noncompliance, crying, insomnia, pacing, jumping up and down, and refusing to cooperate in the morning with staff at the group home where he lived. Information from staff suggested escalation of Mr. C.'s self-injurious behavior during the morning period secondary to panic attacks when he had to leave his residence. The diagnosis of major depression with panic attacks was made and paroxetine was prescribed, but it had to be discontinued, as Mr. C. developed a severe rash on his face, which intensified his self-injurious behavior (i.e., scratching his face). To avoid the risk of developing a rash with another SSRI, trazodone was prescribed. He responded very well to a combination of trazodone 200 mg daily and alprazolam 0.5 mg three times a day. Thioridazine was gradually tapered and discontinued. The dose of trazodone was tapered to 150 mg daily after 3 months, due to his sexual touching of female staff and observed frequent penile erections. Mr. C. has been attending his day program without any problem since then and his self-injurious behavior is controlled.

Lithium has been noted in a review of the literature to reduce aggressivity in people with ID (169) through stabilizing unrecognized mood disorders (101,170). Valproate and carbamazepine were effective in reducing agitation and aggressivity in elderly people with ID (101), as well as paranoid thinking in elderly persons with DS and dementia (57). An attempt to taper and discontinue neuroleptic medication in older adults with severe or profound ID and diagnoses of schizophrenia or psychotic disorder NOS was found to be only partially successful because agitation, behavior problems, psychotic symptoms, and severe dyskinesias re-emerged in some patients during the process (171).

Acetylcholinesterase inhibitors have been used in older people with ID and dementia to modify cognitive decline, but studies to evaluate the benefits and risks have not been done. One 24-week, double-blind placebo control study evaluated donepezil in 30 persons with DS and mild-to-moderate AD, and suggested mild, but not significant, improvement as measured by the Dementia Questionnaire for Mentally Retarded Persons (172). Another study (173) discussed the adverse effects of donepezil in treating AD in persons with DS. A non-randomized, controlled trial of donepezil for 6.5 months in nine patients with DS and moderate dementia found that the treatment was associated with significant cognitive improvement compared to six untreated control patients with similar pathology. Side effects were minimal (174).

In our own clinical experience of 60 persons with DS and AD receiving acetylcholinesterase inhibitors (mainly donepezil) from different clinicians, all but 20 discontinued medication. Side effects (bradycardia, nausea, weight loss, increased irritability, and insomnia) or lack of benefit were reasons for discontinuation (Tsiouris and Patti, unpublished data). An ongoing study of donepezil in younger adults with DS is being conducted to assess its cognitive benefits. Another multicenter double-blind, placebo-controlled study of adults 50 years and older with DS, with or without AD, is assessing vitamin E (2000 IU QD) in delaying cognitive decline (175).

CASE EXAMPLE

Mr. V. was a 56-year-old male with mild ID, living in a small group home and working as a messenger for a manufacturing company. He was a friendly, outgoing person who interacted with everybody and was well-liked. He used to spend every weekend at his father's house, often joined by his brothers. Staff observed that he gradually was becoming withdrawn, not sleeping well, and spending time closing the windows of his room and checking the locks of his room door, something he had not been doing before. When he was questioned by the staff, he said, "I think they try to get into my room and hurt me!" He was taken to his primary physician, who prescribed lorazepam for anxiety and insomnia; but after 2 weeks, his condition did not improve. One day, he tried to open the passenger's door of the moving car he was riding in. He was brought to our office for consultation. When seen, Mr. V. was anxious, agitated with depressed mood and constricted affect, and exhibited sparse speech, paranoid ideation, and a congruent mood. His attempt to open the car door was explained as an attempt to kill himself and get rid of the people who were bothering him. He could not elaborate further on this issue. He was oriented to person, place, and time. His memory was intact, but insight and judgment were impaired.

Mr. V. had never previously had any similar episodes and had never been on psychotropics for psychiatric illness or challenging behaviors. The diagnosis of major depression, single episode, severe with psychotic features, was given. He responded very well and quickly to olanzapine 2.5 mg at bedtime and lorazepam 0.5 mg twice a day. The precipitating factor for this depression was traced to his father's stroke 1 month before the onset of his symptoms. Two years after this episode, Mr. V. had to stop working: he became incontinent at work a few times and defecated in his pants. In his attempt to clean himself, he made a mess in the bathroom and in the offices where he worked, and the cleaning staff would not tolerate it. Three months after he lost his job, he became depressed again, but his depression was reversed when sertraline was added to the olanzapine. Olanzapine was replaced soon after with quetiapine because of his 15-pound weight gain. On sertraline, he became very animated, over-talkative, and social without any paranoid thinking or fear of being attacked. His father died and over the next few months he was able, with the help of his brothers, to mourn appropriately, without a relapse.

CASE EXAMPLE

Mr. G. was a nonverbal 65-year-old male with severe ID of unknown etiology and history of seizures. He had been a resident of a small group home for many years and was attending a related day program regularly. He carried a diagnosis of psychotic disorder NOS for which he received mesoridazine 50 mg daily. He liked to go for rides in the van, smoke, and dance the tango. He was friendly, social, and cooperative. He had to give up smoking due to chronic bronchitis. The mesoridazine had to be tapered due to the signs of a tardive dyskinesia. Mr. G. developed polydipsia and polyuria when mesoridazine was tapered. An inability to restrict his fluid intake caused low serum sodium and precipitated explosive episodes during which Mr. G. attacked everybody around and appeared confused, paranoid, and unable to recognize the staff. Mr. G. was observed in between these episodes mentioning the name of his dead sister, pointing to the ground, and gesturing that he wanted to die.

It was recognized that the explosive episodes were partial complex seizures with random aggressive behavior, reactivated because of low serum sodium levels. Affective lability and paranoid ideation were observed when the mesoridazine was finally discontinued. Olanzapine 5 mg before bedtime was started for his affective lability and paranoid ideations, and was gradually increased to 15 mg daily. Cognitive evaluations and memory testing ruled-out dementia, which had been suspected initially. Phenytoin was prescribed by Mr. G.'s neurologist for seizures, but was replaced with lamotrigine because of side effects. Strict fluid restriction was implemented as part of his behavioral plan. He was stabilized on lamotrigine 500 mg daily and olanzapine 15 mg daily. His final diagnosis was personality changes due to electrolyte disturbances secondary to serum increased anti-diuretic hormone (SIADH). His good response to mesoridazine in the past, although in small doses, and to olanzapine later on, suggested a psychotic disorder NOS. However, schizo-affective disorder (rule out bipolar II) was the diagnosis given to Mr. G., as it has been observed that persons with severe/profound ID very often exhibit psychotic features during the manic or depressed phase of bipolar disorders or unipolar depression.

The following cases reflect misdiagnosis and an unrecognized etiological diagnosis in two elderly persons with ID. In select individuals, careful evaluation and karyotyping can change a past diagnosis that had never been confirmed by the physician.

CASE EXAMPLE

Ms. K. was a 60-year-old female with profound ID referred for evaluation as a result of insomnia, lack of appetite, confusion, and constantly making sounds as she "babbled to herself" in an agitated state. A provisional diagnosis of dementia of Alzheimer's type was given by the referring physician, as she was carrying the diagnosis of DS. Cognitive testing, memory testing, and information did not reveal any drop in ADL skills in the preceding years. Chromosomal analysis revealed a karyotype of 46 XX, which indicated that the diagnosis of DS given because of her short stature and some facial features of DS was incorrect. The diagnosis of dementia was ruled out, but major depression, moderate, and anxiety disorder were seen as

---

the reasons for her insomnia, agitation, and inability to concentrate on tasks, as before. Her babbling was diagnosed as vocal tics, and many motor tics also were observed and thought to be part of a chronic tic disorder. She responded well to a combination of trazodone 50 mg at bedtime and quetiapine 25 mg twice a day. Ms. K.'s sleep and appetite improved, she gained weight, and the agitation and confusion that she had previously demonstrated were eliminated. Her vocal tics, but not the motor tics, subsided.

CASE EXAMPLE

Mr. Z. was a 62-year-old male with moderate ID who was referred to our clinic by his physician at a developmental center. Mr. Z. was a resident because of his poor response to different psychotropics and behavior plans. Non-compliance and screaming were his main challenging behaviors. Destructive, self-injurious, and aggressive behaviors were exhibited as part of an explosiveness displayed when he was cornered by others, or in order to avoid demands or escape certain situations. Irritability, hyperarousability, gaze aversion, and social anxiety were the main characteristics of his presentation. No signs of psychosis, depression, or dementia were reported or observed. His behavioral characteristics and his elongated face, large low-set ears, and large testicles suggested fragile X syndrome, for which he had never been tested and which no one had suspected. Fragile X syndrome was confirmed through testing as the etiology of his ID and as the reason for his behavioral profile. Suggestions for tapering his neuroleptics and adding a β-blocker were made.

Personality Disorders

A few individuals with developmental disabilities, especially those with higher cognitive abilities, cannot be diagnosed with Axis I psychiatric disorders. On close examination of their behaviors through the years, traits of an underlying personality disorder may be recognized in many of these individuals. (176–178).

An established Axis II diagnosis of personality disorder will guide the knowledgeable clinician in the development of additional plans of treatment and action. The standard behavior modification plans often do not work with these individuals and psychotropics, when carefully chosen, may decrease the frequency and the intensity of the challenging behavior. A specially structured environment, increased responsibility, involvement of the community and parents/guardians in the plan, and individual and group counseling have been found to be helpful. Legal accountability for their behaviors, especially in individuals with developmental disabilities for which competency has been established, is another deterrent.

Once a comprehensive functional assessment of problem behavior has been conducted and one or more working hypotheses have been developed, an individualized treatment plan addressing the problem should be selected. In many cases, a problem behavior will have different contributing factors and also serves different functions.

In general, every intervention or treatment should: 1) protect the health and safety of the individual; 2) reduce the frequency and/or severity of the behavior; 3) increase adaptive behaviors; and 4) help in the development of appropriate levels of physical, emotional, cognitive, and social integration, as well as varied activity patterns.

Miscellaneous Behaviors

Akathisia (motor restlessness, pacing), a potential side effect of most neuroleptics, is often perceived by caretakers as hyperactivity, agitation, and excitement, and it has been associated with increased aggressive and self-injurious behavior, noncompliance, running away, or jumping from high places.

Pica can be initiated or exacerbated by iron and zinc deficiency. Treatment and reduction of its frequency through supplementation of these minerals has been reported. Controlling caffeine intake and cigarette or tobacco availability in certain cases, while using them as positive reinforcement at the same time, may reduce the frequency of pica and maladaptive behaviors.

Fecal smearing and rectal digging can be caused by constipation. Also, weight gain is a side effect of many psychotropics. A weight-reducing diet may exacerbate the maladaptive behaviors, and the risk/benefit ratio of the diet must be evaluated and corrective action taken.

Psychogenic polydipsia is a rare symptom of an underlying major psychiatric disorder (schizophrenia or mood disorder), a behavior observed in persons with autistic disorder and/or mental retardation, and a rare side effect of some psychotropics (phenothiazines, other neuroleptics, or lithium). Polydipsia can cause a medical emergency through severe hyponatremia, triggering seizures or water intoxication (vomiting, agitation, incoordination, and rarely, coma). Structural changes, kidney failure, heart failure, and gastrointestinal system problems have been observed with chronic polydipsia. Treatment approaches include: 1) treating the underlying psychiatric disorder; 2) tapering, discontinuing, or switching to a different neuroleptic; or 3) using behavior approaches such as restricting water intake and using a token economy.

Aerophagia is a rare behavior observed in persons with autistic disorder and/or mental retardation. Excessive or prolonged air swallowing results in abdominal distention, excessive flatus, and frequent belching. If aerophagia becomes chronic, it may cause structural changes in the gastrointestinal system and compression of the diaphragm. Although a difficult problem to treat, aerophagia has responded to behavioral treatment approaches (179).

The Use of Psychotropics in Persons with Intellectual Disabilities

ID and other developmental disabilities are not psychiatric disorders, *per se*, and are not indications for the use of drugs. Any medication should be administered only as indicated by person-specific needs, be it a generalized medical problem, a preventive program, or a mental disorder. At no time should any drug be administered without the clear knowledge and documentation of both its purpose and the effects it is expected to achieve. Also to be considered in prescribing a drug, are the size and age of the individual, possible interactions with the other drugs he or she may be receiving, sensitivities, and the individual's capacity to absorb, distribute, metabolize, and excrete the proposed drug.

People with ID often have concomitant physical disorders, organ abnormalities, and/or chronic diseases that might influence the dosage and effects of a particular drug. A drug should always be used in the smallest effective dose, should never exceed maximal doses recommended as safe, and should be used for as short a period of time as necessary. Drugs should be used as part of an overall treatment plan, including behavioral interventions.

Psychotropic drugs should not be used in persons with ID unless, in addition to the basic diagnosis of ID, there is a specifically diagnosed condition for which such agents are indicated. These conditions might include, but are not limited to: acute psychosis; schizophrenia; schizoaffective and other psychotic disorders; delusional, mood, or anxiety disorders; dementia with associated behavioral and psychological symptoms; impulse control and tic disorders; attention deficit hyperactivity disorder; conduct disorders; and stereotypic movement disorder with severe destructive behavior, either self-directed or other-directed.

A comprehensive psychiatric evaluation must be performed before psychotropics are prescribed, except in emergency situations. A definite or tentative psychiatric diagnosis has to be documented, and the drugs prescribed must be within the accepted practice of psychopharmacology corresponding to the diagnosis.

Psychotropics are sometimes prescribed in ID persons for aggressive, destructive, self-injurious, and sexually inappropriate behaviors, as well as temper tantrums and stereotypies, despite there being no diagnosable psychiatric disorder. Psychotropic agents should never be used as a quick substitute for a carefully planned, systematic intervention; but they may be useful for target behaviors when there is documentation that behavior modification plans have been made, implemented, and revised, but have failed to address or decrease the frequency and the intensity of target behaviors.

Consent forms for psychotropics, when required, must be obtained from parents/guardians. Psychotropic agents should be tapered or discontinued on a trial basis in a variety of circumstances including: 1) when they have been prescribed for adjustment disorders and recently exhibited maladaptive behaviors; 2) when history and observations of the individual do not justify the given diagnosis and the medication prescribed; or 3) when drugs given in an optimum dose and period of time have not been sufficiently effective. and substitution is planned. Periodic evaluation and documentation of continued need and benefit of long-term treatment is necessary.

Drug withdrawal trials or drug holidays should be considered at least once in persons with chronic psychiatric disorders who have been stabilized on medication, depending upon diagnosis, clinical state, past history, and risk/benefit base. Drug holidays are not required in all cases, especially if previous attempts have had detrimental effects for the person or others.

ACKNOWLEDGMENTS

The authors extend their sincere thanks to Valerie Mazza and Maureen Marlow for help in typing, editing, and preparing this chapter.

The first author (John A. Tsiouris) was supported in part by the New York State Office of Mental Retardation and Developmental Disabilities.

REFERENCES

1. Malone Q. Mortality and survival of the Down's syndrome population in Western Australia. *J Ment Defic Res.* 1988;32:59–65.
2. Carter G, Jancar J. Mortality in the mentally handicapped: a 50-year survey at the Stoke Park group of hospitals (1930–1980). *J Ment Defic Res.* 1983;27:143–156.
3. Baird PA, Sadovnick AD. Life expectancy in Down syndrome. *J Pediatrics.* 1987;110:849–854.
4. Janicki MP, Dalton AR, Henderson CM, Davidson PW. Mortality and morbidity among older adults with intellectual disabilities: health services considerations. *Disabil and Rehab.* 1999;21:284–294.
5. Patja K, Iivanainen M, Vesala H, Oksanen H, Ruoppila I. Life expectancy of people with intellectual disability: a 35-year follow-up study. *J Intellect Disabil Res.* 2000;44:591–599.
6. Davidson PW, Prasher VP, Janicki MP, eds. *Mental Health, Intellectual Disabilities and the Aging Process.* London: Blackwell Publishing; 2003.
7. Torr J, Chiu E. The elderly with intellectual disability and mental disorder: a challenge for old age psychiatry. *Psychiatry.* 2002;15:383–385.
8. Voelker R. Putting mental retardation and mental illness on health care professionals' radar screen. *JAMA.* 2002;288:433–435.
9. Cooper S-A. The psychiatry of elderly people with mental handicaps. *Interna J Geria Psychiatry.* 1992;7:865–874.
10. Cooper S-A. The relationship between psychiatric and physical health in elderly people with intellectual disability. *J Intellect Disabil Res.* 1999;43:54–60.
11. Davidson PW, Cain N, Sloane-Reeves J, et al. Characteristics of community-based individuals with mental retardation and aggressive behavioral disorders. *Am J Ment Retard.* 1994;98: 704–716.
12. Day K, Jancar J. Mental and physical health and ageing in mental handicap: a review. *J Intellect Disabil Res.* 1994;38:241–256.
13. Jacobson J. Problem behavior and psychiatric impairment within a developmentally disabled population I: behavior frequency. *Appl Res Ment Retard.* 1982;3:121–139.
14. Lunsky Y, Havercamp SM . Women's mental health. In: Walsh P, Heller T, eds. *Health of Women with Intellectual Disabilities.* Oxford, England: Blackwell; 2002:59–75.
15. Reiss S. Prevalence of dual diagnosis in community-based day programs in the Chicago metropolitan area. *Am J Ment Retard.* 1990;94:578–585.
16. Davidson PW, Morris D, Cain NN. Community services for people with dual diagnosis and psychiatric or severe behaviour disorders. In: Bouras N, ed. *Psychiatric and Behavioural Disorders in Developmental Disabilities and Mental Retardation.* Cambridge: Cambridge University Press; 1999:359–372.
17. Cooper, S-A. Clinical study of the effects of age on the physical health of adults with mental retardation. *Am J Ment Retard.* 1998;102:582–589.
18. Kapell D, Nightingale B, Rodriguez A, Lee JH, Zigman WB, Schupf N. Prevalence of chronic medical conditions in adults with mental retardation: comparison with the general population. *Ment Retard.* 1998;36:269–279.
19. van Schrojenstein Lantman-de Valk HMJ. *Health Problems in People with Intellectual Disability: Aspects of Morbidity in Residential Settings and in Primary Health Care.* Maastricht, The Netherlands: Maastricht University; 1995.
20. Evenhuis HM. Medical aspects of ageing in a population with intellectual disability: I. Visual impairment. *J Intellect Disabil Res.* 1995;39:19–26.
21. Evenhuis HM. Medical aspects of ageing in a population with intellectual disability: II. Hearing impairment. *J Intellect Disabil Res.* 1995;39:27–33.
22. Evenhuis HM. Associated medical aspects. In: Janicki MP, Dalton AJ, eds. *Dementia, Aging, and Intellectual Disabilities: A Handbook.* Philadelphia: Brunner-Mazel; 1999:103–118.
23. Evenhuis HM, Henderson CM, Beange H, Lennox N, Chicoine B. *Healthy Aging—Adults with Intellectual Disabilities—Physical Health Issues.* Geneva, Switzerland: World Health Organization; 2000.
24. Janicki MP, Dalton AJ. Sensory impairments among older adults with intellectual disability. *J Intellect Diabil Res.* 1998;23:3–11.
25. Janicki MP, Davidson PW, Henderson CM, et al. Health characteristics and health services utilization in older adults with intellectual disabilities living in community residences. *J Intellect Disabil Res.* 2002;46:287–298.
26. Henderson CM, Davidson PW. Comprehensive adult and geriatric assessment. In Janicki MP, Ansello E, eds. *Community Supports for Aging Adults with Lifelong Disabilities.* Baltimore: Paul Brookes Publishing Inc.; 2000:373–386.
27. Fernald CD. When in London. . . : differences in disability language preferences among English-speaking countries. *Ment Retard.* 1995;33:99–103.
28. Carlsen WR, Galliuzzi KE, Forman LF, Cavalieri TA. Comprehensive geriatric assessment: applications for community-residing, elderly people with mental retardation/developmental disabilities. *Ment Retard.* 1994;32:334–340.
29. Chicoine B, McGuire D, Hebein S, Gilly D. Development of a clinic for adults with Down syndrome. *Ment Retard.* 1994;32:100–106.
30. Gambert SR, Crimmins D, Cameron DJ, et al. Geriatric assessment of the mentally retarded elderly. *NY Medi Quart.* 1988;8:144–147.
31. McCreary BD, Fotheringham JB, Holden JJA, Ouellette-Kuntz H, Robertson DM. Experiences in an Alzheimer clinic for persons with Down syndrome. In: Berg JM, Karlinsky H, Holland AJ, eds. *Alzheimer's Disease, Down Syndrome, and Their Relationship.* Oxford: Oxford University Press; 1993:115–131.
32. World Health Organization. *The International Classification of Mental and Behaviour Disorders—Clinical Descriptions and Diagnostic Guidelines.* 10th rev (ICD-10). Geneva: World Health Organization; 1992.
33. American Psychiatric Association. *Diagnostic and Statistical Manual of Mental Disorders,* 4th Edition, Text Revision. Washington, DC: American Psychiatric Association; 2000.
34. Cooper S-A. Psychiatry of elderly compared to younger adults with intellectual disability. *J App Res Intellect Disabil.* 1997;10:303–311.
35. Collacott RA, Cooper S-A, McGrother C. Differential rates of psychiatric disorders in adults with Down's syndrome compared with other mentally handicapped adults. *Br J Psychiatry.* 1992; 161:671–674.
36. Zigman W, Schupf N, Haveman M, Silverman W. The epidemiology of Alzheimer's disease in mental retardation: results and recommendation from an international conference. *J Intellect Disabil Res.* 1997;41:76–80.
37. Service KP, Hahn JE. Issues in aging. The role of the nurse in the care of older people with intellectual and developmental disabilities. *Nurs Clin North Am.* 2003;38:291–312. Review.

38. Tuffrey-Wijne I. The palliative care needs of people with intellectual disabilities: a literature review. *Palliat Med.* 2003;17:55–62.

39. Thorpe L, Davidson P, Janicki MP. Healthy aging—adults with intellectual disabilities: biobehavioral issues. *J Appl Res Intellect Disabil.* 2001;14:218–228.

40. Thorpe L, Davidson P, Janicki MP. Healthy aging—adults with intellectual disabilities: summative report 2002; World Health Organization, Geneva, Switzerland.

41. Linaker OM. Frequency of and determinants for psychotropic drug use in an institution for the mentally retarded. *Br J Psychiatry.* 1990;156:525–530.

42. Brylewski J, Duggan L. Antipsychotic medication for challenging behaviour in people with intellectual disability: a systematic review or randomized controlled trials. *J Intellect Disabil Res.* 1999;43:504–512.

43. Tsiouris JA, Cohen IL, Patti P, Korosh WM. Treatment of previously undiagnosed psychiatric disorders in persons with developmental disabilities decreased or eliminated self-injurious behavior. *J Clin Psychiatry.* 2003;64:1081–1090.

44. Eaton LF, Menolascino FJ. Psychiatric disorders in the mentally retarded: types, problems and challenges. *Am J Psychiatry.* 1982; 139:1297–1303.

45. Benson BA. Behavior disorders and mental retardation: associations with age, sex, and level of functioning in an outpatient clinic sample. *Appl Res Ment Retard.* 1985;6:79–85.

46. Day K. Psychiatric disorder in the middle-aged and elderly mentally handicapped. *Br J Psychiatry.* 1985;147:660–667.

47. Deb S. Epidemiology of psychiatric illness in adults with intellectual disability. In: Hamilton-Kirkwood Z, Ahmed S, Deb S, et al., eds. *Health Evidence Bulletins—Learning Disabilities (Intellectual Disability).* Cardiff: NHS; 2001:14–17.

48. Deb S, Matthews T, Holt G, Bouras N, eds. *Practice Guidelines for the Assessment and Diagnosis of Mental Health Problems in Adults with Intellectual Disability.* Brighton: Pavilion; 2001.

49. Patel P, Goldberg D, Moss S. Psychiatric morbidity in older people with moderate and severe learning disability II: the prevalence study. *Br J Psychiatry.* 1993;163:481–491.

50. Zigman WB, Schupf N, Sersen E, Silverman W. Prevalence of dementia in adults with and without Down syndrome. *Am J Ment Retard.* 1996;100:403–412.

51. Holland AJ, Hon J, Huppert FA, Stevens F, Watson P. Population-based study of the prevalence and presentation of dementia in adults with Down's syndrome. *Br J Psychiatry.* 1998;172:493–498.

52. Shprintzen RJ, Goldberg R, Golding-Kushner KJ, Marion RW. Late-onset psychosis in the velo-cardio-facial syndrome. *Am J Med Genet.* 1992;42:141–142.

53. Murphy KC, Jones LA, Owen MJ. High rates of schizophrenia in adults with velo-cardio-facial syndrome. *Arch Gen Psychiatry.* 1999;56:940–945.

54. Boer H, Holland A, Whittington J, Butler J, Webb T, Clarke D. Psychotic illness in people with Prader-Willi syndrome due to chromosome 15 maternal uniparental disomy. *Lancet.* 2002; 359:135–136.

55. Nordin V, Gillberg C. The long-term course of autistic disorders: update on follow-up studies. *Acta Psychiat Scand.* 1998;97: 99–108.

56. Tranebjaerg L, Orum A. Major depressive disorder as a prominent but underestimated feature of fragile X syndrome. *Compr Psychiatry.* 1991;32:83–87.

57. Tsiouris JA, Patti PJ. Drug treatment of depression associated with dementia or presented as "pseudodementia" in older adults with Down syndrome. *J Appl Res Intellect Disabil.* 1997;10:312–322.

58. Tsiouris JA, Mann R, Patti PJ, Sturmey P. Challenging behaviours should not be considered as depressive equivalents in individuals with intellectual disability. *J Intellect Disabil Res.* 2003;47:14–21.

59. Cooper S-A. High prevalence of dementia among people with learning disabilities not attributable to Down's syndrome. *Psychol Medicine* 1997b;27:609–616.

60. Urv TK, Zigman WB, Silverman W. Maladaptive behaviors related to adaptive decline in aging adults with mental retardation. *Am J Ment Retard.* 2003;108:327–339.

61. Prasher VP, Chung MC. Causes of age-related decline in adaptive behavior of adults with Down syndrome: differential diagnoses of dementia. *Am J Ment Retard.* 1996;101:175–183.

62. Moss S, Patel P. Dementia in older people with intellectual disability: symptoms of physical and mental illness, and levels of adaptive behaviour. *J Intellect Disabil Res.* 1997;41:60–69.

63. Cosgrave MP, Tyrrell J, McCarron M, Gill M, Lawlor BA. Determinants of aggression, and adaptive and maladaptive behavior in older people with Down's syndrome with and without dementia. *J Intellect Disabil Res.* 1999;43:393–399.

64. Cooper S-A, Prasher VP. Maladaptive behaviors and symptoms of dementia in adults with Down's syndrome compared to adults with intellectual disability of other etiologies. *J Intellect Disabil Res.* 1998;42:293–300.

65. Collacott RA, Cooper S-A, Brandford D, McGrother C. Behaviour phenotype for Down's syndrome. *Br J Psychiatry.* 1998;172:85–89.

66. Chapman RS, Hesketh LJ. Behavioral phenotype of individuals with Down syndrome. *Ment Retard and Dev Disabil.* 2000;6:84–95.

67. Patti P, Tsiouris J. Emotional and behavioral disturbances in adults with Down syndrome. In: Davidson PW, Prasher VP, Janicki MP, eds. *Mental Health, Intellectual Disabilities and the Aging Process.* Oxford: Blackwell Publishing; 2003:81–93.

68. Rojahn J, Polster LM, Mulick JA, Wisniewski JJ. Reliability of the Behavior Problems Inventory. *Multihandicapped Person.* 1989; 2:283–293.

69. Aman MG, Singh NN. *Aberrant Behavior Checklist Manual.* New York: Slosson Educational Publications; 1986.

70. Aman MG, Singh NN, Stewart AW. The aberrant behavior checklist: a behavior rating scale for the assessment of treatment effects. *Am J Ment Defic.* 1985;89:485–491.

71. Yudofsky SC, Silver JM, Jackson W, Endicott J, Williams D. The overt aggression scale for the objective rating of verbal and physical aggression. *Am J Psychiatry.* 1986;143:35–39.

72. Cohen IL, Tsiouris JA, Pfadt A. Effects of long-acting propranolol on agonistic and stereotyped behaviors in a man with pervasive developmental disorder and fragile X syndrome: a double-blind, placebo-controlled study. *J Clin Psychopharmacol.* 1991;11:398–399.

73. Aman MA. Review and evaluation of instruments for assessing emotional and behavioural disorders. *Aust and New Zealand J of Dev Disabil.* 1991;17:127–145.

74. Sturmey P, Reed J, Corbett J. Psychometric assessment of psychiatric disorders in people with learning difficulties (mental handicap): a review of measures. *Psychol Medicine.* 1991;21: 143–155.

75. Matson JL, Kazdin AE, Senatore V. Psychometric properties of the psychopathology instrument for mentally retarded adults. *Appl Res in Ment Retard.* 1984;5:81–89.

76. Reiss, S. *Test Manual for the Reiss Screen for Maladaptive Behavior.* Ohio: International Diagnostic Systems; 1988.

77. Matson JL, Gardner WI, Coe DA, Sovner R. A scale for evaluating emotional disorders in severely and profoundly mentally retarded persons: development of the Diagnostic Assessment for the Severely Handicapped (DASH) scale. *Br J Psychiatry.* 1991; 159:404–409.

78. Sireling L. Depression in mentally handicapped patients: diagnostic and neuroendocrine evaluation. *Br J Psychiatry.* 1986;149: 274–278.

79. Kazdin AE, Matson JL, Senatore V. Assessment of depression in mentally retarded adults. *Am J Psychiatry.* 1983;140: 1040–1043.

80. Helsel WJ, Matson JL. The relationship of depression to social skills and intellectual functioning in mentally retarded adults. *J Ment Defic Res.* 1988;32:411–418.

81. Mindham J, Espie CA. Glasgow Anxiety Scale for people with an intellectual disability (GAS-ID): development and psychometric properties of a new measure for use with people with mild intellectual disability. *J Intellect Disabil Res.* 2003;47:22–30.

82. Lindsay WR, Michie AM. Adaptation of the Zung self-rating anxiety scale for people with a mental handicap. *J Ment Defic Res.* 1988;32:485–490.

83. Feurer ID, Dimitropoulos A, Stone WL, Roof E, Butler MG. The latent variable structure of the Compulsive Behaviour Checklist in people with Prader-Willi syndrome. *J Intellect Disabil Res.* 1998;42:472–480.

84. Reynolds WK, Baker JA. Assessment of depression in persons with mental retardation. *Am J Ment Retard.* 1988;93:93–103.

85. Meins W. Prevalence and risk factors for depressive disorders in adults with intellectual disability. *Aust and New Zealand J Dev Disabil.* 1993;18:147–156.

86. Meins W. A new depression scale designed for use with adults with mental retardation. *J Intellect Disabil Res.* 1996;40:222–226.

87. Matson JL, Rush KS, Hamilton M, Anderson SJ, Bamburg JW, Baglio S. Characteristics of depression as assessed by the Diagnostic Assessment for the Severely Handicapped-II (DASH). *Res Dev Disabil.* 1999;20:305–313.

88. Davis JP, Judd FK, Herrman H. Depression in adults with intellectual disability. Part 1: a review. *Australian and New Zealand J Psychiatry.* 1997a;311:232–242.

89. Davis JP, Judd FK, Herrman H. Depression in adults with intellectual disability. Part 2: a pilot study. *Australian and New Zealand J Psychiatry.* 1997b;31:243–251.

90. Meins W. Symptoms of major depression in mentally retarded adults. *J Intellect Disabil Res.* 1995;39:41–45.

91. Marston GW, Perry DW, Roy A. Manifestations of depression in people with intellectual disability. *J Intellect Disabil Res.* 1997;41:476–480.

92. Clarke DJ, Gomez GA. Utility of modified DCR-10 criteria in the diagnosis of depression associated with intellectual disability. *J Intellect Disabil Res.* 1999;43:413–420.

93. Hurley AD. Identifying psychiatric disorders in persons with mental retardation: a model illustrated by depression in Down syndrome. *J Rehab.* 1996;15:6–31.

94. McBrien JA. Assessment and diagnosis of depression in people with intellectual disabilities. *J Intellect Disabil Res.* 2003;47:1–13.

95. Holland AJ, Koot HM. Mental health and intellectual disability: an international perspective. *J Intellect Disabil Res.* 1998;42: 505–512.

96. Sovner R, Lowry M. A behavioral methodology for diagnosing affective disorders in individuals with mental retardation. *Hab Ment Heal News.* 1990;9:55–61.

97. Moss S, Goldberg DP, Simpson N, et al. Psychiatric assessment schedule, modified for use in adults with developmental disabilities (PAS-ADD) ICD-10 version. Hester Adrian Research Centre, University of Manchester; 1993.

98. Prosser H, Moss SC, Costello H, Simpson N, Patel P. *The Mini-PAS-ADD: A Preliminary Assessment Schedule for the Detection of Mental Health Needs in Adults with Learning Disabilities.* Manchester: Hester Adrian Research Centre; 1996.

99. Royal College of Psychiatrists. *DC-LD (Diagnostic Criteria for Psychiatric Disorders for Use with Adults with Learning Disabilities/Mental Retardation).* London: Gaskell Press; 2001.

100. Szymanski LS, King B, Goldberg B, et al. Diagnosis of mental disorders in people with mental retardation. In: Reiss S, Amann MG, eds. *Psychotropic Medications and Developmental Disabilities: The International Consensus Handbook.* Ohio: Ohio State University Nisonger Center; 1998:3–17.

101. Myers BA. Major depression in persons with moderate to profound mental retardation: clinical presentation and case illustrations. *Ment Health Aspect Dev Disabil.* 1998;3:57–68.

102. Tsiouris JA. Diagnosis of depression in people with severe/profound intellectual disability. *J Intellect Disabil Res.* 2001;45: 115–120.

103. Burt DB, Loveland KA, Lewis KR. Depression and the onset of dementia in adults with mental retardation. *Am J Ment Retard.* 1992;96:502–511.

104. Prasher VP. Age-specific prevalence, thyroid dysfunction and depressive symptomatology in adults with Down syndrome and dementia. *Inter J Geria Psychiatry.* 1995;10:25–31.

105. Burt DB. Dementia and depression. In: Janicki MP, Dalton AJ, eds. *Dementia, Aging and Intellectual Disabilities: A Handbook.* Philadelphia: Taylor & Francis; 1999:198–216.

106. Walters RM. Suicidal behavior in severely mentally handicapped patients. *Br J Psychiatry.* 1990;157:444–446.

107. Walters AS, Barrett RP. Suicidal behavior in children and adolescents with mental retardation. *Res Dev Disabil.* 1995;16:85–96.

108. Masi G, Favilla L, Mucci M. Generalized anxiety disorder in adolescents and young adults with mild mental retardation. *Psychiatry.* 2000;63:54–64.

109. Stavrakaki C, Mintsioulis G. Anxiety disorders in persons with mental retardation: diagnostic, clinical and treatment issues. *Psychiatric Ann.* 1997;27:182–189.

110. Ryan R. Posttraumatic stress disorder in persons with developmental disabilities. *Networker.* 1994;3:1–5.

111. Cherry KE, Matson JL, Paclawskyj TR. Psychopathology in older adults with severe and profound mental retardation. *Am J Ment Retard.* 1997;101:445–458.

112. Lund J. The prevalence of psychiatric morbidity in mentally retarded adults. *Acta Psychiat Scandinavia.* 1985;7:563–570.

113. Sovner R, Hurley AD. Do the mentally retarded suffer from affective illness? *Arch Gen Psychiatry.* 1983;40:61–67.

114. Craddock N, Owen M. Is there an inverse relationship between Down's syndrome and bipolar affective disorder? Literature review and genetic implications. *J Intellect Disabil Res.* 1994;38: 613–620.

115. Pary RJ, Loschen EL, Tomkowiak SB. Mood disorders and Down's syndrome. *Seminars in Clinical Neuropsychiatry.* 1996;1:148–153.

116. Reid AH. Psychoses in adult mental defectives: schizophrenic and paranoid psychoses. *Br J Psychiatry.* 1972;120:213–218.

117. Cherry K, Penn D, Matson J, Bamburg J. Characteristics of schizophrenia among persons with severe or profound mental retardation. *Psych Serv.* 2000;51:922–924.

118. Prasher VP. Psychotic features and effect of severity of learning disability on dementia in adults with Down syndrome. Review of literature. *Br J Dev Disabil.* 1997;43:85–92.

119. Patti P. Depression, dementia and Down syndrome. In: Sturmey P, ed. *Mood Disorders in People with Mental Retardation.* Kingston, NY: NADD Press, (in press).

120. Meadows G, Turner T, Campbell L, Lewis SW, Reveley MA, Murray RM. Assessing schizophrenia in patients with mental retardation: a comparative study. *Br J Psychiatry.* 1991;158: 103–105.

121. Glenn SM, Cunningham CC. Parents' reports of young people with Down syndrome talking out loud to themselves. *Ment Retard.* 2000;38:498–505.

122. McGuire D, Chicoine B, Greenbaum E. Self-talk in adults with Down syndrome. *Disabil Solutions.* 1997;2:1–4.

123. Wing L, Shah A. Catatonia in autistic spectrum disorder. *B J Psychiatry.* 2000;176:357–362.

124. Aylward EH, Burt DB, Thorpe LU, Lai F, Dalton AJ. Diagnosis of dementia in individuals with intellectual disability. *J Intellect Disabil Res.* 1997;41:152–164.

125. Janicki MP, Dalton AJ, eds. *Dementia, Aging and Intellectual Disabilities: A Handbook.* Philadelphia: Taylor & Francis; 1999.

126. Burt DB, Aylward EH. Test battery for the diagnosis of dementia in individuals with intellectual disability. *J Intellect Disabil Res.* 2000;44:175–180.

127. Percy MF, Dalton AJ, Markovic DV et al. Autoimmune thyroiditis associated with mild "subclinical" hypothyroidism in adults with Down syndrome: a comparison of patients with and without manifestations of Alzheimer disease. *Am J Med Genet.* 1990a; 36: 148–154.

128. Percy MF, Dalton AJ, Markovic DV et al. Red cell superoxide dismutase, glutathione peroxidase and catalase in Down syndrome patients with and without manifestations of Alzheimer disease. *Am J Med Genet.* 1990b;35:459–467.

129. Mehta PD, Dalton AJ, Mehta SP, Percy ME, Sersen EA, Wisniewski H. Immunoglobulin G subclasses in older persons with Down syndrome. *J Neuro Sci.* 1993;117:186–191.

130. Evenhuis HM. Associated medical aspects. In: Janicki MP, Dalton AJ, eds. *Dementia, Aging, and Intellectual Disabilities: A Handbook.* Philadelphia: Taylor & Francis,1998;103–118.

131. Haveman M, Maaskant MA, Sturmans F. Older Dutch residents of institutions, with and without Down's syndrome: comparison of mortality and morbidity trends and motor/social functioning. *Australia & New Zealand J Develop Disabil.* 1989;15: 241–255.

132. Holland AJ, Karlinsky H, Berg JM. Alzheimer disease in persons with Down syndrome: diagnostic and management considerations. In: Berg JM, Karlinsky H, Holland AJ, eds. *Alzheimer Disease, Down Syndrome and Their Relationship.* Oxford: Oxford Medical Publications; 1993:95–114.

133. Visser FE, Aldenkamp AP, van Huffelen AC, Kullman M, Overweg J, van Wijk J. Prospective study of the prevalence of Alzheimer-type dementia in institutionalized individuals with Down syndrome. *Am J Ment Retard.* 1997;101:400–412.

134. Lai F, Williams RS. A prospective study of Alzheimer disease in Down's syndrome. *Arch Neuro.* 1989;46:849–853.

135. Dalton AJ, Crapper-McLachlan DR. Clinical expression of Alzheimer's disease in Down syndrome. *Psych Clinics No Amer.* 1986;9:659–670.

136. Dalton AJ, Mehta PD, Fedor BL, Patti PJ. Cognitive changes in memory precede those in praxis in aging persons with Down syndrome. *J Intellect Disabil Res.* 1999;24:169–187.

137. Evenhuis HM. The natural history of dementia in Down's syndrome. *Arch Neuro.* 1990;47:263–267.

138. Holland AJ, Hon J, Huppert FA, Stevens F. Incidence and course of dementia in people with Down's syndrome: findings from a population-based study. *J Intellect Disabil Res.* 2000;44:138–146.

139. Dalton AJ, Fedor BL. Onset of dyspraxia in aging persons with Down syndrome: longitudinal studies. *J Intellect Develop Disabil.* 1998;23:13–24.

140. Prasher VP, Corbett JA. Onset of seizures as a poor indicator of longevity in people with Down syndrome and dementia. *Int J Geriatr Psychiatry.* 1993;8:923–927.

141. Tsiouris JA, Patti PJ, Tipu O, Raguthu S. Adverse effects of phenytoin given for late-onset seizures in adults with Down syndrome. *Neurology.* 2002;59:779–780.

142. Gedye A. *Dementia Scale for Down Syndrome (Manual).* Vancouver: Gedye Research and Consulting; 1995.

143. Evenhuis HM, Kengen MMF, Eurlings HAL. *Dementia Questionnaire for Mentally Retarded Persons.* Zwamerdam, the Netherlands: Hooge Burch Institute for Mentally Retarded People; 1990.

144. Dalton AJ, Fedor BL. The Multi-Dimensional Observation Scale for Elderly Subjects (MOSES) applied for persons with Down syndrome. In: *Proceedings of the International Congress III on the Dually Diagnosed.* Washington DC: National Association for the Dually Diagnosed. 1997:173–175.

145. Dalton AJ, McMurray K. *Dalton/McMurray Visual Memory Test.* Waterloo, Ontario: Bytecraft Ltd.; 1995.

146. Dalton AJ. Dementia in Down syndrome: methods of evaluation. In: Nadel L, Epstein CJ, eds. *Down Syndrome and Alzheimer Disease.* New York: Wiley-Liss; 1992:51–76.

147. Warren AC, Holroyd S, Folstein MF. Major depression in Down's syndrome. *Br J Psychiatry.* 1989;155:202–205.

148. Dowling S, Hollins S. Coping with bereavement: the dynamics of intervention. In: Davidson PW, Prasher VP, Janicki MP, eds. *Mental Health, Intellectual Disabilities, and the Aging Process.* London: Blackwell Publishing; 2003:166–178.

149. Oswin M. *Am I Allowed to Cry? A Study of Bereavement Amongst People Who Have Learning Disabilities.* London: Souvenir Press Ltd; 1991.

150. Botsford AL, Force LT. *End of Life Care: A Guide for Supporting Older People with Intellectual Disabilities and Their Families.* Albany, NY: NYSARC Inc.; 2000.

151. Ludlow BL. Life after loss: legal, ethical and practical issues. In: Herr SS, Weber G, eds. *Aging, Rights and Quality of Life: Prospects for Older People with Developmental Disabilities.* Baltimore: Paul H. Brookes Publishing Co.,1999;189–221.

152. Janicki MP, Dalton AJ. Alzheimer disease in a select population of older adults with mental retardation. *Irish J Psychol.* 1993;14:37–46.

153. Koenig BR. *Aged and Dementia Care Issues of People with Intellectual Disability: Literature Review and Survey of Carers.* Brighton, S.A.: MINDA Inc.; 1995.

154. Hammond B, Benedetti P. Perspectives of a care provider. In: Janicki MP, Dalton AJ, eds. *Dementia, Aging, and Intellectual Disabilities: A Handbook.* Philadelphia: Taylor & Francis,1998; 32–41.

155. Udell L. Supports in small group home settings. In: Janicki MP, Dalton AJ, eds. *Dementia, Aging, and Intellectual Disabilities: A Handbook.* Philadelphia: Taylor & Francis,1998;316–329.

156. Marler R, Cunningham C. *Down's Syndrome and Alzheimer's Disease.* London: Down's Syndrome Association; 1994.

157. The Arc. *Developmental Disabilities and Alzheimer's Disease: What You Should Know.* Arlington, Tx: Author; 1995.

158. Janicki MP, Heller T, Seltzer GB, Hogg J. Practice guidelines for the clinical assessment and care management of Alzheimer's disease among adults with intellectual disability. *J Intellect Disabil Res.* 1996;40:374–382.

159. Tsiouris JA. Psychotropic medications. In: Janicki MP, Dalton AJ, eds. *Dementia, Aging, and Intellectual Disabilities: A Handbook.* Philadelphia: Taylor & Francis,1998;232–253.

160. Barron J, Sandman CA. Paradoxical excitement to sedative-hypnotic drugs in mentally retarded clients. *Am J Ment Defici.* 1985;90:124–129.

161. Cooper S-A, Collacott RA. Prognosis of depression in Down's syndrome. *J Nerv Ment Dis.* 1993;181:204–205.

162. Storm W. Differential diagnosis and treatment of depressive features in Down's syndrome: a case illustration. *Res Dev Disabil.* 1990;11:131–137.

163. Thorpe L. Psychiatric disorders. In: Janicki MP, Dalton AJ, eds. *Dementia, Aging and Intellectual Disabilities: A Handbook.* Philadelphia: Taylor & Francis; 1999:217–231.

164. Howland RH. Fluoxetine treatment of depression in mentally retarded adults. *J Nerv Ment Disease.* 1992;180:202–205.

165. McGuire DE, Chicoine BA. Depressive disorders in adults with Down syndrome. *Hab Ment Heal News.* 1996;15.

166. Bhaumik S, Branford D, Naik BI, Biswas AB. A retrospective audit of selective serotonin re-uptake inhibitors (fluoxetine and paroxetine) for the treatment of depressive episodes in adults with learning disabilities. *Br J Dev Disabil.* 2000;46:131–139.

167. Intagliata J, Rinck C. Psychoactive drug use in public and community facilities for mentally retarded persons. *Psychopharm Bulletin.* 1985;21:268–278.

168. Lipman RS, DiMascio A, Reatig N, Kirson T. Psychotropic drugs and mentally retarded children. In: Lipton MA, DiMascio A, Killam KF, eds. *Psychopharmacology: A Generation of Progress.* New York: Raven Press; 1978:1437–1439.

169. Corrigan PW, Yudofsky SC, Silver JM. Pharmacological and behavioral treatments for aggressive psychiatric inpatients. *Hosp Commu Psych.* 1993;44:125–133.

170. Cain NN, Davidson PW, Burhan AM, et al. Identifying bipolar disorders in individuals with intellectual disability. *J Intellect Disabil Res.* 2003;47:31–38.

171. Gualtieri CT, Schroeder SR. Tardive dyskinesia in young mentally retarded individuals. *Arch Gen Psychiatry.* 1986;43: 333–340.

172. Prasher VP, Huxley A, Haque MS, Down Syndrome Ageing Study Group. A 24-week, double-blind, placebo-controlled trial of donepezil in patients with Down syndrome and Alzheimer's disease—pilot study. *Int J Geriatr Psychiatry.* 2002; 17:270–278.

173. Hemingway-Eltomey JM, Lerner AJ. Adverse effects of donepezil in treating Alzheimer's disease associated with Down's syndrome. *Am J Psychiatry.* 1999;156:1470.

174. Lott IT, Osann K, Doran E, Nelson L. Down syndrome and Alzheimer diseasse: response to donepezil. *Arch Neurol.* 2002; 59:1133–1136.

175. Dalton AJ, Sano MC, Aisen PS, Andrews HF, Tsai W-Y. Design and implementation of a multicenter trial of vitamin E in aging individuals with Down syndrome. *J Intel Dis Res.* 2004; 48:428.

176. Reid AH, Ballinger BR. Personality disorder in mental handicap. *Psychological Medicine.* 1987;17:983–987.

177. Deb S, Hunter D. Psychopathology in mentally handicapped patients with epilepsy. III: Personality Disorders. *Br J Psychiatry.* 1991;159:830–834.

178. Khan A, Cowan C, Roy A. Personality disorders in people with learning disabilities: a community study. *J Intellect Disabil Res.* 1997;41:324–330.

179. Holburn CS. Aerophagia. In Konarski EA, Favell JE, Favell J, eds. *Manual for the Assessment and Treatment of the Behavior Disorders of People with Mental Retardation.* Morganton, NC: Western Carolina Center Foundation; 1997:BD14, 1–7.

180. Tsiouris JA, Adelman SA. Guidelines and General Information on the Use of Psychotropic and Antiepileptic Drugs for Individuals with Developmental Disabilities. Staten Island, NY; New York State Institute for Basic Research in Developmental Disabilities; 1997.

181. Sutton E, ed. A Resource Guide for the Training of Specialists in Developmental Disabilities and Aging (Revised). Akron, OH: Rehabilitation Research Training Consortium on Aging and Mental Retardation; 1993.

Associated Psychiatric
Issues

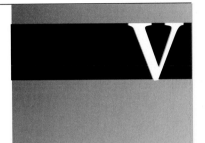

Psychosis and Agitation Associated with Dementia

37

Ashok J. Bharucha   *Bruce G. Pollock*

Psychosis and agitation associated with dementia is prevalent and persistent, and contributes significantly to patient and caregiver suffering, accelerated functional and cognitive decline, and premature institutionalization (1–3). While psychosis often leads to agitation, the latter entity encompasses a much broader range of behavioral disturbances, and the heterogeneity of both has inspired various empirical classification approaches in recent years aimed at subtyping of relatively homogenous symptom clusters (4,5). The paramount importance of this effort lies in the fact that a refined behavioral taxonomy would not only advance basic and clinical research, but also the ability to seek treatment indications from the Food and Drug Administration (FDA) for specific neuropsychiatric syndromes associated with dementia, as exemplified by the development of diagnostic criteria for the psychosis of Alzheimer's disease (AD) (6). This chapter reviews separately the epidemiology, phenomenology, and clinical correlates of the two constructs—psychosis of dementia and agitation—given the heterogeneity of the syndromes. Thereafter, an assessment and treatment approach that is broadly applicable to both and consistent with clinical practice is described, incorporating evidence-based treatment recommendations from the extant literature.

EPIDEMIOLOGY OF PSYCHOSIS IN DEMENTIA

Methodologically rigorous studies using data collected largely from clinical samples report a 30% to 50% frequency of psychotic symptoms in AD (7–9). A range from 10% to 80% is reported, however, when all studies, including those with small sample sizes, varying definitions of dementia and individual psychotic symptoms, and use of different assessment instruments are included (6,10). In addition, a cumulative 51% 4-year incidence of new-onset psychotic symptoms of AD has recently been reported (11). Once present, the psychotic symptoms of dementia often persist over several years until the advanced stages of dementia, when the individual may no longer be able to articulate his or her inner experience (12,13).

Population-based samples also note high prevalence of psychotic symptoms in those with dementia. The first such study of psychosis in AD reported the prevalence of delusions to be 16%, with another 20% of subjects experiencing paranoid ideation that did not reach the level of delusions (14). Visual and auditory hallucinations were present in 13% and 10% of the subjects, respectively. In addition, 30% of the subjects experienced misidentification syndromes. More recently, the Cache County Study of Memory in Aging (CCSMA) reported the prevalence of delusions to be 23% for those with AD and 8% for those with vascular dementia (VaD) (15). Hallucinations were present in 13% of subjects with either type of dementia. Taken together, the high prevalence of psychosis in both population-based and clinical samples of people with dementia, and its strong association with aggression and agitation, highlights the scope and clinical importance of the problem (1,2,16).

PHENOMENOLOGY OF PSYCHOSIS IN DEMENTIA

Delusions, hallucinations and, to a lesser extent, misidentification syndromes constitute the most frequently observed psychotic symptoms associated with dementia. In fact, the diagnostic criteria for psychosis of Alzheimer's disease that were articulated by a consensus conference of experts require only the presence of either delusions *or* hallucinations for the diagnosis of a psychotic syndrome (Table 37-1) (6). These criteria have been criticized, however, for their lack of an empirical basis, and neglect of significant co-occurrence and interrelationships with other neuropsychiatric symptoms of dementia (5). To address these shortcomings, Lyketsos et al. subjected the neuropsychiatric symptoms data from their CCSMA cohort to latent class analysis (5). The authors identified three classes of people with AD based on their neuropsychiatric symptom profiles: unaffected or minimally symptomatic, predominantly affective, and predominantly psychotic. Further analysis of the data revealed hallucinations to be predictive of membership in the psychosis group irrespective of the presence or absence of delusions, while patients with delusions were present in all three groups (17). Similarly, Cook et al. (4) have recently identified two subtypes of psychosis in AD—those with either misidentification/hallucinations or those with persecutory delusions—in their exploratory factor and cluster analysis of Consortium to Establish a Registry for Alzheimer's Disease—Behavioral Rating Scale data collected in an AD research center (18). The findings from the above studies refute the notion of psychosis of AD as a unitary syndrome, and lend clinical credence to studies that posit distinct genetic, neuropathological, and postmortem neurochemical findings between AD patients with psychosis compared to those without psychosis (19,20).

Delusions, defined as fixed false beliefs that are not attributable to membership in a social or cultural group,

---

TABLE 37-1

DIAGNOSTIC CRITERIA FOR PSYCHOSIS OF ALZHEIMER'S DISEASE

1. Characteristic symptoms
Presence of one (or more) of the following symptoms:
   Visual or auditory hallucinations
   Delusions

2. Primary diagnosis
All the criteria for dementia of the Alzheimer type are met.

3. Chronology of the onset of symptoms of psychosis versus onset of symptoms of dementia
There is evidence from the history that the symptoms in criterion 1 have not been present continuously since prior to the onset of the symptoms of dementia.

4. Duration and severity
The symptom(s) in criterion 1 have been present, at least intermittently, for 1 month or longer.
Symptoms are severe enough to cause some disruption in patients' and/or others' functioning.

5. Exclusion of schizophrenia and related psychotic disorders
Criteria for schizophrenia, schizoaffective disorder, delusional disorder, or mood disorder with psychotic features have never been met.

6. Relationship to delirium
The disturbance does not occur exclusively during the course of a delirium.

7. Exclusion of other causes of psychotic symptoms
The disturbance is not better accounted for by another general medical condition or direct physiological effects of a substance (e.g., a drug of abuse, a medication).
Associated features (specify if associated):
   With agitation: when there is evidence, from history or examination, of prominent agitation with or without physical or verbal aggression
   With negative symptoms: when prominent negative symptoms, such as apathy, affective flattening, avolition, or motor retardation are present
   With depression: when prominent depressive symptoms, such as depressed mood, insomnia or hypersomnia, feelings of worthlessness or excessive or inappropriate guilt, or recurrent thoughts of death are present

Adapted from Reference 6.

affect 16% to 70% (median 36.5%) of people with AD, according to a review of 35 studies (17). In the only population-based study of the incidence of delusions and hallucinations in AD, 28% of the sample experienced new-onset delusions over 18 months (21). Unlike the delusions of schizophrenia, those of people with dementia tend to be simple, nonbizarre, and often reflective of their misinterpretation of the environment. Among delusional AD patients, the delusion of stealing is most prevalent, followed by persecutory delusions, delusions of reference, infidelity, grandiosity, and occasionally somatic delusions (17). While uncommon in both the very early and late stages of AD, once present, the delusions of AD tend to recur and persist over time (12,13). No consistent association has been reported between the stage and duration of illness or sociodemographic variables such as age, race, gender, or education level (17). In contrast, there is strong evidence linking more severe cognitive impairment with delusions in AD (3,22).

Hallucinations, defined as false sensory perceptions, affect 4% to 76% (median 23%) of people with AD (17). The CCSMA study has recently reported an incidence of hallucinations of 16% over 18 months (21). When present, visual (range 4–59%; median 19%) and auditory (range 1–29%, median 12%) hallucinations are far more prevalent than tactile, olfactory, or somatic hallucinations (17). Unlike delusions, which appear to be more common in the moderate stages of the illness and are consistently associated with greater cognitive impairment, hallucinations are thought to be rare in the early stages of AD, but may be more common in the later stages of AD (23). Like delusions, no consistent association has been found between hallucinations and sociodemographic variables; however, isolated hallucinosis of AD appears to be more common amongst African Americans (17,24).

Misidentification phenomena have been poorly studied as a separate construct in AD. Nonetheless, a prevalence of 23% to 50% has been reported in two studies that have examined these phenomena (25,26). The most common presentations involve the failure to recognize one's home ("this is not my home" phenomenon), belief that strangers are living in the house (phantom boarder syndrome), or that loved ones are impostors (Capgras phenomenon) (10). Misidentification phenomena are difficult to distinguish from delusions, hallucinations, illusions, or visual agnosia, and remain poorly examined in the dementia literature.

The clinical phenomenology and natural course of psychotic symptoms in AD described so far represent a syndrome that is clearly distinct from schizophrenia in elderly patients, as summarized in Table 37-2 (6). Antipsychotic treatment of psychosis of AD is characterized by considerably lower doses, shorter durations of treatment, and greater vulnerability to extrapyramidal symptoms than in elderly patients with schizophrenia (27,28). In addition to these clinical observations, converging evidence from neurobiological, neuropathological, and genetic studies also strongly supports the notion of psychosis of AD being an entity distinct from schizophrenia in elderly patients (19,29,30).

TABLE 37-2

COMPARISON OF PSYCHOSIS OF ALZHEIMER'S DISEASE WITH SCHIZOPHRENIA IN ELDERLY PATIENTS

	Psychosis in AD	Schizophrenia
Incidence	30–50%	Less than 1%
Bizarre or complex delusions	Rare	Frequent
Misidentification of caregivers	Frequent	Rare
Common form of hallucinations	Visual	Auditory
Schneiderian first-rank symptoms	Rare	Frequent
Active suicidal ideation	Rare	Frequent
Past history of psychosis	Rare	Very common
Eventual remission of psychosis	Frequent	Uncommon
Need for many years of maintenance on antipsychotics	Uncommon	Very common
Average optimal daily dose of an antipsychotic	15–25% of that in a young adult with schizophrenia	40–60% of that in a young adult with schizophrenia

AD, Alzheimer's disease.
Adapted from Reference 6.

AGITATION OF DEMENTIA: EPIDEMIOLOGY AND PHENOMENOLOGY

Agitation is most commonly defined as "inappropriate verbal, vocal, or motoric activity that is not judged by an outside observer to result directly from the needs or confusion of the agitated individual" (31). Those who question the ability of an outside observer to judge the causality of agitation have proposed an alternative definition: "behavior that is disruptive, unsafe or interferes with care in a given environment" (32). *Problem behaviors* and *disruptive behaviors* are other terms commonly used to refer to agitation in clinical settings. With the growing emphasis on measuring behavior (and not cognition alone) as an efficacy outcome in dementia treatment studies, the International Psychogeriatric Association began to address these nosological challenges in its 1st International Consensus Conference on Behavioral Disturbances of Dementia in 1996 (33). An immediate outcome of this conference was the adoption of an equally nonspecific term—behavioral and psychological symptoms of dementia (BPSD)—to describe "a heterogeneous range of psychological reactions, psychiatric symptoms, and behaviors occurring in people with dementia of any etiology" (33). In the absence of empirical data regarding specific symptom clusters that demonstrate differential treatment response, however, the FDA declined to offer a therapeutic claim for the BPSD entity (34). In this regard, the recent articulation of specific diagnostic criteria for both psychosis of AD and depression of AD represents a step forward, though these criteria await empirical validation as well (6,35).

As many as 90% of people with dementia experience agitation at some point during the course of the illness (36). The wide prevalence range of agitation as a global category, and the specific behaviors it encompasses, reflects differences in the populations and settings sampled, varying inclusion criteria pertaining to dementia, disparate definitions of the particular behaviors and symptoms, and differences in the assessment and rating instruments used. To date, the CCSMA is the only population-based epidemiological study of dementia in the United States to estimate the point-prevalence of dementia-associated mental and behavioral disturbances (15). According to the CCSMA, 61% of participants with dementia exhibited one or more mental or behavioral disturbances in the past month as measured by the Neuropsychiatric Inventory (NPI) (37). Apathy (27%), depression (24%), and agitation/aggression (24%) were the most common symptoms, affecting those with dementia four times more frequently than those without dementia. The prevalence of mental or behavioral disturbances varied only modestly by type of dementia or severity of illness. More recently, the CCSMA has reported a 69% incidence rate for one or more mental or behavioral symptoms over an 18-month follow-up (21). Delusions were

the most common (28%), followed by apathy (21%) and aberrant motor behavior (21%).

As demonstrated by the FDA's reluctance to grant a therapeutic claim for the BPSD entity, there is a pressing clinical and research need to subtype agitation into distinct syndromes that demonstrate differential treatment response. While a number of factor analytical studies have been performed using rating instruments designed to measure disruptive behaviors, the domains identified by Cohen-Mansfield and Billig from the Cohen-Mansfield Agitation Inventory (CMAI) have particular clinical utility, because the behaviors described are directly observable (31). According to their analysis, agitated behaviors can be classified into one of the following categories: aggressive behaviors, physically nonaggressive behaviors, and verbal/vocal agitated behaviors.

Aggressive behaviors include hitting, biting, kicking, spitting, pushing, grabbing, scratching, tearing things, hurting self or others, and physical sexual advances. Correlates of aggressive behaviors include male gender, severe cognitive impairment, premorbid aggressive personality, psychosis, and the perception that others are intruding into one's personal space (16,38–41). Although the relationship between physical health and aggressive behavior is unclear, those with greater neurological brain damage may demonstrate more severe behavioral dyscontrol (39,42).

Physically nonaggressive behaviors identified by the CMAI include hiding objects, hoarding objects, general restlessness, intentional falling, pacing, aimless wandering, trying to get to a different place, handling things inappropriately, eating inappropriate substances, inappropriate dressing and disrobing, and performing repetitious mannerisms. People with dementia who manifest physically nonaggressive behaviors tend to have fewer medical conditions and may have been more active throughout their lives (42,43). In addition, individuals with dementia may be particularly prone to develop akathisia as a result of the underlying neurodegenerative condition or treatment with psychoactive agents, particularly antipsychotics.

Verbal and vocal agitated behaviors tend to occur most frequently, and include repetitive sentences or questions, unwarranted requests for attention or help, complaining, negativism, making strange noises, screaming, verbal sexual advances, and cursing and verbal aggression. Correlates of verbally agitated behaviors include female gender, poor health, pain, and depression (42).

BIOLOGICAL BASES OF PSYCHOSIS AND AGITATION OF DEMENTIA

Neurochemical Evidence

The cholinergic hypothesis of AD posits deficits in cholinergic neurotransmission to be central to the cognitive and functional impairment of the disease. It is now well recognized that the cholinergic deficits also contribute to the emergence of neuropsychiatric symptoms. Indirect evidence includes the following:

- Anticholinergic agents produce neuropsychiatric symptoms that are similar to those of AD.
- Anticholinergic medications exacerbate the neuropsychiatric symptoms of AD.
- Cholinergic agents reduce these symptoms to varying extents, as demonstrated most recently by acetylcholinesterase inhibitors (AChEI) (44).

In contrast to psychoses associated with schizophrenia, neurochemical investigations of AD consistently point to widespread dopaminergic deficits (45). These age and/or Alzheimer's-associated reductions in nigrostriatal D2 receptors and dopamine almost certainly contribute to increased adverse effects found when dopamine antagonists are given to older patients. Even in the absence of D2 antagonists, extrapyramidal symptoms are not uncommon in AD, particularly as it progresses (46). This suggests that loss of dopaminergic function in patients with dementia also renders them more prone to extrapyramidal effects of antipsychotic medication than older patients with other psychiatric illness (47).

Considerable evidence has associated serotonergic deficits with aggressive and impulse-control disorders (48). In AD, cell loss frequently occurs in the dorsal raphe nucleus, causing loss of serotonergic (5-HT) innervation to the forebrain (49). Interestingly, 5-HT2 cortical neurons have been found to be relatively preserved in AD patients who were assessed, *antemortem*, to be free of aggressive symptoms (50). Biochemical data have accumulated suggesting serotonergic deficits in AD contribute to aggressive verbal and physical outbursts, sleep disturbance, depression, and psychosis (51). Citalopram has been shown to dramatically increase concentrations of cerebrospinal fluid serotonin in AD patients (52). Serotonergic modulation may also influence psychoses through inhibition of dopamine production or release. Serotonergic projections from the raphe nuclei to the midbrain and basal ganglia can inhibit dopamine neurons, thus decreasing dopamine availability at their terminals by a 5-HT2-mediated synaptic mechanism (53).

Chronic deficits in presynaptic serotonergic function could also lead to postsynaptic up-regulation of 5-HT2 receptors. AD patients have been found to have marked neuroendocrine responses to acute serotonergic challenges, suggesting a relative hyperreactivity in postsynaptic 5-HT2 receptors (54). The degree of this reactivity appears to be more marked in agitated as opposed to nonagitated AD patients (55), and is correlated with response to sertraline treatment (51).

Neuroimaging Evidence

A relationship between agitation and frontal and temporal lobe hypometabolism has been demonstrated, and is consistent with neuroanatomic areas that experience the greatest cholinergic deficits in AD (19). Neuroimaging findings concerning psychosis of dementia are more heterogeneous. AD patients with paranoid delusions have hypoperfusion in the left dorsolateral prefrontal and medial temporal cortex, while AD patients with hallucinations have additional hypoperfusion in the right parietal cortex (56). AD patients with psychosis also have lower perfusion in the right and left dorsolateral frontal, left anterior cingulate, left dorsolateral parietal, left ventral striatal, and left pulvinar regions as documented by single positron emission computerized tomography (57).

Neuropathological Evidence

Tekin et al. have examined the postmortem neuropathological correlates of agitation, controlling for other neuropsychiatric symptoms with a subgroup analysis (58). The authors found significantly higher neurofibrillary tangle counts in the left and right orbitofrontal and left anterior cingulate regions, while no such relationship was established with senile plaque burden. Moreover, increased muscarinic M2 receptor density has been demonstrated in the orbitofrontal cortex in AD patients with psychosis (59). The same group found higher M2 receptor density in the midtemporal cortex of AD patients with hallucinations.

Genetic Evidence

Holmes et al. report subjects with late-onset AD and the DRD1 B1/B2 dopamine receptor genotype to be more likely to present with aggressive behavior or hallucinations than those with the B1/B1 genotype (60). Those with the DRD3 2/2 allele experienced delusions at significantly lesser frequency than those with the DRD3 1/1 genotype. Such association between neurotransmitter receptor gene polymorphism and neuropsychiatric symptoms has also been demonstrated with the serotonin transporter. Sukonick et al. conducted a case-control study comparing 58 AD subjects exhibiting aggressive behavior with 79 nonaggressive AD subjects, and found that those who expressed the L/L (long) genotype for the serotonin transporter promoter region were more likely to be aggressive (61). The same relationship held with greater L allele frequency.

AGITATION: ASSESSMENT AND MEASUREMENT CHALLENGES

Agitation is the leading trigger for psychiatric consultation in nursing homes (62). Yet in the absence of objective, psychometrically sound assessment and measurement methodologies, the clinician is left to rely on disparate, often conflicting cross-sectional observations of events that triggered the consultation. Common patient-related factors that impede the evaluation process include:

- Perceptual deficits such as hearing and visual loss
- Cognitive deficits that impair communication and recall of event(s) in question

- Aggressive behavior that limits the examination
- Large intraindividual and interindividual variability in the frequency and expression of agitated behaviors
- Low frequency (but often high impact) of behavioral disturbances by an individual as measured over time (63)

Clinical staff-related impediments include:

- Inadequate training in the assessment and documentation of behavioral problems
- Poor staff: patient ratios
- Therapeutic nihilism about agitated behaviors
- Other clinical duties that are seen as priorities (e.g., toileting)
- Stress and burnout
- Negative personal reactions that interfere with objectivity

The assessment challenge is particularly paramount in institutional settings with frequent staff and administrative turnovers.

ASSESSMENT OF PSYCHOSIS AND AGITATION

A well-informed assessment of agitation and psychosis necessitates a systematic team approach that begins with collection of history from multiple informants, review of the medical record, direct patient interview, and focused physical, neurological, and mental status examinations. The assessment can be pursued from two classical approaches described in the literature. The first approach, labeled the *ABCs* of dementia management, posits *Antecedents* that trigger the *Behavior* in question, leading to *Consequences* that positively or negatively reinforce the disruptive behavior. The problematic behavior is characterized in detail based on whether it is verbal or physical, and whether it is aggressive or nonaggressive. The frequency, severity, timing, location, level of disruptiveness, and the people involved are also taken into consideration. Most importantly, the key question is whether the behavior is truly disruptive, unsafe, or interfering with the provision of care, or simply repetitive and annoying.

The process of characterizing behavioral disturbances of dementia can be greatly enhanced by the use of a psychopathology rating instrument that has established psychometric properties for the target population and is sensitive to clinical changes over time. A plethora of rating scales designed to characterize neuropsychiatric symptoms of dementia have emerged in recent years (more than 52 between 1985 and 1994 alone). They differ in the choice of respondent, time period of assessment, whether they measure frequency and/or severity, and psychometric performance characteristics (64). Table 37-3 provides an overview of the symptom domains covered by some of the more commonly used psychopathology rating instru-

ments, and their unique advantages/disadvantages or specific applications. These instruments assist in identifying not only more homogeneous cluster(s) of symptoms that may be differentially responsive to specific interventions, but also in monitoring response to those interventions over time.

Once the behavior has been characterized, antecedents to the behavior are sought. The antecedent may be principally medical (e.g., urinary tract infection, pain), environmental (e.g., noise, ambient temperature), psychiatric (e.g., new onset delusions), social (e.g., recent housing relocation), or related to the caregiver's approach to the patient (e.g., impatience in providing intimate care, not paying attention to the patient's affective responses). More commonly, however, a number of factors are simultaneously at play and a temporal relationship is difficult to establish, particularly in institutional settings where knowledgeable informants are scarce.

Not uncommonly, the consequences of the disruptive behavior itself reinforce its propagation. For example, inconsistent limit setting with respect to smoking privileges off a dementia unit often leads to escalating demands for more smoking visits off the unit. Hence, caregiver education and training pertaining to behavioral disturbances of dementia is critical in minimizing inadvertent reinforcement of problematic behaviors. Equally important is the identification of life-long habits, personality traits, unusual life experiences, and characteristic patterns of coping that may contribute to problem behaviors.

An alternative assessment approach uses the strategy of identifying stimuli that are thought to contribute to the disruptive behavior(s). The use of the term "stimulus" avoids the temporal connotation of an antecedent–a timeline that is characteristically difficult to establish in the assessment process. According to this model, behaviors are simply responses to stimuli that may be internal (e.g., depression, paranoia, boredom) or external (e.g., noise, poor lighting). Internal stimuli generally fall into one of three domains: medical, psychiatric, or cognitive. External stimuli are most often the result of environmental factors or caregiver approach. The following case examples and Table 37-4 exemplify these concepts in greater depth.

CASE EXAMPLE

COGNITIVE IMPAIRMENT AND AGITATION

Mrs. S, an 80-year-old retired teacher with no pre-existing cognitive deficits, is admitted to a skilled nursing facility after a large left cerebral hemisphere cerebrovascular accident that has resulted in frontal lobe damage and nonfluent aphasia. She characteristically strikes out at caregivers only during intimate care. When her husband is questioned about these events, he notes that the aides

TABLE 37-3
COMMONLY USED DEMENTIA BEHAVIORAL RATING INSTRUMENTS

Scale	Dimensions	Reference Period	Respondent	Population Studied	Advantages
Cohen-Mansfield Agitation Inventory (99)	29 items: • Physical aggression • Physically nonaggressive behaviors • Verbal aggression • Verbally nonaggressive behaviors	Past 2 weeks	Caregiver/nursing home staff interview by trained rater	• Nursing home patients • Community-dwelling elders	• Established construct validity and interrater reliability • Sensitive to change over time in clinical trials
Neuropsychiatric Inventory (37)	12 items: • Delusions • Hallucinations • Agitation/aggression • Depression/dysphoria • Anxiety • Elation/euphoria • Apathy/indifference • Irritability • Nighttime behaviors • Disinhibition • Aberrant motor behavior • Appetite/eating behaviors	Variable	Caregiver interview by trained rater	Older adults with dementia	• Sensitive to change in randomized clinical trials • Follow-up questions within a category are only asked if the response to the screening question is positive, thus reducing time of administration • Demonstrates ability to discriminate among dementia types
Behavioral Pathology in Alzheimer Disease Rating Scale (100)	25 items: • Paranoid delusions • Hallucinations • Activity disturbance • Aggressiveness • Affective disturbance • Anxiety/phobias • Diurnal disturbances • Global rating scale	Past 2 weeks	Caregiver interview by trained rater	• Nursing home patients • Community-dwelling elders	• Internal consistency • Content validity • Sensitive to change over time in clinical trials
Dementia Behavior Disturbance Scale (101)	28 items, 6 factors: • Passivity • Agitation • Eating disturbance • Aggressiveness • Diurnal disturbance • Sexual misdemeanor	Past week	Caregiver interview or self-report	Community-dwelling elders with dementia	• Does not address depression, anxiety, delusions, hallucinations, or apathy

(continued)

TABLE 37-3 (continued)

Scale	Dimensions	Reference Period	Respondent	Population Studied	Advantages
Pittsburgh Agitation Scale (102)	4 factors: ■ Aberrant vocalization ■ Motor agitation ■ Aggressiveness ■ Resisting care	Past 1–8 hours	Observations by clinical staff or family	■ Inpatient geriatric psychiatry unit ■ Nursing home patients	■ Requires no formal training ■ Positive association with OBRA regs guidelines for antipsychotics ■ Takes less than a minute to complete ■ 17-item version under development
CERAD-BRSD (18)	51 items, 8 factors: ■ Depressive features ■ Psychotic features ■ Defective self-regulation ■ Irritability/agitation ■ Vegetative features ■ Apathy ■ Aggression ■ Affective lability	Past month	Patient and caregiver interview by trained rater	303 patients and caregivers in 16 medical centers	
Neurobehavioral Rating Scale (103)	28 items, 6 factors: ■ Cognition/insight ■ Agitation/disinhibition ■ Behavioral retardation ■ Anxiety/depression ■ Verbal output disturbance ■ Psychosis	Trained rater observes behavior during the interview	Patient interview by trained rater	Alzheimer's and vascular dementia patients	■ Sensitive to change over time in clinical trials

CERAD-BRSD, Consortium to Establish a Registry for Alzheimer's Disease—Behavioral Rating Scale for Dementia; OBRA, Omnibus Budget Reconciliation Act
Adapted from Reference 119.

are quite hurried and impatient and do not allow his wife to verbalize her wishes, which frustrates her. This is an example of a situation where conflicting staff needs (e.g., to get the patient's care done quickly) and the resident's cognitive limitations (aphasia and the resultant inability to refuse care verbally) lead to aggression.

CASE EXAMPLE

MEDICAL CONDITION(S) AND AGITATION

Mrs. J is a 94-year-old widowed resident in an assisted-living facility. She had been free of psychiatric symptoms, but approximately 3 months ago she began to report severe anxiety and was observed incessantly pacing on the unit. Her primary care physician prescribed an antidepressant that did not relieve the symptoms. A psychiatric consultation was ordered. The psychiatrist noted during his visit that Mrs. J was exceptionally distressed, and that her pattern of cognitive and psychiatric deficits did not fall into any clear syndromic pattern. Although the primary care physician was reluctant to admit the resident to a geropsychiatry unit because of her age and his personal ideology (e.g., *what will we do differently even if we find an organic cause at her age?*), Mrs. J was hospitalized after a discussion with her daughter. A magnetic resonance image of her brain revealed a small left frontal lobe tumor. A short-acting benzodiazepine was prescribed, which relieved the anxiety. More importantly, the inpatient evaluation helped the daughter understand and accept her mother's distressing behavior, and prepare for future care needs.

CASE EXAMPLE

PSYCHIATRIC DISORDER(S) AND AGITATION

Mr. M is an 85-year-old gentleman who was admitted to a dementia care unit with functional and cognitive decline consistent with AD. A psychiatric consultation was ordered to address Mr. M's combativeness during daily showers. Upon speaking with Mr. M's wife, it was learned that he was a Holocaust survivor and had often experienced flashbacks, both before and after being diagnosed with dementia. Mrs. M surmised that the showers were increasingly reminding her husband of the Nazi gas chambers. Discontinuing showers in favor of sponge baths eliminated the aggression.

CASE EXAMPLE

ENVIRONMENTAL FACTOR(S) AND AGITATION

Mrs. W, a 90-year-old resident of a dementia unit, suffers from Lewy body dementia. In the past few months she has become increasingly aggressive during meal times. She is disinhibited and will throw food and objects onto staff and other residents. An astute nursing aide who had spoken to Mrs. W's sister made the observation that Mrs. W was a very solitary person who valued her time alone, and preferred one-on-one interactions over group activities. Based on this account, Mrs. W now has supervised meals in her room, with complete resolution of the aggression.

CASE EXAMPLE

CAREGIVER APPROACH AND AGITATION

Mr. T is an 80-year-old gentleman who was admitted to a dementia unit by his depressed and guilt-ridden wife. She had been very conflicted about admitting him to the unit because her daughters did not feel their father was disabled enough to warrant placement. The daughters lived at a distance and had no firsthand knowledge of their father's care needs. In an effort to cope with her depression and guilt, Mrs. T tried to take her husband home for short visits, where he would become bewildered and verbally aggressive. A psychiatric consultation was ordered to comment on whether Mr. T really benefited from going on visits with his wife. After individual and joint meetings with the couple, recommendations were made for Mrs. T to be in supportive psychotherapy. The therapy helped relieve Mrs. T's depression and guilt, and educated Mrs. T and her daughters about the nature and extent of Mr. T's cognitive deficits. With this intervention, the family was able to set reasonable expectations for Mr. T's capabilities, which led to their organizing activities with him on the unit rather than taking him off the unit for short visits.

Table 37-4 provides an outline of contributory factors that are broadly applicable to both psychosis and agitation associated with dementia, and should be thoroughly investigated. For a more complete differential diagnosis, please refer to the chapter on delirium in this textbook.

Internal stimuli, especially those suggesting the presence of acute medical problems such as pain and other causes of delirium, must be addressed first since they can signal a life-threatening emergency. The acuity of onset of the agitation should also lower the threshold for a more urgent, thorough medical evaluation. Other internal stimuli, such as psychosis and depression, especially when accompanied by physical aggression, merit comprehensive assessment and treatment. Inpatient psychiatric evaluation should be promptly sought for individuals who are suicidal, physically aggressive, or demonstrate notable decline in functioning. External stimuli, such as caregiver approach and environmental distractions, should be explored in all cases, and should be considered as contributory factors even in the presence of clear-cut internal stimuli. A form of agitation that can be called *bewilderment* results when the environmental conditions or demands can no longer be comprehended due to cognitive decline. Behaviors of bewilderment can result from both internal and external stimuli; thus, treatment should likely involve manipulations to reduce the environmental demands on the patient, as well as pharmacotherapy in the form of a cognitive enhancer, which may promote greater awareness.

TABLE 37-4

INTERNAL AND EXTERNAL STIMULI IN THE ASSESSMENT OF AGITATION

INTERNAL STIMULI	Medical status	▪ Delirium ▪ Infection ▪ Pain
	Psychiatric status	▪ Psychosis ▪ Depression ▪ Anxiety/phobias ▪ Pre-existing personality disorder
	Cognition/ bewilderment	▪ Memory impairment ▪ Aphasia ▪ Agnosia ▪ Apraxia ▪ Executive dysfunction
EXTERNAL STIMULI	Environmental factors	▪ Lighting ▪ Noise ▪ Ambient temperature ▪ Lack of structure ▪ Boredom ▪ Loneliness, social isolation ▪ Excessive stimulation ▪ Understimulation
	Caregiver approach	▪ Insufficiently educated about dementia? ▪ Confrontational or argumentative? ▪ Demanding? ▪ Minimizing/denying patient's deficits? ▪ Unrealistic expectations? ▪ Intrudes patient's space? ▪ Ineffectively coping with own grief? Depression? ▪ Also cognitively impaired?

TREATMENT OF PSYCHOSIS AND AGITATION ASSOCIATED WITH DEMENTIA: NONPHARMACOLOGICAL INTERVENTIONS

Nonpharmacological interventions designed to curb agitation are based on a combination of the following theoretical considerations:

▪ Addressing unmet physical, emotional, and psychosocial needs
▪ Application of behavior modification principles
▪ Accommodation of reduced stress tolerance as a result of cognitive and physical decline (65)

To date, over 80 nonpharmacological intervention studies have been conducted in people with dementia, including sensory interventions such as music therapy (23 studies), real or simulated social contact (nine studies), behavior therapy (16 studies), staff training (six studies), activities (seven studies), environmental modification (six

studies), medical/nursing interventions (12 studies), and combination therapies (five studies) (65). The vast majority (>75%) of these studies were conducted in residential facilities with methodological limitations that are discussed in the next section.

Efficacy of Nonpharmacological Interventions

Defining efficacy in terms of change from baseline to the intervention condition, a majority of studies report at least modest improvement (>91% of studies), with some reporting significant benefits. The findings must be interpreted, however, in light of the severe methodological limitations, which include:

▪ Sample size less than 25 in over 60% of the studies
▪ Lack of control group or condition
▪ Diverse screening, assessment, and treatment protocols precluding direct comparisons among studies
▪ Inclusion of subjects who were on psychoactive medications or had failed trials of pharmacological interventions
▪ Measurement of agitation as a global entity (i.e., no subclassification according to specific behaviors)
▪ Failure to take the cost and implementability of such interventions into account (65)

These limitations notwithstanding, the Omnibus Budget Reconciliation Act of 1987 mandates nonpharmacological treatment(s) for agitated behaviors in skilled nursing facilities prior to resorting to pharmacotherapy (66). More importantly, nonpharmacological interventions avoid the significant medical morbidities often associated with psychoactive medications, whose modest efficacy is accompanied by potentially detrimental adverse effects such as excessive sedation, falls, drug-drug interactions, and metabolic dysregulation.

TREATMENT OF PSYCHOSIS AND AGITATION ASSOCIATED WITH DEMENTIA: PHARMACOLOGICAL INTERVENTIONS

Pharmacological interventions are extensively used in a variety of clinical settings to manage psychosis and agitation associated with dementia; however, the evidence base is quite limited. In a systematic review of pharmacological treatment, Kindermann et al. identified 48 studies that met their inclusion criteria (67). These included:

▪ Age ≥60 years
▪ Diagnosis of dementia
▪ Behavioral or psychotic disturbance of dementia as the study's primary focus
▪ Sample size >10
▪ Exclusion of dementias related to movement disorders

These studies suffered from many of the methodological limitations previously cited for nonpharmacological intervention studies. For example, 19 (40%) of the studies contained fewer than 30 subjects, 12 (25%) had a treatment duration of less than 6 weeks, one-third did not include a control or comparator group, and more than 20 different instruments were employed to assess treatment effectiveness, not to mention heterogeneity in the definition(s) of response and data analysis strategies. Moreover, as few as one in 10 geriatric subjects approached actually participate in pharmacological intervention trials (68). The recruitment challenges posed by these studies limit the generalizability of efficacy and safety findings to real-world clinical settings.

Table 37-5 summarizes all randomized, double-blind, placebo-controlled trials of psychoactive agents that have been conducted specifically to treat psychosis or agitation in patients with dementia. Pooling the results of these trials, Kindermann et al. report a mean (standard deviation in brackets) improvement rate of 61% (18%) for typical and atypical antipsychotics combined, compared with 35% (20%) for placebo (67). The improvement rate with atypical antipsychotics appears to be slightly higher 72% (24%), while the placebo response rate remains the same.

Although antipsychotics are the most frequently prescribed psychoactive agents to manage psychosis and agitation associated with dementia, converging evidence from neuropathological and neurochemical studies points to relative preservation of dopaminergic neurotransmission, and more profound dysregulation of serotonin neurotransmission in the etiopathogenesis of psychotic and agitated behaviors of AD (51). Based on this premise, Pollock et al. conducted a 17-day pilot study to examine the comparative efficacy, safety, and tolerability of citalopram, perphenazine, and placebo in the acute treatment of psychosis and behavioral disturbances in 85 hospitalized patients with AD who were not depressed (69). Citalopram significantly lowered the total Neurobehavioral Rating Scale score, as well as the agitation/aggression and tension/lability factors compared with placebo. The efficacy of citalopram was highlighted by an effect size of 0.64 compared with 0.36 for perphenazine, though there were no differences in side-effect burden on either medication. A 12-week study is currently in progress that examines the comparative efficacy, safety, and tolerability of citalopram, compared with the atypical antipsychotic risperidone (Pollock et al., personal communication). In addition, the National Institute of Mental Health has sponsored a multicenter 36-week study of the effectiveness of antipsychotics (CATIE: Clinical Antipsychotic Trials of Intervention Effectiveness) that is currently in progress, and which also employs citalopram as a second-line agent (70).

Treatment Recommendations: General Principles of Pharmacotherapy

The most critical step in determining appropriate treatment is the identification of specific causative factors as outlined in the assessment section. Nonpharmacological interventions should always be explored and implemented, even when pharmacotherapy is unavoidable due to the patient's imminent dangerousness to self or others. As with all psychiatric conditions, the choice of a specific psychoactive agent is dictated largely by the adverse event profile and tolerability, rather than efficacy when it is similar for all agents within a particular therapeutic class. The importance of identifying specific target symptoms is particularly salient in the treatment of agitation, since pharmacological treatment of nonspecific behaviors that are annoying, but not truly disruptive, is likely to expose the patient to unwarranted treatment risks and cause frustration for the caregivers. Once a decision to initiate pharmacotherapy has been made, the oft-cited geriatric adage *start low, go slow* should be heeded. The risks of treatment must always be weighed and frequently reassessed in the context of the evolving clinical scenario, and appropriately discussed with the patient and/or their substitute decision-maker.

Figure 37-1 outlines a management approach that targets various clusters of neuropsychiatric symptoms labeled as agitation. Although these first-line recommendations are intended to integrate and reflect findings from the limited evidence base, it should be borne in mind that deviations from such a scheme are often necessary to optimize treatment response in specific individuals. A null or partial response to one agent within a therapeutic class does not rule out the possibility of response to another agent within that class. Moreover, certain individuals will require adult doses of psychoactive medications, even though a prudent course would dictate initiation of therapy at low dosages. The guiding principle should always be clear identification of specific target symptoms, and vigilant weighing of therapeutic response with potential toxicities. For more information, see the chapter on pharmacotherapy in this textbook. Dosing strategies for recommended pharmacologic agents are summarized in Table 37-6.

Atypical Antipsychotics: Efficacy

Antipsychotics are the most commonly prescribed psychotropic agents to manage agitation, aggression, and psychosis associated with dementia, in spite of the fact that they have not been approved by the FDA for these treatment indications.

Risperidone

To date, three large-scale studies of risperidone have been conducted that merit discussion (Table 37-5). Katz et al. assigned 625 long-term care facility patients (mean age = 82.7 years) with dementia and behavioral disturbance to placebo or 0.5, 1.0, or 2.0 mg/day of risperidone in a randomized, double-blind fashion for 12 weeks (71). Defining response as a ≥50% reduction in Behavioral Pathology in Alzheimer's Disease Rating Scale (BEHAVE-AD) score, the primary outcome measure, the authors

TABLE 37-5

PUBLISHED RANDOMIZED, DOUBLE-BLIND, PLACEBO-CONTROLLED TRIALS FOR PSYCHOSIS OR AGITATION IN PATIENTS WITH DEMENTIA

Study	Medication	Sample Size	Drop-Out Rate (%)[a]	Trial Duration (weeks)	Treatment Target	Primary Outcome Measures	Subjects Improved (%)	Primary Adverse Effects[b]
Haloperidol								
Sugarman et al. (104)	Haloperidol	18	NR	6	Chronic brain syndrome; psychosis, agitation	Psychiatric symptom checklist	89%	Akathisia, sedation
Petrie et al. (105)	Haloperidol vs. Loxapine	64	42	10	Dementia; psychosis, agitation	CGI, BPRS, SCAG, NOSIE	65% 58%	Sedation, EPS, hypotension
Devanand et al. (106)	Haloperidol	19	0	6–8	Dementia; psychosis, aggression	Change from baseline BPRS score	NA	EPS
Auchus and Bissey-Black (107)	Haloperidol vs. Fluoxetine	15	20	6	Dementia; agitation	Mean change in CMAI, BEHAVE-AD, CSI	NR	EPS with haloperidol
Devanand et al. (108)	Haloperidol	60	15	6	AD (DSM-III-R); psychosis, aggression, agitation	Mean change in BPRS total, aggression and agitation	NA	EPS
Teri et al. (109)	Haloperidol vs. Trazodone vs. Behavior management	149	39	16	AD (NINCDS-ADRDA) agitation	ADCS-CGIC Secondary measures: CERAD-BRSD, RMBPC, CMAI, ABID	34% of subjects improved compared to baseline; no differences between treatment arms	Haloperidol: parkinsonism and sedation Trazodone: dizziness, sedation, dry mouth
Other Conventional Antipsychotics								
Barnes et al. (110)	Thioridazine	60	43	8	Dementia; behavioral disturbance	CGI	59%	Sedation, EPS, hypotension
Rada and Kellner (111)	Thiothixene	63	11	4	Organic brain syndrome	CGI, BPRS, NOSIE	59%	Sedation, EPS
Finkel et al. (112)	Thiothixene	30	9	11	Dementia; agitation	CMAI	69%	Sedation
Stotsky (113)	Thioridazine vs. Diazepam	610	NR	4	Elderly nonpsychotic patients with emotional and behavioral disorders	HARS, NOSIE	Thioridazine significantly superior global improvement compared to placebo and diazepam	Tremors, drowsiness
Atypical Antipsychotics								
De Deyn et al. (72)	Risperidone vs. Haloperidol	344	35	13	Dementia (DSM-IV); agitation, aggression	Mean change in CMAI, BEHAVE-AD	NA NA	EPS with both drugs

Study	Drug	N	Dropout	Duration	Outcome measures	Results	Adverse events
Katz et al. (71)	Risperidone	625	30	12	50% change in BEHAVE-AD; mean change in CMAI verbal and physical aggression	1 mg: 45% 2 mg: 50%	EPS, sedation, peripheral edema
Street et al. (75)	Olanzapine	206	NR	6	50% change in NPI-NH; mean change in BPRS, CGI	5 mg: 65% 10 mg: 57% 15 mg: 43%	Sedation, abnormal gait
Brodaty et al. (73)	Risperidone	345	27	12	Mean change in CMAI total aggression score; BEHAVE-AD, CGI-S, CGI-C	NA; risperidone significantly superior to placebo in reducing aggression	Sedation, urinary tract infection, EPS
De Deyn et al. (76)	Olanzapine (several fixed doses)	652	25–34%[c]	10	Mean change in NPI-NH Psychosis Total scores, change in CGI-C scores	Olanzapine 7.5 mg/day was superior to placebo on NPI-NH; Olanzapine 2.5 mg/day superior to placebo on CGI-C	Weight gain, anorexia, urinary incontinence, abnormal behavior (none statistically greater than placebo)
Fontaine et al. (85)	Olanzapine vs. Risperidone (no placebo group)	39	15%	2	Mean change in NPI and CGI	Both treatments produced significant reductions in NPI and CGI scores, but no differences between the drugs	Drowsiness and falls; increase in EPS from baseline (not statistically significant)
Meehan et al. (90)	Olanzapine IM vs. lorazepam IM	272	6–11%[c]	24 hours	Change from baseline in PANSS-EC and ACES	At 2 hours post-injection, olanzapine and lorazepam superior to placebo on both measures; at 24 hours, only olanzapine superior to placebo on PANSS-EC	Adverse events not significantly different from placebo

(continued)

TABLE 37-5 (continued)

Study	Medication	Sample Size	Drop-Out Rate (%)[a]	Duration (weeks)	Treatment Target	Primary Outcome Measures	Subjects Improved (%)	Primary Adverse Effects[b]
Selective Serotonin Re-uptake Inhibitors								
Nyth and Gottfries (114)	Citalopram; combined double-blind and open technique	98	38	16 (8 double-blind, 8 open)	AD, (DSM-III), VaD	GBS	Citalopram-treated AD patients showed significant improvement from baseline in confusion, irritability, anxiety, fear panic, depressed mood, and restlessness Only irritability and depressed mood significantly improved compared to placebo; no changes in VaD group	Orthostasis, sexual dysfunction, concentration difficulties, emotional indifference
Olafsson et al. (115)	Fluvoxamine	46	37	6	AD (DSM-III) or VaD	GBS; picture recall and recognition, trail-making test, finger-tapping	Fluvoxamine did not improve cognitive or behavioral functioning; trends favoring fluvoxamine over placebo on confusion, irritability, fear-panic, mood, restlessness	Nausea
Pollock et al. (69)	Citalopram vs. Perphenazine	85	54	17 days	Dementia; psychosis, behavioral disturbances	Mean change in NBRS total score, and agitation/aggression, psychosis, lability/tension factor scores	NA; Citalopram effect size 0.64; Perphenazine effect size 0.36	No change on either medication in UKU Side Effect Rating Scale

Lanctot et al. (116)	Sertraline (double-blind, placebo-controlled cross-over study)	22	4.5	4 weeks each on sertraline and placebo	AD; (DSM-IV, NINCDS-ADRA), behavior problems	Responder = decrease of ≥4 points on NPI total score	8 (38%) completers responded to sertraline; significant improvement on agitation/aggression, irritability, and aberrant motor behavior. Trend for decreased aggression with sertraline versus placebo (p = 0.08)	Decreased memory, flattened affect, sedation, tremor
Anticonvulsants								
Tariot et al. (117)	Carbamazepine (research team blind except for physician-monitor and pharmacist)	51	7.8	6	AD (DSM-III-R, NINCDS-ADRDA), VaD, mixed dementia; agitation, aggression	BPRS, CGI	Significantly greater reductions on BPRS total score with active drug; CGI global improvement of 77% active drug vs. 21% placebo	Ataxia, disorientation and tic (one patient)
Olin et al. (118)	Carbamazepine	21	24	6	AD (NINCDS-ADRDA); behavioral symptoms	CGI-C, BPRS total score	Significant improvement on BPRS total score	Diarrhea, vomiting
Porsteinsson et al. (93)	Divalproex sodium	56	11	6	Dementia; agitation	BPRS (modified)	Significant improvement in BPRS agitation factor score	Sedation, nausea, vomiting, diarrhea

[a]Combined drop-out rate from all treatment arms.
[b]Adverse events on primary study medication.
[c]Discontinuation rates differed depending upon dosage of the active treatment.
ABID, Agitated Behavior Inventory for Dementia; ACES, Agitation-Calmness Evaluation Scale; AD, Alzheimer's disease; ADCS-CGIC, Alzheimer Disease Cooperative Study Clinical Global Impression of Change; BEHAVE-AD, Behavioral Pathology in Alzheimer's Disease Rating Scale; BPRS, Brief Psychiatric Rating Scale; CERAD-BRSD, Consortium to Establish a Registry for Alzheimer's Disease—Behavioral Rating Scale for Dementia; CGI, Clinical Global Impression; CGI-C, Clinical Global Impression—Change; CGI-S, Clinical Global Impression—Severity of illness; CMAI, Cohen-Mansfield Agitation Inventory; CSI, Caregiver Stress Inventory; DSM (III, III-R, IV), Diagnostic and Statistical Manual of Mental Disorders (3rd Edition, 3rd Edition Revised, 4th Edition); EPS, extrapyramidal symptoms; GBS, Gottfries-Brane-Steen scale; HARS, Hamilton Anxiety Rating Scale; IM, intramuscular; NA, not applicable; NBRS, Neurobehavioral Rating Scale; NINCDS-ADRDA, National Institute of Neurological and Communicative Disorders and Stroke and Alzheimer's Disease and Related Disorders Association; NOSIE, Nurse's Observation Scale for Inpatient Examination; NPI, Neuropsychiatric Inventory; NPI-NH, Neuropsychiatric Inventory—Nursing Home version; NR, not reported; PANSS-EC, Positive and Negative Symptom Scale—Excited Component; RMBPC, Revised Memory and Behavior Problem Checklist; SCAG, Sandoz Clinical Assessment—Geriatric; UKU, Udvalg for Kliniske Undersogelser; VaD, vascular dementia.
Adapted from Reference 67.

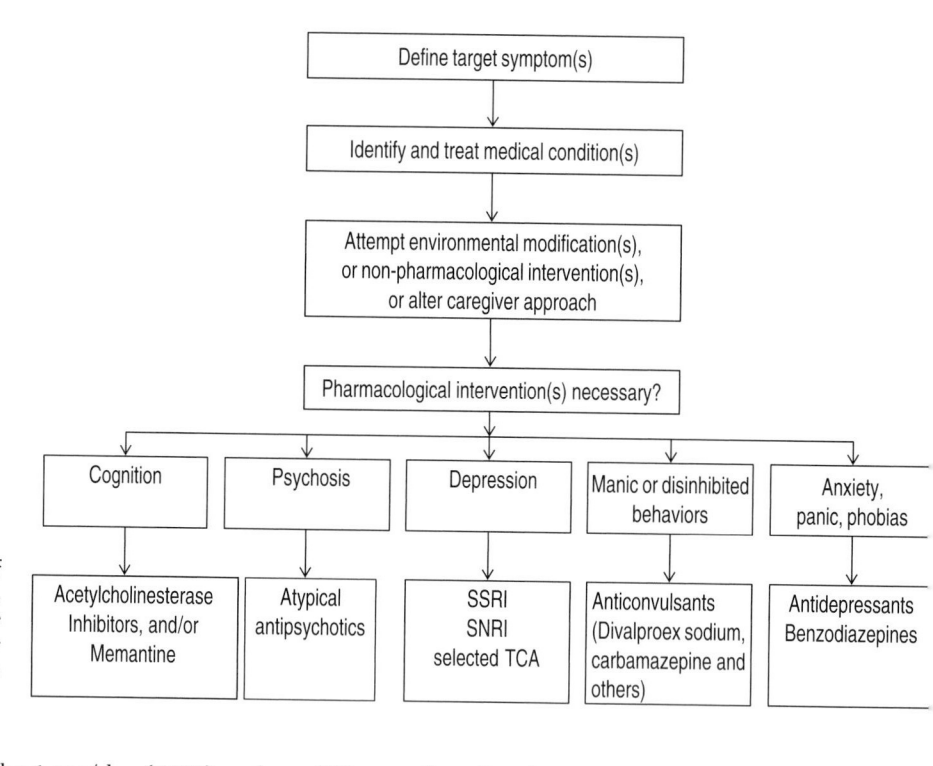

Figure 37-1 Management of agitation and psychosis. SSRI, selective serotonin reuptake inhibitor; SNRI; serotonin-norepinephrine reuptake inhibitor; TCA, tricyclic antidepressant.

found higher response rates in the 1 mg/day (45%) and 2 mg/day (50%) risperidone groups versus the placebo group (33%; p = .02 and .002, respectively). Also, all three risperidone groups produced significant reductions in the aggressiveness subscale of the BEHAVE-AD; separating from placebo as early as week 2. Moreover, the reduction of aggressiveness was not associated with a decrease in psychosis or sedative effects of the medication. Although 30.4% of patients had dropped out of the study, there was no significant difference between the placebo and active treatment groups.

De Deyn and colleagues assigned 334 institutionalized patients (median age = 81 years) with dementia and behavioral disturbance to risperidone (mean dose 1.1 mg/ day), haloperidol (mean dose 1.2 mg/day), or placebo in their 12-week randomized, double-blind study (72). Response rate, defined as a ≥30% reduction in the BEHAVE-AD total score, was not statistically significant amongst the three groups at week 12 or endpoint. However, there was a significant reduction in total BEHAVE-AD score (and the aggressiveness subscale) when comparing risperidone to placebo (p = .05). Furthermore, *post hoc* analysis found risperidone to be superior to haloperidol in decreasing the scores on the BEHAVE-AD aggressiveness (p = .05) and CMAI total (p = .02), as well as verbal aggressiveness (p = .01) scales. The primary reason for patient discontinuation in this study (35.2%) was lack of efficacy, with no significant differences in discontinuation rates amongst the three groups.

Brodaty et al. assigned 345 nursing home patients (mean age = 83 years) with aggression, agitation, or psychosis of dementia to risperidone (mean dose = 0.95 mg/ day) or placebo in their 12-week randomized, double-blind trial (73). The primary endpoint of the study—the

difference from baseline to endpoint in CMAI total aggression score—was significantly superior for the risperidone group versus placebo (p < .001). The authors also reported significant reductions in the CMAI total nonaggression subscale (p < .002), BEHAVE-AD total (p < .001), and psychosis subscale (p = .004) scores. This study is particularly notable for its emphasis on aggressive behaviors, since demonstration of such symptom specificity is critical to seeking the FDA's indication for neuropsychiatric symptom clusters observed in patients with dementia.

Olanzapine

Satterlee et al. conducted a placebo-controlled, flexible-dose study of olanzapine in 238 outpatients with dementia complicated by agitation or psychosis, with the primary aim of characterizing tolerability relative to dose (74). At endpoint, olanzapine therapy did not demonstrate greater efficacy relative to placebo; however, the finding was likely related to suboptimal dosing (mean dose = 2.7 mg/day).

Building on the findings from the Satterlee et al. study, Street and colleagues assigned 206 nursing home patients (mean age = 82.8 years) with AD and behavioral disturbances to 5, 10, or 15 mg/day of olanzapine or placebo under randomized, double-blind conditions (75). Primary response was defined as ≥50% decrease in the Neuropsychiatric Inventory—Nursing Home version (NPI-NH) core total psychosis and agitation/aggression subscale score. The 5 mg/day and 10 mg/day olanzapine groups produced significantly greater reductions than placebo in the primary outcome measure (p < .001 and p = .006, respectively). Interestingly, the 15 mg/day olanzapine group did not separate from placebo, demonstrating a curvilinear dose-response relationship with this antipsychotic. Significant reductions were also noted in a measure of caregiver distress in the 5 mg/day olanzapine group (p = .008). Treatment effects were unrelated to increase in somnolence, and completion rates were similar in all four treatment arms.

Finally, De Deyn et al. published their findings from a 10-week double-blind study of fixed dose olanzapine (1.0, 2.5, 5.0, 7.5 mg/day) versus placebo in 652 AD patients with psychotic symptoms (mean age = 76.6 years), irrespective of the presence of behavioral disturbances, residing in long-term care settings (76). The NPI-NH Psychosis Total scores (sum of delusions and hallucinations items—primary efficacy measure) declined significantly from baseline in all five treatment groups, but no pairwise treatment differences were noted at the 10-week endpoint. The olanzapine 7.5 mg/day dose appeared to produce the greatest improvement relative to placebo on the NPI-NH Psychosis Total scores, while olanzapine 2.5 mg/day produced the greatest improvement on the Clinical Global Impression–Change (CGI-C) scores. Of considerable significance, each dose of olanzapine resulted in significantly reduced scores on the agitation/aggression item of the NPI-NH, compared to placebo. Olanzapine treatment was well-tolerated, with no adverse events occurring with an incidence greater than 8% in any group. Although the incidence of increased weight, anorexia, and urinary incontinence was higher among individual olanzapine treatment groups, there were no significant pairwise differences versus placebo.

Quetiapine

Considerably less data are available regarding the efficacy and safety of the atypical antipsychotics quetiapine, ziprasidone, and aripiprazole in patients with dementia complicated by psychosis or behavioral disturbances. Tariot et al. conducted an open-label, 52-week study of quetiapine (dose range 12.5–800 mg/day) in 184 patients (mean age = 76 years) with various psychotic disorders to preliminarily estimate efficacy, safety, dosing, and titration (77). The authors noted significant declines from baseline in the mean Brief Psychiatric Rating Scale (BPRS) total score and mean Clinical Global Impression–Severity of Illness score by week 2, which were then maintained throughout the study period. However, only 48% of the patients completed the study. Analysis of a subset of 78 patients with AD from this mixed psychotic disorders population revealed significant, sustained reductions in symptoms of psychosis and hostility throughout the 52-week study period.

Tariot and colleagues have conducted a 10-week, double-blind, placebo-controlled study of flexibly dosed quetiapine or haloperidol in 378 nursing home residents with various psychotic disorders (78). Quetiapine demonstrated significant improvements in the BPRS agitation factor (p < 0.05), anergia factor (p < .01), and improved functional status as measured by the Physical Self-Maintenance Scale (p = 0.004) and the Multidimensional Observation Scale for Elderly

Subjects (p < 0.001) compared with haloperidol or placebo in the subset of patients with AD (N = 284). No difference was seen, however, on measures of psychosis across the three treatment groups.

Finally, Zhong et al. have reported the findings from their 10-week randomized, double-blind trial of fixed dose quetiapine for the treatment of agitation in elderly institutionalized patients with mixed dementia diagnoses (79). A total of 333 patients (mean age = 83, mean baseline Mini-Mental State Examination (MMSE) = 6) were randomized in 3:3:2 allocation to quetiapine 200 mg/day (N = 117), 100 mg/day (N = 124), and placebo (N = 92). A total of 219 patients (66%) completed the 10-week study, with no differences in completion rates across the three treatment arms. Defining response as the percentage of patients with at least a 40% reduction in the Positive and Negative Syndrome Scale–Excited Component (PANSS-EC) score (primary outcome measure) and Clinical Global Impression–Change (CGI-C) rating of *much improved* or *very much improved* as a secondary outcome measure, a significantly higher proportion of patients in the quetiapine 200 mg/day group achieved response (42%) compared to those in the placebo group (27%, p < 0.05). The decline in PANSS-EC and CGI-C scores for those receiving quetiapine 100 mg/day did not reach statistical significance compared with placebo. Aside from greater somnolence/sedation, quetiapine's adverse events profile was similar to that of placebo.

Ziprasidone

Ziprasidone is an atypical antipsychotic that exhibits antagonism of D2, 5HT2a, 5HT2c, and 5HT1d receptors while functioning as an agonist at the 5HT1a receptor. Ziprasidone inhibits re-uptake of serotonin and norepinephrine with moderate affinity for the H1 receptor and negligible antimuscarinic effects. In a multiple-dose (8 days of treatment) study involving 32 subjects, there was no difference in pharmacokinetics of ziprasidone between men and women or between elderly (>65 years) and young (18–45 years) subjects (80). Population pharmacokinetic evaluation of patients in controlled trials has revealed no evidence of clinically significant age or gender-related differences in the pharmacokinetics of ziprasidone. Dosage modifications are therefore not recommended by the manufacturer. Ziprasidone intramuscular has not been systematically evaluated in elderly patients (≥65 years).

To our knowledge, only one study has examined the efficacy of ziprasidone for psychosis associated with dementia. Berkowitz examined 62 elderly patients with various diagnoses involving mood and behavior disturbance as a result of major depression, bipolar disorder, schizoaffective disorder, AD, and VaD (81). Retrospective analysis of the charts of 10 randomly chosen patients revealed significant declines in the mean Neuropsychiatric Inventory (NPI) scores (from 76 to 33), with no cases of prolonged QTc interval, postural hypotension, or syncope. The most common side effect was sedation.

Aripiprazole

Aripiprazole is thought to exhibit a unique mechanism of action, namely D2 partial agonism. It also has moderate affinity for H1 and α1 receptors. Three posters have described the use of aripiprazole in patients with AD: De Deyn et al. conducted a 10-week, placebo-controlled study of 208 outpatients with AD (mean age = 81.5 years, baseline MMSE ≥ 14, NPI score ≥ 6) flexibly dosed with 2 to 15 mg/day of aripiprazole for the treatment of psychosis (82). There was no statistically significant difference at endpoint on the NPI-Psychosis score between aripiprazole (mean dose = 10 mg/day) and placebo. However, significant improvement was noted on the BPRS psychosis subscore (secondary outcome measure) compared with placebo. The adverse events profile was similarly benign in both groups, with somnolence being more common in the aripiprazole group.

Breder and colleagues randomized 487 institutionalized patients (mean age = 82.5 years, mean baseline MMSE = 12) with psychotic symptoms associated with AD to treatment with fixed doses of aripiprazole (2, 5, or 10 mg/day) or placebo for 10 weeks (83). Fifty-eight percent of the subjects completed 10 weeks of double-blind therapy. Efficacy measures included the NPI-NH Psychosis subscale (primary variable) and Total score, BPRS, Clinical Global Impression (CGI), and CMAI score. Aripiprazole-treated patients (10 mg/day) showed significant improvement relative to placebo in the NPI-NH Psychosis subscale at endpoint (p = 0.013). Aripiprazole (10 mg/day) also showed significant improvements at endpoint in the NPI Psychosis response rate (65% versus 50%, p = 0.019), changes in CGI severity (−0.72 versus −0.46, p = 0.031), and BPRS total score (−7.12 versus −4.17, p = 0.030). Both 5 mg/day and 10 mg/day doses of aripiprazole were efficacious for reduction of nonspecific agitation as measured by the CMAI. The occurrence of adverse events was comparable between aripiprazole and placebo.

Finally, Streim et al. randomized 256 institutionalized patients (mean age = 83, mean baseline MMSE = 13) with psychosis of AD to placebo or flexible dose of aripiprazole (range 2–15 mg/day) for 10 weeks (84). The authors observed significant improvement in aripiprazole-treated patients (mean dose = 8.6 mg/day) compared with placebo in NPI-NH Total scores (−16.4 versus −10.0, p = 0.009) and BPRS total (−7.7 versus −5.1, p = 0.031) scores. However, aripiprazole-treated patients did not separate from placebo according to the NPI-NH Psychosis subscore, which was the primary outcome measure. Significant improvements in agitation and mood symptoms were observed using the CMAI, Cornell Depression Scale and CGI improvement scores. Aside from somnolence, which was more common in the aripiprazole group (14% versus 4% with placebo), the adverse event profiles were similarly benign for both groups.

Comparative Studies of Atypical Antipsychotics

Fontaine et al. conducted a double-blind parallel study involving 39 extended care facility residents with DSM-IV dementia diagnoses and acute behavioral disturbances (mean age = 83 years, mean MMSE = 8) (85). Olanzapine (N = 20) or risperidone (N = 19) dosing was titrated over 14 days starting with olanzapine 2.5 mg/day ranging to 10 mg/day, and risperidone 0.5 to 2.0 mg/day. At mean doses for olanzapine of 6.65 mg/day and risperidone of 1.47 mg/day, significant reductions were observed on the primary outcome measures, CGI, and NPI scores (p < 0.0001). The most frequent adverse events were drowsiness and falls (risperidone one patient, olanzapine two patients), with mild increase in extrapyramidal symptoms (EPS) over baseline.

Results from the CATIE trials are pending. This 36-week National Institute of Mental Health-sponsored study compares placebo, risperidone, olanzapine, and quetiapine as treatments for patients with AD complicated by delusions, hallucinations, and/or agitation (70).

Intramuscular Preparations of Atypical Antipsychotics

Intramuscular atypical antipsychotics have an important role to play in the management of both acute behavioral emergencies and maintenance treatment of psychosis and agitation. The lower incidence of EPS and tardive dyskinesia, as well as lower relapse rates of schizophrenics treated with atypical antipsychotics, suggests these agents would be better tolerated by cognitively impaired elders with psychosis or agitation than the intramuscular preparations of typical antipsychotics (86). Not uncommonly, a patient's noncompliance with oral antipsychotics will necessitate an intramuscular injection for acute (olanzapine IM) or maintenance (Risperdal Consta) treatment.

Depot Risperidone

Risperdal Consta is a depot formulation consisting of an aqueous suspension of microencapsulated risperidone. Degradation at the injection site results in release of risperidone over several weeks. After intramuscular gluteal injection, there is a small initial release of the drug (<1% of the dose), followed by a lag time of 3 weeks. The main release of the drug starts from 3 weeks onward, is maintained from 4 to 6 weeks, and subsides by 7 weeks following the intramuscular injection. Therefore, oral antipsychotic supplementation should be given during the first 3 weeks of treatment with Risperdal Consta to maintain therapeutic levels. Steady-state plasma concentrations are reached after four injections and are maintained for 4 to 6 weeks after the last injection. Plasma concentrations of risperidone, 9-hydroxyrisperidone (the major metabolite), and both combined are linear over the dosing range of 25 mg to 50 mg.

Gharabawi et al. have examined the use of long-acting risperidone in stable elderly patients with psychotic disorders (mean age = 71 years) (87). Patients received long-acting risperidone 25 mg (N = 24), 50 mg (N = 17), or 75 mg (N = 2) for a period up to 50 weeks. Forty-nine percent of patients demonstrated a ≥20% improvement in total PANSS, and 54.5% improved according to the CGI ratings (88). The most common adverse events were insomnia (10.5%), constipation (10.5%), and bronchitis (12.3%). No cases of tardive dyskinesia were identified by research criteria after up to 50 weeks of treatment (89).

Olanzapine Intramuscular

Intramuscular olanzapine (Zyprexa IntraMuscular) results in rapid absorption with peak plasma concentrations occurring within 15 to 45 minutes. Based upon pharmacokinetic study in healthy volunteers, a 5 mg dose of intramuscular olanzapine produces, on average, a maximum plasma concentration approximately five times higher than that produced by a 5 mg dose of oral olanzapine. The half-life observed after intramuscular injection is similar to that observed after oral dosing (21–54 hours, mean 30 hours). The pharmacokinetics are linear over the clinical dosing range. Metabolic profiles after intramuscular administration are qualitatively similar to the metabolic profiles after oral administration.

Meehan et al. have investigated the efficacy and safety of rapid-acting intramuscular olanzapine in treating agitation associated with AD and/or VaD (90). Two hundred and seventy-two subjects (mean age = 77.6 years, mean MMSE score = 11.8) were randomized to olanzapine 2.5 mg, olanzapine 5.0 mg, lorazepam 1.0 mg, or placebo. At 2 hours, all three active treatments produced significant improvement over placebo on the PANSS-EC and Agitation-Calmness Evaluation Scale (ACES). Olanzapine 5.0 mg and lorazepam were also superior to placebo on the CMAI. At 24 hours, only olanzapine (2.5 mg or 5.0 mg) was superior to placebo. Treatment-emergent adverse events were not significantly different from placebo in any active treatment group.

Ziprasidone Intramuscular

Intramuscular ziprasidone attains peak exposure within approximately 30 minutes, exposure is dose-related, and there is negligible drug accumulation with multiple dose administration. However, ziprasidone intramuscular has not been systematically evaluated in elderly patients (>65 years), and the risk of prolonging the QTc interval should be carefully weighed in this frail population.

Atypical Antipsychotics: Safety and Tolerability

Pooling the data from the three large-scale risperidone trials, the most common side effects were peripheral edema and dose-dependent changes in somnolence and extrapyramidal symptoms. Specifically, the rate of parkinsonism and hypokinesia was significantly higher in the 2 mg/day

risperidone group compared with placebo (p < .001). No significant difference has been found when lower doses of risperidone have been used. In addition, there were no significant changes in vital signs, electrocardiogram (ECG), or laboratory measures. While Brodaty et al. reported serious cerebrovascular events in six patients receiving risperidone, all had pre-existing risk factors such as hypertension, atrial fibrillation, or diabetes mellitus (73).

Olanzapine did not separate from placebo in producing EPS in the Street and colleagues study at any dosage (75). However, dose-dependent differences were found in somnolence and abnormal gait compared with placebo. In addition, peripheral anticholinergic side effects were more common with olanzapine 15 mg/day than with placebo (p = .008). No changes in vital signs, laboratory measures, or ECG were apparent in any treatment arm.

In summary, the atypical antipsychotics risperidone and olanzapine do demonstrate modest efficacy for treatment of behavioral and psychotic disturbances of dementia, and they do so with significantly improved side-effect profiles compared with the conventional antipsychotics, particularly in terms of reduced anticholinergic and extrapyramidal side effects. The incidence of the most concerning adverse event, development of tardive dyskinesia, is thought to be reduced by a factor of 10 or more with these two atypical antipsychotics (91). Additional large-scale, randomized, controlled trials of quetiapine, aripiprazole, and ziprasidone are needed in this population to make more meaningful treatment recommendations for each agent.

Non-Antipsychotic Pharmacotherapy of Agitation

Considerably less is known about nonantipsychotic pharmacotherapy of agitation associated with dementia, and whether psychotic symptoms of dementia would respond to such therapies. In the absence of data, the use of these agents (anticonvulsants, antidepressants, anxiolytics, sedative/hypnotics) has been guided largely by well-characterized syndromes (e.g., mania, depression, etc.) in nondemented adult patients. Hence, anticonvulsants are often utilized for behavioral symptoms and disinhibition of dementia that resemble mania (in the absence of psychosis), while antidepressants target depressive symptoms (hopelessness, worthlessness, guilty ruminations, etc.) that contribute to behavioral disturbances. Although the Pollock et al. study suggests a role for citalopram in the management of agitation in nondepressed patients with dementia, the results should be considered preliminary pending further larger scale investigations (69). Table 37-5 summarizes the limited data regarding nonantipsychotic pharmacotherapy of agitation of dementia. Dosing strategies are presented in Table 37-6.

Acetylcholinesterase Inhibitors

The role of AChEI in the treatment of neuropsychiatric symptoms of AD is being explored. In a systematic review and

TABLE 37-6

RECOMMENDED PHARMACOLOGICAL AGENTS FOR TREATING PSYCHOSIS AND AGITATION ASSOCIATED WITH DEMENTIA[a]

Medication	Starting Dose (mg/day)	Therapeutic Dose (mg/day)	Main Adverse Effects[b]	Special Precautions
Atypical Antipsychotics[c]				
Risperidone	0.25–0.5	1–2	Sedation, EPS, orthostasis, peripheral edema	Active 9-hydroxy metabolite accumulates with renal failure
Olanzapine	2.5–5	5–15	Sedation, orthostasis, EPS	Dysregulation of glucose and lipid metabolism; anticholinergicity
Quetiapine	12.5–25	100–400	Sedation, orthostasis	—
Aripiprazole	2.5–5	5–15	Sedation	—
Selective Serotonin Re-uptake Inhibitors				
Sertraline	25	100–200	Nausea, diarrhea, insomnia	Hyponatremia; EPS
Escitalopram	5–10	10–20	Nausea, headache, constipation	Hyponatremia; EPS
Benzodiazepines				
Lorazepam	0.25	1–2	Sedation, ataxia, cognitive impairment	Avoid chronic use
Oxazepam	15	15–30	Sedation, ataxia, cognitive impairment	Avoid chronic use
Anticonvulsants				
Divalproex sodium	125–250	250–1000	Nausea, sedation	Thrombocytopenia; liver function abnormalities, pancreatitis
Carbamazepine	50–100	200–1000	Sedation, ataxia, nausea	Hyponatremia; pancytopenia
Acetylcholinesterase Inhibitors				
Donepezil	5	5–15	Nausea, diarrhea, transient confusion	Bradycardia possible
Rivastigmine	3	6–12	Nausea, diarrhea, transient confusion	Bradycardia possible
Galantamine	8	16–24	Nausea, diarrhea, transient confusion	Bradycardia possible
Others				
Trazodone	50	50–150	Sedation, orthostasis	Priapism (rare) Arrythmia (at higher doses)
Memantine	5	20	Sedation	—

Behavioral Emergency

If PO administration possible:
Risperidone 0.5 mg (range 0.25–1 mg) *OR*
Olanzapine 5 mg (range 2.5–5 mg) *OR*
Quetiapine 25 mg (range 25–50 mg)

If IM administration necessary:
Olanzapine 5 mg *OR*
Haloperidol 0.5 mg (range 0.5–1 mg); monitor for EPS with haloperidol

If IV access available:
   Haloperidol 0.5 mg (range 0.5–1 mg) with cardiac monitoring for QTc interval prolongation and/or ventricular arrythmias at high doses

For severe agitation, augment any of the above preparations with:
   Lorazepam 0.5–1 mg PO/IM

[a]Only the atypical antipsychotics are recommended for the treatment of psychosis.
[b]Intensity of adverse effects varies with individual medications and individual patients.
[c]Clinicians prescribing atypical antipsychotics in dementia patients should review FDA-mandated warnings on hyperglycemia, potential cerebrovascular adverse events, and findings regarding increased mortality.

EPS, extrapyramidal symptoms, IM, intramuscular; IV, intravenous; PO, oral.

meta-analysis of 16 studies of AChEI that measured neuropsychiatric outcomes, patients randomized to AChEI improved 1.72 points on the NPI (six studies; 95% confidence interval [CI], 0.87–2.57 points), and 0.03 points on the ADAS-noncog (10 studies; 95% CI 0.00–0.05 points) compared with placebo (92). The effect size observed with the NPI in these trials is comparable to that reported with other agents used for neuropsychiatric symptoms in dementia, such as risperidone and valproic acid (71,93). Major limitations of this meta-analysis include the fact that not all patients in these trials had neuropsychiatric symptoms, some patients were on other psychoactive medications, separate meta-analyses could not be performed for each AChEI due to limited power, and individual behaviors were not examined.

Memantine

In addition to dysfunction of cholinergic neurotransmission, overstimulation of the N-methyl-D-aspartate (NMDA) receptor by the excitatory neurotransmitter glutamate is believed to be responsible for cognitive and behavioral symptoms in AD. Conversely, physiologic activation of the NMDA receptor appears to be critical for learning and memory processes. Memantine is a low-to-moderate affinity, uncompetitive NMDA-receptor antagonist that displays voltage-dependent, fast blocking/unblocking kinetics (94). Memantine thereby blocks the effects of abnormal glutamate activity that may lead to neuronal cell damage/loss, while preserving physiological activation of the NMDA receptor required for learning and memory. Memantine has a half-life of 60 to 80 hours and displays linear, dose-proportional kinetics at dosages of 10 to 40 mg/day (95). It is eliminated mostly in urine as parent drug, has minimal or no effects on CYP450 isoenzymes, and has no major pharmacokinetic or pharmacodynamic interactions with donepezil.

The efficacy and safety of memantine has been evaluated in three pivotal trials: monotherapy in moderate-to-severe AD, combination therapy with donepezil in moderate-to-severe AD, and nursing home patients with mixed dementia diagnoses (96–98). The NPI was included as a primary behavioral efficacy measure in the first two studies, but not in the nursing home study. Reisberg et al. examined the efficacy and safety of memantine as monotherapy in 252 moderate-to-severe AD outpatients (operationally defined as MMSE 3–14, Functional Assessment Staging $\geq$ 6a, Global Deterioration Scale stages 5 or 6) (96). At endpoint, there was no statistically significant separation from placebo for total NPI scores. However, when specific items from the NPI were examined, memantine demonstrated statistically significant reductions in delusionality ($p = 0.0386$) and agitation/aggression ($p = 0.0083$). Tariot and colleagues noted statistically significant improvement in total NPI scores in 404 outpatients with moderate-to-severe AD, stably maintained on donepezil for over 2 years, whose treatment was augmented with memantine (97). The authors did not, however, report findings on specific items of the NPI. A behavioral rating instrument was not included as an efficacy measure in the nursing home study (98).

Behavioral Emergencies

Behavioral emergencies in elderly patients with dementia pose considerable treatment challenges given their frailty, medical comorbidities, polypharmacy and, in advanced stages of dementia, their inability to clearly communicate their needs or comprehend caregivers' instructions. Not uncommonly, the acute onset of such emergencies precludes adequate consideration of nonpharmacological management approaches. The safety of the agitated resident and those in their immediate environment takes precedence. While there are no definitive guidelines for

management of acute agitation in persons with dementia, Table 37-6 outlines several options based largely on clinical experience. Initiation of pharmacotherapy to manage acute agitation, particularly via the intramuscular or intravenous route, necessitates active monitoring of the patient's condition. For example, intravenous administration of haloperidol would be contraindicated in the absence of cardiac monitoring. Admission to an inpatient geropsychiatry ward should be sought for any patient with acutely unstable medical conditions, significant risk of harm to self or others, or suboptimal response to behavioral and pharmacotherapeutic measures to curb the agitation.

ETHICAL ISSUES

Two critical ethical issues that arise in the management of patients with psychosis or agitation of dementia are the ability to give informed consent, and balancing patient needs versus system needs. While many people with dementia have identified substitute decision-makers, the nature of consent to pharmacotherapy is often quite cursory. As a result, important side effects and potential long-term consequences of psychoactive medications often remain only partially discussed. For example, the common side effect of diarrhea on selective serotonin reuptake inhibitors could lead to dehydration, falls, and fractures. In this case, it would not be enough to simply report diarrhea as a side effect without explaining its potential consequences in layman's terms to ensure truly informed consent. This issue is particularly important when discussing the potential for extrapyramidal side effects of antipsychotics, since some of these movement abnormalities may be potentially irreversible. In addition, it is critical for clinicians to understand and be able to explain to patients and/or caregivers in laymen's terms new FDA warnings for antipsychotic agents. When possible, written documentation of informed consent to psychoactive medications should be obtained.

Individualizing patient care in inflexible residential environments that demand efficiency is often problematic. For example, residential care facilities will often request pharmacotherapeutic interventions when resources for recreational and social engagement are lacking. Similarly, some residents of assisted living facilities are kept in that environment far longer than their optimal care would dictate, as long as they are not behaviorally disturbed. When these same residents experience acute agitation, there is often an urgency to move them to a more restrictive level of care.

A geriatric psychiatrist is in an ideal position to not only treat the cognitive and mental disorders of later life, thereby maintaining the highest possible level of patient functioning, but also to prime and assist the family in preparing advance directives, to improve communication amongst the multidisciplinary treatment team members, and to plan for optimal living arrangements.

REFERENCES

1. Rabins PV, Mace NL, Lucas MJ. The impact of dementia on the family. *JAMA.* 1982;248:333–335.
2. Steele C, Rovner B, Chase GA, et al. Psychiatric symptoms and nursing home placement of patients with Alzheimer's disease. *Am J Psychiatry.* 1990;147:1049–1051.
3. Drevets WC, Rubin EH. Psychotic symptoms and the longitudinal course of senile dementia of the Alzheimer type. *Biol Psychiatry.* 1989;25:39–48.
4. Cook SE, Miyahara S, Bacanu SA, et al. Psychotic symptoms in Alzheimer disease: evidence for subtypes. *Am J Geriatr Psychiatry.* 2003;11:414–426.
5. Lyketsos CG, Breitner JCS, Rabins PV. An evidence-based proposal for the classification of neuropsychiatric disturbance in Alzheimer's disease. *Int J Geriatr Psychiatry.* 2001;16:1037–1042.
6. Jeste DV, Finkel SI. Psychosis of Alzheimer's disease and related dementias. *Am J Geriatr Psychiatry.* 2000;8:29–34.
7. Wragg R, Jeste DV. Overview of depression and psychosis in Alzheimer's disease. *Am J Psychiatry.* 1989;146:577–587.
8. Mendez M, Martin R, Smyth KA, et al. Psychiatric symptoms associated with Alzheimer's disease. *J Neuropsychiatry Clin Neurosci.* 1990;2:28–33.
9. Hirono N, Mori E, Yasuda M, et al. Factors associated with psychotic symptoms in Alzheimer's disease. *J Neurol Neurosurg Psychiatry.* 1998;64:648–652.
10. Leroi I, Voulgari A, Breitner JCS, Lyketsos CG. The epidemiology of psychosis in dementia. *Am J Geriatr Psychiatry.* 2003;11:83–91.
11. Paulsen JS, Salmon DP, Thal L, et al. Incidence of and risk factors for hallucinations and delusions in patients with probable Alzheimer's disease. *Neurology.* 2000;54:1965–1971.
12. Levy ML, Cummings JL, Fairbanks LA, et al. Longitudinal assessment of symptoms of depression, agitation, and psychosis in 181 patients with Alzheimer's disease. *Am J Psychiatry.* 1996;153:1438–1443.
13. Devanand DP, Jacobs DM, Tang MX, et al. The course of psychopathologic features in mild-to-moderate Alzheimer's disease. *Arch Gen Psychiatry.* 1997;54:257–263.
14. Burns A, Jacoby R, Levy R. Psychiatric phenomena in Alzheimer's disease, I: disorders of thought content. *Br J Psychiatry.* 1990;157:72–76.
15. Lyketsos CG, Steinberg M, Tschantz J, Norton MC, Steffens DC, Breitner JCS. Mental and behavioral disturbances in dementia: findings from the Cache County Study on Memory in Aging. *Am J Psychiatry.* 2000;157:708–714.
16. Gilley DW, Wilson RS, Beckett LA, et al. Psychotic symptoms and physically aggressive behavior in Alzheimer's disease. *J Am Geriatr Soc.* 1997;45:1074–1079.
17. Bassiony MM, Lyketsos CG. Delusions and hallucinations in Alzheimer's disease: review of the brain decade. *Psychosomatics.* 2003;44:388–401.
18. Tariot PN, Mack JL, Patterson MB, Behavioral Pathology Committee of the Consortium to Establish a Registry for Alzheimer's Disease, et al. The behavior rating scale for dementia of the consortium to establish a registry for Alzheimer's disease. *Am J Psychiatry.* 1995;152:1349–1357.
19. Sultzer DL, Mahler ME, Mandelkern MA, et al. The relationship between psychiatric symptoms and regional cortical metabolism in Alzheimer's disease. *J Neuropsychiatry Clin Neurosci.* 1995;7:476–484.
20. Sweet RA, Nimgaonkar VL, Devlin B, et al. Increased familial risk of the psychotic phenotype of Alzheimer disease. *Neurology.* 2002;58:907–911.
21. Steinberg M, Sheppard JM, Tschanz JT, et al. The incidence of mental and behavioral disturbances in dementia: the Cache County Study. *J Neuropsychiatry Clin Neurosci.* 2003;15:340–345.
22. Jeste DV, Wragg RE, Salmon DP, et al. Cognitive deficits of patients with Alzheimer's disease with and without delusions. *Am J Psychiatry.* 1992;149:184–189.
23. Devanand DP, Brockington CD, Moody BJ, et al. Behavioral syndromes in Alzheimer's disease. *Int Psychogeriatr.* 1992;4(Suppl 2):161–184.
24. Bassiony MM, Warren A, Rosenblatt A, et al. Isolated hallucinosis in Alzheimer's disease is associated with African-American race. *Int J Geriatr Psychiatry.* 2002;17:205–210.
25. Rubin E, Drevets W, Burke A. The nature of psychotic symptoms in senile dementia of the Alzheimer type. *J Geriatr Psychiatry Neurol.* 1988;1:16–20.
26. Merriam A, Aronson N, Gaston P, et al. The psychiatric symptoms of Alzheimer's disease. *J Am Geriatr Soc.* 1988;36:7–12.
27. Stern Y, Albert M, Brandt J, et al. Utility of extrapyramidal signs and psychosis as predictors of cognitive and functional decline, nursing home admission, and death in Alzheimer's disease: prospective analyses from the predictors study. *Neurology.* 1994;44:2300–2307.
28. Jeste DV, Rockwell E, Harris MJ, et al. Conventional antipsychotics in elderly patients. *Am J Geriatr Psychiatry.* 1999;7:70–76.
29. Sweet RA, Hamilton RL, Healy MT, et al. Alterations of striatal dopamine receptor binding in Alzheimer's disease are associated with Lewy body pathology and with antemortem psychosis. *Arch Neurol.* 2001;58:466–472.
30. Sweet RA, Nimgaonkar VL, Kamboh MI, et al. Dopamine receptor genetic variation, psychosis, and aggression in Alzheimer's disease. *Arch Neurol.* 1998;55:1335–1340.
31. Cohen-Mansfield J, Billig N. Agitated behaviors in the elderly: a conceptual review. *J Am Geriatr Soc.* 1986;34:711–721.
32. Rosen J, Burgio L, Kollar M, et al. The Pittsburgh Agitation Scale: a user-friendly instrument for rating agitation in dementia patients. *Am J Geriatr Psychiatry.* 1994;2:52–59.
33. International Psychogeriatric Association. Behavioral and psychological signs and symptoms of dementia: implications for research and treatment. *Int Psychogeriatr.* 1996;8(Suppl 3): 215–552.
34. Division of Neuropharmacological Drug Products of the Food and Drug Administration. Position paper. March 9, 2000.
35. Olin JT, Schneider LS, Katz IR, et al. Provisional diagnostic criteria for depression of Alzheimer disease. *Am J Geriatr Psychiatry.* 2002;10:125–128.
36. International Psychogeriatric Association. Behavioral and psychological symptoms of dementia (BPSD): a clinical and research update. *Int Psychogeriatr.* 2000;12(suppl 1):1–424.
37. Cummings JL, Mega M, Gray K, et al. The Neuropsychiatric Inventory: comprehensive assessment of psychopathology in dementia. *Neurology.* 1994;44:2308–2314.
38. Cohen-Mansfield J, Marx MS, Rosenthal AS. Dementia and agitation in nursing home residents: how are they related? *Psychol Aging.* 1990;5:3–8.
39. Ryden M, Bossenmaier M. Aggressive behaviors in cognitively impaired nursing home residents. *Gerontologist.* 1988;28:179A.
40. Spector DW, Jackson ME. Correlates of disruptive behaviors in nursing homes, a reanalysis. *J Aging Health.* 1994;6:173–184.
41. Bridges-Parlet S, Knopman D, Thompson T. A descriptive study of physically aggressive behavior in dementia by direct observation. *J Am Geriatr Soc.* 1994;42:192–197.
42. Cohen-Mansfield J, Billig N, Lipson S, Rosenthal AS, Pawlson LG. Medical correlates of agitation in nursing home residents. *Gerontology.* 1990;36:150–158.
43. Monsour N, Robb SS. Wandering behavior in old age: a psychosocial study. *Social Work.* 1982;27:411–416.
44. Cummings JL, Back C. The cholinergic hypothesis of neuropsychiatric symptoms in Alzheimer's disease. *Am J Geriatr Psychiatry.* 1998;6(Suppl 1):64–78.
45. Palmer AM, Dekosky ST. Neurochemistry of aging. In: Albert M, Knoefel J, eds. *Clinical Neurology of Aging.* New York: Oxford University Press; 1994:79–101.
46. Funkenstein HH, Albert MS, Cook NR, et al. Extrapyramidal signs and other neurologic findings in clinically diagnosed Alzheimer's disease. A community-based study. *Arch Neurol.* 1993;50:51–56.
47. Sweet RA, Mulsant BH, Pollock BG, Rosen J, Altieri LP. Neuroleptic-induced parkinsonism in elderly patients diagnosed with psychotic major depression and dementia of the Alzheimer type with psychotic features. *Am J Geriatr Psychiatry.* 1996;4:311–319.
48. Lesch KP, Merschdorf U. Impulsivity, aggression, and serotonin: a molecular psychobiological perspective. *Behav Sci Law.* 2000;18:581–604.

49. Gottfries CG. Disturbance of the 5-hydroxytryptamine metabolism in brains from patients with Alzheimer's dementia. *J Neural Transm.* 1990;30(Suppl):33–43.

50. Procter AW, Francis PT, Stratmann GC, Bowen DM. Serotonergic pathology is not widespread in Alzheimer patients without prominent aggressive symptoms. *Neurochem Res.* 1992;17:917–922.

51. Lanctot KL, Hermann N, van Reekum R, Eryavec G, Naranjo CA. Gender, aggression and serotonergic function are associated with response to sertraline for behavioral disturbances in Alzheimer's disease. *Int J Geriatr Psychiatry.* 2002;17:531–541.

52. Tohgi H, Abe T, Takahashi S, Saheki M, Kimura M. Indoleamine concentrations in cerebrospinal fluid from patients with Alzheimer type and Binswanger type dementias before and after administration of citalopram, a synthetic serotonin uptake inhibitor. *J Neural Transm.* 1995;9:121–131.

53. Baldessarini RJ, Marsh ER, Kula NS. Interactions of fluoxetine with metabolism of dopamine and serotonin in rat brain regions. *Brain Res.* 1992;579:152–156.

54. McLoughlin DM, Lucey JV, Dinan TG. Central serotonergic hyperresponsivity in late-onset Alzheimer's disease. *Am J Psychiatry.* 1994;151:1701–1703.

55. Mintzer J, Brawman-Mintzer O, Mirski DF, et al. Fenfluramine challenge test as a marker of serotonin activity in patients with Alzheimer's dementia and agitation. *Biol Psychiatry.* 1998;44:918–921.

56. Lopez OL, Smith G, Becker JT, et al. The psychotic phenomenon in probable Alzheimer's disease: a positron emission tomography study. *J Neuropsychiatry Clin Neurosci.* 2001;13:50–55.

57. Mega MS, Lee L, Dinov ID, et al. Cerebral correlates of psychotic symptoms in Alzheimer's disease. *J Neurol Neurosurg Psychiatry.* 2000;69:167–171.

58. Tekin S, Mega MS, Masterman D, et al. Orbitofrontal and anterior cingulate cortex neurofibrillary tangle burden is associated with agitation in Alzheimer's disease. *Ann Neurol.* 2001;49:355–361.

59. Lai MK, Lai OF, Keene J, et al. Psychosis of Alzheimer's disease is associated with elevated muscarinic M2 binding in the cortex. *Neurology.* 2001;57:805–811.

60. Holmes C, Smith H, Ganderton R, et al. Psychosis and aggression in Alzheimer's disease: the effect of dopamine receptor gene variation. *J Neurol Neurosurg Psychiatry.* 2001;71:777–779.

61. Sukonick DL, Pollock BG, Sweet RA, et al. The 5-HTTPR *S/*L polymorphism and aggressive behavior in Alzheimer's disease. *Arch Neurol.* 2001;58:1425–1428.

62. Moak G, Borson S. Mental health services in long-term care: still an unmet need. *Am J Geriatr Psychiatry.* 2000;8:96–100.

63. Cohen-Mansfield J. Approaches to the assessment of disruptive behaviors. In: Lawton MP, Rubinstein RL, eds. *Interventions in Dementia Care: Toward Improving Quality of Life.* New York: Springer Publishing Company; 2000:39–64.

64. Mulsant BH, Mazumdar S, Pollock BG, et al. Methodological issues in characterizing treatment response in demented patients with behavioral disturbances. *Int J Geriatr Psychiatry.* 1997;12: 537–547.

65. Cohen-Mansfield J. Nonpharmacologic interventions for inappropriate behaviors in dementia: a review, summary, and critique. *Am J Geriatr Psychiatry.* 2001;9:361–382.

66. Health Care Financing Administration. Medicare and Medicaid: requirements for long term care facilities final registration. *Federal Register.* 1991;56:48865–48921.

67. Kindermann SS, Dolder CR, Bailey A, Katz IR, Jeste DV. Pharmacological treatment of psychosis and agitation in elderly patients with dementia: four decades of experience. *Drugs Aging.* 2002;19:257–276.

68. Cohen-Mansfield J. Recruitment rates in gerontological research: the situation for drug trials in dementia may be worse than previously reported. *Alzheimer Dis Assoc Disord.* 2002;16:279–282.

69. Pollock BG, Mulsant BH, Rosen J, et al. Comparison of citalopram, perphenazine, and placebo for the acute treatment of psychosis and behavioral disturbances in hospitalized, demented patients. *Am J Psychiatry.* 2002;159:460–465.

70. Schneider LS, Tariot PN, Lyketsos CG, et al. National Institute of Mental Health clinical antipsychotic trials of intervention effectiveness (CATIE): Alzheimer disease trial methodology. *Am J Geriatr Psychiatry.* 2001;9:346–360.

71. Katz IR, Jeste DV, Mintzer JE, et al. Comparison of risperidone and placebo for psychosis and behavioral disturbances associated with dementia: a randomized, double-blind trial. *J Clin Psychiatry.* 1999;60:107–115.

72. De Deyn PP, Rabheru K, Rasmussen A, et al. A randomized trial of risperidone, placebo, and haloperidol for behavioral symptoms of dementia. *Neurology.* 1999;53:946–955.

73. Brodaty H, Ames D, Snowdon J, et al. A randomized placebo-controlled trial of risperidone for the treatment of aggression, agitation, and psychosis of dementia. *J Clin Psychiatry.* 2003;64: 134–143.

74. Satterlee WG, Reams SG, Burns PR, et al. A clinical update on olanzapine treatment in schizophrenia and in elderly Alzheimer's disease patients [abstract]. *Psychopharmacol Bull.* 1995;31:534.

75. Street JS, Clark WS, Gannon KS, et al. Olanzapine treatment of psychotic and behavioral symptoms in patients with Alzheimer disease in nursing care facilities: a double-blind, randomized, placebo-controlled trial. *Arch Gen Psychiatry.* 2000;57:968–976.

76. De Deyn PP, Carrasco MM, Deberdt W, et al. Olanzapine versus placebo in the treatment of psychosis with or without associated behavioral disturbances in patients with Alzheimer's disease. *Int J Geriatr Psychiatry.* 2004;19:115–126.

77. Tariot PN, Salzman C, Yeung PP, et al. Long-term use of quetiapine in elderly patients with psychotic disorders. *Clin Ther.* 2000;22:1068–1084.

78. Tariot P, Schneider L, Katz I, et al. Quetiapine in nursing home residents with Alzheimer's dementia and psychosis. Presented at the 15th Annual Meeting of the American Association for Geriatric Psychiatry; February 24–27, 2002; Orlando, FL.

79. Zhong K, Tariot P, Minkwitz MC, et al. Quetiapine for the treatment of agitation in elderly institutionalized patients with dementia: a randomized, double-blind trial. Presented at the 9th International Conference on Alzheimer's Disease and Related Disorders; July 17–22, 2004; Philadelphia, PA.

80. Pfizer, Inc. Data on file.

81. Berkowitz A. Ziprasidone for elderly dementia: a case series. Presented at the 2003 Annual Meeting of the American Psychiatric Association; San Francisco, CA.

82. De Deyn PP, Jeste D, Mintzer J. Aripiprazole in dementia of the Alzheimer's type. Presented at the 16th Annual Meeting of the American Association for Geriatric Psychiatry; March 1–4, 2003; Honolulu, Hawaii.

83. Breder C, Swanink R, Marcus R, et al. Dose-ranging study of aripiprazole in patients with Alzheimer's dementia. Presented at the 157th American Psychiatric Association Meeting; May 1–6, 2004; New York, NY.

84. Streim J, Breder C, Swanink R, et al. Flexible dose aripiprazole in psychosis of Alzheimer's dementia. Presented at the 157th American Psychiatric Association Meeting; May 1–6, 2004; New York, NY.

85. Fontaine CS, Hynan LS, Koch K, et al. A double-blind comparison of olanzapine versus risperidone in the acute treatment of dementia-related behavioral disturbances in extended care facilities. *J Clin Psychiatry.* 2003;64:726–730.

86. Masand PS, Gupta S. Long-acting injectable antipsychotics in the elderly: guidelines for effective use. *Drugs Aging.* 2003;20(15):1099–1110.

87. Gharabawi G, Erdekens M, Zhu Y, et al. Long-acting risperidone for the management of elderly patients with psychotic disorders: a favorable benefit/risk ratio [abstract/poster]. Presented at the 2001 Annual Meeting of the International College of Geriatric Psychoneuropharmacology.

88. Lasser R, Bossie C, Eerdenkens M, et al. Stable elderly patients with psychotic disorders improve with long-acting risperidone microspheres [poster]. Presented at the 16th Annual Meeting of the American Association for Geriatric Psychiatry; March 1–4, 2003; Honolulu, Hawaii.

89. Lasser R, Bossie C, Zhu Y, et al. A long-term assessment of dyskinesia and other movement disorders in elderly patients receiving long-acting risperidone microspheres [abstract]. *J Clin Psychiatry.* 2002;63:1070.

90. Meehan KM, Wang H, David SR. Comparison of rapidly acting intramuscular olanzapine, lorazepam, and placebo: a double-blind, randomized study in acutely agitated patients with dementia. *Neuropsychopharmacology*. 2002;26:494–504.

91. Jeste DV, Okamoto A, Napolitano J, Kane JM, Martinez RA. Low incidence of persistent tardive dyskinesia in elderly patients with dementia treated with risperidone. *Am J Psychiatry*. 2000;157: 1150–1155.

92. Trinh NH, Hoblyn J, Mohanty S, Yaffe K. Efficacy of cholinesterase inhibitors in the treatment of neuropsychiatric symptoms and functional impairment in Alzheimer disease. *JAMA*. 2003;289: 210–216.

93. Porsteinsson AP, Tariot PN, Erb R, et al. Placebo-controlled study of divalproex sodium for agitation in dementia. *Am J Geriatr Psychiatry*. 2001;9:58–66.

94. Danysz W, Parsons CG, Quack G. NMDA channel blockers: memantine and amino-alkylcyclohexanes—in vivo characterization. *Amino Acids*. 2000;9:167–172.

95. Forest Pharmaceuticals, Inc. Data on file.

96. Reisberg B, Doody R, Stoffler A, et al. Memantine in moderate-to-severe Alzheimer's disease. *N Engl J Med*. 2003;348:1333– 1341.

97. Tariot PN, Farlow MR, Grossberg GT, et al. Memantine treatment in patients with moderate to severe Alzheimer's disease already receiving donepezil: a randomized controlled trial. *JAMA*. 2004;291:317–324.

98. Winblad B, Poritis N. Memantine in severe dementia: results of the 9M-Best Study (Benefit and efficacy in severely demented patients during treatment with memantine). *Int J Geriatr Psychiatry*. 1999;14:135–146.

99. Cohen-Mansfield J. Agitated behaviors in the elderly: II. Preliminary results in the cognitively deteriorated. *J Am Geriatr Soc*. 1986;34:722–727.

100. Reisberg B, Borenstein J, Salob SP, et al. Behavioral symptoms in Alzheimer's disease: phenomenology and treatment. *J Clin Psychiatry*. 1987;48:9–15.

101. Baumgarten M, Becker R, Gauthier S. Validity and reliability of the Dementia Behavior Disturbance Scale. *J Am Geriatr Soc*. 1990;38:221–226.

102. Rosen J, Bobys PD, Mazumdar S, et al. OBRA regulations and neuroleptic use: defining agitation using the Pittsburgh Agitation Scale and the Neurobehavioral Rating Scale. *Ann Long-Term Care*. 1999;7:429–436.

103. Levin H, High W, Goethe K, et al. The Neurobehavioral Rating Scale: assessment of the behavioral sequelae of head injury by the clinician. *J Neurol Neurosurg Psychiatry*. 1987;50:183–193.

104. Sugarman AA, Williams BH, Adlerstein AM. Haloperidol in the psychiatric disorders of old age. *Am J Psychiatry*. 1964;120: 1190–1192.

105. Petrie WM, Ban TA, Berney S, et al. Loxapine in psychogeriatrics: a placebo and standard-controlled clinical investigation. *J Clin Psychopharmacol*. 1982;2:122–126.

106. Devanand DP, Cooper T, Sackheim HA, et al. Low dose oral haloperidol and blood levels in Alzheimer's disease: a preliminary study. *Psychopharmacol Bull*. 1992;28:169–173.

107. Auchus AP, Bissey-Black C. Pilot study of haloperidol, fluoxetine, and placebo for agitation in Alzheimer's disease. *J Neuropsychiatry Clin Neurosci*. 1997;9:591–593.

108. Devanand DP, Marder K, Michaels KS, et al. A randomized, placebo-controlled dose-comparison trial of haloperidol for psychosis and disruptive behaviors in Alzheimer's disease. *Am J Psychiatry*. 1998;155:1512–1520.

109. Teri L, Logsdon RG, Peskind E, et al. Treatment of agitation: a randomized, placebo-controlled clinical trial. *Neurology*. 2000; 55:1271–1278.

110. Barnes R, Veith R, Okimoto J, et al. Efficacy of antipsychotic medications in behaviorally disturbed dementia patients. *Am J Psychiatry*. 1982;139:1170–1174.

111. Rada RT, Kellner R. Thiothixene in the treatment of geriatric patients with chronic organic brain syndrome. *J Am Geriatr Soc*. 1976;24:105–107.

112. Finkel SI, Lyons JS, Anderson RL, et al. A randomized, placebo-controlled trial of thiothixene in agitated, demented nursing home patients. *Int J Geriatr Psychiatry*. 1995;10:129–136.

113. Stotsky B. Multicenter study comparing thioridazine with diazepam and placebo in elderly, nonpsychotic patients with emotional and behavioral disorders. *Clin Ther*. 1984;6: 546–559.

114. Nyth AL, Gottfries CG. The clinical efficacy of citalopram in treatment of emotional disturbances in dementia disorders: a Nordic multicentre study. *Br J Psychiatry*. 1990;157: 894–901.

115. Olafsson K, Jorgensen S, Jensen HV, Bille A, Arup P, Andersen J. Fluvoxamine in the treatment of demented elderly patients: a double-blind, placebo-controlled study. *Acta Psychiatr Scand*. 1992;85:453–456.

116. Lanctot KL, Herrmann N, van Reekum R, Eryavec G, Naranjo CA. Gender, aggression and serotonergic function are associated with response to sertraline for behavioral disturbances in Alzheimer's disease. *Int J Geriatr Psychiatry*. 2002;17:531–541.

117. Tariot PN, Erb R, Podgorski CA, Cox C, Patel S, Jakimovich L, Irvine C. Efficacy and tolerability of carbamazepine for agitation and aggression in dementia. *Am J Psychiatry*. 1998;155: 54–61.

118. Olin JT, Fox LS, Pawluczyk S, Taggart NA, Schneider LS. A pilot randomized trial of carbamazepine for behavioral symptoms in treatment-resistant outpatients with Alzheimer disease. *Am J Geriatr Psychiatry*. 2001;9(4):400–405.

119. Davis LL, Buckwalter K, Burgio L. Measuring problem behaviors in dementia: developing a methodological agenda. *Adv Nurse Sci*. 1997; 20:40–55.

Depression and Anxiety Associated with Dementia

38

Natalie Sachs-Ericsson   *Dan G. Blazer*

Symptoms of depression and anxiety are common among individuals with dementia, complicating both diagnosis and treatment, and are often associated with a more severe clinical course, higher cost of treatment, poorer quality of life, and worse outcomes (1–3). Furthermore, psychiatric symptoms that occur in individuals with dementia are often the primary cause of family burden and distress (4,5).

Depression in late life has repeatedly been shown to adversely influence the outcome of comorbid health disorders and is associated with significant functional impairment, further complicating the course of dementia by increasing disability (6–9). Even so, depression in dementia often goes unrecognized, resulting, at times, in less effective therapeutic intervention (10,11). The identification and effective treatment of depressive disorder in individuals with dementia may substantially augment treatment outcome and improve the quality of life for the patient and family. The following example illustrates one such case (12).

CASE EXAMPLE

Mrs. S was a 70-year-old woman diagnosed by her doctor with severe Alzheimer's disease (AD). Her family reluctantly considered placing her in a residential facility.

During consultation, the psychiatrist obtained the following history from the patient's family. Mrs. S experienced a relatively sudden onset of symptoms over 4 months. She had retired a few years earlier from her job because she found workplace stress increasingly difficult. Following retirement, she cared for her invalid husband. He died 5 months before the assessment. A few weeks before his death, Mrs. S' daughter helped care for her father because it had become too difficult for Mrs. S to provide full-time care for her husband. A few weeks after his death, Mrs. S' condition deteriorated dramatically. She ate little, was agitated, paced continually, and could not sleep. When her family attempted to obtain information from Mrs. S about her husband's will, she simply responded, "I do not know." She ruminated about being of no value to anybody.

Mrs. S was diagnosed as suffering from a major depressive episode with psychotic features. Treatment with antidepressant medication was not effective (it had been attempted by her local physician), but after receiving electroconvulsive therapy (six treatments, unilateral nondominant) she showed marked improvement. She was able to return to the community, living with one of her daughters (who had planned for her mother to live with her after the death of her father). Mrs. S helped around the house and gained weight. Nevertheless, her memory continued to show some impairment. In retrospect, her family believed that she had shown some memory difficulties for at least 2 years before her hospitalization.

Mrs. S experienced a severe episode of major depression (MD) with psychotic features, comorbid with a slowly progressive dementia of the Alzheimer's type. The severe cognitive impairment experienced during the depressive episode exacerbated the symptoms of AD. However, treatment of the depression allowed her to remain with her family, and substantially improved her quality of life.

Anxiety can also complicate the management of the older adult experiencing dementia. The following case illustrates the comorbidity of anxiety and dementia.

CASE EXAMPLE

Mr. J, an 80-year-old man with a 3-year history of progressive dementia, lived with his wife near the coast of North Carolina. Though his cognitive impairment was moderate, behavioral problems had been minimal. During the hurricane season, the family decided to ride out a storm heading for the coast. They had rarely left their home during a hurricane, and this particular storm was predicted to make landfall over 100 miles south. During the height of the storm, however, the wind blew a tree onto the carport of their home and caused major damage, though no one was hurt.

Mr. J was sitting in his easy chair when he heard the crash. He went into a panic, according to his wife. He began to pace the room, kept asking what had happened, and looked very frightened. His wife had great difficulty calming him down. Finally, after the storm had abated, Mr. J went to sleep and slept soundly. The next morning he seemed his old self until he heard a sharp noise outside the house. His wife reported that he panicked again. Thereafter, whenever he heard a loud noise outside the house, he jumped from his chair, paced the room, asked his wife repeatedly what had happened, and required some time to calm down.

When this new problem was reported to the patient's psychiatrist (who had been following him for the memory loss), a low dose of alprazolam (0.25 mg by mouth twice daily) was prescribed, but this medication was of little benefit. The patient appeared to be more sedated most of the day, but continued to react to loud noises with symptoms of anxiety. The psychiatrist then switched the patient to paroxetine, 10 mg daily. The patient gradually improved and experienced no adverse side effects from this drug. The family, however, was concerned that he might again become too sedated, and withdrew the medication. The patient again lapsed into the episodes of panic. Once the medication was restored, the patient experienced only occasional episodes of panic, though his cognitive function continued to gradually decline.

EPIDEMIOLOGY

The prevalence of depression, anxiety, and comorbid depression and anxiety in elderly population samples will be reviewed, as well as the prevalence of dementia and the prevalence of depression, anxiety, and comorbid anxiety among populations with dementia.

In community surveys of the elderly, estimates of the prevalence of MD range between 1% and 3% (13,14). Reports of clinically significant depressive symptoms in community-dwelling elderly have been approximately 8%

to 16% (7). The prevalence of anxiety disorders among elderly community samples is estimated to range from approximately 5.5% (15) to 10% (16). The frequency of clinically significant anxiety-related symptoms among community-dwelling elders has been reported to be as high as 24.2% (17).

In the general population, depression and anxiety are frequently comorbid. Approximately 43% of individuals with a mood disorder also have an anxiety disorder. Among those with anxiety disorders, approximately 25% have a comorbid depressive disorder (18). Similar rates of comorbidity have been found in elderly population samples. In one study, 47.5% of individuals with depressive disorder experienced comorbid anxiety, and 26.1% of individuals with anxiety disorder experienced comorbid depression (19). Lenze and colleagues found that among depressed elderly patients, 23% had a current anxiety diagnosis (20).

The prevalence of dementia in the elderly is approximately 10% to 15%, usually of the Alzheimer's type (21,22). Cerebrovascular disease is another common cause of dementia (23,24). In one study, researchers found stroke patients to be 1.5 times more likely to suffer cognitive impairment than nonstroke patients (25). Desmond and colleagues found the incidence rate of dementia to be 8.49 cases per 100 person-years in the stroke cohort, compared to 1.37 cases per 100 person-years in the control cohort (26). Parkinson's disease is another disorder associated with cognitive impairment, with dementia occurring in approximately one-third to almost one-half of individuals with Parkinson's disease (27,28). In a community sample of individuals with Parkinson's disease, Aarsland and colleagues found that 27.7% of participants had dementia (29).

Prevalence of Depression and Anxiety in Dementia

Rates of depression and anxiety are much higher among individuals with dementia compared to general elderly population samples. Among individuals with some form of dementia, the prevalence of anxiety disorders is approximately 35% to 50% (2,30–32). Two studies estimated the average rate of agitation in demented patients to be 44% (33,34). The prevalence of depression in dementia ranges between 30% to 50% (35,36).

In one study, the prevalence of MD among individuals with AD was found to vary considerably across the recruitment sites, ranging from 22.5% to 54.4% (37). Variability in findings, however, may be due to differences in the definitions of AD and depression (35,36). However, among the most severely demented, researchers have found rates of depression to be around 50% (1,37).

Depression among individuals with dementia may be more frequent in those with vascular diseases compared to those with AD (38–40). Sultzer et al. found patients with vascular dementia (VaD) to have more frequent and more severe symptoms of depression and anxiety than those with AD (after controlling for levels of cognitive impairment) (41). Similarly, Porter and colleagues also found anxiety to be more common in patients with VaD (51%) than with AD (26%) (2). Ballard et al. found that among patients with dementia, 25% had MD and 27.4% had minor depression (40). MD occurred significantly more often and was significantly more severe in patients with VaD than in patients with AD.

In a community sample of stroke patients, Wade and colleagues found that at 3 weeks, 6 months, and 12 months after stroke, 25% to 30% of patients were depressed, and over 50% of patients who were depressed at 3 weeks remained so at 1 year (42). Robinson and colleagues found that nearly 50% of patients studied in the acute stroke period had clinically significant depression (43).

Elevated rates of depression have also been found among individuals with dementia secondary to Parkinson's disease (29,44). In a retrospective chart review of patients with Parkinson's disease, Sano and colleagues found that 10.9% met the criteria for dementia, 51% met the diagnosis of MD, and 5.4% had a comorbid depression and dementia diagnosis (45). While elevated rates of depression have been found among Parkinson's patients in general (46,47), in a community sample of individuals with Parkinson's disease, Aarsland and colleagues found that MD was more common among those with dementia (23%) than those without dementia (2.3%) (29).

The prevalence of co-occurring anxiety and depression in dementing disorders has not been well-studied. However, the frequent comorbidity of depression and anxiety, as well as the comorbidity of both with dementia, suggests a relatively high prevalence. In one study of dementia patients, rates of comorbid anxiety and depression symptoms were quite elevated (48). Specifically, 10 months after diagnosis of AD, the presence of irritability, agitation, and aggression were found to have occurred in the vast majority of patients (81%). Mega and colleagues found behavioral changes had occurred in most patients after the onset of AD (80%), including apathy (72%), agitation (60%), anxiety (48%), irritability (42%), dysphoria, and aberrant motor behavior (38%) (49). Porter et al. examined the comorbidity of depression among individuals with both dementia and anxiety (2). They found that 63.3% of AD patients with anxiety also had depression, while 81.8% of patients with VaD and anxiety also had depression.

ETIOLOGY OF DEPRESSION AND ANXIETY IN DEMENTIA

There are two common theories as to the etiology of depression and anxiety in dementia. One is that the psychiatric symptoms occur in response to the multitude of psychosocial stresses involved with dementia. The other theory proposes that neurological disorders (e.g., AD, Parkinson's, vascular disease) affect cortical structures, which may lead to depression, anxiety, and cognitive impairment (12,47,50). Furthermore, it may be possible that depression unmasks a dementia—such as when an episode of moderate-to-severe depression is accompanied by significant cognitive dysfunction. The cognitive dysfunction remits when the depression improves, yet recurs later as full-fledged dementia (51). Of course, none of these theories is mutually exclusive. Furthermore, it should be noted that research in the area of dementia and neurological correlates of psychiatric symptoms is expanding rapidly, and there are likely to be many important discoveries in upcoming years.

Etiology of Depressive Symptoms in Alzheimer's Disease

The etiology of depressive symptoms in AD remains undetermined, but some believe there is likely to be a common neuropathology of AD that plays a role in the development of depression (36,52). Zubenko and Moossy found that patients with MD had significantly more degenerative findings in the locus ceruleus and substantia nigra than demented patients who were not depressed (53). Tsai's research suggests that a decrease in brain-derived neurotrophic factor (BDNF) is related to both AD and MD (54). The author suggests that BDNF could be a bridge between AD and MD, explaining both the depressive symptoms in AD and cognitive impairment in MD.

There is also some evidence of a genetic link between AD and depression. For example, Pearlson and colleagues found that the lifetime risk of MD was greater in first-degree relatives of index cases of AD (55). In their epidemiological study of the association of depression to dementia, Fahim and colleagues found that the familial aggregation of depression with dementia and perhaps Parkinson's disease suggests there may be shared susceptibility genes underlying these diseases (56). Heun et al. concluded from their research that dementia and early-onset depression represent clinical entities with distinct inheritance, and while late-onset depression does not have substantial inheritance in common with dementia, there is modest familial clustering (57). In one study, both a family history and personal history of depression was found to confer increased risk for depression in AD (58). However, conjointly neither family nor personal history accounted for a substantial amount of the variance in syndromal depression after the onset of AD. Moreover, the researchers found that most depressed AD patients in their sample did not have a positive family history or a previous episode of depression. In contrast, Rovner and colleagues found that the vast majority (70%) of their patients with comorbid AD and depression had a past history of depression (59).

Depression as a Prodromal Indicator or Risk Factor for Alzheimer's Disease

Depression may be a prodromal indicator or risk factor for later development of AD. As noted above, Alexopoulos and colleagues suggest that severe depression may either unmask a dementia, or that the pathophysiological changes in depression and dementia are similar (51). Green et al. found that depressive symptoms were a risk factor for later development of AD (60), while Jost and Grossberg found that for more than 2 years before diagnosis, 72% of dementia patients experienced depression, changes in mood, social withdrawal, or suicidal ideation (48). In a 3-year longitudinal study conducted in Sweden, Berger et al. found that AD patients had more depressive symptoms at baseline (before the diagnosis of AD) than nondemented patients (61). Moreover, these symptoms were predominately comprised of motivational-related depressive symptoms (e.g., lack of interest, loss of energy, and concentration difficulties) rather than mood-related symptoms. The authors suggest that these symptoms represent disease-related changes in the brain rather than a reaction to self-perceived cognitive changes.

Chen and colleagues concluded from their community study of the temporal relationship between depressive symptoms and dementia that depressive symptoms were an early manifestation rather than a predictor of AD (62). In a community sample, Bassuk et al. found that depressive symptoms foreshadowed future cognitive losses among elderly people with moderate cognitive impairments, but not among cognitively intact elderly people (63).

Depressive symptoms in late life can be indicative of the onset of AD (64–68). Even the presence of mild cognitive impairment during an episode of MD in late life that subsequently remits may still be an indicator of the impending development of irreversible dementia. This is more likely to be the case if the depression is severe and characterized by psychomotor retardation or psychosis (51,69).

Etiology of Depressive Symptoms in Vascular Disease

Cerebrovascular disease is thought to be the second most common cause of acquired cognitive impairment and dementia (23). Vascular lesions in selected regions of the brain may contribute to a unique variety of late-life depression (7). Magnetic resonance imaging (MRI) has shown that depressed patients have structural abnormalities of the brain (50,70–73). In one study, patients with late-onset depression had an increased rate of C677T mutation of the methylene tetrahydrofolate reductase enzyme, which may place elderly individuals at an increased risk for vascular depression (74). In addition, *cerebral autosomal dominant arteriopathy with subcortical infarcts and leukoencephalopathy* is a disease of the notch 3 gene. Depression is one of the initial symptoms of this condition, suggesting that genetic polymorphisms or mutations may predispose older individuals to vascular-related depression (75,76).

Robinson and colleagues found the occurrence of depression in stroke victims to vary with the location of the brain lesion (43). The authors found that 25% of patients with left hemispheric lesions met the criteria for MD, while 39% met criteria for minor depression. About 60% of the patients with left anterior lesions had MD, but only 12% with posterior lesions had MD. In addition, 37% of the patients with brainstem lesions were depressed. None of the patients with right anterior lesions were depressed, and approximately 17% with right posterior lesions had depression. Herrmann and colleagues found that lesions in the vicinity of the left hemisphere basal ganglia play a crucial role in the development of MD after the acute stage of stroke (77). The research of Beblo et al. supports the theory that poststroke depression is related to the dysfunction of cortico-striato-pallido-thalamic-cortical projections that modulate cortico-thalamo-cortical loop systems (78).

However, it is important to note that while the common occurrence of depression among individuals with strokes is not questioned, researchers have found the frequency of depression in stroke patients to be quite similar to that of other individuals with chronic medical conditions (79,80). Thus, the individual's experience of having a severe medical problem and the disabilities associated with such problems may have a substantial impact on the occurrence of depression.

Etiology of Depression in Parkinson's Disease

Using data from a general practice registry of 105,416 patients, researchers found that at the time of their diagnosis of Parkinson's disease, 9.2% of the patients had a history of depression, compared with 4% of the control population (81). Leentjens and colleagues concluded that the higher lifetime prevalence of depression in those patients later diagnosed with Parkinson's disease is indicative of a biological risk-factor for depression in these patients (81). The association between depressive illness and Parkinson's disease may indicate that affective symptoms predict Parkinson's disease in some patients, or that depressive illness may be a part of the prodromal phase of Parkinson's disease (82).

Some studies have found differences in Parkinson's patients who become depressed compared to those who do not become depressed. In a prospective study of patients with Parkinson's disease, Sano et al. found that patients who were either depressed or demented had lower cerebrospinal fluid (CSF) concentrations of the serotonin metabolite, 5-hydroxyindoleacetic acid (5-HIAA) concentrations than other patients with Parkinson's disease (45). But, patients who were depressed and demented had the lowest levels. They concluded that the coexistence of dementia and depression represents a unique clinical entity in Parkinson's disease. In his review of the literature, Cummings found that lower CSF levels of 5-HIAA, a past history of depression, and greater functional disability are associated with a greater risk of depression in Parkinson's disease (83). Furthermore, he concluded that studies support the involvement of frontal dopaminergic projections in patients with Parkinson's disease and depression. Finally, Becker and colleagues concluded that a morphological alteration of the brainstem raphe nucleus might be involved in the pathogenesis of depression in Parkinson's disease, possibly reflecting involvement of the basal limbic system in the pathogenesis of secondary depression (84).

In a recent review, McDonald et al. suggest that depression is correlated with changes in central serotonergic function and neurodegeneration of specific cortical and subcortical pathways (85). Furthermore, they describe accumulating evidence that depression in Parkinson's disease is secondary to the underlying neuroanatomical degeneration, rather than simply a reaction to the psychosocial stress and disability. However, others have pointed out that the patient's response to Parkinson's disease is likely to affect the occurrence of depression. Schrag and colleagues found that depression in Parkinson's disease patients is more strongly influenced by the patients' perceptions of handicap than by actual disability (86).

Etiology of Anxiety and Agitation in Dementia

While cognitive impairment has been found to be predictive of agitation (87), the etiology of anxiety disorders in dementia has not been well-studied. Porter suggests that the greater level of anxiety associated with cerebrovascular disease compared to AD may reflect greater involvement of the frontal lobes in these conditions (2). Furthermore, among AD patients, anxiety may be related to cholinergic deficits in the brain. Researchers have found that acetyl-cholinesterase inhibitors have psychotropic effects and may play an important role in controlling neuropsychiatric and behavioral disturbances in patients with AD (88). Lanctot and colleagues suggest there is a complex link between aggression in AD and central serotonergic dysfunction (52).

Porter and colleagues found that among individuals with AD, anxiety symptoms were associated with more severe dementia, younger age of onset of the AD, and more disability (2). Orrell and Bebbington found anxiety symptoms in individuals with dementia to be associated with age, physical dependency, female gender, low socio-economic status, and cognitive impairment (31). Some researchers have found that anxiety symptoms may be more frequent in the earlier stages of dementia (89,90). This may be due to the individual's initial awareness of growing difficulties in completing tasks that were previously easy to do. However, anxiety (as well as other psychiatric disorders) also may simply be difficult to measure in the later, more severe stages of dementia (47).

PSYCHOLOGICAL AND SOCIAL CONSEQUENCES OF DEMENTIA

Individuals with dementia may be particularly sensitive to social stresses (e.g., loss of loved ones, relocation) (91,92). Orrell and Bebbington demonstrated that life-threatening events among individuals with dementia were strongly associated with depressive symptoms (92). They also suggest that dementia itself is a risk-factor for anxiety and depression, predisposing individuals to develop symptoms due to the individual's more limited capacity to deal with stress. As cognitive impairment increases, coping strategies and general functioning become more impaired, leaving the individuals more vulnerable to stress. However, as the dementia progresses, the individual also may be less aware of difficulties (and family members may have taken over responsibilities) and, paradoxically, depressive and anxiety symptoms may diminish. Thus, it is not uncommon for anxiety and depressive symptoms to be more prominent in the initial stages of dementia. The memory and functional impairments associated with the onset of dementia may be extremely distressing to an individual who may still be attempting to manage responsibilities, finances, or other such activities.

While social support has clearly been proven a protective factor against depression among the elderly (93), individuals with dementia may be less able to participate in meaningful social interactions (94). While Orrell and colleagues (95) found that having social support was associated with increased survival among dementia patients, in another study, Orrell and Bebbington found that dementia sufferers with higher social support were actually more anxious than those with less social support (31). They suggest this may be due to conflict among relatives, or possibly the behavior of the relatives toward the individual with dementia. Alternatively, more serious impairment in the individuals may in turn elicit more support from family.

DIAGNOSTIC ISSUES

Distinguishing between Depression and Dementia

Dementia and depression have considerable overlap in symptoms (47). Thus, distinguishing between late-life depression and dementing disorders is one of the more challenging problems facing healthcare professionals treating the elderly (96). There are a cluster of cognitive deficits common to both dementia and depression. Memory impairment is the most frequent symptom that is common to both (12,97). Apathy is also a common symptom among individuals with dementia, including those with and without comorbid depression, as well as among non-demented elderly individuals with depression (98).

As described elsewhere, clinicians often have difficulty when attempting to distinguish a primary mood disorder from other problems associated with depressed mood, in particular what some have referred to as *pseudodementia*. Pseudodementia is a syndrome in which dementia is mimicked, but the underlying cause is a psychiatric disorder that is typically, but not always, depression, (99).

Memory problems accompanying depression in older age may appear quite similar in form to symptoms of dementia. However, depressed elderly patients (without dementia) tend to focus on their memory problems. In contrast, patients with dementia are typically unaware of the extent and severity of their cognitive dysfunction, and may use strategies to conceal their dysfunction from others (35,36,100,101).

Wells compared the clinical features of patients with pseudodementia to those with dementia, and his conclusions are summarized in Table 38–1 (99).

Reynolds and colleagues found that patients with pseudodementia had more neurovegetative symptoms, such as early morning awakening, and more impaired libido (102). Lazarus et al. characterized the depressive symptoms of patients with primary degenerative dementia as being more intrapsychic (e.g., anxiety, helplessness, hopelessness, and worthlessness) rather than neurovegetative in nature (103). Reynolds and colleagues also found that patients with dementia showed more disorientation to time, greater difficulty finding their way around, and more impairment in dressing (102).

In general, individuals with dementia perform more poorly than individuals with depression alone on most cognitive tasks. However, pseudodementia patients more frequently respond to questions by replying, "I do not know," whereas demented patients typically try to answer, but the answer is often incorrect (99). Demented patients are generally less aware of their cognitive difficulties.

In distinguishing between dementia and pseudodementia, it is important for the clinician to keep in mind that persistent, nonremitting depression in the elderly may be a prodromal indicator of dementia. The original conceptualization of pseudodementia represented the hypothesis that the apparent biological abnormalities of depression were the unitary cause of reversible dementia occurring in the context of depression (9). However, some of the patients with pseudodementia may have a preclinical or an early stage dementing disorder (9). In fact, follow-up studies of patients diagnosed with pseudodementia have demonstrated that many of these patients progress into irreversible dementia (64).

Differential Diagnosis of Depression and Alzheimer's Disorders

Temporary mood disturbance is common in individuals with AD, and should be distinguished from the more pervasive and persistent expression of mood disturbance that characterizes individuals with comorbid depression in AD. However, there is an overlap in the symptoms of AD and depression. This overlap includes diminished emotional reactivity, loss of interest, withdrawal, and apparent apathy. Affective dysregulation is also common to both depression and AD. However, in AD, such emotional fluctuations are more typically expressed with minimal provocation and more rapid resolution. Unless such episodes are frequent (e.g., many times a day and many times a week), it is most likely that this is an indication of dysregulation due to dementia rather than depression (36).

The most common symptoms of depression in AD are dysphoria, loss of interest, apathy, and disinhibition (104). Other common symptoms are anxiety, irritability, agitation, motor retardation, lack of energy, sleep disturbance, and suicidal thoughts (40). However, it is not uncommon for individuals with AD who are not depressed to show some indications of this symptomology.

Some researchers have investigated differences in the depressive symptoms of individuals with AD and depression, and nondemented depressed elderly. In general, more vegetative signs are found among the nondemented depressed patients, and less ability to function is found among those with depression and dementia. Zubenko et al. found

TABLE 38-1

CHARACTERISTICS DISTINGUISHING DEMENTIA FROM PSEUDODEMENTIA

Clinical Characteristics	Dementia	Pseudodementia
Onset	Insidious and indeterminate	Rapid
Duration of symptoms	Long	Short
Mood	Consistent	Fluctuates
Mental status exam	Tries to answer, but typically incorrect	"I do not know" answers
Presentation	Tries to conceal disabilities	Highlights disabilities
Cognitive impairment	Stable	Fluctuates

(Adapted from reference 99.)

depressed patients with AD were more likely than nondemented depressed patients to report indecisiveness or a diminished ability to concentrate, and to have more deficits in language, but were less likely to experience sleep disturbances, feelings of worthlessness, or excessive guilt during their major depressive episodes (37). Chemerinski and colleagues found loss of appetite, weight loss, suicidal ideation, and anxiety to be more severe in the nondemented depressed patients than among those with AD and depression (105).

Depression is often seen early in the course of AD. In the initial stages, patients may look quite similar in presentation to elderly depressed patients. Thus, observation over an extended period of time and consultation with family may be crucial in determining an accurate diagnosis. Again, persistent depressive symptoms in the elderly may in fact be prodromal symptoms of AD (106).

There is no laboratory test that identifies depression (7). However, for some subtypes of depression associated with dementia, such as depression associated with AD and VaD, laboratory tests, such as MRI and positron emission tomography (PET), are reasonably sensitive for diagnosing dementia (12,107). In a recent study, Buerger and colleagues suggest that CSF p-tau should be evaluated as a potential biological marker for differentiation of geriatric depression from AD (108).

New Classification of Depression in Alzheimer's Disease

Olin and colleagues suggest that the depression that may co-occur with AD is different from other depressive disorders (35). These investigators propose a diagnosis of *depression of AD* (35). The researchers derived the diagnostic criteria from those for major depressive disorder (MDD) (109); however, there are important differences, which they delineated.

- Depression of AD requires the presence of three or more symptoms, rather than the five or more needed for the diagnoses of MDD.
- Depression of AD does not require the presence of symptoms nearly every day.
- Criteria for the presence of irritability and for social isolation or withdrawal are added.
- The criteria for loss of interest or pleasure are revised to reflect decreased positive affect or pleasure in response to social contact and usual activities.

Differential Diagnosis of Depression and Stroke

There is an overlap in some patients of depression and stroke symptoms that may make it difficult for clinicians to distinguish the origin. Symptoms in common with these disorders include pain, sleep disturbance, psychomotor retardation, or agitation (12). However, cognitive and physical impairment tends to be greater in stroke patients (110). Similarly, emotional dysregulation is common to both depression and stroke (e.g., outbursts of crying or even uncontrollable laughter) (111).

Bolla-Wilson and colleagues compared left and right hemispheric stroke patients who had depression (112). They found those with left-sided lesions exhibited a greater decline in cognitive functioning or a dementia of depression syndrome, while people with right-sided lesions and depression did not exhibit such cognitive decline.

Vascular-related depression symptoms are more likely to be characterized by an absence of psychosis, less family history of depression, more anhedonia, and greater functional disability (74,113–115). Additionally, in vascular depression, subcortical white matter hyperintensities can be found with MRI (12).

Differential Diagnosis of Depression and Parkinson's

Parkinsonism is a clinical syndrome most often exemplified by Parkinson's disease, and is comprised of motor problems (e.g., bradykinesia, resting tremor, rigidity, flexed posture, freezing, loss of postural reflexes) (116,117). However, nonmotor symptoms that also characterize patients with parkinsonism are similar to depression, making differential diagnosis more difficult (118). These include lack of emotional responsiveness, lack of motivation, and passivity (116,118). Brown and MacCarthy found that the symptoms most common in depressed parkinsonian patients included depressed mood, loss of interest, and decreased concentration (119). Additionally, sadness, moodiness, irritability, tension, worry, pessimism, indecision, and an inability to "get started" were common symptoms of the depressed parkinsonian patient. The depressed Parkinson's patient may be more likely to express symptoms of anxiety than patients with equally disabling disorders, such as multiple sclerosis (120).

Cummings found that depression in Parkinson's disease is distinguished from other depressive disorders by greater anxiety and less self-punitive ideation (83). Leentjens and colleagues concluded that nonsomatic symptoms of depression are more common and appear to be the most important for distinguishing between depressed and nondepressed patients with Parkinson's disease, along with reduced appetite and early-morning awakening (118).

Starkstein et al. found in their longitudinal study that parkinsonism was present in 20% of patients with primary depression (98). Furthermore, this syndrome was significantly associated with older age, more severe depression, and more severe cognitive impairment. In a subgroup of depressed patients, parkinsonism was reversible upon recovery from the mood disorder.

Apathy is a symptom common to both Parkinson's disease and depression. Researchers concluded that apathy in Parkinson's disease is more likely to be a direct consequence of disease-related physiological changes than a psychological reaction or adaptation to disability, and that apathy in Parkinson's disease is closely associated with cognitive impairment (121).

Differential Diagnosis of Anxiety or Agitation and Dementia

Many people with dementia also experience significant agitation (122). Lyketsos and colleagues found that aggressive behavior in dementia was closely associated with moderate-to-severe depression, male gender, and greater impairment in activities of daily living (ADL) (123). Moreover, both vascular-related dementia and AD might contribute to suspiciousness and agitation in late life. In a longitudinal study of nondemented individuals with memory changes, Copeland and colleagues found that those diagnosed with AD at 3-year follow-up were more likely to have shown agitation and apathy at baseline than those who did not develop AD (124). They also found that symptoms of apathy and agitation at baseline were related to progression of functional impairment, whereas depressive symptoms were not.

COURSE OF DEMENTIA WITH COMORBID DEPRESSION AND ANXIETY

Dementia alone imposes a great burden on the individual, his or her family, and the community. Kinosian and colleagues found that the degree of cognitive impairment associated with dementia was linked to increased mortality, higher number of years spent in institutions, more hours of required care, and more community, institutional, and medical costs (125).

Dementia associated with agitation and depression has been associated with multiple psychiatric and medical needs, intensive pharmacological treatment, and use of high-cost services (1). In a study of frail elderly nursing home residents, Bartels and colleagues found those with dementia and comorbid anxiety and depression were the most challenging group to manage in long-term care (1).

In one study, longitudinal changes in four subtypes of agitated behaviors were examined in the elderly (126). Generally, greater cognitive impairment and depression at baseline and increases in cognitive impairment and depression over time was associated with increases in agitation-related behaviors.

Devanand and colleagues found that agitation increased over the course of AD (65). Porter et al. found the addition of anxiety to AD contributed to increased disability in social functioning and increased dependence (2). Moreover, others have found that the behavioral symptoms of agitation are one of the most common causes for placement of individuals in nursing homes (127).

Depression is often seen early in the course of AD. One report suggests that as cognitive impairment increases, depression increases, although in more severe dementia depression may decrease (90). However, this latter finding may represent difficulty in assessing depression in individuals with severe dementia, rather than a true decrease in depression associated with more severe cognitive impairment.

Re-occurrence of depression among those with AD has been found to be quite high—up to 85% over a 12-month period (128). However, in a follow-up study of dementia and depression, AD patients were found to have higher rates of spontaneous resolution of depressive symptoms than individuals with VaD. Among VaD patients, depressive symptoms have been found to be more persistent and more refractory to drug treatment (129).

In one longitudinal study of AD patients with depression, Garre-Olma and colleagues found the prevalence, persistence, and emergence of depressive symptoms over 12 months among AD patients to be 51%, 55%, and 20% (130). In addition, they found that remission of depressive symptoms led to a slight increase in functioning. However, some studies have found that depression does not affect the rate of progression of AD (131,132).

There may be a slight, but significant increased risk of mortality among individuals who have AD and are depressed, compared to those with AD without depression (63). However, in one study dementia appeared to confer a greater risk for mortality than depression, and the addition of depression to dementia conferred no added risk (133).

COURSE OF DEPRESSION AMONG STROKE PATIENTS

Depression in poststroke patients has been associated with impaired recovery of ADL during the first 2 years after stroke. In a study examining the effect of remission of depression in poststroke patients, researchers found that patients whose depressive disorder remitted at follow-up had significantly greater recovery in ADL functions compared to patients whose depression did not remit (98). Robinson and Price found that the duration of untreated depression after stroke was approximately 7 to 8 months (134). Moreover, they found that the prevalence of depression increased at 6 months to 2 years after stroke.

TREATMENT

Guidelines for the treatment of comorbid depression and/or anxiety with dementia are outlined in Table 38–2. Treatment begins with a careful differential diagnosis. If symptoms of anxiety or depression emerge, they may be secondary to a physical illness or adverse drug reaction. For example, a demented patient may be experiencing anxiety

TABLE 38-2

TREATMENT GUIDELINES FOR COMORBID DEPRESSION AND/OR ANXIETY WITH DEMENTIA

Take a careful history

Few laboratory studies are currently of benefit to specify the exact etiology of comorbid anxiety and depression with dementia. A careful history, with special attention paid to symptom onset, fluctuation, physical illnesses, and situations that precipitate the complicating symptom, will usually enable the clinician to establish a working diagnosis upon which treatment can be based.

Review current medications

Medications can often cause both anxiety and depression in the demented older adult.

Explore psychosocial interventions

Though individual psychotherapy is of little value in treating the moderately to severely demented elder with depression and anxiety, psychosocial interventions, such as avoidance of situations or places that precipitate the comorbid symptoms, can be of importance in managing the demented elder. In addition, such therapies, if administered by the family, provide the family with a greater sense of control and decreased frustration with the complicating depression and/or anxiety.

Use medications judiciously

Anxiolytic and antidepressant medications may provide significant relief to the depressed or demented older adult. Nevertheless, the medications should be prescribed in low doses initially, and changes in behavior should be monitored carefully. If possible, one medication at a time should be used to treat comorbid depression and/or anxiety.

Maintain contact with the family

During visits with the patient, make certain enough time is allowed for careful review with the family of the outcome of the treatment plan. Discussions in the office and discussions of possible future issues can save the psychiatrist many phone calls during the follow-up period.

secondary to shortness of breath from congestive heart failure. Or, he may be experiencing depressive side effects from an antihypertensive medication. Many medications used by the elderly, such as clonidine or steroid preparations, may cause or exacerbate depression and/or anxiety. In addition, both anxiety and depression may be transient symptoms secondary to a change in environment, such as a move from the community to a nursing home or assisted-living facility.

In addition, the clinician must carefully assess the history from both patient and family, for the patient often cannot provide accurate historical information. If symptoms of depression and anxiety are brief, occurring once or twice a day, these symptoms are much less likely to respond to usual therapies, including pharmacologic therapy. If the symptoms are not particularly disturbing to the patient for most of the day, then they may best go untreated, with careful attention to their progression over time. Clinicians must take care, however, for patients may at times experience brief but extremely severe symptoms that warrant treatment.

Given that older adults with dementia are not as responsive to many psychotherapeutic interventions, treatment should be focused on a combination of environmental interventions and medication management. The types of effective environmental approaches cover a wide range, including physical activity, keeping a light on in the room, sitting quietly with the elder, changing seating arrangements in a long-term care facility, and redirecting elders toward activities that change the focus of their concentration away from anxiety-provoking or depression-provoking stimuli. These interventions are usually initiated by family members and/or nursing personnel, if the elder is in a long-term care facility. Nursing staff should develop care plans that address the problems when they arise. Unfortunately, nursing staff are often pressed beyond their capabilities and may not have the time for comprehensive planning, much less the time to implement these plans. Physicians can assist by suggesting to family members means of interacting with the depressed or anxious elder still living at home (135). In fact, most clinical visits with depressed or anxious and demented elders should include enough time with the family alone to discuss such interventions. The patient will rarely prohibit the family from talking with the physician.

The extant literature contains virtually no studies that specifically address the control of anxiety apart from agitation in double-blind, placebo-controlled trials. Rather, a number of studies document improvement in anxiety, along with a number of other symptoms, when using antidepressant medications in patients with dementia. For example, a small study found fluvoxamine improved confusion, anxiety, fear-panic, and depression in demented elders (136). Citalopram has also been shown in a controlled trial to improve a number of symptoms, including anxiety, fear and panic (137). Some herbal medicines, especially gingko biloba, have been shown to improve symptoms across a number of domains, including the improvement of anxiety and depression (138).

For the most part, however, anxiety in dementia is often very difficult to distinguish from agitation. The treatment of agitation in dementia will not be covered here, except to note that agitation is treated with a wide variety of agents, including both antipsychotic and antianxiety agents. The doses used are lower than in younger people or in elders without dementia. Dosing, however, must be tailored to the patient.

The efficacy of pharmacologic treatment for depression in dementia with antidepressant therapy has been established for over 15 years (139,140), yet the number of conclusive studies remains limited. In one study, sertraline (in doses starting at 25 mg daily and increased to up to 150 mg per day) was found efficacious in treating depression in

AD. In addition to improving mood, the drug treatment was accompanied by lessened behavioral disturbances and improved ADL. Cognition, however, did not improve (141).

The sertraline study is typical, in that mood improves with antidepressant therapy in comorbid depression and dementia, though usually less dramatically than with depression alone. In addition, other behaviors that may accompany both depression and dementia, such as agitation and other behavioral disturbances, also improve. Cognition, however, does not typically improve. In contrast, when cognitive impairment is a direct symptom of the depression (not the dementia), both mood and cognition can improve (142). In one study, the investigators found that conceptualization and initiation/perseveration improved with antidepressant treatment of depression, but that overall cognitive functioning—particularly memory—did not improve (143). This suggests that antidepressants have little impact on cognition, other than cognitive dysfunction directly related to the depressive affect. Other antidepressants, including imipramine, citalopram, and mianserin, have been found effective in the treatment of depression in mild-to-moderate dementia (144,145). Nevertheless, the use of tricyclic antidepressants, such as imipramine, often cause increased cognitive dysfunction due to their greater frequency of anticholinergic side effects. More appropriate options include SSRIs, venlafaxine, mirtazapine, and bupropion.

Other agents have been used to treat depression in dementia. In one uncontrolled study, the calcium channel antagonist, nimodipine, was shown to have some antidepressant effect (146). As noted previously, gingko biloba has also shown some benefit in improving both mood and cognitive function, but larger studies are needed (138).

Psychotherapy has been shown to be an effective treatment of depression in late life, both alone and in combination with pharmacotherapy (147,148). No controlled trials of the efficacy of psychotherapy for the treatment of anxiety disorders in late life could be found in a MedLine search of the literature over the past 10 years. The efficacy of psychotherapy in anxiety and/or depression among the demented has not been documented. Some have argued that psychotherapy should be explored more extensively as a therapy among patients in long-term care facilities, yet warn that careful assessment of cognitive status and function will be critical in determining whether the older adult can benefit from either group or individual psychotherapy (135). Well-trained volunteers may be the most appropriate therapists for the demented in long-term care.

Though dementing illness compromises higher intellectual processes, some evidence has emerged of continued activity of affective life in midbrain areas (135,149). One cognitive strategy is that memory training may improve mood, perhaps through the social interaction as much as anything (150). Cognitive techniques, however, may be less effective, although affectively-oriented strategies may

be effective (151). This type of subvocal therapy may require more, not less, skill on the part of the therapist.

Group therapy may be of particular value in long-term care. Patients can usually be easily encouraged to join the groups, and the logistics of arranging a time and place are much easier to manage (135). Groups can also serve as vital settings to form and nourish relationships, even among the moderately demented.

REFERENCES

1. Bartels SJ, Horn SD, Smout RJ, et al. Agitation and depression in frail nursing home elderly patients with dementia: treatment characteristics and service use. *Am J Geriatr Psychiatry.* 2003; 11(2):231–238.
2. Porter VR, Buxton WG, Fairbanks LA, et al. Frequency and characteristics of anxiety among patients with Alzheimer's disease and related dementias. *J Neuropsychiatry Clin Neurosci.* 2003;15(2):180–186.
3. Ganguli M, Dodge H, Mulsant B. Rates and predictors of mortality in an aging, rural, community-based cohort: the role of depression. *Arch Gen Psychiatry.* 2002;59(11):1046–1052.
4. Aarsland D, Larsen J, Karlsen K, Lim N, Tandberg E. Mental symptoms in Parkinson's disease are important contributors to caregiver distress. *Int J Geriatr Psychiatry.* 1999;14(10):866–874.
5. Reisberg B, Auer S, Monteiro I, Boksay I, Sclan S. Behavioral disturbances of dementia: an overview of phenomenology and methodologic concerns. *Int Psychogeriatr.* 1996;8(2):169–180.
6. Cole MG, Dendukuri N. Risk factors for depression among elderly community subjects: a systematic review and meta-analysis. *Am J Psychiatry.* 2003;160:1147–1156.
7. Blazer DG. Depression in late life: review and commentary. *J Gerontol A Biol Sci Med Sci.* 2003;58(3):M249–M265.
8. Finkel SI, Costa e Silva J, Cohen GD, Miller S, Sartorius N. Behavioral and psychological symptoms of dementia: a consensus statement on current knowledge and implications for research and treatment. *Am J Geriar Psychiatry.* 1998;6:97–100.
9. Alexopoulos GS. Clinical and biological interactions in affective and cognitive geriatric syndromes. *Am J Psychiatry.* 2003;160(5): 811–814.
10. Evers MM, Purohit D, Perl D, Khan K, Marin DB. Palliative and aggressive end-of-life care for patients with dementia. *Psychiatr Serv.* 2002;53(5):609–613.
11. Starkstein SE, Merello M. *Psychiatric and Cognitive Disorders in Parkinson's Disease.* Cambridge, U.K.: University Press; 2002.
12. Blazer D. *Depression in Late Life.* 3rd ed. New York: Springer; 2002.
13. NIH Consensus Conference. Diagnosis and treatment of depression of late life. *JAMA.* 1992;268:1018–1024.
14. Cole MG, Yaffe K. Pathway to psychiatric care of the elderly with depression. *Int J Geriatr Psychiatry.* 1996;11:157–161.
15. Regier D, Boyd J, Burke J, et al. One-month prevalence of mental disorders in the United States. Based on five epidemiologic catchment area sites. *Arch Gen Psychiatry.* 1988;45:977–986.
16. van Balkom A, Beekman A, de Beurs E, Deeg D, van Dyck R, van Tilburg W. Comorbidity of the anxiety disorders in a community-based older population in the Netherlands. *Acta Psychiatr Scand.* 2000;101:37–45.
17. Forsell V, Winblad B. Incidence of major depression in a very elderly population. *Int J Geriatr Psychiatry.* 1999;14:368–372.
18. Regier D, Farmer M, Rae D, et al. Comorbidity of mental disorders with alcohol and other drug abuse. Results from the Epidemiologic Catchment Area (ECA) Study. *JAMA.* 1990;264:2511–2518.
19. Beekman ATF, de Beurs E, van Balkom AJLM, Deeg DJH, van Dyck R, van Tilburg W. Anxiety and depression in later life: co-occurrence and communality of risk factors. *Am J Psychiatry.* 2000;157(1):89–95.
20. Lenze EJ, Mulsant BH, Shear MK, et al. Comorbid anxiety disorders in depressed elderly patients. *Am J Psychiatry.* 2000;157: 722–728.

21. Evans D, Funkenstein H, Albert M. Prevalence of Alzheimer's disease in a community population of older persons: higher than previously reported. *JAMA.* 1989;262:2551–2556.
22. Jorm A, Korten A, Henderson A. The prevalence of dementia: a quantitative integration of the literature. *Acta Psychiatr Scand.* 1987;76:465–479.
23. O'Brien J, Erkinjuntti T, Reisberg B, et al. Vascular cognitive impairment. *Lancet Neurol.* 2003;2(2):89–98.
24. McPherson SE, Cummings JL. Neuropsychological aspects of vascular dementia. *Brain Cogn.* 1996;31(2):269–282.
25. Srikanth VK, Thrift AG, Saling MM, et al. Increased risk of cognitive impairment 3 months after mild to moderate first-ever stroke: a community-based prospective study of nonaphasic English-speaking survivors. *Stroke.* 2003;34(5):1136–1143.
26. Desmond DW, Moroney JT, Sano M, Stern Y, Merino JG. Incidence of dementia after ischemic stroke: results of a longitudinal study [editorial comment]. *Stroke.* 2002;33(9):2254–2262.
27. Korczyn A. Dementia in Parkinson's disease. *J Neurol.* 2001;248(3):1–4.
28. Korczyn A. Dementia in Parkinson's disease. In: Fisher A, Hanin I, Lachman C, eds. *Alzheimer's and Parkinson's Disease: Strategies for Research and Development.* New York: Plenum Press; 1986:177–189.
29. Aarsland D, Tandberg E, Larsen JP, Cummings JL. Frequency of dementia in Parkinson disease. *Arch Neurol.* 1996;53:538–542.
30. Absher JR, Cumming E. Cognitive and noncognitive aspects of dementia syndromes: an overview. In: Burns A, Levy R, eds. *Dementia.* London: Chapman and Hall; 1994:59–76.
31. Orrell M, Bebbington P. Psychosocial stress and anxiety in senile dementia. *J Affect Disord.* 1996;39(3):165–73.
32. Wands K, Merskey H, Hachinski V, Fisman M, Fox H, Boniferro M. A questionnaire investigation of anxiety and depression in early dementia. *J Am Geriatr Soc.* 1990;38(5):535–538.
33. Tariot P. Treatment strategies for agitation and psychosis in dementia. *J Clin Psychiatry.* 1996;57(14):21–29.
34. Tariot P, Blazina L. The psychopathology of dementia. In: Morris J, ed. *Handbook of Dementing Illnesses.* New York: Marcel Dekker, Inc.; 1994:461–475.
35. Olin J, Katz I, Meyers B, Schneider L, Lebowitz B. Provisional diagnostic criteria for depression of Alzheimer disease: rationale and background. *Am J Geriatr Psychiatry.* 2002;10:129–141.
36. Olin J, Schneider L, Katz I, et al. Provisional diagnostic criteria for depression of Alzheimer Disease. *Am J Geriatr Psychiatry.* 2002;10:125–128.
37. Zubenko GS, Zubenko WN, McPherson S, et al. A collaborative study of the emergence and clinical features of the major depressive syndrome of Alzheimer's disease. *Am J Psychiatry.* 2003;160(5):857–866.
38. Cummings JL, Miller B, Hill MA, Neshkes R. Neuropsychiatric aspects of multi-infarct dementia and dementia of the Alzheimer type. *Arch Neurol.* 1987;44(4):389–393.
39. Kim J, Lyons D, Shin I, Yoon J. Differences in the behavioral and psychological symptoms between Alzheimer's disease and vascular dementia: are the different pharmacologic treatment strategies justifiable? *Hum Psychopharmacol.* 2003;18(3):215–220.
40. Ballard C, Bannister C, Solis M, Oyebode F, Wilcock G. The prevalence, associations and symptoms of depression amongst dementia sufferers. *J Affect Disord.* 1996;36(3–4):135–144.
41. Sultzer D, Levin H, Mahler M, High W, Cummings J. A comparison of psychiatric symptoms in vascular dementia and Alzheimer's disease. *Am J Psychiatry.* 1993;150(12):1806–1812.
42. Wade D, Legh-Smith J, Hewer R. Depressed mood after stroke. A community study of its frequency. *Br J Psychiatry.* 1987;151(2):200–205.
43. Robinson R, Starr L, Kubos K, Price T. A two-year longitudinal study of post-stroke mood disorders: findings during the initial evaluation. *Stroke.* 1983;14(5):736–741.
44. Blazer D. *Depression in Late Life.* St. Louis, MO: Mosby; 1994.
45. Sano M, Stern Y, Williams J, Cote L, Rosenstein R, Mayeux R. Coexisting dementia and depression in Parkinson's disease. *Arch Neurol.* 1989;46:1284–1286.
46. Cole S, Woodard J, Juncos J, Kogos J, Youngstrom E, Watts R. Depression and disability in Parkinson's disease. *J Neuropsychiatry Clin Neurosci.* 1996;8(1):20–25.
47. Aarsland D, Larsen JP, Lim N, et al. Range of neuropsychiatric disturbances in patients with Parkinson's disease. *J Neurol Neurosurg Psychiatry.* 1999;67:492–496.
48. Jost B, Grossberg G. The evolution of psychiatric symptoms in Alzheimer's disease: a natural history study. *J Am Geriatr Soc.* 1996;44(9):1078–1081.
49. Mega M, Cummings J, Fiorello T, et al. The spectrum of behavioral changes in Alzheimer's disease. *Neurology.* 1996;46:130–135.
50. Krishnan K, McDonald W, Doraiswamy P, et al. Neuroanatomical substrates of depression in the elderly. *Eur Arch Psychiatry Clin Neurosci.* 1993;243:41–46.
51. Alexopoulos G, Meyers B, Young R, Mattis S, Kakuma T. The course of geriatric depression with "reversible dementia": a controlled study. *Am J Psychiatry.* 1993;150:1693–1699.
52. Lanctot K, Herrmann N, Eryavec G, van Reekum R, Reed K, Naranjo C. Central serotonergic activity is related to the aggressive behaviors of Alzheimer's disease. *Neuropsychopharmacology.* 2002;27(4):646–654.
53. Zubenko G, Moossy J. Major depression in primary dementia. Clinical and neuropathologic correlates. *Arch Neurol.* 1988;45:1182–1186.
54. Tsai S. Brain-derived neurotrophic factor: a bridge between major depression and Alzheimer's disease? *Med Hypotheses.* 2003;61(1):110–113.
55. Pearlson G, Ross C, Lohr W, Rovner B, Chase G, Folstein M. Association between family history of affective disorder and the depressive syndrome of Alzheimer's disease. *Am J Psychiatry.* 1990;147(4):452–456.
56. Fahim S, van Duijn C, Baker F, et al. A study of familial aggregation of depression, dementia and Parkinson's disease. *Eur J Epidemiol.* 1998;14(3):233–238.
57. Heun R, Papassotiropoulos A, Jessen F, Maier W, Breitner J. A family study of Alzheimer disease and early- and late-onset depression in elderly patients. *Arch Gen Psychiatry.* 2001;58:190–196.
58. Butt ZA, Strauss ME. Relationship of family and personal history to the occurrence of depression in persons with Alzheimer's disease. *Am J Geriatr Psychiatry.* 2001;9(3):249–254.
59. Rovner B, Broadhead J, Spencer M, Carson K, Folstein M. Depression and Alzheimer's disease. *Am J Psychiatry.* 1989;146(3):350–353.
60. Green RC, Cupples LA, Kurz A, et al. Depression as a risk factor for Alzheimer disease: the MIRAGE study. *Arch Neurol.* 2003;60(5):753–759.
61. Berger A, Small B, Forsell Y, Winblad B, Backman L. Preclinical symptoms of major depression in very old age: a prospective longitudinal study. *Am J Psychiatry.* 1998;155:1039–1043.
62. Chen P, Ganguli M, Mulsant B, DeKosky S. The temporal relationship between depressive symptoms and dementia: a community-based prospective study. *Arch Gen Psychiatry.* 1999;56:261–266.
63. Bassuk SS, Berkman LF, Wypij D. Depressive symptomatology and incident cognitive decline in an elderly community sample. *Arch Gen Psychiatry.* 1998;55(12):1073–1081.
64. Alexopoulos G, Young R, Meyer B. Geriatric depression: age of onset and dementia. *Biol Psychiatry.* 1993;34:141–145.
65. Devanand D, Sano M, Tang M-X, et al. Depressed mood and the incidence of Alzheimer's disease in the elderly living in the community. *Arch Gen Psychiatry.* 1996;53:175–182.
66. Steffens D, Plassman B, Helms M, et al. A twin study of late-onset depression and apolipoprotein epsilon 4 as a risk factor for Alzheimer's disease. 1997;41:851–856.
67. Geerlings M, Schoevers R, Beekman A, et al. Depression and the risk of cognitive decline and Alzheimer's disease: results of two prospective community-based studies in the Netherlands. *Br J Psychiatry.* 2000;176:568–575.
68. Ritchie K, Gilham C, Ledesert B, Touchon J, Kotzki P-O. Depressive illness, depressive symptomology and regional cerebral blood flow in elderly people with sub-clinical cognitive impairment. *Age Ageing.* 1999;28:385–391.
69. Speck C, Kukull W, Brenner D, et al. History of depression as a risk factor for Alzheimer's disease. *Epidemiology.* 1995;6:366–369.
70. Krishnan K, McDonald W, Escalona P, et al. Magnetic imaging of the caudate nuclei in depression: preliminary observation. *Arch Gen Psychiatry.* 1992;49:553–557.

71. Husain M, McDonald W, Doraiswamy P, et al. A magnetic resonance imaging study of putamen nuclei in major depression. *Psychiatry Res.* 1991;40:95–99.

72. Lai T, Payne M, Byrum C, Steffens D, Krishnan K. Reduction of orbital frontal cortex volume in geriatric depression. *Biol Psychiatry.* 2000;48:971–975.

73. Steffens D, Payne M, Greenberg D, et al. Hippocampal volume and incident dementia in geriatric depression. *Am J Geriatr Psychiatry.* 2002;10:62–71.

74. Hickie I, Scott E, Naismith S, et al. Late-onset depression: genetic, vascular and clinical contributions. *Psychol Med.* 2001; 31:1403–1412.

75. Desmond D, Moroney J, Lynch T, Chan S, Chin S, Mohr J. The natural history of CADASIL: a pooled analysis of previously published cases. *Stroke.* 1999;30:1230–1233.

76. Krishnan K. Biological risk factors in late life depression. *Biol Psychiatry.* 2002;52:185–192.

77. Herrmann M, Bartels C, Schumacher M, Wallesch C-W. Poststroke depression: is there a pathoanatomic correlate for depression in the postacute stage of stroke? *Stroke.* 1995;26:850–856.

78. Beblo T, Wallesch C, Herrmann M. The crucial role of frontostriatal circuits for depressive disorders in the postacute stage after stroke. *Neuropsychiatry Neuropsychol Behav Neurol.* 1999;12(4):236–246.

79. Robins A. Are stroke patients more depressed than other disabled subjects? *J Chronic Dis.* 1976;29:479–482.

80. Aben I, Verhey F, Strik J, Lousberg R, Lodder J, Honig A. A comparative study into the one year cumulative incidence of depression after stroke and myocardial infarction. *J Neurol Neurosurg Psychiatry.* 2003;74(5):581–585.

81. Leentjens A, Van den Akker M, Metsemakers J, Lousberg R, Verhey F. Higher incidence of depression preceding the onset of Parkinson's disease: a register study. *Mov Disord.* 2003;18(4): 414–418.

82. Flemming M, Nilsson FM, Kessing LV. Depression as a risk factor for Parkinson's disease? [e-letter to the Editor]. *Neurology.* Online 2002. Available at: http://www.neurology.org/cgi/eletters/58/10/1501. Accessed August 2003.

83. Cummings J. Depression and Parkinson's disease: a review. *Am J Psychiatry.* 1992;149(4):443–454.

84. Becker T, Becker G, Seufert J, et al. Parkinson's disease and depression: evidence for an alteration of the basal limbic system detected by transcranial sonography. *J Neurol Neurosurg Psychiatry.* 1997;63:590–595.

85. McDonald W, Richard I, DeLong M. Prevalence, etiology, and treatment of depression in Parkinson's disease. *Biol Psychiatry.* 2003;54(3):363–375.

86. Schrag A, Jahanshahi M, Quinn N. What contributes to depression in Parkinson's disease? *Psychol Med.* 2001;31(1):65–73.

87. Vance DE, Burgio LD, Roth DL, Stevens AB, Fairchild JK, Yurick A. Predictors of agitation in nursing home residents. *J Gerontol B Psychol Sci Soc Sci.* 2003;58(2):P129–P137.

88. Cummings JL. Cholinesterase inhibitors: a new class of psychotropic compounds. *Am J Psychiatry.* 2000;157:4–15.

89. Reisberg B, Ferris S, Franssen E. An ordinal functional assessment tool for Alzheimer's-type dementia. *Hosp Community Psychiatry.* 1985;36(6):593–595.

90. Forsell Y, Jorm A, Winblad B. Variation in psychiatric and behavioural symptoms at different stages of dementia: data from physicians' examinations and informants' reports. *Dementia.* 1993;4(5):282–286.

91. Orrell M, Bebbington P. Life events and senile dementia. I. Admission, deterioration and social environment change. *Psychol Med.* 1995;25(2):373–386.

92. Orrell M, Bebbington P. Life events and senile dementia. Affective symptoms. *Br J Psychiatry.* 1995;166(5):613–620.

93. Blazer D. Impact of late-life depression on the social network. *Am J Psychiatry.* 1983;140:162–166.

94. Orrell M, Bebbington P. Social factors and psychiatric admission for senile dementia. *Int J Geriatr Psychiatry.* 1995;10(4): 313–323.

95. Orrell M, Butler R, Bebbington P. Social factors and the outcome of dementia. *Int J Geriatr Psychiatry.* 2000;15(6): 515–520.

96. Karlawish J, Clark C. Diagnostic evaluation of elderly patients with mild memory problems. *Ann Intern Med.* 2003;138(5): 411–419.

97. Knott P, Fleminger J. Presenile dementia: the difficulties of early diagnosis. *Acta Psychiatr Scand.* 1975;51:210–217.

98. Starkstein SE, Petracca G, Chemerinski E, Merello M. Prevalence and correlates of parkinsonism in patients with primary depression. *Neurology.* 2001;57(3):553–555.

99. Wells C. Pseudodementia. *Am J Psychiatry.* 1979;136:895–900.

100. Kahn R. The mental health system and the future aged. *Gerontologist.* 1975;15:24–31.

101. Feehan M, Knight RG, Partridge FM. Cognitive complaint and test performance in elderly patients suffering depression or dementia. *Int J Geriatr Psychiatry.* 1991;6(5):287–293.

102. Reynolds C, Hoch C, Kupfer D, et al. Bedside differentiation of depressive pseudodementia from dementia. *Am J Psychiatry.* 1988;145:1099–1103.

103. Lazarus L, Newton N, Cohler B, Lesser J. Frequency in presentation of depressive symptoms in patients with primary degenerative dementia. *Am J Psychiatry.* 1987;144:41–45.

104. Ready RE, Ott BR, Grace J, Cahn-Weiner DA. Apathy and executive dysfunction in mild cognitive impairment and Alzheimer disease. *Am J Geriatr Psychiatry.* 2003;11(2):222–228.

105. Chemerinski E, Petracca G, Sabe L, Kremer J, Starkstein S. The specificity of depressive symptoms in patients with Alzheimer's disease. *Am J Psychiatry.* 2001;(158):68–72.

106. Paterniti S, Verdier-Taillefer MH, Dufouil C, Alperovitch A. Depressive symptoms and cognitive decline in elderly people: longitudinal study. *Br J Psychiatry.* 2002;181(5):406–410.

107. Kraaij V, de Wilde E. Negative life events and depressive symptoms in the elderly: a life span perspective. *Aging Ment Health.* 2001;5:84–91.

108. Buerger K, Zinkowski R, Teipel SJ, et al. Differentiation of geriatric major depression from Alzheimer's disease with CSF tau protein phosphorylated at threonine 231. *Am J Psychiatry.* 2003;160(2):376–379.

109. American Psychiatric Association. *Diagnostic and Statistical Manual of Mental Disorders.* 4th ed. Text Revision. Washington, D.C.: American Psychiatric Association; 2000.

110. Lipsey J, Spencer W, Rabins P, Robinson R. Phenomenological comparison of poststroke depression and functional depression. *Am J Psychiatry.* 1986;143(4):527–529.

111. Horne A. Mood disorders after stroke: a review of the evidence. *Int J Geriatr Soc.* 1987;2:211–221.

112. Bolla-Wilson K, Robinson R, Starkstein S, Boston J, Price T. Lateralization of dementia of depression in stroke patients. *Am J Psychiatry.* 1989;146(5):627–634.

113. Alexopoulos G, Meyers B, Young R, Campbell S, Silbersweig D, Charlson M. "Vascular depression" hypothesis. *Arch Gen Psychiatry.* 1997;54:915–922.

114. Krishnan K, Hays J, Blazer D. MRI-defined vascular depression. *Am J Psychiatry.* 1997;154:497–501.

115. Salloway S, Malloy P, Kohn R, et al. MRI and neuropsychological differences in early- and late-life-onset geriatric depression. *Neurology.* 1996;46:1567–1574.

116. Fahn S. Description of Parkinson's disease as a clinical syndrome. *Ann NY Acad Sci.* 2003;991(1):1–14.

117. Rao G, Fisch L, Srinivasan S, et al. Does this patient have Parkinson disease? *JAMA.* 2003;289(3):347–353.

118. Leentjens AFG, Marinus J, Van Hilten JJ, Lousberg R, Verhey FRJ. The contribution of somatic symptoms to the diagnosis of depressive disorder in Parkinson's disease: a discriminant analytic approach. *Neuropsychiatry Clin Neurosci.* 2003;15:74–77.

119. Brown R, MacCarthy B. Psychiatric morbidity in patients with Parkinson's disease. *Psychol Med.* 1990;20(1):77–87.

120. Schiffer R, Kurlan R, Rubin A, Boer S. Evidence for atypical depression in Parkinson's disease. *Am J Psychiatry.* 1988;145(8): 1020–1022.

121. Pluck GC, Brown RG. Apathy in Parkinson's disease. *J Neurol Neurosurg Psychiatry.* 2002;73:636–642.

122. Cohen-Mansfield J, Billig N. Agitated behaviors in the elderly: a conceptual review. *J Am Geriatr Soc.* 1986;34(10):711–721.

123. Lyketsos CG, Steele C, Galik E, et al. Physical aggression in dementia patients and its relationship to depression. *Am J Psychiatry.* 1999;156:66–71.

124. Copeland M, Daly E, Hines V, et al. Psychiatric symptomatology and prodromal Alzheimer's disease. *Alzheimer Dis Assoc Disord.* 2003;17(1):1–8.

125. Kinosian BP, Stallard E, Lee JH, Woodbury MA, Zbrozek AS, Glick HA. Predicting 10-year care requirements for older people with suspected Alzheimer's disease. *J Am Geriatr Soc.* 2000;48(6): 631–638.

126. Cohen-Mansfield J, Werner P. Longitudinal changes in behavioral problems in old age: a study in an adult day care population. *J Gerontol A Biol Sci Med Science.* 1998;53(1):65–71.

127. O'Donnell B, Drachman D, Barnes H, Peterson K, Swearer J, Lew RA. Incontinence and troublesome behaviors predict institutionalization in dementia. *J Geriatr Psychiatry Neurol.* 1992;5(1): 45–52.

128. Levy M, Cummings J, Fairbanks L, Bravi D, Calvani M, Carta A. Longitudinal assessment of symptoms of depression, agitation, and psychosis in 181 patients with Alzheimer's disease. *Am J Psychiatry.* 1996;153(11):1438–1443.

129. Williams S. Reason, emotion and embodiment: is 'mental' health a contradiction of terms? In: Bushfield J, ed. *Rethinking the Sociology of Mental Health.* London: Blackwell; 2001:17–38.

130. Garre-Olmo J, Lopez-Pousa S, Vilalta-Franch J, et al. Evolution of depressive symptoms in Alzheimer disease: one-year follow-up. *Alzheimer Dis Assoc Disord.* 2003;17(2):77–85.

131. Reynolds C, Kupper L, Hoch C, Stack J, Houck P. Two-year follow-up of elderly patients with mixed depression and dementia: clinical electroencephalographic sleep findings. *J Am Geriatr Soc.* 1986;34:793–799.

132. Lopez O, Boller F, Becker J, Miller M, Reynolds C. Alzheimer's disease and depression: neuropsychological impairment and progression of the illness. *Am J Psychiatry.* 1990;147(7): 855–860.

133. Hoch CC, Reynolds CF, Buysse DJ, Fasiczka AL. Two-year survival in patients with mixed symptoms of depression and cognitive impairment: comparison with major depression and primary degenerative dementia. *Am J Geriatr Psychiatry.* 1993;1(1):59–66.

134. Robinson R, Price T. Post-stroke depressive disorders: a follow-up study of 103 patients. *Stroke.* 1982;13:635–641.

135. Lichtenberg P. Psychological assessment and psychotherapy in long-term care. *Clin Psychol Science and Practice.* 2000;7: 317–328.

136. Olafsson K, Jorgensen S, Jensen H, Bille A, Arup P, Andersen J. Fluvoxamine in the treatment of demented elderly patients: a double-blind, placebo-controlled trial. *Acta Psychiatr Scand.* 1992;85:453–456.

137. Nyth A, Gottfries C. The clinical efficacy of citalopram in treatment of emotional disturbances in dementia disorders. A Nordic multicentre study. *Br J Psychiatry.* 1990;157:894–901.

138. Beaubrun G, Gray G. A review of herbal medicines for psychiatric disorders. *Psychiatr Serv.* 2000;51:1130–1134.

139. Reifler B, Larson E, Henley R. Coexistence of cognitive impairment and depression in geriatric outpatients. *Am J Psychiatry.* 1982;139:623–626.

140. Bains J, Birks J, Dening T. The efficacy of antidepressants in the treatment of depression in dementia. *Cochrane Database Syst Rev.* 2002;(4):CD003944.

141. Lyketsos C, DelCampo L, Steinberg M, et al. Treating depression in Alzheimer disease. *Arch Gen Psychiatry.* 2003;60:737–746.

142. Alexopoulos G, Meyers B, Young R, et al. Recovery in geriatric depression. *Arch Gen Psychiatry.* 1996;53:305–312.

143. Butters M, Becker J, Nebes R, Zmuda M, Mulsant B, Pollock B, Reynolds C III. Changes in cognitive functioning following treatment of late-life depression. *Am J Psychiatry.* 2000;157: 1949–1954.

144. Reifler B, Teri L, Raskind M, Veith R, Barnes R. Double-blind trial of imipramine in Alzheimer's disease patients with and without depression. *Am J Psychiatry.* 1989;146:45–49.

145. Karlsson I, Godderis J, Augusto De Mendonca Lima C, et al. A randomized, double-blind comparison of the efficacy and safety of citalopram compared to mianserin in elderly depressed patients with or without mild to moderate dementia. *Int J Geriatr Psychiatry.* 2000;15(4):295–305.

146. De Vry J, Fritze J, Post R. The management of coexisting depression in patients with dementia: potential of calcium channel antagonists. *Clin Neuropharmacol.* 1997;20:22–35.

147. Gallagher D, Thompson L. Treatment of major depressive disorder in older outpatients with brief psychotherapies. *Psychother Theory Res Prac.* 1982;19:482–490.

148. Reynolds C, Frank E, Perel J, et al. Nortriptyline and interpersonal psychotherapy as maintenance therapies for recurrent major depression: a randomized controlled trial in patients older than 59 years. *JAMA.* 1999;281:39–45.

149. van der Kolk B, McFarland A. The black hole of trauma. In: van der Kolk B, McFarlane A, Weisaeth L, eds. *Traumatic Stress: The Effects of Overwhelming Experience on Mind, Body and Society.* New York: Guilford Press; 1996:3–23.

150. Chiu M. Memory training for older adult medical patients in a primary health care setting. In: Duffy M, ed. *Handbook of Counseling and Psychotherapy with Older Adults.* New York: Wiley; 1999:614–631.

151. Duffy M. Reaching the person behind the dementia: treating comorbid affective disorders through subvocal and nonverbal strategies. In: Duffy M, ed. *Handbook of Counseling and Psychotherapy with Older Adults.* New York: Wiley; 1999:577–589.

Psychiatric Manifestations of Medications in the Elderly

39

Michael Kotlyar   **Catherine I. Lindblad**   **Shelly L. Gray**
Joseph T. Hanlon

CASE EXAMPLE

An 82-year-old female is referred to the geriatric clinic by her primary physician and family for evaluation of functional decline and confusion. The patient denies any problems; however, the family reports that she was in her usual state of health until approximately 3 months ago, when they noted that she had difficulty concentrating on tasks and attending to phone conversations, and occasional trouble recognizing familiar faces. As of 1 month ago, she was disoriented to time and had increasing problems with memory. She had become confused about her medication regimen (whereas she had previously managed her own medications). Her medical history includes hypothyroidism, hypertension, insomnia, osteoarthritis, seasonal rhinitis, and chronic constipation. Current medications include chlorpheniramine, levothyroxine, lisinopril, diltiazem, propoxyphene/acetaminophen, hydrochlorothiazide, clorazepate, and docusate sodium. No medical causes for these symptoms could be identified.

This case example illustrates how commonly-used medications (or drugs), when prescribed to the elderly, can lead to symptoms consistent with psychiatric disorders. The cognitive impairment observed in this patient may well have been due, at least in part, to some of the medications being used (i.e., chlorpheniramine, a highly anticholinergic antihistamine; clorazepate, a long half-life benzodi-

azepine; or propoxyphene, an opioid analgesic). Of potential concern is that psychiatric adverse events (cognitive impairment in this case) due to medications are misinterpreted in a patient as a new psychiatric problem, leading to the prescribing of a psychotropic medication. This phenomenon has been referred to as the *prescribing cascade*, and puts the elder at additional risk for adverse drug reactions due to the new psychotropic agent (1).

Nearly 12% of community-dwelling elders report use of antianxiety agents, sedatives, and hypnotics (2). Also in community settings, up to 11% are prescribed an antidepressant (3). The prevalence of antidepressant use by elders residing in long-term care facilities is higher at 35%, whereas the prevalence of antianxiety agents, sedatives, and hypnotics use is similar to that found in the community (4). In these long-term care facilities, 17% of elders are prescribed an antipsychotic agent, often to treat behavioral complications of delirium/dementia (4). The frequency with which these medications are prescribed in response to psychiatric adverse effects due to another medication has not been well-analyzed, but other lines of observational evidence suggest that certain medications are more likely to be associated with psychiatric manifestations than others.

This chapter will address three major types of psychiatric manifestations commonly related to medications in older people: cognitive impairment, insomnia, and depression. Each major section will list implicated drugs commonly used in elders, as identified by comprehensive literature searches. When available, information will be provided regarding possible mechanisms of toxicity, as well as detection, management, and prevention of these psychiatric manifestations of medication use.

DRUG-INDUCED COGNITIVE DISORDERS

Cognitive impairment in the elderly is a major public health problem, particularly in light of the aging of the population. Although the etiology of cognitive disorders is multifactorial, an important cause of reversible cognitive disorders is medication adverse effects (5,6). This review will focus on the role of medications commonly used in the elderly, which cause cognitive impairment, including delirium. Table 39-1 includes medications that have been reported in the literature.

Anticholinergic Agents

The cholinergic system is important for attention and memory processes (7). Age-related decreases in cholinergic function are likely a factor responsible for the increased sensitivity of older patients to medications with anticholinergic activity (7). For example, tests of memory are impaired to a greater extent with scopolamine in older subjects compared to younger subjects (8,9), and in patients with Alzheimer's disease (AD) compared to normal age-matched controls (10).

Medications with anticholinergic properties are a well-known cause of cognitive impairment (8–11). Many

TABLE 39-1
DRUGS/DRUG CLASSES THAT MAY CAUSE COGNITIVE DISORDERS

Anticholinergics (including histamine-H1 receptor antagonists)[a]
Antiepileptics
Antibiotics
Antiparkinsonian drugs
Antipsychotics
Barbiturates
Benzodiazepines[a]
Beta-blockers
Calcium-channel blockers
Acetylcholinesterase inhibitors
Clonidine
Corticosteroids
Cyclosporine
Digoxin
Histamine-2 (H2) receptor antagonists[a]
Lithium
Nonsteroidal anti-inflammatory drugs
Omeprazole
Opioid agonists (especially meperidine, pentazocine)[a]
Tricyclic antidepressants[a]

---

[a]Clinically important based on sufficient information and discussed in text. (Adapted from references 7, 133–135.)

medications with anticholinergic effects are commonly used in older patients, including certain antiarrhythmics, tricyclic antidepressants (TCAs), antipsychotics, first-generation antihistamines, and urinary antispasmodics. Diphenhydramine, a common over-the-counter (OTC) antihistamine medication used by older adults for insomnia, has been found to impair attention, short-term verbal memory, concentration, and reaction time in older volunteers, and to cause delirium in elderly hospitalized patients (11–13). In healthy younger patients, second-generation antihistamines (e.g., loratadine, fexofenadine) cause less sedation and cognitive impairment, and are therefore preferable choices for the elderly, provided no contraindications exist (14,15). Oxybutynin, a medication often used to treat overactive bladder in older adults, has also been found to impair several tests of cognition and to cause delirium (11,16). It is not clear whether newer extended-release or transdermal formulations are more or less likely to cause cognitive impairment. Tolterodine, an alternative to oxybutynin, is less likely to penetrate the central nervous system (CNS); however, this medication may also cause delirium (17). Some agents traditionally not considered to have anticholinergic effects (e.g., histamine-2 receptor antagonists [H2RAs], furosemide, digoxin, and codeine) may have serum anticholinergic activity, and they exhibit reversal of cognitive effects with the administration of physostigmine, a cholinergic agonist (18–22).

Benzodiazepines

Benzodiazepines have a wide range of CNS effects such as sedation, drowsiness, memory difficulties, and lack of coordination. But the sedative properties of benzodiazepines do not fully explain these impairments (23). Older adults are likely to have increased risk for adverse effects of benzodiazepines because of the age-related changes in pharmacokinetic and pharmacodynamic parameters observed for many of these medications.

Short-term clinical studies have indicated that benzodiazepines have acute effects on attention, memory, and psychomotor performance (24–26). The long-term effects of benzodiazepine use on cognition are more difficult to quantify. In a study of 308 patients with suspected dementia, the cognitive impairment was attributed in 13 patients to chronic benzodiazepine use (6). A cohort study of community-dwelling elders found that benzodiazepine users were more likely to have memory problems than nonusers. Those taking higher doses were particularly at risk, and users of both short and long half-life agents were at greater risk (27). Another large epidemiological study has also found that chronic users of benzodiazepines are at higher risk for cognitive decline (28).

Use of benzodiazepines in hospitalized patients has been associated with increased risk for delirium in some, but not all, studies (29–31). In one study, patients taking benzodiazepines were approximately three times more likely to develop delirium after surgery compared to nonusers (29). Users of long-acting benzodiazepines were significantly more likely to experience delirium compared to nonusers or those using short-acting agents. Importantly, risk of delirium was higher in those taking higher doses of benzodiazepines (29). Delirium may also occur in hospitalized patients with the inadvertent sudden withdrawal of short-acting benzodiazepines. Alternative agents for the treatment of anxiety (e.g., buspirone, a selective serotonin reuptake inhibitor [SSRI]) or insomnia (e.g., zolpidem or zaleplon) may therefore be better options for older adults, although case reports of delirium also have been reported for zolpidem (32–34).

Antidepressants

Cognitive impairment can be a manifestation of depression. The treatment of depression often results in improvement in cognitive abilities; however, side effects of antidepressants may mask or blunt this improvement. TCAs cause cognitive dysfunction, including delirium, primarily through their anticholinergic effects (7,35). SSRIs are not generally associated with delirium, but can cause this problem as part of the *serotonergic syndrome*, although this most frequently occurs when SSRIs are used in combination with other serotonergic agents (e.g., TCAs, trazodone, nefazodone) or monoamine oxidase inhibitors (MAOIs).

Of all the antidepressants, TCAs are the most likely to cause impaired cognition. Amitriptyline is associated with reduced reaction time, impaired retrieval from secondary memory (36), and impaired information processing. However, even TCAs with lower anticholinergic properties (e.g., nortriptyline) can cause deficits in cognition (38). SSRIs have minimal effects on cognition and may even improve specific measurements of cognition (7,37,39). SSRIs appear to be well-tolerated in patients with cognitive decline/dementia (40,41). Little is known about the cognitive effects of newer antidepressants (e.g., nefazodone, venlafaxine, mirtazapine, bupropion).

Opioid Analgesics

Patients not receiving effective pain control are more likely to develop delirium, indicating the importance of adequately treating pain (42). Meperidine has an active metabolite, normeperidine (half-life of 15 to 30 hours), which can accumulate in elderly patients with renal insufficiency and is associated with CNS toxicity. Meperidine also has weak anticholinergic activity (7). The route of opioid administration may play a role in the risk for delirium. In two studies, epidural (29) and intramuscular administration (43) of opioids resulted in higher risk of confusion/delirium when compared to patient-controlled analgesia.

Opioid use was associated with delirium in three of six large prospective studies of hospitalized patients (29,30,42). In two studies, meperidine was the only opioid that increased risk for delirium, resulting in twofold to threefold greater risk in patients post hip fracture (42) or following surgery (29). Pentazocine, a partial agonist-antagonist, can precipitate psychiatric reactions in as many as 10% of patients (44). Therefore, it is prudent to avoid the use of meperidine and pentazocine for pain control in elders.

Antiepileptics

Patients with epilepsy have impaired cognitive performance compared to healthy controls matched for age and education. Multiple factors may adversely affect cognitive function in patients with epilepsy, including the underlying pathology of epilepsy, severity and frequency of seizures, and adverse events from the antiepileptic drugs (AEDs) (45). AEDs probably result in cognitive impairment by reducing neuronal excitability.

AEDs may impair attention, vigilance, and psychomotor speed. Successful management of seizure disorders will actually improve cognition, which may partially offset any untoward effects of the therapy. Many studies have assessed the cognitive effects of AEDs in patients and healthy volunteers; however, many of the patient studies are difficult to interpret because of flaws in the study design. A large Veterans Affairs (VA) Cooperative study that compared carbamazepine, phenytoin, primidone, and phenobarbital in adult patients with new-onset epilepsy found no consistent pattern on tests of cognition, and little change between pre-AED and post-AED treatment (46). A second VA Cooperative study found no difference in cognitive effects between carbamazepine and valproate after 1 year of therapy (47). Well-conducted studies in healthy volunteers have demonstrated modest negative cognitive effects (e.g., reaction time, motor speed, memory) of carbamazepine, phenytoin, and valproate (48,49); however, the effects of phenobarbital seem to be more pronounced. Although few head-to-head comparisons have been conducted with the newer AEDs, gabapentin and lamotrigine seem to result in fewer cognitive deficits when compared to carbamazepine (50–52). In general, use of monotherapy and maintaining serum levels within the therapeutic range will minimize cognitive problems in most patients (45). Nonetheless, all AEDs have dose-related adverse effects and should be monitored appropriately.

Antihypertensives

Hypertension is associated with increased risk for both vascular dementia and AD (53,54). Moreover, a number of studies suggest an inverse relationship between hypertension and cognitive functioning (55–57). Use of alpha-methyldopa, clonidine, or reserpine may be related to cognitive impairment by affecting the catecholamine system (58,59). Diuretics may result in delirium if the patient becomes dehydrated.

The evidence for a negative effect of antihypertensives on dementia is less compelling because much of it is derived from case reports and observational studies. Case reports suggest that antihypertensives may be a cause of cognitive impairment, with beta-blockers (e.g., propranolol), diuretics (e.g., hydrochlorothiazide), and alpha blockers (e.g., methyldopa) most commonly cited (6). Initial reports suggested that lipophilic beta-blockers (e.g., propranolol) had a greater risk of CNS effects than hydrophilic agents (e.g., atenolol) because of greater penetration into the CNS; however, other studies have disputed these findings (58,59) and the overall incidence of beta-blocker-induced cognitive impairment is rare (59–62).

The effect of calcium-channel blockers on cognition is unclear. Evidence from epidemiological surveys suggests that these medications decrease cognitive function (63,64). However, a large randomized, double-blind, placebo-controlled trial found that use of a long-acting dihydropyridine calcium-channel blocker (e.g., nitrendipine) resulted in lower risk for dementia (65), and a randomized, double-blind, crossover trial comparing atenolol and nifedipine reported no gross effects on cognitive function among elderly hypertensive patients (61). Data from a large randomized, long-term, controlled trial found minimal effects on cognition of commonly used antihypertensives (e.g., atenolol, diuretics) (60,66). Short-term trials did not find detrimental effects associated with angiotensin converting enzyme (ACE) inhibitors (62,67). Thus, it appears that agents currently recommended for first-line and second-line treatment of hypertension (e.g., diuretics, beta-blockers, ACE inhibitors) are unlikely to impair cognition for most older adults.

Histamine-2 Receptor Antagonists

The mechanism by which H2RAs result in cognitive impairment is not known. Evidence exists for full or partial reversal of symptoms with physostigmine administration, suggesting that an indirect effect on cholinergic transmission may be involved in mediating drug-induced effects on cognition (18–20).

Delirium has been reported with all H2RAs, but is relatively rare (68–70). A large prospective study did not find an increased risk of delirium with H2RAs (30); however, a possible relationship may have been obscured if only a subset of patients were at increased risk. A recent cohort study found nonstatistically significant trends compatible with an increased risk of cognitive decline associated with use of H2RAs, particularly in those taking these agents short-term and at higher doses (71). Cimetidine has received the most attention, likely because of its widespread use as the first available agent in this class (70). Some patients can tolerate change to a different H2RA without re-emergence of symptoms, whereas cross-sensitivity between agents has also been described (68–70). One approach to preventing this problem is to appropriately reduce the daily dose, taking into account age and the disease-related decline in renal function present in many older individuals.

Detection and Management or Prevention of Drug-Induced Delirium

The ultimate goal is to prevent delirium, but this may be difficult in frail older adults. General principles to minimize onset of this problem include the avoidance of medication likely to cause delirium if alternative medications exist, and using the lowest effective dose. Patients should be monitored carefully when multiple agents with CNS effects are required. These principles are particularly important for patients with baseline cognitive impairment, who are at an increased risk for delirium.

Early resolution of delirium hinges on accurate and prompt identification of the syndrome. If delirium is suspected, a comprehensive history and physical exam should be conducted to identify all precipitating factors (e.g., infection). Delirium often is caused by multiple concurrent factors, and management should address each suspected factor. As part of this workup, reviewing medication use will assist in determining if the delirium is drug-related. First, new medications or dosage increases should be identified, and an appropriate temporal relationship should be established between these changes and onset of symptoms. If a medication is suspected in the etiology of the delirium, it should be discontinued, if warranted, or the dose reduced. Supportive care, such as ensuring adequate sleep, nutrition, and hydration, and providing cueing and emotional reassurance is important for managing the patient with delirium. If symptoms cannot be managed with supportive care, pharmacological strategies may be needed to control severe agitation and psychosis.

Detection and Management or Prevention of Drug-Induced Cognitive Impairment

It is important for clinicians to have an awareness that subtle changes in cognition in their elderly patients may be caused by drug therapy. Thoughtful provider-prescribing may avoid some cases of drug-induced cognitive decline. It is important for prescribers to know all medications their patients are taking. Patients often receive medications from multiple prescribers or take OTC medications or herbal products, making it difficult for providers to be aware of all medication use. Medications that are not documented may be responsible for drug-related cognitive decline. For example, recent worsening of dementia caused by an over-the-counter antihistamine may be overlooked if the clinician is not the prescriber of this agent, and the patient does not inform the clinician of its use. Thus, patients should be encouraged to bring a list of all their medications—prescribed and other—to each clinic visit.

Recognition of drug-induced cognitive impairment, especially if deficits are subtle, may be difficult in the older adult. Symptoms often appear insidiously, and patients may not bring the deficits to the attention of their provider. Thus, patients should be assessed for changes in cognition with each addition to, or increase in, medication dosages. If a change in cognition is suspected, elimination *one at a time* of the suspected drug(s) and follow-up evaluation may be the only way to identify drug-induced cognitive impairment.

DRUG-INDUCED INSOMNIA

Sleep complaints, including insomnia, are a common problem in the elderly. Approximately 40% to 50% of older adults report problems with initiating or maintaining sleep (72,73). There are a number of factors that may contribute to insomnia in elderly patients, including medical and psychiatric disorders and/or the treatment of these conditions. Various aspects of sleep are affected by a number of neurotransmitters (e.g., dopamine, acetylcholine, histamine, norepinephrine, serotonin) (74). Altering their activity can cause wakefulness (e.g., dopamine, acetylcholine, histamine, norepinephrine), affect the rapid eye movement (REM) stage of sleep (e.g., acetylcholine, serotonin, norepinephrine), or otherwise affect sleep regulation or induction (e.g., serotonin) (74). Medications affecting these neurotransmitters are among the most likely to have been associated with insomnia in case reports and observational studies. There are currently little data, however, from controlled studies. The following sections review the most common classes of agents involved in drug-induced insomnia, with a focus on the specific neurotransmitters involved. Additionally, drug withdrawal as a cause of insomnia is briefly discussed. Table 39-2 provides a more comprehensive list of medications that have been shown to cause sleep problems.

Acetylcholinesterase Inhibitors

These agents increase acetylcholine by inhibiting the activity of the enzyme acetylcholinesterase. Cholinergic pathways are thought to play a role in the quality of sleep as well as onset and duration of dream sleep (75).

Donepezil, the most commonly-used acetylcholinesterase inhibitor, has been reported to cause nightmares in patients, resulting in insomnia (76). Rates of insomnia in trials comparing placebo, 5 mg donepezil, and 10 mg donepezil were 5%, 8%, and 18%, respectively. Furthermore, Stahl and colleagues found that sedative-hypnotic use was significantly more common in patients with AD taking donepezil than in those not taking donepezil (9.8% versus 3.9%) (75). Since insomnia appears to be a dose-related adverse event, lowering the dose of donepezil may be an effective approach to limit the severity of adverse effects (although efficacy may be affected as well). This is also likely to be the case with other

TABLE 39-2
DRUGS/DRUG CLASSES THAT MAY CAUSE INSOMNIA

Acetylcholinesterase inhibitors
Alcohol (acute ingestion and withdrawal)
Antibiotics (e.g., ciprofloxacin, clarithromycin)
Antidepressants (e.g., selective serotonin reuptake inhibitors, tricyclic antidepressants, bupropion, venlafaxine)[a]
Antihypertensives (e.g., beta-blockers, clonidine, methyldopa, reserpine, diuretics administered at bedtime)
Central nervous system stimulants (e.g., amphetamine, methylphenidate, pseudoephedrine, beta-adrenergic agonists)[a]
Sedative/hypnotic use, chronic
Digoxin
Dopamine enhancers (e.g., ropinirole, levodopa)
Drug withdrawal (e.g., clozapine, opioids, benzodiazepines, antihistamines, sedative/hypnotic agents)[a]
Hormonal agents (e.g., anabolic steroids, corticosteroids, oral contraceptives)
Methylxanthines (e.g., caffeine, theophylline)[a]
Methyldopa
Naproxen
Nicotine
Phenytoin
Thyroid preparations

[a]Clinically important based on sufficient information and discussed in text. (Adapted from references 81, 135.)

acetylcholinesterase inhibitors (e.g., galantamine, rivastigmine).

Antidepressants

Insomnia is a common symptom experienced by depressed patients. Therefore, it can be difficult to differentiate whether the insomnia is a symptom of the disease or a side effect of the medications. Antidepressant effects on the neurotransmitter serotonin are thought to be the cause of sleep problems.

Amphetamines, methylphenidate, MAOIs, TCAs, SSRIs, venlafaxine, and bupropion are all associated with a variety of sleep problems, including insomnia (77,78). SSRIs have also been reported to cause visual dreaming and nightmares (77,79), while mirtazapine has been associated with REM-sleep behavior disorder in Parkinson's patients (80).

Antiparkinsonian Agents

Increased dopamine neurotransmission has been associated with sleep disturbances (e.g., insomnia, vivid dreaming, nightmares). Antiparkinson medications that affect this neurotransmitter (e.g., levodopa, pergolide, ropinirole, and pramipexole) have been associated with various sleep disturbances, including insomnia (77).

Levodopa has been reported to cause insomnia, vivid dreams, nightmares, and changes in sleep architecture (81). In a safety and efficacy study comparing levodopa and ropinirole (a direct dopamine-receptor agonist), Rascol and colleagues found that insomnia was the third most commonly reported adverse event (25% in the ropinirole group and 24% in the levodopa group) (82). Despite a high prevalence of insomnia in both groups, lack of a placebo arm makes it difficult to assess whether these symptoms were caused by the medication, the disease state, or other factors.

Methylxanthines

Two common methylxanthines associated with insomnia include theophylline and caffeine. Both agents, via their CNS stimulatory effects, can interfere with sleep by increasing sleep latency and decreasing the duration of deep sleep (72).

There is evidence to suggest the elderly have an enhanced sensitivity to caffeine and potentially have a lower clearance of the drug (83). Ninety percent of caffeine intake comes from coffee, tea, and soft drinks (72). Other sources of caffeine intake include food, cocoa, and over-the-counter analgesic and migraine medications. Theophylline's effect on sleep may be more pronounced in the elderly due to decreased clearance (84). Additionally, drug interactions have been identified that may further inhibit the clearance of theophylline, thereby leading to increased plasma concentrations and toxicity. To avoid risks associated with theophylline in the elderly, the inhaled bronchodilators are appropriate alternatives to help with breathing.

Sympathomimetics

Sympathomimetic agents increase norepinephrine concentrations, leading to wakefulness and possibly alterations in sleep architecture.

Commonly used oral decongestants, such as pseudoephedrine, can affect older adults' ability to sleep (81). Other sympathomimetic agents sometimes used in the elderly include stimulants such as methylphenidate. Avoiding these agents when possible (e.g., using nasal spray in lieu of systemic decongestants) or timing the administration of these agents to occur in the morning is the most effective approach to minimize their effects on sleep.

Drug-Withdrawal as a Cause of Insomnia

Unfortunately, drugs used to treat insomnia can also cause rebound insomnia once withdrawn (85). Rebound insomnia is worse than the original insomnia in most cases, and may promote long-term use and possibly dependence on the drug (86). A postulated mechanism for rebound insomnia is that receptors may upregulate during therapy with these agents, and when therapy is withdrawn, the patient is more sensitive to effects from the neurotransmit-

ters (86,87). Clozapine is also associated with rebound insomnia (87).

Detection and Management or Prevention of Drug-Induced Insomnia

Normal changes in sleep architecture associated with aging include decreased total sleep time and increased number of awakenings (74). It is therefore important for the healthcare professional to differentiate between drug-induced insomnia and age-related changes in sleep pattern. Every patient complaining of sleep problems should have a complete physical exam and medication history, and have the opportunity to complete a sleep questionnaire, which may include 1 to 2 weeks of a sleep diary. Healthcare professionals need to inquire about all potential sources of caffeine in a patient's diet (not just coffee), and advise patients that caffeine use should be minimized, and avoided entirely after 4 PM. Strategies to minimize medication-induced insomnia include changing the administration time, lowering the dose and, if possible, discontinuation of the offending medication or substitution with an agent less likely to cause insomnia. Additional strategies, such as improving sleep "hygiene" (e.g., going to sleep at the same time every night, reducing daytime naps, using the bed for sleep only) have also been found effective. For agents that tend to cause insomnia during medication withdrawal, slow tapering is recommended.

DRUG-INDUCED DEPRESSIVE SYMPTOMS

Medications have long been reported as a potential cause of depressive symptoms. Early observations that reserpine (an antihypertensive drug that depletes biogenic amines from CNS neurons) caused depressive symptoms in a number of patients led, in part, to the recognition that biogenic amines play an important role in depression (88). Additional early reports linked other antihypertensive agents (e.g., methyldopa, clonidine) with symptoms of depression (89). Reports for these and other medications associated with depressive symptoms are generally based on uncontrolled observations, and relatively few prospective studies have addressed this issue. Because many medical conditions are associated with an increased likelihood of the occurrence of depressive symptoms (90), the lack of prospective-controlled studies leads to difficulties in ascertaining a cause-effect relationship between drug exposure and symptoms of depression.

The following sections examine the drugs commonly used in the elderly that are most associated with depressive symptoms. Table 39-3 includes additional drugs that have been reported in the literature to be associated with depressive symptoms.

TABLE 39-3

DRUGS/DRUG CLASSES REPORTED TO CAUSE SYMPTOMS OF DEPRESSION

Antiepileptics
Antihypertensives (e.g., angiotensin converting enzyme inhibitors, beta-blockers, calcium-channel blockers, clonidine, methyldopa, reserpine)[a]
Barbiturates
Benzodiazepines
Central nervous system stimulants
Corticosteroids[b]
Digoxin
Fluoroquinolones
Histamine-H2 receptor blockers
Hormone replacement therapy
Interferon-alpha
Levodopa
Lipid-lowering agents
Mefloquine
Metoclopramide
Nonsteroidal anti-inflammatory drugs
Tamoxifen

[a]Particularly with sympatholytic agents (e.g., reserpine, methyldopa).
[b]Clinically important based on sufficient information and discussed in text.
(Adapted from references 91, 134,135).

Beta-Blockers

Beta-blockers have received a great deal of attention as a possible cause of drug-induced depression. A number of studies suggest that chronic treatment with antidepressants results in reduced beta-adrenergic receptor-density in cortical tissues (88). Chronic treatment with beta-blockers appears to have the opposite effect on beta-adrenergic receptors, leading to hypotheses that beta-blockers may induce symptoms of depression or could interfere with the actions of antidepressants (91).

Although the focus of much attention, the role of beta-blockers as contributors to symptoms of depression is still unclear. Multiple case reports and case series describe the onset of symptoms of depression shortly after beta-blocker initiation (including topical beta-blocker exposure) (92), with some reports suggesting that the more lipophilic beta-blockers (e.g., propranolol) are more likely to induce symptoms of depression than those that are less lipophilic (e.g., atenolol). A number of studies have evaluated the association between beta-blockers and depression, and although conflicting results have been reported, most did not find an association (93–95). These data suggest that if there is an association between beta-blockers and depressive symptoms, it is likely not as strong as initially believed.

Other Antihypertensives

The mechanisms by which antihypertensives other than beta-blockers might cause symptoms of depression are

unclear. However, as with beta-blockers (and most other medications), when analyzing associations between these agents and depressive symptoms, it is necessary to distinguish whether the medication is responsible for the observed symptoms or if the underlying disease state being treated is a contributing factor.

Case reports have implicated the use of ACE inhibitors and calcium-channel blockers as potential causes of depressive symptoms (96–98), but results of studies examining these relationships have been contradictory (99–102). Conflicting data have also been reported regarding an association between the use of these agents and suicide. Whereas Lindberg et al. found that calcium-channel blockers but not ACE inhibitors were associated with suicide (103), Sorensen et al. did not find this association (104). The interpretation of these studies as a whole is difficult due to the variety of measures used to assess symptoms of depression, and by the known relationship between depression and cardiovascular disease, which may confound the results. Based on the conflicting data currently available, it is not clear whether ACE inhibitors or calcium-channel blockers are associated with symptoms of depression. However, due to the known association between cardiovascular disease and depression, and the possible association between these classes of antihypertensives and symptoms of depression, it is prudent to assess those with cardiovascular disease for symptoms of depression prior to and during antihypertensive treatment.

Corticosteroids

Abnormalities in the hypothalamic-pituitary-adrenal (HPA) axis have been observed in depressive disorders. Many patients with major depressive disorder (MDD) have elevated cortisol concentrations, and fail to suppress cortisol production after the administration of the corticosteroid dexamethasone (105). Furthermore, patients with Cushing's disorder have reported depressive episodes similar to those seen in MDD, further confirming the relationship between HPA axis activity and depressive symptoms (91).

Severe depressive episodes have been reported in case reports following systemic corticosteroid initiation (106, 107). Follow-up studies have generally confirmed an association between corticosteroid use and symptoms of depression, although it is not clear if these effects are dose-related. Two cross-sectional surveys found that among patients with chronic obstructive pulmonary disease, those using corticosteroids had greater symptoms of depression (108,109). A prospective cohort study found that those exposed to corticosteroids had a greater incidence of depressive symptoms, as measured by a modified version of the Center for Epidemiological Studies Depression Rating Scale (risk ratio = 3.1), although this difference did not reach statistical significance (110). Not all studies, however, found a positive association between corticosteroids and depressive symptoms. In the Boston Collaborative Drug Surveillance Program, depression was reported by only two of 676 individuals receiving prednisone (111). A case-control study by Patten et al. found no association between corticosteroid use and a diagnosis of depression (112). This study, however, did not assess for symptoms of depression. Overall, research evidence suggests there is likely an association between use of corticosteroids and symptoms of depression.

Lipid-Lowering Agents

There is some evidence that changes in cholesterol concentrations can alter brain serotonergic activity, leading to increased impulsivity or depression (113).

A number of studies have found an association between lowered cholesterol and higher mortality due to suicide, murder, or accidents. These associations have been reported after both pharmacological and lifestyle modification interventions for cholesterol lowering; however, the evidence supporting these associations is limited and recent studies, many of which assessed the effect of hydroxymethylglutaryl-coenzyme A reductase inhibitors ("statins"), found no relationship between cholesterol concentrations and suicide (or other violent death) (114–119). The impact of cholesterol on mood or impulsivity is therefore still unclear; however, the beneficial effects of lowering cholesterol have been well-established.

Tamoxifen

Hormone replacement therapy, when used in postmenopausal women, has been associated with reducing symptoms of depressed mood, and this effect is thought to be due to the effects of estrogen (120,121). Tamoxifen, a selective estrogen-receptor modulator, can act as an estrogen antagonist (122), thereby potentially having negative effects on mood.

The data concerning the relationship between tamoxifen and depressive symptoms are inconsistent. Reports suggesting a positive association have shown that symptoms of depression increase over time in women taking tamoxifen (123). These symptoms of depression are more common among elderly women taking tamoxifen than among those not taking the drug (124). This is also true when comparing women with breast cancer taking tamoxifen relative to those who are not (125). Conversely, efficacy studies of tamoxifen, in which symptoms of depression or other measures of psychosocial well-being were also assessed, did not find that treatment with tamoxifen was associated with such adverse effects (126–128). Despite the inconsistent data with this agent, it is prudent to monitor women taking tamoxifen for the emergence of (or worsening of) depressive symptoms.

Management or Prevention of Drug-Induced Depressive Symptoms

In the depressed elderly, mood may be a less prominent feature than other symptoms (e.g., changes in appetite or sleep, withdrawal) or somatic symptoms (129,130). If symptoms of depression emerge, the clinician should conduct a review of the patient's medication regimen to determine if any of them might be contributing to the observed symptoms. These medications should then be substituted, if possible, with agents less likely to cause depression. If symptoms occur despite these actions, appropriate therapy may be necessary. The use of antidepressants to prevent or reverse medication-associated depression has been best studied in conjunction with the use of interferon-alpha (an agent with substantial evidence suggesting it may cause symptoms of depression). When used in this manner, antidepressants appear useful in decreasing symptoms (131,132). The use of antidepressants in the treatment of depressive symptoms caused by other medications has not been adequately assessed, but should be considered if other approaches are not successful.

CONCLUSION

Numerous medications have been associated with psychiatric manifestations. Although the data supporting these associations in many cases are not based on well-controlled studies, the elderly are likely more susceptible to many of these medication-induced symptoms. It is therefore particularly important in elderly patients to assess whether medications may be contributing to problems with cognition, sleep, or mood, especially if changes have been noted. Although not discussed here, medications may also initiate or contribute to problems with psychosis, anxiety, or agitation in the elderly. Care should be taken, whenever possible, to avoid initiating new drug therapy to treat side-effects of previously prescribed medications. Instead, preventive strategies directed at avoiding high-risk medication, appropriately adjusting doses based on age-related changes in physiology, and close monitoring should be used.

REFERENCES

1. Rochon PA, Gurwitz JH. Optimising drug treatment for elderly people: the prescribing cascade. *BMJ.* 1997;315:1096–1099.
2. Blazer D, Hybels C, Simonsick E, Hanlon JT. Sedative, hypnotic, and antianxiety medication use in an aging cohort over ten years: a racial comparison. *J Am Geriatr Soc.* 2000;48:1073–1079.
3. Blazer DG, Hybels CF, Simonsick EM, Hanlon JT. Marked differences in antidepressant use by race in an elderly community sample: 1986–1996. *Am J Psychiatry.* 2000;157:1089–1094.
4. Tobias D, Sey M. General and psychotherapeutic medication use in 328 nursing facilities: a year 2000 national survey. *Consult Pharm.* 2001;16:54–64.
5. Francis J, Martin D, Kapoor WN. A prospective study of delirium in hospitalized elderly. *JAMA.* 1990;263:1097–1101.
6. Larson EB, Kukull WA, Buchner D, Reifler BV. Adverse drug reactions associated with global cognitive impairment in elderly persons. *Ann Intern Med.* 1987;107:169–173.

7. Gray SL, Lai KV, Larson EB. Drug-induced cognition disorders in the elderly: incidence, prevention and management. *Drug Saf.* 1999;21:101–122.

8. Molchan SE, Martinez RA, Hill JL, et al. Increased cognitive sensitivity to scopolamine with age and a perspective on the scopolamine model. *Brain Res Rev.* 1992;17:215–226.

9. Ray PG, Meador KJ, Loring DW, Zamrini EW, Yang XH, Buccafusco JJ. Central anticholinergic hypersensitivity in aging. *J Geriatr Psychiatry Neurol.* 1992;5:72–77.

10. Sunderland T, Tariot PN, Weingartner H, et al. Pharmacologic modelling of Alzheimer's disease. *Prog Neuropsychopharmacol Biol Psychiatry.* 1986;10:599–610.

11. Katz IR, Sands LP, Bilker W, DiFilippo S, Boyce A, D'Angelo K. Identification of medications that cause cognitive impairment in older people: the case of oxybutynin chloride. *J Am Geriatr Soc.* 1998;46:8–13.

12. Tejera CA, Saravay SM, Goldman E, Gluck L. Diphenhydramine-induced delirium in elderly hospitalized patients with mild dementia. *Psychosomatics.* 1994;35:399–402.

13. Agostini JV, Leo-Summers LS, Inouye SK. Cognitive and other adverse effects of diphenhydramine use in hospitalized older patients. *Arch Intern Med.* 2001;161:2091–2097.

14. McCue JD. Safety of antihistamines in the treatment of allergic rhinitis in elderly patients. *Arch Fam Med.* 1996;5:464–468.

15. Kay GG, Berman B, Mockoviak SH, et al. Initial and steady-state effects of diphenhydramine and loratadine on sedation, cognition, mood, and psychomotor performance. *Arch Intern Med.* 1997;157:2350–2356.

16. Donnellan CA, Fook L, McDonald P, Playfer JR. Oxybutynin and cognitive dysfunction. *BMJ.* 1997;315:1363–1364.

17. Edwards KR, O'Connor JT. Risk of delirium with concomitant use of tolterodine and acetylcholinesterase inhibitors. *J Am Geriatr Soc.* 2002;50:1165–1166.

18. Goff DC, Garber HJ, Jenike MA. Partial resolution of ranitidine-associated delirium with physostigmine: case report. *J Clin Psychiatry.* 1985;46:400–401.

19. Mogelnicki SR, Waller JL, Finlayson DC. Physostigmine reversal of cimetidine—induced mental confusion. *JAMA.* 1979;241:826–827.

20. Jenike MA, Levy JC. Physostigmine reversal of cimetidine-induced delirium and agitation. *J Clin Psychopharmacol.* 1983;3:43–44.

21. Eisendrath SJ, Goldman B, Douglas J, Dimatteo L, Van Dyke C. Meperidine-induced delirium. *Am J Psychiatry.* 1987;144:1062–1065.

22. Tune L, Carr S, Hoag E, Cooper T. Anticholinergic effects of drugs commonly prescribed for the elderly: potential means for assessing risk of delirium. *Am J Psychiatry.* 1992;149:1393–1394.

23. Vgontzas AN, Kales A, Bixler EO. Benzodiazepine side effects: role of pharmacokinetics and pharmacodynamics. *Pharmacology.* 1995;51:205–223.

24. Pomara N, Deptula D, Medel M, Block RI, Greenblatt DJ. Effects of diazepam on recall memory: relationship to aging, dose, and duration of treatment. *Psychopharmacol Bull.* 1989;25:144–148.

25. Nikaido AM, Ellinwood EH Jr, Heatherly DG, Gupta SK. Age-related increase in CNS sensitivity to benzodiazepines as assessed by task difficulty. *Psychopharmacology.* 1990;100:90–97.

26. Curran HV. Benzodiazepines, memory and mood: a review. *Psychopharmacology.* 1991;105:1–8.

27. Hanlon JT, Horner RD, Schmader KE, et al. Benzodiazepine use and cognitive function among community-dwelling elderly. *Clin Pharmacol Ther.* 1998;64:684–692.

28. Paterniti S, Dufouil C, Alperovitch A. Long-term benzodiazepine use and cognitive decline in the elderly: the Epidemiology of Vascular Aging Study. *J Clin Psychopharmacol.* 2002;22:285–293.

29. Marcantonio ER, Juarez G, Goldman L, et al. The relationship of postoperative delirium with psychoactive medications. *JAMA.* 1994;272:1518–1522.

30. Schor JD, Levkoff SE, Lipsitz LA, et al. Risk factors for delirium in hospitalized elderly. *JAMA.* 1992;267:827–831.

31. Inouye SK, Charpentier PA. Precipitating factors for delirium in hospitalized elderly persons. Predictive model and interrelationship with baseline vulnerability. *JAMA.* 1996;275:852–857.

32. Toner LC, Tsambiras BM, Catalano G, Catalano MC, Cooper DS. Central nervous system side effects associated with zolpidem treatment. *Clin Neuropharmacol.* 2000;23:54–58.

33. Brodeur MR, Stirling AL. Delirium associated with zolpidem. *Ann Pharmacother.* 2001;35:1562–1564.

34. Mahoney J, Webb M, Gray SL. Zolpidem prescribing and adverse drug reactions in hospitalized general medicine patients. *Am J Geriatr Pharmacother.* 2004;2(1):66–74.

35. Oxman TE. Antidepressants and cognitive impairment in the elderly. *J Clin Psychiatry.* 1996;57(Suppl 5):38–44.

36. Branconnier RJ, Cole JP. Effects of acute administration of trazodone and amitriptyline on cognition, cardiovascular function, and salivation in the normal geriatric subjects. *J Clin Psychopharmacol.* 1981;1(Suppl 6):82S–88S.

37. Kerr JS, Fairweather DB, Hindmarch I. Effects of fluoxetine on psychomotor performance, cognitive function and sleep in depressed patients. *Int Clin Psychopharmacol.* 1993;8:341–343.

38. Meyers BS, Mattis S, Gabriele M, Kakuma T. Effects of nortriptyline on memory self-assessment and performance in recovered elderly depressives. *Psychopharmacol Bull.* 1991;27:295–299.

39. Hindmarch I. The behavioural toxicity of the selective serotonin reuptake inhibitors. *Int Clin Psychopharmacol.* 1995;9(Suppl 4):13–17.

40. Taragano FE, Lyketsos CG, Mangone CA, Allegri RF, Comesana-Diaz E. A double-blind, randomized, fixed-dose trial of fluoxetine vs. amitriptyline in the treatment of major depression complicating Alzheimer's disease. *Psychosomatics.* 1997;38:246–252.

41. Nyth AL, Gottfries CG, Lyby K, et al. A controlled multicenter clinical study of citalopram and placebo in elderly depressed patients with and without concomitant dementia. *Acta Psychiatr Scand.* 1992;86:138–145.

42. Morrison RS, Magaziner J, Gilbert M, et al. Relationship between pain and opioid analgesics on the development of delirium following hip fracture. *J Gerontol A Biol Sci Med Sci.* 2003;58:76–81.

43. Egbert AM, Parks LH, Short LM, Burnett ML. Randomized trial of postoperative patient-controlled analgesia vs intramuscular narcotics in frail elderly men. *Arch Intern Med.* 1990;150:1897–1903.

44. Weiner DK, Hanlon JT. Pain in nursing home residents: management strategies. *Drugs Aging.* 2001;18:13–29.

45. Meador KJ. Cognitive outcomes and predictive factors in epilepsy. *Neurology.* 2002;58:S21–S26.

46. Smith DB, Mattson RH, Cramer JA, Collins JF, Novelly RA, Craft B. Results of a nationwide Veterans Administration Cooperative Study comparing the efficacy and toxicity of carbamazepine, phenobarbital, phenytoin, and primidone. *Epilepsia.* 1987;28(Suppl 3):S50–S58.

47. Prevey ML, Delaney RC, Cramer JA, Cattanach L, Collins JF, Mattson RH. Effect of valproate on cognitive functioning. Comparison with carbamazepine. The Department of Veterans Affairs Epilepsy Cooperative Study 264 Group. *Arch Neurol.* 1996;53:1008–1016.

48. Meador KJ, Loring DW, Allen ME, et al. Comparative cognitive effects of carbamazepine and phenytoin in healthy adults. *Neurology.* 1991;41:1537–1540.

49. Meador KJ, Loring DW, Moore EE, et al. Comparative cognitive effects of phenobarbital, phenytoin, and valproate in healthy adults. *Neurology.* 1995;45:1494–1499.

50. Meador KJ, Loring DW, Ray PG, et al. Differential cognitive and behavioral effects of carbamazepine and lamotrigine. *Neurology.* 2001;56:1177–1182.

51. Meador KJ, Loring DW, Ray PG, et al. Differential cognitive effects of carbamazepine and gabapentin. *Epilepsia.* 1999;40:1279–1285.

52. Brodie MJ, Overstall PW, Giorgi L. Multicentre, double-blind, randomised comparison between lamotrigine and carbamazepine in elderly patients with newly diagnosed epilepsy. The UK Lamotrigine Elderly Study Group. *Epilepsy Res.* 1999;37:81–87.

53. Strub R. Vascular dementia. *South Med J.* 2003;96:363–366.

54. Skoog I, Gustafson D. Hypertension and related factors in the etiology of Alzheimer's disease. *Ann N Y Acad Sci.* 2002;977:29–36.

55. Elias MF, Wolf PA, D'Agostino RB, Cobb J, White LR. Untreated blood pressure level is inversely related to cognitive functioning: the Framingham Study. *Am J Epidemiol.* 1993;138:353–364.

56. Tzourio C, Dufouil C, Ducimetiere P, Alperovitch A. Cognitive decline in individuals with high blood pressure: a longitudinal study in the elderly. EVA Study Group. Epidemiology of Vascular Aging. *Neurology.* 1999;53:1948–1952.

57. Glynn RJ, Beckett LA, Hebert LE, Morris MC, Scherr PA, Evans DA. Current and remote blood pressure and cognitive decline. *JAMA.* 1999;281:438–445.

58. Muldoon MF, Manuck SB, Shapiro AP, Waldstein SR. Neurobehavioral effects of antihypertensive medications. *J Hypertens.* 1991;9:549–559.

59. Goldstein G, Materson BJ, Cushman WC, et al. Treatment of hypertension in the elderly: II. Cognitive and behavioral function. Results of a Department of Veterans Affairs Cooperative Study. *Hypertension.* 1990;15:361–369.

60. Prince MJ, Bird AS, Blizard RA, Mann AH. Is the cognitive function of older patients affected by antihypertensive treatment? Results from 54 months of the Medical Research Council's trial of hypertension in older adults. *BMJ.* 1996;312:801–805.

61. Skinner MH, Futterman A, Morrissette D, Thompson LW, Hoffman BB, Blaschke TF. Atenolol compared with nifedipine: effect on cognitive function and mood in elderly hypertensive patients. *Ann Intern Med.* 1992;116:615–623.

62. Applegate WB, Phillips HL, Schnaper H, et al. A randomized controlled trial of the effects of three antihypertensive agents on blood pressure control and quality of life in older women. *Arch Intern Med.* 1991;151:1817–1823.

63. Heckbert SR, Longstreth WT Jr, Psaty BM, et al. The association of antihypertensive agents with MRI white matter findings and with Modified Mini-Mental State Examination in older adults. *J Am Geriatr Soc.* 1997;45:1423–1433.

64. Maxwell CJ, Hogan DB, Ebly EM. Calcium-channel blockers and cognitive function in elderly people: results from the Canadian Study of Health and Aging. *CMAJ.* 1999;161:501–506.

65. Forette F, Seux ML, Staessen JA, et al. The prevention of dementia with antihypertensive treatment: new evidence from the Systolic Hypertension in Europe (Syst-Eur) study. *Arch Intern Med.* 2002;162:2046–2052.

66. Applegate WB, Pressel S, Wittes J, et al. Impact of the treatment of isolated systolic hypertension on behavioral variables. Results from the systolic hypertension in the elderly program. *Arch Intern Med.* 1994;154:2154–2160.

67. Starr JM, Whalley LJ, Deary IJ. The effects of antihypertensive treatment on cognitive function: results from the HOPE study. *J Am Geriatr Soc.* 1996;44:411–415.

68. Catalano G, Catalano MC, Alberts VA. Famotidine-associated delirium. A series of six cases. *Psychosomatics.* 1996;37:349–355.

69. Yuan RY, Kao CR, Sheu JJ, Chen CH, Ho CS. Delirium following a switch from cimetidine to famotidine. *Ann Pharmacother.* 2001;35:1045–1048.

70. Cantu TG, Korek JS. Central nervous system reactions to histamine-2 receptor blockers. *Ann Intern Med.* 1991;114:1027–1034.

71. Hanlon JT, Landerman LR, Artz MA, Fillenbaum GG, Gray SL, Schmader KE. Histamine-2 receptor antagonist use and decline in cognitive function among community dwelling elderly [abstract]. *Drug Saf.* 2003;12:S157.

72. Brown SL, Salive ME, Pahor M, et al. Occult caffeine as a source of sleep problems in an older population. *J Am Geriatr Soc.* 1995;43:860–864.

73. Cohen-Zion M, Ancoli-Israel S. Sleep disorders. *Principles of Geriatric Medicine and Gerontology.* New York: McGraw-Hill; 2003.

74. Curtis J, Jermain D. Sleep disorders. In: Posey L, ed. *Pharmacotherapy: A Pathophysiologic Approach.* New York: McGraw Hill; 2002:1323–1333.

75. Stahl SM, Markowitz JS, Gutterman EM, Papadopoulos G. Co-use of donepezil and hypnotics among Alzheimer's disease patients living in the community. *J Clin Psychiatry.* 2003;64: 466–472.

76. Ross JS, Shua-Haim JR. Aricept-induced nightmares in Alzheimer's disease: 2 case reports. *J Am Geriatr Soc.* 1998;46: 119–120.

77. Pagel JF, Helfter P. Drug induced nightmares—an etiology based review. *Hum Psychopharmacol.* 2003;18:59–67.

78. Vanderkooy JD, Kennedy SH, Bagby RM. Antidepressant side effects in depression patients treated in a naturalistic setting: a study of bupropion, moclobemide, paroxetine, sertraline, and venlafaxine. *Can J Psychiatry.* 2002;47:174–180.

79. Asnis GM, Chakraburtty A, DuBoff EA, et al. Zolpidem for persistent insomnia in SSRI-treated depressed patients. *J Clin Psychiatry.* 1999;60:668–676.

80. Onofrj M, Luciano AL, Thomas A, Iacono D, D'Andreamatteo G. Mirtazapine induces REM sleep behavior disorder (RBD) in parkinsonism. *Neurology.* 2003;60:113–115.

81. Foral P, Hopkins H, Holstein S, Wright C, Malesker M. Medications as a cause of sleep disturbances. *Consult Pharm.* 2002;17:417–426.

82. Rascol O, Brooks DJ, Korczyn AD, De Deyn PP, Clarke CE, Lang AE. A five-year study of the incidence of dyskinesia in patients with early Parkinson's disease who were treated with ropinirole or levodopa. 056 Study Group. *N Engl J Med.* 2000;342:1484–1491.

83. Curless R, French JM, James OF, Wynne HA. Is caffeine a factor in subjective insomnia of elderly people? *Age Ageing.* 1993;22: 41–45.

84. Hendeles L, Jenkins J, Temple R. Revised FDA labeling guideline for theophylline oral dosage forms. *Pharmacotherapy.* 1995;15: 409–427.

85. Hajak G, Clarenbach P, Fischer W, et al. Rebound insomnia after hypnotic withdrawal in insomniac outpatients. *Eur Arch Psychiatry Clin Neurosci.* 1998;248:148–156.

86. Roth T, Hajak G, Ustun TB. Consensus for the pharmacological management of insomnia in the new millennium. *Int J Clin Pract.* 2001;55:42–52.

87. Staedt J, Stoppe G, Hajak G, Ruther E. Rebound insomnia after abrupt clozapine withdrawal. *Eur Arch Psychiatry Clin Neurosci.* 1996;246:79–82.

88. Musselman DL, DeBattista C, Nathan KI, Kilts CD, Schatzberg AF, Nemeroff CB. Biology of mood disorders. In: Nemeroff CB, ed. *Textbook of Psychopharmacology.* Washington DC: American Psychiatric Press; 1998:549–588.

89. Long TD, Kathol RG. Critical review of data supporting affective disorder caused by nonpsychotropic medication. *Ann Clin Psychiatry.* 1993;5:259–270.

90. Evans DL, Charney DS. Mood disorders and medical illness: a major public health problem. *Biol Psychiatry.* 2003;54:177–180.

91. Patten SB, Love EJ. Drug-induced depression. *Psychother Psychosom.* 1997;66:63–73.

92. Schweitzer I, Maguire K, Tuckwell V. Antiglaucoma medication and clinical depression. *Aust NZ J Psychiatry.* 2001;35:569–571.

93. Kohn R. Beta-blockers an important cause of depression: a medical myth without evidence. *Med Health R I.* 2001;84:92–95.

94. Ried LD, McFarland BH, Johnson RE, Brody KK. Beta-blockers and depression: the more the murkier? *Ann Pharmacother.* 1998;32:699–708.

95. Ko DT, Hebert PR, Coffey CS, Sedrakyan A, Curtis JP, Krumholz HM. Beta-blocker therapy and symptoms of depression, fatigue, and sexual dysfunction. *JAMA.* 2002;288:351–357.

96. Biriell C, McEwen J, Sanz E. Depression associated with diltiazem. *BMJ.* 1989;299:796.

97. Hullett FJ, Potkin SG, Levy AB, Ciasca R. Depression associated with nifedipine-induced calcium channel blockade. *Am J Psychiatry.* 1988;145:1277–1279.

98. Patterson JF. Depression associated with enalapril. *South Med J.* 1989;82:402–403.

99. Hallas J. Evidence of depression provoked by cardiovascular medication: a prescription sequence symmetry analysis. *Epidemiology.* 1996;7:478–484.

100. Patten SB, Williams JV, Love EJ. Case-control studies of cardiovascular medications as risk factors for clinically diagnosed depressive disorders in a hospitalized population. *Can J Psychiatry.* 1996;41:469–476.

101. Rathmann W, Haastert B, Roseman JM, Giani G. Cardiovascular drug prescriptions and risk of depression in diabetic patients. *J Clin Epidemiol.* 1999;52:1103–1109.

102. Dhondt TD, Beekman AT, Deeg DJ, Van Tilburg W. Iatrogenic depression in the elderly. Results from a community-based study in the Netherlands. *Soc Psychiatry Psychiatr Epidemiol.* 2002;37: 393–398.

103. Lindberg G, Bingefors K, Ranstam J, Rastam L, Melander A. Use of calcium channel blockers and risk of suicide: ecological findings confirmed in population based cohort study. *BMJ.* 1998;316: 741–745.

104. Sorensen HT, Mellemkjaer L, Olsen JH. Risk of suicide in users of beta-adrenoceptor blockers, calcium channel blockers and angiotensin converting enzyme inhibitors. *Br J Clin Pharmacol.* 2001;52:313–318.

105. Glassman A, Arana G, Baldessarini R, et al. The dexamethasone suppression test: an overview of its current status in psychiatry. The APA Task Force on Laboratory Tests in Psychiatry. *Am J Psychiatry.* 1987;144:1253–1262.

106. Grigg JR. Prednisone mood disorder with associated catatonia. *J Geriatr Psychiatry Neurol.* 1989;2:41–44.

107. Lewis DA, Smith RE. Steroid-induced psychiatric syndromes. A report of 14 cases and a review of the literature. *J Affect Disord.* 1983;5:319–332.

108. Gift AG, Wood RM, Cahill CA. Depression, somatization and steroid use in chronic obstructive pulmonary disease. *Int J Nurs Stud.* 1989;26:281–286.

109. Patten SB, Lavorato DH. Medication use and major depressive syndrome in a community population. *Compr Psychiatry.* 2001; 42:124–131.

110. Patten SB, Williams JV, Love EJ. Self-reported depressive symptoms following treatment with corticosteroids and sedative-hypnotics. *Int J Psychiatry Med.* 1996;26:15–24.

111. Program BCDS. Acute adverse reactions to prednisone in relation to dosage. *Clin Pharmacol Ther.* 1972;13:694–698.

112. Patten SB, Williams JV, Love EJ. A case-control study of corticosteroid exposure as a risk factor for clinically-diagnosed depressive disorders in a hospitalized population. *Can J Psychiatry.* 1995;40:396–400.

113. Manfredini R, Caracciolo S, Salmi R, Boari B, Tomelli A, Gallerani M. The association of low serum-cholesterol with depression and suicidal behaviours: new hypotheses for the missing link. *J Int Med Res.* 2000;28:247–257.

114. Young-Xu Y, Chan KA, Liao JK, Ravid S, Blatt CM. Long-term statin use and psychological well-being. *J Am Coll Cardiol.* 2003; 42:690–697.

115. Golomb BA. Cholesterol and violence: is there a connection? *Ann Intern Med.* 1998;128:478–487.

116. Muldoon MF, Manuck SB, Mendelsohn AB, Kaplan JR, Belle SH. Cholesterol reduction and non-illness mortality: meta-analysis of randomised clinical trials. *BMJ.* 2001;322:11–15.

117. Muldoon MF, Barger SD, Ryan CM, et al. Effects of lovastatin on cognitive function and psychological well-being. *Am J Med.* 2000;108:538–546.

118. Stewart RA, Sharples KJ, North FM, Menkes DB, Baker J, Simes J. Long-term assessment of psychological well-being in a randomized placebo-controlled trial of cholesterol reduction with pravastatin. The LIPID Study Investigators. *Arch Intern Med.* 2000;160:3144–3152.

119. Tanskanen A, Vartiainen E, Tuomilehto J, Viinamaki H, Lehtonen J, Puska P. High serum cholesterol and risk of suicide. *Am J Psychiatry.* 2000;157:648–650.

120. Bjorn I, Sundstrom-Poromaa I, Bixo M, Nyberg S, Backstrom G, Backstrom T. Increase of estrogen dose deteriorates mood during progestin phase in sequential hormonal therapy. *J Clin Endocrinol Metab.* 2003;88:2026–2030.

121. Zweifel JE, O'Brien WH. A meta-analysis of the effect of hormone replacement therapy upon depressed mood. *Psychoneuroendocrinology.* 1997;22:189–212.

122. Riggs BL, Hartmann LC. Selective estrogen-receptor modulators—mechanisms of action and application to clinical practice. *N Engl J Med.* 2003;348:618–629.

123. Shariff S, Cumming CE, Lees A, Handman M, Cumming DC. Mood disorder in women with early breast cancer taking tamoxifen, an estradiol receptor antagonist. An expected or unexpected effect? *Ann N Y Acad Sci.* 1995;761:365–368.

124. Breuer B, Anderson R. The relationship of tamoxifen with dementia, depression, and dependence in activities of daily living in elderly nursing home residents. *Women Health.* 2000;31:71–85.

125. Cathcart CK, Jones SE, Pumroy CS, Peters GN, Knox SM, Cheek JH. Clinical recognition and management of depression in node negative breast cancer patients treated with tamoxifen. *Breast Cancer Res Treat.* 1993;27:277–281.

126. Day R, Ganz PA, Costantino JP. Tamoxifen and depression: more evidence from the National Surgical Adjuvant Breast and Bowel Project's Breast Cancer Prevention (P-1) Randomized Study. *J Natl Cancer Inst.* 2001;93:1615–1623.

127. Fallowfield L, Fleissig A, Edwards R, et al. Tamoxifen for the prevention of breast cancer: psychosocial impact on women participating in two randomized controlled trials. *J Clin Oncol.* 2001;19: 1885–1892.

128. Love RR, Cameron L, Connell BL, Leventhal H. Symptoms associated with tamoxifen treatment in postmenopausal women. *Arch Intern Med.* 1991;151:1842–1847.

129. Charney DS, Berman RM, Miller HL. Treatment of depression. In: Nemeroff CB, ed. *Textbook of Psychopharmacology.* Washington DC: American Psychiatric Press; 1998.

130. Nelson JC. Diagnosing and treating depression in the elderly. *J Clin Psychiatry.* 2001;62(Suppl 24):18–22.

131. Kraus MR, Schafer A, Faller H, Csef H, Scheurlen M. Paroxetine for the treatment of interferon-alpha-induced depression in chronic hepatitis C. *Aliment Pharmacol Ther.* 2002;16:1091–1099.

132. Musselman DL, Lawson DH, Gumnick JF, et al. Paroxetine for the prevention of depression induced by high-dose interferon alfa. *N Engl J Med.* 2001;344:961–966.

133. Anonymous. Drugs that may cause cognitive disorders in the elderly. *Med Lett Drugs Ther.* 2000;42:111–112.

134. Anonymous. Drugs that may cause psychiatric symptoms. *Med Lett Drugs Ther.* 2002;44:59–62.

135. Fick DM, Cooper JW, Wade WE, Waller JL, Maclean JR, Beers MH. Updating the Beers criteria for potentially inappropriate medication use in older adults: results of a US consensus panel of experts. *Arch Intern Med.* 2003;163:2716–2724.

Parkinson's Disease

40

Tsao-Wei Liang   Stacy Horn

Idiopathic Parkinson's disease (PD) is a neurodegenerative disorder seen frequently in clinical practice. Idiopathic PD is a clinical diagnosis based on signs and symptoms including tremor, bradykinesia (slowness of movement), rigidity, and postural instability. The disorder typically starts unilaterally and progresses over time to involve both sides, but even late in the course asymmetry is present. The following chapter will discuss PD's epidemiology, genetics, pathology, clinical features, differential diagnosis, associated features, and treatment options.

EPIDEMIOLOGY AND RISK FACTORS

PD is the second most common age-related neurodegenerative disorder in the US, affecting 1.5% to 2.5% of adults over the age of 70 (1). The estimated annual incidence of 13 per 100,000 will no doubt rise as the elderly population increases (2). There is a modest male predominance and a predilection for Caucasians as compared to Blacks, Hispanics, and Asians (2,3).

Large-scale epidemiological studies have identified a number of possible environmental risk factors for PD, including head trauma (4), industrial pollutants, well-water drinking, rural living (1), pesticide exposure (5), and plantation work (6). Mitochondrial toxins such as 1-methyl-4-phenyl-1, 2,3,6-tetrahydropyridine (MPTP (7), a heroin contaminant), rotenone (8) (a pesticide), and cyanide (9) can cause parkinsonism in humans and animals, suggesting that symptoms of PD may arise from defective oxidative phosphorylation.

Intriguingly, cigarette smoking and coffee consumption have consistently been found to be protective for PD. A meta-analysis by Hernan et al. summarizes the data for both of these factors (10). While it has been argued that these behaviors may be genetically or biologically driven, thus confounding the association, twin studies have argued against this possibility. A cohort study of twins from the World War II Veterans Registry showed that, among twins discordant for PD, the twin without PD had smoked significantly more than the other (11). This difference was more pronounced in monozygotic than dizygotic twins and was seen up to 10 years before the onset of disease, arguing against the possibility that early subclinical disease led to the behavior. Longitudinal data collected on 8,004 Japanese-American men enrolled in the prospective Honolulu Heart Program showed that the risk of developing PD was significantly lower for coffee drinkers than for non–coffee drinkers, and even less in those reporting heavy coffee intake (seven cups or more a day) (12). Whether either of these factors has a direct protective role, or represent epiphenomena, remains debatable.

GENETICS

PD occurring after the age of 50 is not typically associated with a genetic predisposition. On the other hand, concordance for PD among monozygotic twins under 50 years of age is significantly greater than in dizygotic twins, suggesting that genetic factors may play a larger role in young-onset PD (13). Rare kindreds of familial parkinsonism offer insight into the interaction of genetic and environmental factors and the pathophysiology of neurodegeneration. Study of these kindreds has converged on the common pathological processes of neuronal inclusion formation, protein aggregation, and altered protein degradation via the ubiquitin-proteasomal system. There are now three major gene products associated with hereditary parkinsonism and several other genetic loci with unknown gene products. Mutations in the *parkin* gene, on the long arm of chromosome 6, were first identified in Japanese families with autosomal recessive juvenile parkinsonism (ARJP) (14). Pathologically, degeneration of pigmented neurons in the substantia nigra and locus ceruleus occurs without Lewy bodies (LB), the hallmark feature of PD. The parkin protein product was subsequently identified as a ligase of ubiquitin (15). In 1997, a missense mutation in the *α-synuclein* gene was identified in a large Italian kindred with autosomal dominant, levodopa responsive parkinsonism with LB (16). α-Synuclein was later found to be the major component of LB, further implicating this protein in the pathogenesis of PD. A third gene mutation associated with autosomal dominant parkinsonism was recently discovered in a small German pedigree (17). The protein product was found to be ubiquitin carboxy-terminal hydroxylase, or UCH-L1, a deubiquitinating enzyme involved in protein degradation and clearance (18).

PATHOLOGY

The pathological hallmark of PD is loss of pigmented dopaminergic neurons in the substantia nigra pars compacta (SNpc). Grossly, this is evident as depigmentation of the midbrain substantia nigra (Figure 40-1). Within the remaining neurons are LB, large eosinophilic cytoplasmic inclusions (Figure 40-2). LB may be easily identified with immunohistochemical techniques using α-synuclein or ubiquitin antibodies. Whether these inclusions are the cause or the end result of neuronal degeneration is debatable. LB are specific for sporadic PD and are characteristically absent in other forms of parkinsonism, such as progressive supranuclear palsy (PSP), multiple system atrophy (MSA), postencephalitic parkinsonism, parkin-related ARJP, and dementia pugilistica. The pathology of PD is now known to extend beyond the SN and dopaminergic system, explaining the various bulbar, autonomic, and neuropsychiatric symptoms. Cranial nerve nuclei such as the dorsal vagal nucleus (19), brainstem and forebrain centers such as the locus ceruleus and the nucleus basalis of Meynert (20), and even peripheral intestinal ganglion (21) are affected.

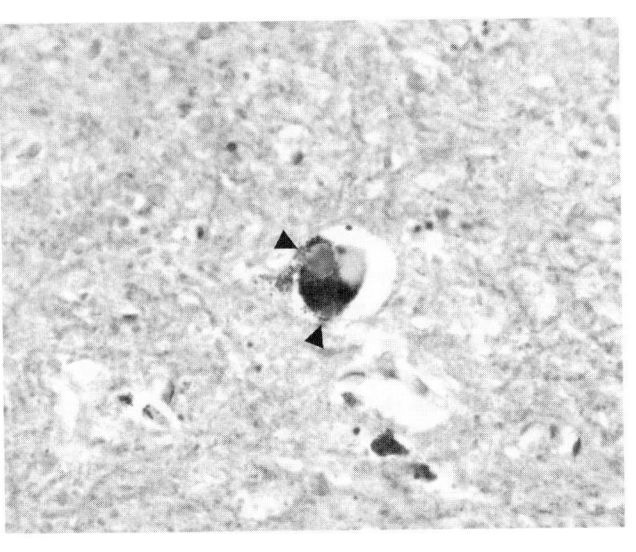

Figure 40-2 40×photomicrograph of a surviving melanin-containing neuron within the SN of a patient with PD. Immunohistochemistry with monoclonal antibody to α-synuclein (syn202) reveals two spherical cytoplasmic inclusions, or Lewy bodies (arrowheads).

Cortical LB, dystrophic neurites (Figure 40-3), and Alzheimer's pathology are seen in neocortical and limbic regions of pathologically proven cases of PD (19,22).

CLINICAL FEATURES AND DIAGNOSIS

The diagnosis of PD is still made purely by clinical examination. No radiological or laboratory study can confirm the diagnosis. Thus, pathological examination remains the gold standard for the diagnosis of PD (Table 40-1).

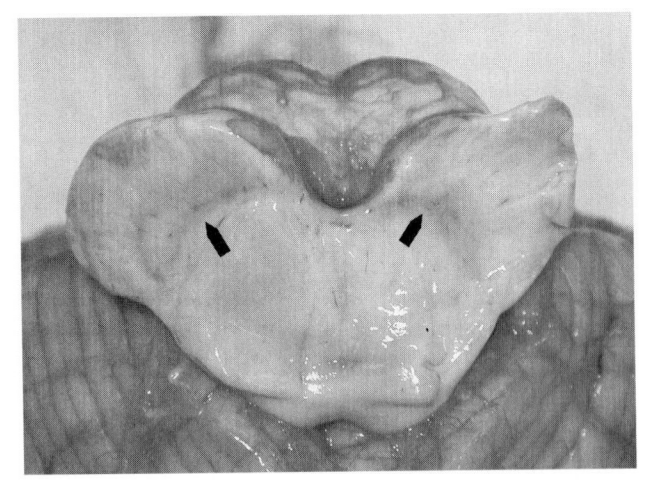

Figure 40-1 Gross section of the midbrain of a patient with PD. The normally dark linear staining of the substantia nigra (SN) is markedly depigmented in this patient (arrowheads). (Courtesy of Paul Kotzbauer, MD, PhD, Department of Neurology, University of Pennsylvania School of Medicine).

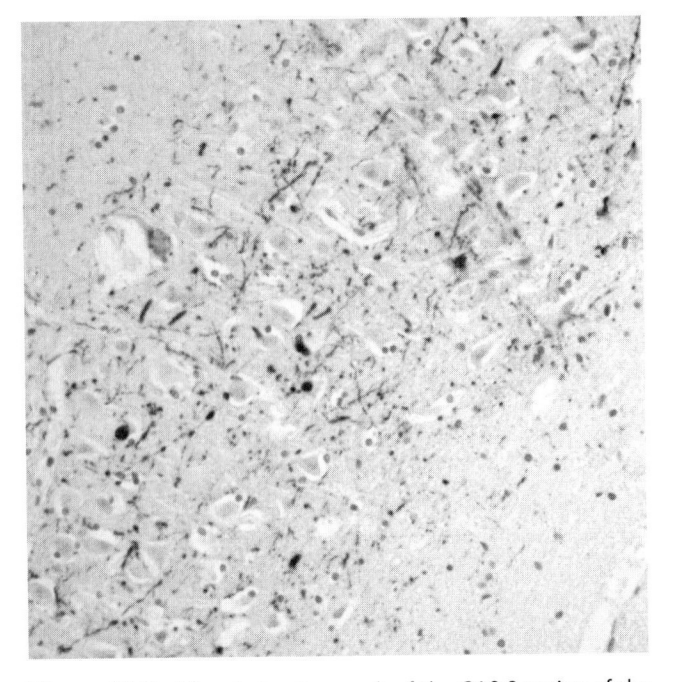

Figure 40-3 20× photomicrograph of the CA2-3 region of the hippocampus, showing dense neuritic pathology in a patient with PD and dementia (anti-α-synuclein and syn303).

TABLE 40-1

COMMON FEATURES OF PARKINSON'S DISEASE

Cardinal features
- Rest tremor
- Rigidity
- Bradykinesia
- Postural instability

Secondary features
- Dystonia
- Dysphagia
- Dysarthria, palilalia, hypophonia
- Hypomimia
- Micrographia
- Festination, retropulsion, freezing, start hesitation, en bloc turning
- Stooped posture, kyphosis, scoliosis
- Drooling/sialorrhea
- Constipation
- Overactive bladder
- Erectile dysfunction
- Seborrheic dermatitis
- Pain/paresthesias

Currently accepted clinical diagnostic criteria for probable PD include at least two out of four cardinal symptoms: tremor typically resting in nature, bradykinesia, cogwheel rigidity, and postural reflex impairment. Asymmetric symptom onset persisting throughout the disease course and a prolonged, robust response to levodopa further support the diagnosis. Even in the best hands, up to 20% of patients have an alternative diagnosis at autopsy, while cases with atypical features may prove to have PD (19). When cardinal symptoms are present, the diagnosis is fairly obvious. Diagnostic difficulty usually arises when intermittent and subtle symptoms predominate in early stages.

Cardinal Features

Tremor occurs in the majority (70%) of pathologically proven PD patients (19). Tremor is generally tested in three conditions: rest, sustained posture, and during active movements or intention. The typical tremor of PD is a low-to-medium-frequency (4–6 Hz) rest tremor affecting the hands, legs, jaw, or tongue. The term *pill-rolling* is used to describe the pronation–supination at the wrist and flexion–extension of the fingers typical of the parkinsonian tremor. Action will often dampen the tremor, while mental concentration and anxiety typically enhance the tremor.

Tone is tested in a relaxed patient using passive, multidirectional movements of the extremities. The increase in tone associated with basal ganglia or extrapyramidal lesions is present and constant throughout the range of movement, leading to the descriptive term *lead-pipe rigidity*. Active movements of the contralateral limb will cause an increase in tone *(Froment's sign)* and may be used to confirm subtle hypertonicity.

In addition to referring to slowed movements, the term bradykinesia refers to hesitancy, arrests, poverty of movement, and decreased amplitude of movements. The clinical expressions of akinesia or bradykinesia are myriad. Impaired finger dexterity, loss of facial expression *(hypomimia)*, and small handwriting *(micrographia)* are some of the earliest signs of parkinsonism. Reduction in stride length, step height, and arm swing lead to the characteristic shuffling gait. The voice can be hypophonic and monotone with a loss of diction. The combination of rigidity and bradykinesia leads to difficulty with ordinary tasks such as turning in bed, rising from a chair, or getting in and out of a car. Because of the loss of dexterity and range of motion, dressing and routine hygiene can become laborious.

Postural instability is one of the later cardinal manifestations of idiopathic PD. Nonetheless, in the elderly with comorbidities such as diabetic neuropathy or arthritis, baseline balance may already be tenuous. Postural stability is tested using the *pull test*, in which the examiner firmly tugs the patient from behind (with warning) and assesses the ability to maintain an upright stance. Retropulsion, or toppling backwards, occurs when the ability to adjust or maintain the center of gravity is lost.

Secondary Features

Gait abnormalities in early PD are often subtle. The initial exam findings may consist only of decreased arm swing or dragging of one leg. Patients often report that walking feels unnatural. A characteristic stooped posture develops with forward flexion of the trunk, neck, elbows, shoulders, and knees. Stride height and length are reduced, leading to a shuffling gait. The stooped posture and shift in the center of gravity contributes to a tendency to fall forward *(propulsion)* and an inability to stop *(festination)*. Turning occurs en bloc, as the head, neck, torso, and extremities no longer rotate independently due to rigidity and bradykinesia.

Patients may describe *freezing*, as though the feet are transiently stuck or "glued" to the ground. The phenomenon typically occurs in doorways, narrow hallways, or near obstacles. Patients often find that visual cues such as floor or sidewalk markings and thresholds will release them from freezing. Due to the combination of freezing, propulsion, and postural instability, forward falls are typical of PD. *Start hesitation* causes difficulty rising from a chair or initiating walking. Freezing is one of the more debilitating symptoms encountered in parkinsonian states and often leads to immobility and falls. Unfortunately, freezing is, more often than not, refractory to levodopa therapy.

At least half of patients on dopaminergic therapy develop motor or response fluctuations within 5 years (23). Fluctuations refer to the shortened and sometimes unpredictable responses that develop after chronic treatment with levodopa. Differences in the *on* state (i.e., when levodopa is working) and the *off* state (i.e., when levodopa is not working) become noticeable as symptoms and the disease process progress. The etiology of fluctuations is unclear, but most experts believe that they result from progressive loss of both presynaptic dopamine storage capacity and postsynaptic striatal nerve terminals. Common types of response fluctuations include wearing-off, on–off phenomena, dyskinesias, and dystonia. Wearing-off occurs several hours after a levodopa dose and is usually the first type of response fluctuation to develop. Later, the duration of response may progressively shorten, responses may become unpredictable, or choreoathetoid dyskinesias may develop. Dosing intervals may need to be shortened to every 1 to 2 hours to prevent the off state. Levodopa may fail to work altogether or may suddenly stop working in the middle of a dosing cycle. Painful limb dystonia or cramping can be one of the most troubling symptoms of PD in the off state.

PD is often associated with dysphagia, excess saliva or drooling (sialorrhea), constipation, overactive bladder, erectile dysfunction, seborrheic dermatitis, orthostatic hypotension, pain, paresthesias, and sleep disturbances including rapid eye movement sleep behavior disorder, periodic limb movement of sleep, restless legs syndrome, insomnia, and obstructive sleep apnea. Numbness, tingling, and aching are frequent symptoms of PD. Fatigue and weakness are common complaints of PD patients that may be dismissed early in the diagnosis or mistaken for somatic symptoms of depression. Neuropsychiatric manifestations will be discussed in a subsequent section.

The Modified Hoehn and Yahr Staging System (Table 40-2) is the most widely used system in clinical and research practice for the staging of motor disability in PD (24). Major determinants of stage, and ultimately prognosis, include unilateral versus bilateral disease, impairment of balance, and functional disability.

The Unified Parkinson's Disease Rating Scale, or UPDRS, is the most widely used scoring system in clinical research and practice (25). The instrument contains 42 items in four separate sections encompassing mental function, activities of daily living (ADL), motor examination, and side effects of therapy.

DIFFERENTIAL DIAGNOSIS

Many conditions can mimic PD, but only idiopathic PD displays a prolonged and robust response to levodopa followed by the development of response fluctuations (Table 40-3). Red flags alerting the clinician to an alternate diagnosis include: ocular motor palsy, cerebellar signs, vocal cord paresis, early and prominent gait dysfunction, cranial nerve or bulbar symptoms, orthostatic hypotension, pyramidal signs, or amyotrophy. Early drooling, speech disturbance, or falls can be a sign of PSP. Prominent cognitive or behavioral changes beginning before or coincident with motor symptoms suggests Alzheimer's disease with extrapyramidal features, dementia with Lewy bodies (DLB), or vascular parkinsonism. It is very unusual for PD to present with a primary gait disorder, falls, or postural instability and should alert the physician to alternate forms of parkinsonism.

TABLE 40-2
MODIFIED HOEHN AND YAHR STAGING

Stage 0	No signs of disease
Stage 1	Unilateral disease
Stage 1.5	Unilateral plus axial involvement
Stage 2	Bilateral disease without impairment of balance
Stage 2.5	Mild bilateral disease with recovery on pull test
Stage 3	Mild-to-moderate bilateral disease, some postural instability; physically independent
Stage 4	Severe disability, still able to walk or stand unassisted
Stage 5	Wheelchair bound or bedridden unless aided

Cerebrovascular disease, or the multi-infarct state, is a relatively common cause of parkinsonism. Strategically placed lacunar infarctions are probably less common than diffuse white matter disease that results from untreated vascular risk factors. Patients may present with abrupt onset of gait disorder or lower body parkinsonism. A stepwise pattern of progression is often a clue to recurrent small vessel ischemic events. Levodopa treatment is not typically effective, but should be attempted for both diagnostic and therapeutic purposes. Cerebrovascular risk factors, a history of stroke or transient

---

TABLE 40-3
DIFFERENTIAL DIAGNOSIS OF PARKINSONISM

Sporadic neurodegenerative
- Idiopathic Parkinson's disease
- Dementia with Lewy bodies (DLB)
- Progressive supranuclear palsy (PSP)
- Multiple system atrophy (formerly Shy-Drager syndrome, olivopontocerebellar atrophy, and striatonigral degeneration)
- Alzheimer's disease with extrapyramidal features
- Corticobasal ganglionic degeneration (CBGD)
- ALS-parkinsonism dementia complex of Guam (ALS-PDC)

Secondary
- Cerebrovascular disease/multi-infarct state
- Drug induced (neuroleptics, antiemetics such as metoclopramide or prochlorperazine, presynaptic dopamine depleters such as reserpine and tetrabenazine)
- Toxin induced (MPTP, carbon monoxide, manganese)
- Posttraumatic parkinsonism
- Postencephalitic parkinsonism (Von Economo's disease)
- Normal pressure hydrocephalus
- Basal ganglia neoplasm, infarct, hemorrhage, infection

Hereditary neurodegenerative
- Parkin, α-synuclein, UCH-L1 kindreds
- Wilson's disease
- Juvenile Huntington's disease
- Neurodegeneration with brain iron accumulation (Hallervorden-Spatz syndrome)
- Dentatorubral pallidoluysian atrophy (DRPLA)
- Spinocerebellar ataxia type 3 (Machado-Joseph disease)

Psychogenic

MPTP, 1-methyl-4-phenyl-1, 2,3,6-tetrahydropyridine; UCH, ubiquitin carboxy-terminal hydrolase.

neurological events, cognitive disturbance, or gait apraxia may be present (26).

Post-encephalitic parkinsonism (PEP) is a rare cause of parkinsonism in this day and age. From 1916 to 1927, epidemic encephalitis (also known as Von Economo's disease, encephalitis lethargica, or sleeping sickness) spread across Europe and the US. The acute phase of the illness, characterized by fever, somnolence, and ophthalmoparesis, was followed with variable latency by a syndrome of young-onset, levodopa-responsive parkinsonism with oculogyric crises, neuropsychiatric symptoms, dystonia, tics, or chorea (27). Although geographically and temporally linked to an influenza pandemic, no definite evidence of influenza infection or other specific etiology has been discovered (28,29). Pathologically, cases have demonstrated periventricular and midbrain inflammation with Alzheimer-type neurofibrillary tangles (30), leading to comparisons to progressive supranuclear palsy and parkinsonism-dementia complex of Guam (31). Rare sporadic cases similar to classic PEP have since been reported in the literature (32,33). Some investigators propose the possibility that the disorder is still prevalent and may result from a neurotrophic autoimmune reaction (34).

Parkinsonism due to chronic antipsychotic treatment is common and potentially reversible. The blockade of dopamine receptors by these agents may cause a clinical picture identical to idiopathic PD. The risk of parkinsonism due to antipsychotic medications is dose-dependent and increased in the elderly (35). With the exception of clozapine, no antipsychotic is free of this risk (36). Other medications that potentially may induce parkinsonism include antiemetics such as metoclopramide or prochlorperazine due to their dopamine-blocking capabilities, dopamine depleters such as reserpine or tetrabenazine, and lithium. In addition to MPTP and cyanide, other toxins associated with include manganese (37) and carbon monoxide (38).

Magnetic resonance imaging is useful in excluding hydrocephalus, lacunar infarcts, or ischemic white matter disease, all of which may cause secondary parkinsonism. Although no imaging finding is diagnostic for PD, putaminal hypointensity and increased diffusion-weighted signal have been used to distinguish PD from atypical parkinsonian syndromes such as PSP and MSA (39–41).

NEUROPSYCHIATRIC MANIFESTATIONS OF PARKINSON'S DISEASE

PD is now known to be associated with a wide range of neuropsychiatric symptoms (Table 40-4). Symptoms such as depression, dementia, hallucinations, or psychosis can be just as, if not more, disabling than the motor symptoms of PD. Although anxiety or depression may simply be seen as a reaction to a chronic illness, studies using comparably disabled patients as controls have challenged this notion (42,43). Our current understanding of these features is that they are a result of an interaction between both environmental (including treatment) and biological factors.

TABLE 40-4
COMMON NEUROPSYCHIATRIC MANIFESTATIONS OF PARKINSON'S DISEASE

- Cognitive and intellectual impairment
- Dementia
- Visual hallucinations
- Delusions
- Depression
- Anxiety or akathisia
- Apathy or amotivation
- Sleep disorders such as insomnia, excessive daytime somnolence, REM behavior disorder, and periodic leg movements of sleep
- Addictive or compulsive behaviors

REM, rapid eye movement.

Dementia and Cognitive Decline

Prevalence, Incidence, and Risk Factors
Dementia occurs in up to 40% of PD patients, while an additional 30% to 40% of PD patients manifest intellectual and cognitive impairment not meeting diagnostic criteria for dementia (3,19,44,45). Estimates of incidence vary from 42.6 to 95.3/1000 person-years of observation, which is as much as six times greater than age-matched controls (46,47). Cognitive impairment and dementia are among the most distressing symptoms reported by caregivers and strong predictors of nursing home placement (44,48,49).

Older age of onset (>60 years), longer disease duration, akinetic-rigid disease, postural instability and gait dysfunction, depression, hallucinations, and atypical features for PD (e.g., autonomic failure, symmetric disease onset, poor response to dopaminergic agents) often portend the development of dementia (44,50). Cognitive function correlates with both motor function and symptoms refractory to levodopa therapy, suggesting that both dopaminergic and nondopaminergic pathways are affected (51,52).

Phenomenology of Cognitive Dysfunction
PD patients frequently develop cognitive and intellectual decline not fulfilling criteria for dementia. The most frequent cognitive domain affected is executive function, the higher-order initiation, organization, and planning of goal-oriented behaviors in response to environmental and inner stimuli. Commonly, patients and their caregivers report forgetfulness, poor attention, absent-mindedness, or disorganization. Bradyphrenia refers to the slowing of mental processing and responses and can be thought of as the cognitive correlate of bradykinesia.

The term subcortical dementia has been used to differentiate PD-related dementia (PDD) and other disorders from cortical dementias such as Alzheimer's disease or frontotemporal dementia. Subcortical dementias are characterized by relative preservation of functions such as language, memory, and praxis. Although the Folstein Mini-Mental State Exam (MMSE) is useful as a general screen for cognitive dysfunction, a normal-range score does not exclude dementia, particularly one involving frontal or executive function. If suspicion remains high, formal neuropsychological testing may help to sort out the pattern of dysfunction. More practical instruments for the assessment of cognitive dysfunction in PD are currently in development (53).

Pathogenesis of Cognitive Dysfunction

From a neuropharmacological standpoint, dysfunction of mesolimbic monoaminergic and cholinergic pathways is the primary mechanism of cognitive dysfunction in PD (54). Functional imaging demonstrates specific patterns of cortical hypoperfusion (55), decreases in cortical cholinergic binding (56), and focal decreased metabolic activity using [^{18}F] dopa positron emission tomography (PET) (57). Pathologically, neuronal loss and synuclein inclusions occur in neocortical and limbic regions, the locus ceruleus, raphe nuclei, nucleus basalis of Meynert, and striatum. Because cortical LB (CLB) and Alzheimer's-type neurofibrillary tangles are associated with PDD, investigators have placed PDD on a spectrum with DLB and the LB variant of Alzheimer's disease (58,59). In PDD, CLB have been shown to more sensitive and specific predictors of cognitive impairments than either Alzheimer's-type plaques or tangles (60–62). For more information, see the chapter on DLB in this textbook.

Visual Hallucinations

Prevalence, Incidence, and Risk Factors

Visual hallucinations (VH) are a common and prominent feature in middle-to-later stages of PD, affecting approximately 20% of patients in population-based studies and 40% of patients in hospital-based series (63–65). In a cohort study by Goetz et al., the prevalence of hallucinations increased from 33% at baseline to 63% at 48 months, despite best medical therapy, attesting to the chronic, progressive, and refractory nature of VH (66). Patients at risk for VH tend to be older, have a longer disease duration, and are more likely to suffer from motor and cognitive impairments, depression, and excessive daytime somnolence (65,67). VH in the elderly PD patient have been shown to be an independent risk factor for nursing home placement (48,68).

Phenomenology

In PD, minor hallucinations may occur shortly after the initiation of levodopa treatment. Patients may describe sensations of a person or animal in close proximity to the patient (presence hallucinations), brief sensations of a person or animal passing sideways (passage hallucinations), or misperceptions (illusions). In most instances, the sensations are brief, lasting seconds to minutes, easily dismissed, and rarely mentioned spontaneously by the patient. These events often occur without any major psychological consequence or underlying psychosis. Complex

VH occur in up to 25% of patients with PD (65). They are often described as vivid scenes of people or animals with or without voices and action. Most episodes are typically brief (<5 minutes). Vague auditory hallucinations may accompany formed VH, but almost never have the persecutory quality seen in schizophrenia. Insight usually remains intact and delusions are a rare occurrence in the nondemented PD patient. Early onset of formed VH (within 2 years of initial symptoms) in the setting of cognitive dysfunction and parkinsonism suggests a diagnosis of DLB rather than idiopathic PD (69). Routine questioning and explanation of VH uncovers these phenomena, and may serve to alleviate anxiety or embarrassment.

Pathogenesis

Hallucinations in PD invariably begin in association with dopaminergic therapy. All antiparkinsonian agents (levodopa, dopamine agonists, amantadine, and anticholinergic agents) have a tendency to induce hallucinations in predisposed PD patients. The course of hallucinosis is typically chronic and progressive, although some patients have remissions with medication reductions or addition of antipsychotic treatment. However, no consistent relationship has been demonstrated between VH and medication dosage or motor function (66). In fact, even high-dose levodopa infusions in patients with chronic daily VH do not reliably induce these phenomena (70).

Similar to PD hallucinosis, VH in the visually impaired (the so-called *Charles Bonnet syndrome*) and in patients with midbrain lesions *(peduncular hallucinosis)* are well-formed, occur in psychologically normal individuals, and are prominent in evening hours or in low light. Thus, investigators have speculated that PD hallucinosis may arise from impaired visual perception or brainstem-mediated release of cortical visual centers. Pathology in ventral-temporal regions involved in visual imagery may lead to hallucinations in PD (71).

Recent attention has focused on the association between VH and disordered sleep. A long-held belief has been that vivid dreams often represent a precursor to VH. Decreased rapid eye movement (REM) sleep has been associated with the presence of PD-related hallucinations (72,73). REM intrusion into daytime wakefulness, similar to what occurs in narcolepsy, has been considered a possible mechanism (74).

Thought Disorders/Delusions

Delusions occur less frequently than VH (in roughly 6%–10% of PD patients) (75). When present, they often are accompanied by formed VH. Typical scenarios include intrusive or threatening neighbors who may be stealing, spying, or plotting against them. Patients may report that a family member has been replaced by an identical imposter (the so-called *Capgras syndrome*). Another common theme is the suspicion of spousal infidelity. Delusional PD patients are often more depressed and have more advanced cognitive and motor impairment, particularly akinesia and rigidity (75,76). VH and delusions are more typical of Lewy body disorders (PD and DLB), rather than Alzheimer's disease, and may occur as a result of presynaptic cholinergic deficiency (77–79).

Depression

Depression and mood disorders are very common in PD. The lifetime risk of major depression and dysthymia in PD is approximately 30% to 60%, with an annual estimated incidence of 2% (43,80,81). Nevertheless, depression is underrecognized and undertreated in this population (82). Depression may predate the onset of motor disability in as many as 25% of patients, and a case-control study has identified a higher likelihood of premorbid anxiety and depression in those subsequently diagnosed with PD (83,84). Early onset of PD, male sex, hallucinations or delusions, and the akinetic-rigid form of PD have been identified as risk factors for depression (85–89). Depression has also been associated with right-sided predominant symptoms that may be a result of more severe left cerebral pathology (85,90).

Symptoms common to PD, such as emotional blunting, fatigue, excessive daytime somnolence, insomnia, and sexual dysfunction may suggest to the clinician a diagnosis of major depressive disorder. Mood swings, dysphoria, and anxiety may be induced by response fluctuations to levodopa. Moreover, PD patients often present with atypical features of depression such as generalized anxiety, panic attacks, and social phobias (91). Dysthymia is common as well (81,89). Clinical features differentiating PD-related depression from major depressive disorder include increased pessimism, hopelessness, apathy, increased concern for health, and suicidal ideation without action or plan. Levels of guilt, self blame, and worthlessness tend to be lower (80,92,93). Suicide rates in the PD population are no different or lower when compared to the general population (94,95). However, depressed PD patients may progress faster and have greater cognitive decline and loss of independent function compared to PD controls (96,97).

Both biological and psychological factors have been implicated. The reaction to a chronic neurodegenerative disease without cure is an obvious but incomplete explanation. Compared to chronically ill patients with similar levels of disability, PD patients score higher on psychiatric rating scales such as the Beck Depression Inventory (83). Multiple studies have demonstrated that severity of depression is independent of motor disability, suggesting an etiology separate from the nigrostriatal dopaminergic system (43,88,90,97–99). [^{18}F] deoxyglucose PET studies have revealed caudate, limbic, and frontal hypometabolism in depressed and dysphoric PD patients (100,101). In keeping with current biological theories of depression, cerebrospinal fluid serotonin metabolites are reduced in depressed PD patients compared to controls (102).

Sleep

Excessive daytime somnolence (EDS), insomnia, periodic limb movements of sleep (PLMS), narcolepsy-like sleep attacks, and obstructive sleep apnea are all highly prevalent in PD. It has recently been suggested that PD hallucinosis may be a manifestation of altered sleep architecture (74,103–105). EDS is one of the more common complaints of PD patients and has been measured quantitatively using the Epworth Sleep Scale (106) and nocturnal polysomnograms (PSG). Arnulf et al. evaluated possible factors for EDS by performing PSG in 54 consecutive PD patients complaining of sleepiness (107). A narcolepsy-like phenotype with sleep-onset REM periods and short mean sleep latencies has been described. Furthermore, severity of EDS did not correlate with dopamine agonist treatment, PLMS, arousals, or apneas–hypopneas, suggesting an inherent pathochemical alteration as an etiology.

REM sleep behavior disorder (RBD) is the acting-out of dreams with complex motor and vocal behaviors, such as screaming, walking, thrashing, and even hitting. The disorder is characterized by loss of muscle atonia during REM sleep leading to complex motor behaviors. According to the International Classification of Sleep Disorders, RBD is defined by limb or body movements associated with dream mentation and at least one of the following: harmful or potentially harmful sleep behaviors, dreams that are acted out, or sleep behaviors that disrupt sleep continuity (108). The behavior causes injury in at least one-third of patients with the disorder (72). RBD is prevalent in otherwise-normal elderly males, in PD, and in other neurodegenerative disorders, such as DLB or multiple system atrophy associated with α-synuclein pathology. Approximately 33% of unselected PD patients have RBD as measured by nocturnal PSG. Only half of those patients report a history suggestive of the diagnosis; so, an overnight sleep study is often necessary to make a diagnosis (109). Treatment with clonazepam is often very effective in controlling the behavior.

Other Neuropsychiatric Manifestations

Anxiety

Anxiety may occur in isolation, as a feature of depression, or as a manifestation of levodopa response fluctuations (42,110). Approximately 25% to 40% of PD outpatients meet DSM criteria for an anxiety disorder (42,111). Other pathways besides the nigrostriatal dopamine pathway may be involved in the pathogenesis of anxiety, since levodopa dosage and motor function have not been shown to correlate with symptoms (111).

Akathisia

Akathisia may coexist with or be mistaken for anxiety. True akathisia is described as an inner sensation of restlessness in the absence of rigidity or pain. The sensations are often accompanied by repetitive, automatic behaviors, such as rocking, shifting, or pacing. In a series of 100 PD patients, 26% reported true akathisia (112). Akathisia may be a prominent off state symptom in PD as a result of relative dopamine deficiency, and can be one of the most distressing symptoms in PD. Likewise, akathisia related to dopamine receptor blocking agents may be identical. However, in individual patients, akathisia may respond to anticholinergics, β-adrenergic or α-adrenergic blockers, or opiates, suggesting a complex neurochemical alteration.

Apathy

Apathy, or lack of interest, is common in PD and may be difficult to differentiate from anhedonia, the lack of the ability to experience pleasure. There is a body of evidence suggesting that, both premorbidly and during illness, PD patients display a specific personality subtype characterized by lack of novelty-seeking behaviors (113,114). Novelty-seeking or risk taking in humans may be the correlate of exploratory behavior in animals, which is thought to be dopamine-mediated. Other terms used to describe this personality type include: rigid, stoic, slow-tempered, frugal, and orderly. When compared to similarly disabled controls with osteoarthritis, PD patients show higher levels of apathy and a strong correlation between apathy and executive dysfunction (114). The origin of apathy may be linked to ventral tegmental dopamine deficiency. Methylphenidate and similar stimulants may be useful in the treatment of PD-related apathy (115,116).

Addictive and Compulsive Behaviors

Addictive and compulsive behaviors may occur as a complication of PD treatment. *Punding*, a rare stereotypical motor behavior characterized by intense fascination and repetitive handling of inanimate objects, has been associated with levodopa treatment in PD patients (117). Excessive levodopa intake associated with compulsive spending may also occur. Recently pathological gambling has been reported in association with dopamine-agonist therapy (118). These behaviors are often diminished with withdrawal of the suspected agent.

TREATMENT OF PARKINSON'S DISEASE

Nonpharmacological, pharmacological, and surgical therapies exist for PD, each designed to diminish disability and improve patients' quality of life. Pharmacological treatment of PD is further divided by disease severity into neuroprotective, early disease, and advanced disease treatments.

Nonpharmacological Therapies

Nonpharmacological therapies in PD can be another tool for the clinician to improve function and quality of life, although these modalities have not been studied extensively. Educational resources and support groups are designed to help patients cope with their illness. Because of the potential distress that may occur when early disease patients meet with advanced disease patients, support groups are

TABLE 40-5

NATIONAL PARKINSON'S DISEASE ORGANIZATIONS

The National Parkinson Foundation
1-800-327-4545
www.parkinson.org

Parkinson's Disease Foundation
1-800-457-6676
www.pdf.org

American Parkinson Disease Association
1-888-400-2732
www.apdaparkinson.org

often divided into stages and age of onset. Some areas even offer gender-specific groups. More information on support groups and other resources can be obtained through the many regional or national organizations dedicated to supporting PD patients (Table 40-5).

Physical and occupational therapy can be important in early stages by encouraging physical activity and exercise, and during advanced stages when balance and gait can lead to major disability. A blinded trial randomizing patients to either normal physical activity versus intensive physical therapy showed improvements in the latter group in UPDRS motor and ADL scores, which returned to baseline at the cessation of the trial (119). Occupational therapy can be useful to determine home safety and the need for assistive devices in improving activities of daily living.

Speech therapy with exercises such as the *Lee Silverman technique* has been shown to improve hypophonia and hypokinetic dysarthria. The technique is taught through an intensive program administered by specially certified therapists. Several studies have shown that the technique produces sustained improvement in vocal intensity, inflection, as well as control of oral musculature as compared to placebo and traditional techniques (120–125). At the same time, a swallowing evaluation can also help to diagnose and classify dysphagia types and identify subclinical aspiration.

Pharmacologic Therapies

Possible Neuroprotective Therapy

Neuroprotective treatments are designed to slow or arrest the progression of neuronal loss. To date, no agent has been clearly shown to be neuroprotective, despite extensive study of multiple agents. Potential agents are sought that reduce oxidative stress, mitochondrial dysfunction, and free radical formation. The oxidative hypothesis is derived from the understanding that dopamine is oxidatively metabolized in the central nervous system and by the fact that mitochondrial toxins have been shown to lead to parkinsonian states (126). Unfortunately, determining whether or not an agent is neuroprotective is inherently difficult due to the lack of specific clinical endpoints, confounding due to a symptomatic benefit, and the lengthy follow-up required.

Selegiline, an irreversible monoamine oxidase (MAO) type B inhibitor with antioxidant properties, was shown in DATATOP (Deprenyl and Tocopherol Antioxidative Therapy of Parkinsonism), a large-scale double-blind placebo-controlled trial, to have previously unrecognized clinical benefits (127). Untreated PD patients received either placebo, selegiline (10 mg a day), tocopherol (a vitamin E component at 2000 IU a day), or a combination of tocopherol and selegiline. Degree of neuroprotection was measured as the time to disability and initiation of levodopa therapy. Tocopherol had no clinical effect, while a significant benefit was seen in subjects treated with selegiline during the first 12 months. The benefit observed was the same with or without tocopherol treatment. Unfortunately, because selegiline was found to exert a mild symptomatic benefit of undetermined duration, a clear neuroprotective benefit was not demonstrated. Subsequent follow-up accounting for the symptomatic benefit of selegiline found that selegiline- and nonselegiline-treated patients had comparable levels of disability after several years (128).

Coenzyme Q10 (CoQ) is an electron acceptor for complexes I and II of the mitochondrial electron transport chain (129). A pilot study of 15 subjects showed that CoQ was well tolerated and safe at a dose of 800 mg a day. Secondary measurement of the UPDRS showed no change (130). A subsequent multi-center blinded, randomized trial of 80 patients with early untreated PD demonstrated significantly less decline in UPDRS scores with higher doses of CoQ (1200 mg) as compared to placebo (131). Although suggestive of a neuroprotective benefit, a larger-scale study needs to be undertaken.

In addition to their proven symptomatic benefits, dopamine agonists have been proposed to be neuroprotective through various mechanisms, including decreased dopamine metabolism, free radical scavenging, and protection against neurotoxins (132). Functional imaging with PET and single photon emission computed tomog-raphy (SPECT) have served as surrogate markers of neuron loss. The REAL-PET study (ReQuip as Early Therapy versus Levodopa PET Study) followed [^{18}F] dopa PET scans in newly diagnosed PD patients treated with either levodopa or ropinirole for 2 years (133). Blinded evaluations of the imaging showed that patients treated with ropinirole had less decline in [^{18}F] dopa uptake as compared to levodopa patients. The CALM-PD trial (Comparison of the Agonist Pramipexole versus Levodopa on Motor Complications of PD) compared the effects of initial pramipexole versus levodopa treatment in *de novo* patients. Changes in the SPECT ligand [^{123} β]-CIT ([N-(3-fluoropropyl)-2 β-carbomethoxy-3 β-(4-iodo-phenyl)nortropane]) were studied in a subset of the randomized patients (134). The imaging portion of the study demonstrated less decline in striatal [^{123} β]-CIT uptake in subjects treated with pramipexole as compared to levodopa. Again, it is unclear whether the imaging changes represent an actual neuroprotective effect or regulatory postsynaptic changes induced by the agonist, unrelated to the degree of neuron loss.

Early Symptomatic Therapy

Treatment of PD is typically initiated when patients begin to experience social or functional disability. Factors to take into consideration when deciding upon treatment include the problematic symptoms, age, functional status, comorbid medical conditions, and cognitive status. A wide range of medications with proven symptomatic effects exists for PD. These include MAO inhibitors, anticholinergic agents, amantadine, dopamine agonists, and levodopa (Table 40-6).

Both selegiline and rasagiline irreversibly inhibit MAO type B, resulting in modest enhancement of striatal dopamine levels. As mentioned previously, selegiline has been shown in the DATATOP study to delay the need for levodopa therapy, at a dose of 10 mg a day. In practice, insomnia is the most commonly reported side effect, making daytime administration

TABLE 40-6
MEDICATIONS FOR THE SYMPTOMATIC TREATMENT OF PARKINSON'S DISEASE

Medication	Mechanism of Action	Typical Therapeutic Dosage
Selegiline	MAO-B inhibitor	5–10 mg a day
Rasagiline	MAO-B inhibitor	1–2 mg a day
Benztropine	Anticholinergic	0.5–4 mg a day
Trihexyphenidyl	Anticholinergic	2–8 mg a day
Amantadine	NMDA antagonist	200–400 mg a day
Pergolide	Dopamine agonist	0.75–5 mg a day
Bromocriptine	Dopamine agonist	10–40 mg a day
Pramipexole	Dopamine agonist	1.5–4.5 mg a day
Ropinirole	Dopamine agonist	7.5–24 mg a day
Levodopa		150–600 mg a day
Entacapone	COMT inhibitor	200 mg a day

COMT, catechol-o-methyltransferase; MAO-B, monoamine oxidase type B; NMDA, N-methyl-D-aspartate.

more appropriate. Rasagiline at 1 or 2 mg a day in early untreated PD patients has been shown to improve UPDRS scores from baseline, relative to placebo (135). Both agents also have theoretical neuroprotective properties but further studies are needed to help clarify this potential benefit.

Anticholinergic agents such as benztropine and tri-hexyphenidyl were among the original drugs used to treat PD. They have moderate effects on tremor, rigidity, and dystonia; however, side effects such as urinary retention, cognitive impairment, dry mouth, and blurred vision limit their use in the elderly (136).

Amantadine, originally developed for use against influenza, is a tricyclic amine with multiple putative mechanisms, including enhanced dopamine release, inhibition of dopamine reuptake, antimuscarinic effects, and N-methyl D-aspartate receptor antagonism (137). In addition to its use in early PD, its antidyskinetic properties make it useful for advanced-staged patients with motor fluctuations. Amantadine is generally well tolerated, but lower extremity edema, mental confusion, and hallucinations may complicate treatment.

Dopamine agonists have become the mainstay of treatment in early PD patients with mild symptoms, and are a useful adjunct in advanced patients with motor fluctuations. Bromocriptine, pergolide, ropinirole, and pramipexole are available in the US. Apomorphine, a potent D2 agonist, has multiple routes for administration, including intravenous, subcutaneous, sublingual, and intranasal, making it ideal for rescue therapy. Subcutaneous apomorphine has recently been FDA-approved for the treatment of refractory off periods. Dopamine agonists directly stimulate striatal dopamine receptors and, in general, all have greater affinity for the D_2 subfamily of receptors than the D_1 subfamily. Compared to placebo, all of the agonists have demonstrated similar efficacy and improvements in function as measured by UPDRS scores (138–140). Common side effects of all agonists include nausea, lightheadedness, pedal edema, hallucinations, and sedation (Table 40-7). Most of these adverse effects are dose-related and can be avoided by slow titration of the drug. The ergot agonists, bromocriptine and pergolide, carry the additional risk of retroperitoneal fibrosis and Raynaud's phenomenon. Cardiac valvular abnormalities have recently been attributed to pergolide use (141).

Two large-scale trials comparing initial levodopa to ropinirole and pramipexole therapy have demonstrated decreased motor fluctuations and dyskinesias over long-term follow-up (23 months for pramipexole and 5 years for ropinirole) (142,143). Although levodopa therapy was associated with higher UPDRS scores, subjects were able to maintain agonist monotherapy for prolonged periods with similar ADL scores and without more adverse events.

Despite the recent advances in pharmacotherapy, levo-dopa remains the most time-honored and effective treatment for symptoms of PD. The majority of PD patients will

TABLE 40-7
COMMON SIDE EFFECTS OF TREATMENT

- Hallucinations
- Insomnia
- Sedation
- Nausea, vomiting, anorexia
- Dyskinesias (chorea, athetosis)
- Dystonia
- Wearing-off, on–off phenomena, medication failures

attain significant, long-lasting benefit from levodopa, superior to any of the previously mentioned agents. It is well tolerated and effective across a large dose range, as long as administered with a peripheral decarboxylase inhibitor (e.g., carbidopa). Without such an inhibitor, the dramatic peripheral effects of dopamine, such as orthostatic hypotension, nausea, and emesis, prevent its tolerance, and availability to the brain. In the US, carbidopa is combined with levodopa in various formulations (10/100, 25/100, 25/250), marketed as Sinemet, allowing for flexible dosing. The half-life of Sinemet is approximately 90 minutes, so multiple daily doses are usually necessary. Typical dosing starts with $1/2$ of a 25/100 tablet three times daily, increasing over a few weeks to 1 to 2 tablets three times daily, watching for dose-dependent peripheral side effects. Central nervous system side effects such as sedation, insomnia, VH, confusion, or psychosis may also occur, especially in the elderly or in later stages of PD, but are generally infrequent in early stages.

For convenience, medication dosing is often scheduled around meal times. However, because levodopa absorption occurs in the duodenum through a saturable amino acid transporter, bioavailability may be limited by meals containing large protein content. To maximize bioavailability, patients should be instructed to take levodopa on an empty stomach (at least 45 minutes before a meal or 1–2 hours after a meal).

TABLE 40-8
MANAGEMENT OF PSYCHOSIS AND HALLUCINATIONS

- Exclude infection or other intercurrent illness that may cause a delirium
- Obtain detailed medication history with emphasis on recent additions (dosage changes, withdrawals, or possible ingestions)
- Withdraw medications in this order: anticholinergics, amantadine, selegiline, dopamine agonists, COMT inhibitors. If troubling hallucinations persist, consider decreasing levodopa dosage.
- Treatment with an atypical antipsychotic, e.g., quetiapine
- Clozapine for refractory psychosis

COMT, catechol-o-methyltransferase.

Controlled-release (CR) Sinemet has a half-life of approximately 3 hours, but with a slower onset of action and decreased bioavailability. Sinemet CR comes in 25/100 and 50/200 formulations. In early disease, Sinemet CR can be dosed twice a day, and is often used at bedtime to prevent wearing-off upon awakening. Physicians should be aware that less Sinemet CR is required than regular Sinemet during conversion from one to the other (100 mg regular Sinemet is equivalent to 133 mg of Sinemet CR).

Medical Treatment of Advanced Disease

Initially, the dose range and therapeutic window of levodopa is very wide. Small doses of levodopa have sustained and robust clinical benefit for several years. However, levodopa-responsive patients almost invariably require increasing doses (up to 1000–1500 mg) to maintain a stable level of function. With time, motor complications develop in virtually all PD patients as a result of a narrowing therapeutic window. As the disease progresses, the dose–response curve of levodopa evolves from a relatively smooth, long response curve to one with wider, and hence clinically apparent, variation from *on* (levodopa is working) to *off* (levodopa is not working). In other words, the dose–response curve in later disease mirrors the actual short half-life of levodopa. Strategies at this point focus on maximizing on time and minimizing off time and dyskinesias, fluctuations, and side effects while in the on state. The development of fluctuations may be related not only to progressive loss of the striatal dopamine storage capacity, but also to pulsatile stimulation of a declining number of striatal receptors (144). Therefore, it follows that strategies aimed at minimizing pulsatile stimulation may prevent the development of motor complications.

More frequent dosing is the most basic therapeutic maneuver, but is limited by the patient's ability to handle round-the-clock dosing and levodopa failures. Use of a controlled-release drug, e.g., Sinemet CR, may prolong on time but, in our experience, the decreased bioavailability often causes unpredictable responses in advanced patients. Furthermore, direct comparison of Sinemet CR to regular Sinemet has shown no major difference in the incidence of dyskinesia and motor complications (145).

The effects of the dopamine agonists pergolide, ropinirole, and pramipexole as adjunctive therapy in advanced PD with motor fluctuations have been independently studied in large-scale, controlled trials (146–148). All studies have shown decreased off time and improved on time function in association with a reduction of levodopa dosages. However, adverse effects such as dyskinesias and hallucinations were more common in treated groups.

The catechol-o-methyltransferase (COMT) inhibitors, tolcapone and entacapone, inhibit the peripheral catabolism of levodopa, leading to enhanced central nervous system availability of levodopa. Since the action of COMT inhibitors is dependent on the presence of levodopa, they have no effect on parkinsonian symptoms if levodopa is not co-administered. Entacapone significantly increases the area under the curve and the half-life of levodopa without increasing maximal plasma concentrations (149). Side effects are primarily dopaminergic, but both agents can also cause severe diarrhea and an orange urine discoloration. Both entacapone and tolcapone have been shown to improve motor fluctuations by decreasing wearing-off symptoms, increasing on time, and decreasing off time in randomized, controlled trials (150,151). Tolcapone is not currently in use due to the significant risk of developing fulminant hepatitis.

MAO inhibitors and amantadine have also shown utility in advanced stages of PD. In a blinded, controlled crossover study of 14 patients with dyskinesias, amantadine was shown to reduce dyskinesias by 60% over placebo, without affecting the antiparkinsonian effects of levodopa (152). Patients also noticed a beneficial effect on motor fluctuations. In patients with renal insufficiency, dose adjustments need to be made based on creatinine clearance, since amantadine is renally excreted. As an adjunctive agent, selegiline has been shown to decrease motor fluctuations, albeit transiently, in open-label studies (153,154). Similarly, rasagiline may reduce off time by controlling PD symptoms (155).

Management of Dementia

The efficacy of current acetylcholinesterase inhibitors donepezil, rivastigmine, and galantamine has been proven in Alzheimer's disease, and to a lesser extent in DLB. Case reports suggest that acetylcholinesterase inhibitors may potentially exacerbate parkinsonism (156,157). A small, blinded 10-week crossover study of donepezil in PDD showed improvement in MMSE and clinician and caregiver's impression of change without change in UPDRS motor score (158). A second short-term study showed similar cognitive benefits in the memory subscale of the Mattis Dementia Rating Scale (159). Open-label studies of rivastigmine show improvement in cognition and behavior without adversely affecting motor function (160,161). Recently, a multi-center blinded study of rivastigmine in PDD showed moderate improvement in subjective and objective measures of cognitive function; however, the treated patients were more likely to suffer from nausea, vomiting, and tremor than placebo group (162). Given that there are no current alternatives for PDD, we tend to use acetylcholinesterase inhibitors cautiously and promptly taper or withdraw the medication with the development of side effects.

Management of Psychosis and Hallucinations

VH in PD are unique in that they commonly occur in the absence of psychosis, delusions, or alteration in consciousness and attention. When VH occur infrequently in a patient with good cognition, insight, and judgment, there is not always an urgent need to treat them. On the other hand, psychosis and delusions tend to develop insidiously, are more likely to occur in a hallucinating patient, and may not be apparent until a catastrophic event such as an acute confusional episode, fall, or hospitalization brings the events to the physician's or caregiver's attention. We therefore advocate treating hallucinations once they become regular and frequent events, before they lead to complications.

Management of VH, psychosis, or altered mental status should be approached in a systematic manner. (Table 40-8). An abrupt change in mental function should always prompt a search for intercurrent infection or toxic–metabolic causes for altered mental status. Medication additions or withdrawals need to be carefully considered. At a certain point in the disease process, treatment of motor symptoms may be at odds with the mental stability of the patient. In other words, treating the thought disorder may be more critical than maximizing motor function and overmedication with dopaminergic agents should be avoided. It may be prudent to withdraw medications that have a tendency to induce hallucinations, starting with anticholinergics, amantadine, and selegiline, and then the dopamine agonists. Levodopa is relatively less likely to induce hallucinations and psychosis, but nevertheless may need to be withdrawn in certain patients.

The addition of antipsychotic medication is often necessary in order to avoid complete withdrawal of levodopa. Few safe options for the treatment of PD-related psychosis existed before the advent of the newer atypical agents, clozapine, risperidone, olanzapine, quetiapine, ziprasidone, and aripiprazole. To this day, only clozapine remains free of extrapyramidal side effects. Numerous retrospective and prospective studies have demonstrated that low-dose clozapine is effective in treating PD-related psychosis (reviewed by Friedman (163) and Factor (36)). Two multi-center blinded placebo-controlled trials from the US Parkinson Study Group and the French Clozapine Parkinson Study Group showed that low doses of clozapine are effective in treating PD-related psychosis. Effective daily doses are one-tenth the typical dosages used to treat schizophrenia. Furthermore, clozapine may in fact have beneficial effects on tremor (164–167), levodopa-induced dyskinesia (168–170), and nocturnal akathisia (171). Clozapine use is limited by the 1% to 2% risk of idiosyncratic leukopenia and agranulocytosis and the need for frequent blood count monitoring. In a 5-year follow-up study of 32 PD patients on low-dose clozapine, no patients developed neutropenia and withdrawal was most commonly due to remission of psychosis (172). In the US, a patient must be entered into a national registry and weekly blood counts are required for the first 6 months and then biweekly afterwards. Only a one-week supply of the medication can be dispensed at a time.

Risperidone was the second atypical antipsychotic approved in the US. Open-label studies in PD-related psychosis have shown conflicting and inconclusive results due to the small numbers of patients studied. While most studies have demonstrated improvement in psychosis, concern arose regarding reports of worsening parkinsonism (173–175). The initial open-label study of risperidone by Meco et al.

was promising in that all treated patients experienced improvement in psychosis without any observable change in motor function (176). However, after long-term follow-up (up to 1 year), risperidone was discontinued in seven out of ten patients, in two due to worsening of parkinsonism (173). In a larger cohort followed over 26 weeks, 16 of the 39 patients completed the study and showed no worsening of UPDRS motor scores, while six others had rapid and pronounced deterioration of parkinsonism, resulting in early termination. The author explained that these six patients had probable Lewy body dementia rather than PD (177). Similarly, a 12-week study of 17 patients showed similar benefits at low doses without worsening of UPDRS (178). However, hypokinesia, drooling, falls, and gait abnormalities were among the most common adverse events in this study. A small, randomized head-to-head study of risperidone and clozapine showed similar effect on psychosis severity after 12 weeks. However, the agents tended to have opposing effects on UPDRS motor scores (decreasing scores in the risperidone group and increasing scores in the clozapine group), though not reaching clinical significance (179). Based on concern for potential parkinsonian side effects, risperidone is usually used less often in PD-related psychosis (175,180,181), and at doses of 0.25 to 1 mg/day.

Initial studies of olanzapine treatment in PD showed improvement in psychosis without worsening of parkinsonism (182,183). A study by Graham et al. showed early worsening of motor function prompting study withdrawal (184). Other open-label studies suggested that olanzapine was less well tolerated by PD patients due to adverse effects and worsening of motor function, even when compared to the frequent blood work associated with clozapine (185–190). In a placebo-controlled trial, olanzapine did not significantly improve hallucinations and had adverse effects on motor function (191). A comparative trial of clozapine and olanzapine was terminated early due to significant decline in motor function from baseline in the olanzapine group (192). When it is used, it's at doses of 2.5 to 10 mg/day.

In open-label studies, quetiapine has shown to be effective for PD-related psychosis with minimal risk of inducing extrapyramidal side effects (193–195). Its efficacy was comparable to clozapine's in one preliminary head-to-head study (196). Clozapine had the additional advantage of improving motor function while quetiapine had no major beneficial or deleterious effects on motor function. Switching from clozapine to quetiapine may be desirable for some patients and in two studies has been accomplished with success (197,198).

Given quetiapine's relative balance of efficacy and safety as compared to other atypical antipsychotics, although with limited data supporting its antipsychotic effect at less than 200 mg/day, it is used often in PD patients. Dosing usually starts at 12.5 mg at bedtime and is increased by 12.5 mg every 3 to 5 days until a dose of 50 mg at bedtime is reached; dosing may be slowly increased further until psychosis is controlled or side effects–particularly sedation–develop. Typically, doses between 50 and 150 mg/day are adequate in controlling symptoms. When necessary, 50 mg or less of clozapine added is usually adequate to control symptoms.

At the time of writing, very little evidence exists for the use of ziprasidone or aripiprazole in PD-related psychosis (199). Improvement in behavior, hallucinations, and delusions have also been reported with acetylcholinesterase inhibitors (161,200–203).

Management of Depression and Mood Symptoms in Parkinson's Disease

In the elderly PD population, tricyclic antidepressants may be effective for depression but poorly tolerated due to anticholinergic side effects, such as sedation, cognitive effects, constipation, dry mouth, and blurred vision. In practice, selective serotonin-reuptake inhibitors (SSRI) are well tolerated and just as effective. However, parkinsonism may theoretically worsen. Open-label studies of SSRIs have all shown improvement in depressive scores and symptoms without any worsening of parkinsonism (204). Electroconvulsive therapy has been shown to have beneficial effects on not only depression, but also psychosis and motor function in PD (205).

A Clinical Algorithm

In summary, the medical treatment of PD has advanced dramatically in the last decade but is limited by the relentless progression of the disease. To date, no effective disease-modifying therapies have been discovered. The current state of treatment rests primarily on a symptom-based approach.

Although levodopa remains the most effective therapy for symptoms of PD, we typically begin treatment of mild or early PD in younger patients with a dopamine agonist alone. The rationale behind this approach is to delay the onset of response fluctuations and dyskinesias. Mild symptoms can often be adequately controlled for several months to years on these agents. Any possible neuroprotective benefit is secondary in this decision. Concerns over levodopa toxicity and eventual lack of efficacy are unfounded.

For patients above the age of 65, the risk for development of motor complications is low and agonist tolerability is often decreased. In such cases, we advocate starting with low doses of carbidopa/levodopa (25/100 TID) and maintaining a dose adequate to alleviate disability. There is no fixed dosage ceiling, although 1000 mg of levodopa is generally considered more than adequate to control symptoms in PD. The dose may be increased by one-half- to whole-tablet increments per dose as needed.

If end-of-dose wearing-off occurs, it is important to assess not only the length of the levodopa response, but also the frequency and predictability. Mild predictable wearing-off is easily addressed by increasing the frequency of dosing from the typical 5-to-6-hour cycle of mealtime dosing to 3-to-4-hour dosing cycles. As the duration

between wearing-off and the next dose increases, frequent dosing becomes impractical. Entacapone (200 mg) can be added to each dose of levodopa to increase the duration of the response, thus increasing daily on time. A concomitant reduction in levodopa dosage by 15% to 30% is recommended if the patient is at the high end of the therapeutic window.

Response to levodopa may become more unpredictable with advancing disease. Response failure may occur with absent or delayed onset of action, or sudden or unpredictable turning off. Addition of a dopamine agonist is often useful in patients with complex or unpredictable motor complications, as long as dyskinesias, VH, and other levodopa-related side effects are manageable.

In a certain subset of patients, the secondary symptoms of PD can become quite disabling. Often increasing dopaminergic therapy is not effective. Table 40-9 outlines some of the most common secondary symptoms of PD and the accepted therapeutic strategies. These strategies have been adopted by our center and are taken from consensus guidelines published by the American Academy of Neurology (206).

Surgical Therapy

Surgical therapy has become the mainstay of therapy in patients with medically refractory PD. Like all medical therapies, no surgical therapy has been shown to modify or alter the course of the disease. In recent years, lesioning surgery, or the selective destruction of basal ganglia targets (e.g., pallidotomy) has fallen out of favor and deep brain stimulation (DBS) has become the surgical treatment of choice. DBS is performed by stereotactically implanting microelectrodes into one of two locations in the basal ganglia: the globus pallidus interna (GPi) or the subthalamic nucleus (STN). The electrodes are connected to a small adjustable stimulator implanted in the chest wall. The effect of stimulation approximates temporary inhibition of the target. Voltage, frequency, and pulse width are adjusted to decrease symptoms. The main advantages of DBS over lesioning therapy include decreased brain trauma, modifiability, and reversibility of effects. Compared to bilateral ablative procedures that are often fraught with complications, bilateral DBS is both safe and effective.

The first open-label studies of DBS in both brain targets occurred in parallel in the late 1990s. Stimulation of either site revealed dramatic improvement in the motor symptoms of PD, particularly in patients with pronounced fluctuations between on and off medication states. Reduction of on-period dyskinesias have demonstrated improved on function (207–212). Stimulation of the STN also was associated with a significant reduction in levodopa dosage (212,213). Recent 5-year follow-up of 49 patients with bilateral STN DBS showed sustained improvement in tremor, rigidity, and independent function in the majority of patients. Fluctuations, dyskinesia, and levodopa dosage were significantly reduced. However, akinesia, speech, postural stability, and

TABLE 40-9
SECONDARY SYMPTOMS OF PARKINSON'S DISEASE AND THERAPEUTIC STRATEGIES

Symptom	Nonpharmacologic	Pharmacologic
Constipation	Increasing dietary fiber and fluid intake Regular exercise Discontinue anticholinergics	Stool softeners (docusate) Osmotic laxatives (lactulose, milk of magnesia) Stimulant laxative (bisacodyl) Enemas
Drooling	Speech evaluation and therapy	Botulinum toxin injections Peripheral anticholinergic agent (glycopyrrolate)
Dysarthria/hypophonia	Speech therapy (Lee Silverman technique)	If off symptom, increase dopaminergic therapy
Dysphagia	Dysphagia evaluation Soft-mechanical diet Schedule meals with on time Gastrostomy	If off symptom, increase dopaminergic therapy
Freezing	Physical–occupational therapy for gait training. Visual cues	If off symptom, increase dopaminergic therapy
Postural instability/falls	Physical–occupational therapy for gait training or home-safety evaluation care, walker, wheelchair, or other form of assistance Evaluation for orthostasis	If off symptom, increase dopaminergic therapy
Male impotence	Review medications	Trial of an oral erectogenic drug Alprostadil (intracavernous injections or intraurethral suppository)
Orthostasis	Evaluate for diabetes or underlying endocrine disorder Urological evaluation Elevate head of bed 10–30 degrees Encourage dietary salt intake Compression stockings	Discontinue potential hypotensive drugs Salt-retaining mineralocorticoid (e.g., fludrocortisone) Pressors (e.g., midodrine, ephedrine)
Overactive bladder	Avoid bedtime fluid intake Exclude infection, prostatism, or other urological problems	Antimuscarinic agents (oxybutynin, tolteridine, imipramine)
Seborrheic dermatitis		Coal tar or selenium-based shampoos Topical steroids

freezing measured while on levodopa continued to decline in parallel with the expected progression of disease (214). The question arises as to which is the superior DBS site. A nonrandomized blinded crossover study of stimulation at the GPi versus STN showed very similar benefits in both groups of patients (215). A large-scale randomized, double-blinded trial is currently underway to address the question of whether one site of stimulation is superior to the other.

Complications unique to DBS include electrical malfunction, lead fracture, battery replacement (every 1–5 years), lengthy initial stimulator programming, infection, skin erosion, intracerebral hemorrhage, and infarct. The appropriate candidate should have idiopathic PD with disabling symptoms responsive to levodopa, be free of cognitive or neuropsychological illness, and have the emotional capabilities and social support to cope with potentially life-altering surgery and the often-frequent and involved visits required after surgery. No firm age requirement has been recommended, although it is generally believed that patients above 75 years of age may respond less well to the rigors of surgery and incur greater risk due to medical comorbidities and cognitive status.

REFERENCES

1. Tanner CM, Goldman SM. Epidemiology of Parkinson's disease. *Neurol Clin.* 1996;14:317–335.
2. Mayeux R, Marder K, Cote LJ, et al. The frequency of idiopathic Parkinson's disease by age, ethnic group, and sex in northern Manhattan, 1988–1993. *Am J Epidemiol.* 1995;142:820–827.
3. Mayeux R, Denaro J, Hemenegildo N, et al. A population-based investigation of Parkinson's disease with and without dementia. Relationship to age and gender. *Arch Neurol.* 1992;49:492–497.
4. Taylor CA, Saint-Hilaire MH, Cupples LA, et al. Environmental, medical, and family history risk factors for Parkinson's disease: a New England-based case control study. *Am J Med Genet.* 1999; 88:742–749.
5. Seidler A, Hellenbrand W, Robra BP, et al. Possible environmental, occupational, and other etiologic factors for Parkinson's disease: a case-control study in Germany. *Neurology.* 1996;46:1275–1284.
6. Petrovitch H, Ross GW, Abbott RD, et al. Plantation work and risk of Parkinson disease in a population-based longitudinal study. *Arch Neurol.* 2002;59:1787–1792.
7. Langston JW, Ballard P. Parkinsonism induced by 1-methyl-4-phenyl-1,2,3,6-tetrahydropyridine (MPTP): implications for treatment and the pathogenesis of Parkinson's disease. *Can J Neurol Sci.* 1984;11:160–165.
8. Betarbet R, Sherer TB, MacKenzie G, Garcia-Osuna M, Panov AV, Greenamyre JT. Chronic systemic pesticide exposure reproduces features of Parkinson's disease. *Nat Neurosci.* 2000;3:1301–1306.
9. Uitti RJ, Rajput AH, Ashenhurst EM, Rozdilsky B. Cyanide-induced parkinsonism: a clinicopathologic report. *Neurology.* 1985;35:921–925.
10. Hernan MA, Takkouche B, Caamano-Isorna F, Gestal-Otero JJ. A meta-analysis of coffee drinking, cigarette smoking, and the risk of Parkinson's disease. *Ann Neurol.* 2002;52:276–284.
11. Tanner CM, Goldman SM, Aston DA, et al. Smoking and Parkinson's disease in twins. *Neurology.* 2002;58:581–588.
12. Ross GW, Abbott RD, Petrovitch H, et al. Association of coffee and caffeine intake with the risk of Parkinson disease. *JAMA.* 2000;283:2674–2679.
13. Tanner CM, Ottman R, Goldman SM, et al. Parkinson disease in twins: an etiologic study. *JAMA.* 1999;281:341–346.
14. Lucking CB, Durr A, Bonifati V, et al. Association between early-onset Parkinson's disease and mutations in the parkin gene. French Parkinson's Disease Genetics Study Group. *N Engl J Med.* 2000;342:1560–1567.
15. Shimura H, Hattori N, Kubo S, et al. Familial Parkinson disease gene product, parkin, is a ubiquitin-protein ligase. *Nat Genet.* 2000;25:302–305.
16. Polymeropoulos MH, Lavedan C, Leroy E, et al. Mutation in the alpha-synuclein gene identified in families with Parkinson's disease. *Science.* 1997;276:2045–2047.
17. Leroy E, Boyer R, Auburger G, et al. The ubiquitin pathway in Parkinson's disease. *Nature.* 1998;395:451–452.
18. Mouradian MM. Recent advances in the genetics and pathogenesis of Parkinson disease. *Neurology.* 2002;58:179–185.
19. Hughes AJ, Daniel SE, Blankson S, Lees AJ. A clinicopathologic study of 100 cases of Parkinson's disease. *Arch Neurol.* 1993;50:140–148.
20. Nakano I, Hirano A. Parkinson's disease: neuron loss in the nucleus basalis without concomitant Alzheimer's disease. *Ann Neurol.* 1984;15:415–418.
21. Kupsky WJ, Grimes MM, Sweeting J, Bertsch R, Cote LJ. Parkinson's disease and megacolon: concentric hyaline inclusions (Lewy bodies) in enteric ganglion cells. *Neurology.* 1987;37:1253–1255.
22. Duda JE, Giasson BI, Mabon ME, Lee VM, Trojanowski JQ. Novel antibodies to synuclein show abundant striatal pathology in Lewy body diseases. *Ann Neurol.* 2002;52:205–210.
23. Rinne UK, Rinne JO, Rinne JK, Laakso K, Laihinen A, Lonnberg P. Brain receptor changes in Parkinson's disease in relation to the disease process and treatment. *J Neural Transm Suppl.* 1983;18:279–286.
24. Hoehn MM, Yahr MD. Parkinsonism: onset, progression and mortality. *Neurology.* 1967;17:427–442.
25. The Unified Parkinson's Disease Rating Scale (UPDRS): status and recommendations. *Mov Disord.* 2003;18:738–750.
26. Winikates J, Jankovic J. Clinical correlates of vascular parkinsonism. *Arch Neurol.* 1999;56:98–102.
27. Krusz JC, Koller WC, Ziegler DK. Historical review: abnormal movements associated with epidemic encephalitis lethargica. *Mov Disord.* 1987;2:137–141.
28. Lo KC, Geddes JF, Daniels RS, Oxford JS. Lack of detection of influenza genes in archived formalin-fixed, paraffin wax-embedded brain samples of encephalitis lethargica patients from 1916 to 1920. *Virchows Arch.* 2003;442:591–596.
29. McCall S, Henry JM, Reid AH, Taubenberger JK. Influenza RNA not detected in archival brain tissues from acute encephalitis lethargica cases or in postencephalitic Parkinson cases. *J Neuropathol Exp Neurol.* 2001;60:696–704.
30. Ishii T, Nakamura Y. Distribution and ultrastructure of Alzheimer's neurofibrillary tangles in postencephalitic Parkinsonism of Economo type. *Acta Neuropathol (Berl).* 1981;55:59–62.
31. Geddes JF, Hughes AJ, Lees AJ, Daniel SE. Pathological overlap in cases of parkinsonism associated with neurofibrillary tangles. A study of recent cases of postencephalitic parkinsonism and comparison with progressive supranuclear palsy and Guamanian parkinsonism-dementia complex. *Brain.* 1993;116(Pt 1):281–302.
32. Kiley M, Esiri MM. A contemporary case of encephalitis lethargica. *Clin Neuropathol.* 2001;20:2–7.
33. Howard RS, Lees AJ. Encephalitis lethargica. A report of four recent cases. *Brain.* 1987;110 (Pt 1):19–33.
34. Dale RC, Church AJ, Surtees RA, et al. Encephalitis lethargica syndrome: 20 new cases and evidence of basal ganglia autoimmunity. *Brain.* 2004;127:21–33.
35. Hardie RJ, Lees AJ. Neuroleptic-induced Parkinson's syndrome: clinical features and results of treatment with levodopa. *J Neurol Neurosurg Psychiatry.* 1988;51:850–854.
36. Factor SA, Friedman JH. The emerging role of clozapine in the treatment of movement disorders. *Mov Disord.* 1997;12:483–496.
37. Olanow CW. Manganese-induced parkinsonism and Parkinson's disease. *Ann N Y Acad Sci.* 2004;1012:209–223.
38. Klawans HL, Stein RW, Tanner CM, Goetz CG. A pure parkinsonian syndrome following acute carbon monoxide intoxication. *Arch Neurol.* 1982;39:302–304.
39. Stern MB, Braffman BH, Skolnick BE, Hurtig HI, Grossman RI. Magnetic resonance imaging in Parkinson's disease and parkinsonian syndromes. *Neurology.* 1989;39:1524–1526.
40. Schocke MF, Seppi K, Esterhammer R, et al. Diffusion-weighted MRI differentiates the Parkinson variant of multiple system atrophy from PD. *Neurology.* 2002;58:575–580.
41. Seppi K, Schocke MF, Esterhammer R, et al. Diffusion-weighted imaging discriminates progressive supranuclear palsy from PD, but not from the Parkinson variant of multiple system atrophy. *Neurology.* 2003;60:922–927.
42. Menza MA, Robertson-Hoffman DE, Bonapace AS. Parkinson's disease and anxiety: comorbidity with depression. *Biol Psychiatry.* 1993;34:465–470.
43. Tandberg E, Larsen JP, Aarsland D, Cummings JL. The occurrence of depression in Parkinson's disease. A community-based study. *Arch Neurol.* 1996;53:175–179.
44. Aarsland D, Tandberg E, Larsen JP, Cummings JL. Frequency of dementia in Parkinson disease. *Arch Neurol.* 1996;53:538–542.
45. Tison F, Dartigues JF, Auriacombe S, Letenneur L, Boller F, Alperovitch A. Dementia in Parkinson's disease: a population-based study in ambulatory and institutionalized individuals. *Neurology.* 1995;45:705–708.
46. Aarsland D, Andersen K, Larsen JP, Lolk A, Nielsen H, Kragh-Sorensen P. Risk of dementia in Parkinson's disease: a community-based, prospective study. *Neurology.* 2001;56:730–736.
47. Hughes TA, Ross HF, Musa S, et al. A 10-year study of the incidence of and factors predicting dementia in Parkinson's disease. *Neurology.* 2000;54:1596–1602.
48. Aarsland D, Larsen JP, Tandberg E, Laake K. Predictors of nursing home placement in Parkinson's disease: a population-based, prospective study. *J Am Geriatr Soc.* 2000;48:938–942.
49. Aarsland D, Larsen JP, Karlsen K, Lim NG, Tandberg E. Mental symptoms in Parkinson's disease are important contributors to caregiver distress. *Int J Geriatr Psychiatry.* 1999;14:866–874.

50. Aarsland D, Andersen K, Larsen JP, Lolk A, Kragh-Sorensen P. Prevalence and characteristics of dementia in Parkinson disease: an 8-year prospective study. *Arch Neurol.* 2003;60:387–392.
51. Marder K, Tang MX, Cote L, Stern Y, Mayeux R. The frequency and associated risk factors for dementia in patients with Parkinson's disease. *Arch Neurol.* 1995;52:695–701.
52. Pillon B, Dubois B, Bonnet AM, et al. Cognitive slowing in Parkinson's disease fails to respond to levodopa treatment: the 15-objects test. *Neurology.* 1989;39:762–768.
53. Marinus J, Visser M, Verwey NA, et al. Assessment of cognition in Parkinson's disease. *Neurology.* 2003;61:1222–1228.
54. Taylor AE, Saint-Cyr JA, Lang AE. Frontal lobe dysfunction in Parkinson's disease. The cortical focus of neostriatal outflow. *Brain.* 1986;109 (Pt 5):845–883.
55. Sawada H, Udaka F, Kameyama M, et al. SPECT findings in Parkinson's disease associated with dementia. *J Neurol Neurosurg Psychiatry.* 1992;55:960–963.
56. Kuhl DE, Minoshima S, Fessler JA, et al. In vivo mapping of cholinergic terminals in normal aging, Alzheimer's disease, and Parkinson's disease. *Ann Neurol.* 1996;40:399–410.
57. Vander Borght T, Minoshima S, Giordani B, et al. Cerebral metabolic differences in Parkinson's and Alzheimer's diseases matched for dementia severity. *J Nucl Med.* 1997;38:797–802.
58. Hakim AM, Mathieson G. Basis of dementia in Parkinson's disease. *Lancet.* 1978;2:729.
59. Gaspar P, Gray F. Dementia in idiopathic Parkinson's disease. A neuropathological study of 32 cases. *Acta Neuropathol (Berl).* 1984;64:43–52.
60. Mattila PM, Roytta M, Torikka H, Dickson DW, Rinne JO. Cortical Lewy bodies and Alzheimer-type changes in patients with Parkinson's disease. *Acta Neuropathol (Berl).* 1998;95:576–582.
61. Apaydin H, Ahlskog JE, Parisi JE, Boeve BF, Dickson DW. Parkinson disease neuropathology: later-developing dementia and loss of the levodopa response. *Arch Neurol.* 2002;59:102–112.
62. Hurtig HI, Trojanowski JQ, Galvin J, et al. Alpha-synuclein cortical Lewy bodies correlate with dementia in Parkinson's disease. *Neurology.* 2000;54:1916–1921.
63. Aarsland D, Larsen JP, Cummins JL, Laake K. Prevalence and clinical correlates of psychotic symptoms in Parkinson disease: a community-based study. *Arch Neurol.* 1999;56:595–601.
64. Aarsland D, Cummings JL, Larsen JP. Neuropsychiatric differences between Parkinson's disease with dementia and Alzheimer's disease. *Int J Geriatr Psychiatry.* 2001;16:184–191.
65. Fenelon G, Mahieux F, Huon R, Ziegler M. Hallucinations in Parkinson's disease: prevalence, phenomenology and risk factors. *Brain.* 2000;123 (Pt 4):733–745.
66. Goetz CG, Leurgans S, Pappert EJ, Raman R, Stemer AB. Prospective longitudinal assessment of hallucinations in Parkinson's disease. *Neurology.* 2001;57:2078–2082.
67. Aarsland D, Ballard C, Larsen JP, McKeith I. A comparative study of psychiatric symptoms in dementia with Lewy bodies and Parkinson's disease with and without dementia. *Int J Geriatr Psychiatry.* 2001;16:528–536.
68. Goetz CG, Stebbins GT. Mortality and hallucinations in nursing home patients with advanced Parkinson's disease. *Neurology.* 1995;45:669–671.
69. McKeith IG, Galasko D, Kosaka K, et al. Consensus guidelines for the clinical and pathologic diagnosis of dementia with Lewy bodies (DLB): report of the consortium on DLB international workshop. *Neurology.* 1996;47:1113–1124.
70. Goetz CG, Pappert EJ, Blasucci LM, et al. Intravenous levodopa in hallucinating Parkinson's disease patients: high-dose challenge does not precipitate hallucinations. *Neurology.* 1998;50:515–517.
71. Harding AJ, Broe GA, Halliday GM. Visual hallucinations in Lewy body disease relate to Lewy bodies in the temporal lobe. *Brain.* 2002;125:391–403.
72. Comella CL, Nardine TM, Diederich NJ, Stebbins GT. Sleep-related violence, injury, and REM sleep behavior disorder in Parkinson's disease. *Neurology.* 1998;51:526–529.
73. Comella CL, Tanner CM, Ristanovic RK. Polysomnographic sleep measures in Parkinson's disease patients with treatment-induced hallucinations. *Ann Neurol.* 1993;34:710–714.
74. Nomura T, Inoue Y, Mitani H, Kawahara R, Miyake M, Nakashima K. Visual hallucinations as REM sleep behavior disorders in patients with Parkinson's disease. *Mov Disord.* 2003;18:812–817.
75. Aarsland D, Larsen JP, Lim NG, et al. Range of neuropsychiatric disturbances in patients with Parkinson's disease. *J Neurol Neurosurg Psychiatry.* 1999;67:492–496.
76. Naimark D, Jackson E, Rockwell E, Jeste DV. Psychotic symptoms in Parkinson's disease patients with dementia. *J Am Geriatr Soc.* 1996;44:296–299.
77. Klatka LA, Louis ED, Schiffer RB. Psychiatric features in diffuse Lewy body disease: a clinicopathologic study using Alzheimer's disease and Parkinson's disease comparison groups. *Neurology.* 1996;47:1148–1152.
78. Ballard C, Piggott M, Johnson M, et al. Delusions associated with elevated muscarinic binding in dementia with Lewy bodies. *Ann Neurol.* 2000;48:868–876.
79. Burn DJ, McKeith IG. Current treatment of dementia with Lewy bodies and dementia associated with Parkinson's disease. *Mov Disord.* 2003;18(Suppl 6):S72–S79.
80. Cummings JL. Depression and Parkinson's disease: a review. *Am J Psychiatry.* 1992;149:443–454.
81. Dooneief G, Mirabello E, Bell K, Marder K, Stern Y, Mayeux R. An estimate of the incidence of depression in idiopathic Parkinson's disease. *Arch Neurol.* 1992;49:305–307.
82. Weintraub D, Moberg PJ, Duda JE, Katz IR, Stern MB. Recognition and treatment of depression in Parkinson's disease. *J Geriatr Psychiatry Neurol.* 2003;16:178–183.
83. Ehmann TS, Beninger RJ, Gawel MJ, Riopelle RJ. Depressive symptoms in Parkinson's disease: a comparison with disabled control subjects. *J Geriatr Psychiatry Neurol.* 1990;3:3–9.
84. Shiba M, Bower JH, Maraganore DM, et al. Anxiety disorders and depressive disorders preceding Parkinson's disease: a case-control study. *Mov Disord.* 2000;15:669–677.
85. Cole SA, Woodard JL, Juncos JL, Kogos JL, Youngstrom EA, Watts RL. Depression and disability in Parkinson's disease. *J Neuropsychiatry Clin Neurosci.* 1996;8:20–25.
86. Cubo E, Bernard B, Leurgans S, Raman R. Cognitive and motor function in patients with Parkinson's disease with and without depression. *Clin Neuropharmacol.* 2000;23:331–334.
87. Tandberg E, Larsen JP, Aarsland D, Laake K, Cummings JL. Risk factors for depression in Parkinson disease. *Arch Neurol.* 1997;54:625–630.
88. Starkstein SE, Berthier ML, Bolduc PL, Preziosi TJ, Robinson RG. Depression in patients with early versus late onset of Parkinson's disease. *Neurology.* 1989;39:1441–1445.
89. Starkstein SE, Petracca G, Chemerinski E, et al. Depression in classic versus akinetic-rigid Parkinson's disease. *Mov Disord.* 1998;13:29–33.
90. Starkstein SE, Preziosi TJ, Bolduc PL, Robinson RG. Depression in Parkinson's disease. *J Nerv Ment Dis.* 1990;178:27–31.
91. Schiffer RB, Kurlan R, Rubin A, Boer S. Evidence for atypical depression in Parkinson's disease. *Am J Psychiatry.* 1988;145:1020–1022.
92. Brown RG, MacCarthy B, Gotham AM, Der GJ, Marsden CD. Depression and disability in Parkinson's disease: a follow-up of 132 cases. *Psychol Med.* 1988;18:49–55.
93. Gotham AM, Brown RG, Marsden CD. Depression in Parkinson's disease: a quantitative and qualitative analysis. *J Neurol Neurosurg Psychiatry.* 1986;49:381–389.
94. Stenager EN, Wermuth L, Stenager E, Boldsen J. Suicide in patients with Parkinson's disease. An epidemiological study. *Acta Psychiatr Scand.* 1994;90:70–72.
95. Myslobodsky M, Lalonde FM, Hicks L. Are patients with Parkinson's disease suicidal? *J Geriatr Psychiatry Neurol.* 2001;14:120–124.
96. Starkstein SE, Mayberg HS, Preziosi TJ, Andrezejewski P, Leiguarda R, Robinson RG. Reliability, validity, and clinical correlates of apathy in Parkinson's disease. *J Neuropsychiatry Clin Neurosci.* 1992;4:134–139.
97. Starkstein SE, Bolduc PL, Mayberg HS, Preziosi TJ, Robinson RG. Cognitive impairments and depression in Parkinson's disease: a follow up study. *J Neurol Neurosurg Psychiatry.* 1990;53:597–602.
98. Starkstein SE, Bolduc PL, Preziosi TJ, Robinson RG. Cognitive impairments in different stages of Parkinson's disease. *J Neuropsychiatry Clin Neurosci.* 1989;1:243–248.

99. Starkstein SE, Preziosi TJ, Berthier ML, Bolduc PL, Mayberg HS, Robinson RG. Depression and cognitive impairment in Parkinson's disease. *Brain.* 1989;112 (Pt 5):1141–1153.

100. Mayberg HS, Starkstein SE, Sadzot B, et al. Selective hypometabolism in the inferior frontal lobe in depressed patients with Parkinson's disease. *Ann Neurol.* 1990;28:57–64.

101. Mentis MJ, McIntosh AR, Perrine K, et al. Relationships among the metabolic patterns that correlate with mnemonic, visuospatial, and mood symptoms in Parkinson's disease. *Am J Psychiatry.* 2002;159:746–754.

102. Mayeux R, Stern Y, Cote L, Williams JB. Altered serotonin metabolism in depressed patients with parkinson's disease. *Neurology.* 1984;34:642–646.

103. Manni R, Pacchetti C, Terzaghi M, Sartori I, Mancini F, Nappi G. Hallucinations and sleep-wake cycle in PD: a 24-hour continuous polysomnographic study. *Neurology.* 2002;59:1979–1981.

104. Pappert EJ, Goetz CG, Niederman FG, Raman R, Leurgans S. Hallucinations, sleep fragmentation, and altered dream phenomena in Parkinson's disease. *Mov Disord.* 1999;14:117–121.

105. Arnulf I, Bonnet AM, Damier P, et al. Hallucinations, REM sleep, and Parkinson's disease: a medical hypothesis. *Neurology.* 2000;55:281–288.

106. Ondo WG, Dat Vuong K, Khan H, Atassi F, Kwak C, Jankovic J. Daytime sleepiness and other sleep disorders in Parkinson's disease. *Neurology.* 2001;57:1392–1396.

107. Arnulf I, Konofal E, Merino-Andreu M, et al. Parkinson's disease and sleepiness: an integral part of PD. *Neurology.* 2002;58:1019–1024.

108. Abad VC, Guilleminault C. Review of rapid eye movement behavior sleep disorders. *Curr Neurol Neurosci Rep.* 2004;4:157–163.

109. Gagnon JF, Bedard MA, Fantini ML, et al. REM sleep behavior disorder and REM sleep without atonia in Parkinson's disease. *Neurology.* 2002;59:585–589.

110. Witjas T, Kaphan E, Azulay JP, et al. Nonmotor fluctuations in Parkinson's disease: frequent and disabling. *Neurology.* 2002;59:408–413.

111. Stein MB, Heuser IJ, Juncos JL, Uhde TW. Anxiety disorders in patients with Parkinson's disease. *Am J Psychiatry.* 1990;147:217–220.

112. Lang AE, Johnson K. Akathisia in idiopathic Parkinson's disease. *Neurology.* 1987;37:477–481.

113. Menza MA, Golbe LI, Cody RA, Forman NE. Dopamine-related personality traits in Parkinson's disease. *Neurology.* 1993;43:505–508.

114. Pluck GC, Brown RG. Apathy in Parkinson's disease. *J Neurol Neurosurg Psychiatry.* 2002;73:636–642.

115. Chatterjee A, Fahn S. Methylphenidate treats apathy in Parkinson's disease. *J Neuropsychiatry Clin Neurosci.* 2002;14:461–462.

116. Jansen IH, Olde Rikkert MG, Hulsbos HA, Hoefnagels WH. Toward individualized evidence-based medicine: five "N of 1" trials of methylphenidate in geriatric patients. *J Am Geriatr Soc.* 2001;49:474–476.

117. Fernandez HH, Friedman JH. Punding on L-dopa. *Mov Disord.* 1999;14:836–838.

118. Driver-Dunckley E, Samanta J, Stacy M. Pathological gambling associated with dopamine agonist therapy in Parkinson's disease. *Neurology.* 2003;61:422–423.

119. Comella CL, Stebbins GT, Brown-Toms N, Goetz CG. Physical therapy and Parkinson's disease: a controlled clinical trial. *Neurology.* 1994;44:376–378.

120. Ramig LO, Countryman S, O'Brien C, Hoehn M, Thompson L. Intensive speech treatment for patients with Parkinson's disease: short- and long-term comparison of two techniques. *Neurology.* 1996;47:1496–1504.

121. Ramig LO, Sapir S, Countryman S, et al. Intensive voice treatment (LSVT) for patients with Parkinson's disease: a 2-year follow up. *J Neurol Neurosurg Psychiatry.* 2001;71:493–498.

122. Ramig LO, Sapir S, Fox C, Countryman S. Changes in vocal loudness following intensive voice treatment (LSVT) in individuals with Parkinson's disease: a comparison with untreated patients and normal age-matched controls. *Mov Disord.* 2001;16:79–83.

123. Sapir S, Ramig LO, Hoyt P, Countryman S, O'Brien C, Hoehn M. Speech loudness and quality 12 months after intensive voice treatment (LSVT) for Parkinson's disease: a comparison with an alternative speech treatment. *Folia Phoniatr Logop.* 2002;54:296–303.

124. Sharkawi AE, Ramig L, Logemann JA, et al. Swallowing and voice effects of Lee Silverman Voice Treatment (LSVT): a pilot study. *J Neurol Neurosurg Psychiatry.* 2002;72:31–36.

125. de Swart BJ, Willemse SC, Maassen BA, Horstink MW. Improvement of voicing in patients with Parkinson's disease by speech therapy. *Neurology.* 2003;60:498–500.

126. Olanow CW. Attempts to obtain neuroprotection in Parkinson's disease. *Neurology.* 1997;49:S26–S33.

127. Effects of tocopherol and deprenyl on the progression of disability in early Parkinson's disease. The Parkinson Study Group. *N Engl J Med.* 1993;328:176–183.

128. Impact of deprenyl and tocopherol treatment on Parkinson's disease in DATATOP subjects not requiring levodopa. Parkinson Study Group. *Ann Neurol.* 1996;39:29–36.

129. Ernster L, Dallner G. Biochemical, physiological and medical aspects of ubiquinone function. *Biochim Biophys Acta.* 1995;1271:195–204.

130. Shults CW, Beal MF, Fontaine D, Nakano K, Haas RH. Absorption, tolerability, and effects on mitochondrial activity of oral coenzyme Q10 in parkinsonian patients. *Neurology.* 1998;50:793–795.

131. Shults CW, Oakes D, Kieburtz K, et al. Effects of coenzyme Q10 in early Parkinson disease: evidence of slowing of the functional decline. *Arch Neurol.* 2002;59:1541–1550.

132. Schapira AH. Neuroprotection and dopamine agonists. *Neurology.* 2002;58:S9–S18.

133. Whone AL, Watts RL, Stoessl AJ, et al. Slower progression of Parkinson's disease with ropinirole versus levodopa: The REAL-PET study. *Ann Neurol.* 2003;54:93–101.

134. Dopamine transporter brain imaging to assess the effects of pramipexole vs levodopa on Parkinson disease progression. *JAMA.* 2002;287:1653–1661.

135. A controlled trial of rasagiline in early Parkinson disease: the TEMPO Study. *Arch Neurol.* 2002;59:1937–1943.

136. Calne DB. The role of various forms of treatment in the management of Parkinson's disease. *Clin Neuropharmacol.* 1982;5(Suppl 1):S38–S43.

137. Goetz CG. New lessons from old drugs: amantadine and Parkinson's disease. *Neurology.* 1998;50:1211–1212.

138. Barone P, Bravi D, Bermejo-Pareja F, et al. Pergolide monotherapy in the treatment of early PD: a randomized, controlled study. Pergolide Monotherapy Study Group. *Neurology.* 1999;53:573–579.

139. Adler CH, Sethi KD, Hauser RA, et al. Ropinirole for the treatment of early Parkinson's disease. The Ropinirole Study Group. *Neurology.* 1997;49:393–399.

140. Shannon KM, Bennett JP, Jr., Friedman JH. Efficacy of pramipexole, a novel dopamine agonist, as monotherapy in mild to moderate Parkinson's disease. The Pramipexole Study Group. *Neurology.* 1997;49:724–728.

141. Pritchett AM, Morrison JF, Edwards WD, Schaff HV, Connolly HM, Espinosa RE. Valvular heart disease in patients taking pergolide. *Mayo Clin Proc.* 2002;77:1280–1286.

142. Rascol O, Brooks DJ, Korczyn AD, De Deyn PP, Clarke CE, Lang AE. A five-year study of the incidence of dyskinesia in patients with early Parkinson's disease who were treated with ropinirole or levodopa. 056 Study Group. *N Engl J Med.* 2000;342:1484–1491.

143. Pramipexole vs levodopa as initial treatment for Parkinson disease: A randomized controlled trial. Parkinson Study Group. *JAMA.* 2000;284:1931–1938.

144. Mouradian MM, Heuser IJ, Baronti F, Chase TN. Modification of central dopaminergic mechanisms by continuous levodopa therapy for advanced Parkinson's disease. *Ann Neurol.* 1990;27:18–23.

145. Block G, Liss C, Reines S, Irr J, Nibbelink D. Comparison of immediate-release and controlled release carbidopa/levodopa in Parkinson's disease. A multicenter 5-year study. The CR First Study Group. *Eur Neurol.* 1997;37:23–27.

146. Olanow CW, Fahn S, Muenter M, et al. A multicenter double-blind placebo-controlled trial of pergolide as an adjunct to Sinemet in Parkinson's disease. *Mov Disord.* 1994;9:40–47.

147. Lieberman A, Olanow CW, Sethi K, et al. A multicenter trial of ropinirole as adjunct treatment for Parkinson's disease. Ropinirole Study Group. *Neurology.* 1998;51:1057–1062.

148. Lieberman A, Ranhosky A, Korts D. Clinical evaluation of pramipexole in advanced Parkinson's disease: results of a double-blind, placebo-controlled, parallel-group study. *Neurology.* 1997; 49:162–168.

149. Nutt JG, Woodward WR, Beckner RM, et al. Effect of peripheral catechol-O-methyltransferase inhibition on the pharmacokinetics and pharmacodynamics of levodopa in parkinsonian patients. *Neurology.* 1994;44:913–919.

150. Entacapone improves motor fluctuations in levodopa-treated Parkinson's disease patients. Parkinson Study Group. *Ann Neurol.* 1997;42:747–755.

151. Rajput AH, Martin W, Saint-Hilaire MH, Dorflinger E, Pedder S. Tolcapone improves motor function in parkinsonian patients with the "wearing-off" phenomenon: a double-blind, placebo-controlled, multicenter trial. *Neurology.* 1997;49:1066–1071.

152. Verhagen Metman L, Del Dotto P, van den Munckhof P, Fang J, Mouradian MM, Chase TN. Amantadine as treatment for dyskinesias and motor fluctuations in Parkinson's disease. *Neurology.* 1998;50:1323–1326.

153. Golbe LI. Long-term efficacy and safety of deprenyl (selegiline) in advanced Parkinson's disease. *Neurology.* 1989;39:1109–1111.

154. Waters CH, Sethi KD, Hauser RA. Selegiline reduces "off" time in Parkinson's disease patients with motor fluctuations: a 3-month, randomized, placebo-controlled study. *Mov Disord.* In press.

155. Schwid S. A randomized placebo-controlled trial of rasagiline in Parkinson's disease patients with levodopa-related motor fluctuations (The PRESTO Study). Personal communication, 2005.

156. Richard IH, Justus AW, Greig NH, Marshall F, Kurlan R. Worsening of motor function and mood in a patient with Parkinson's disease after pharmacologic challenge with oral rivastigmine. *Clin Neuropharmacol.* 2002;25:296–299.

157. Bourke D, Druckenbrod RW. Possible association between donepezil and worsening Parkinson's disease. *Ann Pharmacother.* 1998;32:610–611.

158. Aarsland D, Laake K, Larsen JP, Janvin C. Donepezil for cognitive impairment in Parkinson's disease: a randomised controlled study. *J Neurol Neurosurg Psychiatry.* 2002;72:708–712.

159. Leroi I, Brandt J, Reich SG, et al. Randomized placebo-controlled trial of donepezil in cognitive impairment in Parkinson's disease. *Int J Geriatr Psychiatry.* 2004;19:1–8.

160. Giladi N, Shabtai H, Gurevich T, Benbunan B, Anca M, Korczyn AD. Rivastigmine (Exelon) for dementia in patients with Parkinson's disease. *Acta Neurol Scand.* 2003;108:368–373.

161. Bullock R, Cameron A. Rivastigmine for the treatment of dementia and visual hallucinations associated with Parkinson's disease: a case series. *Curr Med Res Opin.* 2002;18:258–264.

162. Emre M, Aarsland D, Albanese A, et al. Rivastigmine for dementia associated with Parkinson's disease. *N Engl J Med.* 2004; 351:2509–2518.

163. Friedman JH, Factor SA. Atypical antipsychotics in the treatment of drug-induced psychosis in Parkinson's disease. *Mov Disord.* 2000;15:201–211.

164. Bonuccelli U, Ceravolo R, Salvetti S, et al. Clozapine in Parkinson's disease tremor. Effects of acute and chronic administration. *Neurology.* 1997;49:1587–1590.

165. Friedman JH, Koller WC, Lannon MC, Busenbark K, Swanson-Hyland E, Smith D. Benztropine versus clozapine for the treatment of tremor in Parkinson's disease. *Neurology.* 1997;48: 1077–1081.

166. Friedman JH, Lannon MC. Clozapine-responsive tremor in Parkinson's disease. *Mov Disord.* 1990;5:225–229.

167. Jansen EN. Clozapine in the treatment of tremor in Parkinson's disease. *Acta Neurol Scand.* 1994;89:262–265.

168. Bennett JP, Jr., Landow ER, Schuh LA. Suppression of dyskinesias in advanced Parkinson's disease. II. Increasing daily clozapine doses suppress dyskinesias and improve parkinsonism symptoms. *Neurology.* 1993;43:1551–1555.

169. Bennett JP, Jr., Landow ER, Dietrich S, Schuh LA. Suppression of dyskinesias in advanced Parkinson's disease: moderate daily clozapine doses provide long-term dyskinesia reduction. *Mov Disord.* 1994;9:409–414.

170. Durif F, Vidailhet M, Assal F, Roche C, Bonnet AM, Agid Y. Low-dose clozapine improves dyskinesias in Parkinson's disease. *Neurology.* 1997;48:658–662.

171. Linazasoro G, Marti Masso JF, Suarez JA. Nocturnal akathisia in Parkinson's disease: treatment with clozapine. *Mov Disord.* 1993;8:171–174.

172. Klein C, Gordon J, Pollak L, Rabey JM. Clozapine in Parkinson's disease psychosis: 5-year follow-up review. *Clin Neuropharmacol.* 2003;26:8–11.

173. Meco G, Alessandri A, Giustini P, Bonifati V. Risperidone in levodopa-induced psychosis in advanced Parkinson's disease: an open-label, long-term study. *Mov Disord.* 1997;12:610–612.

174. Rich SS, Friedman JH, Ott BR. Risperidone versus clozapine in the treatment of psychosis in six patients with Parkinson's disease and other akinetic-rigid syndromes. *J Clin Psychiatry.* 1995;56:556–559.

175. Ford B, Lynch T, Greene P. Risperidone in Parkinson's disease. *Lancet.* 1994;344:681.

176. Meco G, Alessandria A, Bonifati V, Giustini P. Risperidone for hallucinations in levodopa-treated Parkinson's disease patients. *Lancet.* 1994;343:1370–1371.

177. Leopold NA. Risperidone treatment of drug-related psychosis in patients with parkinsonism. *Mov Disord.* 2000;15:301–304.

178. Mohr E, Mendis T, Hildebrand K, De Deyn PP. Risperidone in the treatment of dopamine-induced psychosis in Parkinson's disease: an open pilot trial. *Mov Disord.* 2000;15:1230–1237.

179. Ellis T, Cudkowicz ME, Sexton PM, Growdon JH. Clozapine and risperidone treatment of psychosis in Parkinson's disease. *J Neuropsychiatry Clin Neurosci.* 2000;12:364–369.

180. Friedman JH, Ott BR. Should risperidone be used in Parkinson's disease? *J Neuropsychiatry Clin Neurosci.* 1998;10:473–475.

181. Factor SA, Molho ES, Friedman JH. Risperidone and Parkinson's disease. *Mov Disord.* 2002;17:221–222.

182. Wolters EC, Jansen EN, Tuynman-Qua HG, Bergmans PL. Olanzapine in the treatment of dopaminomimetic psychosis in patients with Parkinson's disease. *Neurology.* 1996;47:1085–1087.

183. Aarsland D, Larsen JP, Lim NG, Tandberg E. Olanzapine for psychosis in patients with Parkinson's disease with and without dementia. *J Neuropsychiatry Clin Neurosci.* 1999;11:392– 394.

184. Graham JM, Sussman JD, Ford KS, Sagar HJ. Olanzapine in the treatment of hallucinosis in idiopathic Parkinson's disease: a cautionary note. *J Neurol Neurosurg Psychiatry.* 1998;65:774–777.

185. Marsh L, Lyketsos C, Reich SG. Olanzapine for the treatment of psychosis in patients with Parkinson's disease and dementia. *Psychosomatics.* 2001;42:477–481.

186. Gimenez-Roldan S, Mateo D, Navarro E, Gines MM. Efficacy and safety of clozapine and olanzapine: an open-label study comparing two groups of Parkinson's disease patients with dopaminergic-induced psychosis. *Parkinsonism Relat Disord.* 2001;7: 121–127.

187. Friedman JH, Goldstein S, Jacques C. Substituting clozapine for olanzapine in psychiatrically stable Parkinson's disease patients: results of an open-label pilot study. *Clin Neuropharmacol.* 1998;21:285–288.

188. Breier A, Sutton VK, Feldman PD, et al. Olanzapine in the treatment of dopamimetic-induced psychosis in patients with Parkinson's disease. *Biol Psychiatry.* 2002;52:438–445.

189. Molho ES, Factor SA. Worsening of motor features of parkinsonism with olanzapine. *Mov Disord.* 1999;14:1014–1016.

190. Jimenez-Jimenez FJ, Tallon-Barranco A, Orti-Pareja M, Zurdo M, Porta J, Molina JA. Olanzapine can worsen parkinsonism. *Neurology.* 1998;50:1183–1184.

191. Ondo WG, Levy JK, Vuong KD, Hunter C, Jankovic J. Olanzapine treatment for dopaminergic-induced hallucinations. *Mov Disord.* 2002;17:1031–1035.

192. Goetz CG, Blasucci LM, Leurgans S, Pappert EJ. Olanzapine and clozapine: comparative effects on motor function in hallucinating PD patients. *Neurology.* 2000;55:789–794.

193. Reddy S, Factor SA, Molho ES, Feustel PJ. The effect of quetiapine on psychosis and motor function in parkinsonian patients with and without dementia. *Mov Disord.* 2002;17:676–681.

194. Brandstadter D, Oertel WH. Treatment of drug-induced psychosis with quetiapine and clozapine in Parkinson's disease. *Neurology.* 2002;58:160–161.

195. Juncos JL, Roberts VJ, Evatt ML, et al. Quetiapine improves psychotic symptoms and cognition in Parkinson's disease. *Mov Disord.* 2004;19:29–35.
196. Morgante L, Epifanio A, Spina E, et al. Quetiapine versus clozapine: a preliminary report of comparative effects on dopaminergic psychosis in patients with Parkinson's disease. *Neurol Sci.* 2002;23(Suppl 2):S89–S90.
197. Fernandez HH, Friedman JH, Jacques C, Rosenfeld M. Quetiapine for the treatment of drug-induced psychosis in Parkinson's disease. *Mov Disord.* 1999;14:484–487.
198. Menza MM, Palermo B, Mark M. Quetiapine as an alternative to clozapine in the treatment of dopamimetic psychosis in patients with Parkinson's disease. *Ann Clin Psychiatry.* 1999;11:141–144.
199. Lopez Del Val LJ, Santos S. [Quetiapine and ziprasidone in the treatment of the psychotic disorders in Parkinson's disease]. *Rev Neurol.* 2004;39:661–667.
200. Bergman J, Lerner V. Successful use of donepezil for the treatment of psychotic symptoms in patients with Parkinson's disease. *Clin Neuropharmacol.* 2002;25:107–110.
201. Kurita A, Ochiai Y, Kono Y, Suzuki M, Inoue K. The beneficial effect of donepezil on visual hallucinations in three patients with Parkinson's disease. *J Geriatr Psychiatry Neurol.* 2003;16:184–188.
202. Fabbrini G, Barbanti P, Aurilia C, Pauletti C, Lenzi GL, Meco G. Donepezil in the treatment of hallucinations and delusions in Parkinson's disease. *Neurol Sci.* 2002;23:41–43.
203. Aarsland D, Hutchinson M, Larsen JP. Cognitive, psychiatric and motor response to galantamine in Parkinson's disease with dementia. *Int J Geriatr Psychiatry.* 2003;18:937–941.
204. McDonald WM, Richard IH, DeLong MR. Prevalence, etiology, and treatment of depression in Parkinson's disease. *Biol Psychiatry.* 2003;54:363–375.
205. Aarsland D, Larsen JP, Waage O, Langeveld JH. Maintenance electroconvulsive therapy for Parkinson's disease. *Convuls Ther.* 1997;13:274–277.
206. Olanow CW, Watts RL, Koller WC. An algorithm (decision tree) for the management of Parkinson's disease (2001): treatment guidelines. *Neurology.* 2001;56:S1–S88.
207. Pahwa R, Wilkinson S, Smith D, Lyons K, Miyawaki E, Koller WC. High-frequency stimulation of the globus pallidus for the treatment of Parkinson's disease. *Neurology.* 1997;49:249–253.
208. Kumar R, Lozano AM, Kim YJ, et al. Double-blind evaluation of subthalamic nucleus deep brain stimulation in advanced Parkinson's disease. *Neurology.* 1998;51:850–855.
209. Limousin P, Krack P, Pollak P, et al. Electrical stimulation of the subthalamic nucleus in advanced Parkinson's disease. *N Engl J Med.* 1998;339:1105–1111.
210. Volkmann J, Sturm V, Weiss P, et al. Bilateral high-frequency stimulation of the internal globus pallidus in advanced Parkinson's disease. *Ann Neurol.* 1998;44:953–961.
211. Kumar R, Lang AE, Rodriguez-Oroz MC, et al. Deep brain stimulation of the globus pallidus pars interna in advanced Parkinson's disease. *Neurology.* 2000;55:S34–S39.
212. Rodriguez-Oroz MC, Gorospe A, Guridi J, et al. Bilateral deep brain stimulation of the subthalamic nucleus in Parkinson's disease. *Neurology.* 2000;55:S45–S51.
213. Herzog J, Volkmann J, Krack P, et al. Two-year follow-up of subthalamic deep brain stimulation in Parkinson's disease. *Mov Disord.* 2003;18:1332–1337.
214. Krack P, Batir A, Van Blercom N, et al. Five-year follow-up of bilateral stimulation of the subthalamic nucleus in advanced Parkinson's disease. *N Engl J Med.* 2003;349:1925–1934.
215. Deep-brain stimulation of the subthalamic nucleus or the pars interna of the globus pallidus in Parkinson's disease. *N Engl J Med.* 2001;345:956–963.

Neuroleptic-Induced Movement Disorders

41

David Naimark   *Elizabeth Collumb*
Ansar M. Haroun   *Dilip V. Jeste*

Modern geriatric psychiatry presents physicians with choices of numerous medications to treat various ailments. Although these medications offer considerable benefits to elderly patients, the risks are significant as well. Many psychotropic medications can produce side effects in the elderly that are disturbing and, in some cases, dangerous. This places significant responsibility on the treating psychiatrist; careful and reasoned thought must go into the analysis of whether the benefit of treatment exceeds the risk to the patient. The need to obtain informed consent may present additional issues for the geriatric psychiatrist with demented and/or psychotic patients (1). Finally, when a psychiatrist prescribes a medication that may induce significant side effects, the physician–patient relationship becomes particularly important. However, the patients who may benefit most from these medications (e.g., demented or paranoid patients) are sometimes the least amenable to establishing a trusting relationship with their physician.

Among the most common, and most uncomfortable, side effects from psychotropic medications (especially *conventional* or *typical* antipsychotics or neuroleptics) are the acute and chronic movement disorders (MDs). Any psychiatrist in clinical practice has witnessed the intense distress that medication-induced MDs can bring to patients. Perhaps most disturbing is that, unlike many other medications, neuroleptics can produce *tardive* (late-occurring) MDs that can be persistent, progressive, and irreversible. While these MDs are significantly less common with the newer atypical antipsychotics including clozapine, risperidone, olanzapine, quetiapine, ziprasidone, and aripiprazole, they are seen when the atypicals (or at least some of

them) are used in higher doses, particularly in vulnerable populations such as elderly patients.

MDs are generally divided into those that occur acutely or subacutely, and those that occur late in treatment (tardive). In this chapter, MDs will be discussed in these two groups:

- The relatively acute neuroleptic-induced disorders (acute dystonias, parkinsonism, and extrapyramidal symptoms [EPS], akathisia, and neuroleptic malignant syndrome [NMS])
- The later-onset tardive dyskinesias (TDs) and dystonias

This reflects the diagnostic groupings contained within the *Diagnostic and Statistical Manual of Mental Disorders*, Fourth Edition, Text Revision (DSM-IV-TR) (2). A time line for the emergence of these iatrogenic MDs is provided in Table 41-1. The main goal of this chapter is to provide updated and clinically relevant information about medication-induced MDs.

HISTORICAL BACKGROUND

The presence of extrapyramidal motor reactions to drugs was first noticed in the 1940s with reserpine. With the discovery of the antipsychotic effect of chlorpromazine in the early 1950s, attention focused on the motor effects of these new drugs. In 1952, Delay and Deniker reported EPS in patients being treated with chlorpromazine (3). Many of these cases of EPS appeared similar to Parkinson's disease (PD), and some psychiatrists proposed that the onset of antipsychotic benefit only occurred in the presence of EPS. It was further noted that neuroleptic-induced parkinsonism

TABLE 41-1

TIME-LINE FOR NEUROLEPTIC-INDUCED MOVEMENT DISORDERS

Condition	Highest Risk of Emergence
Acute dystonia	Days 0–7
Neuroleptic malignant syndrome	Days 0–7 (continues at lesser degree until end of first month)
Akathisia	Days 7–14 (continues at lesser degree until 2–3 months)
Parkinsonism	First month (continues at lesser degree until 2–3 months)
Tardive dyskinesia	>3 months (risk increases with increasing time on neuroleptic); >1 month in elderly
Nonneuroleptic movement disorders	Days 0–14

(NIP) generally reversed upon discontinuation of the medication (4).

In 1957, Schonecker noted the onset of orobuccal dyskinesias that occurred after prolonged treatment with chlorpromazine. In marked contrast to the reversible PD-like EPS, these abnormal, late-onset movements persisted even after discontinuation of the medication. Other reports soon followed from around the world of various persistent abnormal movements in patients treated with neuroleptics (5). The term *tardive dyskinesia* was first defined in 1964 to describe these abnormal movements (6). The number of reports grew rapidly, and many cases were reported to be irreversible. The clinical relevance of TD is underscored by the formation of two American Psychiatric Association task forces (in 1980 and 1992). It was not until 1994, however, that TD was included in the DSM (2). This reflected recognition that TD nomenclature needed to be standardized in order to prevent underdiagnosis and inadequate documentation of the disorder. Though neuroleptics are the class of medications historically most associated with medication-induced MDs, other classes of psychotropic medications have also been noted to produce MDs as an unwelcome side effect.

Extensive research efforts have been undertaken to unravel the intricacies of these MDs. Advances in research have led to improved knowledge of the epidemiology, phenomenology, risk factors, and courses of these disorders. However, precise explanations of the pathophysiology, as well as satisfactory long-term treatments, remain elusive. Furthermore, there has been a dramatic increase in malpractice litigation initiated against psychiatrists and hospitals by patients suffering from these iatrogenic MDs (7). As discussed later, the MDs are less of a problem with the atypical antipsychotics.

GENERAL CONSIDERATIONS

MDs associated with the use of neuroleptics (especially the older, typical agents) can occur acutely and with prolonged exposure to these drugs. As a group, older people are generally more sensitive to such disorders. Thus, careful and slow titration of neuroleptics, with maintenance on the minimum dosage required for effective treatment, is particularly important. In addition, geriatric patients show increased sensitivity to side effects of other medications often used to treat these MDs, such as anticholinergics. Polypharmacy (with its concomitant risks for drug–drug interactions, altered drug levels, and adverse effects) is also more likely to occur in elderly patients. Hence, the geropsychiatric clinician should take care to monitor patients' medication regimens, including those drugs prescribed by nonpsychiatric physicians. The clinician should keep in mind that the elderly are more likely to suffer from noniatrogenic as well as iatrogenic MDs (8). When evaluating a patient with an MD, careful examination and consideration of etiologies—pharmacologic and otherwise—should be kept in mind. Consultation with a neurologist colleague can be useful.

ACUTE NEUROLEPTIC-INDUCED MOVEMENT DISORDERS

Though the temporal boundary between acute and nonacute is blurry, we will consider acute neuroleptic-induced MDs as those most likely to occur during the first month of treatment with any given neuroleptic, or during the month following an increase in dose. Practitioners should be aware, however, that acute MDs may develop at any point during treatment. Acute neuroleptic-induced MDs include dystonias, parkinsonism/EPS, akathisia, and NMS. A summary of treatment of these disorders is provided in Table 41-2.

ACUTE DYSTONIA

Definition and Diagnosis

Acute dystonia presents as sustained and painful muscle spasms, with twisting, squeezing, and pulling movements of the muscle groups involved. A sensation of tongue thickening or difficulty swallowing may precede the frank dystonic reaction by 3 to 6 hours (1). Though any muscle group in the body can be affected, the most commonly involved muscles are those in the eyes, jaw, tongue, and neck.

TABLE 41-2

TREATMENT OPTIONS FOR NEUROLEPTIC-INDUCED MOVEMENT DISORDERS

	First-Line Treatments	Second-Line Treatments	Third-Line Treatments
Acute dystonia	■ 50 mg diphenhydramine IM or IV; repeat in 30 minutes PRN, then can usually switch to PO medications	■ 50 mg diphenhydramine PO, or 2 mg benztropine PO; repeat in 1 hour PRN	■ Lorazepam 1 mg IV/IM/PO, especially if pharyngeal or laryngeal involvement
Parkinsonism/EPS	■ If on typical neuroleptic, switch to atypical ■ If already on atypical, switch to different atypical with lower D2 affinity ■ Decrease atypical neuroleptic dose if feasible and patient does not wish to change medications	■ If on typical antipsychotic and switch to atypical not feasible, change to lower-potency typical ■ Lower dose if on typical antipsychotic and patient does not wish to change medications ■ Low-dose anticholinergics (e.g., benztropine 0.5–1 mg PO BID), and monitor for side effects ■ Increase dose of anticholinergic medications as needed, with frequent attempts at weaning	■ If EPS is mild, consider not treating, especially if patient cannot tolerate anticholinergic medications ■ Discontinue neuroleptic treatment altogether, then start another neuroleptic in slow titration ■ Dopamine agonists such as amantadine ■ Experimental treatments such as Vitamin E, calcium, gingko biloba, acupuncture
Akathisia	■ If on typical neuroleptic, switch to atypical ■ If already on atypical, switch to different atypical with lower D2 affinity ■ Decrease atypical neuroleptic dose if feasible and patient does not wish to change medications	■ Low-dose β-blockers such as propranolol 10 mg PO TID with cautious titration ■ Low-dose anticholinergics as above, especially if EPS also present ■ Switch to low-potency typical neuroleptic	■ Low-dose benzodiazepines (not recommended for use with β-blockers) such as clonazepam 0.5 mg BID ■ Benzodiazepine plus anticholinergic ■ Clonidine ■ Opioids
Neuroleptic malignant syndrome	■ Discontinue offending neuroleptic ■ Supportive care and inpatient monitoring	■ Dantrolene 1–3 mg/kg per day, divided QID or continuous IV infusion ■ Bromocriptine 5–10 mg PO TID	■ ECT ■ Levodopa/carbidopa ■ Steroids ■ NMDA antagonists

BID, twice daily; ECT, electroconvulsive therapy; EPS, extrapyramidal symptoms; IM, intramuscular; IV, intravenous; NMDA, N-methyl-D-aspartate; PO, by mouth; PRN, as needed; QID, four times daily; TID, three times daily.

A variety of names describe dystonias affecting particular muscle groups:

- Trismus (forced jaw closure)
- Blepharospasm (forced eye closures)
- Oculogyric crisis (deviation of the eyes in one direction)
- Torticollis (pulling of the head to one side)
- Retrocollis (pulling back of the head)
- Anterocollis (pulling of the head forward)
- Opisthotonos (arching of the back like a bow)

If the larynx or pharynx is involved, rapid respiratory compromise can occur, making acute dystonia a potentially life-threatening drug reaction, particularly in those elderly patients who may already have some degree of respiratory impairment or disease. Acute dystonias can induce tremendous fear and anxiety in patients, especially if the patient was not informed of the possibility of such a reaction or is unable to obtain immediate treatment. Acute dystonias, and fear of acute dystonias, are associated with medication noncompliance (9).

Neuroleptic-induced acute dystonias are dramatic and distinctive in their presentation, and are usually fairly easy to diagnose, especially when a clinician has knowledge of the antecedent of a recent initiation or dose increase of neuroleptic medication. There are a few other conditions that can present similarly, however, that must be considered before making a definitive diagnosis.

Spontaneously occurring focal or segmental dystonias may persist in the absence of neuroleptic medication. Conditions of the central nervous system (CNS), including temporal lobe epilepsy, infections, trauma, and tumors, have been noted to produce symptoms similar to neuroleptic-induced acute dystonia. Recreational drugs such as MDMA (ecstasy) may rarely cause dystonia. Although use of these illicit drugs may be less common among geriatric populations, the clinician must also consider if another prescribed medication might be causing the dystonia (10). Many non-neuroleptic medications, including various anticonvulsants, mood stabilizers, and antidepressants (particularly selective serotonin-reuptake inhibitors [SSRIs]), are known to cause dystonias.

NMS can produce sustained muscle contractions that look similar to acute dystonia, but NMS is distinguished by its characteristic "lead pipe" rigidity, fever, delirium, and vital sign instability. Catatonia associated with an affective or psychotic disorder can be difficult to distinguish on physical examination from dystonia; however, catatonia does not respond to the administration of anticholinergic medications and will usually persist and worsen upon the discontinuation of neuroleptic medications. In addition, catatonic patients are typically not concerned about their stiffness, whereas a patient with an acute dystonia is nearly always distressed and anxious (1).

On occasion, acute dystonia may be confused with new-onset TD. Again, administration of anticholinergic medications can be expected to quickly resolve the dystonia, whereas anticholinergic medications will not affect—or may even worsen—TD. The differential diagnosis between acute dystonia and tardive dystonia (a variant of TD) can be very difficult. It is important to remember that tardive dystonia occurs late in the course of neuroleptic treatment and is a chronic condition, compared with acute dystonia, which occurs early in the course of medication treatment and generally responds briskly to treatment with anticholinergics.

Epidemiology and Risk Factors

Neuroleptic-induced dystonia usually begins 12 to 36 hours after a neuroleptic—usually a high-potency conventional one—is started or the dosage of a pre-existing neuroleptic is increased. Approximately 90% of acute dystonic reactions occur within the first 5 days of neuroleptic treatment; it is unusual for acute dystonia to appear after 2 weeks of treatment on a given dose (1).

The incidence of neuroleptic-induced dystonia is far less than that of parkinsonian EPS, and has declined even more with the widespread acceptance of the atypical antipsychotics as a first-line treatment for psychosis. The frequency of acute dystonia has been reported to range from negligible (for patients on atypicals such as clozapine and quetiapine) to 50% (for patients given high doses of high-potency typical agents). Indeed, high doses of high-potency neuroleptics appear to be the most consistent risk factor for acute dystonia (11). Other factors that predispose to dystonia include male gender, concurrent hyperthyroidism, concurrent treatment with lithium, and a primary diagnosis of an affective rather than a psychotic disorder. For unknown reasons, older age is a protective factor; acute dystonic reactions occur far less frequently in geriatric pop-

ulations. A prior dystonic reaction is a good predictor of a repeated episode when the same neuroleptic is rechallenged (12). The incidence of acute dystonic reactions can be minimized (likely to less than 2%) by the strategy of slow dose titration and the use of atypical antipsychotic medications.

Pathophysiology

During the 1950s and 1960s, dystonia was often regarded as a disorder of psychogenic origin; there is, however, no evidence to support this notion. Similarly, there is no support for the hypothesis that dystonia in different muscle groups results from different pathophysiologic mechanisms.

The exact pathophysiology of neuroleptic-induced acute dystonia is still unknown, although several hypotheses have been advanced over the past 25 years, some of which are at odds with each other. In neuroleptic-induced acute dystonia, anticholinergic medication consistently reverses the dystonia, suggesting that a hypercholinergic state is a correlate of dystonia, and that abnormalities in the dopamine-acetylcholine balance in the brain may be the possible mechanism (13).

Dopaminergic agonists also generally seem to improve dystonias (though frequently worsening psychosis) in many patients, suggesting that a hypodopaminergic state, as well as the hypercholinergic state, may be implicated (14). This hypothesis is further strengthened by the fact that neuroleptics, particularly the high-potency typical antipsychotic medications, are strong dopamine antagonists. Other nonneuroleptic dopamine antagonists also seem to exacerbate dystonia (15).

In contrast, other investigators have proposed that dopaminergic excess may be the responsible factor (16). This hypothesis posits that neuroleptic administration produces postsynaptic dopamine receptor blockade, resulting in increased dopamine turnover in the brain. When the level of the neuroleptic decreases, which occurs during a dosing trough or in the wake of a single dose of antipsychotic medication given to control agitation, there is still increased dopamine turnover. According to this hypothesis, therefore, this increased dopaminergic release on now-unblocked receptors results in a hyperdopaminergic state that causes the dystonia.

Other hypotheses suggest a possible correlation of dystonia with changing blood–brain levels of neuroleptics. It is further possible that dystonia is related to changes in the ratio of dopamine D2 and D1 receptors (17). The fact that these receptor ratios appear to change normally over the aging process may explain why neuroleptic-induced acute dystonia occurs more commonly in younger people. Another theory posits that predisposition to dystonia occurs in people with certain genetic polymorphisms, such as at the locus for the enzyme GTP cyclohydrolase, involved in dopamine synthesis, on chromosome 14 (18). Clearly, more research is needed to satisfactorily explain the precise pathophysiologic mechanisms of acute dystonia.

Treatment and Course

Although a neuroleptic-induced acute dystonia typically subsides spontaneously within hours of onset, treatment should be started as soon as the dystonia is diagnosed, because the experience is intensely distressing to the patient.

Standard treatment of acute dystonia is the immediate administration of anticholinergic medication followed by the immediate discontinuation of the offending neuroleptic. Although anticholinergic medication may be administered orally in mild cases of dystonia, it is usually preferable to administer the medication intravenously (IV) or intramuscularly (IM). Since acute dystonia frequently involves the tongue, throat, jaw, and facial muscles, IM and IV administration of anticholinergic medication reduces the risk of aspiration. Just as importantly, however, such IM or IV administration provides far more rapid relief to the patient. Oral medication takes longer to work and is likely to result in unnecessarily prolonged distress to the patient.

There is consensus that the first dose of medication should be the equivalent of 50 mg of diphenhydramine or 2 mg of benztropine. This should be repeated if the first dose does not produce a robust response within 30 minutes (5). This standard one-dose or two-dose approach is usually successful in resolving the acute dystonia. In an unusually refractory case, IM or IV anticholinergic drugs should be used at repeated, frequent dosing intervals, and consideration should be given to adding an IV or IM injection of a short-acting benzodiazepine such as lorazepam for sedation and anxiolysis.

In cases of laryngeal or pharyngeal dystonias, anticholinergic medications should always be administered IV or IM, and strong consideration should be given to a higher starting dose of anticholinergic medication (the equivalent of 100 mg of diphenhydramine or 4 mg of benztropine) (19). If airway compromise occurs, immediate consultation and support should be obtained from an anesthesiologist, and the patient should receive general anesthesia with intubation and airway protection. Fortunately, this very rarely occurs.

It should be kept in mind that the half-lives of most antipsychotics are much longer than the half-lives of commonly used anticholinergic medications. Thus, after a neuroleptic-induced dystonia has resolved, the patient should be maintained on anticholinergic medication for at least 48 hours; it is acceptable to switch to oral administration at this time if the patient is able to swallow without difficulty. If there is a history of previous dystonias, anticholinergic treatment should be continued for 2 weeks (1).

Treatment with anticholinergic drugs is particularly problematic in geriatric patients, because the elderly can be exquisitely sensitive to the anticholinergic and antihistaminergic effects of these medications. Delirium, hypotension, tachycardia, and urinary retention are only a few of the side effects that must be anticipated, particularly when using these drugs in an elderly patient. Close monitoring of vital signs and mental status is of the essence, and inpatient hospitalization, particularly for psychotic or demented patients who may be unable to articulate how they are feeling, is frequently necessary. The incidence of acute dystonia can be minimized, as mentioned earlier, by the use of atypical or low-potency typical antipsychotics, as well as by cautious and slow dose titration (20).

An acute dystonic reaction, although usually easily treated, can be a terrifying experience for a patient, particularly if there is airway compromise. The damage to the physician–patient relationship may be significant, and the patient may become noncompliant with future treatment recommendations. Careful attention should be paid to patient education and to obtaining full and informed consent from the patient. The psychiatrist should always try to discuss with the patient and, when appropriate, with family members and caretakers, the possibility of acute dystonia. The patient should also be reassured that dystonia, although unpleasant, can be treated rapidly and generally does not produce any lasting harm.

PARKINSONISM AND EXTRAPYRAMIDAL SYMPTOMS

Definition and Diagnosis

NIP, frequently referred to as EPS, is defined as the development of parkinsonian signs or symptoms in association with the use of a neuroleptic medication. The three cardinal parkinsonian symptoms are tremor, muscle rigidity, and bradykinesia.

Parkinsonian tremor is a steady, rhythmic, oscillatory motion. It occurs at a frequency of 3 to 6 hertz. The hands and arms are most frequently affected, but the tremor may also involve the head, neck, jaw, face, tongue, legs, and trunk. It is a resting tremor that is typically suppressed during action, although it is also suppressed during sleep. The tremor increases in prominence during times of anxiety, stress, and fatigue (2).

Parkinsonian muscle rigidity is noted on physical examination as firmness or spasm of muscles at rest. This rigidity may affect all skeletal muscles, or be confined to a few specific muscle groups. The physician can check for muscle rigidity by placing his or her hands over the patient's limbs and moving the joints; the patient should not offer any resistance, and passively allow the joints to be moved by the examiner. Parkinsonian rigidity may appear as a diffuse and continuous lead-pipe stiffness that resists movement, or as "cogwheel" ratcheting-type stiffness around a joint. Cogwheeling may actually be a high-frequency (8–12 hertz) action tremor that is superimposed on stiffness (20). Rather than complain of stiffness, the patient may note muscle pain, generalized body aches, and discoordination. The treating physician must be alert to these complaints as possible EPS, particularly in elderly patients who may have pre-existing arthritis or noniatrogenic MDs (1).

Finally, the bradykinesia of parkinsonian EPS is seen clinically as a diminution of spontaneous motor activity and as global slowness in the initiation and execution of voluntary movements. The physician should look for such slowness, as well as drooling, hunched shoulders or bent neck, and the classic *masked facies*.

The differential diagnosis of NIP can be difficult, particularly in elderly patients. Parkinsonism occurs in numerous medical and neurological conditions and can be caused by medications other than neuroleptics. Idiopathic PD can be difficult to distinguish from NIP, and both may coexist in an elderly patient. Observation of the timing of onset of symptoms is crucial. In NIP, most symptoms occur within the first month of treatment with a neuroleptic; symptoms beginning after that time, particularly after the first 3 months of treatment, should raise suspicions for idiopathic PD. Clinical course must also be closely observed, because neuroleptic-induced EPS tends to plateau or even diminish over time, whereas the course of idiopathic PD is one of progressive decline and increasing impairment. There are also more subtle differences between the two disorders: idiopathic PD exhibits unilaterality of signs in the early stages of the disease, whereas NIP is usually bilateral from the start. The resting tremor also tends to be more prominent in idiopathic PD. Finally, the response to anticholinergic medication tends to be far more robust in NIP than in PD (21).

Careful attention should be paid to a new-onset tremor in an elderly patient, because the differential diagnosis for tremor is wide, and the tremor of NIP must be distinguished from tremors caused by other conditions. In general, nonparkinsonian tremors are finer, faster, and worse on intention, whereas parkinsonian tremors diminish on intention. The tremor of alcohol or benzodiazepine withdrawal typically presents with associated hyperreflexia, increased blood pressure, and tachycardia. Cerebellar disease produces a tremor with associated nystagmus and ataxia. Strokes and other brain lesions may produce a parkinsonian tremor, but frequently have associated focal neurological symptoms; magnetic resonance imaging (MRI) or computed tomography can help localize such lesions. Distinguishing TD from NIP can be very difficult, particularly since both conditions can coexist in the same patient (22). One observation that may be useful is that the tremor of TD does not typically have the steady rhythm of the parkinsonian tremor. Finally, it is important to distinguish NIP from life-threatening NMS; both can present with bradykinesia and rigidity. NMS has other associated findings, however, which include elevated creatine kinase, fever, and delirium.

A number of primary psychiatric illnesses may mimic the symptoms of NIP and further compound the difficulties in making an accurate diagnosis. It can be easy to confuse the negative symptoms of schizophrenia and the neurovegetative signs of major depression with the bradykinesia and rigidity of NIP. Catatonia and NIP may also be difficult to distinguish, and there is some evidence that the two conditions are related to each other (23). Often, the diagnosis of NIP must be made provisionally and then clarified by observing the patient's response to treatment.

Epidemiology and Risk Factors

The reported frequency of neuroleptic-induced EPS varies from less than 5% to greater than 90%, depending on the antipsychotic used and the study reviewed. This wide variation is due to the different definitions of parkinsonism (e.g., the inclusion of very mild bradykinesia as a sign of NIP) used in various studies, the demographics (age, gender, diagnosis) of the patients included in these studies, and the medications used (24).

A number of patient-related and medication-related risk factors have been delineated. Older age, any history of prior episodes of neuroleptic-induced EPS, and a concomitant history of organic brain injury is thought to predispose patients to the development of NIP (2). In addition, patients with dementia appear more vulnerable to EPS than do patients with schizophrenia. A higher-than-expected (though still low) percentage of patients who have experienced NIP are subsequently diagnosed with idiopathic PD. This may suggest that subclinical PD is a risk factor for NIP or, conversely, that NIP may somehow influence the development of PD in certain patients (25).

As with acute dystonia, rapid neuroleptic dose titration represents another risk factor for the development of NIP, particularly for the elderly (26). Administration of higher absolute doses of antipsychotics is another risk factor. Highly anticholinergic low-potency neuroleptics such as thioridazine or chlorpromazine are less likely to cause NIP. Similarly, coadministration of anticholinergic medications with high-potency neuroleptics such as haloperidol and fluphenazine reduces the incidence of NIP. However, most elderly patients are unable to tolerate the anticholinergic effects of such treatment strategies. The newer atypical antipsychotics are less likely to cause NIP, particularly when used at low doses, and again are considered the first-line treatment for most patients (27). At increasing doses, risperidone and, to a lesser degree, olanzapine, are more likely to cause NIP than clozapine, quetiapine, ziprasidone, or aripiprazole.

Pathophysiology

Neuroleptic-induced EPS is presumed to result from a blockade of postsynaptic dopaminergic (D2) receptors in the corpus striatum, causing a functional state that clinically resembles the pathological state of idiopathic PD, with destruction of dopaminergic cells in the striatum. The depletion of dopaminergic neurons that occurs with normal aging may explain, at least in part, why elderly patients are more likely to develop EPS. However, it is not clear whether loss of dopaminergic function in the nigrostriatal tracts is adequate to explain the clinical symptoms seen in both NIP and PD (5). It is likely that other neurochemical abnormalities coexist with dopaminergic depletion. Abnormalities in serotonin and norepinephrine have also been reported to be involved in the mechanism (28). This may explain the high incidence of mood symptoms, particularly dysphoria, associated with PD and NIP (29).

Early studies posited that the neuroleptic threshold—the dose of a neuroleptic at which bradykinesia or rigidity becomes evident—was the marker for the lowest effective dose of the medication (4). This suggested that the development of EPS was related to the therapeutic antipsychotic effect of neuroleptic medications. This concept has been hotly disputed through the years, with other investigators failing to observe a consistent association between EPS and improved control of psychiatric symptoms. Notably, the atypical antipsychotics produce potent effects in the absence of significant EPS, again implicating the roles of other neurotransmitters.

Treatment and Course

Untreated, NIP symptoms will continue unchanged or, in some cases, diminish over several months following onset. Treatment, in the form of dose reduction, addition of anticholinergic medication, or switching to an atypical or lower-potency antipsychotic medication, will almost always lead to improvement in NIP symptoms. However, as noted earlier, a small percentage of patients with NIP may go on to develop idiopathic PD (25).

Given the considerations above, the first goal of treatment should be prevention. The atypical agents are associated with a lower incidence of NIP, and should be used as first-line treatments. However, among the atypical antipsychotics, risperidone and, to a lesser extent, olanzapine are more likely to cause EPS than clozapine, quetiapine, ziprasidone, and aripiprazole (30). In fact, quetiapine and clozapine are associated with almost negligible rates of EPS, particularly at lower doses. Risperidone at higher doses, given its strong binding affinity for D2 receptors, causes the highest incidence of EPS among the atypical agents (31). Aripiprazole, with its mixed D2 agonism-antagonism, has a low incidence of EPS, but is not free of this troublesome side effect for some patients. High-potency typical neuroleptics are the most likely to cause EPS, with the low-potency agents being significantly less likely to do so. Many elderly people are unable to tolerate the anticholinergic effects of the low-potency typical neuroleptics.

Since EPS is at least in part dose-dependent, the clinician should always treat a patient with the lowest possible dose needed for good clinical effect, regardless of drug class. Sometimes lowering the neuroleptic dose slightly can be enough to relieve parkinsonian symptoms. Switching to another medication may also relieve symptoms, particularly if the switch is from a typical to an atypical antipsychotic, or from a high-potency to a low-potency typical possessing more intrinsic anticholinergic activity (1).

The treating provider must work with the patient in assessing the risks and benefit of treatment. Many mild cases of EPS are not bothersome to the patient and do not require treatment. Some elderly patients, especially if they have experienced significant side effects from anticholinergic medications or low-potency typicals, or if they have experienced significant improvements in their psychiatric conditions from a particular neuroleptic, may prefer to live with untreated EPS rather than add an anticholinergic treatment or switch neuroleptics. Here again, issues of informed consent, patient education, and the physician–patient relationship come to the forefront.

If NIP symptoms become problematic, and decreasing the dose of a particular neuroleptic or changing to a different neuroleptic is not feasible or has failed, the next step is to add a low dose of an anticholinergic medication. Though 1 mg of benztropine twice a day may relieve or significantly ameliorate most EPS symptoms, the geropsychiatrist may prefer to treat even more cautiously, initiating treatment with as little as 0.5 mg of benztropine daily, and titrating up as needed and according to patient tolerance. Especially for elderly patients, periodic attempts should be made to wean the patient from the anticholinergic agent. Studies have shown, even when high-potency typical neuroleptics are used at relatively high doses, that the majority of patients do not require adjunctive anticholinergic medication at the end of 3 months (32,33). Anticholinergic medication should always be tapered slowly, to avoid the rapid re-emergence of parkinsonian symptoms as well as the possibility of cholinergic rebound, which can be extremely uncomfortable for the patient. Elderly patients should be closely monitored, either with frequent outpatient follow-up or inpatient observation.

Refractory cases of NIP do occur, and some elderly patients may be extremely sensitive and prone to developing severe EPS. These cases may require even more aggressive management. While higher doses of anticholinergic agents may provide relief from EPS, they should be used for the shortest possible time, with rigorous attention being paid to untoward anticholinergic effects such as urinary retention, fecal impaction, and delirium. Though some young and healthy patients with NIP can tolerate anticholinergic medication doses as high as 20 mg/day of benztropine, most elderly patients cannot (1).

Another treatment approach for the refractory case is to discontinue the offending neuroleptic completely, wait until EPS resolves entirely, and then begin a very cautious and slow titration of a different neuroleptic. This treatment strategy frequently requires observation in an inpatient setting to monitor for re-emergence of psychiatric symptoms as well as medication side effects. Consideration may also be given to starting a dopamine agonist such as amantadine. A major concern with this treatment approach is the possibility of exacerbating psychosis. Therefore, this is usually a treatment of last resort, and may be best attempted in an inpatient setting.

A number of experimental treatment strategies have been proposed for the treatment of EPS. These include calcium, vitamin E and other antioxidants, herbal supplements such as gingko biloba, and complementary medicine treatments such as acupuncture (34,35). Though the evidence for the utility of such treatments is mixed, it may be reasonable for some patients to try these approaches. Vitamin E, the most widely used of these alternative treatments, is generally safe at doses less than 2,000 IU/day. Open communication between the treating physician and the patient is essential.

AKATHISIA

Definition and Diagnosis

Akathisia is a subjective and unpleasant feeling of restlessness with an intense need to move that occurs secondary to treatment with neuroleptics. Patients with akathisia complain of inner restlessness and the feeling that they must keep in motion, most frequently in their lower extremities. Many patients, however, have difficulty describing these feelings. On clinical examination, the psychiatrist should be alert for fidgeting, frequent changes in posture, crossing and uncrossing of the legs, tapping of the feet, rocking while sitting, and shuffling while walking (2).

Akathisia, like EPS and dystonia, tends to occur soon after initiating or increasing the dose of neuroleptic medication. It most commonly develops during the first 2 to 4 weeks of treatment, and rarely develops more than 3 months into treatment.

Akathisia is often associated with significant dysphoria, anxiety, and irritability. When akathisia is severe, aggressive and violent behavior, including suicide attempts, may occur (36,37). Akathisia in a psychotic or demented patient can easily be mistaken for a worsening of the primary psychiatric illness, resulting in an increase in the neuroleptic dose and a subsequent worsening of the akathisia. Hence, mistaking akathisia for a primary psychiatric disorder results in an intervention that is the exact opposite of what is appropriate. Conversely, onset of agitation before the initiation or increase of neuroleptic medication, lack of increase in agitation or aggression following treatment with a neuroleptic, and lack of relief (or exacerbation of symptoms) following a decrease in neuroleptic dose are all clues that suggest the problem is a primary mental disorder rather than neuroleptic-induced akathisia (2). Obtaining a good history from the patient and other sources is particularly important in making a correct diagnosis.

The strange subjective discomfort associated with acute akathisia is also the feature that is most useful in making a differential diagnosis between neuroleptic-induced akathisia and other MDs. TD and tardive akathisia are often associated with a lack of sensory perception of the movements; this contrasts with acute akathisia, in which the patient is intensely aware and very distressed. Acute akathisia commonly involves the legs, whereas TD is more likely to involve the arms, face, and trunk. The tremors of EPS and PD may be mistaken for akathisia, especially if the legs are involved, because the rhythmic appearance of akathisia sometimes suggests a tremulous condition (1).

The clinician should also keep in mind that a number of other medications, including the SSRIs, may produce akathisia that is clinically indistinguishable from neuroleptic-induced akathisia (38). Since polypharmacy is common among psychiatric patients and especially among the elderly, this makes proper diagnosis and treatment all the more important for the geriatric psychiatrist.

Finally, iron-deficiency anemia is a condition common in elderly patients that may present with symptoms similar to neuroleptic-induced akathisia. Since anemia can coexist with akathisia, and may even predispose to akathisia and TD, it is important to diagnose, workup, and treat both conditions appropriately (39).

Epidemiology and Risk Factors

Akathisia is a very common—perhaps the most common—side effect of high-potency typical neuroleptic treatment. It is estimated to occur in between 2% and 75% of patients treated with neuroleptics (1). The wide discrepancy in reported prevalence results from lack of consistency in the definition of akathisia, different medications and dosing strategies used in studies, different study designs, and differences in population demographics. Akathisia is thought to be a leading cause of noncompliance with treatment and refusal of neuroleptic medication by patients.

As with EPS and dystonia, higher doses and rapid dose escalation of neuroleptics, particularly high-potency medications, are most frequently associated with the development of acute akathisia. Previous episodes of neuroleptic-induced akathisia are also a risk factor (2). The middle aged and elderly are more susceptible to akathisia than are the young, and some studies suggest that women may be more vulnerable than men. There is also some suggestion in the literature that persistent acute akathisia may be a precursor to TD (40–43).

Pathophysiology

The pathophysiology of akathisia remains unknown, although a number of theories have been advanced. Early theories that presented akathisia as a subjective response to the objective rigidity and akinesia of NIP have been largely discarded (44). Akathisia has also been suggested to be a primary sensory disturbance with an unknown mechanism, in which motor disturbance occurs as a direct response to the sensory disturbance (45).

Many researchers have suggested that akathisia is simply another expression of NIP, with the same etiology. This theory is bolstered by the fact that akathisia frequently develops along the same time course and occurs in conjunction with EPS. However, this theory begs the question as to why anticholinergic drugs, though an appropriate treatment, are less effective at relieving akathisia than they are at ameliorating tremor, rigidity, and bradykinesia.

Recent research suggests that dopamine blockade in the mesocortical system, rather than in the nigrostriatal pathways, may cause the restlessness and dysphoria of akathisia (16). Mesocortical dopaminergic neurons in the prefrontal cortex seem to be resistant to depolarization induced by long-term neuroleptic treatment, suggesting an explanation for why akathisia, unlike EPS, often does not improve over time (5). Excess noradrenergic activity likely plays a role in the development of akathisia. This hypothesis is supported by the efficacy of β-blockers in improving many cases of akathisia. Opioid (46) and γ-aminobutyric acid (47) mechanisms have also been proposed to contribute to akathisia.

Treatment and Course

Akathisia is difficult to treat effectively. As such, attempts to prevent or minimize its presentation are especially desirable. Once again, atypical antipsychotics should be used as first-line treatment whenever neuroleptics are needed; however, it should be noted that although atypicals are less likely than typical neuroleptics to produce akathisia, the reduction in incidence is not as dramatic as it is for other neuroleptic-induced MDs (48). Low-potency typical neuroleptics are somewhat less likely than high-potency agents to be associated with akathisia, although, as previously noted, many elderly patients cannot tolerate their strong anticholinergic effects. Dose titration should be done slowly and cautiously.

If akathisia persists after these initial steps, the clinician should consider the addition of an anti-akathisia medication. Agents that have been reported effective and that are commonly used include β-blockers, anticholinergics, and benzodiazepines (19). Less frequently used, and more controversial, are clonidine and opioids. Unfortunately, neuroleptic-induced akathisia frequency lasts as long as neuroleptic treatment is continued, and treatment of the akathisia may not always alter its course.

For treatment of akathisia due to use of a high-potency typical neuroleptic, or with higher doses of a higher affinity D2-blocking atypical agent, the best initial approach is a β-blocker such as propranolol, especially if the clinical picture is not complicated by the presence of other neuroleptic-induced MDs such as parkinsonism. Dosing may be started conservatively at 10 mg three times a day, and titrated up slowly to effect. Anticholinergic medications may be added or substituted if full relief is not obtained, if there are other EPS present, or if the patient cannot tolerate high doses of β-blockers due to adverse cardiovascular symptoms such as bradycardia. As a final resort, a benzodiazepine such as clonazepam or lorazepam may also be of use, especially in conjunction with an anticholinergic (1).

In akathisia caused by a low-potency typical neuroleptic or an atypical with high affinity for muscarinic cholinergic receptors, a β-blocker is also the treatment of choice, followed by benzodiazepines. Anticholinergic medications increase the risk of toxicity, and should be reserved for situations where other EPS are present; the combination of anticholinergic and β-blocking medications may be effective. In general, the use of benzodiazepines with β-blockers is not recommended, particularly in medically at-risk elderly populations.

The clinician must consider polypharmacy, drug–drug interactions, and side effects from these various classes of medication. As noted previously, anticholinergics are not well tolerated in the elderly, particularly in those with dementia, and using these drugs prophylactically is not recommended (49). Benzodiazepines may cause marked sedation in the elderly, even at low doses, and increase the risk of falls. Some elderly patients, especially those suffering from dementia, may also exhibit marked disinhibition as well. β-Blockers are generally well tolerated, especially at low doses, but the psychiatrist must closely monitor vital signs and be keenly aware of the patient's other medical conditions and medications.

NEUROLEPTIC MALIGNANT SYNDROME

Definition and Diagnosis

This potentially fatal reaction to neuroleptic medication is characterized by muscle rigidity, fever, autonomic instability, and alterations in level of consciousness. Diffuse lead-pipe muscle rigidity and hyperthermia are considered by many to be the cardinal diagnostic features.

Many other features may or may not be present, as noted in the DSM-IV-TR criteria, including confusion, delirium, coma, tachycardia, labile blood pressure, laboratory evidence of muscle damage (such as elevated creatine kinase levels and myoglobinuria), and leukocytosis (2). Other clinical presentations include diaphoresis, tachypnea, tremor, incontinence, mutism, sialorrhea, dystonias, and dysphagia (50).

Prompt and accurate diagnosis of NMS is crucial, yet the variability in presentation complicates the differential diagnosis. Numerous general medical and neurological conditions (e.g., CNS infections and tumors, status epilepticus, tetanus, porphyria, heat stroke) can present with symptoms that mimic NMS. It is crucial, therefore, to rule out other acute illnesses when patients receiving neuroleptics become acutely ill. Because medical illness is a likely predisposing factor, it is important to note that NMS may be present even if another disease is found that explains the patient's symptoms (51). The presence of significantly elevated temperature and severe muscle rigidity makes a diagnosis of NMS more likely. The most important point to keep in mind is that the psychiatrist must always start by suspecting NMS, and then carefully rule out other possible problems.

Other psychiatric conditions can mimic NMS, although it is again important to remember that these conditions may coexist with NMS. Catatonia, seen most frequently in manic and schizophrenic patients, can present with hyperthermia, autonomic instability, and elevated creatine kinase. Obviously, it is important to determine whether the patient is being treated with a neuroleptic. Unlike a patient with NMS, however, a catatonic patient may have periods of catatonic excitement. A history of catatonia is important in making the differential diagnosis. Since catatonia may respond to lorazepam treatment, and NMS does not, a brief trial of lorazepam may provide a useful but not definitive method of distinguishing the two conditions (52,53).

Reactions to other classes of medications may also mimic NMS. The common clinical characteristics of the *serotonin syndrome* include hyperthermia, rigidity, myoclonus, and tremor (54). Since patients receiving neuroleptics may also be treated with serotonergic agents, and since many of the newer atypical antipsychotics act on serotonin as well as on dopamine, the clinical picture can be very confusing (55). Lithium intoxication, anticholinergic delirium, anticholinergic withdrawal delirium, and stimulant intoxication can all present with symptoms resembling NMS.

Epidemiology and Risk Factors

The incidence of NMS is not well known, although it is commonly believed to be much less than that of the other acute neuroleptic-induced MDs. A number of studies, both retrospective and prospective, have found that between 0.02% and 1.9% of patients treated with neuroleptics are affected with NMS. This large variability in frequency is likely a result of differences in study methodologies and the use of varying diagnostic criteria (56).

Many factors are thought to lead to or facilitate the development of NMS, including dehydration, physical exhaustion, a hot and humid environment, excessive sympathetic discharge, use of long-acting depot antipsychotics, high doses of neuroleptics, the abrupt discontinuation of antiparkinsonian agents, and concurrent lithium therapy (57,58). Patients with organic CNS disease and HIV-positive patients may also be at higher risk for developing NMS (59).

NMS usually presents in the first month of neuroleptic treatment; approximately two-thirds of cases manifest within the first week of treatment. NMS has occurred as soon as 45 minutes and as late as 65 days after initiation of neuroleptic treatment (60). A prior episode of NMS appears to predispose to future episodes of NMS; however, the longer the time elapsed after an episode of NMS, the lower the risk of recurrence becomes (61). Rapid loading and dose escalation are also risk factors for the development of NMS.

NMS is more frequently reported in men, and is less frequently seen in the elderly, although morbidity and mortality are higher in elderly patients with NMS. Patients with mood disorders may also be at higher risk for developing NMS when treated with neuroleptics (62).

With the advent of the atypical antipsychotics, NMS is much less frequently observed. Its importance when it occurs, however, cannot be underestimated.

Pathophysiology

The pathophysiologic mechanism of NMS remains unclear. Reduced dopaminergic activity secondary to neuroleptic-induced dopaminergic blockade has been put forth as a likely hypothesis. This reduced dopaminergic activity in various areas of the brain may also serve to explain the myriad clinical features of NMS. For example, reduced dopaminergic activity in the hypothalamus may cause fever and autonomic instability. Rigidity may be explained by hypodopaminergia in the nigrostriatal system. A reduction in corticolimbic dopaminergic activity may lead to altered consciousness (56). This theory is supported by the fact that most neuroleptics, particularly the high-potency typical neuroleptics (which are most frequently implicated in NMS), are strong dopamine-blocking agents. However, this does not explain why patients treated with the atypical neuroleptics, which have much lower affinity for dopamine receptors, have also developed NMS. The dopaminergic blockade theory also does not explain why NMS develops in some patients, but not others, and at varying times in the course of treatment. Alteration of dopaminergic and serotonergic transmission in the body, enhanced synthesis and action of prostaglandin E1 and E2, and a modification of calcium-mediated signal transduction has also been suggested as playing a role in the development of NMS (57).

In addition to the constitutional, environmental, and pharmacologic factors that interact to produce the syndrome, there are likely to be genetic factors as well. Possibly, a predisposition similar to that seen in malignant hyperthermia may be involved. Genetic polymorphisms are associated with individual differences in drug responses, both for efficacy and adverse reactions. Genetic association studies have sought to identify polymorphisms influencing susceptibility to NMS, especially with respect to dopamine, serotonin, and GABA receptors, and cytochrome P450 2D6 (63,64). While a few candidate polymorphisms have been tentatively associated with NMS, it must be noted that the studies were not large, and there are no clinical applications at this time.

Treatment and Course

The most important step in treatment is to recognize the clinical features of the syndrome and rapidly discontinue the neuroleptic. Once the neuroleptic has been stopped, supportive care remains the mainstay of treatment. This care, especially for elderly patients with pre-existing medical illnesses, often requires hospitalization in a medical intensive care unit. Supportive interventions are targeted to specific symptoms and include cooling blankets and antipyretics for fever, cardiac monitoring for arrhythmias, IV fluids for dehydration, and dialysis for acute renal failure (1).

Several specific treatments for NMS are widely used, although not without controversy. Most investigators advocate initial supportive measures for a day or two, followed by the use of specific treatments if the patient does not improve. Dantrolene, a muscle relaxant, is used to treat rigidity, hyperthermia, and tachycardia. Dantrolene can be given orally or by IV, four times per day, at doses of 1 to 3 mg/kg per day, although some investigators advocate continuous IV infusion (57). Dopamine agonists may also provide relief of symptoms, especially rigidity. Bromocriptine is commonly used, in doses of 5 to 10 mg orally, three times a day, in conjunction with dantrolene. Levodopa/carbidopa is used less frequently.

Electroconvulsive therapy (ECT) is another treatment option, and is thought to work by increasing dopamine turnover in the brain. Some psychiatrists have reported rapid and dramatic success in treating NMS with ECT; however, the high rate of mortality reported in some studies generally makes ECT a second-line or third-line treatment. ECT is particularly indicated when there is difficulty in distinguishing between NMS and catatonia (65,66). Experimental treatments include the use of steroids and N-methyl-D-aspartate antagonists (67,68).

The course of NMS is variable. Some cases follow a mild, self-limited course, whereas others may progress rapidly to death. Mortality in most case series ranges between 4% and 25%. Delays in diagnosis typically lead to poorer outcomes. Myoglobulinemia, renal failure requiring dialysis, and respiratory failure requiring ventilation is also linked to poor outcomes, with mortality up to 50% (69). Mortality is high in vulnerable populations, including elderly patients with pre-existing medical complications. Once the syndrome is recognized and the offending neuroleptic medication is discontinued, NMS usually resolves between 2 weeks and 1 month later.

Atypical antipsychotics appear to have a reduced liability in inducing NMS, just as they are less likely overall to be associated with other neuroleptic-induced MDs. However, NMS can still occur in patients taking these drugs, and the physician must be alert to this possibility (70). Initially, clozapine was thought to be free of the risk of NMS; however, case reports implicated clozapine as a cause of NMS in conjunction with other medications such as lithium and carbamazepine (50,71). More recently, there have been case reports of NMS in patients on clozapine monotherapy (72,73).

A particular difficulty for psychiatrists and patients with NMS is that rechallenge with neuroleptics can instigate a recurrence. Successful rechallenge is positively related to the length of time elapsed after resolution of NMS (61). Many physicians and patients prefer to rechallenge with a different neuroleptic after an episode of NMS, substituting a lower-potency or atypical drug for the offending agent. Rechallenge with the same neuroleptic can be done successfully in some cases (74). Extremely slow titration, close observation, and careful patient education is essential.

NONACUTE (TARDIVE) NEUROLEPTIC-INDUCED MOVEMENT DISORDERS

As noted previously, the temporal boundary between acute and nonacute is blurry. However, the tardive (or late-occurring) MDs usually occur after long-term exposure to neuroleptics. The time to onset of these disorders is usually measured in years, rather than days or weeks.

TARDIVE DYSKINESIA

Definition and Diagnosis

TD is a syndrome consisting of abnormal involuntary movements, usually choreoathetoid and stereotyped in nature, associated with long-term treatment with neuroleptics. The diagnostic criteria proposed in DSM-IV-TR specify that a minimum of 3 months' exposure to neuroleptics is required to make a diagnosis of TD in most patients; however, recognizing the increased risk of TD in the elderly, only 1 month of exposure is required in patients over 60 years of age. The diagnostic criteria also require that the abnormal movements develop during neuroleptic treatment or within 2 months of exposure to neuroleptics (2).

TD occurs most commonly in the tongue, neck, and face muscles, with a slow and insidious onset. Less common are involuntary movements of the trunk and limbs. Rarely, even the muscles of chewing, swallowing, and breathing may be involved (75). The earliest symptoms typically involve repetitive chewing, lip smacking, grimacing, or licking movements of the facial, jaw, lip, and tongue muscles. These are frequently referred to as buccolingual-masticatory movements. Clinical wisdom suggests that the earliest place to detect TD is in the tongue, specifically with the observation of vermiform movements. Limb movements may be choreiform (rapid and jerky, with a flinging quality), athetoid (slow and sinuous, with a writhing quality), or stereotypical (rhythmic and repetitive). Frequency and amplitude of the movements can vary greatly from patient to patient. TD can be classified as mild, moderate, or severe, not only in terms of the number of muscle groups involved, but also in terms of the disability it may cause the patient (76).

The differential diagnosis of TD is extensive. The major, and most difficult, task for the treating psychiatrist is to rule out other causes of the abnormal movements.

In many patients, TD is comorbid with acute neuroleptic-induced MDs such as parkinsonism, dystonia, and akathisia, making accurate diagnosis and treatment a formidable challenge (77). Other medications, psychiatric and nonpsychiatric, can cause acute and tardive MDs, again confounding accurate diagnosis in this era of polypharmacy. Amphetamines, tricyclic antidepressants, mood stabilizers (notably lithium), SSRIs, and bupropion can induce tremors, akathisia, stereotypies, and dyskinesia (78,79). These medications can also worsen neuroleptic-induced TD, as can certain nonpsychiatric medications and drugs of abuse such as methamphetamine, cocaine, and alcohol (80–82). Taking comprehensive, accurate, and regularly updated medication and substance use histories is essential.

Other MDs are part of the differential diagnosis, especially with elderly patients, who are more likely to suffer from noniatrogenic MDs such as PD, strokes of the basal ganglia, Huntington's chorea, essential tremor, cerebellar disease, and spontaneous dyskinesias. These may be difficult clinically to distinguish from TD (83). Sydenham's chorea, Tourette's disorder, and Wilson's disease are less likely to be diagnosed in geriatric patients. Family history, the presence or absence of dementia, other neurological symptoms, and the results of imaging tests may be useful in making a definitive diagnosis.

Psychiatric disorders may present with abnormalities of movement. Anxiety states, substance intoxication and withdrawal, conversion disorders, tics, compulsions, and malingering may need to be considered in the differential diagnosis. Endocrine disorders such as hyperthyroidism and hypoparathyroidism can also produce dyskinesia; judicious laboratory testing will help clarify the diagnosis (1). Especially in elderly patients, dental problems and ill-fitting dentures commonly mimic TD.

Epidemiology and Risk Factors

The reported prevalence and incidence of TD has been variable, likely as a result of different study populations, different medications and doses used, and different study methodologies. A meta-analysis done before the introduction of the commonly used atypical antipsychotics showed a prevalence of TD of 24.2% in a total population of 40,000 neuroleptic-treated patients (84). Another review reported a prevalence rate of 30% (85). A prospective study, again done before the introduction of the atypical

agents, found the incidence of TD after cumulative exposure to neuroleptics in young adults to be approximately 5% per year of exposure, with an incidence of 5% after 1 year, 18.5% after 4 years, and 40% after 8 years (86). In contrast, the cumulative annual incidence of TD is approximately 30% in middle-aged and elderly patients treated with typical neuroleptics (27,87). Other studies have offered similar conclusions. Thus, the cumulative length of exposure to neuroleptics and older age are major risk factors for the development of TD.

There is considerable evidence that the type of antipsychotic medication used is an important risk factor. In particular, the use of atypical antipsychotics is consistently associated with a much lower risk of developing TD, although higher doses of these drugs that produce EPS are associated with an increased risk of TD (88–90). Overall, it is difficult to estimate a specific reduction in risk, given that atypical antipsychotics are relatively new, many patients currently on atypical drugs have been on typical antipsychotics in the past, and the doses used in clinical practice and in studies vary greatly.

For patients on typical antipsychotics, there is some evidence that high-potency neuroleptics, especially at high doses, may be associated with a higher frequency of TD (91). Thus, the type of antipsychotic taken by the patient, the length of exposure to antipsychotic medications, and the cumulative dose of antipsychotics are likely all iatrogenic risk factors for developing TD.

There are many other risk factors. Female gender appears to be a risk factor for TD, although it is unclear if this represents a true biological difference or if this is a reflection of gender-based treatment differences (84). Interestingly, studies of older patients do not show a higher incidence in female patients (92). There are conflicting reports regarding ethnicity. Some studies report a higher incidence in African Americans and a lower incidence in Asians and Asian Americans than in White patients (93,94). Other studies of patients treated with neuroleptics show no significant differences in TD prevalence among various ethnic groups (95).

Mood disorders, particularly unipolar depression, have been reported as risk factors for TD, but this finding is not consistent (96,97). A positive family history of affective disorder in first-degree relatives of schizophrenic patients may also be a risk factor for the development of TD (98). Other comorbid neurological and psychiatric disorders, such as dementia, mental retardation, substance abuse (particularly alcohol and stimulants), a history of subdural hematoma, and stroke may be risk factors as well, but the evidence is mixed and, at times, contradictory (91,92,99). Patients who experience acute neuroleptic-induced MDs, such as parkinsonism and akathisia, may be at higher risk for the development of TD in the future (100). Some evidence exists that diabetics may have an increased risk of developing TD (101,102). This is of particular concern given both the significant endocrine effects of the atypical neuroleptics and the increasing prevalence of diabetes in the United States and elsewhere in the world.

The most important patient-related risk factor for the development of TD, however, is age (97). Both the prevalence and severity of TD generally increases with age, and the practicing geriatric psychiatrist must keep this in mind when prescribing neuroleptics to older patients. Studies estimate that elderly patients have a five- to six-fold increased risk as compared to young patients, even when duration of treatment with neuroleptics is relatively brief and the dose is relatively low (103). One study reported an incidence of 31% after only 43 weeks of conventional neuroleptic treatment in elderly patients; another study found that almost 60% of elderly psychiatric patients had TD after 3 years of study treatment (91,92).

Pathophysiology

Historically, striatal dopamine receptor (D2) supersensitivity was proposed to account for the development of TD. However, it is apparent that this hypothesis is inadequate as an explanation. Dopamine receptor hypersensitivity occurs rapidly in patients treated with neuroleptics, whereas TD develops slowly in some patients, and not at all in others. In some patients, TD may lessen or remit over time, even if antipsychotic treatment is continued (100). A modification of the D2-receptor hypersensitivity hypothesis incorporates a role for D1 dopamine receptors. The core of this hypothesis is based on the observation that clozapine and other atypical neuroleptics are active at both D1 and D2 receptors, and that patients on these atypicals are less likely to develop TD. These observations have led to the theory that TD results from an imbalance between D1-mediated and D2-mediated effects in the basal ganglia (104).

Some researchers propose that neuroleptic-induced striatal degeneration may be the mechanism of TD. It is hypothesized that long-term neuroleptic use generates toxic free radicals that oxidize and damage neurons in the basal ganglia, resulting in the persistent MD of TD (105). The basal ganglia, with their high oxidative metabolism, are particularly vulnerable to membrane lipid peroxidation as a result of the increased catecholamine turnover induced by neuroleptic drugs. Other researchers propose a *double hit hypothesis,* viewing schizophrenia itself as resulting at least in part from accumulated toxins secondary to lipid membrane abnormalities. The addition of neuroleptics may cause more damage in an already susceptible brain (106).

Many other neurochemical imbalances have been proposed to explain the pathophysiology of TD. Given that the disease differs from patient to patient, and that there are so many different risk factors, it is likely there are multiple pathologies at work. GABA, acetylcholine, serotonin, norepinephrine, estrogen, fatty acids, and various neuropeptides have all been postulated to play a role in TD, as

has dysregulation of glucose, protein, and mineral metabolism (104). Reasoned arguments can be made for a critical interaction between patient and drug parameters; the specific contributions of individual factors are unknown. The search for genetic markers and polymorphisms that might predispose patients to TD has not been fruitful to date (107–109).

Treatment and Course

There are many different treatments for TD, but none has proven consistently effective. Thus, the psychiatrist must focus primarily on prevention of the disease. Management of risk factors and amelioration of symptoms if the disease is present is also important.

First and foremost, neuroleptic use, in dose and duration, should be minimized in *all* patients. Although patients with chronic psychotic disorders may need long-term treatment with neuroleptics, only the minimum dose needed to treat their condition and control their symptoms should be used. Tapers and dose reductions should be attempted in stable, elderly, schizophrenic patients (110). Despite the widely accepted use of neuroleptics in treating nonpsychotic psychiatric conditions, such as behavioral disturbances and dementia, careful consideration should be given to using nonneuroleptic medications, behavioral programs, and environmental modifications for these patients whenever possible. For patients with psychotic depressions or manias, neuroleptics should be used at low doses and for brief periods of time whenever possible, with tapering doses and eventual discontinuation once the psychosis is resolved (1).

In general, there must be enough clinical evidence to show that the benefits of treatment with a particular neuroleptic agent outweigh the potential risks, especially the risk of TD. These risks and benefits must be discussed with the patient, and the patient's family if appropriate, on an ongoing basis. It is recommended that the physician document these discussions in the patient's chart (111).

Atypical antipsychotics are considered first-line treatment for psychosis, and should be used preferentially over the typical medications to minimize the risk for TD. All of the atypical agents have a lower risk for TD compared to the typicals, provided they are used in appropriately low (non–EPS-inducing) doses. One study (89) compared the risk of TD with haloperidol versus risperidone in 132 patients aged 45 and older. Most of these patients had either schizophrenia or dementia with psychosis or agitation. Both risperidone-treated and haloperidol-treated patients received a median daily dose of 1 mg/day; however, the cumulative incidence of TD was significantly higher in the haloperidol group than in the risperidone group (p = .05). Another study (90) compared the risk of developing definitive TD after treatment with either a conventional antipsychotic or an atypical antipsychotic in 240 middle-aged and older patients (130 treated with conventional agents and 110 treated with

Instructions: Rate greatest severity of abnormality observed.

Code: 0 = none; 1 = minimal; 2 = mild; 3 = moderate; 4 = severity

Choreoathetoid and Dystonic Movements

1.	Muscles of facial expression		0	1	2	3	4
2.	Lips and perioral		0	1	2	3	4
3.	Jaw		0	1	2	3	4
4.	Tongue		0	1	2	3	4
5.	Upper extremities	R	0	1	2	3	4
		L	0	1	2	3	4
6.	Lower extremities	R	0	1	2	3	4
		L	0	1	2	3	4
7.	Trunk		0	1	2	3	4

Total (1–7) _____

Global Judgements

8.	Severity of abnormal movements	0	1	2	3	4
9.	Incapacitation due to abnormal movements	0	1	2	3	4
10.	Patients awareness of abnormal movements (rate only patient's report)	0	1	2	3	4

Dental Status

11.	Current problems with teeth and/or dentures?	Yes ____	No ____
12.	Does patient usually wear dentures?	Yes ____	No ____

Subject has *clinical* diagnosis of tardive dyskinesia   Yes ____   No ____

Pt. Name _____ Pt. # _____ Rater _____ Date _____

Figure 41-1 Abnormal Involuntary Movement Scale (AIMS).

atypical agents including risperidone, olanzapine, and quetiapine). Patients treated with conventional antipsychotics were significantly more likely to develop TD than those treated with atypical antipsychotics (p <.001).

Patients who require treatment with neuroleptics should have periodic evaluations every 3 to 6 months to assess TD symptoms. Rating scales can be useful. One commonly used scale is the *Abnormal Involuntary Movement Scale* or *AIMS* (Figure 41-1). Although not the most accurate measure for TD-specific symptoms, this scale is easy to administer and

has good interrater reliability. A positive score indicates that TD may be developing, even in the absence of other overt symptoms (91). Scores over time can be monitored to track the progression or remission of a patient's TD.

Obviously, certain risk factors such as age cannot be controlled, but other risk factors can and should be modified. Medical conditions such as diabetes that may play a role in the development of TD should be closely managed. Patients should be advised that the use of alcohol, nicotine, cocaine, and amphetamines exacerbates TD and may increase the

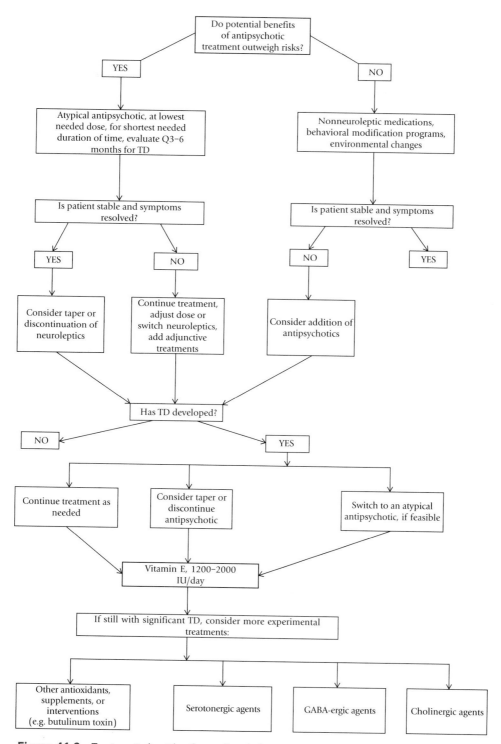

Figure 41-2   Treatment algorithm for tardive dyskinesia. GABA, γ-aminobutyric acid; IU, international units; Q3–6, every three to six; TD, tardive dyskinesia.

risk of developing TD. Other nonneuroleptic medications should be monitored and may need to be minimized; for example, anticholinergic medications tend to worsen the symptoms of TD, although there is no strong evidence that they are a causative factor (112). Emotional arousal, stress, and fatigue also exacerbate TD, so exercise, relax-

ation techniques, and good sleep hygiene should be encouraged.

Many other treatments for TD have been suggested, based on various hypotheses of pathophysiology. A number of antioxidant medications and supplements have been tried as treatments for TD. Vitamin E is perhaps the most well known of these alternative treatments, with evidence for possible benefit at doses of 1,200 to 2,000 IU/day. This has been supported in a number of studies, with the most significant benefits for patients who have had TD of brief duration. Some researchers suggest using vitamin E at the first sign of TD; others suggest using it prophylactically at the onset of psychosis or simultaneously with the initiation of neuroleptic treatment (113–115). The long-term safety of high doses of vitamin E in the prevention or treatment of neurological and psychiatric diseases is unknown (116). Other antioxidants that have been used experimentally in the treatment of TD include vitamin B6 at 100 mg/day and melatonin at up to 10 mg/day, with the latter also being an inhibitor of dopaminergic activity in the striatum and hypothalamus (117,118). Results have been suggestive of benefit, but larger studies are needed. Coenzyme Q, vitamin B12, and omega fatty acids may also hold promise. Hormonal treatments may include estrogen (109), although their longer-term use may be associated with other adverse effects.

Given that many neurotransmitters have been posited to play a role in the development of TD, treatments that affect these neurotransmitters have also been tried. Noradrenergic antagonists such as β-blockers and clonidine may be helpful, as may serotonin receptor modulators such as ondansetron and nefazodone, but the evidence is both preliminary and mixed (119–122). GABA-ergic medications such as the benzodiazepines and valproate, may be beneficial in some cases, and some preliminary evidence exists for the treatment benefits of acetylcholinesterase inhibitors such as donepezil (123,124). However, it should be stressed that all of these treatments have their own side effects, and their overall efficacy for TD is uncertain. If such experimental and alternative treatments are to be tried, it is important for the treating psychiatrist to have an open discussion with the patient or the patient's caregiver.

Other treatments that have been used, particularly in cases of severe TD, include botulinum toxin injections and neurosurgical interventions (125,126). These should be considered treatments of last resort. A suggested treatment algorithm is offered in Figure 41-2.

Time itself may be the most significant factor in the treatment of TD. Up to one-third of TD patients experience significant remission within 3 months of discontinuation of neuroleptics, with approximately 50% of patients in remission within 18 months of discontinuation (2). However, elderly patients have been reported to have lower rates of remission (1). Even in patients with TD who are maintained on neuroleptics, symptoms of TD may lessen in approximately 50% (100). However, this finding is not to suggest that the treating physician take TD lightly.

Severe TD can lead to numerous physical complications and psychosocial problems in the elderly. Dental problems are common sequelae of buccomandibular and oral dyskinesia, as are ulcerations of the tongue, cheeks, and lips (127). Dysarthria, swallowing dysfunction, and respiratory

difficulties may also occur, although these are rare (128). Subjective distress is also common, leading to dysphoria, depression, and suicidality in some cases. Aggressive prevention and informed treatment is essential.

OTHER TARDIVE MOVEMENT DISORDERS

A variety of other tardive MDs exist, including tardive dystonia, tardive akathisia, tardive parkinsonism, and tardive Tourette's disorder. Though these may represent variants of classical TD, some researchers suggest different pathophysiologies and different classification systems (8). However, at this time treatments remain similar to those for TD.

ACKNOWLEDGMENTS

This work was supported in part by NIMH grants MH-43693, MH-49671, and MH-59101, by the National Alliance for Research on Schizophrenia and Depression, and by the Department of Veterans Affairs.

REFERENCES

1. Jeste DV, Naimark D. Medication-induced movement disorders. In: Tasman A, Lieberman J, Kay J, eds. *Psychiatry*. Philadelphia: WB Sanders Company; 1997;1334–1354.
2. American Psychiatric Association. *Diagnostic and Statistical Manual of Mental Disorders*. 4th Ed, Text Revision. Washington, DC: American Psychiatric Association; 2000.
3. Delay J, Deniker P. Drug-induced extrapyramidal syndromes. In: Vinken PJ, Bruyn GW, eds. *Diseases of the Basal Ganglia*. Amsterdam: North-Holland; 1968;248–266.
4. Haase HJ. Extrapyramidal system and neuroleptics: a "conditio sine qua non." In: Bordeleau LM, ed. *Systeme Extra-Pyramidal et Neuroleptiques (Extrapyramidal System and Neuroleptics)*. Montreal: Editions Psychiatriques; 1961;329–353.
5. Lohr JB, Jeste DV. Neuroleptic-induced movement disorders: acute and subacute disorders. In: Michels R, Cavenar JO Jr, Brodie NKH, et al., eds. *Psychiatry*. Revised Edition. Philadelphia: J.B. Lippincott Co.; 1988;1–19.
6. Faurbye A, Rasch PJ, Petersen PB, Brandborg G, Pakkenberg H. Neurological symptoms in pharmacotherapy of psychoses. *Acta Psychiatr Scand*. 1964;40:10–27.
7. Tancredi LR. Malpractice and tardive dyskinesia: a conceptual dilemma. *J Clin Psychopharmacol*. 1988;8:71S–76S.
8. Lauterbach EC, Carter WG, Rathke KM, et al. Tardive dyskinesia-diagnostic issues, subsyndromes, and concurrent movement disorders: a study of state hospital inpatients referred to a movement disorder consultation service. *Schizophr Bull*. 2001;27:601–613.
9. Patterson TL, Klapow JC, Eastham J, et al. Correlates of functional status in older patients with schizophrenia. *Psychiatry Res*. 1998;80:41–52.
10. Patterson TL, Lacro JP, Jeste DV. Abuse and misuse of medications in the elderly. *Psychiatric Times*. 1999;16:54–57.
11. Rupniak NMJ, Jenner P, Marsden CD. Acute dystonia induced by neuroleptic drugs. *Psychopharmacology*. 1986;88:403–419.
12. Keepers GA, Casey DE. Prediction of neuroleptic-induced dystonia. *J Clin Psychopharmacol*. 1986;7:342–344.
13. Stahl SM, Berger PA. Bromocriptine, physostigmine, and neurotransmitter mechanisms in the dystonias. *Neurology*. 1982;32:889–892.
14. Lang AE. Dopamine agonists in the treatment of dystonia. *Clin Neuropharmacol*. 1985;8:38–57.

15. Burke RE, Reches A, Traub MM, Ilson J, Swash M, Fahn S. Tetrabenazine induces acute dystonic reactions. *Ann Neurol.* 1985;17:200–202.
16. Marsden CD, Jenner P. The pathophysiology of extra-pyramidal side-effects of neuroleptic drugs. *Psychol Med.* 1980;10: 55–72.
17. Wong DF, Wagner HN Jr, Dannals RF, et al. Effects of age on dopamine and serotonin receptors measured by positron emission tomography in the living human brain. *Science.* 1984;226: 1393–1396.
18. Scott BL. Evaluation and treatment of dystonia. *South Med.* 2000;176:746–751.
19. Arana GW, Rosenbaum JF. *Handbook of Psychiatric Drug Therapy.* 4th Ed. Philadelphia: Lippincott Williams & Wilkins; 2000.
20. Lance JW, McLeod JG. *A Physiological Approach to Clinical Neurology.* London: Butterworth & Co.; 1981.
21. Hausner RS. Neuroleptic-induced parkinsonism and Parkinson's disease: differential diagnosis and treatment. *J Clin Psychiatry.* 1983;44:13–16.
22. Caligiuri MP, Lohr JB, Bracha HS, Jeste DV. Clinical and instrumental assessment of neuroleptic-induced parkinsonism in patients with tardive dyskinesia. *Biol Psychiatry.* 1991;29: 139–148.
23. Lohr JB, Lohr MA, Wasli E, et al. Self-perception of tardive dyskinesia and neuroleptic-induced parkinsonism: a study of clinical correlates. *Psychopharmacol Bull.* 1987;23:211–214.
24. Miller LG, Jankovic J. Drug-induced movement disorders: an overview. In: Joseph AB, Young RR, eds. *Movement Disorders in Neurology and Neuropsychiatry.* Boston: Blackwell Scientific Publications; 1992;7.
25. Peabody CA, Warner D, Whiteford HA. Neuroleptics and the elderly. *J Am Geriatr Soc.* 1987;35:233–238.
26. Byne W, Stamu C, White L, Parella M, Harvey PD, Davis KL. Prevalence and correlates of parkinsonism in an institutionalized population of geriatric patients with chronic schizophrenia. *Int J Geriatric Psychiatry.* 2000;15:7–13.
27. Jeste DV, Rockwell E, Harris MJ, Lohr JB, Lacro J. Conventional vs. newer antipsychotics in elderly patients. *Am J Geriatr Psychiatry.* 1999;7:70–76.
28. Langston JW, Irwin I. MPTP: current concepts and controversies. *Clin Neuropharmacol.* 1986;9:485–507.
29. Barnes TR, McPhillips MA. How to distinguish between the neuroleptic-induced deficit syndrome depression and disease-related negative symptoms in schizophrenia. *Int Clin Psychopharmacol.* 1995;10:115–121.
30. Taylor D. Ziprasidone: an atypical antipsychotic. *Pharmaceutical J.* 2001;266:396–401.
31. Barnes TR, McPhillips MA. Critical analysis and comparison of the side-effect and safety profiles of the new antipsychotics. *Br J Psychiatry.* 1999;174:34–43.
32. Coleman JH, Hays PE. Drug-induced extrapyramidal effects—a review. *Dis Nerv Syst.* 1975;36:591–593.
33. Johnson DAW. Prevalence and treatment of drug-induced extrapyramidal symptoms. *Br J Psychiatry.* 1978;132:27–30.
34. Osser DN. Neuroleptic-induced pseudoparkinsonism. In: Joseph AB, Young RR, eds. *Movement Disorders in Neuropsychiatry and Neuropsychiatry.* Boston: Blackwell Scientific Publications; 1992; 73–74.
35. Zhang XY, Zhou DF, Zhang PY, Wu GY, Su JM, Cao LY. A double-blind, placebo-controlled trial of extract of ginkgo biloba added to haloperidol in treatment-resistant patients with schizophrenia. *J Clin Psychiatry.* 2001;62:878–883.
36. Tandon R, Jibson MD. Suicidal behavior in schizophrenia: diagnosis, neurobiology, and treatment implications. *Curr Opin Psychiatry.* 2003;16:193–197.
37. Siris SG. Suicide and schizophrenia. *J Psychopharmacol.* 2001;15: 127–135.
38. Caley CF. Extrapyramidal reactions and the selective serotonin-reuptake inhibitors. *Ann Pharmacother.* 1997;31:1481–1489.
39. Hofmann M, Seifritz E, Botschev C, Krauchi K, Muller-Spahn F. Serum iron and ferritin in acute neuroleptic akathisia. *Psychiatry Res.* 2000;93:201–207.
40. Barnes TRE, Braude WM. Persistent akathisia associated with early tardive dyskinesia. *Postgrad Med J.* 1984;60:359–361.
41. Barnes TRE, Braude WM. Akathisia variants and tardive dyskinesia. *Arch Gen Psychiatry.* 1985;42:874–878.
42. Munetz MR, Cornes CL. Akathisia, pseudoakathisia and tardive dyskinesia: clinical examples. *Compr Psychiatry.* 1982;23: 345–352.
43. Muscettola G, Barbato G, Pampallona S, Casiello M, Bollini P. Extrapyramidal syndromes in neuroleptic-treated patients: prevalence, risk factors, and association with tardive dyskinesia. *J Clin Psychopharmacol.* 1999;19:203–208.
44. Tarsy D. Akathisia. In: Joseph AB, Young RR, eds. *Movement Disorders in Neurology and Neuropsychiatry.* Boston: Blackwell Scientific Publications; 1992;88–99.
45. Sovner R, Dimascio A. Extrapyramidal syndromes and other neurological side effects of psychotropic drugs. In: Lipton MA, Dimascio A, Killam KF, eds. *Psychopharmacology: a Generation of Progress.* New York: Raven Press; 1978;1021–1032.
46. Walters A, Hening W, Chokroverty S, Fahn S. Opioid responsiveness in patients with neuroleptic-induced akathisia. *Mov Disord.* 1986;1:119–127.
47. Hirose S, Ashby CR. Immediate effect of intravenous diazepam in neuroleptic-induced acute akathisia: an open-label study. *J Clin Psychiatry.* 2002;63:524–527.
48. Bowles TM, Levin GM. Aripiprazole: a new atypical antipsychotic drug. *Ann Pharmacother.* 2003;37:687–694.
49. Raleigh FR Jr. Reducing unnecessary antiparkinsonian medication in antipsychotic therapy. *J Am Pharm Assoc.* 1977;17:101–105.
50. Pope HG, Keck PE, McElroy SL. Frequency and presentation of neuroleptic malignant syndrome in a large psychiatric hospital. *Am J Psychiatry.* 1986;143:1227–1233.
51. Sewell DD, Jeste DV. Distinguishing neuroleptic malignant syndrome (NMS) from NMS-like acute medical illnesses: a study of 34 cases. *J Neuropsychiat Clin Neurosci.* 1991;4:265–269.
52. Carroll BT. Catatonia on the consultation-liaison service. *Psychosomatics.* 1992;33:310–315.
53. Salam SA, Kilzieh N. Lorazepam treatment of psychogenic catatonia: an update. *J Clin Psychiatry.* 1988;49:16–21.
54. Sternbach H. The serotonin syndrome. *Am J Psychiatry.* 1991;148: 705–713.
55. Ener RA, Meglathery SB, Van Decker WA, Gallagher RM. Serotonin syndrome and other serotonergic disorders. *Pain Med.* 2003;4:63–74.
56. Sewell DD, Jeste DV. Neuroleptic malignant syndrome: clinical presentation, pathophysiology, and treatment. In: Stoudemire A, Fogel BS, eds. *Medical Psychiatric Practice.* Washington, DC: American Psychiatric Press; 1992:425–452.
57. Ebadi M, Pfeiffer RF, Murrin LC. Pathogenesis and treatment of neuroleptic malignant syndrome. *Gen Pharmacol.* 1990;21: 367–386.
58. Keck PE, Pope HG, Cohen BM. Risk factors for neuroleptic malignant syndrome: a case-control study. *Arch Gen Psychiatry.* 1989;46:914–918.
59. Harris MJ, Jeste DV, Gleghorn A, Sewell DD. New-onset psychosis in HIV-infected patients. *J Clin Psychiatry.* 1991;52:369–376.
60. Shalev A, Munitz H. The neuroleptic malignant syndrome: agent and host interaction. *Acta Psychiatr Scand.* 1986;73:337–347.
61. Rosebush PI, Stewart TD, Gelenberg AJ. Twenty neuroleptic rechallenges after neuroleptic malignant syndrome in 15 patients. *J Clin Psychiatry.* 1989;50:295–298.
62. Addonizio G, Susman VL, Roth SD. Neuroleptic malignant syndrome: review and analysis of 115 cases. *Biol Psychiatry.* 1987;22: 1004–1020.
63. Kawanishi C. Genetic predisposition to neuroleptic malignant syndrome: implications for antipsychotic therapy. *Am J Pharmacogenomics.* 2003;3:89–95.
64. Yamawaki S, Yanagawa K, Morio M. Possible central effect of dantrolene sodium in neuroleptic malignant syndrome. *J Clin Psychopharmacol.* 1986;6:378–379.
65. Scheftner WA, Shulman RB. Treatment choice in neuroleptic malignant syndrome. *Convuls Ther.* 1992;8:267–279.
66. Susman VL. Clinical management of neuroleptic malignant syndrome. *Psychiatr Q.* 2001;72:325–336.
67. Sato Y, Asoh T, Metoki N, Satoh K. Efficacy of methylprednisolone pulse therapy on neuroleptic malignant syndrome in Parkinson's disease. *J Neurol Neurosurg Psychiatry.* 2003;74:574–576.

68. Weller M, Kornhuber J. A rationale for NMDA receptor antagonist therapy of the neuroleptic malignant syndrome. *Med Hypotheses.* 1992;38:329–333.

69. Shalev A, Hermesh H, Munitz H. Mortality from neuroleptic malignant syndrome. *J Clin Psychiatry.* 1989;50:18–25.

70. Caroff SN, Mann SC, Campbell EC, Sullivan KA. Movement disorders associated with atypical antipsychotic drugs. *J Clin Psychiatry.* 2002;63:12–19.

71. Muller T, Becker T, Fritze J. Neuroleptic malignant syndrome after clozapine plus carbamazepine. *Lancet.* 1988;2:1500.

72. Bottlender R, Jager M, Hofschuster E, Dobmeier P, Moller HJ. Neuroleptic malignant syndrome due to atypical neuroleptics: three episodes in one patient. *Pharmacopsychiatry.* 2002;35:119–121.

73. Thornberg SA, Ereshefsky L. Neuroleptic malignant syndrome associated with clozapine monotherapy. *Pharmacotherapy.* 1993;13:510–514.

74. Weller M, Kornhuber J. Clozapine rechallenge after an episode of neuroleptic malignant syndrome. *Br J Psychiatry.* 1992;161:855–856.

75. Burn DJ, Coulthard A, Connolly S, Cartlidge NE. Tardive diaphragmatic flutter. *Mov Disord.* 1998;13:190–192.

76. Gardos G, Cole JO, Schniebolk S, Salomon M. Comparison of severe and mild tardive dyskinesia: implications for etiology. *J Clin Psychiatry.* 1987;48:359–362.

77. Bitton V, Melamed E. Coexistence of severe parkinsonism and tardive dyskinesia as side effects of neuroleptic therapy. *J Clin Psychiatry.* 1984;45:28–30.

78. Mann SC, Greenstein RA, Eilers R. Early onset of severe dyskinesia following lithium-haloperidol treatment. *Am J Psychiatry.* 1983;140:1385–1386.

79. Muthane UB, Prasad BN, Vasanth A, Satishchandra P. Tardive parkinsonism, orofacial dyskinesia, and akathisia following brief exposure to lithium carbonate. *J Neurol Sci.* 2000;176:78–79.

80. Dixon L, Weiden PJ, Haas G, Sweeney J, Frances AJ. Increased tardive dyskinesia in alcohol-abusing schizophrenic patients. *Compr Psychiatry.* 1992;33:121–122.

81. Marti-Masso JF, Poza JJ. Cinnarizine-induced parkinsonism: ten years later. *Mov Disord.* 1998;13:486–489.

82. Sewell DD, Jeste DV. Metoclopramide-associated tardive dyskinesia: an analysis of 67 cases. *Arch Fam Med.* 1992;1:271–278.

83. Jeste DV, Wyatt RJ. *Understanding and Treating Tardive Dyskinesia.* New York: Guilford Press, Inc.; 1982.

84. Yassa R, Jeste DV. Gender differences in tardive dyskinesia: a critical review of the literature. *Schizophr Bull.* 1992;18:701–715.

85. Llorca PM, Chereau I, Bayle FJ, Lancon C. Tardive dyskinesias and antipsychotics: a review. *Eur Psychiatry.* 2002;17:129–138.

86. Kane JM, Woerner M, Lieberman J. Tardive dyskinesia: prevalence, incidence, and risk factors. *J Clin Psychopharmacol.* 1988;8(Suppl):S52–S56.

87. Jeste DV, Gilbert PL, McAdams LA, Harris MJ. Considering neuroleptic maintenance and taper on a continuum: need for individual rather than dogmatic approach. *Arch Gen Psychiatry.* 1995;52:209–212.

88. Davidson M. Long-term safety of risperidone. *J Clin Psychiatry.* 2001;62:26–28.

89. Jeste DV, Lacro JP, Bailey A, Rockwell E, Harris J, Caligiuri MP. Lower incidence of tardive dyskinesia with risperidone compared with haloperidol in older patients. *J Am Geriatr Soc.* 1999;47:716–719.

90. Dolder CR, Jeste DV. Incidence of tardive dyskinesia with typical versus atypical antipsychotics in very high risk patients. *Biol Psychiatry.* 2003;53:1142–1145.

91. Jeste DV, Caligiuri MP, Paulsen JS, et al. Risk of tardive dyskinesia in older patients: a prospective longitudinal study of 266 patients. *Arch Gen Psychiatry.* 1995;52:756–765.

92. Saltz BL, Woerner MG, Kane JM, et al. Prospective study of tardive dyskinesia incidence in the elderly. *JAMA.* 1991;266:2402–2406.

93. Lacro JP, Jeste DV. The role of ethnicity in the development of tardive dyskinesia. In: Yassa R, Nair NVP, Jeste DV, eds. *Neuroleptic-Induced Movement Disorders.* New York: Cambridge University Press; 1997:298–310.

94. Morgenstern H, Glazer WM. Identifying risk factors for tardive dyskinesia among long-term outpatients maintained with neuroleptic medications: results of the Yale Tardive Dyskinesia Study. *Arch Gen Psychiatry.* 1993;50:723–733.

95. Sramek J, Roy S, Ahrens T, Pinanong P, Cutler NR, Pi E. Prevalence of tardive dyskinesia among three ethnic groups of chronic psychiatric patients. *Hosp Community Psychiatry.* 1991;42:590–592.

96. Casey DE. Affective disorders and tardive dyskinesia. *L'Encephale.* 1988;14:221–226.

97. Smith JM, Baldessarini RJ. Changes in prevalence, severity, and recovery in tardive dyskinesia with age. *Arch Gen Psychiatry.* 1980;37:1368–1373.

98. Wegner JT, Catalano F, Gibralter J, Kane JM. Schizophrenics with tardive dyskinesia. *Arch Gen Psychiatry.* 1985;42:860–865.

99. Yassa R, Nair V, Schwartz G. Tardive dyskinesia: a two-year follow-up study. *Psychosomatics.* 1984;25:852–855.

100. Kane JM, Jeste DV, Barnes TRE, et al. *Tardive Dyskinesia: A Task Force Report of the American Psychiatric Association.* Washington, DC: American Psychiatric Association; 1992.

101. Ganzini L, Heintz RT, Hoffman WF, Casey DE. The prevalence of tardive dyskinesia in neuroleptic-treated diabetics: a controlled study. *Arch Gen Psychiatry.* 1991;48:259–263.

102. Woerner MG, Saltz BL, Kane JM, Lieberman JA, Alvir MJ. Diabetes and development of tardive dyskinesia. *Am J Psychiatry.* 1993;150:966–968.

103. Jeste DV. Tardive dyskinesia in older patients. *J Clin Psychiatry.* 2000;61:27–32.

104. Casey DE. Tardive dyskinesia: pathophysiology and animal models. *J Clin Psychiatry.* 2000;6:5–9.

105. Lohr JB, Jeste DV. Neuroleptic-induced movement disorders: tardive dyskinesia and other tardive syndromes. In: Michels R, Cavenar JO Jr, Brodie NKH, et al., eds. *Psychiatry.* Revised Edition. Philadelphia: J.B. Lippincott Co.; 1988:1–17.

106. Brown K, Reid A, White T, et al. Vitamin E, lipids, and lipid peroxidation products in tardive dyskinesia. *Biol Psychiatry.* 1998;43:863–867.

107. Garcia-Barcelo MM, Lam LC, Ungvari GS, Lam VK, Tang WK. Dopamine D3 receptor gene and tardive dyskinesia in Chinese schizophrenic patients. *J Neural Transmission.* 2001;108:671–677.

108. Kaiser R, Tremblay PB, Klufmoller F, Roots I, Brockmoller J. Relationship between adverse effects of antipsychotic treatment and dopamine D2 receptor polymorphisms in patients with schizophrenia. *Mol Psychiatry.* 2002;7:695–705.

109. Turrone P, Seeman MV, Silvestri S. Estrogen receptor activation and tardive dyskinesia. *Can J Psychiatry.* 2000;45:288–290.

110. Gilbert PL, Harris MJ, McAdams LA, Jeste DV. Neuroleptic withdrawal in schizophrenic patients. *Arch Gen Psychiatry.* 1995;52:173–188.

111. Jeste DV, Naimark D, Halpain MC, et al. Neuropsychiatric and mental health services aspects of tardive dyskinesia. In: Ovsiew F, ed. *Neuropsychiatry and Mental Health Services.* Washington DC: American Psychiatric Press; 1999:335–361.

112. Jeste DV, Krull AJ, Kilbourn K. Tardive dyskinesia: managing a common neuroleptic side effect. *Geriatrics.* 1990;45:49–58.

113. Adler L, Peselow E, Rosenthal M, et al. Vitamin E treatment of tardive dyskinesia. *Biol Psychiatry.* 1992;21:230A.

114. Elkashef AM, Ruskin PE, Bacher N, Barrett D. Vitamin E in the treatment of tardive dyskinesia. *Am J Psychiatry.* 1990;147:505–506.

115. Sajjad SH. Vitamin E in the treatment of tardive dyskinesia: a preliminary study over 7 months at different doses. *Int Clin Psychopharmacol.* 1998;13:147–155.

116. Vantassery GT, Bauer T, Dysken M. High doses of vitamin E in the treatment of disorders of the central nervous system in the aged. *Am J Clin Nutr.* 1999;70:793–801.

117. Lerner V, Miodownik C, Kaptsan A, et al. Vitamin B6 in the treatment of tardive dyskinesia: a double-blind, placebo-controlled, crossover study. *Am J Psychiatry.* 2001;158:1511–1514.

118. Shamir E, Barak Y, Shalman I, et al. Melatonin treatment for tardive dyskinesia: a double-blind, placebo-controlled, crossover study. *Arch Gen Psychiatry.* 2001;58:1049–1052.

119. Casey DE. Tardive dyskinesia: nondopaminergic treatment approaches. *Psychopharmacology.* 1985;2:137–144.

120. de Angelis L. 5-HT2A antagonists in psychiatric disorders. *Curr Opin Investig Drugs.* 2002;3:106–112.

121. Sirota P, Mosheva T, Shabtai H, Korczyn AD. Treating tardive dyskinesia with ondansetron. *J Clin Psychopharmacol.* 2001;21:355–356.
122. Wynchank D, Berk M. Efficacy of nefazodone in the treatment of neuroleptic-induced extrapyramidal side effects: a double-blind randomized parallel group placebo-controlled trial. *Hum Psychopharmacol.* 2003;18:271–275.
123. Caroff SN, Campbell EC, Havey J, Sullivan DA, Mann SC, Gallop R. Treatment of tardive dyskinesia with donepezil: a pilot study. *J Clin Psychiatry.* 2001;10:772–775.
124. Egan MF, Apud J, Wyatt RJ. Treatment of tardive dyskinesia. *Schizophr Bull.* 1997;23:583–609.
125. Kanovsky P, Streitova H, Bares M, et al. Treatment of facial and orolinguomandibular tardive dystonia by botulinum toxin A: evidence of long-lasting effect. *Mov Disord.* 1999;14:886–888.
126. Trottenberg T, Paul G, Meissner W, et al. Pallidal and thalamic neurostimulation in severe tardive dystonia. *J Neurol Neurosurg Psychiatry.* 2001;70:557–559.
127. Yassa R, Jones BD. Complications of tardive dyskinesia: a review. *Psychosomatics.* 1985;26:305–313.
128. Jackson IV, Volavka J, James B, et al. The respiratory components of tardive dyskinesia. *Biol Psychiatry.* 1980;15:485–487.

Psychiatric Care of the Older Adult with Persistent Pain

42

Jordan F. Karp   *Debra K. Weiner*

The inclusion of a chapter on pain in a textbook of geriatric psychiatry reflects the strides our field has made in recognizing the significance pain plays in the lives of our patients. If this textbook had been prepared 10 years ago, it is unlikely that the editors would have considered allocating space to this topic. However, given that the life expectancy of humans in developed nations continues to increase, so too has the prevalence of frailty and chronic medical conditions such as arthritis, spinal stenosis, osteoporosis-associated fractures, postherpetic neuralgia, myofascial pain disorders, and diabetic neuropathy. Adults over 75 years of age represent the fastest growing segment of the total population (1), so these painful disorders have particular importance for both geriatricians and psychiatrists who treat older adults. Since our practices reflect our communities, psychiatrists will continue to see increasing numbers of aging baby boomers and their parents who have pain syndromes as well as emotional and cognitive disorders. Pain has ceased to be an area that psychiatrists—especially those who treat older adults—can ignore.

Both acute and persistent pain have significant health implications for older adult patients. This chapter, however, is primarily concerned with pain that is persistent in nature, because of the common occurrence of psychiatric, cognitive, and functional disability associated with persistent pain conditions. In addition, patients rarely present to a psychiatrist while suffering from or seeking treatment for acute pain symptoms. These patients usually seek care from their primary care provider or the emergency room. Mental health practitioners, however,

frequently care for patients with chronic health and pain disorders, although typically pain is not the presenting symptom.

CASE EXAMPLE

Mrs. RC is a 74-year-old widowed woman who had been seeing you, her psychiatrist, for the past 8 months for treatment of a bereavement-associated depression. Combination therapy with an antidepressant and twice-monthly supportive psychotherapy has led to a moderate improvement in her low mood, weight loss, insomnia, and generalized anxiety.

Mrs. RC's daughter, her primary caretaker who usually accompanies Mrs. RC to her many physician appointments, is now expressing concern that her mother's memory and ability to manage medications is deteriorating. She is not remembering to take her medications as prescribed, especially the oral hypoglycemics for diabetes and the nonsteroidal anti-inflammatory agents that she takes for advanced hip osteoarthritis and spinal stenosis. As a result of her difficulty with maintaining medication compliance, her pain symptoms recently flared, and she has also developed neuropathic pain in her feet. Mrs. RC is now spending more time in bed, saying it is too painful for her to leave the house, and "what do I have to live for anyway."

You tell Mrs. RC that you take her pain problems very seriously, and that you think her pain and depression are "feeding each other." You increase the dose of antidepressant, and ask her daughter to approach other family members about providing practical support. You then provide Mrs. RC with a referral to the community hospital-based pain clinic with which you have a good working relationship. You also assess her daughter for depression. In the medical record, you make a note to more completely assess Mrs. RC's cognition once her depression and pain symptoms are better controlled.

PREVALENCE OF PERSISTENT PAIN IN OLDER ADULTS

Persistent pain, i.e., pain that persists at least 3 to 6 months, is common in older people (2), and increases with each decade of life. Studies have determined that 25% to 50% of community-dwelling older adults suffer important pain problems (3,4). A Harris telephone survey found that one in five older Americans takes analgesics several times a week, and 63% of those had taken prescription pain medications for more than 6 months (5). The consequences of persistent pain among older adults are numerous, and include depression, anxiety, decreased socialization, sleep and appetite disturbance, impaired ambulation, and increased healthcare utilization and costs (6). Although less thoroughly described, other conditions such as gait disturbances, slow rehabilitation, and adverse effects from polypharmacy are potentially worsened by the presence of pain in older adults (7).

Interface Between Pain and Mental Illness in Older Adults

Besides poorly controlled pain in older adults leading to depression, anxiety, sleep and appetite disturbance, increased utilization of health care, and impaired activities of daily living, it may also be associated with cognitive dysfunction, although well-controlled studies that definitively demonstrate this association are lacking. A strong relationship between depression and persistent pain has been consistently reported (8,9). Psychological barriers to pain control in older adults include a sense of fatalism, denial, and the desire to be "the good patient." Studies have shown that between 30% and 100% of persistent pain patients are diagnosed with depression (8). In addition, depressed patients frequently complain of pain symptoms (10). Among patients with rheumatoid arthritis (RA), it has been shown that an episode of major depression, even if it occurs prior to the onset of RA, leaves patients at risk for higher levels of pain when depressive symptoms persist, even 11 years after the depressive episode (11). Fishbain et al. reviewed 83 studies on pain and depression (12), which consistently showed a statistically significant relationship between the presence of persistent pain and depression. Fishbain concluded that this rela-

tionship is not in doubt, and that depression may be more common in patients with pain than in any of the other clinical populations examined in the meta-analysis. These studies were conducted with mixed-age groups, but because the majority of ambulatory healthcare utilization in the United States is by patients older than 65 years (13), these results are also representative of older adults.

Nondepressive psychopathology also has been shown to be associated with pain. Patients with persistent pain frequently have high levels of fear and vigilance (14). This anxiety has been associated with concerns about functional disability (15), as well as fears that physical activity and movement may increase both pain and the likelihood of (re)injury (16,17). Fear is also a common symptom of patients with dementia (18). Fear in demented patients with pain may be contributed to by a variety of factors. Many of these adults, for example, suffer from word-finding difficulties or other aphasias as part of their cognitive disorder, and are unable to verbally express their physical distress. These patients may also misinterpret their pain as originating from an external source. Such scenarios may lead to paranoia, depression, and behavioral disturbance, including agitation, resistiveness, and even assaultive behavior.

Many community-dwelling older adults live with an intense fear of falling (19), often as a result of gait instability or musculoskeletal pain. This frequently leads to immobility, increased functional disability, social isolation, depression, and more pain. In addition to these movement-related anxieties, Asmundson et al. reported a high incidence of phobic responses such as the fear of social interaction, leaving secure environments, blood, illness, and death, among this group of patients (20). It appears that anxiety and fear may transcend the pain experience and generalize to other areas of concern.

Substance abuse is also associated with persistent pain. Hoffman et al. described a sample of 414 patients with persistent pain, of whom 97 (23.4%) met criteria for active alcohol, analgesic, or sedative misuse or dependency (21). Current dependency was most common for analgesics (12.6%), followed by alcohol (9.7%), and sedatives (7.0%). Again, this was a mixed-age group. However, the use of narcotic analgesics, alcohol, and sedative-hypnotics by an older adult population may worsen current memory complaints or other cognitive dysfunction. In addition, a substantial number of hospitalized Medicare patients have diagnosed substance use disorders (22,23). Given our aging society, with the associated increased prevalence of painful disorders and current substance use trends, the size of this group with comorbid syndromes is expected to grow (24).

Finally, somatoform disorder has been shown to be prevalent among patients with persistent pain. The rates for somatoform disorders for these patients have been found to be as high as 53% (25). There is a paucity of research on somatoform disorders in older adults. This may partially be a result of the discriminatory quality of the diagnostic criteria, which require that symptoms of somatization disorder begin before age 30 and be persistent. Memory deficits among older adults may artificially lower rates of this disorder, as patients may not recall the onset of their symptoms (26). However, given that patients often develop psychologically mediated physical symptoms similar to their medical syndromes, it is likely that older adults with persistent pain also may suffer from somatoform illness.

Clearly, these disorders are a significant health dilemma for all patient populations. How persistent pain impacts these disorders in older adults, however, has yet to be determined. The unique medical, cognitive, psychosocial, economic, and functional qualities of the older adult are often in limited reserve compared to their younger counterparts. The added burden of persistent pain likely is underreported in the current literature.

UNDERSTANDING PAIN

The International Association for the Study of Pain (IASP) defines pain as "an unpleasant sensory and emotional experience which we primarily associate with tissue damage or describe in terms of such damage, or both" (27). This definition is broad, but remains the benchmark, attesting to the complexity of pain. The statement also allows for patient subjectivity, different causes of pain, and for the multidimensional quality (e.g., sensory and emotional) of the pain experience. Table 42-1 illustrates Melzack's conceptualization of pain, which is composed of three hierarchical levels (*gate control model*), postulating that nociception is the result of the simultaneous integration of motivational-affective, cognitive-evaluative, and sensory-discriminative factors (28,29). The gate control theory places equal weight on sensory and psychological processes in the unique perceptual process of nociception.

TABLE 42-1
MELZACK'S HIERARCHICAL CONCEPTUALIZATION OF PAIN

Multidimensional Categories of Pain	Components
Sensory-discriminatory	• Location • Intensity • Quality
Motivational-affective	• Depression • Anxiety
Cognitive-evaluative	• Thoughts concerning the cause and significance of pain

TABLE 42-2
COMMON CAUSES OF PAIN IN THE OLDER ADULT

Musculoskeletal disorders
- Osteoarthritis
- Myofascial pain
- Low back pain
- Osteoporosis
- Regional musculoskeletal disorders

Neuropathic disorders
- Peripheral neuropathy
- Postherpetic neuralgia
- Vasogenic claudication

Mixed/unspecified disorder
- Fibromyalgia syndrome

This model of persistent pain reflects current training in psychiatry, which is to treat patients utilizing a biopsychosocial approach. A multidimensional understanding of persistent pain is particularly useful when treating older adults, because of the physiological, cognitive, and psychological aspects of aging, all of which affect the experience of pain. To assist with treatment planning and prognosis, determining the cause of pain is crucial with older adults. Some of the common causes of pain are listed in Table 42-2. These conditions are understood to result from either 1) nociceptive, 2) neuropathic, 3) mixed/unspecified pain syndromes, or 4) idiopathic/psychological mechanisms.

Nociceptive Pain

All pain is modulated by specialized receptors (*nociceptors*). Nociceptive pain is categorized as a unique form of pain, both to differentiate it from neuropathic pain, as well as to describe its result from a disruptive stimulus. Nociceptive pain involves the activation of the nociceptive system by noxious stimuli such as pressure, temperature, tissue inflammation, mechanical deformation, distention of a hollow organ, or disruption of membrane integrity. Nociceptors are found in skin, muscle, joints, and viscera (29). Older adults frequently complain of nociceptive pain. Traditional approaches to pain management, including common analgesic medications and nonpharmacologic strategies, are often effective treatments.

Patients often describe nociceptive pain as aching, squeezing, stabbing, or throbbing. Common examples among older adults are arthritis and metastatic bone pain. Chronic inflammation with a nociceptive stimulus may be the cause of persistent pain. Nociceptive sensitization may be involved in the development of some types of persistent pain syndromes, which occurs within the site of injury.

Neuropathic Pain

Neuropathic pain is defined by the IASP as pain initiated or caused by a primary lesion or dysfunction in the nervous system (27). Many of the initiating incidents that may cause neuropathic pain are degenerative or age related, so it is not surprising that these syndromes are common in older adults. A history that suggests damage to the nervous system, together with the patient's use of language that describes the burning, paroxysmal, stabbing, or electric shock-like sensations, typical of neuropathic pain, should be sought (30). Older adults may complain of "pins and needles" or "burning feet." Neuropathic pain occurs most commonly in the lower extremities. Typical etiologies seen among older adults include trauma, vascular insufficiency, diabetes mellitus and other metabolic disorders, hereditary neuropathies, motor neuron disease, paraproteinemia, nutritional deficiencies, connective tissue disease, toxins, medications, and malignancies. As patients with HIV disease and AIDS live longer, physicians will see more older adults with HIV-associated neuropathy. The most prevalent neuropathic pain syndromes seen are diabetic neuropathy and postherpetic neuralgia. Anticonvulsants, tricyclic antidepressants, and opioids are commonly used in the treatment of this type of pain.

Mixed or Unspecified Pain

Some pain disorders are neither purely nociceptive nor purely neuropathic, but have features of both. An example of such a disorder is fibromyalgia syndrome (FMS). While patients with FMS experience muscular pain, muscle biopsies do not support intrinsic pathology. Increasing data supports primary central nervous system dysregulation of pain-processing as the underlying etiology of FMS.

Psychiatrists are likely to see older adults with FMS, as it is fairly common in this age group, and psychological/psychiatric comorbidities are a common part of the syndrome. A large epidemiologic study estimated that as many as 7% of older women suffer from FMS (31). Typical features include generalized pain, nonrestorative sleep, fatigue, and morning stiffness. Patients with FMS also frequently experience depression, anxiety, and poor coping skills. Physical exam is remarkable only for characteristic tender points. Treatment consists of aerobic exercise, analgesics, antidepressant therapy, and a variety of nonpharmacologic interventions.

Idiopathic Pain

Persistent symptoms that defy etiologic understanding but cause significant suffering are common in both outpatient medical and psychiatric practices. Idiopathic pain is also known as "psychological pain," a term which should be avoided, as it connotes a pain experience inherently less severe than nociceptive or neuropathic pain. While idiopathic pain frequently is associated with psychiatric symptoms, the distress experienced by these patients is generally similar to those patients with nociceptive or neuropathic pain. Diagnostic testing frequently fails to reveal a discrete disease that has a specific therapy. For many of these patients the increased psychiatric comorbidity involves depressive and anxiety disorders (32–34). The vast majority of patients with depression in primary care present with physical complaints such as pain, not emotional problems (35–37). Examples of unspecified pain disorders include recurrent headaches and some pelvic pain syndromes. Treatment selection and response is often unpredictable, and may require sequential trials or combination therapies.

Comorbid depression, anxiety, and somatoform disorders generally worsen the experience of pain, independent of the etiology. The patient with idiopathic pain presents a challenge to health care providers, who are often stymied by a lack of explanation for the pain. Physicians need to be willing to believe the older adult's self-report of pain, and investigate the cause. However, the presence of comorbid anxiety, depression, or somatization disorders, in the absence of an objective cause, should guide the treatment in the direction of psychiatric care and supportive psychotherapy.

PRIMER ON PAIN PATHWAYS AND SIGNIFICANT NEUROTRANSMITTERS

The Sensory Pathway

For a comprehensive explanation of the pathophysiology of pain, the reader is referred to a textbook on pain (38,39). A basic understanding of sensory pathways and neurotransmitters is necessary, however, for the psychiatrist to rationally approach the older adult with persistent pain.

Pain pathways can be broken down into three basic sets of neurons: *first-order*, *second-order*, and *third-order neurons*. First-order neurons relay noxious stimuli from the periphery or viscera to the spinal cord. First-order neurons have at one end *transducers* (the free nerve ending), which convert energy in the environment into action potentials in neurons. These tracts, comprised of A-δ and C neurons, have long dendrites with fine terminal arborizations present in skin, viscera, joints, bone, and muscle. When stimulated, action potentials extend from the dendrites to the cell body, which is located in the dorsal root ganglion of the spinal cord. A-δ fiber information is well-localized, sharp, pricking, and pulsating. However, it is relatively short-lived. Shortly thereafter, C fibers relay information that is less definitive or localized, but of a more persistent, dull, aching, and burning quality (40). Both A-δ and C fibers synapse directly, or indirectly, through interneurons, on second-order neurons (29).

Second-order neurons are located in the spinal column, and comprise the spinothalamic tract. Most of these fibers cross-over to the contralateral cord and ascend in the anterolateral aspect of the white matter. Ascending uninterrupted, they terminate in the contralateral thalamus. A small number of fibers project to the ipsilateral thalamus (40).

The thalamus is the primary relay station for sensory information from the periphery (via first-order and second-order neurons) to the cortex. Second-order neurons terminate in the ventral posterior nucleus (VPN) of the thalamus. From the VPN, the thalamus projects to the somatosensory cerebral cortex in the posterior lobe. Via this pathway, discriminative aspects of pain such as localization, and the coordination of motor responses to pain, can be coordinated (42). For older adults with a history of cerebrovascular accident, these projections may be disrupted (especially if the stroke involves the thalamus), resulting in poststroke or thalamic pain syndromes. In addition to projections to the somatosensory cortex, thalamic information is relayed to the reticular formation, medial thalamus, hypothalamus, prefrontal cortex, hypothalamic-pituitary axis, and the autonomic nervous system (43). Through these spinothalamocortical projections, the noxious stimulus influences affect, attention, memory, cognition and the endocrine/stress-response systems (44). All of these systems may already be compromised as a result of concurrent disease processes such as dementia, so further disruption or activation of these systems may be of particular concern for the older adult.

Among factors that influence sensitivity to, and perception of, pain in later life are: 1) loss of receptors for pain (nociceptors); 2) changes in conduction properties of primary nociceptive afferents; 3) changes in central mechanisms coding the sensation and perception of pain; 4) changes in segmental nociceptive reflexes and autonomic nervous system response to nociceptive input; 5) changes in descending modulation of pain; 6) psychosocial influences affecting the meaning of pain to the individual; and 7) altered interpersonal relationships and degree of self-efficacy to manage the tasks of daily life (41).

Significant Neurotransmitters

Psychiatrists are well aware of the role neurotransmitters such as serotonin, norepinephrine, γ-aminobutyric acid (GABA), and acetylcholine have in depression, anxiety, cognitive dysfunction, and other mental disorders. These neurotransmitters are also involved in nociceptive pathways, and their modulation by reuptake inhibitors has been documented (45); tricyclic antidepressants (norepinephrine and serotonin reuptake inhibitors) and selective serotonin reuptake inhibitors both have been observed to offer relief from persistent pain for some patients. This

may be due to an increase in the duration and concentration of neurotransmitters in synapses associated with central pain regulation (46).

Areas of central pain regulation, also known as supraspinal analgesia, have been identified in the midbrain, pons, and the medulla (especially around the cerebral aqueduct, i.e., the periaqueductal gray matter) (47). These areas of the brain are rich in endogenous opioids and opioid receptors, and they also give rise to fiber tracts that project to the dorsal horn of the spinal cord, where serotonin, norepinephrine, and acetylcholine are released. The action of these tracts is to inhibit nociceptive input from afferents and/or output by nociceptive second-order neurons. These neurotransmitters, especially serotonin, result in inhibition on dorsal horn nociceptive structures, which is mediated by the activation of opioid-releasing interneurons. The spinal actions of norepinephrine on the dorsal horn nociceptive mechanisms are mediated by α-2 receptors and are inhibitory. The action of serotonin in the dorsal horn is mediated by several 5-hydroxytryptamine (5-HT) receptor subtypes, including 5-HT_{1A}, 5-HT_2, and 5-HT_3, with both excitatory and inhibitory effects. GABA, enkephalin, and substance P also have corticospinal projections that are involved in the regulation of nociception (48).

Medications that increase the levels of these neurotransmitters also have extra-corticospinal mechanisms of action. For example, serotonin is released from platelets when tissue is injured and plays several roles in pain. The serotonin released from platelets activates the ion-channel-coupled 5-HT_3 receptors on primary afferents, producing brief pain. However, tachyphylaxis develops within minutes, so 5-HT_3 antagonists are not practical analgesics. Peripheral 5-HT_2 receptors may be important for some types of pain, acting indirectly to enhance the effects of other inflammatory mediators such as prostaglandin E2 or bradykinin (49).

ACUTE VERSUS PERSISTENT PAIN

While the primary concern with older adults is persistent pain, it is useful to understand the differences between acute and persistent pain. This distinction is especially relevant in the selection of effective analgesia and prognosis. Acute pain is characteristically of recent onset lasting no more than days or weeks. Pain is by convention considered to be persistent if it lasts more than 3 to 6 months. In older adults, especially those who are cognitively impaired, paying attention to associated pain-related behaviors or features of pain may be of more use in making this distinction than a verbal history. While feelings of anxiety may be expressed by patients experiencing acute or persistent pain, those with persistent pain more often describe irritability and/or depression. In addition, patients with persistent pain may or may not have vegetative signs, such as lassitude, anorexia, weight loss, insomnia, and loss of libido, which may be seen with acute pain. These signs may be difficult to distinguish from other disease-related effects.

THE ROLE OF THE PSYCHIATRIST

Because many older adults suffer from persistent pain, the role of the psychiatrist, particularly the geriatric psychiatrist, in the treatment of pain is emerging, but is still poorly defined. According to the program requirements for psychiatric residency education as outlined by the Accreditation Council for Graduate Medical Education, psychiatric residents should attain a "comprehension of the diagnosis and treatment of neurologic disorders commonly encountered in psychiatric practice such as . . . . intractable pain, and other related disorders." This requirement went into effect in January 2001. To our knowledge, no surveys of pain education during psychiatric residency are yet available, so the actual implementation of this requirement may not be universal. In addition, there is an enormous cohort of otherwise well-trained psychiatrists who graduated from their residencies before this requirement was instituted that have received no formal training in assessing and treating persistent pain. Our goal as psychiatrists and pain specialists is to fill this gap in the education of many psychiatrists, and provide an overview of how clinicians should approach their older adult patients with persistent pain.

WHERE DO PSYCHIATRISTS SEE OLDER ADULT PAIN PATIENTS?

Psychiatrists see patients with pain at every treatment site. For numerous reasons, however, they do not always know that their patients are suffering from pain. Chief among the reasons for not knowing is failure to ask, which results in an incomplete assessment of the psychiatric patient. As stated earlier, not inquiring about pain is most likely due to a lack of training during both psychiatric residency and postresidency education.

In the Office

The most common site to see older adult patients with persistent pain is in private practice or the outpatient clinic. Research has shown that patients with persistent pain symptoms have both an increased point prevalence and lifetime prevalence of psychopathologic disorders, compared with normative populations, and thus are more likely to present to a psychiatrist for treatment. Examples of the increased prevalence of mental illness include work done by Magni et al. who used the Center for Epidemiologic Studies Depression Scale in a study of 416 patients with

persistent pain (50). He found that 18.3% of these patients scored in the clearly depressed range (score of greater than 20), compared with only 8.8% of patients without persistent pain (n = 2388).

In another study, Fishbain et al. noted that almost 30% of a group of 283 patients with persistent pain had concurrent depression (51). Finally, Von Korff et al. reported that relative to nondepressed individuals, patients with moderate-to-severe depressive symptoms were more likely to develop headaches and chest pain (52,53). They also reported that depressive symptoms were more frequent in patients with persistent pain than in a control group. The most common complaints included feeling that everything was an effort, disturbed sleep, worry, and low energy. Those described in these studies were patients with persistent pain—not psychiatric patients. In addition, the studies were of mixed ages. However, it can be surmised that with rates of depression of up to 30% among patients with persistent pain, a substantial number of them are either already in psychiatric treatment or eventually will be.

In the Hospital

Psychiatrists frequently see patients with both acute and persistent pain when providing consultations in the hospital for their medical and surgical colleagues. Pain is frequent and often severe in both seriously ill and older patients during hospitalization, as well as at follow-up, and before death, even in those with diseases not traditionally associated with pain. In a study of 205 hospitalized inpatients, despite analgesia, approximately 79% of subjects reported pain during the 24-hour period prior to data collection (54). Over 33% of subjects who reported pain rated it as distressing, horrible, or excruciating. This level represents a lower proportion than in previous studies where as many as 58% of patients reported excruciating pain, and fewer than half of these patients reported having a member of the health care team ask them about their pain or noted the pain in the record (55). In the Yates et al. study, a large proportion of patients indicated that pain affected their movement and made them feel worried and exhausted (54). Pain was also found to affect patients' eating, and made them feel angry and alone. Another significant finding was that pain affected sleep for more than half of the sample. This finding that pain interferes with sleep is consistent with work reported by Cohen who found that 67% of patients reported their sleep was affected by pain (56).

The emotional and somatic symptoms reported in these studies are similar to those of depression. Indeed, insomnia, irritability, loneliness, exhaustion, anorexia, and anxiety are all frequently seen in late-life depression. When conducting a consultation on a patient with pain in the hospital, the consultation-liaison (C/L) psychiatrist should determine if the prescribed analgesic is appropriate and effective for the clinical situation. The C/L psychiatrist need not write new analgesic orders; however, introducing the need for improved analgesia, if pain is present and undertreated, will be a useful recommendation. The primary treatment team may have overlooked pain as the possible source of the symptoms prompting the psychiatric consultation.

While it is difficult to distinguish a primary depression or anxiety disorder from pain-related emotional symptoms, the C/L psychiatrist should treat psychiatric symptoms that are comorbid with the pain as if they were primary. These treatments can include supportive psychotherapy, family therapy, education about coping skills while in the hospital, and prescribing symptom-specific medications. If patients are delirious, demented (often with limited communication skills), or are agitated, recommending symptom-specific treatments to keep the patient and staff safe are indicated. Importantly, the C/L psychiatrist should educate his or her medical and nursing colleagues about the emotional and behavioral sequelae of undertreated pain in older adults.

In Nursing Homes and Long-Term Care Facilities

Psychiatrists have increased their presence in nursing homes and long-term care facilities over the past 15 years. The reasons for this are (1) an increased awareness of the need for psychiatric care—given the patient population—in these environments, and (2) government regulations, such as the Omnibus Budget Reconciliation Act of 1987, which requires regular monitoring and attempts to decrease the doses of antipsychotic and tranquilizer medications (57). Despite these advances, there is still a significant shortage of mental health services in these facilities. For example, Smyer et al. showed that although more than three quarters of residents with a mental disorder resided at a nursing home that provided counseling services, less than one-fifth actually received any mental health services within the year (58).

Psychiatrists are generally asked to evaluate patients in these settings for depression, anxiety, psychosis, paranoia, agitation and other disruptive behaviors, delirium, and to review psychiatric medications. These requests for consultation are similar to those in the medical/surgical setting. It is rare that psychiatrists are consulted about analgesia. However, it is important to keep in mind that up to 80% of older adults who live in nursing homes may experience pain (59–63). These individuals may have been suffering from untreated or undertreated pain for months or even years (63,64), and may subsequently be plagued by depression and anxiety (8,50,65–68), compromised cognitive function (69–71), sleep disturbance (72,73), functional disability (60,67,72), and compromised quality of life. Verbal agitation (e.g., constant complaints, yelling out) is a frequent reason for psychiatric consultation in the long-term care setting. It has been shown that verbal agitation is more common among nursing home residents who have multiple physical diagnoses, mental disease (other than schizophrenia and affective disorders), more reported pain, and higher cognitive functioning than the nursing home population as a whole (74).

THE PSYCHIATRIC ASSESSMENT OF THE OLDER ADULT WITH PERSISTENT PAIN

In the current age of medicine, most older adults seeking treatment for persistent pain are not treated solely by a psychiatrist, if at all. However, it is imperative that mental health professionals working with these patients understand the cause of the pain, how it is being treated, and the role pain plays in their lives. While it is not necessary to repeat work-ups performed by other physicians, psychiatrists do need to interview patients about their pain. If they begin to treat a patient referred because of *idiopathic* (e.g., "psychological") pain, they must be comfortable with eliminating an organic basis for the pain. Accepting this "diagnosis of exclusion" should not be taken at face value. It is doing the patient a disservice to not evaluate medical records and review current and past medications. For example, although there is poor correlation between symptoms and radiographs or other imaging modalities in patients with back pain (75,76), non-pychiatric causes still must be ruled out. Most psychiatrists do not perform physical exams. However, with older adults, a simple examination of bony deformities, skin integrity, extremity range of motion, and muscular or dermatomal asymmetry, contributes valuable information to the initial assessment.

In addition to the physical suffering caused by persistent pain, older adults often suffer from a variety of psychosocial and cognitive pain-related consequences. Thus, the pain assessment needs to have a wide focus to be able to formulate optimal treatment. Successful diagnosis or understanding of the pathology is only part of the assessment necessary for the psychiatrist treating the older adult with persistent pain. According to Weiner, assessment must also include an evaluation of physical, psychosocial, and cognitive function (64). These domains are outlined in Table 42-3.

While there are numerous instruments available to assess pain, the most accurate and reliable evidence of the existence of pain and its intensity is the report by the patient (77). In the care of older adults with persistent pain, it is crucial that clinicians, as well as family members and caregivers, believe the reports of pain and take them seriously. Failure to do so may result in anxiety, depression, and interpersonal problems.

Caring for an older adult with persistent pain can cause emotional distress for family and caregivers. In many

TABLE 42-3		
DOMAINS TO BE ASSESSED IN THE OLDER ADULT WITH PERSISTENT PAIN		
Physical Function	**Psychosocial Function**	**Cognitive Function**
▪ Ability to perform ADLs ▪ Ability to perform IADLs ▪ Ability to perform AADLs ▪ Sleep ▪ Appetite	▪ Mood ▪ Interpersonal interactions ▪ Fear of pain and pain-related activity ▪ Self-efficacy ▪ Coping skills	▪ Acute or subacute confusion ▪ Beliefs about pain

AADLs, advanced activities of daily living; ADLs, activities of daily living; IADLs, instrumental activities of daily living.

respects this is similar to providing care to a loved one with dementia. Caregivers often feel overwhelmed with their responsibilities, ill-prepared to provide the type of care required, and feel helpless when they see a loved one in persistent distress. Assessing how the patient's pain affects the caregiver, and providing emotional and practical support to improve coping mechanisms or providing a referral to another mental health provider if indicated, is frequently useful in helping families successfully cope.

A brief screening questionnaire that can be used to identify key elements of the pain signature of older adult patients is listed in Table 42-4. Since many older adults present to the psychiatrist with an informant such as a family member or other caregiver, the final five probes of this assessment are directed at assessing how the patient's pain affects the functioning of the caregiver and of the patient-caregiver dyad.

ASSESSING PAIN IN COGNITIVELY IMPAIRED PATIENTS

Cognitively impaired older adults suffer from the same range of illnesses and pain experience as their cognitively intact counterparts. Difficulties in obtaining reliable reports in patients with cognitive impairment and dementia, such as Alzheimer's disease, presents a challenge in performing a pain assessment. Recent studies have shown that in the nursing home, poor assessments put these individuals at risk of under-recognition and undertreatment of pain and its psychiatric sequelae (78,79). Executive functions that govern the expression of pain are significantly reduced by dementia, leading to atypical behaviors and reactions with pain (80).

Table 42-5 describes common pain behaviors in cognitively impaired older adults. Direct observation, reviewing nurse and other staff notes in the medical record, and speaking with family about any new or unusual behaviors, especially those associated with movement, are excellent

TABLE 42-4
BRIEF PAIN IMPACT ASSESSMENT FOR VERBAL PATIENTS (AND THEIR CAREGIVERS)

Questions for Patient
1. How strong is your pain (right now, worst, average over past week)?
2. How many days over the past week have you been unable to do what you would like to do because of your pain?
3. Over the past week, how often has pain interfered with your ability to take care of yourself, for example with bathing, eating, dressing, and going to the toilet?
4. Over the past week, how often has pain interfered with your ability to take care of your home-related chores such as going grocery shopping, preparing meals, paying bills, and driving?
5. How often do you participate in pleasurable activities such as hobbies, socializing with friends, and travel? Over the past week, how often has pain interfered with these activities?
6. How often do you do some type of exercise? Over the past week, how often has pain interfered with your ability to exercise?
7. Does pain interfere with your ability to think clearly?
8. Does pain interfere with your appetite? Have you lost weight?
9. Does pain interfere with your sleep? How often over the past week?
10. Has pain interfered with your energy, mood, personality, or relationships with other people?
11. Over the past week, how often have you taken pain medications?
12. How would you rate your health at the present time?

Questions for Caregiver
13. How has the patient's pain affected your life?
14. Have you had to change your routine or activities as a result of the pain?
15. Do you believe the severity of the patient's pain?
16. Are you angry with the patient for being in pain?
17. Do you find yourself depressed or irritable as a result of the situation in which the patient's pain has placed you (and your family)?

Adapted and reprinted with permission from Reference 127.

TABLE 42-5

COMMON PAIN BEHAVIORS IN COGNITIVELY IMPAIRED OLDER ADULTS

Facial Expressions
- Slight frown, sad, frightened face
- Grimacing, wrinkled forehead, closed or tightened eyes
- Any distorted expression
- Rapid blinking

Verbalizations, Vocalizations
- Sighing, moaning, groaning
- Grunting, chanting, calling out
- Noisy breathing
- Asking for help
- Verbally abusive

Body Movements
- Rigid, tense body posture, guarding
- Fidgeting
- Increased pacing, rocking
- Restricted movement
- Gait or mobility changes

Changes in Interpersonal Interactions
- Aggressive, combative, resisting care
- Decreased social interactions
- Socially inappropriate, disruptive
- Withdrawn

Changes in Activity Patterns or Routines
- Refusing food, appetite change
- Increase in rest periods
- Sleep, rest pattern changes
- Sudden cessation of common routines
- Increased wandering

Mental Status Changes
- Crying or tears
- Increased confusion
- Irritability or distress

Reprinted with permission from Reference 6.

---

ways to make an informed pain assessment of these individuals. Nonverbal and facial expressions of pain have been found to be consistent across all levels of cognition and related to the intensity of pain (78). As stated earlier, psychiatrists are generally not directly consulted about pain or analgesia in the long-term care facility setting. However, knowledge about the presentation of pain in cognitively impaired older adults will inform the consultation differential diagnosis and help to focus the psychiatric recommendations.

MEASURES USED IN THE ASSESSMENT OF PAIN IN OLDER ADULTS

As stated earlier, an individual's description of his or her pain experience, independent of cognitive status, is generally the best way to understand pain (77). Direct observation can help in the distinction between acute and persistent pain, and is imperative in the assessment of the older adult with cognitive impairment. Quantitative instruments are frequently used in addition to observation and subjective reports as a means to organize the pain experience for the patient, clinician, and researcher. These instruments provide patients with a construct and vocabulary with which to describe their pain experience. This transformation of their experience into words can then provide data to the clinician to help develop a diagnosis and treatment plan.

Both *unidimensional* and *multidimensional* scales are used in the assessment of pain in the older adult. The Numeric

Rating Scale (NRS), Verbal Descriptor Scale (VDS), and the Faces Pain Scale (FPS) are among the commonly used unidimensional scales. These measures are relatively simple to use. Patients are instructed to document on the instrument the relative intensity of their pain, either at the present time or during some other time period. For the NRS, patients indicate their pain intensity on a scale of 0 to 10 or 0 to 20, with "no pain" (i.e., 0) at one end of the scale and "worst pain possible" at the other, and equally spaced hatch marks in between. For the VDS, responses range from "no pain," "mild pain," "moderate pain," "severe pain," "very severe pain," to "the most intense pain imaginable." Both the NRS and the VDS have been shown to be valid and reliable in older adults (81,82). The FPS consists of a series of progressively distressed facial expressions that represent the severity or intensity of the individual's current pain. Like the NRS or BDS, the FPS has been shown to be valid and reliable for use with older adults, both in cognitively intact and mild-to-moderately impaired older adults (81). The VDS is preferred for many older adults, and has been used successfully with many cognitively impaired individuals (83,84).

Studies suggest that older adults prefer verbal descriptor scales and numeric rating scales among the unidimensional measures (85). In our university-based clinical and research center, a variation of the VDS is used, called the Pain Thermometer (86). A pain thermometer that has been evaluated for use with older adults is illustrated in Figure 42-1. The Pain Thermometer is preferred for patients with moderate-to-severe cognitive deficits or patients who have

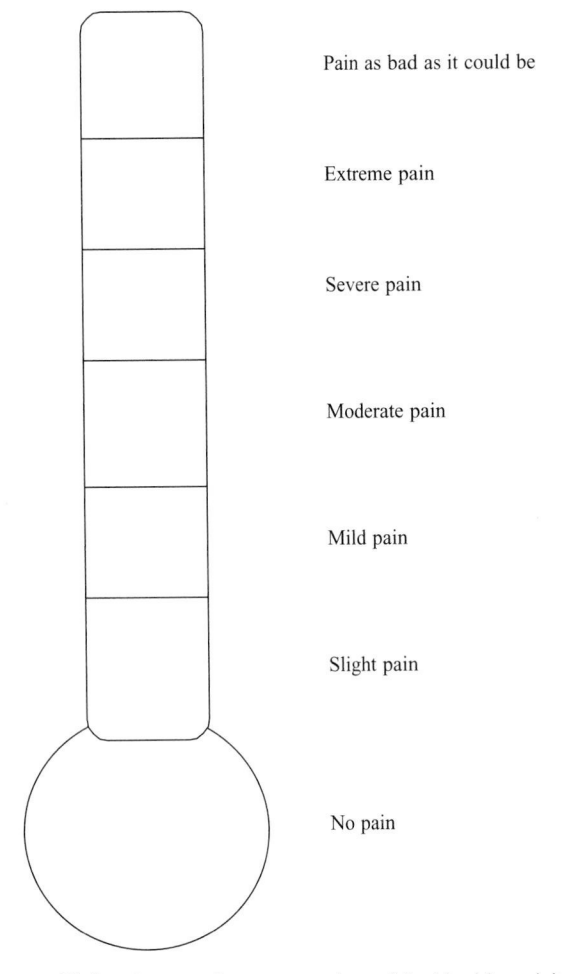

Pain as bad as it could be

Extreme pain

Severe pain

Moderate pain

Mild pain

Slight pain

No pain

Figure 42-1   The pain thermometer is useful with older adults.

difficulty with abstract thinking and verbal communication (64,83).

While unidimensional scales are simple to use and a quick method to quantify pain, multidimensional scales collect more information about the pain experience. These more comprehensive assessments determine both the quality of the pain as well as its effect on mood, cognition, and function. These scales are more difficult to administer to older adult patients who are cognitively impaired, but may still be of value, especially if a family member or other informant is available to assist with their completion.

Scales such as the short form version of the McGill Pain Questionnaire or Brief Pain Inventory may be useful in patients who are verbal but cognitively impaired (87–89). The McGill Pain Questionnaire assesses the sensory, affective, and evaluative aspects of the pain experience, and enhances the information obtained from unidimensional scales. Although most psychiatrists do not use multidimensional scales in the assessment of their older adult patients with persistent pain, acknowledging that pain is both highly personal and subjective and is experienced on many levels and influenced by numerous factors will facilitate the care of these individuals. Table 42-6 lists the various

elements often included in formal multidimensional assessments that should be a part of the psychiatric assessment of the older adult with pain. These features have been alluded to in other sections of this chapter, but because of their importance, are repeated here.

TREATING THE OLDER ADULT PSYCHIATRIC PATIENT WITH PERSISTENT PAIN

The Role of the Psychiatrist

Up to now this chapter has been concerned with the definition and assessment of pain, and identifying the locations where psychiatrists treat older adult pain patients. General recommendations for care have been provided. The goal of the next section is to provide specifics for the care that should be offered to older adults with persistent pain.

The role of psychiatrists in the care of patients with persistent pain has been poorly defined. In addition, historically there have been conflicting views between the pain community and psychiatry. These conflicts have generally resulted from differing theories about pain between dynamically-informed psychiatrists (e.g., Freudian psychiatrists, who led the field from the late 1940s until the mid-1970s) and the behavioral psychologists, internists, and anesthesiologists working in general medical settings and in tertiary referral pain centers.

For example, Freud felt that (90):

"Pain, in general, is considered as one of the dominating conversion symptoms, which means that an unconscious conflict is symbolized by a somatic symptom to keep the conflict unconscious . . . In one of his female patients with hysteria, he assumed that 'in place of the mental pains which she avoided, physical pains made their appearance'. Within the psychoanalytical process, he made the experience that the initial uncovering of unconscious conflicts provokes pain and the analytical processing of this conflict relieves the patient of the pain."

Freud revolutionized psychiatry, and there is much truth to his writing. Conversion symptoms do occur in patients who cannot *psychologically metabolize* negative affect or trauma, and these symptoms may manifest as physical pain. In addition, pain symptoms are often worsened by affective illness. This is especially true for older adults whose depression might not present as sadness, but more as fatigue, neurovegetative disturbance, and aches and pains. Indeed, question 13 of the 21-item Hamilton Rating Scale for Depression assesses somatic symptoms by inquiring about backache, headache, and muscle aches (91).

However, Freud's approach to the pain patient disregards the multidimensional quality of pain. In addition, purely

TABLE 42-6
DOMAINS INCLUDED IN MULTIDIMENSIONAL ASSESSMENTS OF PAIN IN OLDER ADULTS

Pain location	Pain quality	Effect of pain on functional status	Current psychological state
Pain intensity	Pain duration/ temporal course	Personal meaning of pain	Personality structure (e.g., internal or external locus of control, degree of dependence/independence, problem-solving abilities)

psychoanalytic treatments are not recommended for the treatment of persistent pain. Instead, other psychological therapies such as cognitive-behavioral therapy (CBT), relaxation training, and biofeedback are conventionally chosen because they have been shown to be useful in improving analgesia (92). Finally, nonpsychiatric practitioners working with pain patients tend to view them as psychologically normal people struggling with the extraordinary circumstance of persistent pain. The pronouncement of unresolved neurotic conflicts as the cause of persistent pain has at times been viewed as both dogmatic and actually unhelpful by those working in the pain community.

Earlier we identified the different sites where psychiatrists treat older adults with persistent pain and psychiatric illness. When the patient with persistent pain is referred to the psychiatrist, he or she generally assumes the role of consultant. This is especially true in a hospital or long-term care facility. However, when the psychiatrist is the physician of record (e.g., the patient is self-referred, or has been a patient for many years because of a primary psychiatric illness), and persistent pain begins to negatively affect the life of the individual, the psychiatrist now must decide between treating this pain on his or her own, or seeking consultation from a pain specialist.

The decision to treat persistent pain in the older adult depends on how comfortable the psychiatrist is with caring for this type of disorder. Also of concern is his or her degree of facility with prescribing medications such as opioids, which are not a routine part of the psychiatrist's formulary. While some psychiatrists are comfortable treating mild arthritis pain with acetaminophen and nonsteroidal anti-inflammatory drugs (NSAIDS), migraine with valproate, or diabetic neuropathy with gabapentin or antidepressants, many more seek the counsel and recommendations of specialists to help with symptoms they consider to be outside their area of expertise. The near impossibility of staying current with the literature makes some clinicians concerned that they are not providing state-of-the-art care and/or are putting themselves at risk of liability if they venture into the realm of treating persistent pain.

The dilemma when confronted with an older adult patient with persistent pain, however, is that it is not perfectly clear these symptoms should be considered outside the area of psychiatric expertise. Most of the persistent pain problems outlined in Table 42-2 are non-life-threatening disorders that are closely linked with mood, anxiety, and cognitive disorders in older adults. As recommended by the ACGME's residency training requirements, there should be a certain degree of facility in the management of these common disorders.

This does not mean that the psychiatrist should work in a clinical vacuum. To optimize the care of older adults with persistent pain and psychiatric illness, the psychiatrist functions best by viewing his or her role as part of a treatment team. This does not need to be a formal unit of practitioners, but should involve a collaborative approach that includes frequent consultation with internists, pain specialists, and neurologists. Although not available in every area, becoming familiar with the referral pathway of local pain clinics, and developing collegial relationships with the pain specialists at these centers, will facilitate the care of older adult psychiatric patients with persistent pain.

This multidisciplinary approach will both provide optimal care for the patient, as well as offer protection for the psychiatrist from possible legal repercussions.

Treatment: Providing Care Using an Algorithmic Approach

The treatment of persistent pain is as varied as the complex of conditions that combine to generate it. It is rare that the older adult has a single pathologic factor causing symptoms. Low back pain, for example, is typically caused by a variety of musculoskeletal factors such as degenerative facet disease, lumbar spinal stenosis, sacroiliac strain contributed by spinal curvature and/or pelvic asymmetry as well as hip and knee osteoarthritis, myofascial pain, and leg length discrepancy. These patients often have difficulty performing activities of daily living, as well as psychological distress caused by mood disturbance, poor coping skills, and decreased self-efficacy. Patients with dementia add another layer of complexity because of the fear that often surrounds pain in these individuals.

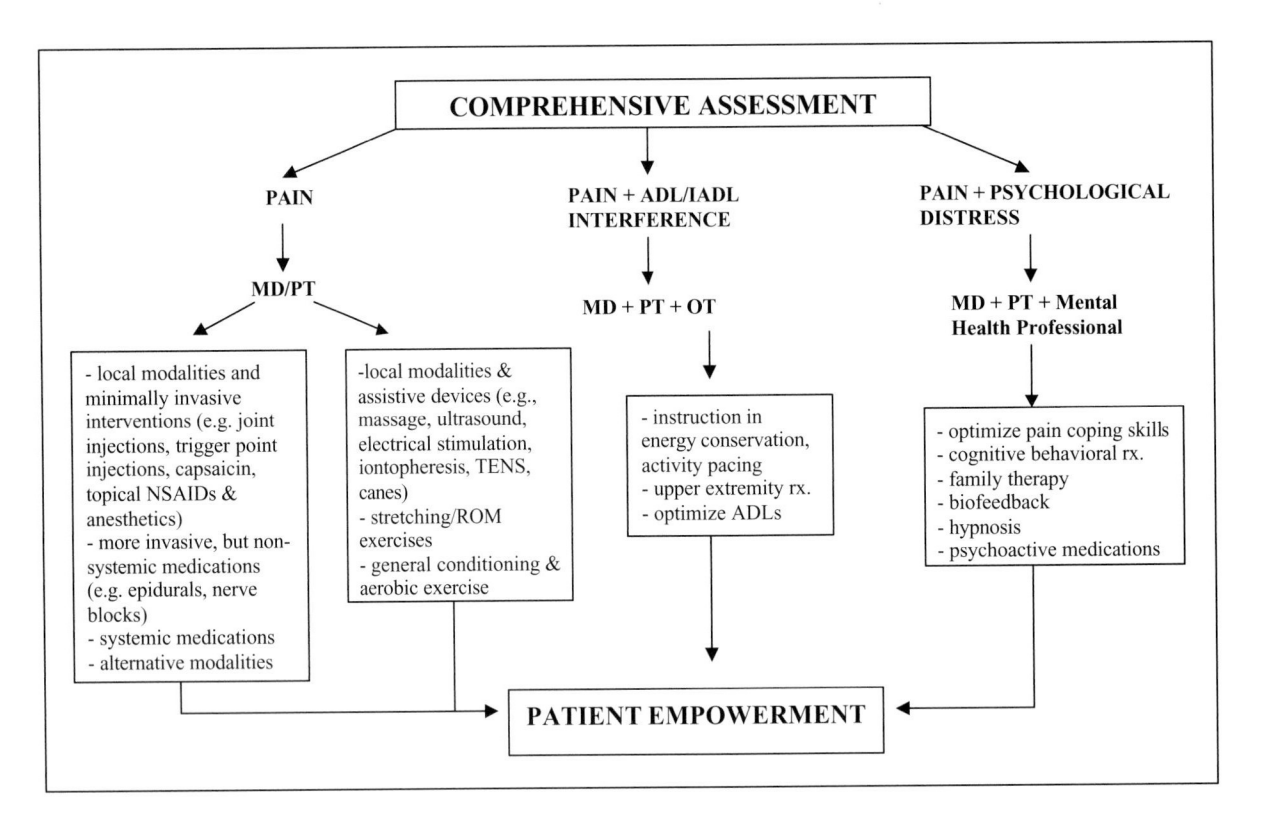

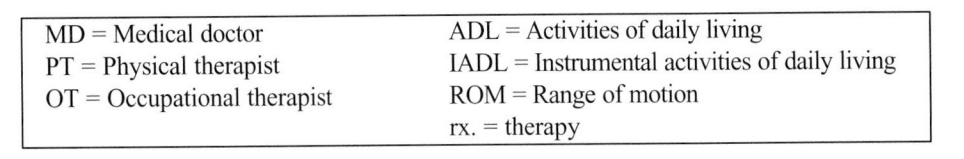

Figure 42-2   Algorithmic approach to the treatment of persistent pain in older adults.

When treating the older adult patient with persistent pain, it is important to create realistic treatment expectations. Studies have shown that patients referred to interdisciplinary pain clinics can expect to experience at least 35% reduction in pain intensity and at least 50% improvement in functional capacity (93). Complete pain relief is rare, but patients can typically look forward to significant improvement in their quality of life.

Because of the varied physical, psychological, and cognitive factors that often underlie persistent pain in older adults, medications alone may not adequately control symptoms. A practical framework for the comprehensive team treatment of older adults with persistent pain is shown in Figure 42-2. Clearly the first step toward effective treatment is optimum assessment, which serves to define the individual contributors to the pain syndrome. In addition to analgesia, a primary goal of pain treatment is patient empowerment, that is, a sense of autonomy and control over the pain condition. Because musculoskeletal disorders cause persistent pain in the vast majority of older adult sufferers, a physical therapist who is experienced in treating frail people with persistent pain should almost always be involved in the patient's care. A variety of techniques might be offered, including localized modalities such as ultrasound, electrical stimulation, iontophoresis (i.e., transcutaneous administration of topical medication using low level electrical current), transcutaneous electrical nerve stimulation (TENS), stretching, range of motion exercises, as well as general conditioning, and aerobic exercise. Recommendation of assistive devices such as canes and rolling walkers to enhance mobility and unload painful lower extremity joints is also under the auspices of the physical therapist. The occupational therapist should be involved with patients that have significant dysfunction of their upper extremities or that have difficulty in performing their activities of daily living. Instructions in how to pace activities, enhance leisure activities (i.e., advanced activities of daily living [94]), and conserve energy are all very useful techniques typically taught by an occupational therapist. It is worth mentioning that a patient's report of failure of physical and/or occupational therapy in the past should not preclude prescribing these modalities again, as therapists have different backgrounds and experience. The therapist that is relatively inexperienced in treating patients with myofascial pain might inadvertently administer overly aggressive treatment, causing exacerbation of pain, and lack of patient follow-up. We see this scenario often in patients referred to our older adult pain program.

A wide variety of pain treatment modalities can be prescribed and/or administered by a physician. Because of potential side effects, as well as drug-drug and drug-disease interactions, systemic medications should be used as a last resort. All medications should be viewed as a means of promoting successful rehabilitation and optimization of functional status. Depending upon the pain condition that is being treated, a variety of nonsystemic medications initially should be considered. For example, the patient with back and leg pain that is ultimately caused by knee osteoarthritis might first be treated with joint injection (95) and/or topical capsaicin (96) before considering acetaminophen. The patient with severe myofascial pain might well benefit from trigger-point injections. The individual with a herniated lumbar disc and radicular pain should be given an epidural corticosteroid if there are no contraindications to this approach (97).

When nonsystemic pain management modalities provide inadequate relief, and systemic medications are initiated, older adults must be monitored very carefully for adverse drug reactions. Mild-to-moderate pain should be treated with non-opioid medications, while opioids are appropriate for the treatment of moderate-to-severe pain. Table 42-7 summarizes the appropriate dose and rate of titration of common non-opioid and opioid medications. For a more detailed discussion of pharmacokinetics, pharmacodynamics, drug-drug, and drug-disease interactions, a textbook of pain management should be consulted (38).

A common question that arises among patients and providers when considering opioids, is that of addiction. True addiction, as defined by the DSM-IV, and notable for both clinically significant impairment or distress and functional impairment, is uncommon, and estimated to occur in less than one in 200 individuals with chronic nonmalignant pain (98). Indeed, appropriate medical use of opioids rarely leads to drug abuse or addiction (99).

Physical dependence, on the other hand, is a not uncommon physiologic state that occurs when opioids are prescribed in a chronic, continuous fashion. When these medications are abruptly discontinued, patients may experience withdrawal that is characterized by restlessness, tachycardia, hypertension, fever, tremors, and/or lacrimation. This type of reaction can be avoided by slowly tapering opioids over a period of days to weeks. The phenomenon of tolerance, that is, requirement for increasing doses of opioids over time, is controversial, as many conditions that opioids are used to treat may be associated with increasingly severe pain as the underlying pathology progresses.

The Interface Between Pain Medications and Psychiatric Medications: Can Two Birds Be Killed with One Stone?

Because of the morbidity and mortality associated with inappropriate polypharmacy in older adults, the fewer the medications prescribed, the better. This principal should be applied to the older adult with persistent pain. For example, the patient with fibromyalgia syndrome (FMS) or neuropathic pain who is also depressed might be effectively treated both for the pain and the mood disorder with a tricyclic antidepressant such as nortriptyline or desipramine. Small daily doses (e.g., 10–30 mg at bedtime) of these medications might be effective for the frail older adult, and serum levels should be monitored carefully. An adequate trial of a tricyclic should last 6 to 8 weeks with at least 1 to 2 weeks at the maximum tolerated dosage. In general, the analgesic effects of tricyclics have been found to occur at lower doses than their antidepressant effects. Cyclobenzaprine, which has intrinsic tricyclic properties, may be effective to promote sleep and relieve pain in patients with FMS (100), but practitioners who prescribe this agent must be vigilant for oversedation.

Gabapentin may also have a dual purpose for the patient with persistent pain. Trials examining the efficacy of gabapentin for peripheral neuropathy and postherpetic neuralgia indicate that one of the salient effects of this drug is enhanced pain tolerance and mood (101,102). We have had successful clinical experience with gabapentin, in doses ranging from 300 mg to approximately 2,400 mg daily, as an adjunct to other analgesics or antidepressants in pain patients with significant sleep disturbance. With higher doses, patients need to be monitored closely for dizziness, oversedation, ataxia, and delirium. Gabapentin can also be used as monotherapy for peripheral neuropathy.

Psychiatric Side Effects of Pain and Pain Medications

The older adult pain patient with multiple medical comorbidities, taking multiple medications, and presenting with new onset psychiatric symptoms may present a diagnostic dilemma. It is incumbent upon the mental health practitioner to decide whether the new symptoms are attributable to medical illness (e.g., cardiac ischemia, infection, nonmotoric status epilepticus), nonanalgesic medication side effects (especially medications with anticholinergic side effects), the pain itself, or analgesic medication side effects. The first step in this diagnostic process is determining the temporal association between the new psychiatric symptoms and other symptoms or timing of medications.

The psychiatric side effects of pain itself, particularly mood disorders, were addressed earlier. However, the relationship between pain and cognitive dysfunction is unclear. Several studies have been done in younger individuals that indicate a relationship between pain intensity and

TABLE 42-7

SYSTEMIC PHARMACOTHERAPY FOR MANAGEMENT OF PERSISTENT PAIN

Recommended Selected Non-opioid Analgesics

Chemical Class and Agents	Total Daily Dose	Dosing Interval	Terminal Disposition Half-Life (Hr.)
Nonacetylated salicylate			
salsalate	1.0–3.0 gm	BID–TID	2–20
Propionic acid	1.2–3.2 gm	TID–QID	1–3
Nonsteroidal anti-inflammatory drug			
ibuprofen	400–800 mg	BID	
naproxen	125–250 mg	BID	—
Seratonin/norepinephrine reuptake inhibitor (useful if depression is comorbid)			
duloxetine	60–90 mg	QD	12
Benzodiazepine			
clonazepam	0.25–0.5 mg	BID	
Cytochrome oxygenase II inhibitor			
celecoxib	100 mg	QD or BID	—
Acetaminophen[a]	2.6–4.0 gm	QID	1–3

Recommended Selected Opioid Analgesic Starting Regimens[b]

Drug	Dosage Regimen	Half-Life (Hr.)
Codeine 30 mg and acetaminophen 325 mg combination tablets	1 tablet Q6h	3–4
Oxycodone 5 mg and acetaminophen 325 mg combination tablets	1 tablet Q6h	3–4
Liquid morphine (various strengths) alone, or in combination with acetominophen 325 mg tablets; 10 mg/5 mL–500 mL	2.5 mg Q4h	2–3.5

Recommended Selected Adjunctive Analgesics

Agent	Daily Dosing Guidelines	Half-Life (Hr.)
Carbamazepine[c]	50–600 mg BID	12–17
Desipramine[d]	10–75 mg QD	14–25
Gabapentin[d]	100–900 mg BID–QID	5–7
Nortriptyline[d]	10–75 mg QD	15–39

[a]Drug of choice for noninflammatory disorders.
[b]Dosage regimens approximately equianalgesic—assumes patient is opioid naïve. Medications are listed in sequential order of their use in terms of increasing pain severity.
[c]Drug of choice for trigeminal neuralgia.
[d]Drug of choice for diabetic neuropathy and postherpetic neuralgia.
Oral dosing unless otherwise specified

BID, twice a day; Q4h, every 4 hours; Q6h, every 6 hours; QD, once a day; QID, four times a day; TID, three times a day.
Reprinted with permission from Reference 128.

impaired attention (71,103,104), with improvement in cognitive function upon administration of successful analgesia (105). Some studies suggest that pain may cause acute confusion in older adults, particularly those with pre-existing dementia (106,107), but a variety of methodologic constraints prevent definitive conclusions from being drawn.

Clearly, pain should be high on the differential diagnostic list in the older adult presenting with delirium. Medications used to treat pain also may be associated with adverse cognitive and psychiatric side effects. A summary of common pain medication classes associated with these reactions is provided in Table 42-8.

TABLE 42-8

PAIN MEDICATIONS WITH PSYCHIATRIC SIDE EFFECTS

Medication Class	Potential Psychiatric Side Effects
Nonsteroidal antiinflammatory drugs	• Depression, anxiety • Impaired concentration • Hypertension (if severe, and associated with hypertensive crisis, may cause mental status changes) • Meningitis, especially individuals with SLE
Corticosteroids	• Delirium • Dementia • Depression • Mania • Mood Lability • Psychosis
Opioids	• Delirium • Anxiety/Agitation • Depression • Sedation • Irritability
Tricyclic antidepressants	• Somnolence • Sedation • Anxiety • Insomnia

SLE, systemic lupus erythematosus.

The Role of Psychotherapy

Psychotherapy should play a central role in the psychiatric treatment of the older adult with persistent pain. In general, empirically-based manualized psychotherapies are recommended, such as CBT, relaxation training, problem-solving therapy (PST), and biofeedback. A common goal of these treatments, and of physician-patient interactions in the context of pain, is to facilitate both self-efficacy and a sense of mastery over the unpredictable nature of persistent pain. Unfortunately, older adults often have negative preconceived attitudes towards psychotherapy. Putting the talking therapies in a medical context makes these treatments more palatable. For example, a clinician can say to their older adult patient that they are "prescribing" a certain number of counseling sessions as part of their treatment for chronic pain. Explaining that pain affects thoughts and emotions, and that psychotherapy is frequently prescribed specifically to help treat the persistent pain can normalize the experience and reduce stigma. In a study of middle-aged and older adults with rheumatoid arthritis, those patients who received CBT appeared to have a less progressive worsening of their illness (108). This study reported that the core effects of the treatment pertained more to improved coping, emotional stabilization, and reduced impairment than to an actual reduction in pain intensity. Passive, emotion-focused coping, helplessness, depression, anxiety, affective pain, and fluctuation of pain were reduced in those patients who received CBT, while acceptance of illness was improved. This report mirrors the experience at our pain clinic.

The CBT approach consists of four interrelated components. These include 1) education, 2) skills acquisition, 3) cognitive and behavioral rehearsal, and 4) generalization and maintenance (109). The educational component of CBT involves presenting to the patient in a simple and direct way the idea that pain and its control (e.g., the role of thoughts, feelings, environment, behavior, and physical factors) will be examined throughout treatment. The educational portion of the CBT approach also should address the unspoken fears that many patients have about their condition, such as concerns about immobility or that their complaints will not be believed by caregivers.

Skills acquisition attempts to change patients' perceptions of their situation and thus their ability to monitor and modify cognition and behavior. These techniques need to be individually tailored and taught in a manner that increases the patient's perceptions of self-efficacy and intrinsic motivation. Turk and Rudy describe two basic sets of skills that are useful in the psychological management of persistent pain in older adults (109). The first of these is relaxation and biofeedback techniques. Relaxation training is generally easier to provide than biofeedback. Both approaches utilize an awareness of bodily sensations in an attempt to create a more relaxed physical state. Relaxation techniques include diaphragmatic breathing, progressive muscle relaxation, visualization, autogenic suggestion, and mental distraction.

While relaxation training focuses on bodily sensations, the other domain of skills acquisition involves cognitive modification. The objective of this intervention is to help patients sort through their accumulated perceptions and thoughts associated with all aspects of their pain experience. This helps identify those that are distorted, maladaptive, and thus counterproductive to effective coping, and reinforces those that are helpful or constructive (110). The pathway of cognitive modification involves: 1) providing a rationale for the intervention including a description of the relationship between cognition and nociception, 2) a discussion of the patient's cognition about all major aspects of their pain to identify key thoughts, emotions, and behaviors that can be modified, and 3) acquisition of self-directed skills to decrease distress and improve effective coping. An example of this type of modification is to challenge *cognitive errors*, which are beliefs about oneself and situations that are distorted in a way that they emphasize negative aspects and imply pessimistic outcomes. One type of cognitive error is *catastrophizing*. This occurs when focusing exclusively on the

TABLE 42-9

THE SIX STAGES OF PROBLEM-SOLVING THERAPY

1) Identification and clarification of the problem
2) The setting of clear goals
3) Formulation of alternative solutions
4) Selection of preferred solutions
5) Clarification of the necessary steps to implement the solution
6) Evaluation of progress

worst possibility regardless of the likelihood of occurrence (e.g., "My continued pain means my condition is progressive and my whole body is falling apart. It won't be long before I will be totally incapacitated and bedridden.") (111). Addressing these thought distortions occurs during sessions with the therapist, and then rehearsed through homework assignments until the patient gains enough confidence to use these techniques in a self-directed manner.

The third phase of the CBT approach includes rehearsing the acquired skills in a home environment. These rehearsals can include role playing and mental practice. Role reversal, where the clinician acts as the patient and the patient teaches skills to the clinician, can also be particularly effective (112). As treatment nears termination, the focus shifts to ways of predicting and avoiding, or dealing with pain and pain-related problems, after the therapy ends. The main purposes of maintenance and generalization are to 1) encourage the patient to anticipate and plan for the posttreatment period when symptoms are greatly

improved but not totally removed and 2) to prepare for the conditions necessary for long-term success, in particular the knowledge that minor setbacks are to be expected, and do not signal total failure (110).

Another structured psychotherapy that holds promise for older adults with persistent pain is PST. This approach has been found useful by primary care physicians in the treatment of depression (113), and has successfully been used in the treatment of depression in older adults with executive dysfunction (114). The driving theory of PST for the treatment of persistent pain is that patients should gain skills in dealing with their problems both psychologically as well as practically (115). Patients learn to use their own skills to deal with both present and future problems (116). Table 42-9 describes the six stages of PST. Both PST and CBT are manualized therapies. Most psychiatrists working in the community, however, practice eclectic forms of psychotherapy. To achieve optimal outcome, psychiatrists should become familiar with these empirically proven treatments, and use them to maximize the psychotherapeutic approach to the older adult with persistent pain.

TREATING THE PSYCHIATRIC AND SOCIAL SYMPTOMS ASSOCIATED WITH PAIN

In general, there is little difference in the treatment of psychiatric conditions comorbid with persistent pain than in the pain-free older adult. However, choosing certain psychiatric medications which have been shown to have analgesic

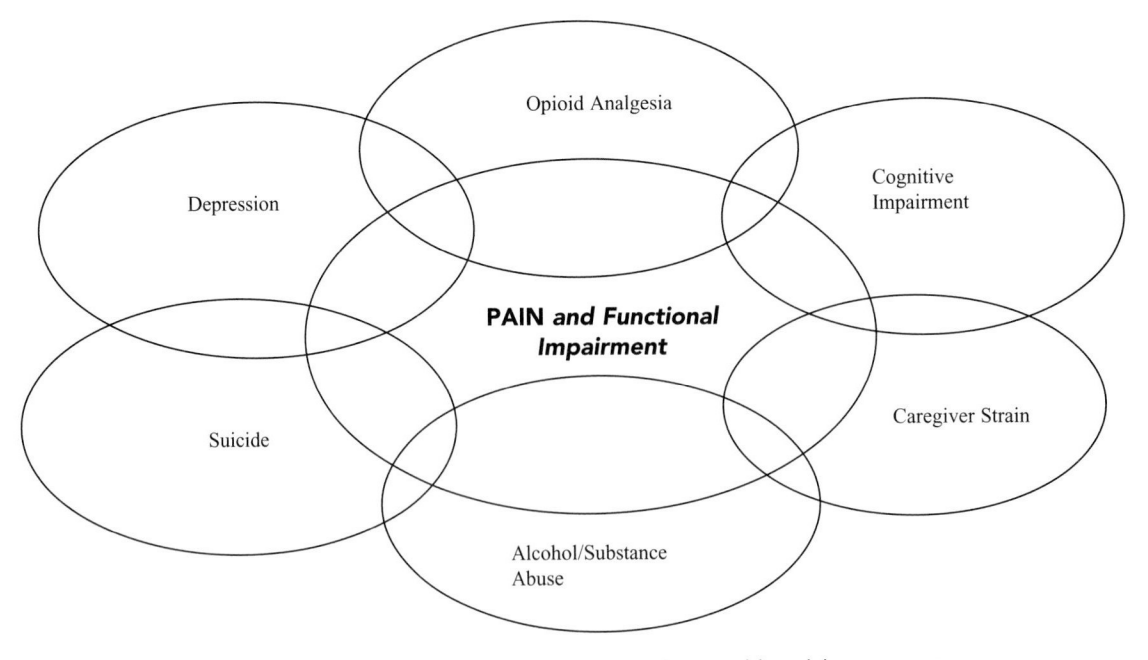

Figure 42-3 Interactions between pain and psychopathology in older adults.

properties (e.g., venlafaxine for depression or generalized anxiety disorder) may provide two benefits with one pill (117). However, certain caveats need to be considered when treating disorders such as depression and anxiety in older adults who also suffer from pain. First, although these patients may be a challenge, they usually respond to methodical, assertive treatment. We have shown that among older adult outpatients being treated for major depression who had comorbid persistent pain, over 78% responded to acute treatment with interpersonal psychotherapy and paroxetine (118). Second, the presence of a chronic general medical disorder, persistent pain, or functional impairment, are major risk factors for recurrence of major depression (119). It is crucial to treat these patients remission, follow them for residual symptoms of depression (another risk factor for recurrence), and aggressively treat their pain.

Figure 42-3 suggests the complex psychiatric comorbidities often present among older adults with persistent pain. Assessing for the presence of other disorders such as substance abuse, functional impairment, and cognitive dysfunction is necessary, as they can slow the remission of a pain-associated depression or anxiety syndrome. Anxiety is often comorbid with depression (120), may be associated with pain (14), and is associated with greater levels of suicidality (121). It is of immense benefit to both our patients and our medical colleagues to assess for complex psychiatric comorbidity and treat accordingly, so the clinical outcome is optimized.

Of the psychiatric comorbidities illustrated in Figure 42-3, suicidality is the area of most concern for older adults with persistent pain. One of the most common demographic correlates of suicide is older age (122). It is well documented that mental health, physical health, and social factors may all play a role in suicide in the elderly (123). Bartels et al. reported that among older primary care patients (who often present with pain as their chief complaint) reporting both depression and anxiety, 18% reported suicidal ideation (124). In addition, depression is often comorbid with alcohol abuse and dependence, and both of these syndromes are independent predictors of suicide (125). Finally, physical illness, a common cause of persistent pain, is frequently comorbid with depression, and is an independent risk factor for suicide (123,126). Minimizing the impact of these comorbidities will go far in achieving analgesia, as well as improving mental health, and reducing the risk of suicide.

REFERENCES

1. Ferrell BA. Overview of aging and pain. In: Ferrell BR, Ferrell BA, eds. *Pain in the Elderly.* Seattle: IASP Press; 1996:1–10.
2. Helme RD, Gibson SJ. Pain in older people. In: Crombie IK, Croft PR, Linton SJ, et al., eds. *Epidemiology of Pain.* Seattle: IASP Press; 1999:103–112.
3. Blyth FM, March LM, Brnabic AJ, Jorm LR, Williamson M, Cousins MJ. Chronic pain in Australia: a prevalence study. *Pain.* 2001;89:127–134.
4. Mantyselka P, Kumpusalo E, Ahonen R, et al. Pain as a reason to visit the doctor: a study in Finnish primary health care. *Pain.* 2001;89:175–180.
5. Cooner E, Amorosi S. *The Study of Pain in Older Americans.* New York: Louis Harris and Associates; 1997.
6. AGS Panel on Persistent Pain in Older Persons. The management of persistent pain in older persons. *J Am Geriatr Soc.* 2002;50(6): S205–S224.
7. AGS Panel on Chronic Pain in Older Persons. The management of chronic pain in older persons. *J Am Geriatr Soc.*1998;46: 635–651.
8. Romano JM, Turner JA. Chronic pain and depression: does the evidence support a relationship? *Psychol Bull.* 1985;97:18–34.
9. Atkinson JH, Slater MA, Patterson TL, Grant I, Garfin SR. Prevalence, onset, and risk of psychiatric disorders in men with chronic low back pain: a controlled study. *Pain.* 1991;45:111–121.
10. Magni G, Moreschi C, Rigatti-Luchini S, Merskey H. Prospective study on the relationship between depressive symptoms and chronic musculoskeletal pain. *Pain.* 1994;56:289–297.
11. Fifield J, Tennen H, Reisine S, McQuillan J. Depression and the long-term risk of pain, fatigue, and disability in patients with rheumatoid arthritis. *Arthritis Rheum.* 1998;41(10):1851–1857.
12. Fishbain DA, Cutler R, Rosomoff HL, Rosomoff RS. Chronic pain associated depression: antecedent or consequence of chronic pain? A review. *Clin J Pain.* 1997;13:116–137.
13. Cherry DK, Burt CW, Woodwell DA. National Ambulatory Medical Care Survey: 2001 summary. *Adv Dat.* 2003;337:1–44.
14. Aldrich S, Eccleston C, Crombez G. Worrying about chronic pain: vigilance to threat and misdirected problem solving. *Behav Res Ther.* 2000;38:457–470.
15. McCracken LM, Zayfert C, Gross RT. The Pain Anxiety Symptoms Scale: development and validation of a scale to measure fear of pain. *Pain.* 1992;50(1):67–73.
16. Kori SH, Miller RP Todd DD. Kinisophobia: a new view of chronic pain behaviour. *Pain Management.* 1990;3(1):35–43.
17. Vlaeyen JW, Kole-Snijders AM, Boeren RG, van Eek H. Fear of movement (re)injury in chronic low-back-pain and its relation to behavioural performance. *Pain.* 1995;62(3):363–372.
18. Lyketsos CG, Lopez O, Jones B, Fitzpatrick AL, Breitner J, DeKosky S. Prevalence of neuropsychiatric symptoms in dementia and mild cognitive impairment: results from the cardiovascular health study. *JAMA.* 2002;288(12):1475–1483.
19. Howland J, Peterson EW, Levin WC, Fried L, Pordon D, Bak S. Fear of falling among the community-dwelling elderly. *J Aging Health.* 1993;5(2):229–243.
20. Asmundson GJ, Norton GR, Jacobson SJ. Social, blood/injury, and agoraphobic fears in patients with physically unexplained chronic pain—are they clinically significant? *Anxiety.* 1996;2(1); 28–33.
21. Hoffmann NG, Olofsson O, Salen B, Wickstrom L. Prevalence of abuse and dependency in chronic pain patients. *Int J Addict.* 1995;30(8):919–927.
22. Adams WL, Yuan Z, Barboriak J, Rimm AA. Alcohol-related hospitalizations of elderly people. Prevalence and geographic variation in the United States. *JAMA.* 1993;270:1222–1225.
23. Brennan PL, Kagay CR, Geppert JJ, Moos RH. Elderly Medicare inpatients with substance use disorders: characteristics and predictors of hospital readmissions over a four-year interval. *J Stud Alcohol.* 2000;61(6):891–895.
24. Hilton ME. Trends in U.S. drinking patterns: further evidence from the past 20 years. *Br J Addict.* 1988;83:269–278.
25. Dworkin RH, Caligor E. Psychiatric diagnoses and chronic pain: DSM-III-R and beyond. *J Pain Symptom Manage.* 1988;3:87–98.
26. Robins LN, Helzer JE, Weissman MM, et al. Lifetime prevalence of specific psychiatric disorders in three sites. *Arch Gen Psychiatry.* 1984;41:949–958.
27. Merskey H, Bogduk N, eds. *Classification of Chronic Pain.* 2nd Ed. Seattle: IASP Press; 1994:xi–xv.
28. Melzack R, Casey KL. Sensory, motivational, and central control determinants of pain: a new conceptual model. In: Kenshalo D, ed. *The Skin Senses.* Springfield, IL: Charles C Thomas; 1968:137–153.
29. Byers MR, Bonica JJ. Peripheral pain mechanisms and nociceptor plasticity. In Loeser JD, Butler SH, Chapman CR, et al., eds.

Bonica's Management of Pain. 3rd Ed. Philadelphia: Lippincott, Williams & Wilkins; 2001:26–72.

30. National Health & Medical Research Council Report. Acute Pain Management: Scientific Evidence. Australia: Commonwealth of Australia, 1999. http://nhmrc.gov.au/publications/_files/cp57.pdf. accessed 18 July 2005.

31. Wolfe F, Ross K, Anderson J, Russell IJ, Hebert L. The prevalence and characteristics of fibromyalgia in the general population. *Arthritis Rheum.* 1995;38:19–28.

32. Cannon RO 3rd, Quyyumi AA, Mincemoyer R, et al. Imipramine in patients with chest pain despite normal coronary angiograms. *N Engl J Med.* 1995;332:1529–1534.

33. O'Malley PG, Wong PW, Kroenke K, Roy M, Wong RK. The value of screening for psychiatric disorders prior to upper endoscopy. *J Psychosom Res.* 1998;44:279–287.

34. O'Malley PG, Jackson JL, Kroenke K, Yoon IK, Hornstein E, Dennis GJ. The value of screening for psychiatric disorders in rheumatology referrals. *Arch Intern Med.* 1998;158:2357–2362.

35. Katon W, Kleinman A, Rosen G. Depression and somatization: a review. *Am J Med.* 1982; 72:127–35, 241–247.

36. Kroenke K, Spitzer RL, Williams JB, et al. Physical symptoms in primary care. Predictors of psychiatric disorders and functional impairment. *Arch Fam Med.* 1994;3:774–779.

37. Smith GR. The epidemiology and treatment of depression when it coexists with somatoform disorders, somatization, or pain. *Gen Hosp Psychiatry.* 1992;14:265–272.

38. Weiner RS. *Pain Management: A Practical Guide For Clinicians.* 6th Ed. Boca Raton, FL: CRC Press; 2002.

39. Wall PD, Melzack R. *Textbook of Pain.* 4th Ed. Edinburgh; New York: Churchill Livingstone; 1999.

40. Besson JM, Chaouch A. Peripheral and spinal mechanisms of nociception. *Physiol Rev.* 1987;67:67–186.

41. Harkins SW. What is unique about the older adult's pain experience? In: Weiner DK, Herr K, Rudy TE, eds. *Persistent Pain in Older Adults: An Interdisciplinary Guide for Treatment.* Springer: New York; 2002.

42. Rome H, Rome J. Limbically augmented pain syndrome (LAPS): kindling, corticolimbic sensitization, and the convergence of affective and sensory symptoms in chronic pain disorders. *Pain Med.* 2000;1:7–23.

43. Giesler GJ, Katter JT, Dado RJ. Direct spinal pathways to the limbic system for nociceptive information. *Trends Neurosci.* 1994;17:244–250.

44. Chudler EH, Bonica JJ. Supraspinal mechanisms of pain and nociception. In Loeser JD, Butler SH, Chapman CR, et al., eds. *Bonica's Management of Pain.* 3rd Ed. Philadelphia: Lippincott, Williams & Wilkins; 2001:153–179.

45. Godfrey RG. A guide to the understanding and use of tricyclic antidepressants in the overall management of fibromyalgia and other chronic pain syndromes. *Arch Intern Med.* 1996;156(10): 1047–1052.

46. Sorkin LS, Wallace MS. Acute pain mechanisms. *Surg Clin North Am.* 1999;79:213–229.

47. Berne RM, Levy MN, ed. *Physiology.* 4th Ed. St. Louis: Mosby; 1998.

48. Strassman AM. Neurotransmitters. In: Warfield CA, Fausett HJ, eds. *Manual of Pain Management.* 2nd Ed. Lippincott, Williams & Wilkins; 2002.

49. Blier P, Abbott FV. Putative mechanisms of action of antidepressant drugs in affective and anxiety disorders and pain. *J Psychiatry Neurosci.* 2001;26(1):37–43.

50. Magni G, Caldieron C, Rigatti-Luchini S, Merskey H. Chronic musculoskeletal pain and depressive symptoms in the general population: an analysis of the 1st National Health and Nutrition Examination Survey data. *Pain.* 1990;43:299–307.

51. Fishbain DA, Goldberg M, Meagher BR, Steele R, Rosomoff H. Male and female chronic pain patients categorized by DSM-III psychiatric diagnostic criteria. *Pain.* 1986;26:181–97.

52. Von Korff M, Le Resche L, Dworkin SF. First onset of common pain symptoms: a prospective study of depression as a risk factor. *Pain.* 1993;55(2):251–258.

53. Von Korff M, Simon G. The relationship between pain and depression. *Br J Psychiatry Suppl.* 1996;30:101–108.

54. Yates P, Dewar A, Edwards H, et al. The prevalence and perception of pain amongst hospital in-patients. *J Clin Nurs.* 1998;7(6):521–530.

55. Donovan M, Dillon P, McGuire L. Incidence and characteristics of pain in a sample of medical-surgical in-patients. *Pain.* 1987; 30:69–78.

56. Cohen FL. Post-surgical pain relief: patients' status and nurses' medication choices. *Pain.* 1980;9:265–274.

57. Stoudemire A, Smith DA. OBRA regulations and the use of psychotropic drugs in long-term care facilities: impact and implications for geropsychiatric care. *Gen Hosp Psychiatry.* 1996;18: 77–94.

58. Smyer MA, Shea DG, Streit A. The provision and use of mental health services in nursing homes: results from the National Medical Expenditure Survey. *Am J Public Health.* 1994;84(2): 284–287.

59. Roy R, Thomas M. A survey of chronic pain in an elderly population. *Can Fam Physician.* 1986;32:513–516.

60. Ferrell BA, Ferrell BR, Osterweil D. Pain in the nursing home. *J Am Geriatr Soc.* 1990;38:409–414.

61. Sengstaken EA, King SA. The problems of pain and its detection among geriatric nursing home residents. *J Am Geriatr Soc.* 1993;41:541–544.

62. Parmelee PA. Assessment of pain in the elderly. In: Lawton MP, Teresi J, eds. *Annual Review of Gerontology and Geriatrics.* New York: Springer; 1994:281–301.

63. Weiner D, Peterson B, Ladd K, McConnell E, Keefe F. Pain in nursing home residents: an exploration of prevalence, staff perspectives and practical aspects of measurement. *Clin J Pain.* 1999;15(2):92–101.

64. Weiner DK, Peterson BL, Logue P, Keefe FJ. Predictors of pain self-report in nursing home residents. *Aging.*1998;10:411–420.

65. Casten RJ, Parmelee PA, Kleban MH, Lawton MP, Katz IR. The relationships among anxiety, depression, and pain in a geriatric institutionalized sample. *Pain.* 1995;61:271–276.

66. Williams AK, Schulz R. Association of pain and physical dependency with depression in physically ill middle-aged and elderly. *Phys Ther.* 1988;68(8):1226–1230.

67. Williamson GM, Schulz R. Pain, activity restriction, and symptoms of depression among community-residing adults. *J Gerontol.* 1992;47:367–372.

68. Cohen-Mansfield J, Marx MS. Pain and depression in the nursing home: corroborating results. *J Gerontol.* 1993;48:96–97.

69. Fordyce WE. Evaluating and managing chronic pain. *Geriatrics.* 1978;33:59–62.

70. Kewman DG, Vaishampayan N, Zald D, Han B. Cognitive impairment in musculoskeletal pain patients. *Int J Psychiatr Med.* 1991;21:253–262.

71. Eccleston C, Crombez G, Aldrich S, Stannard C. Attention and somatic awareness in chronic pain. *Pain.* 1997;72:209–215.

72. Lavsky-Shulan M, Wallace RB, Kohout FJ, Lemke JH, Morris MC, Smith IM. Prevalence and functional correlates of low back pain in the elderly: the Iowa 65+ Rural Health Study. *J Am Geriatr Soc.* 1985;33:23–28.

73. Gentili A, Weiner DK, Kuchibhatil M, Edinger JD. Factors that disturb sleep in nursing home residents. *Aging Clin Exp Res.* 1997;9(3):207–213.

74. Cohen-Mansfield J, Billig N, Lipson S, Rosenthal AS, Pawlson LG. Medical correlates of agitation in nursing home residents. *Gerontology.* 1990;36(3):150–158.

75. Boden SD, Davis DO, Dina TS, Patronas NJ, Wiesel SW. Abnormal magnetic-resonance scans of the lumbar spine in asymptomatic subjects. A prospective investigation. *J Bone Joint Surg Am.* 1990;72(3):403–408.

76. Witt I, Vestergaard A, Rosenklint A. A comparative analysis of x-ray findings of the lumbar spine in patients with and without lumbar pain. *Spine.* 1984;9:298–300.

77. Max MB, Payne R, Edwards WT, et al. *Principles of Analgesic Drug Use in the Treatment of Acute Pain and Cancer Pain.* 4th Ed. Glenville IL: American Pain Society; 1999.

78. Parmelee PA. Pain in cognitively impaired older persons. *Clin Geriatr Med.* 1996;12:473–487.

79. Stein WM. Pain in the nursing home. *Clin Geriatr Med.* 2001;17:575–594.

80. Ward SE, Goldberg N, Miller-McCauley V, et al. Patient-related barriers to management of cancer pain. *Pain.* 1993;52(3):319–324.

81. Chibnall JT, Tait RC. Pain assessment in cognitively impaired and unimpaired older adults: a comparison of four scales. *Pain.* 2001;92:173–186.

82. Herr K, Mobily P, Richardson G, Spratt K. Use of experimental pain to compare psychometric properties and usability of pain scales in the adult and older adult populations [Abstract]. Annual meeting of the American Society for Pain Management in Nursing, Orlando FL, 1998.
83. Herr K, Mobily PR. Comparison of selected pain assessment tools for use with the elderly. *Appl Nurs Res.* 1993;6:39–46.
84. Feldt KS. The checklist of nonverbal pain indicators (CNPI). *Pain Manag Nurs.* 2000;1:13–21.
85. Herr KA, Garand L. Assessment and measurement of pain in older adults. *Clin Geriatr Med.* 2001;17(3):457–478.
86. Roland M, Morris R. A study of the natural history of back pain. Part 1: development of a reliable and sensitive measure of disability in low-back pain. *Spine.* 1983:8;141–144.
87. Melzack R. The short-form McGill Pain Questionnaire. *Pain.* 1987;30:191–197.
88. Cleeland CS. Measurement of pain by subjective report. In: Chapman CR, Loeser JD, eds. *Issues in Pain Measurement.* New York: Raven Press; 1989.
89. Rosenberg SK, Boswell MV. Pain management in geriatrics. In: Weiner RS, ed. *Pain Management: a Practical Guide for Clinicians.* Boca Raton, FL: St. Lucie Press; 1998:683–692.
90. Karwautz A, Wober-Bingol C, Wober C. Freud and migraine: the beginning of a psychodynamically oriented view of headache a hundred years ago. *Cephalalgia.* 1996;16(1):22–26.
91. Hamilton M. A rating scale for depression. *J Neurol Neurosurg Psychiatry.* 1960;23:56–62.
92. Lamberg L. Effective pain treatment promotes activities. *JAMA.* 2002;288(8):948–949.
93. Flor H, Fydrich T, Turk DC. Efficacy of multidisciplinary pain treatment centers: a meta-analytic review. *Pain.* 1992;49:221–230.
94. Reuben DB, Laliberte L, Hiris J, Mor V. A hierarchical exercise scale to measure function at the Advanced Activities of Daily Living (AADL) level. *J Am Geriatr Soc.* 1990;38:855–861.
95. Raynauld JP, Buckland-Wright C, Ward R, et al. Safety and efficacy of long-term intraarticular steroid injections in osteoarthritis of the knee: a randomized, double-blind, placebo-controlled trial. *Arthritis Rheum.* 2003;48:370–377.
96. Zhang W, Li Wan Po A. The effectiveness of topically applied capsaicin. A meta-analysis. *Eur J Clin Pharmacol.* 1994;46:517–522.
97. Watts RW, Silagy CA. A meta-analysis of the efficacy of epidural corticosteroids in the treatment of sciatica. *Anaesth Intensive Care.* 1995;23:564–569.
98. Porter J, Jick H. Addiction rare in patients treated with narcotics. *N Engl J Med.* 1980;302:123.
99. Joranson DE, Ryan KM, Gilson AM, Dahl JL. Trends in medical use and abuse of opioid analgesics. *JAMA.* 2000;283:1710–1714.
100. Bennett RM, Gatter RA, Campbell SM, Andrews RP, Clark SR, Scarola JA. A comparison of cyclobenzaprine and placebo in the management of fibrositis. A double-blind controlled study. *Arthritis Rheum.* 1988;31:1535–1542.
101. Backonja M, Beydoun A, Edwards KR, et al. Gabapentin for the symptomatic treatment of painful neuropathy in patients with diabetes mellitus: a randomized controlled trial. *JAMA.* 1998;280:1831–1836.
102. Rowbotham M, Harden N, Stacey B, Bernstein P, Magnus-Miller L. Gabapentin for the treatment of postherpetic neuralgia: a randomized controlled trial. *JAMA.* 1998;280:1837–1842.
103. Eccleston C. Chronic pain and attention: a cognitive approach. *Br J Clin Psychol.* 1994;33:535–547.
104. Eccleston C. Chronic pain and distraction: an experimental investigation into the role of sustained and shifting attention in the processing of chronic persistent pain. *Behav Res Ther.* 1995;33:391–405.
105. Lorenz J, Beck H, Bromm B. Cognitive performance, mood and experimental pain before and during morphine-induced analgesia in patients with chronic non-malignant pain. *Pain.* 1997;73:369–375.
106. Duggleby W, Lander J. Cognitive status and postoperative pain: older adults. *J Pain Symptom Manage.* 1994;9:19–27.
107. Lynch EP, Lazor MA, Gellis JE, Orav J, Goldman L, Marcantonio ER. The impact of postoperative pain on the development of postoperative delirium. *Anesth Analg.* 1998; 86:781–785.
108. Leibing E, Pfingsten M, Bartmann U, Rueger U, Schuessler G. Cognitive-behavioral treatment in unselected rheumatoid arthritis outpatients. *Clin J Pain.* 1999;15(1):58–66.
109. Turk DC, Rudy TE. A cognitive-behavioral perspective on chronic pain: beyond the scalpel and syringe. In Tollison CD, ed. *Handbook of Pain Management.* Baltimore: Williams & Wilkins; 1994: 136–151.
110. Rudy TE, Hanlon RB, Markham JR. Psychosocial issues and cognitive-behavioral therapy: from theory to practice. In: Weiner DK, Herr K, Rudy TE, eds. *Persistent Pain in Older Adults: An Interdisciplinary Guide for Treatment.* New York, NY: Springer; 2002.
111. Turk DC. The role of psychological factors in chronic pain. *Acta Anaesthesiol Scand.* 1999;43(9):885–888.
112. Holzman AD, Turk DC. *Pain Management: A Handbook of Psychological Treatment Approaches.* Elmsford, NY: Pergamon Press; 1986.
113. Mynors-Wallis LM, Gath DH, Lloyd-Thomas AR, Tomlinson D. Randomised controlled trial comparing problem solving treatment with amitriptyline and placebo for major depression in primary care. *BMJ.*1995;310(6977):441–445.
114. Alexopoulos GS, Raue P, Arean P. Problem-solving therapy versus supportive therapy in geriatric major depression with executive dysfunction. *Am J Geriatr Psychiatry.* 2003;11(1):46–52.
115. Wilkinson P, Mynors-Wallis L. Problem-solving therapy in the treatment of unexplained physical symptoms in primary care: a preliminary study. *J Psychosom Res.* 1994;38(6):591–598.
116. Hawton KH, Kirk JW. Problem-solving. In: Hawton K, Salkovskis PM, Kirk JW, Clark DM, eds. *Cognitive Behavior Therapy for Psychiatric Problems—A Practical Guide.* Oxford: Oxford Medical Publications;1989.
117. Lynch ME. Antidepressants as analgesics: a review of randomized controlled trials. *J Psychiatry Neurosci.* 2001;26(1):30–36.
118. Karp JF, Seligman K, Houck P, Reynolds CF. The effect of bodily pain on time to remission in late life depression. Presented at the Annual Meeting of the American Psychiatric Association. San Francisco, CA, 2003.
119. American Psychiatric Association. Practice guideline for the treatment of patients with major depression (revision). American Psychiatric Association. *Am J Psychiatry.* 2000;157(4 Suppl):1–45.
120. Lenze EJ, Mulsant BH, Shear MK, Alexopoulos GS, Frank E, Reynolds CF III. Comorbidity of depression and anxiety disorders in later life. *Depress Anxiety.* 2001;14(2):86–93.
121. Lenze EJ, Mulsant BH, Shear MK, et al. Comorbid anxiety disorders in depressed elderly patients. *Am J Psychiatry.* 2000;157(5):722–728.
122. Peters KD, Kochanek KD, Murphy SL. Deaths: final data for 1996. *Natl Vital Stat Rep.* 1998;47(9):1–100.
123. Conwell Y, Duberstein PR, Caine ED. Risk factors for suicide in later life. *Biol Psychiatry.* 2002;52:193–204.
124. Bartels SJ, Coakley E, Oxman TE, et al. Suicidal and death ideation in older primary care patients with depression, anxiety, and at-risk alcohol use. *Am J Geriatr Psychiatry.* 2002;10(4):417–427.
125. Szanto K, Gildengers A, Mulsant BH, Brown G, Alexopoulos GS, Reynolds CF 3rd. Identification of suicidal ideation and prevention of suicidal behavior in the elderly. *Drugs Aging.* 2002;19(1):11–24.
126. Thorn H. "Central" pain can raise suicide risk. *Clin Psychiatric News.* 1994:11.
127. Weiner DK, Herr K. Comprehensive interdisciplinary assessment and treatment planning: an integrative overview. In: Weiner DK, Herr K, Rudy TE, eds. *Persistent Pain in Older Adults: An Interdisciplinary Guide for Treatment.* New York, NY: Springer; 2002;21.
128. Guay DR, Lackner TE, Hanlon JT. Pharmacologic management: noninvasive modalities. In: Weiner DK, Herr K, Rudy TE, eds. *Persistent Pain in Older Adults: An Interdisciplinary Guide for Treatment.* New York, NY: Springer; 2002;164–174.

Apathy

43

William B. Orr

The loss of motivation or interest is a common complaint of geriatric patients: such patients are often described as apathetic. *Apathy*, derived from the Greek word, pathos, meaning passions, refers to a lack of interest, pleasure, or emotion. The most widely accepted definition is a lack of motivation or drive. Marin proposed specific criteria for the syndrome of apathy that emphasize three dimensions: diminished goal-directed behavior, diminished cognitive drive (loss of interest or concern), and lack of emotional responsivity (i.e., flat affect) (1). Apathy is strongly associated with impairment in executive functioning, and as a result it is often viewed as a type of frontal lobe syndrome. The presence of apathy leads to increases in functional disability and caregiver burden, and it impairs treatment response in geriatric depression (2–6).

While most experts agree that apathy exists as a distinct syndrome, it most often presents in the elderly as a comorbid feature of other psychiatric or medical conditions. Some epidemiological data suggest that apathy by itself in the elderly may be relatively rare (7). When it occurs as a distinct syndrome, the lack of motivation is not attributable to acute changes in consciousness, cognitive impairment, or emotional distress (8). Most often, apathy is seen clinically within the setting of depression or dementia. Indeed, apathy may be viewed as occupying the middle ground between depression and dementia. As a result, the differential diagnosis of apathy can be extremely challenging because of overlapping features with those two conditions (see Figure 43-1). It is essential, however, for clinicians to learn to accurately identify and manage apathy because, left unchecked, it can significantly interfere with the successful treatment of other conditions.

APATHY VERSUS DEPRESSION

Apathy and depression often coexist in geriatric patients. Geriatric patients who are both apathetic and depressed display not only low mood, irritability, and decreased self-esteem, but also have prominent loss of interest or motivation. Diagnosis of apathy in the presence of late-life depression can be confounded by the effects of comorbid medical conditions or medication side effects. Nevertheless, when careful assessment is made, apathy is found in a great many depressed elderly patients. Starkstein and colleagues found apathy in 32% of nondemented, depressed elderly patients (9). This figure may actually represent an underestimate since apathetic patients often do not present for clinical assessment. Still, this is a much higher rate of apathy associated with depression than is observed in younger patients. It has been suggested that depression with apathy may represent a sub-type of depression that is more common in the elderly.

Recent studies on late-life depression have demonstrated that a great many elderly patients with depression also have disturbances in executive functioning (10–12). Executive functioning refers to the ability to plan, organize, and initiate decisions, and encompasses the concepts of insight and judgement. Deficits in these areas interfere with a person's ability to interact and initiate action in a coherent, goal-directed fashion. In addition, executive dysfunction is associated with poor or slow responses to antidepressant treatment (6), early relapse and recurrence of depression in elderly patients (12), and a greater degree of overall functional impairment (13,14). In this context, however, apathy represents only a sub-type of executive dysfunction, and can be distinguished using selected neuropsychological tests (15,16). Whereas executive dysfunction in general manifests in the impaired ability to plan and initiate action, apathy is represented more strictly through loss of motivation and interest (17). This distinction can be very difficult to make for patients, caregivers, and clinicians alike. Perhaps the most important point is that apathy and executive dysfunction can both be present in late-life depression.

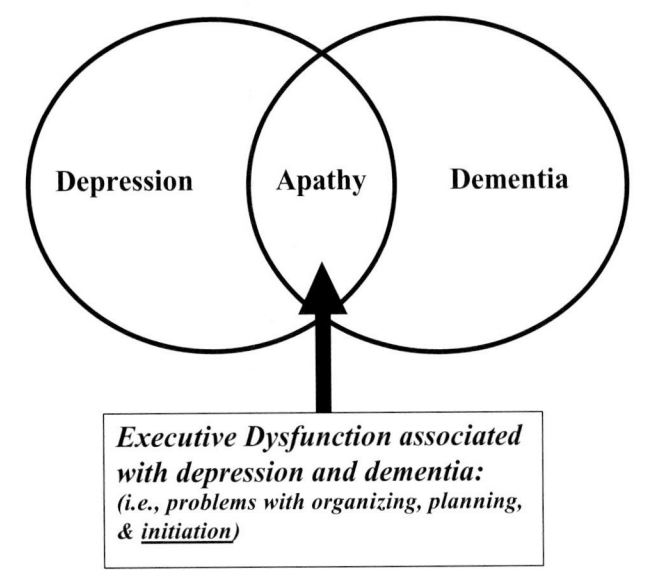

Figure 43-1   Apathy is associated with both depression and dementia in the elderly.

The fact that loss of executive functioning plays such an important role in apathy and depression may also have implications for what experts have come to identify as *vascular depression*. There is a growing body of evidence that subcortical vascular lesions are strongly associated with depression in the elderly (18,19), which supports current thinking that disruption of subcortical connections to cortical regions results in mood dysregulation. In fact, it is hypothesized that disruption of specific subcortical-cortical connections can result in frontal lobe syndromes (20). For example, disruption of subcortical connections to dorsolateral prefrontal cortex produces deficits in organizational strategies and the ability to interpret abstract concepts. Subcortical lesions affecting lateral orbitofrontal cortex are associated with irritability and impulsivity, whereas those affecting medial orbitofrontal cortex are more likely to produce anergic personality changes and depressive moods.

Apathy is believed to be specifically associated with disruption of the connections between the ventral striatum, anteromedial thalamus, and the anterior cingulate cortex. Indeed, a study using functional brain imaging has shown significant hypoperfusion of the anterior cingulate bilaterally in both nondemented and demented patients with apathy (21). Moreover, numerous case reports of apathy following lesions of the thalamus are described in the literature (22). In the most severe cases of this subcortical damage, patients present with *akinetic mutism* (23), which arguably is the most severe form of apathy. Since most subcortical vasculopathies involve lesions in several subcortical domains, patients commonly present with mixed frontal lobe syndromes that may include apathetic features. The fact that problems with executive functioning is a recurrent theme in both apathy and late-life depression is

not surprising given the frequency of subcortical vasculopathy in many of the medically ill elderly patients who present with depression. The clinician must remain mindful of this association and approach all assessments of depression and apathy in the elderly, looking for risks and evidence for subcortical vascular disease.

CASE EXAMPLE: APATHY IN DEPRESSION

Mr. F was a 75-year-old married, Caucasian male who was brought into a geriatric psychiatry clinic by his wife because she suspected that he was depressed. According to Mrs. F, for the past 6 to 12 months, Mr. F had appeared progressively less interested and motivated to do things, which represented a clear change for him. One year prior, he was having unstable angina and underwent triple bypass surgery, with a protracted recovery. His angina resolved after surgery, but he never returned to his previous level of activity. In the 2 months leading up to the appointment, his condition progressed to the point where he tended to sit all day. Mrs. F was constantly prodding him to get up from his chair and do things, and found this task to be the most frustrating. She stated that "there are times when I feel like I am living by myself." There were other times when Mr. F became irritable, with an increasingly "short-fuse." However, he denied feeling depressed. He did seem to understand that his behavior was concerning his wife. Both Mr. and Mrs. F denied that he had any significant memory problems.

Mr. F had no previous psychiatric history. His active medical problems included hypertension, late-onset diabetes, mild chronic obstructive lung disease, benign prostatic hypertrophy, and coronary artery disease. A review of systems revealed only a complaint of low energy during the day and some middle-of-the-night insomnia. A later sleep study was negative. There was no history of transient ischemic attacks or stroke. His medical problems appeared to be under good control and he was compliant with medications, including hydrochlorothiazide, glipizide, tolterodine, and an occasional inhaler. Laboratory studies revealed a very mild anemia. A brain scan from last year showed subcortical vascular ischemic disease. Mr. F was a retired maintenance supervisor and had been happily married for over 50 years. The couple had four children, all of whom were doing well. The patient retired 10 years ago and had several hobbies, including playing golf, gardening, and repairing old juke boxes in his garage.

Physical and mental status exams appeared mostly unremarkable. Mr. F was about 40 pounds overweight, but otherwise appeared fairly healthy. His ambulation and other movements were symmetrical and well-coordinated. His speech was fluent, although he presented as a man of few words. His affect was mostly euthymic and appropriate, although subdued and with a somewhat constricted range. He demonstrated a good rapport with his wife and did not become irritable or defensive when listening to her descriptions of his behavior. Indeed, he indicated regret that his behavior was so concerning to his wife and expressed concern that he had become a burden to her.

Cognitive screening was unremarkable, although later neuropsychological testing revealed mild-to-moderate decreases in visual attention.

After being evaluated, Mr. F was started on sertraline 25 mg at bedtime for 2 weeks and then increased to 50 mg. On follow-up visit 4 weeks later, he denied seeing any difference in himself, although his wife reported that he was noticeably less irritable and his sleep had improved. Still, the major complaint remained of his lack of initiative and interest, particularly evident in the morning. He was then started on methylphenidate 5 mg at 8 AM and at noon as an adjunctive treatment. A phone follow-up was done after another 2 weeks, with Mrs. F reporting some improvement. The dose of methylphenidate was increased to 10 mg at 8 AM and 5 mg at noon. At a follow-up visit 2 weeks later, the wife reported clear improvement: Mr. F appeared more alert and interactive, and was more spontaneous in his interests. Additionally, he was much less irritable, and no longer saw himself as a burden to his wife. Subsequent follow-up visits revealed the same reported improvement. Several months later, Mr. and Mrs. F reported that they had run out of the methylphenidate for a week, resulting in the return of some of the lack of interest. The change in his condition was "like night and day," so Mrs. F had restarted him on the methylphenidate. Since then, Mr. F has remained stable on both sertraline and methylphenidate.

This case is a typical presentation of overlapping apathy and depression in an elderly man. The most prominent feature of this patient's presentation was the apathy, but there also were clues that he was depressed—specifically, the irritability and lowered self-esteem. The fact that he denied any emotional distress is not unusual in depressed, geriatric patients. It is very common for individuals from older generations to grossly underreport depressive feelings because they view depression as a weakness, rather than as a medical problem. Moreover, both patients and families (and sometimes clinicians) often misattribute such symptoms to normal aging, or to medical problems. In the face of a difficult and highly overlapping differential, it usually is best to try an antidepressant first and to see how much overall benefit can be achieved by the one medication alone. If, after an adequate trial, there is resolution of depressive symptoms, but apathy remains, treatment should specifically target the apathy.

APATHY AND DEMENTIA

Apathy is an extremely common phenomenon in various types of dementia; it has been reported in stroke (24), Parkinson's disease (25), Huntington's disease (26), and Alzheimer's disease (AD) (27,28). Starkstein and colleagues reported that apathy was present in 37% of patients with AD (9). One large epidemiological study reported that apathy was the most common neuropsychiatric problem in both vascular dementia (VaD) and AD, with a rate of 27% (29). Both apathetic and demented patients exhibit a decrease in goal-directed behaviors. A distinguishing factor, however, is that demented patients with apathy have a characteristic flattening of emotional responsiveness. In contrast, dementia patients who are not apathetic and do not exhibit emotional distress are often pleasant and able to enjoy experiences. Indeed, they demonstrate a wide range of normal emotional responses. Interestingly, some studies suggest that irritability or disinhibition and apathy are actually commonly associated with one another (30), likely due to disruption of adjacent regions or circuits that subserve both aspects of normal emotional regulation (27,31).

Still, elucidating apathy within dementia can be challenging (32). For example, one cannot count on the presence of emotional reactivity in a demented individual to completely eliminate the presence of apathy. Starkstein and colleagues showed that apathy was more common in AD patients who were depressed (24%) than in AD patients who were not depressed (13%) (9). Kuzis and colleagues showed that AD patients who were both depressed and apathetic produced the most severe deficits in abstract thinking (verbal memory, naming, set shifting, verbal fluency), while AD patients with apathy only had the next lowest scores, and AD patients who were depressed, but not apathetic, had comparable scores to nondepressed AD patients (33). Finally, McPherson and colleagues showed that AD patients with apathy performed significantly worse than nonapathetic AD patients on several tests of executive functioning (16). Combined, these results suggest that patients with dementia and significant executive dysfunction are more likely to appear apathetic. As with depression, this factor again seems to be one of the most reliable indicators of apathy.

As a practical matter to most clinicians, identification of executive dysfunction in patients can be extremely challenging. This is particularly true in patients who have mild cognitive impairment and only exhibit isolated problems with planning, organization, or initiation of tasks or behaviors. In such cases, the deficits are often context-specific, only becoming apparent to family members intermittently when the patient is faced with a particular circumstance requiring executive skills. In all cases, it is critical to obtain information from an informant, particularly a caregiver who is able to observe the individual's performance with a range of daily tasks over time. The informant may also notice subtle changes in personality or in emotional regulation that can indicate executive dysfunction. The caveat here is that if one finds executive dysfunction, apathy quite likely is not far behind, and *vice versa*. Accurate differential diagnosis of apathy in dementia is important for understanding the level of functional impairment seen in the patient (2), as well as having important implications regarding successful treatment.

CASE EXAMPLE: APATHY IN DEMENTIA

Ms. S was an 82-year-old widowed female who presented with her daughter for assessment of depression and behavioral changes seen over the past several months. Ms. S lived alone in a senior apartment complex, where she had moved after her husband's death, 4 years prior. Her daughter visited her regularly, and reported that her mother was not going to her usual social events, and appeared relatively disinterested and lacking in motivation. She also noticed that her mother's apartment was not as clean and organized as usual, and she was not appropriately managing her finances or medications. Most recently, Ms. S appeared less interested in seeing her grandchildren, explaining that it felt like too much effort. Her daughter was concerned that her mother was depressed, but Ms. S denied it. Although Ms. S admitted that she was not socializing as much, she was distinctly unconcerned about it. She reported that her sleep, appetite, and energy were fine.

Ms. S's active medical problems included atrial fibrillation, hypertension, hyperthyroidism, macular degeneration, osteoarthritis, and migraines. She had one previous episode of depression about the time of her husband's death, and had been successfully treated with citalopram 20 mg per day, which she still was taking. There was no other history of psychiatric problems. Her daily medications included digoxin, citalopram, warfarin, atenolol, levothyroxine, and acetaminophen. Laboratory studies were unremarkable. A work-up for dementia 3 years prior had been negative. A brain scan found mild cerebral atrophy, and the neuropsychological report cited the presence of "mild deficits in verbal processing and attention" that were attributed to depression. In terms of social history, Ms. S had retired many years ago from a part-time position as a legal assistant. She was married for 45 years and, together with her husband, raised two children. Previously, she had been very active in her community and local church. She had volunteered at the local senior center until the past year.

On examination, Ms. S was a small-framed, well-groomed, elderly female. She ambulated a bit slowly, consistent with her arthritis, but her movements were generally fluid and symmetrical. Her speech was clear and articulate, although there were rare instances of word-finding problems. She denied feeling depressed, although admitted that at times she has felt lonely. Her affect was pleasant, although with a narrow range, and she was socially quite poised; she presented as rather disengaged from the entire process. Her cognition, on the other hand, was clearly impaired. She exhibited clear difficulty with short-term recall and very poor planning on the clock-drawing test. She could only name six farm animals in 1 minute and did very poorly on recalling current news events. Her score on the Folstein Mini Mental Status Exam was 21 out of 30. It was clear on her presentation that she had very good social skills and a high baseline verbal intelligence, both of which likely helped her cover-up cognitive deficits over the years.

Because the examiner did think depression could be a minor factor in her presentation, the dose of citalopram was increased to 30 mg per day. Repeat neuropsychological testing revealed deficits in delayed verbal and visuospatial recall, as well as poor planning and set-shifting. These results, together with the daughter's unambiguous descriptions of a slowly progressive cognitive and functional decline, led to the diagnosis of probable Alzheimer's disease. No change was perceived on the increased citalopram. Ms. S was then started on the acetylcholinesterase inhibitor (AChEI) donepezil 5 mg at bedtime for 4 weeks, and then increased to 10 mg. Her daughter was referred to a caregiver support group. Through the group, she acquired a better understanding of how cognitive impairment disrupted her mother's behavior and daily function, and she learned how better to manage it. By keeping a journal of her mother's behaviors, she was able to notice improvement on the AChEI after 2 months. Ms. S appeared more likely to initiate activity on her own, such as preparing a simple meal or cleaning her apartment. She continued to exhibit obvious short-term memory deficits and mild aphasia. However, Ms. S also appeared more spontaneous and less apathetic. She remained stable for the next 12 to 18 months, after which there was more noticeable cognitive decline.

This case demonstrates how patients with early dementia can present with apathy. Once again, it is usually family members who observe subtle changes in the patient. Patients who are particularly skilled at covering up the amnestic or aphasic aspects of early dementia may be less able to cover-up problems with executive functioning, particularly when there are losses in the ability to initiate activities. Family members often observe these changes in personality and attribute them entirely to depression. They complain that the patient appears emotionally detached, or has lost all interest in usual activities. Caregivers may feel guilty and frustrated about trying to prompt the patient to do things, and he or she often resents it. In the end, the patient may remain inactive and appear quite apathetic. AChEIs can produce modest improvement on a range of behaviors with both AD and VaD, including abilities related to executive functioning. Caregivers sometimes notice changes in behavior and function, more than in memory. Although the patient may still have difficulty completing certain tasks, due to forgetfulness or problems with organization, a newfound level of interest and initiative may make him or her appear less depressed and less apathetic.

APATHY IN OTHER NEUROPSYCHIATRIC SYNDROMES

As suggested earlier, apathy has been associated with a variety of neuropsychiatric syndromes, medical problems, and medications, many of which are listed in Table 43-1 (34,35). Duffy and Kant provide a detailed summary of

TABLE 43-1

NEUROPSYCHIATRIC SYNDROMES, MEDICAL PROBLEMS, AND MEDICATIONS ASSOCIATED WITH APATHY

Neuropsychiatric Syndromes	Medical Problems	Medications
Alzheimer's disease	Anemia	SSRIs
Parkinson's disease	Anorexia	Antipsychotics
Frontotemporal dementia (Pick disease)	Obstructive sleep apnea	Narcotics/opioids
Huntington's disease	Sleep disorders	Steroids
Progressive supranuclear palsy	Chronic fatigue	Reserpine
Carbon monoxide poisoning	Chronic pain	Sedative/hypnotics
Anoxic brain injury	Hypothyroidism	
Traumatic brain injury	Hyperthyroidism	
Stroke syndromes (aphasia, apraxia, and anosognosia)	Pseudohypoparathyroidism	
	Diabetes mellitus	
Vascular dementia	Chronic fatigue syndrome	
Delirium	Testosterone deficiency	
HIV-associated dementia	Malignancy	
	Congestive heart failure	
	Hepatic or renal failure	
	COPD	
	Cushing's disease	
	Addison's disease	

COPD, chronic obstructive pulmonary disease; SSRIs, selective serotonin-reuptake inhibitors.

many of these syndromes, emphasizing the two frontal cortical regions (mesial-frontal and dorsolateral) that appear to be strongly associated with the presentation of apathy (36). Starkstein and colleagues found in a series of 80 post-stroke patients that 18 (22.5%) exhibited apathy; half of those patients also were depressed (24). The apathy was significantly associated with older age, cognitive impairments, and deficits in activities of daily living. Lesions were often in the posterior limb of the internal capsule. Okada and colleagues (37) found that poststroke apathy was associated with depression and decreased cerebral blood flow in the right dorsolateral frontal and left frontotemporal regions of the cortex. Frontotemporal dementias in general are commonly associated with apathy (38).

Lesions or dysfunction of subcortical regions, such as the thalamus and basal ganglia, frequently produce apathy in elderly patients by disrupting cortical-subcortical connections. An important example of this is the well-recognized association between Parkinson's disease and apathy. Using the Apathy Scale, Starkstein and colleagues found in a series of Parkinson patients that 12% had apathy alone and 30% were both apathetic and depressed (25). Several investigators have shown that this association is not simply a reaction to the disability from the illness, and it appears more often in patients with cognitive impairment (25,39). Indeed, Aarsland and colleagues found, using the Neuropsychiatric Inventory, that the presence of apathy in Parkinson's disease was associated with executive dysfunction, but correlated negatively with the stage of the disease (40, 41).

Another example of subcortical damage resulting in apathy is anoxic injury, which commonly affects the basal ganglia. Such injury is associated with both cognitive and motoric slowing, as well as apathy. These symptoms are commonly observed in subcortical dementia. In subcortical damage (bilateral thalamic lesions), causing *akinetic mutism*, patients have a profound lack of movement and communication, despite the fact that they are still capable of both.

APATHY AND PSYCHOSIS

Apathy comorbid with psychosis is most commonly observed in older patients with chronic schizophrenia. In these cases, the likelihood of apathy being present appears to be related to the age of onset of the illness (42). For example, most patients with early-onset schizophrenia (before age 45) and approximately half of those with late-onset schizophrenia (between age 45 and 65), exhibit both positive (e.g., hallucinations, delusions) and negative (e.g., blunted affect, apathy) symptoms of the illness (43). In contrast, a subset of patients with late-onset schizophrenia and those with very-late-onset schizophrenia-like illness (after age 65) are less likely to develop the blunted affect and apathy (43). As they age, patients with schizophrenia exhibit less positive symptoms, more prominent negative symptoms, including apathy, and nonprogressive cognitive impairment characterized by marked deficits in executive functioning (44).

The conventional antipsychotic medications (e.g., haloperidol, perphenazine, chlorpromazine) are not effective in treating negative symptoms of chronic schizophrenia, and may even exacerbate apathetic symptoms in the elderly. Moreover, there has long been concern that chronic treatment with these older-generation antipsychotics might negatively impact cognition (45), and lead to a drug-induced apathy. Others have speculated that the apathy associated with chronic schizophrenia may be related to long-term institutionalization (46). In contrast, the atypical antipsychotics (clozapine, risperidone, olanzapine, quetiapine, ziprasidone, and aripiprazole) are likely more effective in treating the negative symptoms in chronic schizophrenia (47), and are better tolerated in the elderly. This improved efficacy is thought to be related to combined action on both dopaminergic and serotonergic pathways, which ultimately improves executive functioning.

Thus, elderly patients with apathy in the context of a chronic, psychotic illness are best treated with an atypical antipsychotic. It is often the case that such patients remain apathetic, even when on optimal treatment. In such cases, it may be beneficial to supplement treatment with cognitive enhancers, such as an AChEI (48), or memantine, or even theoretically with a stimulant such as atomoxetine to increase noradrenergic functioning (49). Caution must be exercised when using dopaminergic agents so as not to induce or exacerbate psychotic symptoms.

APATHY AND MEDICAL ILLNESS

There are a number of common late-life medical illnesses that are associated with apathy (50). As listed in Table 43-1, these conditions include major cardiac and pulmonary diseases, sleep disorders, chronic pain, endocrine disorders, and metabolic conditions such as renal and hepatic failure. Common to many of these conditions is daytime fatigue and loss of energy. When these symptoms become chronic, patients may ultimately lose their drive to overcome them, resulting in a loss of motivation and hence apathy.

Although there are no generally agreed-upon criteria, the term *failure-to-thrive* primarily refers to patients who present with persistent anorexia and involuntary weight loss (51). Such patients often exhibit loss of motivation that results in a gradual decline in overall functioning along with social withdrawal. Common underlying illnesses responsible for failure-to-thrive include dementia, depression, and delirium (52). The morbidity and mortality of such patients is quite high. In one study, Hildebrand and colleagues described 132 elderly patients from a Veteran's Administration hospital over a 3-year period: 14% of their subjects died in the hospital, an additional 11% died within 30 days, and 35% died within 1 year after discharge (51). Cancer was the most common underlying diagnosis (30%), followed by infection, dehydration, and depression. It is commonly believed that many of these

patients manifest a particularly malignant form of depression that results in anorexia and/or increasing disability (53). This condition is a particularly difficult treatment challenge, often requiring combinations of antidepressants and psychostimulants to increase both energy and appetite.

ASSESSMENT

Assessment of apathy begins with a careful clinical history. Apathetic patients frequently passively resist coming to appointments and providing much history, so caregiver interviews become paramount, at times even preempting patient interviews. However, clinicians should always endeavor to include the patient from the start, in order to build rapport and trust. When seen together, the clinician can observe how the patient interacts with the caregiver and responds to their concerns. Spontaneous questions, comments, and motor movements are often minimal. Apathetic patients will not struggle to offer much history or to protest the complaints of caregivers; that is the nature of their problem. Apathetic patients are notable for a relative lack of emotional responsiveness and their inability to provide cogent explanations. They are often at a loss for explanations for their own behavioral changes. Although apathetic patients are often pleasant, they continue to be rather matter of fact even when confronted with heartfelt concerns expressed by their family. To aid the clinician, a number of scales have been developed to either differentiate symptoms of apathy from dementia or depression, or to identify apathy as a distinct syndrome. These are listed in Table 43-2.

The differential diagnosis for cases of suspected apathy is quite broad. Quite frequently, the major concern centers on whether or not the patient is depressed, demented, or both. In addition to the clinical history, a complete review of systems is useful to look for symptoms of depression and dementia, as well as identify concerns such as pain, sensory impairment, physical deconditioning, dizziness, sleep disorders, and exacerbation of cardiac or pulmonary conditions. Undetected or undertreated medical or psychiatric problems or medication side-effects must be identified and addressed, since they can impair an individual's ability to care for himself or herself, leading to symptomatic loss of energy, functional impairment, or changes in neurovegetative function. Sometimes a simple lack of energy is confused with apathy. Stress over finances, a change in environment, loss of mobility, or bereavement can contribute to decreased levels of activity that may mimic apathy or trigger it.

The examination of the apathetic patient should parallel a dementia workup, and include a physical and neurological evaluation, a brain scan, and blood tests (complete blood count, electrolytes, calcium, renal, hepatic, and

TABLE 43-2
VALIDATED SCALES FOR APATHY

Scale Name	Description
Irritability-Apathy Scale	Provides a clinical description of irritability, aggression, and apathy in Huntington's and Alzheimer's disease (54)
Apathy Evaluation Scale (AES)	Based on Marin's criteria (1), has been used in several studies, and has been validated (55)
Apathy Scale	Abridged version of AES, less comprehensive, but in validation study authors describe it as less demanding on patients with Parkinson's disease (25)
Apathy-related items of the Hamilton Rating Scale for Depression (ApHRSD)	Used HRSD questions on lack of interest, anergy, lack of insight, and psychomotor retardation (17,56)
Neuropsychiatric Inventory (NPI)	Subsections on apathy ask about loss of interest, motivation, spontaneity, enthusiasm, affectionate behavior, and not caring about doing new things (30,57)
Apathy Inventory	Based on NPI model, but designed to provide separate assessment of emotional, behavioral, and cognitive aspects per criteria (58)

thyroid function, vitamin B12, and folate). The need for additional tests, such as toxicology for specific infectious agents (e.g., syphilis, Lyme disease) can be guided by history or the results of the screening tests. Special attention should be paid to manifestations of subcortical and frontal lobe injury, such as extrapyramidal symptoms (e.g., parkinsonism, dyskinesia) or frontal release signs, given the high association with apathy. Neuropsychological testing can be very helpful to identify executive dysfunction, which is strongly correlated with the presence of apathy. Functional testing may also be useful to determine the practical effects of cognitive impairment on the ability to initiate and organize tasks, which would help in the differential diagnosis of apathy.

TREATMENT

The treatment of apathy depends foremost on treatment of underlying conditions that may be triggering or exacerbating it. Beyond that, both pharmacological and nonpharmacological strategies will vary, depending on comorbid conditions.

Pharmacological Approaches

Unfortunately, there have not been double-blinded, placebo-controlled studies that looked at the treatment of apathy as a distinct syndrome. As a result, there are no medications that have been approved by the Food and Drug Administration (FDA) for the treatment of apathy. Instead, clinicians have based treatment on the findings of numerous case reports—usually involving older individuals—that

have found successful treatments of apathetic symptoms associated with other syndromes, particularly dementia or depression. Marin and colleagues describe seven cases of apathy associated with depression, degenerative dementia, strokes, or traumatic brain injury (TBI) (59). In all cases (age range 23 to 86 years), apathy responded well to methylphenidate, amphetamine, bupropion, levodopa, or selegiline. Campbell and Duffy conducted a comprehensive review of case reports describing the effectiveness of dopaminergic agonists, including bromocriptine, amantadine, and amphetamine (60). They found that the vast majority of cases (age range 13 to 86 years) reported improvement. Again, all of the cases involved apathy in the context of other neuropsychiatric syndromes, such as TBI, stroke, anoxia, or various causes of dementia. The stimulant methylphenidate has been used to successfully treat apathy associated with subcortical infarcts and Parkinson's disease (61,62). In another case series, bupropion, an antidepressant with dopaminergic properties, improved apathy in three patients with depression or organic brain disease (63).

As reflected in these reports, most experts have long recommended use of medications with dopaminergic (and to a lesser extent, noradrenergic) enhancing properties in the treatment of apathy. The three categories of medications include the psychostimulants (methylphenidate, amphetamine, dextroamphetamine, pemoline, and modafinil), specific dopamine agonists (bromocriptine, levodopa, amantadine, pergolide, and selegiline), and stimulating antidepressants, specifically bupropion. The AChEIs have emerged as a fourth, novel pharmacologic category for apathy. Use of all of these medications is considered *off-label*, since none of them have a specific FDA indication for

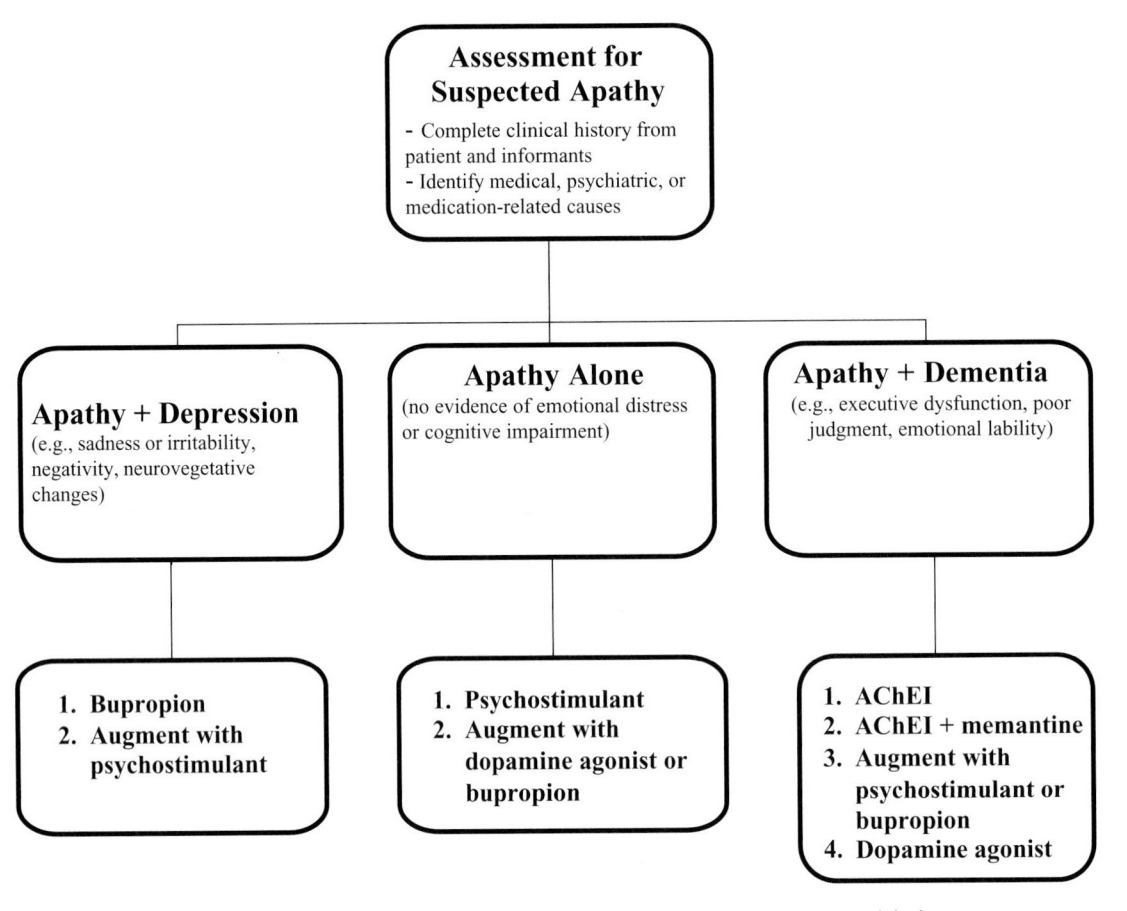

Figure 43-2 Protocol for assessment and treatment of apathy. AChEI, acetylcholinesterase inhibitor.

apathy. In the protocol presented in Figure 43-2, the treatment of apathy is presented within three contexts: apathy alone, apathy plus dementia, and apathy plus depression.

Apathy Alone

For older individuals with apathy, initial treatment commonly involves use of a psychostimulant. Several examples are listed in Table 43-3, along with dosing ranges. With the exception of modafinil, all psychostimulants are structurally similar to amphetamine, and work by enhancing dopaminergic and noradrenergic activity in the brain. Modafinil appears to work by stimulating hypothalamic neurons. Methylphenidate has been the most widely used psychostimulant. When treating apathy, methylphenidate can be started at 5 mg in the morning, with potential benefits including increased energy and activity levels being seen within hours or days. A second 5 mg dose can be added at noontime, and both doses titrated to effect in a range of 5 mg to 10 mg once or twice daily. These doses are usually well-tolerated, but can interfere with sleep if given too late in the day. Potential side effects include irritability, restlessness, tics, increased blood pressure, decreased appetite, or sleep disturbance. Concerns about abuse or addiction are usually

unfounded in the elderly. Other psychostimulants will have similar effects, although they have not been studied as much as methylphenidate.

Although there are a number of specific dopamine agonists that have been shown to benefit some patients with apathy, they are used less often due to an increased potential for side effects in the elderly. For example, side effects of bromocriptine and pergolide include orthostasis, psychosis, dyskinesias, and gastrointestinal discomfort. Levodopa and selegiline are used more commonly in the treatment of Parkinson's disease than with apathy, and can also result in psychosis and dyskinesias. Amantadine is a unique agent used to treat Parkinson's disease, extrapyramidal symptoms, and viral infections, but its clinical effects can take several weeks to manifest and it can also cause psychotic symptoms.

Apathy and Dementia

Recently, investigators have reported that the AChEIs used to treat cognitive and functional symptoms in AD and other dementias may also be useful in the treatment of apathy (64). In a large, double-blind, placebo-controlled trial examining the prevalence of behavioral

TABLE 43-3
PHARMACOLOGICAL TREATMENTS FOR APATHY IN THE ELDERLY

Medication	Dose Range (mg/day)
Psychostimulants	
Methylphenidate	5–40
Dextroamphetamine	5–20
Pemoline	37.5–75
Modafinil	100–400
Dopamine agonists	
Amantadine	50–300
Bromocriptine	2.5–20
Pergolide	1–5
Levodopa/Carbidopa	25/100 tid–25/250 qid
Selegiline	5–10
Stimulating antidepressants	
Bupropion	75–450
Acetylcholinesterase inhibitors	
Donepezil	5–15
Rivastigmine	6–12
Galantamine	16–24
NMDA receptor antagonist	
Memantine	10–20

NMDA, N-methyl-D-aspartate.

symptoms in patients with moderate-to-severe AD, apathy was identified as one of the most common symptoms (seen in 67% of affected individuals) (65). After 24 weeks of treatment with the donepezil, apathy was one of several behavioral indices that improved significantly. Similar beneficial effects on apathy have been demonstrated for rivastigmine and galantamine (66). The mechanism of action is unclear, but may be related neurophysiologically to enhancement of dopaminergic activity in the brain, and neuropsychologically to improvement in executive function. *In vitro* data for both donepezil and galantamine indicate that these agents may enhance the release of dopamine in the brain (67). Memantine, a glutamate-receptor (N-methyl-D-aspartate-receptor) antagonist used to treat AD, may also have benefit for apathy (68).

Psychostimulants or specific dopamine agonists may also be used for apathy with dementia, alone or in combination with AChEIs. Special caution is required in this population, however, because enhanced dopaminergic activity may lead to increased irritability, paranoia, hallucinations, impulsivity, or combativeness. This may be particularly true in frontal lobe dementias, or dementias with movement disorders, such as Lewy body dementia. Psychostimulants also can potentially exacerbate movement disorders, such as dyskinesias or tics. One alternative may be modafinil (FDA-approved for the treatment of narcolepsy) since it lacks specific dopaminergic properties.

Apathy and Depression

If a patient appears to have apathy associated with depression, the best initial strategy is a stimulating antidepressant. Selective serotonin reuptake inhibitors (SSRIs) are typically first-line antidepressants in the elderly, and can have stimulating properties. However, there are a number of case reports of SSRI-induced apathy (69). Bupropion used alone or in combination with other antidepressant agents might be a better choice for depressed individuals with apathy given its dopaminergic properties. Unlike psychostimulants, bupropion and other antidepressants take anywhere from 2 to 3 weeks to start working, and up to 8 weeks for maximum effect for symptoms of depression and apathy. Methylphenidate used alone may help improve certain types of depression (70), or may be added to an SSRI to obtain an accelerated response (71). The selected types of depression examined using stimulants include those associated with medical illness, involuntary weight loss, and malignancy (70). Psychostimulants may play a singular role in stimulating appetite in severely demented, apathetic nursing home patients suffering from failure-to-thrive (72). Similarly, modafinil combined with the antidepressant mirtazapine has been shown useful for these patients (73). In general, monotherapy with methylphenidate has not been established as a consistent antidepressant approach (74,75). Antipsychotic medications combined with antidepressants may also play a role in treating apathy associated with depression (76).

Nonpharmacological Approaches

It is common for caregivers to feel a great deal of stress when dealing with an apathetic individual. Despite their best efforts, the patient has little motivation to interact or spontaneously participate in daily tasks and activities. Caregivers may resort to pestering, pleading, and even threatening to externally motivate the person, and often experience frustration, anger, and anxiety, particularly when the person is not cooperating with needed socialization or physical rehabilitation. Apathetic individuals can become more isolated and physically deconditioned by their lack of motivation. Without understanding the nature of underlying apathy, caregivers may feel disappointed and even rejected. They may assume that the apathetic person is being willfully resistant, or that he or she is depressed. In these circumstances, it is important for clinicians to provide education about apathy as a brain syndrome, along with support for the caregiver role. Caregivers can then form more realistic expectations.

In addition, the use of physical, occupational, and recreational therapy can sometimes stimulate an apathetic patient, or at least counteract social isolation and deconditioning. Adjusting the environment to suit the interests of the patient and correcting for sensory or mobility impairments can remove barriers to increased functioning, e.g., speech therapy can improve communication. Psychotherapy itself is less helpful for apathy *per se* since the fundamental problem is usually organic in origin. However, apathetic patients can experience feelings of depression or anxiety that might be amenable to talk therapy.

REFERENCES

1. Marin RS. Apathy: a neuropsychiatric syndrome. *J Neuropsychiatry Clin Neurosci.* 1991;3:243–254.
2. Zawacki TM, Grace J, Paul R, et al. Behavioral problems as predictors of functional abilities of vascular dementia patients. *J Neuropsychiatry Clin Neurosci.* 2002;14:296–302.
3. Boyle PA, Malloy PF, Salloway S, Cahn-Weiner DA, Cohen R, Cummings JL. Executive dysfunction and apathy predict functional impairment in Alzheimer disease. *Am J Geriatr Psychiatry.* 2003;11:214–221.
4. Norton LE, Malloy PF, Salloway S. The impact of behavioral symptoms on activities of daily living in patients with dementia. *Am J Geriatr Psychiatry.* 2001;9:41–48.
5. Thomas P, Clement JP, Hazif-Thomas C, Leger JM. Family, Alzheimer's disease and negative symptoms. *Inter J Geriatr Psychiatry.* 2001;16:192–202.
6. Kalayam B, Alexopoulos GS. Prefrontal dysfunction and treatment response in geriatric depression *Arch Gen Psychiatry.* 1999;56: 713–718.
7. Steinberg M, Sheppard J, Tschanz J, et al. The incidence of mental and behavioral disturbances in dementia: the Cache County study. *J Neuropsychiatry Clin Neurosci.* 2003;15(3):340–345.
8. Marin RS. Differential diagnosis and classification of apathy. *Am J Psychiatry.* 1990;147:22–30.
9. Starkstein SE, Petracca G, Chemerinski E, Kremer J. Syndromic validity of apathy in Alzheimer's disease. *Am J Psychiatry.* 2001; 158:872–877.
10. Krishnan KR, Hays JC, Tupler LA, George LK, Blazer DG. Clinical and phenomenological comparisons of late-onset and early-onset depression. *Am J Psychiatry.* 1995;152:785–788.
11. Royall DR. Frontal systems impairment in major depression. *Semin Clin Neuropsychiatry.* 1999;4:13–23.
12. Alexopoulos GS, Meyers BS, Young RC, et al. Executive dysfunction and long-term outcomes of geriatric depression. *Arch Gen Psychiatry.* 2000; 57:285–290.
13. Kiosses DN, Alexopoulos GS, Murphy C. Symptoms of striatofrontal dysfunction contribute to disability in geriatric depression. *Int J Geriatr Psychiatry.* 2000;15:992–999.
14. Kiosses DN, Klimstra S, Murphy C, Alexopoulos GS. Executive dysfunction and disability in elderly patients with major depression. *Am J Geriatr Psychiatry.* 2001;9:269–274.
15. Feil D, Razani J, Boone K, Lesser I. Apathy and cognitive performance in older adults with depression. *Int J Geriatr Psychiatry.* 2003;18:479–485.
16. McPherson S, Fairbanks L, Tiken S, Cummings JL, Back-Madruga C. Apathy and executive function in Alzheimer's disease. *J Int Neuropsychol Soc.* 2002;8:373–381.
17. Marin RS, Butters MA, Mulsant BH, Pollock BG, Reynolds CF 3rd. Apathy and executive function in depressed elderly. *J Geriatr Psychiatry and Neurol.* 2003;16:112–116.
18. Coffey CE, Figiel GS, Djang WT, Weiner RD. Subcortical hyperintensity on magnetic resonance imaging: a comparison of normal and depressed elderly subjects. *Am J Psychiatry.* 1990;147: 187–189.
19. Krishnan KR, Hays JC, Blazer DG. MRI-defined vascular depression. *Am J Psychiatry.* 1997;154:497–501.
20. Mega MS, Cummings JL. Frontal-subcortical circuits and neuropsychiatric disorders. *J Neuropsychiatry Clin Neurosci.* 1994;6: 358–370.
21. Migneco O, Benoit M, Koulibaly PM, et al. Perfusion brain SPECT and statistical parametric mapping analysis indicate that apathy is a cingulate syndrome: a study in Alzheimer's disease and nondemented patients. *Neuroimage.* 2001;13:896–902.
22. Engelborghs S, Marien P, Pickut BA, Verstraeten S, De Deyn PP. Loss of psychic self-activation after paramedian bithalamic infarction. *Stroke.* 2000;31:1762–1765.
23. Nagaratnam N, McNeil C, Gilhotra JS. Akinetic mutism and mixed transcortical aphasia following left thalamo-mesencephalic infarction. *J Neurol Sci.* 1999;163:70–73.
24. Starkstein SE, Fedoroff JP, Price TR, Leiguarda R, Robinson RG. Apathy following cerebrovascular lesions. *Stroke.* 1993;24(11): 1625–1630.
25. Starkstein SE, Mayberg HS, Preziosi TJ, Andrezejewski P, Leiguarda R, Robinson RG. Reliability, validity, and clinical correlates of apathy in Parkinson's disease. *J Neuropsychiatry Clin Neurosci.* 1992;4:134–139.
26. Burns A, Folstein S, Brandt J, et al. Clinical assessment of irritability, aggression, and apathy in Huntington and Alzheimer disease. *J Nerv Ment Dis.* 1990;178:20–26.
27. Duffy JD. The neural substrates of motivation. *Psychiatric Annals.* 1997;27:24–29.
28. Landes AM, Sperry SD, Strauss ME, Geldmacher DS. Apathy in Alzheimer's disease. *J Am Geriatr Soc.* 2001;49:1700–1707.
29. Lyketsos CG, Steinberg M, Tschanz JT, Norton MC, Steffens DC, Breitner JC. Mental and behavioral disturbances in dementia: findings from the Cache County Study on Memory in Aging. *Am J Psychiatry.* 2000;157:708–714.
30. Levy ML, Cummings JL, Fairbanks LA, et al. Apathy is not depression. *J Neuropsychiatry Clin Neurosci.* 1998;10:314–319.
31. Mega MS, Cummings JL. Frontal-subcortical circuits and neuropsychiatric disorders. *J Neuropsychiatry Clin Neurosci.* 1994;6:358–370.
32. Marin RS, Firinciogullari S, Biedrzycki RC. Group differences in the relationship between apathy and depression. *J Nerv and Ment Dis.* 1994;182:235–239.
33. Kuzis G, Sabe L, Tiberti C, Dorrego F, Starkstein SE. Neuropsychological correlates of apathy and depression in patients with dementia. *Neurology.* 1999;52:1403–1407.
34. Marin RS. Apathy—who cares? An introduction to apathy and related disorders of diminished motivation. *Psychiatric Annals.* 1997a;27(1):18–23.
35. Marin RS. Differential diagnosis of apathy and related disorders of diminished motivation. *Psychiatric Annals.* 1997b;27(1):30–33.
36. Duffy JD, Kant R. Apathy secondary to neurologic disease. *Psychiatric Annals.* 1997;27(1):39–43.
37. Okada K, Kobayashi S, Yamagata S, Takahashi K, Yamaguchi S. Poststroke apathy and regional cerebral blood flow. *Stroke.* 1997;28:2437–2441.
38. Chow TW, Miller BL, Boone K, Mishkin F, Cummings JL. Frontotemporal dementia classification and neuropsychiatry. *Neurologist.* 2002;8:263–269.
39. Pluck GC, Brown RG. Apathy in Parkinson's disease. *J Neurol Neurosurg Psychiatry.* 2003;73:636–642.
40. Aarsland D, Cummings JL, Larsen JP. Neuropsychiatric differences between Parkinson's disease with dementia and Alzheimer's disease. *Int J Geriatr Psychiatry.* 2001;16:184–191.
41. Aarsland D, Larsen JP, Lim NG, et al. Range of neuropsychiatric disturbances in patients with Parkinson's disease. *J Neurol Neurosurg Psychiatry.* 1999;67:492–496.
42. Jeste DV, Harris MJ, Krull A, Kuck J, McAdams LA, Heaton R. Clinical and neuropsychological characteristics of patients with late-onset schizophrenia. *Am J Psychiatry.* 1995;152:722–730.
43. Howard R, Rabins PV, Seeman MV, Jeste DV. Late-onset schizophrenia and very-late-onset schizophrenia-like psychosis: an international consensus. The International Late-Onset Schizophrenia Group.. *Am J Psychiatry.* 2000;157:172–178.
44. Heaton R, Paulsen JS, McAdams LA, et al. Neuropsychological deficits in schizophrenics. Relationship to age, chronicity, and dementia. *Arch Gen Psychiatry.* 1994;51:469–476.
45. Sharma T. Impact on cognition of the use of antipsychotics. *Curr Med Res Opin.* 2002; 18(Suppl 3):s13–17.
46. Ananth J, Djenderdjian A, Shamasunder P, Costa J, Herrera J, Sramek J. Negative symptoms: psychopathological models. *J Psychiatry Neurosci.* 1991;16(1):12–18.
47. Moller HJ. Management of the negative symptoms of schizophrenia: new treatment options. *CNS Drugs.* 2003;17:793–823.
48. Friedman JI. Cholinergic targets for cognitive enhancement in schizophrenia: focus on cholinesterase inhibitors and muscarinic agonists. *Psychopharmacology* (Berl). 2004;174:45–53.
49. Friedman JI, Stewart DG, Gorman JM. Potential noradrenergic targets for cognitive enhancement in schizophrenia. *CNS Spectr.* 2004;9:350–355.

50. Krupp BH, Fogel BS. Motivational impairment in primary psychiatric and medical illness. *Psychiatric Annals.* 1997;27(1):34–38.
51. Hildebrand JK, Joos SK, Lee MA. Use of the diagnosis "failure to thrive" in older veterans. *J Am Geriatr Soc.* 1997;45:1113–1117.
52. Palmer RM. "Failure to thrive" in the elderly: diagnosis and management. *Geriatrics.* 1990;45(9):47–50, 53–55.
53. Katz IR, DiFilippo S. Neuropsychiatric aspects of failure to thrive in late life. *Clin Geriatr Med.* 1997;13:623–638.
54. Burns A, Folstein S, Brandt J, Folstein M. Clinical assessment of irritability, aggression, and apathy in Huntington and Alzheimer disease. *J Nerv Ment Dis.* 1990;178:20–26.
55. Marin RS, Biedrzycki RC, Firinciogullari S. Reliability and validity of the Apathy Evaluation Scale. *Psychiatry Res.* 1991;38:143–162.
56. Marin RS, Biedrzycki RC, Firinciogullari S. The sources of convergence between measures of apathy and depression. *J Affect Disord.* 1993;28:117–124.
57. Cummings JL, Mega M, Gray K, Rosenberg-Thompson S, Carusi DA, Gornbein J. The Neuropsychiatric Inventory: comprehensive assessment of psychopathology in dementia. *Neurology.* 1994;44:2308–2314.
58. Robert PH, Clairet S, Benoit M, et al. The Apathy Inventory: assessment of apathy and awareness in Alzheimer's disease, Parkinson's disease and mild cognitive impairment. *Int J Geriatr Psychiatry.* 2002;17:1099–1105.
59. Marin RS, Fogel BS, Hawkins J, Duffy J, Krupp B. Apathy: a treatable syndrome. *J Neuropsychiatry Clin Neurosci.* 1995;7(1):23–30.
60. Campbell JJ, Duffy JD. Treatment strategies in amotivated patients. *Psychiatric Annals.* 1997;27(1):44–49.
61. Watanabe MD, Martin EM, DeLeon OA, Gaviria M, Pavel DG, Trepashko DW. Successful methylphenidate treatments of apathy after subcortical infarcts. *J Neuropsychiatry Clin Neurosci.* 1995;7:502–504.
62. Chatterjee A, Fahn S. Methylphenidate treats apathy in Parkinson's disease. *J Neuropsychiatry Clin Neurosci.* 2002;14:461–462.
63. Corcoran C, Wong ML, O'Keane V. Bupropion in the management of apathy. *J Psychopharmacol.* 2004;18:133–135.
64. Boyle PA, Malloy PF. Treating apathy in Alzheimer's disease. *Dement Geriatr Cogn Disord.* 2004;17(1–2):91–99.
65. Gauthier S, Feldman H, Hecker J, et al. Efficacy of donepezil on behavioral symptoms in patients with moderate to severe Alzheimer's disease. *Int Psychogeriatr.* 2002;14:389–404.
66. Wynn ZJ, Cummings JL. Cholinesterase inhibitor therapies and neuropsychiatric manifestations of Alzheimer's disease. *Dement Geriatr Cogn Disord.* 2004;17(1–2):100–108.
67. Zhang L, Zhou FM, Dani JA. Cholinergic drugs for Alzheimer's disease enhance in vitro dopamine release. *Mol Pharmacol.* 2004;66:538–544.
68. Grutzner L. [Case report. Dementia with apathy] *MMW Fortschr Med.* 2002;144(31–32):56.
69. Barnhart WJ, Makela EH, Latocha MJ. SSRI-induced apathy syndrome: a clinical review. *J Psychiatr Prac.* 2004;10:196–199.
70. Challman TD, Lipsky JJ. Methylphenidate: its pharmacology and uses. *Mayo Clin Proc.* 2000;75:711–721.
71. Lavretsky H, Kim MD, Kumar A, Reynolds CF III. Combined treatment with methylphenidate and citalopram for accelerated response in the elderly: an open trial. *J Clin Psychiatry.* 2003;64:1410–1414.
72. Maletta GJ, Winegarden T. Reversal of anorexia by methylphenidate in apathetic, severely demented nursing home patients. *Am J Geriatr Psychiatry.* 1993;1:234–243.
73. Schillerstrom JE, Seaman JS. Modafinil augmentation of mirtazapine in a failure-to-thrive geriatric inpatient. *Int J Psychiatry Med.* 2002;32(4):405–410.
74. Mattes JA. Methylphenidate in mild depression: a double-blind controlled trial. *J Clin Psychiatry.* 1985;46:525–527.
75. Satel SL, Nelson JC. Stimulants in the treatment of depression: a critical overview. *J Clin Psychiatry.* 1989;50:241–249.
76. Marangell LB, Johnson CR, Kertz B, Zboyan HA, Martinez JM. Olanzapine in the treatment of apathy in previously depressed participants maintained with selective serotonin reuptake inhibitors: an open-label, flexible-dose study. *J Clin Psychiatry.* 2002;63:391–395.

APPENDIX A

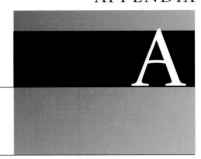

Guide to Psychotropic Pharmacotherapy in the Elderly

Kimberly M. Mattox Shane A. Fishco Gabe J. Maletta

Pharmacotherapy is an important tool in the treatment of psychiatric conditions in the elderly. Drug discovery, development, and approval in the United States is a complex, expensive, and time consuming process. Fewer than 1-in-5,000 compounds entering preclinical testing are ultimately approved (Figure A-1) (1). Growth in the number and type of psychotropic medications continues despite the rigorous approval process. The Food and Drug Administration (FDA) has approved over 60 psychotropic medications since lithium, chlorpromazine, and imipramine were first introduced in the 1940s and 1950s (2). Still more psychotropic medications remain in the development process. An understanding of the pharmacokinetics and pharmacodynamics of available agents is important in selecting an appropriate psychotropic medication for use in an elderly patient.

PSYCHOTROPIC MEDICATION PRESCRIBING GUIDELINES

Pharmacokinetic and pharmacodynamic changes associated with aging should be considered before initiating psychotropic medications. Absorption, distribution, metabolism, and elimination are pharmacokinetic parameters that characterize movement of the medication through the body. Another important pharmacokinetic consideration is the medication half-life. A medication's half-life is the time required after a given dose to decrease peak serum concentration by 50%, and is important in determining the appropriate dosing interval. The steady-state concentration of a medication is approached in three to five half-lives. During titration, dose adjustments should be made only after steady-state concentrations have been reached to maximize benefit and minimize adverse effects. In patients with normal organ function, a medication should be completely metabolized or "washed out" in three to five half-lives after the medication has been discontinued. Clinically significant pharmacokinetic changes of psychotropic medications associated with aging include altered drug distribution due to changes in body composition, decreased metabolism due to decreased hepatic blood flow and reduced oxidative metabolism, and decreased renal elimination due to decreased glomerular filtration rate (3–5).

Pharmacodynamics describes the body's response to medications, including clinical response and adverse drug reactions (ADRs). The World Health Organization defines an adverse reaction as "a response to a drug which is noxious and unintended, and which occurs at doses normally used in man for the prophylaxis, diagnosis, or therapy of disease, or for the modification of physiological function" (6). Older patients are often more sensitive to the effects of psychotropic medications and may experience more ADRs. The risk of experiencing an ADR increases with the number of medications used. Because chronic diseases are more common in the elderly, these patients are more likely to be treated with multiple medications. Thirty percent of hospital admissions in elderly patients may be

FIGURE A.1

The drug discovery, development, and approval process

It takes 12–15 years on average for an experimental drug to travel from the lab to US patients. Only five in 5,000 compounds that enter preclinical testing make it to human testing. One of these five tested in people is ultimately approved.

	Discovery/ Preclinical Testing		Phase I	Phase II	Phase III		FDA		Phase IV
Years	6.5		1.6	2	3.5		1.5	15 Total	
Test Population	Laboratory and animal studies	File NDA at FDA	20 to 100 healthy volunteers	100 to 500 patient volunteers	1000 to 5000 patient volunteers	File NDA at FDA	Review and approval process		Additional post marketing testing required by FDA
Purpose	Assess safety, biological activity, and formulations		Determine safety and dosage	Evaluate effectiveness, look for side effects	Confirm effectiveness, monitor adverse reactions from long-term use				
Success Rate	5,000 compound evaluated		5 enter trials				1 approved		

Figure A-1. Drug discovery, development and approval process. FDA, US Food and Drug Administration. (Reprinted with permission from Phrma.org from Kelly JT. The drug development and approval process. *New Medicines in Development for 2005.* A report.) IND, investigational new drug application; NDA, new drug approval application.

linked to drug-related problems (7). The Institute of Medicine estimated that deaths due to ADRs cost the United States economy eight billion dollars annually (8). Unfortunately, the therapeutic window for many drugs is narrower in the elderly, resulting in a tenuous balance between their risks and pharmacological benefits, often resulting in an increased incidence of toxicity. ADRs can often be avoided through proper prescribing practices and patient evaluation.

The Beers Criteria provide an excellent guide for clinicians to avert inappropriate prescribing practices in the geriatric population (9). Clinicians should be cognizant of such recommendations for use of medications in the elderly. Utilizing the criteria can minimize drug-related problems and costs.

Tables A-1 to A-4 list psychotropic medications with their dosing range, half-life, FDA-approved indications for psychiatric conditions, and common non–FDA-approved (off-label) uses in psychiatry. Guidelines for use in the elderly, including adverse effects and available alternative dosage forms are provided (10–20). When a manufacturer provides no specific dosing guidelines for elderly patients, dosing ranges based on clinical experience are listed. In general, a conservative approach to initiating therapy in elderly patients is to start at one-half the normal adult dose and titrate based on the patient's individual pharmacokinetic and pharmacodynamic response. Table A-5 lists psychotropic medications that are considered inappropriate for use in the elderly due to their high potential for ADRs.

HERBAL MEDICATIONS COMMONLY USED BY THE ELDERLY FOR PSYCHIATRIC INDICATIONS

Herbal medicine is the fastest-growing form of complementary and alternative medicine in the United States (21). Herbal medicines and nutrient supplements are not regulated as drugs by the FDA. Manufacturers are required to meet less stringent standards according to the Dietary Supplement and Health Education Act of 1994 (22). Herbal medicines have been associated with potentially severe adverse events (23). Frequently, patients receiving prescription medications also use herbal medicines or other nutrient supplements which may increase the risk for ADRs (21,24). Unfortunately, many patients using herbal medicines do not openly discuss their use with their physicians or other members of the health care team (21,25,26). It is important for clinicians to ask in a nonjudgmental manner which herbal medicine and nutrient supplements patients are using, in order to identify potential ADRs and drug interactions. Herbal medicines and other nutrient supplements commonly used in the elderly for the treatment of psychiatric conditions are listed in Table A-6.

OBRA REGULATIONS FOR USE OF PSYCHOTROPIC MEDICATIONS IN NURSING HOMES

Psychiatric disorders are common problems in residents of long-term care facilities, particularly in those residents with

TABLE A-1

ANTIPSYCHOTIC MEDICATIONS

Drug (Trade Name)	Dosing Range in the Elderly (mg/day)	Half-Life (hours)	FDA Psychiatric Indications	Common Off-Label Uses in Psychiatry	Comments
Atypical Antipsychotics*[a,b,c]					
Aripiprazole (Abilify)	5–30	75–146	▪ Schizophrenia ▪ Bipolar mania (acute and mixed)	▪ Psychosis and/or agitation in dementia	Partial dopamine agonist activity **Adverse effects:** orthostatic hypotension, headache, insomnia
Clozapine (Clozaril)	6.25–100	4–66	▪ Treatment-resistant schizophrenia	▪ Psychosis in Parkinson's disease	Requires weekly CBC for first 6 months and biweekly thereafter, due to its association with serious blood dyscrasias **Adverse effects:** FDA warning regarding cardiac toxicity leading to potentially fatal myocarditis, sedation, anticholinergic effects, weight gain, agranulocytosis, excessive drooling **Additional dosage form:** rapidly disintegrating tablet (Fazaclo®)
Olanzapine (Zyprexa)	2.5–20	21–54	▪ Schizophrenia ▪ Bipolar disorder (acute, mixed and maintenance) ▪ Agitation associated with schizophrenia and bipolar mania (IM form)	▪ Psychosis and/or agitation in dementia	LFTs should be done periodically during therapy **Adverse effects:** orthostatic hypotension, oversedation, gait instability, weight gain, elevated triglyceride levels, transaminase elevations **Additional dosage form:** injection, rapidly disintegrating tablets (Zydis), also available in combination with fluoxetine for treatment of bipolar depression (Symbyax)
Quetiapine (Seroquel)	12.5–450	6	▪ Schizophrenia ▪ Bipolar mania (acute and mixed)	▪ Psychosis and/or agitation in dementia	Dose adjustment may be necessary for patients with hepatic impairment Give in divided doses (BID) **Adverse effects:** oversedation, orthostatic hypotension, weight gain
Risperidone (Risperdal)	0.25–4	3–20	▪ Schizophrenia ▪ Bipolar mania (acute and mixed)	▪ Psychosis and/or agitation in dementia	Doses should be reduced in patients with renal or hepatic impairment **Adverse effects:** extrapyramidal symptoms **Additional dosage forms:** liquid, rapidly disintegrating tablets (M-Tab), long-acting injection (Consta)

(continued)

TABLE A-1 (continued)

Drug (Trade Name)	Dosing Range in the Elderly (mg/day)	Half-Life (hours)	FDA Psychiatric Indications	Common Off-Label Uses in Psychiatry	Comments
Ziprasidone (Geodon)	40–160	4–10	■ Schizophrenia ■ Bipolar mania (acute and mixed) ■ Acute agitation in schizophrenia (IM dosage form)	■ Psychosis and/or agitation in dementia	Little experience in geriatric population Baseline ECG and follow up ECG recommended Give in divided doses (BID) with food **Adverse effects:** FDA warning regarding propensity to prolong the QTc interval, potentially leading to cardiac arrhythmias, orthostatic hypotension, somnolence, rash **Additional dosage form:** injection
Conventional (Typical) Antipsychotics[d]					
Chlorpromazine (Thorazine)	Not recommended for use	7–119	■ Schizophrenia ■ Preop restlessness/apprehension ■ Manic-type behavior	■ Anxiety	Dose adjustment may be necessary for patients with hepatic impairment **Adverse effects:** QT distortions, hypotension, sedation, extrapyramidal effects, TD, NMS, anticholinergic effects, leukopenia **Additional dosage forms:** liquid, injection
Fluphenazine (Prolixin)	Not recommended as a new medication	13–58	■ Psychotic disorders	■ Psychosis and/or agitation in dementia	**Adverse effects:** extrapyramidal effects, TD, NMS, elevated prolactin **Additional dosage forms:** liquid, injection, long-acting injection (decanoate)
Haloperidol (Haldol)	0.25–4	10–20	■ Psychotic disorders ■ Pediatric behavioral problems ■ Tourette's disorder	■ Psychosis and/or agitation in dementia	**Adverse effects:** extrapyramidal effects, TD, NMS **Additional dosage forms:** liquid, injection, long-acting injection (decanoate) **Drug–drug interaction:** report of encephalopathic syndrome resulting when taken with lithium (rare)

Drug (Trade Name)	Dosing Range in the Elderly (mg/day)	Half-Life (hours)	FDA Psychiatric Indications	Common Off-Label Uses in Psychiatry	Comments
Loxapine (Loxitane)	Not recommended as a new medication	3–4	▪ Schizophrenia	▪ Psychosis and/or agitation in dementia ▪ Psychotic depression	**Adverse effects:** extrapyramidal effects, sedation, hypotension, TD, NMS
Mesoridazine (Serentil)	Not recommended as a new medication	9–31	▪ Schizophrenia	▪ Tourette's disorder	Active metabolite of thioridazine **Black box warning:** prolonged QTc interval **Adverse effects:** hypotension, sedation, TD, NMS **Additional dosage forms:** liquid, injection
Molindone (Moban)	Not recommended as a new medication	2	▪ Schizophrenia	▪ Premenstrual tension	**Adverse effects:** ECG changes, hypotension, extrapyramidal effects, TD, NMS
Perphenazine (Trilafon)	Not recommended as a new medication	8–12	▪ Psychotic disorders	▪ Psychosis and/or agitation in dementia	**Adverse effects:** sedation, anticholinergic effects, ECG changes, hypotension, weight gain, extrapyramidal effects, TD, NMS **Additional dosage forms:** injection, liquid, also available in combination with amitriptyline (Triavil, Etrafon)
Pimozide (Orap)	Not recommended as a new medication	53–55	▪ Tourette's disorder	▪ Schizophrenia	Dose reductions should be considered in severe hepatic impairment **Adverse effects:** extrapyramidal effects, TD, NMS prolonged QTc **Drug–food interaction:** increased plasma concentrations when taken with grapefruit juice
Thioridazine (Mellaril)	Not recommended as a new medication	21–24	▪ Schizophrenia	▪ Psychosis and/or agitation in dementia	Baseline ECG and follow up ECG recommended **Black box warning:** prolonged QTc interval **Adverse effects:** extrapyramidal effects, TD, NMS, hypotension, anticholinergic effects **Additional dosage form:** liquid

(continued)

TABLE A-1 (continued)

Drug (Trade Name)	Dosing Range in the Elderly (mg/day)	Half-Life (hours)	FDA Psychiatric Indications	Common Off-Label Uses in Psychiatry	Comments
Thiothixene (Navane)	Not recommended as a new medication	34	• Schizophrenia	• None	**Adverse effects:** extrapyramidal effects, TD, NMS **Additional dosage form:** injection
Trifluoperazine (Stelazine)	Not recommended for use	7–21	• Anxiety, nonpsychotic • Schizophrenia	• Psychosis and/or agitation in dementia	**Adverse effects:** drowsiness, dizziness, anticholinergic effects, extrapyramidal effects, TD, NMS **Additional dosage forms:** injection, oral

* FDA Public Health Advisory April 11, 2005. The FDA has determined that some elderly patients with dementia-related psychosis treated with atypical anti-psychotic drugs are at an increased risk of death compared to placebo. The deaths are mostly due to heart-related events, or infections. This is thought by the FDA to be a probable "class effect"; the warning includes the olanzapine/fluoxetine combination drug.

[a] Hyperglycemia and diabetes mellitus, in some cases associated with ketoacidosis, have been reported in some patients treated with atypical antipsychotics. This is thought by the FDA to be a probable "class effect".

[b] Cerebrovascular adverse events (CAE), including stroke, have been reported in some elderly demented patients treated with atypical antipsychotics. This is thought by the FDA to be a probable "class effect".

[c] Prescribing in individual elderly patients should be consistent with the need to minimize the potential risk of tardive dyskinesia, neuroleptic malignant syndrome, and seizures.

[d] Use cautiously in patients with seizure history or with conditions that lower seizure threshold.

Compiled from: Maletta G, Mattox KM, Dysken M. Update 2000: guidelines for prescribing psychoactive drugs. *Geriatrics.* 2000;55(March):65–79; Jacobson SA, Pies RW, Greenblatt DJ, eds. *Handbook of Geriatric Psychopharmacology.* Washington, DC: American Psychiatric Publishing, Inc.; 2002; Salzman C, Satlin A, Burrows AB. Geriatric psychopharmacology. In: Schatzberg AF, Nemeroll CB, eds. *Textbook of Psychopharmacology.* Washington, DC: American Psychiatric Publishing, Inc.; 1998; Hutchison TA, Shahan DR, eds. *DRUGDEX® System.* Greenwood Village, Colorado: MICROMEDEX; (Edition expires 3/2004).

ECG, electrocardiogram; FDA, US Food and Drug Administration; LFTs, liver-function tests; QTc, corrected QT interval; TD, tardive dyskinesia; NMS, neuroleptic malignant syndrome; BID, twice daily.

Drug (Trade Name)	Dosing Range in the Elderly (mg/day)	Half-Life (hours)	FDA Psychiatric Indications	Comments
Anxiolytics				
Alprazolam (Xanax)	0.125–2	9–20	• Anxiety • Panic disorder	Not a drug of first choice in elderly Potential for dependence and abuse Dose reductions should be considered in severe hepatic impairment **Adverse effects:** CNS depression, potential for paradoxical reactions **Additional dosage forms:** XR tablet, oral solution, rapidly disintegrating tablets (Niravam®)
Buspirone (Buspar)	10–45	1–11	• Anxiety	Less sedation and psychomotor impairment than benzodiazepines. Lacks potential for physical dependence or abuse. **Adverse effects:** dizziness, light-headedness, diarrhea, nausea, vomiting **Drug–drug interaction:** with MAOI, may result in hypertensive crisis **Drug–food interaction:** decreased peak concentrations when taken with grapefruit juice
Chlordiazepoxide (Librium)	Not recommended as new medication in the elderly	9–30	• Alcohol withdrawal • Anxiety	Active metabolites desmethylchlordiazepoxide and demoxepam with prolonged half-lives (50–100 hours) lead to accumulation in the elderly Dose reductions should be considered in hepatic impairment potential for respiratory depression—use with caution in patients with compromised respiratory function **Adverse effects:** CNS depression, potential for paradoxical reactions **Additional dosage forms:** available in combination with amitriptyline (Limbitrol) and the antispasmodic clidinium bromide (Librax)
Clonazepam (Klonopin)	0.25–4	30–40	• Panic disorders	Avoid abrupt withdrawal Dose reductions should be considered in hepatic impairment **Adverse effects:** CNS depression, potential for paradoxical reactions **Additional dosage forms:** rapidly dissolving wafers
Clorazepate (Tranxene)	Not recommended as new medication in the elderly	Prodrug for nor-diazepam 40–50	• Alcohol withdrawal • Anxiety	Avoid abrupt withdrawal Dose reductions should be considered in hepatic impairment Active metabolites nordiazepam and DMDZ with prolonged half-lives (64–120 hours) may lead to accumulation in the elderly **Adverse effects:** CNS depression, potential for paradoxical reactions
Diazepam (Valium)	Not recommended as new medication in the elderly	20–80	• Alcohol withdrawal • Anxiety	Avoid abrupt withdrawal Dose reductions should be considered in hepatic impairment Active metabolite DMDZ with prolonged half-lives may lead to accumulation in the elderly Use with caution in patients with compromised respiratory function due potential for respiratory depression **Adverse effects:** CNS depression, potential for paradoxical reactions **Additional dosage forms:** injection, oral solution, rectal gel

(continued)

TABLE A-2 (continued)

Drug (Trade Name)	Dosing Range in the Elderly (mg/day)	Half-Life (hours)	FDA Psychiatric Indications	Comments
Halazepam (Paxipam)	Not recommended as new medication in the elderly	9–28	■ Anxiety	**Drug–food interaction:** increased plasma concentrations when taken with grapefruit juice Dose reductions should be considered in hepatic impairment Active metabolite DMDZ with prolonged half-lives may lead to accumulation in the elderly **Adverse effects:** CNS depression, potential for paradoxical reactions
Lorazepam (Ativan)	0.25–2	10–20	■ Anxiety ■ Preanesthesia	Less risk of accumulation in the elderly due to shorter half-life and lack of active metabolites **Adverse effects:** CNS depression, potential for paradoxical reactions **Additional dosage forms:** injection, oral solution
Oxazepam (Serax)	10–45	3–25	■ Alcohol withdrawal ■ Anxiety	Less risk of accumulation in the elderly due to shorter half-life and lack of active metabolites **Adverse effects:** CNS depression, potential for paradoxical reactions
Prazepam (Centrax)	Not recommended as new medication in the elderly	78	■ Anxiety	Active metabolite DMDZ with prolonged half-lives may lead to accumulation in the elderly **Adverse effects:** CNS depression, potential for paradoxical reactions
Sedative/Hypnotics Estazolam (ProSom)	0.5	8–28	■ Insomnia	Indicated for short-term (7–10 days) treatment of insomnia Dose reductions should be considered in hepatic impairment Use with caution in patients with compromised respiratory function due potential for respiratory depression **Adverse effects:** CNS depression, potential for paradoxical reactions
Flurazepam (Dalmane)	Not recommended for use in the elderly	Prodrug	■ Insomnia	Active metabolite desalkylflurazepam with prolonged half-live may lead to accumulation in the elderly **Adverse effects:** CNS depression, potential for paradoxical reactions
Eszopiclone (Lunesta)	1–2	6–9	■ Insomnia	Non-benzodiazepine hypnotic agent Approved for long-term use Indicated for the treatment of patients who experience difficulty falling asleep as well as for the treatment of patients who are unable to sleep through the night **Adverse Effects:** unpleasant taste, headache, drowsiness and dizziness
Quazepam (Doral)	Not recommended for use in the elderly	25–41	■ Insomnia	Dose reductions should be considered in hepatic impairment **Adverse effects:** CNS depression, potential for paradoxical reactions

TABLE A-2 (continued)

Drug (Trade Name)	Dosing Range in the Elderly (mg/day)	Half-Life (hours)	FDA Psychiatric Indications	Comments
Temazepam (Restoril)	7.5–30	5–20	▪ Insomnia	Tolerance and dependence can occur with nightly use for more than a few weeks **Adverse effects:** CNS depression, potential for paradoxical reactions **Additional dosage forms:** rapidly dissolving tablets
Triazolam (Halcion)	0.125–0.25	2–4	▪ Insomnia	Tolerance and dependence can occur with nightly use for more than a few weeks Dose reductions should be considered in hepatic impairment **Adverse effects:** CNS depression, potential for paradoxical reactions **Drug–food interaction:** increased plasma concentrations when taken with grapefruit juice
Zaleplon (Sonata)	5–10	1	▪ Insomnia	Indicated for short-term (7–10 days) treatment of insomnia. May be useful in reducing sleep latency Dose reductions should be considered in hepatic impairment and severe renal impairment **Adverse effects:** somnolence, dizziness, dry mouth
Zolpidem (Ambien)	5–10	2–3	▪ Insomnia	Indicated for short-term (7–10 days) treatment of insomnia Dose reductions should be considered in hepatic impairment **Adverse effects:** drowsiness, dizziness

Compiled from: Maletta G, Mattox KM, Dysken M. Update 2000: guidelines for prescribing psychoactive drugs. *Geriatrics*. 2000;55(March):65–79; Jacobson SA, Pies RW, Greenblatt DJ, eds. *Handbook of Geriatric Psychopharmacology*. Washington, DC: American Psychiatric Publishing, Inc.; 2002; Salzman C, Satlin A, Burrows AB. Geriatric psychopharmacology. In: Schatzberg AF, Nemeroll CB, eds. *Textbook of Psychopharmacology*. Washington, DC: American Psychiatric Publishing, Inc.; 1998; Hutchison TA, Shahan DR, eds. *DRUGDEX*® System. Greenwood Village, Colorado: MICROMEDEX; (Edition expires 3/2004).

CNS, central nervous system; DMDZ, desmethyldiazepam; FDA, US Food and Drug Administration; MAOI, monoamine oxidase inhibitor; XR, extended release.

TABLE A-3
ANTIDEPRESSANTS

Drug (Trade Name)	Dosing Range in the Elderly (mg/day)	Half-Life in Adults (hours)	FDA Psychiatric Indications	Comments
Tricyclic (TCA) Antidepressants				
TCA-Tertiary Amines				
Amitriptyline (Elavil)	Not recommended for the treatment of depression in the elderly 25–50 for treatment of neuropathic pain	9–25	• MDD	Lower doses used for neuropathic pain **Adverse effects:** anticholinergic effects, orthostatic hypotension, sedation, and increased degree of heart block or worsening of pre-existing arrhythmia in patients with cardiac disease **Additional dosage forms:** injection, oral solution, combination product with perphenazine (Etrafon or Trilafon) and chlordiazepoxide (Limbitrol)
Clomipramine (Anafranil)	Not recommended for use in the elderly	19–37	• OCD	Only TCA not approved for depression Contraindicated in recovery phase of acute MI **Adverse effects:** anticholinergic effects, orthostatic hypotension, sedation, and increased degree of heart block or worsening of pre-existing arrhythmia in patients with cardiac disease **Drug–food interaction:** increased plasma concentrations when taken with grapefruit juice
Doxepin (Sinequan)	Not recommended for use in the elderly	16.8 (range: 8–25)	• MDD • Anxiety • Psychotic depressive disorders • Depressive disorders with associated anxiety	Give at bedtime due to sedating properties **Adverse effects:** anticholinergic effects, orthostatic hypotension, sedation, and increased degree of heart block or worsening of pre-existing arrhythmia in patients with cardiac disease **Additional dosage form:** oral solution
Imipramine (Tofranil)	Not recommended for use in the elderly	6–18	• MDD	Half-life significantly extended in elderly (25–30 hours) **Adverse effects:** anticholinergic effects, orthostatic hypotension, sedation, and increased degree of heart block or worsening of pre-existing arrhythmia in patients with cardiac disease **Additional dosage forms:** injection, oral solution
Trimipramine (Surmontil)	Not recommended for use in the elderly	23	• MDD	**Adverse effects:** anticholinergic effects, orthostatic hypotension, sedation, and increased degree of heart block or worsening of pre-existing arrhythmia in patients with cardiac disease
TCA-Secondary Amines				
Desipramine (Norpramin)	10–100	14.3–24.7	• MDD	Recommended serum level: 75–150 ng/mL TCA of choice in geriatric population **Adverse effects:** anticholinergic effects, orthostatic hypotension, sedation, and increased degree of heart block or worsening of pre-existing arrhythmia in patients with cardiac disease

Drug (Trade Name)	Dosing Range in the Elderly (mg/day)	Half-Life in Adults (hours)	FDA Psychiatric Indications	Comments
Nortriptyline (Pamelor)	10–100	15–39	■ MDD	Recommended serum level: 50–100 ng/mL Used for neuropathic pain TCA of choice in geriatric population Half-life significantly extended in elderly (90 hours) **Adverse effects:** anticholinergic effects, weight gain, sedation, and increased degree of heart block or worsening of pre-existing arrhythmia in patients with cardiac disease **Additional dosage form:** oral solution
Protriptyline (Vivactil)	Not recommended for use in the elderly	54–198	■ MDD	**Adverse effects:** anticholinergic effects, orthostatic hypotension, sedation, and increased degree of heart block or worsening of pre-existing arrhythmia in patients with cardiac disease
Amoxapine (Asendin)	Not recommended for use in the elderly	8	■ MDD ■ Psychotic depression	Active metabolite of loxapine lending dopamine antagonist properties Contraindicated in recovery phase of acute MI **Adverse effects:** extrapyramidal side effects including akathisia dyskinetic movements, tardive dyskinesia, dystonic reactions, and neuroleptic malignant syndrome
Tetracyclic antidepressants				
Maprotiline (Ludiomil)	Not recommended for use in the elderly	27–58	■ MDD	Contraindicated in acute MI and seizure disorders Use caution in type 2 diabetics due to altered insulin secretion **Adverse effects:** seizures and exanthematous rash
Mirtazapine (Remeron)	7.5–45	25–40	■ MDD	Sedation resolves at higher doses Appetite stimulant Baseline and periodic LFT monitoring recommended **Adverse effects:** somnolence, weight gain, xerostomia, constipation, and agranulocytosis **Additional dosage form:** orally disintegrating tablets (SolTab) **Drug–drug interactions:** MAOIs
Selective Serotonin-Reuptake Inhibitors (SSRI)[a]				
Citalopram (Celexa)	10–60	33–37	■ MDD	Potential adverse events associated with discontinuation Avoid abrupt discontinuation when possible **Adverse effects:** restlessness, anxiety, dizziness, insomnia, tremor, hyponatremia, nausea/vomiting, anorexia, dry mouth, diaphoresis, and ejaculatory disorder **Drug–drug interactions:** MAOIs
Escitalopram (Lexapro)	5–20	22–32	■ MDD ■ GAD	S(+)-enantiomer of citalopram Potential adverse events associated with discontinuation Avoid abrupt discontinuation when possible **Adverse effects:** nausea, insomnia, somnolence, ejaculation disorder, diaphoresis, and fatigue

(continued)

TABLE A-3 (continued)

Drug (Trade Name)	Dosing Range in the Elderly (mg/day)	Half-Life in Adults (hours)	FDA Psychiatric Indications	Comments
Fluoxetine (Prozac)	10–60 90 (weekly dosing)	1–3 days (acute administration) 4–6 days (chronic administration) Norfluoxetine 4–16 days (acute and chronic administration)	• MDD • Bulimia nervosa • Panic disorder • Premenstrual dysphoric disorder (Sarafem) • OCD	Dose reductions should be considered in hepatic impairment First dose of Prozac weekly should be separated by 7 days after last daily dosing regimen **Adverse effects:** nausea, hypotension, headache, anxiety, nervousness, insomnia, dry mouth, anorexia, visual disturbances, weight loss, and sexual dysfunction **Additional dosage forms:** oral solution, extended-release product, combination product with olanzapine for bipolar depression (Symbyax) **Drug–drug interaction:** MAOIs, thioridazine, drugs metabolized by CYP450
Fluvoxamine (Luvox)	50–300	15.6	• OCD	Only SSRI not approved for depression Dose reductions should be considered in hepatic impairment **Adverse effects:** headache, insomnia, somnolence, nervousness, dizziness, dry mouth, diarrhea, and dyspepsia **Drug–drug interactions:** MAOIs
Paroxetine (Paxil, Paxil CR)	10–60 25 to 75 (CR)	15–22	• MDD • OCD • Social anxiety disorder • GAD • Panic disorder • PTSD	Dose adjustment may be necessary for patients with renal and hepatic impairment Potential adverse events associated with discontinuation Avoid abrupt discontinuation when possible **Adverse effects:** GI symptoms, sexual dysfunction, weight gain and sedation **Additional dosage form:** controlled release tablet **Drug–drug interactions:** MAOIs, drugs metabolized by CYP450
Sertraline (Zoloft)	25–200	22–32	• MDD • OCD • Panic disorder • PTSD • Premenstrual dysphoric disorder • Social anxiety disorder	Dose adjustment may be required with hepatic impairment Potential adverse events associated with discontinuation Avoid abrupt discontinuation when possible **Adverse effects:** GI symptoms, sexual dysfunction **Drug–drug interaction:** MAOIs **Drug–food interaction:** increased plasma concentrations when taken with grapefruit juice
Monoamine Oxidase Inhibitors (MAOI)[b,c] **Phenelzine (Nardil)**	Not recommended for use in the elderly	1.5–4	• Atypical depression	Contraindicated with pheochromocytoma, CHF, history of liver disease or abnormal LFTs **Adverse effects:** orthostatic hypotension, sedation, anticholinergic effects, weight gain, hepatocellular damage, sexual dysfunction, and hypertensive crisis **Drug–drug interactions:** multiple contraindicated concomitant medications **Drug–food interactions:** tyramine-containing foods or caffeine containing beverages

[a]Class of choice for depression in geriatric population

Drug (Trade Name)	Dosing Range in the Elderly (mg/day)	Half-Life in Adults (hours)	FDA Psychiatric Indications	Comments
Selegiline (Eldepryl)	5–30	1.2	• Parkinson's disease	Not approved for depression, but used off-label **Adverse effects:** sleep disturbances, dizziness, nausea, headache, psychosis, agitation, confusion, and dyskinesias **Drug–drug interactions:** multiple contraindicated concomitant medications **Drug–food interactions:** caution about the consumption of tyramine-containing foods with doses of 20 mg daily or more of selegiline
Tranylcypromine (Parnate)	Not recommended for use in the elderly	1.5–3.5	• Major depressive episode without melancholia	Psychological dependence and tolerance reported Contraindicated with pheochromocytoma, CHF **Adverse effects:** orthostatic hypotension, insomnia, anticholinergic effects, sexual dysfunction, and hypertensive crisis **Drug–drug interactions:** multiple contraindicated concomitant medications **Drug–food interactions:** tyramine-containing foods or caffeine containing beverages
Isocarboxazid (Marplan)	Not recommended for use in the elderly	Not available	• MDD • Atypical depression	Contraindicated with pheochromocytoma, CHF, history of liver disease or abnormal LFTs **Adverse effects:** orthostatic hypotension, anticholinergic effects, sexual dysfunction and hypertensive crisis **Drug–drug interactions:** multiple contraindicated concomitant medications **Drug–food interactions:** tyramine containing foods or caffeine-containing beverages

[b]should not be used as first-line antidepressant
[c]separate administration from SSRIs, SNRIs and TCAs by 14 days

Aminoketone antidepressants

Drug (Trade Name)	Dosing Range in the Elderly (mg/day)	Half-Life in Adults (hours)	FDA Psychiatric Indications	Comments
Bupropion (Wellbutrin, Wellbutrin SR, Wellbutrin XL)	100–450	14	• MDD	Lower incidence of sexual side effects compared to SSRIs May cause generalized seizures in a dose-dependent manner. Maximum daily dose should not exceed 450 mg. Best given in divided doses Wellbutrin SR initial dose 150 mg QAM then increase to 150 mg BID Wellbutrin XL initial dose 150 mg QAM then increase to 300 mg QAM **Adverse effects:** dizziness, tremor, anxiety, insomnia, skin reactions, nausea, vomiting, constipation, and xerostomia, muscle weakness **Additional dosage forms:** sustained-release tablet, extended-release tablet

Triazolopyridine antidepressants

Drug (Trade Name)	Dosing Range in the Elderly (mg/day)	Half-Life in Adults (hours)	FDA Psychiatric Indications	Comments
Nefazodone (Serzone)	100–400	1.9–5.3	• MDD	Avoid use in hepatic dysfunction, monitor LFTs **Black box warning:** hepatic failure **Adverse effects:** dizziness, orthostatic hypotension, nausea, xerostomia, asthenia, and somnolence **Drug–drug interactions:** concurrent use with simvastatin, cisapride, triazolam, pimozide, or carbamazepine should be avoided
Trazodone (Desyrel)	25–200	7.1	• MDD	More commonly used for sedating properties than as an antidepressant **Adverse effects:** sedation, cognitive slowing, dizziness, orthostatic hypotension, and priapism (rare) resulting in need for surgical intervention and potential impotence if not corrected

(continued)

TABLE A-3
(continued)

Drug (Trade Name)	Dosing Range in the Elderly (mg/day)	Half-Life in Adults (hours)	FDA Psychiatric Indications	Comments
Serotonin Norepinephrine Reuptake Inhibitors (SNRI)				
Duloxetine (Cymbalta)	30–90	11–16	• MDD • Pain associated with diabetic peripheral neuropathy	**Adverse effects:** insomnia, somnolence, headache, nausea, diarrhea, and dry mouth
Venlafaxine (Effexor, Effexor XR)	37.5–375	5	• MDD • GAD • Social anxiety disorder	Dose-dependent increase in diastolic blood pressure Monitor blood pressure regularly and adjust or discontinue accordingly Dosing adjustment may be necessary in renal and hepatic impairment Effexor XR initial dose 37.5 mg daily then increase to 75 mg daily. Titrate as indicated **Adverse effects:** nausea, constipation, xerostomia, dizziness, nervousness, sweating, asthenia, altered orgasm, anorexia **Additional dosage form:** extended-release tablet

Compiled from: Jacobson SA, Pies RW, Greenblatt DJ, eds. *Handbook of Geriatric Psychopharmacology.* Washington, DC: American Psychiatric Publishing, Inc.; 2002; Hutchison TA, Shahan DR, eds. *DRUGDEX® System.* Greenwood Village, Colorado: MICROMEDEX; (Edition expires 3/2004); McEvoy GK, et al., eds. *AHFS Drug Information 2001.* Bethesda, MD: American Society of Health-System Pharmacists, Inc.; 2001; DiPiro JT, et al., eds. *Pharmacotherapy: A Pathophysiologic Approach.* 5th Ed. McGraw-Hill Medical Publishing Division; 2002; Chui HFK. Antidepressants in the elderly. *IJCP.* 1997;51:369–374; Lapid MI, Rumans TA. Evaluation and management of geriatric depression in primary care. *Mayo Clin Proc.* 2003;73:1423–1429.

BID, twice a day; CHF, congestive heart failure; CYP450, cytochrome P450; FDA, US Food and Drug Administration; GI, gastrointestinal; LFT, liver-function test; MAOIs, monoamine oxidase inhibitors; MDD, major depressive disorder; MI, myocardial infarction; OCD, obsessive-compulsive disorder; PTSD, posttraumatic stress disorder; QAM, in the morning; SSRIs, selective serotonin-reuptake inhibitors; TCA, tricyclic antidepressant.

MOOD STABILIZERS, STIMULANTS AND COGNITIVE ENHANCERS

Drug (Trade Name)	Dosing Range in the Elderly (mg/day)	Half-Life, in Adults (hours)	FDA Psychiatric Indications	Common Off-Label Uses in Psychiatry	Comments
Mood Stabilizers					
Carbamazepine (Tegretol)	100–1200	12–17	None	▪ Aggression ▪ Agitation (dementia, and traumatic brain injury related) ▪ Behavioral problems ▪ Bipolar disorder ▪ Depression ▪ PTSD ▪ Psychotic disorder	Baseline and periodic evaluations of CBC and LFTs Contraindicated in patients with bone marrow suppression Used for pain and tic douloureux **Serum concentration:** Bipolar disease: 4–8 μg/mL Agitation in dementia: 2.4–5.2 μg/mL **Black box warning:** aplastic anemia and agranulocytosis **Adverse effects:** dizziness, ataxia, weakness, drowsiness, asthenia, nausea, leukopenia, thrombocytopenia, bradycardia, exacerbation of sinus node dysfunction, and hepatic dysfunction **Additional dosage forms:** chewable tablet, oral suspension, and extended-release tablets **Drug–drug interaction:** MAOIs: induces enzyme activity which may result in altered plasma concentrations of medications **Drug–food interaction:** increased plasma concentrations when taken with grapefruit juice
Valproic acid (Depakene, Depakote)	125–1500	8–17	▪ Bipolar mania	▪ Affective disorders ▪ Bipolar disorder maintenance ▪ Borderline personality disorder ▪ Schizoaffective disorder—bipolar type ▪ Agitation in dementia ▪ Behavior disorders in intellectually disabled	Drug of choice in bipolar disease Baseline and periodic evaluations of CBC, LFTs, and amylase **Serum concentration:** Bipolar disease: 50–100 μg/mL Agitation in dementia: 40–80 μg/mL **Black box warning:** hepatotoxicity and pancreatitis **Adverse effects:** GI intolerance, muscle weakness, sedation, thrombocytopenia, leukopenia, rash, alopecia, SIADH, and tremor **Additional dosage forms:** capsule with sprinkles, sustained and extended-release tablets, oral solution, and injectable
Lithium (Lithobid, others)	150–1800	14–36	▪ Bipolar mania ▪ Bipolar disease maintenance	▪ Depression ▪ Depression—post-ECT ▪ Depression—refractory ▪ Bipolar depression ▪ Depression with psychosis	First-line agent in bipolar disease Dose reduction recommended in renal Baseline and/or periodic evaluations of renal function, CBC, TFTs, and ECG **Serum concentration:** Acute mania: 0.4–0.8 mEq/L Maintenance: 0.2–0.6 mEq/L

(continued)

703

TABLE A-4
(continued)

Drug (Trade Name)	Dosing Range in the Elderly (mg/day)	Half-Life, in Adults (hours)	FDA Psychiatric Indications	Common Off-Label Uses in Psychiatry	Comments
					Black box warning: toxicity can occur at doses close to therapeutic levels **Adverse effects:** GI intolerance, muscle weakness, lethargy, polydipsia, polyuria, weight gain, cognitive impairment, headache, tremor, nephrogenic diabetes insipidus, hypothyroidism, T-wave inversion, atrioventricular block, bradycardia, dermatological effects, and leukocytosis **Additional dosage forms:** extended-release tablet and oral solution **Drug–drug interaction:** NSAIDs, potential for multiple drug interactions
Lamotrigine (Lamictal)	12.5–400	31	• Bipolar disorder	• Bipolar depression • Agitation in dementia	Dose adjustment recommended for patients with renal and hepatic dysfunction **Black box warning:** severe life-threatening rashes, Steven-Johnson syndrome, and toxic epidermal necrosis have occurred during therapy in adults (0.3%). With first sign of rash, therapy should be tapered and discontinued if indicated. Titrate dose slowly. **Adverse effects:** GI intolerance, abdominal pain, dizziness, ataxia, somnolence, insomnia, diplopia, blurred vision, and nonserious rash **Additional dosage form:** chewable tablet **Drug–drug interaction:** valproic acid decreases clearance; carbamazepine increases clearance
Gabapentin (Neurontin)	100–3600	5–7	• None	• Anxiety disorder • Behavior problems—dementia related • Bipolar disorder • Mania • OCD—augmentation therapy • Panic disorder	Dose reduction recommended in patients with renal impairment Used for pain **Adverse effects:** GI intolerance, xerostomia, weight gain, peripheral edema, dizziness, ataxia, somnolence, fatigue **Additional dosage form:** oral solution
Oxcarbazepine (Trileptal)	600–1200	1–2.5	• None	• Bipolar disorder • Panic disorder	Little information on its use in the elderly Patients with hypersensitivity to carbamazepine may experience hypersensitivity to oxcarbazepine **Adverse effects:** headache, ataxia, dizziness, nausea, hyponatremia **Additional dosage form:** oral solution

Drug (Trade Name)	Dosing Range in the Elderly (mg/day)	Half-Life, in Adults (hours)	FDA Psychiatric Indications	Common Off-Label Uses in Psychiatry	Comments
Topiramate (Topamax)	25–200	18–24	• None	• Bipolar disorder	Dosing adjustment for renal and hepatic impairment **Adverse effects:** oligohydrosis, hyperthermia, psychomotor slowing, somnolence, fatigue, acute myopia, and secondary angle-closure glaucoma **Additional dosage form:** sprinkle capsules
Stimulants Modafinil (Provigil)	100–200	7.5–15	• Idiopathic hypersomnia • Narcolepsy	• Depression	Morning dosing recommended Used as an augmentation therapy for depression Dose adjustment recommended for patients with renal and hepatic impairment Caution recommended in patients with cardiovascular disease, emotional instability, drug abuse, or psychosis **Adverse effects:** headache, nausea, nervousness, anxiety, infection, hypertension, and insomnia **Drug–drug interaction:** Potential interaction with medications metabolized by CYP450 isozymes
Atomoxetine (Strattera)	40–80	4–5	• ADHD	• Fatigue • Somnolence—drug induced	No data regarding use in elderly Contraindicated in patients with narrow-angle glaucoma Caution recommended in patients with cardiovascular or cerebrovascular disease due to increases in blood pressure and pulse Dose reduction recommended for patients with hepatic impairment **Adverse effects:** xerostomia, insomnia, nausea, decreased appetite, constipation, dysmenorrhea, dizziness, urinary hesitation or retention, decreased libido, erectile disturbance, mydriasis, and hypersensitivity (angioneurotic edema, urticaria, and rash) **Drug–drug interaction:** Potential interaction with medications metabolized by CYP450 isozymes
Methylphenidate (Ritalin, others)	2.5–60	2–7	• ADD • Narcolepsy	• Depression	Caution recommended in patients with seizure history, hypertension, visual disturbances, and severe depression of either exogenous or endogenous origin Contraindicated in patients with marked anxiety, tension, agitation, glaucoma, motor tics, or with a family history of Tourette's syndrome

Additional off-label uses under Methylphenidate:
• Bipolar disorder—adjunctive treatment
• Depression
• OCD
• Schizophrenia
• Cancer-associated fatigue
• Apathetic presentation in elderly

(continued)

TABLE A-4 (continued)

Drug (Trade Name)	Dosing Range in the Elderly (mg/day)	Half-Life, in Adults (hours)	FDA Psychiatric Indications	Common Off-Label Uses in Psychiatry	Comments
Dextroamphetamine and amphetamine mixture (Adderall)	5–40	9–13	• ADHD	• Depression • Apathetic presentation in elderly	**Adverse effects:** nervousness, insomnia, hypersensitivity (including skin rash, urticaria, fever, arthralgia, and thrombocytopenic purpura), anorexia, nausea, abdominal pain, weight loss (during prolonged therapy), dizziness, palpitations, headache, dyskinesia, drowsiness, hypertension, angina, and cardiac arrhythmia **Additional dosage forms:** extended-release and sustained-release tablets **Black box warning:** potential for dependence
Cognitive Enhancers **Acetylcholinesterase Inhibitors**[a] Donepezil (Aricept)	5–15	70	• Mild to moderate dementia of the Alzheimer's type	• Cognitive impairment in multiple sclerosis • Dementia with Lewy bodies • Huntington's disease • Memory dysfunction • Supranuclear palsy progressive • Schizoaffective disorders • ADHD • Vascular dementia	**Adverse effects:** anorexia, insomnia, weight loss, emotional lability, depression **Drug–drug interactions:** lithium, phenytoin, haloperidol, propoxyphene, meperidine **Additional dosage forms:** extended release capsule Take without regard to food **Adverse effects:** nausea, diarrhea, vomiting, anorexia, syncope, dizziness, insomnia, abnormal dreams, and muscle cramps **Drug–drug interaction:** concomitant use with NSAID may increase risk for ulcers **Additional dosage forms:** orally disintegrating tablets (ODT)
Galantamine (Razadyne, Razadyne ER)	8–24	5.7	• Mild to moderate dementia of the Alzheimer's type	• Anticholinergic syndrome • Autism • Vascular dementia • Lewy body dementia	Take with food Formerly Reminyl Dose titration at 4-week intervals Dose reduction recommended in patients with moderate renal or hepatic impairment Use not recommended in severe renal or hepatic impairment **Adverse effects:** nausea, diarrhea, vomiting, anorexia, bradycardia, and tremor **Additional dosage form:** oral solution , extended release tablet (Razadyne ER) **Drug–drug interaction:** concomitant use with NSAID may increase risk for ulcers

Drug (Trade Name)	Dosing Range in the Elderly (mg/day)	Half-Life, in Adults (hours)	FDA Psychiatric Indications	Common Off-Label Uses in Psychiatry	Comments
Rivastigmine (Exelon)	3–12	1.4–1.7	■ Mild to moderate dementia of the Alzheimer's type	■ Dementia with Lewy bodies ■ Huntington's disease ■ Parkinson's disease	Take with food Dose titration at 2-week intervals **Adverse effects:** nausea, diarrhea, vomiting, anorexia, dizziness, fatigue, and malaise **Additional dosage form:** oral solution **Drug–drug interaction:** concomitant use with NSAID may increase risk for ulcers
Tacrine (Cognex)	Not recommended for use in the elderly	2–4	■ Mild to moderate dementia of the Alzheimer's Type		Take with food if upset stomach occurs. 10 mg QID starting dose Dose titration at 4 weeks to 20 mg QID. Titrate to 40 QID if tolerated. LFTs (serum transaminase activity) recommended every other week dose titration and every 3 months thereafter Contraindicated in patients with hepatic dysfunction **Adverse effects:** elevated transaminases, nausea and/or vomiting, diarrhea, dyspepsia, myalgia, anorexia, and ataxia **Drug–drug interaction:** concomitant use with NSAID may increase risk for ulcers

[a]Off-label use for inattentional agitation in patients with severe dementia and/or chronic psychosis.

N-methyl-D-aspartate (NMDA) Receptor Antagonist

Drug (Trade Name)	Dosing Range in the Elderly (mg/day)	Half-Life, in Adults (hours)	FDA Psychiatric Indications	Common Off-Label Uses in Psychiatry	Comments
Memantine (Namenda)	5–20	60–80	■ Moderate to severe dementia of the Alzheimer's type		Dose titration at weekly intervals Dosing adjustment may be necessary in renal dysfunction Contraindicated in severe renal dysfunction as insufficient information is available in this population Can be used in combination with acetylcholinesterase inhibitors **Adverse effects:** dizziness, confusion, headache, and constipation **Drug–drug interaction:** caution when given concomitantly with acetazolamide and sodium bicarbonate, as tubular secretion reduced when urine pH > 8

Compiled from: Jacobson SA, Pies RW, Greenblatt DJ, eds. *Handbook of Geriatric Psychopharmacology.* Washington, DC: American Psychiatric Publishing, Inc.; 2002; Salzman C, Satlin A, Burrows AB. Geriatric psychopharmacology. In: Schatzberg AF, Nemeroll CB. eds. *Textbook of Psychopharmacology.* Washington, DC: American Psychiatric Publishing, Inc.; 1998; Hutchison TA, Shahan DR, eds. *DRUGDEX® System.* Greenwood Village, Colorado: MICROMEDEX; (Edition expires 3/2004); McEvoy GK, et al., eds. *AHFS Drug Information 2001.* Bethesda, MD: American Society of Health-System Pharmacists, Inc.; 2001; DiPiro JT, et al., eds. *Pharmacotherapy: A Pathophysiologic Approach.* 5th Ed. McGraw-Hill Medical Publishing Division; 2002; Chui HFK. Antidepressants in the elderly. *IJCP.* 1997;51:369–374; Lapid MI, Rumans TA. Evaluation and management of geriatric depression in primary care. *Mayo Clin Proc.* 2003;73:1423–1429; Complete prescribing information for Lamictal (lamotrigene). Available from http://www.lamictal.com. Accessed January 29, 2004; Complete prescribing information for Provigil (modafinil). Available from http://www.provigil.com. Accessed January 29, 2004; Complete prescribing information for Strattera (atomoxetine). Available from http://www.strattera.com. Accessed January 29, 2004.

ADD, attention deficit disorder; ADHD, attention deficit hyperactivity disorder; CBC, complete blood count; CYP450, cytochrome P450; ECG, electrocardiogram; ECT, electroconvulsive therapy; FDA, US Food and Drug Administration; GI, gastrointestinal; LFTs, liver-function tests; MAOIs, monoamine oxidase inhibitors; NSAID, nonsteroidal anti-inflammatory drug; OCD, obsessive–compulsive disorder; PTSD, posttraumatic stress disorder; SIADH, syndrome of inappropriate antidiuretic hormone; TFTs, thyroid function tests.

TABLE A-5
PSYCHOTROPIC MEDICATIONS CONSIDERED INAPPROPRIATE FOR USE IN THE ELDERLY

Medication	Comments
Tertiary amine tricyclic antidepressants (e.g., amitriptyline, doxepin)	High anticholinergic and sedating properties—not antidepressant of choice in elderly
Barbiturates (other than phenobarbital)	Addictive—should not be started as new medications in the elderly. High potential for toxicity.
Diphenhydramine	Increased risk for falls and oversedation. Not for use as a hypnotic; for allergies, use lowest dose possible
Ethchlorvynol	Because of newer, safer, and more effective medications for sleep, generally no longer used
Glutethamide	Because of newer, safer, and more effective medications for sleep, generally no longer used
Hydroxyzine	Not for use as a hypnotic; for allergies, use lowest dose possible
Long-acting benzodiazepines (e.g., diazepam, chlordiazepoxide, flurazepam)	Accumulation leading to sedation, ataxia, falls, and increased hip fractures
Methyprylon	Because of newer, safer, and more effective medications for sleep, generally no longer used
Meprobamate	Accumulation leading to sedation, ataxia, and increased hip fractures
Mesoridazine	CNS and extrapyramidal adverse effects
Thioridazine	CNS and extrapyramidal adverse effects

Compiled from: Fick DM, Cooper JW, Wade WE, et al. Updating the Beers Criteria for potentially inappropriate medication use in older adults. *Arch Intern Med.* 2003;163:2; Hutchison TA, Shahan DR, eds. *DRUGDEX® System.* Greenwood Village, Colorado: MICROMEDEX; (Edition expires 3/2004).

CNS, central nervous system.

TABLE A-6
PSYCHOTROPIC HERBAL MEDICINES AND SUPPLEMENTS COMMONLY USED IN ELDERLY

Herbal/Supplement	Traditional Use[a]	Comments and Cautions
Ginkgo	Cognitive impairment, circulation	▪ Potential drug interaction with anticoagulants
St. John's wort	Depression, Anxiety	▪ Potential drug interaction with SSRIs ▪ Phototoxicity
Ginseng	General health and energy	▪ Potential drug interaction with hypoglycemic drugs ▪ May increase blood pressure
Passionflower	Sedative Insomnia	▪ May potentiate other CNS depressants
Kava kava	Insomnia	▪ May potentiate other CNS depressants ▪ Avoid in patients with Parkinson's disease
Ma huang (ephedra)	Stimulant	▪ Likely unsafe, banned in the United States ▪ Potential drug interaction with stimulants, β-blockers, MAOIs, phenothiazines, theophylline
Melatonin	Insomnia	▪ Potential drug interaction with anticoagulants
SAMe	Depression	▪ Caution with concomitant antidepressants
Tarvil	Tardive dyskinesia	▪ Classified as a "medical food;" used for the management of tardive dyskinesia in men ▪ Contraindications include diabetes, thyroid dysfunction, malabsorption, pancreatitis, renal disease, and gout
Valerian	Anxiety Sedative Insomnia	▪ May potentiate other CNS depressants

Compiled from: Hutchison TA, Shahan DR, eds. *DRUGDEX® System.* Greenwood Village, Colorado: MICROMEDEX; (Edition expires 3/2004); Sifton DW, ed. *PDR Drug Guide for Mental Health Professionals.* Montvale, NJ: Thomson Medical Economics; 2002.
[a]Either to improve normal function (eg, circulation, energy), or to treat disease (eg, cognitive impairment, depression).

CNS, central nervous system; MAOIs, monoamine oxidase inhibitors; SSRIs, selective serotonin-reuptake inhibitors.

TABLE A-7
OBRA REGULATIONS FOR USE OF PSYCHOTROPIC MEDICATIONS IN NURSING HOMES

Psychotropic Medication	Indication	Dose, Duration, or Duplication	Monitoring Adverse Reactions
Antidepressant	Depression Pain Insomnia	▪ Dose adjusted for concomitant disease states for clinically accepted duration of use ▪ Lowest possible dose for symptom control	Documentation of common adverse reactions in progress notes or allergy and adverse reaction data as indicated
Anxiolytic	Anxiety disorder PTSD	▪ Short-acting agent preferred ▪ Limit daily use to less than 4 months unless dosage reduction is unsuccessful ▪ Attempt dosage reduction twice in a year unless harmful to the patient ▪ Long-acting benzodiazepine only if resident fails trial of short-acting agent	Documentation of common adverse reactions in progress notes or allergy and adverse reaction data as indicated
Sedative/Hypnotic	Insomnia	▪ Limit daily use to less than 10 days unless dosage reduction is unsuccessful ▪ Attempt dosage reduction three times in 6 months unless harmful to the patient	Documentation of common adverse reactions in progress notes or allergy and adverse reaction data as indicated
Antipsychotic	**Psychiatric diagnosis:** Schizophrenia, schizo-affective disorder, delusional disorder, psychotic mood disorders, acute psychotic episodes, brief reactive psychosis, atypical psychosis, Tourette's disorder, Huntington's disease **Organic mental syndrome:** "Delirium, dementia, and amnestic and other cognitive disorders" *with associated psychotic and/or agitated behavior* ▪ Quantitative, objective documentation of specific behavior warranting antipsychotic medication ▪ The associated psychotic and/or agitated behaviors must be quantitatively and objectively documented ▪ These behaviors should be persistent and not caused by preventable reasons ▪ The behaviors must cause the resident to present a danger to himself/herself, others, or cause impairment in functional capacity **Nausea/Vomiting/Hiccups**	**Attempt dosage reduction unless:** ▪ Dosage reduction has been attempted twice in a year and failed ▪ Psychiatric diagnosis is present and symptoms stabilized without incurring significant adverse effects ▪ Written justification stating dose reduction is clinically contraindicated is provided **PRN only if:** ▪ Titrating doses upward for symptom relief ▪ Titrating dose downward to avoid adverse effects or for dosage reduction ▪ Managing unexpected, harmful behaviors that cannot be managed in other ways **Nausea and vomiting:** ▪ Short-term (7 day) use for treatment of nausea and vomiting ▪ Residents with nausea and vomiting secondary to cancer or chemotherapy can be treated with higher doses for longer periods of time	Documentation of common adverse reactions in progress notes or allergy and adverse reaction data as indicated Specific emphasis on monitoring for: ▪ Parkinsonism ▪ Akathisia ▪ Tardive dyskinesia ▪ Orthostatic hypotension ▪ Cognitive/behavioral impairment

Compiled from the American Geriatrics Society and American Association for Geriatric Psychiatry recommendations for policies in support of quality mental health care in U.S. nursing homes. *J Am Geriatr Soc.* 2003;51:1299–1304.
OBRA, Omnibus Budget Reconciliation Act of 1987; PRN, as necessary; PTSD, posttraumatic stress disorder.

dementing illnesses (27). Psychotropic medications such as antipsychotics, mood stabilizers, sedative/hypnotics, anxiolytics, and antidepressants are commonly prescribed in this setting for the treatment of these disorders (28). Concerns regarding psychotropic medication abuse in long-term care facilities resulted in the Omnibus Budget Reconciliation Act (OBRA) of 1987, which protects residents from medically unnecessary "physical or chemical restraints." Interpretive guidelines from the Centers for Medicare and Medicaid Services for fulfilling the OBRA regulations state that residents "must be free of unnecessary drugs," defined as those medications that are duplicative, excessive in dose or duration, or used in the presence of ADRs without adequate monitoring or indication (29). Specific OBRA guidelines for management of residents receiving psychotropic medications in long-term care facilities are reviewed in Table A-7; the guidelines are also reviewed in detail in chapter 3 of this textbook.

REFERENCES

1. Kelly JT. The drug development and approval process. *New Medicines in Development for 2005*. A report.
2. Ban T. Pharmacotherapy of mental illness—a historical analysis. *Prog Neuro-sychopharmacol & Biol Psychoatr.* 2001;25: 709–727.
3. Herman RJ, Wilkinson GR. Disposition of diazepam in young and elderly subjects after acute and chronic dosing. *Br J Clin Pharmacol.* 1996;42:147–155.
4. Sproule BA, Hardy BG, Shulman KI. Differential Pharmacokinetics of lithium in elderly patients. *Drugs Aging.* 2000;16:165–177.
5. Von Moltke LL, Greenblatt DJ, Shader RI. Clinical pharmacokinetics of antidepressants in the elderly. Therapeutic implications. *Clin Pharmacokinet.* 1993;24:141–160.
6. Hanlon JT, Schmader KE, Kornkowski MJ, et al. Adverse drug events in high-risk older outpatients. *J AM Geriatr Soc.* 1997;45: 945–948.
7. American Society of Health-System Pharmacists. ASHP guidelines on adverse drug reaction monitoring and reporting. *Am J Health-Syst Pharm.* 1995;52:417–419.
8. Kohn L, Corrigan J, Donaldson M, eds. *To Err is Human: Building a Safer Health System.* Washington, DC: National Academy of Press; 1999.
9. Fick DM, Cooper JW, Wade WE, et al. Updating the Beers Criteria for potentially inappropriate medication use in older adults. *Arch Intern Med.* 2003;163:2.
10. Maletta G, Mattox KM, Dysken M. Update 2000: guidelines for prescribing psychoactive drugs. *Geriatrics.* 2000;55(March): 65–79.
11. Jacobson SA, Pies RW, Greenblatt DJ, eds. *Handbook of Geriatric Psychopharmacology.* Washington, DC: American Psychiatric Publishing, Inc.; 2002.
12. Salzman C, Satlin A, Burrows AB. Geriatric psychopharmacology. In: Schatzberg AF, Nemeroll CB, eds. *Textbook of Psychopharmacology.* Washington, DC: American Psychiatric Publishing, Inc.; 1998.
13. Hutchison TA, Shahan DR, eds. *DRUGDEX® System.* Greenwood Village, Colorado: MICROMEDEX; (Edition expires 3/2004).
14. McEvoy GK, et al., eds. *AHFS Drug Information 2001.* Bethesda, MD: American Society of Health-System Pharmacists, Inc.; 2001.
15. DiPiro JT, et al., eds. *Pharmacotherapy: A Pathophysiologic Approach.* 5th Ed. McGraw-Hill Medical Publishing Division; 2002.
16. Chui HFK. Antidepressants in the elderly. *IJCP.* 1997;51:369–374.
17. Lapid MI, Rumans TA. Evaluation and management of geriatric depression in primary care. *Mayo Clin Proc.* 2003;73:1423–1429.
18. Complete prescribing information for Lamictal (lamotrigene). Available from http://www.lamictal.com. Accessed January 29, 2004.
19. Complete prescribing information for Provigil (modafinil). Available from http://www.provigil.com. Accessed January 29, 2004.
20. Complete prescribing information for Strattera (atomoxetine). Available from http://www.strattera.com. Accessed January 29, 2004.
21. Desai AK, Grossberg GT. Herbals and botanicals in geriatric psychiatry. *Am J Geriatr Psychiatry.* 2003;11:498–506.
22. De Smet P. Drug therapy: herbal remedies. *N Engl J Med.* 2002;347(25):2046–2056.
23. Ernst E. Serious psychiatric and neurological adverse effects of herbal medicines—a systematic review. *Acta Psychiatr Scand.* 2003;108:83–91.
24. Kaufman DW, Kelly JP, Rosenberg L, et al. Recent patterns of medication use in the ambulatory adult population of the United States. *JAMA.* 2002;287:337–344.
25. Eisenberg DM, Davis RB, Ettner SL, et al. Trends in alternative medicine use in the United States, 1990–1997. *JAMA.* 1998;280: 1569–1575.
26. Sifton DW, ed. *PDR Drug Guide for Mental Health Professionals.* Montvale, NJ: Thomson Medical Economics; 2002.
27. The American Geriatrics Society and American Association for Geriatric Psychiatry recommendations for policies in support of quality mental health care in U.S. nursing homes. *J Am Geriatr Soc.* 2003;51:1299–1304.
28. Lasser RA, Sunderland T. Newer psychotropic medication use in nursing home residents. *J Am Geriatr Soc.* 1998;46:202–207.
29. Gong J. ed. 2002 Healthcare practitioner reference manual for use in long-term-care facilities. Available from http://www. novartisvin.com/seniorcare/hps/refman/appendixD.pdf. Accessed January 27, 2004.

Review of Human Neuroanatomy for the Practicing Psychiatrist

Britt Sanford

The human nervous system can be divided into four major components: the central nervous system (CNS), the peripheral nervous system (PNS), the autonomic nervous system (ANS), and the somatic nervous system (SNS) (Figure B-1). The CNS comprises the brain and spinal cord; the PNS comprises the peripheral nerves and their innumerable branches. These two components are completely interdependent. Even the simplest of reflexes—the monosynaptic or myotatic reflex, such as the patellar or knee-jerk reflex—depends upon elements of both nervous systems to function. The dendrite of an intramuscular sensory neuron (PNS) courses through a peripheral nerve to reach the spinal cord (CNS), where it synapses with a motor neuron. The axon of this lower motor neuron then exits the CNS and travels distally toward its target muscle fibers through the same peripheral nerve (PNS) that the sensory process coursed through centrally.

The SNS is dependent upon the CNS and PNS for its normal function and innervates only nonvisceral tissues (e.g., striated muscle, bone, joints, and skin of the limbs, trunk, head, and neck). The SNS does not innervate organs, body cavity linings, or blood vessels. The SNS is also called the voluntary nervous system because many of its functions involve conscious sensory reception and voluntary motor responses.

The ANS is as dependent upon the CNS and PNS as the latter are interdependent. Autonomic sensory neurons are located solely within the peripheral reaches of the PNS. Their communicating processes travel centrally through peripheral nerves to reach the spinal cord or brainstem of the CNS. First-order autonomic motor neurons begin in the CNS, and their axons course peripherally through peripheral nerves to reach their specific cellular targets.

EMBRYOLOGIC DEVELOPMENT OF THE HUMAN NERVOUS SYSTEM

There are three primary embryologic tissues: *endoderm*, *mesoderm*, and *ectoderm* (Figure B-2). Endoderm, the innermost of the three embryonic tissues, gives rise to tissues that line the hollow viscera of the gastrointestinal (GI) and respiratory tracts, blood vessels, and urogenital structures, as well as the parenchyma of the liver, pancreas, thyroid, parathyroid, and thymus glands. Mesoderm is located between endoderm and ectoderm. It gives rise to all types of connective tissue, muscle, and the linings of the body cavities, as well as the centrally positioned notochord, around which the three embryologic tissues are

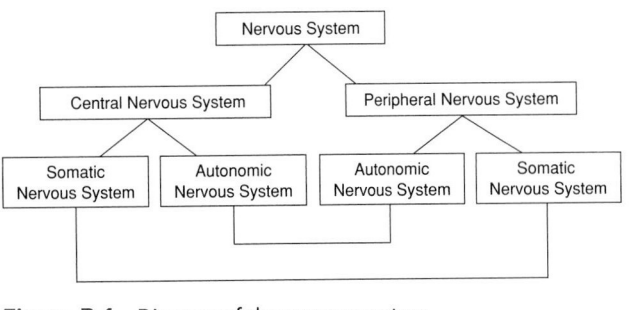

Figure B-1   Diagram of the nervous system.

positioned and develop. Ectoderm, the outermost embryonic tissue, gives rise to the epidermis and its related structures, as well as the entire human nervous system.

After 2 weeks of intrauterine life, the embryologic ectoderm begins differentiating by forming a central neural plate. This neural plate then folds inward to form the longitudinal neural groove, which is capped on each side by a longitudinal neural crest. The neural groove continues its inward folding, ultimately pinching off completely from the remaining superficial ectoderm to form the neural tube; this process is termed *neurulation*.

As neurulation advances, each longitudinal neural crest separates from the underlying neural tube and migrates laterally. These neural crest cells will develop into the peripheral sensory neurons (of the spinal cord and brainstem), the associated dorsal root (or spinal) ganglia, the postganglionic neurons and ganglia of the

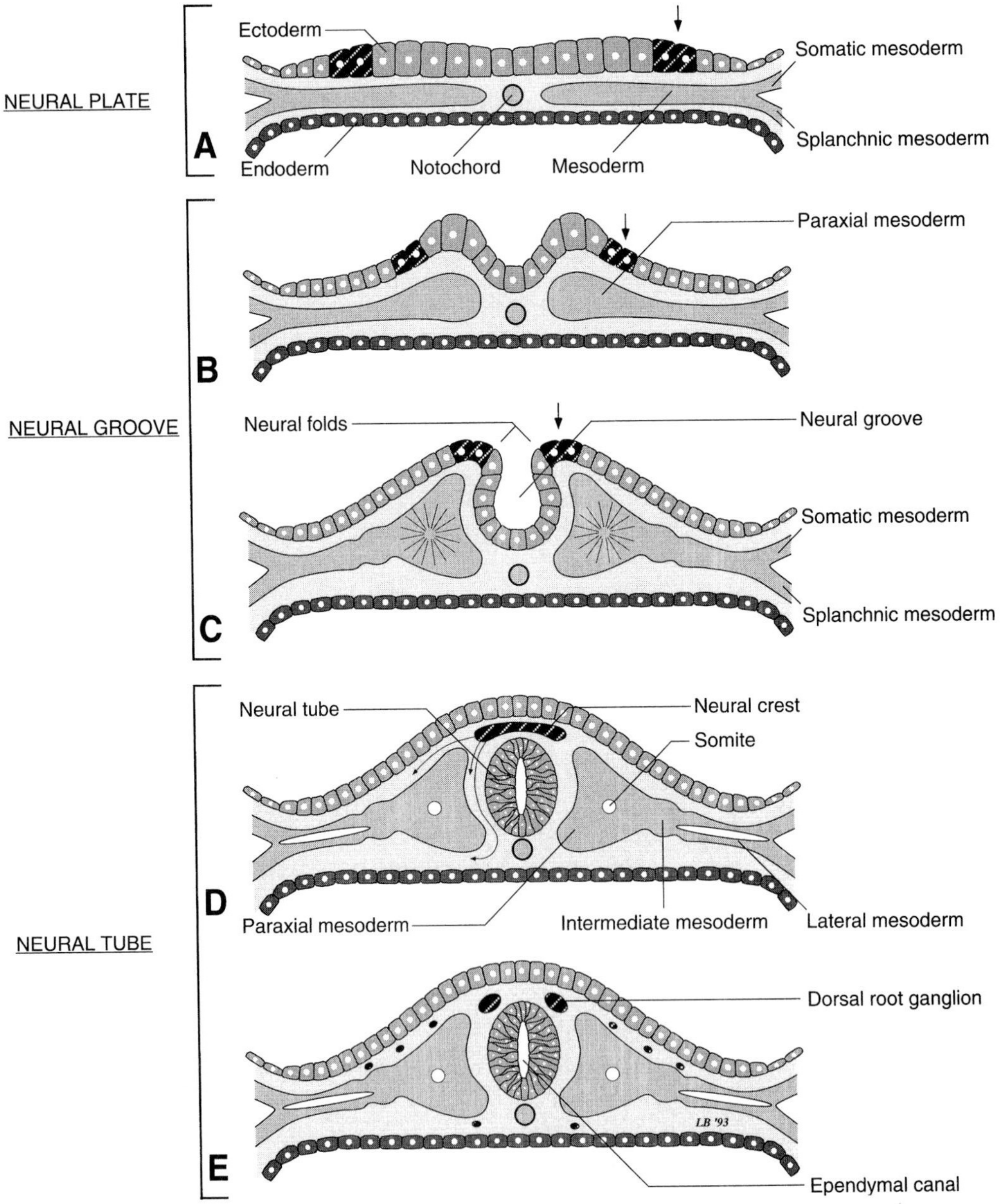

NEURAL PLATE

Ectoderm
Somatic mesoderm
Endoderm
Notochord
Mesoderm
Splanchnic mesoderm

A

NEURAL GROOVE

Paraxial mesoderm

B

Neural folds
Neural groove
Somatic mesoderm
Splanchnic mesoderm

C

NEURAL TUBE

Neural tube
Neural crest
Somite
Paraxial mesoderm
Intermediate mesoderm
Lateral mesoderm

D

Dorsal root ganglion
Ependymal canal

E

Figure B-2   Transverse sections of embryos at different ages to show development of the spinal cord. **A.** Neural plate stage. **B.** Early neural groove stage. **C.** Late neural groove stage. **D.** Early neural tube and neural crest stage. **E.** Neural tube and dorsal root ganglion stage.

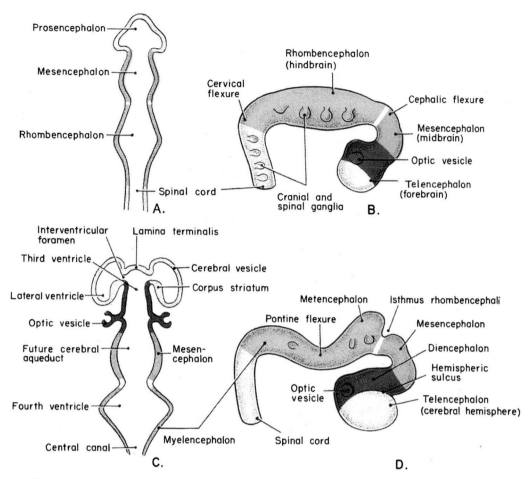

Figure B-3   Developing brain vesicles and ventricular system. **A, B.** Three-brain vesicle stage of a 4-week embryo. **C, D.** Five-brain vesicle stage of a 6-week human embryo. The prosencephalon, telencephalon, and spinal cord are stippled.

ANS, and the Schwann cells that supply myelin to the axons of peripheral neurons.

The rostral end of the hollow neural tube develops into the brain. The remainder develops into the spinal cord; its central cavity will develop into the ventricular system of the brain and the central canal of the spinal cord. A shallow crease, the sulcus limitans, develops along the lateral walls of the length of the neural tube, separating it into dorsal and ventral halves that will persist in the mature spinal cord and brainstem. The dorsal half is concerned only with sensory function, and the ventral half solely with motor function.

Five swellings or vesicles develop at the rostral end of the neural tube, the telencephalon (develops into the cerebrum), the diencephalon (develops into the thalamus and hypothalamus), the mesencephalon (develops into the midbrain portion of the brainstem), the metencephalon (develops into the cerebellum and the pons of the central brainstem), and the myelencephalon (develops into the medulla [or medulla oblongata] of the caudal brainstem) (Figure B-3). Three flexures occur among the five vesicles: the cervical flexure occurs at the junction between the spinal cord and medulla, the pontine flexure occurs between the medulla and the pons, and the cephalic flexure occurs between the midbrain and the diencephalon. The cephalic flexure is great enough—nearly 90 degrees—to cause a change of axes between the brainstem and the telencephalon and diencephalon (collectively termed the prosencephalon). As a result, directional terms describing brainstem structures are not perfectly interchangeable with similar terms describing cerebral structures. For example, the terms superior and dorsal are synonymous when referring to the cerebrum, whereas they are at right angles to one another when describing the brainstem.

The growth of the cerebrum is far greater than the growth of the other components of the brain. The rapidly expanding human cerebrum pursues its growth in the shape of a C, with its two poles curving rostrally. This serves to conserve space and pack as much cortex and cerebral tissue as possible into the confines of the human skull. The significant infolding of its cortical surface into gyri (folds) and sulci (furrows) enables the roughly 2.5 m^2 of cortex to fit within the human neurocranium. This massive growth causes the cerebrum to actually overgrow much of the more ventrally positioned thalamus,

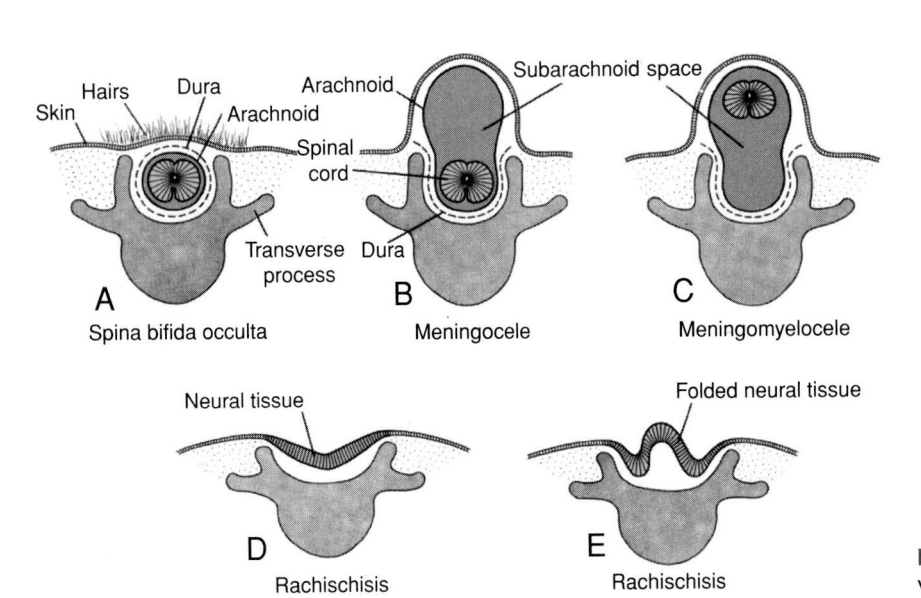

Figure B-4 Schematic drawings to show various types of spina bifida.

hypothalamus, and midbrain. Several deep cerebral structures are also forced to conform to the C-shape growth of the cerebrum. These include the lateral ventricles, corpus callosum, fornices, caudate nuclei, and stria terminalis, which will be considered later in this review.

Understanding the normal embryologic development of the nervous system affords the opportunity to explain developmental defects. Abnormal closure of the neural tube early in the development of the nervous system can result in both spinal cord and cerebral defects. In spina bifida (Figure B-4), a frequent cause of congenital malformations of the central nervous system (1:1000 live births), the bony roof of the sacrum, which is composed of five fused sacral vertebrae, is incompletely formed. In spina bifida occulta, the integrity of the spinal canal is typically intact, although it lacks the protection of a complete bony canal. In many cases, this abnormality may never be detected because there are no neural defects and no obvious structural defects. In some cases, although the etiology is not fully understood, spina bifida occulta is heralded by a patch of hair growing from the skin overlying the defective sacrum. In other cases, a communication occurs between the overlying skin and the spinal canal—a dermal sinus.

In spina bifida complicated with meningocele, a herniation of the meninges that surround the spinal cord protrudes completely through the bony sacrum and overlying connective tissue, and presents as a bulge within the skin overlying the defect. When the meningocele defect includes elements of the spinal cord—usually dorsal and ventral roots of the lower spinal nerves—it is termed a meningomyelocele. Meningomyeloceles are usually accompanied by an Arnold-Chiari malformation, in which the developing cerebellum and caudal brainstem is forced inferiorly through the foramen magnum into the cervical spinal canal. Hydrocephalus commonly occurs as a result of this crowding within the rostral extent of the vertebral column's spinal canal.

If the rostral extent of the neural tube does not close normally, anencephaly (in which much of the cerebrum is absent) usually results. Anencephaly is not compatible with life.

In cases where the neural tube closes normally but the bones of the skull do not, cerebrospinal fluid (CSF)-filled swellings of the brain's meningeal coverings may herniate through the neurocranium's bony defects as an encephalocele.

Neural tube defects are most commonly detected in the developing fetus upon ultrasound examination, and by the measurement of elevated levels of α-fetoprotein in the maternal circulation. Maternal folic acid deficiency is the most common known cause of neural tube defects, and can be effectively treated with folic acid supplements during the early months of gestation.

GROSS ANATOMY OF THE HUMAN BRAIN

The brain consists of two cerebral hemispheres and the underlying diencephalon, brainstem, and cerebellum.

Whole Brain: Dorsal and Lateral Aspects

With its richly undulating surface, the cerebrum comprises five cortical lobes: frontal, parietal, temporal, occipital, and limbic (Figure B-5). It is not necessary to specify each of the many gyri and sulci of the corrugated cerebral cortex; however, a few of these merit consideration. First, the massive longitudinal or interhemispheric fissure that occurs between the two cerebral hemispheres, limited inferiorly by the corpus callosum. The substantial, longitudinal lateral sulcus (or Sylvian fissure) is a significant feature on the lateral aspect of the cerebrum, separating the more inferior temporal lobe from the more superior frontal and

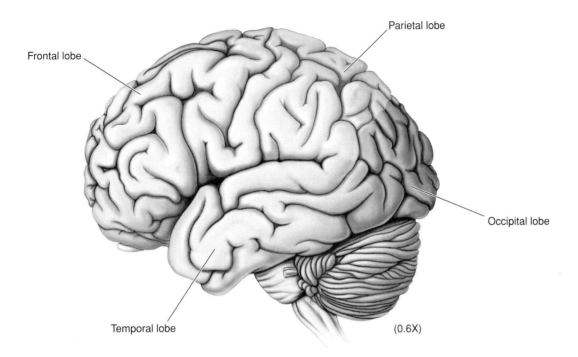

Frontal lobe

Parietal lobe

Occipital lobe

Temporal lobe

(0.6X)

Figure B-5   Cerebral lobes.

parietal lobes. The more subtle central sulcus, which courses horizontally near the center of the cerebral hemisphere, neatly divides the more anterior frontal lobe from the more posterior parietal lobe. The line of demarcation separating the most posterior cerebral lobe—the occipital lobe—from the more anterior temporal and parietal lobes is imaginary and is drawn from the preoccipital notch, inferiorly, to the superior extent of the parietooccipital sulcus, superiorly.

Other features of the lateral aspect of the whole brain include the pons and medulla of the brainstem, and the cerebellum, positioned immediately posterior to the pons and medulla and inferior to the occipital pole of the cerebrum.

An island of cerebral cortex, the aptly named insula, is hidden from view. Tucked behind the areas of cortex from the frontal, parietal, and temporal lobes that border the lateral sulcus, the insula is accessible by prying open the lateral sulcus or removing the overlying cerebral cortex.

Whole Brain: Basal Aspect

On the basal (or ventral) surface of the whole brain, only elements of the frontal and temporal lobes are readily visible (Figure B-6). If the brainstem is removed, the occipital lobe is seen.

The basal surface of each frontal lobe is marked by a gentle impression made by the bony roof of the orbit; the individual gyri located here are the orbital gyri of the frontal lobe. A longitudinal strip of tissue runs along the medial aspect of the basal surface of the frontal lobe. This is the olfactory bulb, distally, and the olfactory tract, proximally (i.e., cranial nerve [CN] I).

CN II, the optic nerve, is typically truncated in the anatomic specimen, leaving only a short stub. The two optic nerves course caudally to reach the optic chiasm, where approximately one-half of their fibers cross before forming the more distal optic tracts. The optic tracts can be identified wrapping around the massive cerebral peduncles of the midbrain as they make their way to the lateral geniculate nuclei of the thalamus, where they synapse.

Immediately posterior to the optic chiasm is the infundibulum of the hypophysis (i.e., the pituitary stalk). Immediately posterior to the infundibulum are the paired mammillary bodies.

Posterior to the mammillary bodies, much of the ventral aspect of the midbrain is obscured by the encroaching temporal lobes and pons. However, the laterally positioned cerebral peduncles can usually be identified, with each optic tract wrapping around their superior margins. The space between the cerebral peduncles, the interpeduncular fossa, is interrupted by the pair of oculomotor nerves (CN III) that project ventrally from the midbrain. The oculomotor nerve innervates four of the six extraocular muscles that move the ocular globe, as well as two smooth muscles located deep within the globe.

The slender trochlear nerve (CN IV) is normally found coursing around the margin of the seam where the midbrain and pons meet. It is usually difficult—indeed, often impossible—to identify this CN on the whole brain. The trochlear nerve innervates one of the six extraocular muscles (i.e., the superior oblique) that move the ocular globe.

Next is the pons, the middle cerebellar peduncles projecting laterally into each cerebellar hemisphere. The large,

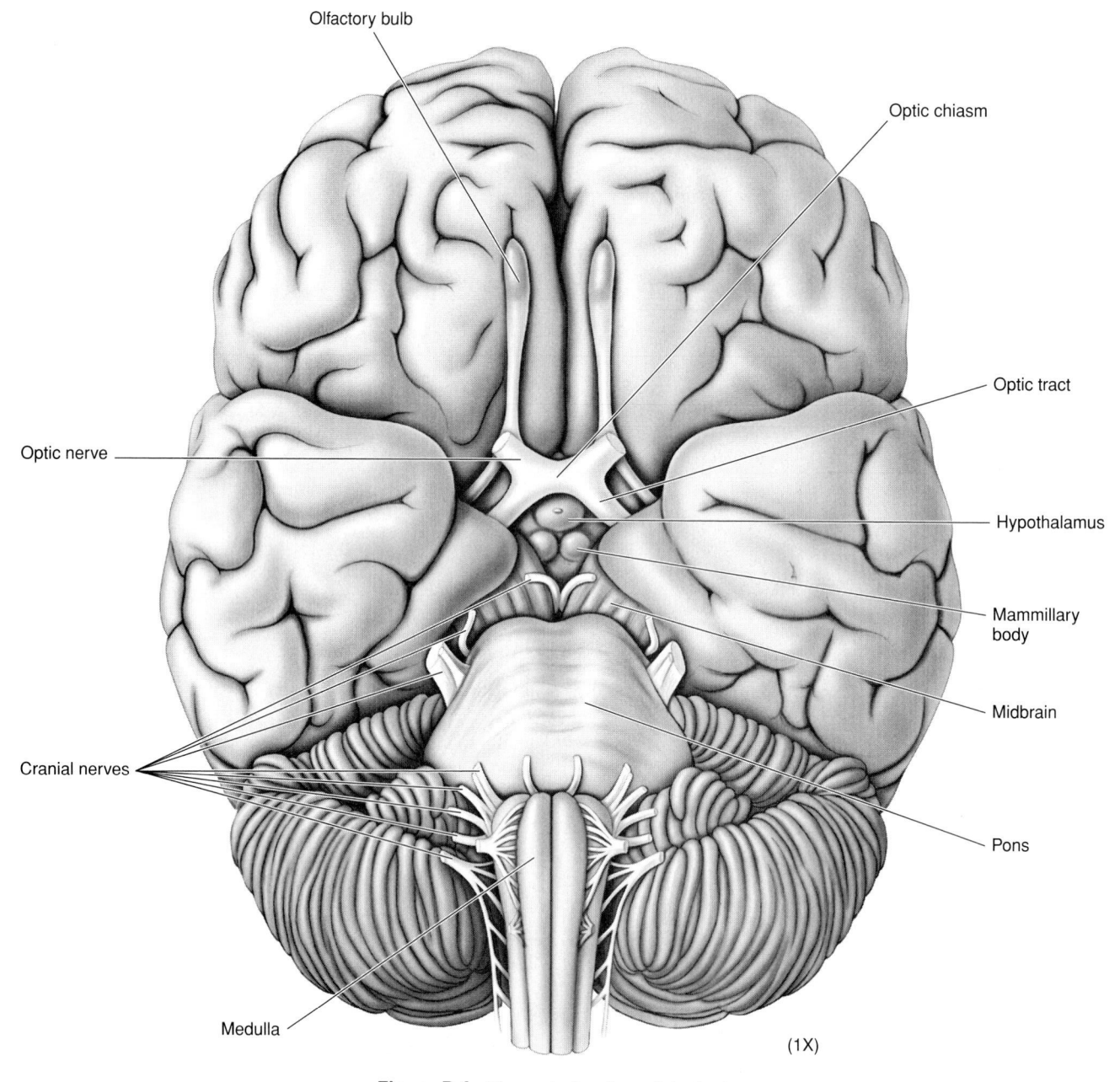

Olfactory bulb

Optic chiasm

Optic tract

Optic nerve

Hypothalamus

Mammillary body

Midbrain

Cranial nerves

Pons

Medulla

(1X)

Figure B-6   The ventral surface of the brain.

unpaired basilar artery runs rostrally along the pontine midline, where it elaborates numerous branches. Located on the lateral aspect of the mid-pons is the largest of the CNs, the trigeminal nerve (CN V). Although it is the fifth CN, it is termed *tri*geminal because it is composed of three major divisions: ophthalmic, maxillary, and mandibular. The largely sensory trigeminal nerve (for the face) has a small motor component (that innervates the muscles of mastication) that can often be differentiated from the sensory components with the unaided eye.

Posteriorly, the pons meets the medulla. At the pontomedullary angle, CN VI, the abducens nerve, exits. The abducens nerve, as its name suggests, innervates the lateral rectus extraocular muscle, which abducts the ocular globe.

Located lateral to the pontomedullary angle and the abducens nerve is the pontocerebellar angle and the facial and vestibulocochlear nerves (CNs VII and VIII, respectively). The more medial facial nerve contains five types of neuronal fibers, and the vestibulocochlear nerve contains specialized sensory neurons responsible for auditory and vestibular sense. The flocculus of the flocculonodular lobe of the cerebellum is found bulging against the middle cerebellar peduncle immediately lateral to CNs VII and VIII. It is often also accompanied by a tuft of choroid plexus that projects from the lateral apertures (of Luschka) of the underlying fourth ventricle. The vermis of the cerebellum interconnects the two cerebellar hemispheres and is not visible on the basal surface of the brain.

Below the pons is the medulla, with its ventrally projecting pyramids; the medulla is continuous with the spinal cord caudally. CNs IX, X, XI, and XII (glossopharyngeal, vagus, spinal accessory, and hypoglossal) emerge from the anterior and anterolateral surfaces of the medulla.

ARTERIAL SUPPLY OF THE BRAIN

The brain receives its arterial supply from two systems: the subclavian and carotid. The arch of the aorta normally elaborates three vessels: the left subclavian, left common carotid, and brachiocephalic arteries. The brachiocephalic artery, in turn, divides into the right subclavian and right common carotid arteries. A major branch of the subclavian artery is the vertebral artery, which ascends along the cervical vertebral column and enters the cranium by passing through the massive foramen magnum in close juxtaposition to the medulla. The internal carotid artery, one of two branches of the common carotid artery, ascends along the deep, anterior aspect of the neck and enters the neurocranium through its own canal. These two pairs of arteries provide the entire arterial supply of the brain (Figure B-7).

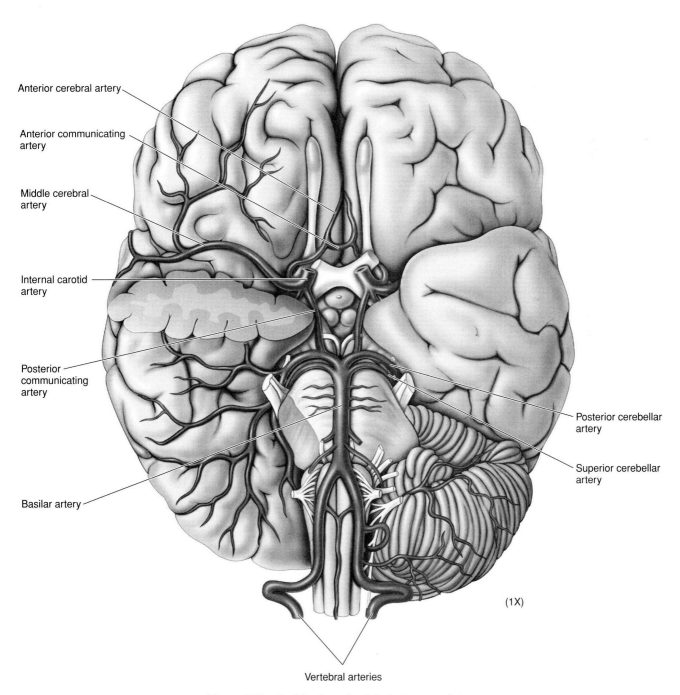

Anterior cerebral artery

Anterior communicating artery

Middle cerebral artery

Internal carotid artery

Posterior communicating artery

Basilar artery

Posterior cerebellar artery

Superior cerebellar artery

(1X)

Vertebral arteries

Figure B-7   The blood supply of the brain, ventral view.

The two vertebral arteries ascend along the anterolateral aspect of the medulla and unite near the pontomedullary junction to form the unpaired basilar artery, which courses along the ventral surface of the pons. Single branches from each vertebral artery unite to form the anterior spinal artery, which, as its name suggests, runs inferiorly along the anterior aspect of the spinal cord. Each vertebral artery also elaborates a posterior spinal artery, which descends along the posterolateral aspect of the spinal cord, and two cerebellar arteries—the posterior inferior and anterior inferior—that, as one might imagine, supply the cerebellum. The basilar artery itself elaborates numerous branches that supply the pons and associated structures, and a pair of superior cerebellar arteries, before giving off its two terminal branches, the posterior cerebral arteries.

The internal carotid artery, which yields no branches in the neck, elaborates a single intracranial branch—the ophthalmic artery—before dividing into the anterior and middle cerebral arteries. The two anterior cerebral arteries, which course anteriorly side by side through the interhemispheric fissure, are linked by a very short vessel, the anterior communicating artery. The massive middle cerebral artery projects laterally through the equally massive lateral sulcus on its way to the lateral surface of the cerebral hemisphere. The middle cerebral artery is joined to the posterior cerebral artery by the slim posterior communicating artery. Thus, the cerebral arterial circle (of Willis) is formed. The posterior cerebral arteries are confluent with one another at the rostral limit of the basilar artery. Each posterior cerebral artery is joined to the ipsilateral middle cerebral artery, which is directly linked to the ipsilateral anterior cerebral artery, and the two anterior cerebral arteries are joined by the slim anterior communicating artery. It is thought that this circle of Willis helps to ensure the continuous flow of arterial blood to the brain. If one of its formative components becomes compromised, arterial blood can be rerouted to maintain a continuous blood supply. Intracranial arterial aneurysms most often occur at branching points in the circle of Willis.

The brainstem itself is supplied by six different arteries. The medulla is supplied by the vertebral, posterior inferior cerebellar, and anterior and posterior spinal arteries. The pons is supplied by the basilar, anterior inferior cerebellar, and superior cerebellar arteries. The midbrain is supplied by the basilar, superior cerebellar, posterior cerebral, and posterior communicating arteries.

Occlusive events involving these arteries result in classic syndromes reflecting damage to the specific anatomic structures supplied. For example, a lesion involving the anterior spinal artery may result in a medial medullary syndrome, in which damage occurs to the hypoglossal nucleus and nerve (that innervates seven of the eight tongue muscles), the corticospinal tract (the major descending motor supply to the spinal cord), and the

medial lemniscus (that carries sensory information regarding fine touch and proprioception). Signs and symptoms include loss of motor function to one side of the tongue, loss of touch and proprioception sensation on one side of the body, and complete paralysis of one side of the body.

The cerebellum is supplied by three different arteries: the posterior inferior, anterior inferior, and superior cerebellar.

The cerebral cortex and neighboring white matter is supplied by the three major cerebral arteries. The anterior cerebral artery curls around the peripheral border of the corpus callosum, where it runs within the callosal sulcus, and supplies the medial and mediodorsal aspects of the frontal and parietal lobes as well as the cingulate gyrus of the limbic lobe. The middle cerebral artery runs laterally through the lateral sulcus to reach the dorsolateral surface of the cerebral hemisphere, where its branches supply the dorsolateral aspect of the frontal and parietal lobes as well as the lateral aspect of the temporal lobe. The posterior cerebral artery supplies the entire basal (or mediobasal) aspect of the temporal lobe as well as nearly the entire occipital lobe.

The three major cerebral arteries also supply deeper structures (i.e., the basal ganglia, diencephalon, and internal capsule). Anteriorly, perforating branches from the anterior and middle cerebral arteries supply the basal ganglia and internal capsule. Posteriorly, deep structures are supplied largely by perforating branches of the posterior cerebral artery, with some contribution laterally by perforating branches of the middle cerebellar artery and posterolaterally by the anterior choroidal artery, a major branch of the medial cerebral artery. Deep structures are also supplied, somewhat equally, by perforating branches of the middle and posterior cerebral arteries and the anterior choroidal artery.

MENINGES

The CNS is completely enclosed within a series of three connective tissue membranes, or mater (Figure B-8). The outer layer, the dura mater, is the only meningeal layer that has its own blood supply and sensory innervation. Within the skull, it is confluent with the inner aspect of the cranium (the endosteum), and only a *potential* space occurs between these two structures. Thus, under normal conditions a distinct anatomic space does not exist here. However, skull trauma that results in a tear of the dura mater and its supplying arteries (e.g., the middle meningeal artery along the lateral cranial wall) can result in the accumulation of arterial blood superficial to the dura mater, forming an epidural hematoma. Regarding the spinal cord, on the other hand, a significant space between its dura mater and the surrounding bony elements of the vertebral column is present, and is filled

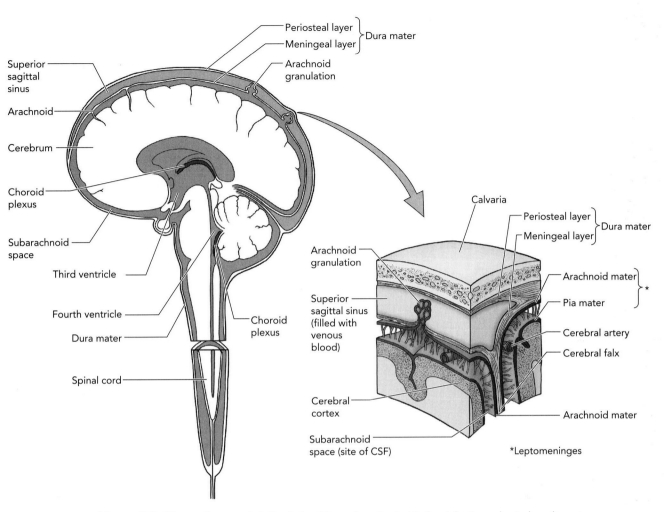

Figure B-8   The meninges and their relationship to the calvaria (skullcap), brain, and spinal cord.

largely by adipose tissue through which local vasculature courses.

Portions of the cranial dura mater are arranged into folds or reflections that serve to separate and support various components of the brain. For example, the falx cerebri is a dural septum that protrudes from the inner surfaces of the frontal, parietal, and occipital bones to divide the two cerebral hemispheres from one another. Similarly, the much smaller falx cerebelli, projecting vertically from the occipital bone, accomplishes the same for the two cerebellar hemispheres. The tentorium cerebelli is a dural shelf that projects horizontally from the occipital and temporal bones, serving to support the occipital cerebral lobe and separate it from the underlying cerebellum. The posteroinferior aspect of the falx cerebri joins the tentorium cerebelli at its midline. The tentorium cerebelli divides the intracranial space into supratentorial and infratentorial compartments. The supratentorial compartment contains the cerebrum, and the infratentorial compartment contains the cerebellum and brainstem. The anterior margin of the tentorium is curved and open to

permit the passage of the brainstem, and this tentorial notch (or incisure) has significant clinical importance. Secondary to an expanding mass, the temporal lobe can herniate medially across the tentorial notch and compress the midbrain, which can lead to coma and death. Furthermore, a large supratentorial lesion involving the diencephalon and internal capsule that induces coma can result in decorticate rigidity, in which the lower limbs and the head and neck are extended and the upper limbs are flexed. If such a lesion extends inferiorly, below the tentorial notch, to involve the brainstem, decerebrate rigidity—in which all four limbs and the head and neck are extended—can develop.

The innermost layer of the meninges, the pia mater, is extremely thin and composed of a single layer of cells. It is closely apposed to the surface of the spinal cord and brain and accompanies blood vessels that penetrate the surfaces of the CNS components. No space exists between the pia mater and the surface of the CNS it invests.

The intermediate meningeal layer is the arachnoid mater. Normally, the arachnoid mater is closely apposed

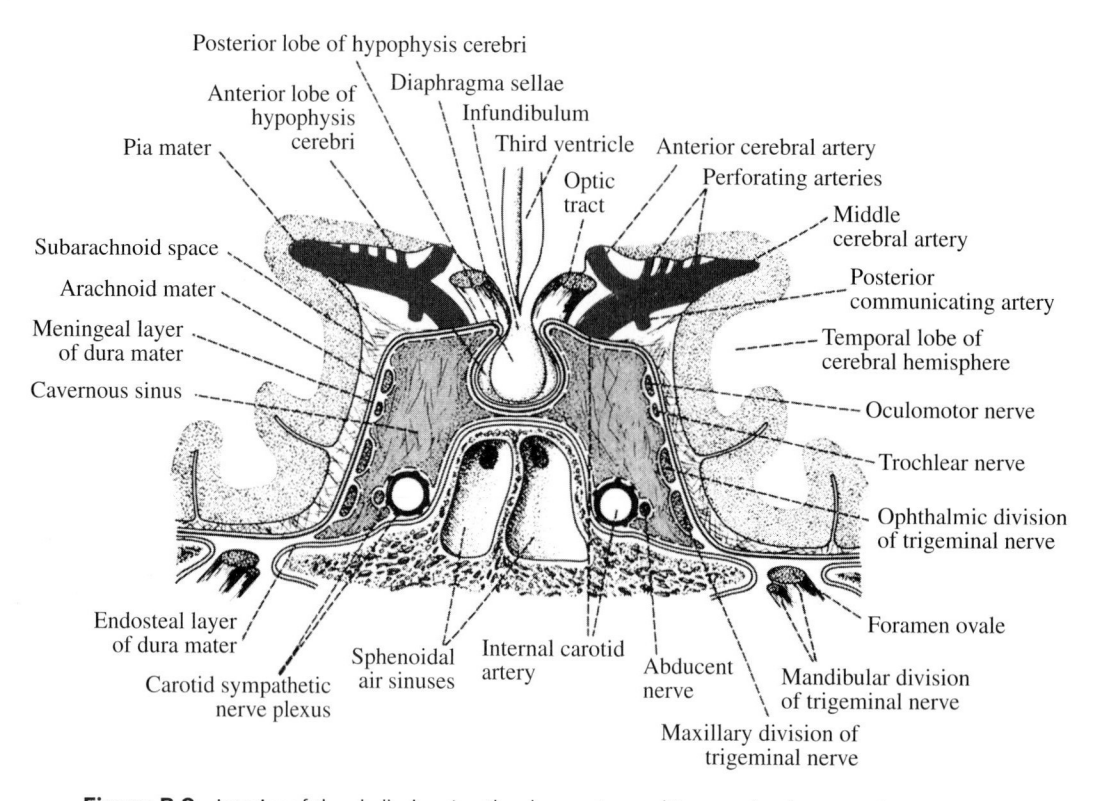

Figure B-9   Interior of the skull, showing the dura mater and its contained venous sinuses.

to the inner surface of the dura mater, leaving only a potential space—the subdural space—between the two. Skull trauma resulting in the disruption of one of the cranial dural venous sinuses can lead to the formation of a subdural hematoma. From the inner surface of the arachnoid mater project collections of collagenous fibers—the trabeculae—that reach across a CSF-filled space (the subarachnoid space) and fuse with the pia mater.

The arachnoid mater is not suspended from the surface of the brain and spinal cord at a simple, fixed, static distance; therefore, there are numerous regions where the subarachnoid space is fairly deep and broad. For example, there are large CSF-filled subarachnoid spaces, or cisterns, surrounding the optic chiasm (the chiasmatic cistern) between the two cerebral peduncles; the interpeduncular cistern, anterior to the pons; the pontine cistern; and the very large space between the cerebellum and the medulla, the cisterna magna. Thus, the brain and spinal cord are literally suspended within this CSF-filled space.

Superficial cerebral arteries and veins course across the surface of the brain within the subarachnoid space. A subarachnoid hematoma is often the result of a laceration to one of these vessels, usually a cerebral artery. An epidural hematoma, secondary to a torn meningeal artery, occurs between the dura mater and the bony cranium. A subdural hematoma, secondary to a torn dural vein, occurs between the dura mater and arachnoid mater. A subarachnoid hematoma, secondary to a lacerated superficial cerebral

artery, occurs between the arachnoid mater and the pia mater.

DURAL VENOUS SINUSES

Many of the edges of the various dural septa separate to form dural venous sinuses (Figure B-9). These triangular spaces receive drainage from the cerebral veins and are lined with the same endothelium that lines all veins. The superior sagittal sinus is located along the superior margin of the falx cerebri where it attaches to the cranium. It receives drainage from the superficial superior cerebral veins, as well as from the greater anastomotic vein (of Trolard), which is linked to the inferior anastomotic vein (of Labbe). The inferior sagittal sinus is found in the free inferior margin of the falx cerebri. The transverse sinus is formed where the tentorium cerebelli attaches peripherally to the cranium, and receives superficial inferior cerebral veins as well as the inferior anastomotic vein (of Labbe). The inferior anastomotic vein also has connections with the superior sagittal, transverse, and cavernous sinuses. The straight sinus is formed where the falx cerebri joins the midline of the tentorium cerebelli. It drains the great cerebral vein (of Galen) and the inferior sagittal sinus posteriorly to where it intersects with the superior sagittal sinus at the so-called confluence of sinuses. From the confluence, each of two bilateral transverse sinuses drains laterally and anteriorly into the S-shaped sigmoid

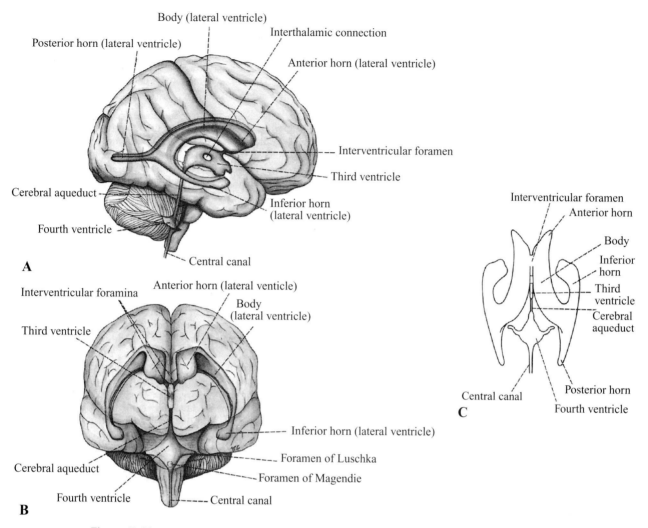

Figure B-10 Cast of the ventricular cavities of the brain as seen from (**A**) lateral view, (**B**) anterior view, and (**C**) superior view.

sinus, which, in turn, empties through the jugular foramen in the base of the skull into the internal jugular vein.

Other dural venous sinuses include the sphenoparietal, cavernous, intercavernous, basilar, superior petrosal, inferior petrosal, and occipital sinuses.

THE VENTRICULAR SYSTEM

The ventricular system comprises two pairs of lateral ventricles and single, unpaired third and fourth ventricles, as well as the conduit (the cerebral aqueduct) that joins the third ventricle with the fourth ventricle (Figure B-10).

Pulled along with the C-shaped growth of the developing cerebrum, the lateral ventricles are also C-shaped. Each lateral ventricle consists of a central body, located largely within the frontal and parietal lobes; an anterior horn, which projects anteriorly into the frontal lobe; a posterior horn, which projects posteriorly into the occipital lobe; and an inferior horn, which projects inferiorly and anteri-

orly into the temporal lobe. The trigone (or atrium) occurs where the body and posterior and inferior horns meet.

The unpaired third ventricle occurs along the midline, between the left and right thalami and hypothalami. It is linked to the two lateral ventricles by the interventricular foramen (of Monro). The third ventricle is linked to the fourth ventricle by the cerebral aqueduct (of Sylvius) that runs immediately posterior to the midbrain and pontine tegmentum.

The fourth ventricle is a tent-shaped space that projects posteriorly into the adjoining cerebellum. The fourth ventricle tapers caudally into the narrow central canal, which passes caudally through the caudal medulla and through the length of the spinal cord. The fourth ventricle also communicates with the subarachnoid space surrounding the cerebellum, medulla, and entire CNS via two lateral apertures (of Luschka) and one unpaired, median aperture (of Magendie).

CSF is produced by the choroid plexus. Choroid plexus occurs within the lateral, third, and fourth ventricles. It passes through the interventricular foramen (of Monro) from the lateral ventricles to the third ventricle, and passes through the three openings of the fourth ventricle, as described earlier. Choroid plexus does not occur within the narrow cerebral aqueduct (of Sylvius) that joins the third ventricle with the fourth ventricle.

CSF circulates throughout the ventricular system as follows. CSF produced by the choroid plexus of the lateral ventricles circulates superiorly and anteriorly from the inferior and posterior horns, and posteriorly from the anterior horn, to reach the interventricular foramen (of Monro) located near where the anterior horn meets the body. Here, the CSF produced within the lateral ventricles flows into the third ventricle, where it joins CSF produced by the choroid plexus of the third ventricle. The CSF then streams down the cerebral aqueduct (of Sylvius) and into the fourth ventricle, where it joins locally produced CSF. CSF then exits the fourth ventricle, through its three apertures, to flow into the subarachnoid space that encloses the cerebellum, medulla, and entire CNS. CSF also exits the fourth

ventricle by entering the central canal of the medulla and spinal cord. After circulating around and through the length of the spinal cord, CNS returns to the subarachnoid space enveloping the cerebrum.

Along the midline of the superior aspect of the subarachnoid space-enclosed cerebrum, circulating CSF is filtered through arachnoid granulations, or villi, which filter CSF back into the superior sagittal sinus. Arachnoid granulations are parcels of arachnoid mater that evaginate superiorly through the neighboring dura mater to enter the superior sagittal sinus; arachnoid granulations are not found in any of the other dural sinuses and veins of the brain.

THE SPINAL NERVE

Each of the 62 different spinal nerves (31 pairs) has a similar composition (Figure B-11). The typical spinal nerve is a component of the PNS; it is composed of innumerable sensory (afferent) and motor (efferent) neural processes

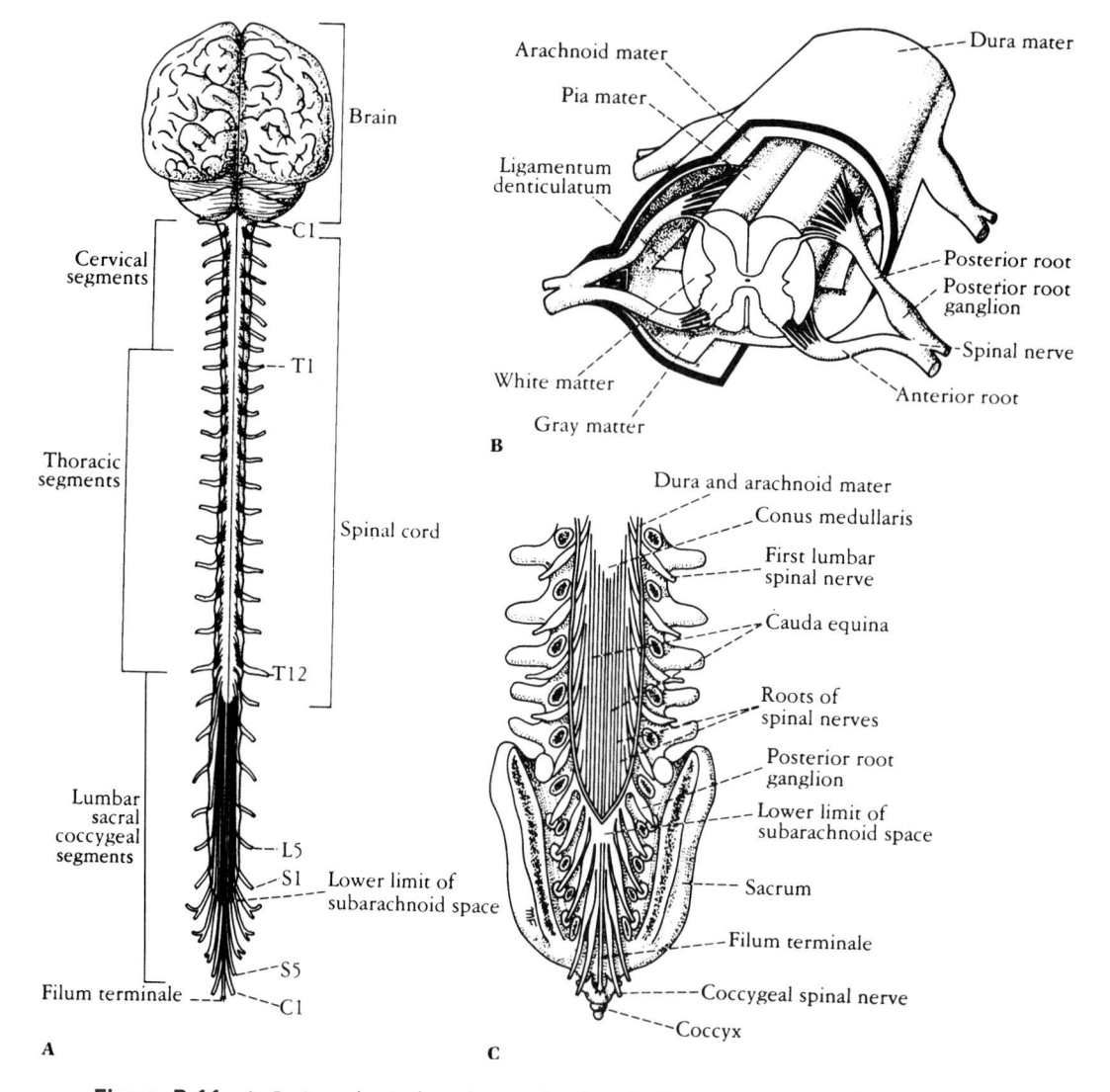

Figure B-11 A. Brain and spinal cord posterior view. B. Transverse section of the spinal cord in the thoracic region, showing anterior and posterior roots of a spinal nerve and the meninges. C. Posterior view of the lower end of the spinal cord and the cauda equina.

that supply a given body region. Fiber types are generally grouped as general somatic or general visceral (or autonomic). Immediately lateral to the spinal cord, the spinal nerve divides into two divisions: the dorsal root and the ventral root. At the junction of the dorsal root and the spinal nerve proper is a small dilatation, the dorsal root ganglion (DRG) (or spinal ganglion), in which the cell bodies of *all* sensory neurons reside. The dorsal root is composed of the axons of these various sensory neurons heading toward the dorsal (sensory) horn of the spinal cord.

The ventral horn, on the other hand, carries information from the spinal cord toward the periphery, and is composed mostly of the cell bodies of primary (or α or lower) motor neurons. The axons of these neurons exit the ventral horn and pass through the ventral root, eventually reaching the spinal nerve at the point where the dorsal and ventral roots merge. These lower motor neurons directly innervate individual skeletal muscle cells.

A spinal nerve, therefore, can also be described as the neural structure formed by the merging of the dorsal and ventral roots, containing general somatic motor and sensory fibers and general visceral motor and sensory fibers. Almost immediately after the spinal nerve is formed, it divides into a small dorsal ramus and a much larger ventral ramus. The former supplies innervation for dorsal structures and regions of the back, whereas the latter supplies the much broader ventral and lateral areas. Dermatomes are regional cutaneous areas innervated by a single spinal nerve (Figures B-12 and B-13).

BRAINSTEM: INTEGRATIVE FUNCTION

The reticular formation runs through the central core of the brainstem. It is filled with neurons that receive input from virtually the entire CNS—the spinal cord, other brainstem nuclei, cerebellum, basal ganglia, diencephalon,

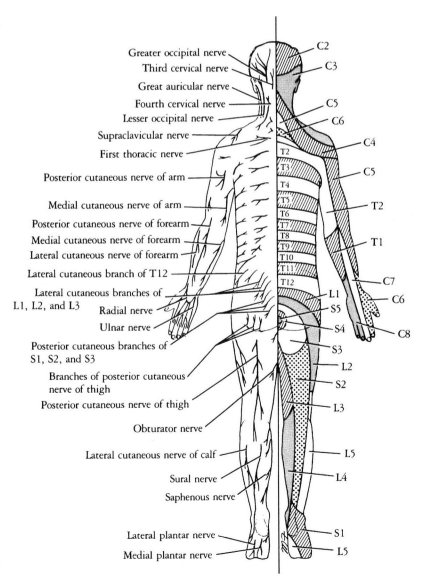

Figure B-12 Posterior aspect of the body, showing the distribution of cutaneous nerves on the left side and dermatomes on the right side.

```
C1 ⇨ NO sensory component
C2 ⇨ posterior scalp
C3 ⇨ a band encompassing the entire neck
C4 ⇨ posterior neck and upper shoulders
C5 ⇨ posterior neck, shoulders, anterior aspect of arm & forearm
C6 ⇨ posterior shoulders & lateral aspect of arm,forearm,& hand
C7 ⇨ posterior shoulders & posterior aspect of arm,forearm, & hand
C8 ⇨ upper back & medial aspect of arm,forearm, & hand

T1-T12 ⇨ successive bands encircling trunk
T10 coverage includes the umbilicus

L1-L5 ⇨ successive bands across the inferior trunk, then descending bands over
the lower limbs
L1 ⇨ groin
L2 ⇨ upper thigh
L3 ⇨ mid thigh
L4 ⇨ lower thigh, anterior knee, anteromedial leg, and medial foot
L5 ⇨ lateral thigh, knee, and leg, and anterior foot

S1 ⇨ band including upper buttock region and lateral aspect of posterior thigh,
     leg, and foot
S2 ⇨ band including mid-buttock region and medial aspect of posterior thigh,leg,
     and foot, external genitalia
S3 ⇨ deep, central buttock region and external genitalia
S4 ⇨ deep perineal region
S5 ⇨ deepest perineal region
```

Figure B-13 Dermatomes.

limbic system, and cerebral cortex—and discharges efferents to an equally wide spread of targets. The reticular formation provides the highest degree of integration of a myriad of information sources. It participates in the regulation of posture as well as trunk and proximal limb movements, modulates the central transmission of pain information, regulates blood pressure homeostasis, and monitors respiration, and it is where the states of consciousness and arousal are regulated.

CRANIAL NERVES

Six different classes of neural fibers compose the 12 CNs (Table B-1): three types of afferent (or sensory) fibers, and three types of efferent (or motor) fibers (Figure B-14).

General somatic afferents (GSA) transmit sensory information (e.g., pain, temperature, touch, and proprioception) drawn from the integument and its related structures, and from connective tissue structures such as skeletal muscle, bone, tendons, and ligaments. GSAs abound in the 31 pairs of spinal nerves and their branches, as well as in CN V (the trigeminal nerve), which provides cutaneous sensation to the face. CNs VII, IX, and X also carry small numbers of GSA fibers that provide cutaneous sensation to the external ear.

General visceral afferents (GVA) transmit sensory information from the body's visceral structures, such as blood vessels, smooth muscle, adipose tissue, glands, many mucus membranes, and, of course, organs. GVA fibers are either sympathetic or parasympathetic and are found throughout the body. For example, sympathetic GVA fibers innervate cardiac muscle, transmitting pain sensation that occurs with angina pectoris; and parasympathetic GVA fibers provide most, if not all, of the conscious sensations

associated with the urge to micturate or defecate, and the sensation of fullness or gastric distress following a meal. All GVAs are anchored in the solitary nucleus, found in the medulla and pons.

A subcategory of GVA fibers is special visceral afferents (SVA), which conduct taste sensation from the tongue and neighboring structures. The facial (CN VII), glossopharyngeal (CN IX), and vagus (CN X) nerves contain SVA fibers. As with all GVAs, the cell bodies of all SVA fibers reside in the brainstem's solitary nucleus.

The third category of sensory neuronal fibers is special sensory. The olfactory (CN I), optic (CN II), and vestibulocochlear (CN VIII) nerves contain special sensory fibers.

General somatic efferents (GSE) innervate skeletal muscle (not cardiac or smooth muscle) and, obviously, run rife in the 31 pairs of spinal nerves and their branches. The oculomotor (CN III), trochlear (CN IV), abducens (CN VI), and hypoglossal (CN XII) nerves contain GSE.

General visceral efferents (GVE) are of two types—sympathetic and parasympathetic—and innervate smooth and cardiac muscle, adipose tissue, and glandular tissue. These will be discussed more fully in a later section dedicated to the ANS. The oculomotor (CN III), facial (CN VII), glossopharyngeal (CN IX), and vagus (CN X) nerves contain (preganglionic) parasympathetic GVE fibers. None of the CNs carries sympathetic GVE fibers.

Special visceral efferents (SVE), also called branchial motor fibers, innervate skeletal muscle developed from the first pharyngeal (or branchial) arch. The trigeminal (CN V), facial (CN VII), glossopharyngeal (CN IX), vagus (CN X), and spinal accessory (CN XI) nerves contain SVE fibers.

Ten of the twelve CNs are elaborated from the brainstem. The first, the olfactory nerve (CN I), is directly connected to the telencephalon, and the second, the optic nerve (CN II), is directly connected to the diencephalon. Of the 10 CNs that are elaborated by the brainstem, nine emerge from its ventral aspect. Only the trochlear nerve emerges from the dorsal surface of the brainstem.

The olfactory nerve (CN I) is actually a misnomer. There are actually thousands of individual olfactory nerves, located in the olfactory epithelium of the nasal cavities, which project through the floor of the anterior cranial fossa (cribriform foramina of the cribriform plate) and synapse with second-order neurons within the olfactory bulb. The olfactory tract carries these fibers to the cerebrum. The olfactory bulb and tract sits directly upon the inferior aspect of the frontal lobe. Olfactory neurons are the only sensory neurons of the human body that do not relay first through the thalamus before reaching cerebral cortex; neurons of the olfactory tract make direct cortical connections without the use of any thalamic nuclei (Table B-1).

As with the olfactory nerve, the optic nerve (CN II) is composed of special sensory neurons (Table B-1)—in this case, neurons sensitive to visual stimulation. After a series of synapses within the ocular retina, the axons of

TABLE B-1

CRANIAL NERVES

Cranial Nerve	Fiber Type	Nucleus	Location	Target
I Olfactory	SS	Olfactory bulb[a]	Telencephalon[b]	Olfactory epithelium
II Optic	SS	Lateral geniculate	Posterior thalamus	Retina: ganglion cell layer
III Oculomotor	① GSE	① Oculomotor	Rostral midbrain	① 4 of 6 Extraocular mm.
	② GVE	② Edinger-Westphal		② a Pupillary sphincter m.[c]
				② b Ciliary m.[d]
IV Trochlear	GSE	Trochlear	Caudal midbrain	Superior oblique muscle
V Trigeminal	① GSA	① a Main sensory	① a Rostral pons	① Face, head, and meninges
	② SVE	① b Mesencephalic	① b Midbrain	② Muscles of mastication[a]
		① c Spinal nucleus	① c Medulla ⇨ rostral pons	
		② Trigeminal motor	② Rostral pons	
VI Abducens	GSE	Abducent	Mid pons	Lateral rectus muscle
VII Facial	① GSA	① Spinal trigeminal	① Medulla ⇨ rostral pons	① External ear
	② SVA	② Solitary	② Rostral medulla ⇨ caudal pons	② Taste—anterior 2/3 of tongue
	③ GVE	③ Superior salivatory	③ Mid pons	③ Salivary glands[e]
	④ SVE	④ Facial motor	④ Mid pons	④ Facial expression mm.[f]
VIII Vestibulocochlear	SS	① Vestibular (4)	① Rostral medulla ⇨ pons	① Vestibular apparatus
		② Cochlear (dorsal and ventral)	② Rostral medulla	② Organ of Corti
IX Glossopharyngeal	① GSA	① Spinal trigeminal	① Medulla ⇨ rostral pons	① External ear
	② SVA	② Solitary	② Rostral medulla ⇨ caudal pons	② Taste—posterior 1/3 of tongue
	③ GVA	③ Solitary	③ Rostral medulla ⇨ caudal pons	③ Mucous membranes[g]
	④ GVE	④ Inferior salivatory	④ Caudal pons	④ Parotid salivary gland
	⑤ SVE	⑤ Nucleus ambiguus	⑤ Medulla	⑤ Stylopharyngeus m.
X Vagus	① GSA	① Spinal trigeminal	① Medulla ⇨ rostral pons	① External ear
	② SVA	② Solitary	② Rostral medulla ⇨ caudal pons	② Taste—epiglottis and esophagus
	③ GVA	③ Solitary	③ Rostral medulla ⇨ caudal pons	③ Thoracic and abdominal viscera
	④ GVE	④ Dorsal motor nucleus	④ Medulla	④ Thoracic and abdominal viscera
	⑤ SVE	⑤ Nucleus ambiguus	⑤ Medulla	⑤ Laryngeal and pharyngeal mm.[h]
XI Spinal Accessory	SVE	① Spinal accessory nucleus	① Rostral cervical spinal cord	① SCM and trapezius mm.
		② Nucleus ambiguus	② Medulla	② ⇨ vagus ⇨ laryngeal/pharyngeal mm.[h]
XII Hypoglossal	GSE	Hypoglossal	Medulla	① 3/4 of extrinsic tongue mm.[i]
				② 4/4 of intrinsic tongue mm.

[a]Primary olfactory sensory fibers synapse here with second-order neurons.
[b]Olfactory bulb and tract are located along basal surface of cerebrum.
[c]GVEs elaborated by the E-W nucleus synapse in ciliary ganglion, second-order neurons innervate these two smooth muscles.
[d]Tensor tympani, tensor veli palatini, mylohyoid, anterior belly of digastric.
[e]Submandibular and sublingual salivary glands, palatine and nasal glands, and lacrimal gland.
[f]Stapedius, stylohyoid, and posterior belly of digastric.
[g]Nasopharynx and eustachian tube, also carotid sinus and body.
[h]Three pharyngeal constrictors, palatoglossus, levator veli palatini, uvular muscle, intrinsic laryngeal muscles.
[i]Does not innervate palatoglossus muscle (innervated by vagus nerve).

m, muscle; mm, muscles; SCM, sternoclitomastoid; SS, special sensory.

Fiber Type	Abbreviation	Cranial Nerve
General somatic afferent	GSA	V (and VII, IX, X)
General visceral afferent	GVA	IX, X (solitary nucleus)
Special visceral afferent	SVA	VII, IX, X (solitary nucleus)
Special sensory	SS	I, II, VIII
General somatic efferent	GSE	III, IV, VI, XII
General visceral efferent	GVE	III, VII, IX, X (preganglionic parasympathetic)
Special visceral (branchial) efferent	SVE	V, VII, & IX, X, XI (N. ambiguus)

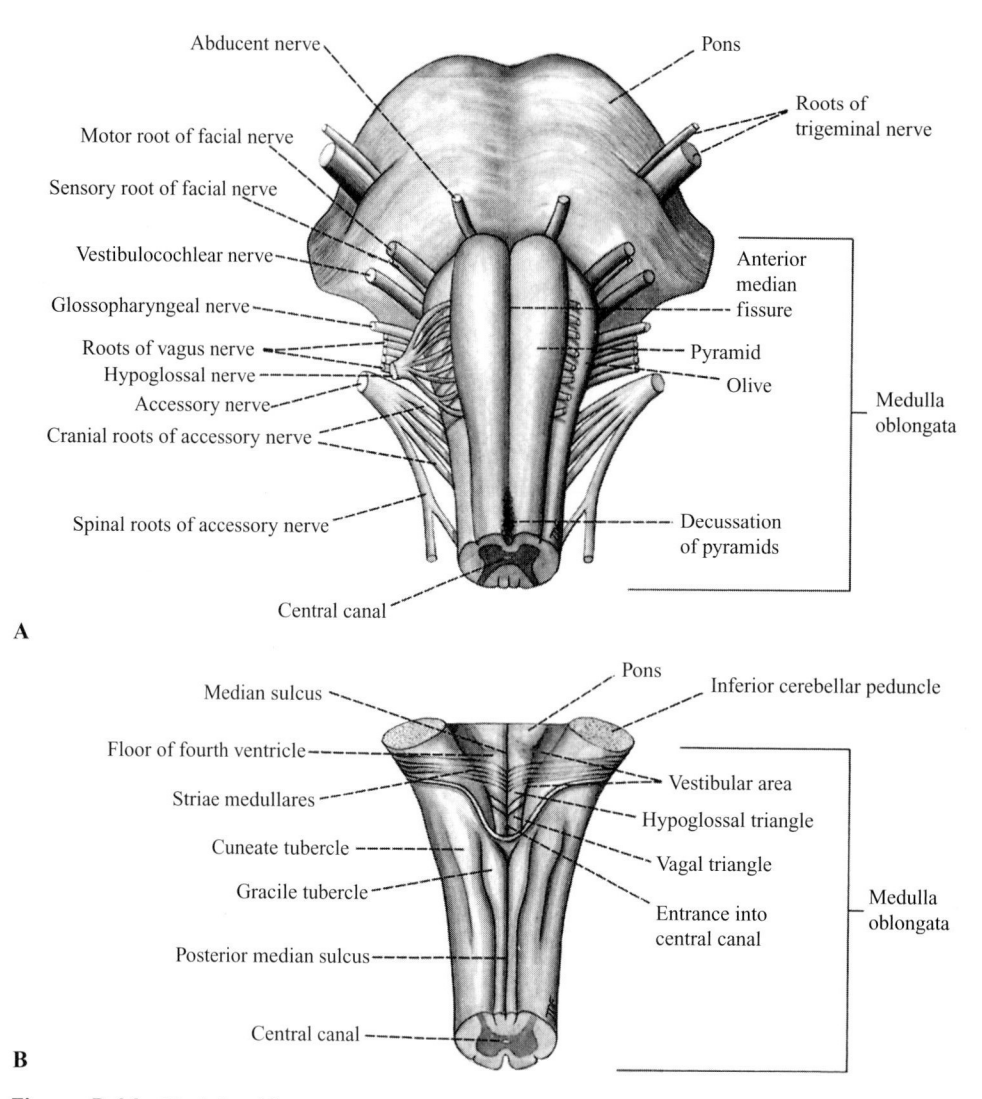

Figure B-14   Medulla oblongata. **A.** Anterior view. **B.** Posterior view. Note that the roof of the fourth ventricle and the cerebellum have been removed.

retinal ganglion cells exit the eye via the optic nerve (Figure B-1). Upon reaching the optic chiasm, fibers representing the lateral (or temporal) retina pass through the chiasm and into the ipsilateral optic tract. Fibers representing the medial (or nasal) retina pass through the chiasm and into the contralateral optic tract. Thus, each optic tract comprises fibers representing the ipsilateral temporal retina and fibers representing the contralateral nasal retina.

The third CN, the oculomotor nerve (CN III), contains two types of neuronal fibers: GSE and GVE (Table B-1). The GSE fibers innervate four of the six extraocular muscles (that move the ocular globe); the medial rectus, superior rectus, inferior rectus, and inferior oblique muscles; as well as the levator palpebrae superioris (a muscle of the upper eyelid). The main oculomotor nucleus is located in the rostral midbrain. The parasympathetic GVE fibers innervate (via the ciliary ganglion) the pupillary constrictor muscle and ciliary muscle of the eye. The

first muscle, as its name suggests, constricts the pupil; the second muscle acts upon the ocular lens, forcing it to change its shape for viewing objects near and far. A separate nucleus from the main oculomotor nucleus, the Edinger-Westphal nucleus, elaborates these GVE fibers and is located in the rostral midbrain alongside the main oculomotor nucleus. CN III projects from the rostral midbrain into the interpeduncular fossa, as described previously.

The fourth CN, the trochlear nerve (CN IV), contains only GSE neurons, innervates the superior oblique muscle, is elaborated by the trochlear nucleus located in the caudal midbrain, and is the only CN to project from the dorsal aspect of the brain—specifically, it springs forth immediately caudal to the inferior colliculus (Table B-1).

The fifth CN, the trigeminal nerve (CN V), contains two neuronal fiber types: GSA and SVE (Table B-1). As its name suggests, the trigeminal nerve is composed of three divisions: ophthalmic (V_1), maxillary (V_2), and mandibular

(V_3). Each of these three divisions provides cutaneous innervation to prescribed areas of facial skin. The SVE fibers are found solely within the third division (V_3) of the trigeminal nerve, and innervate the four muscles of mastication, as well as four other small muscles located deep within the face. The trigeminal nerve originates from no less than four brainstem nuclei. The spinal nucleus and tract is located through the length of the medulla and the caudal pons. The main sensory and motor nuclei are located at the rostral end of the spinal nucleus and tract, in the mid-pons. The fourth nucleus, the mesencephalic nucleus, extends from the mid-pons through the length of the midbrain (as its name—mesencephalic—suggests). The trigeminal nerve emerges from the anterolateral surface of the mid-pons.

The sixth CN, the abducens nerve (CN VI), contains only GSE neurons, innervates the lateral rectus extraocular muscle, is elaborated by the abducens nucleus located within the caudal pons, and projects from the pontomedullary angle (Table B-1).

The seventh CN, the facial nerve (CN VII), contains four types of neuronal fibers: GSA, SVA, GVE, and SVE (Table B-1). The GSA fibers account for a small area of the external ear, and, through a quirk of nature and evolution, actually end up riding the trigeminal nerve into the brainstem. The SVA fibers transmit taste sensation from the anterior two-thirds of the tongue to the solitary nucleus and tract. The GVE fibers are parasympathetic, arise from the superior salivatory nucleus located in the caudal pons, and innervate—via two different cranial parasympathetic ganglia (submandibular and pterygopalatine)—the submandibular and sublingual salivary glands and the lacrimal (tear) gland. Lastly, the SVE fibers, which arise from the facial motor nucleus located in the caudal pons, innervate all of the muscles of facial expression as well as four other small muscles located deep within the face. The facial nerve projects from the medial aspect of the pontocerebellar angle, immediately medial to the vestibulocochlear nerve, which will be discussed next.

The eighth CN, the vestibulocochlear nerve (CN VIII), is composed of two sets of SS fibers; vestibular fibers innervate the vestibular apparatus, and the cochlear fibers innervate the auditory apparatus of the inner ear (Table B-1). There are four pairs of vestibular nuclei, located in the medulla and pons, and two pairs of cochlear nuclei, located in the rostral medulla. The vestibulocochlear nerve projects from the pontocerebellar angle immediately lateral to the aforementioned facial nerve.

The ninth CN, the glossopharyngeal nerve (CN IX), comprises five different neural fiber types: GSA, GVA, SVA, GVE, and SVE (Table B-1). As with the facial nerve, GSA fibers from the glossopharyngeal nerve, through another quirk of evolution, account for a small area of the external ear and ride the trigeminal nerve into the brainstem. The GVA fibers provide general sensory innervation to the mucus membranes of the pharynx; its nucleus, the solitary nucleus and tract, is located throughout the length of the medulla and the caudal pons. The SVA fibers transmit taste sensation from the posterior one-third of the tongue to the solitary nucleus and tract. The GVE fibers are parasympathetic and innervate, via the otic ganglion, the parotid salivary gland. Lastly, the SVE fibers innervate a single pharyngeal muscle and arise from the nucleus ambiguus located through the length of the medulla. The glossopharyngeal nerve projects from the lateral aspect of the medulla (posterior to the olive) from the same sulcus from which the vagus and spinal accessory nerves emerge.

The tenth CN, the vagus nerve (CN X), as with the glossopharyngeal nerve, also carries five different neural fiber types: GSA, GVA, SVA, GVE, and SVE (Table B-1). As with the facial and glossopharyngeal nerves, GSA fibers from the vagus nerve, through another eccentricity of development, account for a small area of the external ear and ride the trigeminal nerve into the brainstem. The GVA fibers provide general sensory innervation to the mucus membranes of the pharynx; its nucleus, the solitary nucleus and tract, is located throughout the length of the medulla and the caudal pons. The SVA fibers transmit taste sensation from the epiglottis and pharynx to the solitary nucleus and tract. The GVE fibers are parasympathetic and provide the lion's share of the parasympathetic innervation of the body's viscera, accounting for the entire parasympathetic innervation of the viscera of the neck and thorax, and most of the abdomen. CN X's nucleus, the dorsal motor nucleus of the vagus, is located throughout most of the length of the medulla. The vagus nerve projects from the lateral aspect of the medulla from the same sulcus (posterior to the olive) from which the glossopharyngeal and spinal accessory nerves emerge.

The eleventh CN, the spinal accessory nerve (CN XI), has two separate components—the cranial and spinal roots—but carries a single neuronal fiber type: SVE (Table B-1). The SVE fibers arise from the nucleus ambiguus, located through the length of the medulla. The spinal accessory nucleus is actually present in the upper four or five cervical spinal cord levels. The spinal accessory nerve projects from the lateral aspect of the medulla from the same sulcus (posterior to the olive) from which the glossopharyngeal and vagus nerves emerge.

Lastly, the twelfth CN, the hypoglossal nerve (CN XII), uses its GSE fibers to innervate seven of the eight muscles of the tongue (Table B-1). The hypoglossal nucleus arises through most of the medulla, immediately medial to the dorsal motor nucleus of the vagus, and the hypoglossal nerve projects from the anterior aspect of the medulla, from the sulcus that separates the pyramid from the olive.

Thus, the nucleus ambiguus provides SVE fibers for three CNs: the glossopharyngeal, vagus, and spinal accessory nerves (the other SVE fibers are carried by the trigeminal nerve and are elaborated by the motor nucleus of the trigeminal nerve). The solitary nucleus and tract receives GVA fibers that innervate the mucus membranes of the pharynx, as well as (SVE) taste fibers from the tongue and neighboring structures. These GVA and SVA fibers are carried by three CNs: the facial, glossopharyngeal, and vagus nerves.

DIENCEPHALON

Continuing rostrally from the midbrain of the brainstem, the diencephalon is next encountered. The diencephalon sits perfectly interpositioned between the midbrain, caudally, and the cerebrum, rostrally. It comprises the thalamus

and the more ventral (and aptly named) hypothalamus, as well as a few other related structures.

Thalamus

The thalamus comprises more than three-quarters of the diencephalon and serves as the entryway to the cerebral cortex for subcortical structures with cortical aspirations (Figure B-15). These include projections from the basal ganglia, from numerous brainstem structures, and sensory fibers from the body's entire system of sensory information collection, with the lone exception of the olfactory system. All CNs carrying sensory fibers, with the exception of CN I,

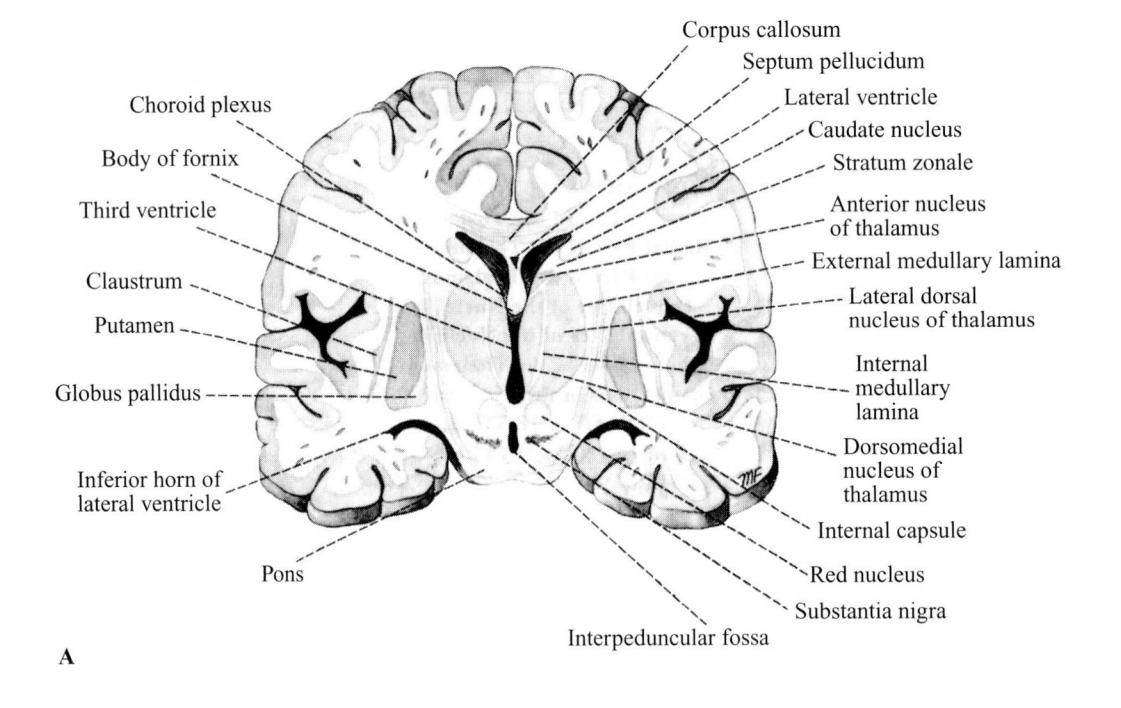

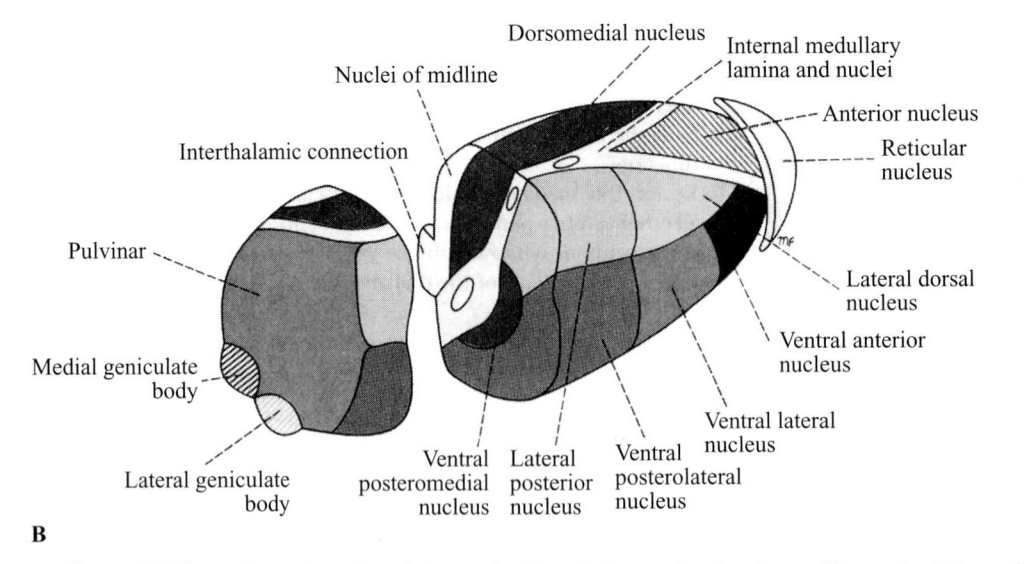

Figure B-15   **A.** Coronal section of the cerebral hemispheres, showing the position and relations of the thalamus. **B.** The nuclei of the thalamus.

communicate directly with thalamic nuclei before their information is distributed to the cerebral cortex.

The optic nerve (CN II), which is a direct extension of the diencephalon, communicates with the lateral geniculate nucleus, which, in turn, projects to the visual cortex located in the occipital lobe. The sensory fibers from the trigeminal nerve (CN V) are relayed to the ventroposteromedial (VPM) nucleus, which, in turn, projects to the somatosensory cortex located in the parietal lobe. Special visceral afferent fibers—taste fibers—from the facial (CN VII), glossopharyngeal (CN IX), and vagus (CN X) nerves are relayed through the VPM nucleus to the gustatory cortex located in the insula. The auditory sensory fibers contained within the cochlear division of the eighth CN are directed to the medial geniculate nucleus, which projects to the auditory cortex located in the temporal lobe. The vestibular sensory fibers contained within the vestibular division of the same eighth CN are directed through the thalamus to the vestibular cortex located in the insula.

The ascending, afferent, sensory projections contained within the spinothalamic tracts and the posterior column–medial lemniscus pathway pass through the spinal cord and brainstem to reach the VPM and ventroposterolateral (VPL) nuclei of the thalamus.

Limbic system information is routed through the mammillary nucleus of the hypothalamus to the anterior nucleus of the thalamus (via the mammillothalamic tract), which, in turn, projects to the cingulate gyrus of the cerebral limbic lobe.

The basal ganglia project to the ventral anterior and ventral lateral nuclei, which, in turn, project to the motor cortex, located in the frontal lobe.

Two thalamic nuclei have extensive interconnections with the two association cortices of the cerebrum: the dorsomedial nucleus with the prefrontal cortex, and the pulvinar and lateral posterior nucleus with the posterior parietal cortex.

The unpaired pineal gland, which arises as a posterior evagination of the roof of the diencephalon and is officially an element of the epithalamus, plays a vital role in the regulation of the body's circadian rhythm and has connections—via the hypothalamus—with the retina.

The subthalamic nucleus and zona incerta comprise the subthalamus. The zona incerta is a rostral continuation of the midbrain reticular formation, and the subthalamic nucleus is also a member of the basal ganglia, which will be examined in the next section.

Internal Capsule

All of the projections between the cerebral cortex and thalamic nuclei course through the internal capsule, as do descending cortical projections to the brainstem (corticobulbar fibers) and to the spinal cord (corticospinal fibers).

The internal capsule is arranged somewhat like a funnel: its inferior aspect, which leads into the cerebral peduncles, is tapered and narrow, whereas its superior aspect fans out to accommodate the expanse of cerebral cortex. The internal capsule is sandwiched between the thalamus and head of the caudate nucleus medially, and the putamen and globus pallidus (i.e., lenticular nucleus) laterally, and is composed of five distinct parts. The anterior limb carries fibers to and from the prefrontal lobe and cingulate gyrus of the limbic lobe, the posterior limb carries fibers to and from the parietal lobe, the intervening genu (knee) carries largely fibers related to the motor cortices, the retrolenticular limb carries visual system fibers to and from the visual cortex of the occipital lobe, and the sublenticular limb carries auditory system fibers to and from the auditory cortex of the temporal lobe.

Hypothalamus

The hypothalamus, positioned immediately ventral to the thalamus, is a complex array of numerous nuclei and a handful of fiber tracts.

On the basal surface of the whole brain specimen, only a small portion of the hypothalamus is visible: the pair of mammillary bodies and the pituitary. The optic chiasm, a projection of the thalamus, is located immediately rostral to the pituitary.

In hemisection, the medial aspect of the hypothalamus is readily visible. The column of the fornix is located immediately posterior to the anterior commissure. It disappears into the substance of the hypothalamus on its way to synapse in the mammillary body, located along the ventral margin of the hypothalamus.

The hypothalamus sits at the center of homeostatic control of the entire organism's physiologic functions, concerning itself with somatic, autonomic, affective, and endocrine functions. Its pituitary gland (or hypophysis) is considered the "master gland," because it releases hormones into the vascular system that serve to regulate the functions of other, peripheral glands. The posterior lobe of the pituitary, the neurohypophysis, produces two hormones: antidiuretic hormone (or vasopressin), and oxytocin. Antidiuretic hormone stimulates the resorption of water in the kidney, and oxytocin stimulates contractions of the uterus and mammary gland. The anterior lobe of the pituitary, the adenohypophysis, releases numerous hormones, including adrenocorticotropic hormone, thyroid-stimulating hormone, luteinizing hormone, follicle stimulating hormone, luteotropic hormone (prolactin), and human growth hormone.

Basal Ganglia

The basal ganglia comprise five telencephalic collections of neuronal cell bodies: the caudate nucleus, the putamen, the globus pallidus (also termed pallidum), the subthalamic nucleus, and the substantia nigra (Figure B-16). Several different collective terms are used to describe these basal ganglia. The term *striatum* refers to the caudate nucleus and

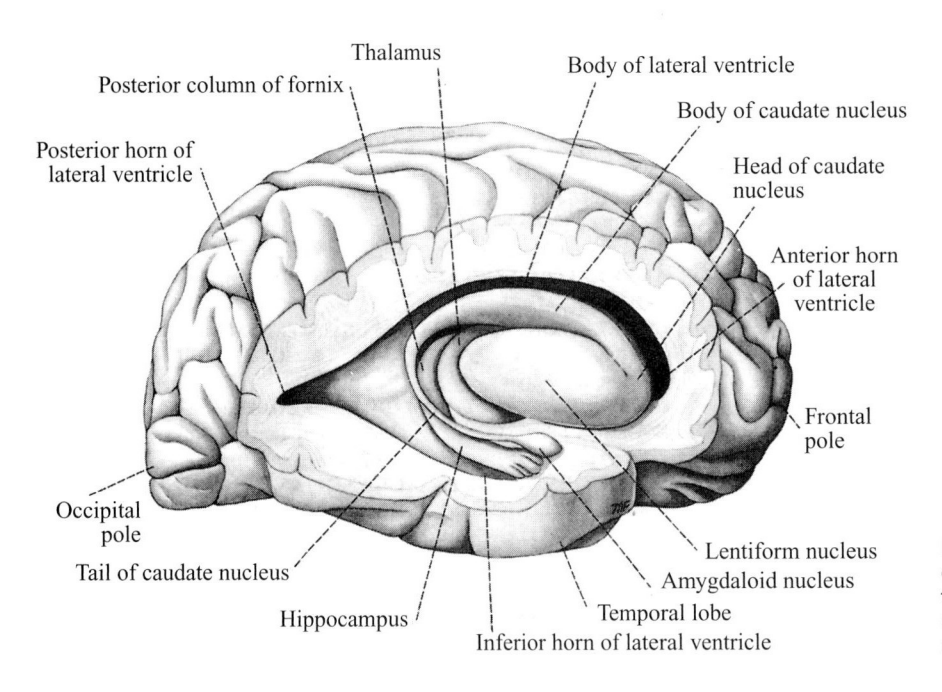

Posterior column of fornix

Thalamus

Body of lateral ventricle

Body of caudate nucleus

Posterior horn of lateral ventricle

Head of caudate nucleus

Anterior horn of lateral ventricle

Frontal pole

Occipital pole

Tail of caudate nucleus

Lentiform nucleus

Amygdaloid nucleus

Hippocampus

Temporal lobe

Inferior horn of lateral ventricle

Figure B-16   Horizontal section of the cerebrum as seen from above, showing the relationship between the lentiform nucleus, the caudate nucleus, the thalamus, and the internal capsule.

putamen, *lenticular* or *lentiform nucleus* refers to the putamen and globus pallidus, *corpus striatum* refers to striatum plus the globus pallidus, and *ventral striatum* refers to the nucleus accumbens and the basal forebrain region.

The best-known function of the basal ganglia is their role in the neural control of the body's motor system. Defects in the basal ganglia lead to a variety of movement disorders, such as parkinsonism and Huntington's chorea. However, the basal ganglia also modulate circuits involving the cerebral cortex and thalamus, and are involved in disparate functions such as affect and cognition.

The caudate nucleus is one of the structures caught up in the massive C-shaped growth of the telencephalon early in its embryologic development. It runs along the lateral wall of the anterior horn, body, and posterior horn of the lateral ventricle. The large head of the caudate nucleus is located within the depths of the frontal lobe. The body follows the contours of the body of the lateral ventricle, and the tail curls inferiorly and anteriorly along with the inferior horn of the lateral ventricle.

The putamen and globus pallidus, the so-called lenticular nucleus, sits across the internal capsule from the head of the caudate nucleus and the thalamus. Embryologically, the caudate nucleus and putamen have the same origin; this is particularly evidenced by the fact that they are joined together, as the nucleus accumbens, at the anteroventral margins of these two structures. The putamen is located just deep to the cortex of the cerebral insula. The two are separated from one another by three slim structures: two fiber tracts that conduct intrahemispheric, corticocortical projections (the external and extreme capsules); and a single area of gray matter, the claustrum (that is thought to have some connections with the visual system). The subthalamic nucleus of the thalamic subdivision, the subthalamus, sits sandwiched between the thalamus proper and

the substantia nigra (the final component of the basal ganglia), and the cerebral peduncle of the midbrain.

There are numerous routes of communication between the five members of the basal ganglia, such as the ansa lenticularis and subthalamic fasciculus, which interconnect the globus pallidus with the subthalamic nucleus; the thalamic fasciculus, which connects the subthalamic nucleus with the ventral anterior and ventral lateral nuclei of the thalamus; and the nigrostriatal fibers, which link the substantia nigra with the caudate nucleus and the putamen.

Multiple parallel neural loops are formed between the basal ganglia, the thalamus, and the cerebral cortex. The cerebral cortex, substantia nigra, and a specific set of thalamic nuclei project to the caudate nucleus and putamen, the striatum; the striatum projects to the substantia nigra and globus pallidus; the globus pallidus projects to a set of specific thalamic nuclei; and these thalamic nuclei project back to the striatum, as well as to most of the cerebral cortex, and the cycle continues. In sum, these loops of neural circuitry all work to perform a single function: to modulate cortical output. Breakdowns among these circuits lead to movement disorders such as Parkinson's disease and Huntington's disease.

CEREBELLUM

As described previously, the cerebellum develops from the metencephalon, which also gives rise to the pons. It comprises two hemispheres that are joined along the midline by the vermis. Further, the cerebellum comprises three lobes, three sets of deep nuclei, three cortical layers, three peduncles, and is supplied by three arteries. The three lobes are the anterior, posterior, and flocculonodular. The three sets of deep nuclei are the dentate, interposed

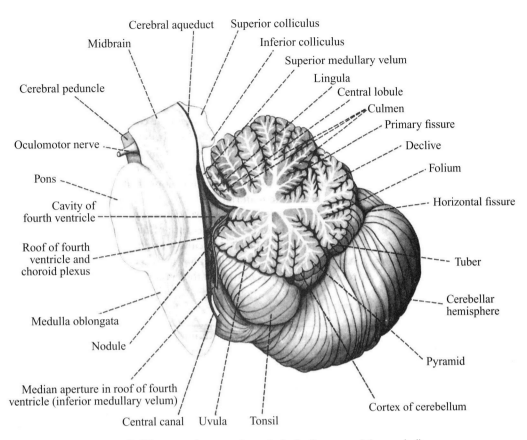

Figure B-17 Sagittal section through the brainstem and the cerebellum.

(composed of the emboliform and globose nuclei), and the fastigial. The three cortical layers are the granular, Purkinje cell, and molecular. The three peduncles are the inferior, middle, and superior. The three arteries are the posterior inferior cerebellar, anterior inferior cerebellar, and superior cerebellar (Figure B-17).

The cerebellum accounts for fully one-half of the total number of neurons located within the CNS. Its appearance is similar to that of the cerebrum; it has a thin cortex that is thrown into folds and crevices, termed folia and fissures, respectively. The cerebrum has its deep nuclei (the basal ganglia), and the cerebellum has its own complement of deep nuclei. The cerebrum has a pair of peduncles that connects fiber tracts between the cerebral cortex and subcortical structures, and the cerebellum has three sets of cerebellar peduncles that connect it to other structures of the brain.

A lateral view of the cerebellum of the whole brain specimen demonstrates its position ventral to the occipital pole of the cerebrum and posterior to the pons and medulla. *In situ*, the dural reflection (the tentorium cerebelli) separates the occipital pole and the cerebellum; in fact, the occipital pole actually rests on this dural shelf.

A medial view afforded by a hemisection of the whole brain specimen demonstrates the sectioned midline vermis. The early anatomists used the term, arbor vitae, to describe the tree-like appearance of the sectioned vermis.

Note that the vermis directly abuts the fourth ventricle, forming its tent-peaked roof. The medial view demonstrates its relationship with the entire brainstem (anteriorly), the cervical spinal cord (caudally), and the occipital lobe of the cerebrum (dorsally).

The anterior lobe is largely hidden beneath the occipital pole of the cerebrum *in situ*. It is divided from the posterior lobe by the primary fissure. The cerebellar tonsil, and medial appendage of each cerebellar hemisphere, is nestled up next to the medulla. Circumstances in which intracranial pressure is increased (e.g., secondary to swelling) can result in tonsillar herniation, in which the tonsil herniates caudally through the foramen magnum and is forced against the medulla, where respiratory centers can be injured. This is, obviously, a life-threatening event. The remaining cerebellar component is the flocculonodular lobe.

The middle peduncle projects laterally from the pons and is the largest of the three peduncles; the substantial trigeminal nerve projects from its anterolateral surface. The superior peduncle is directed rostrally away from the cerebellum, and the inferior peduncle is directed superiorly into the cerebellum.

The cerebellum is perhaps best known for its relationship with the body's motor system; one of its main functions is to coordinate limb movements and help with postural adjustments. However, the cerebellum is also involved in motor learning, eye movements, and even cognitive functions. Thus, cerebellar damage may elicit cognitive deficits as well as motor ataxia.

The inferior cerebellar peduncle conducts only afferent fibers into the cerebellum. This peduncle transmits the posterior spinocerebellar and cuneocerebellar tracts into the cerebellum. The former carries proprioception sensory information from the lower limbs, and the latter, from the upper limbs. The inferior cerebellar peduncle also transmits fibers that originate in the inferior olivary complex, vestibular nuclei, reticular formation, thalamus, and trigeminal nuclei. This peduncle transmits no efferent fibers from the cerebellum; it is strictly used for incoming traffic.

The massive middle cerebellar peduncle, the largest of the three cerebellar peduncles, conducts only a single type of fiber in only a single direction. Pontocerebellar fibers project from pontine nuclei into the cerebellum; nothing else goes into the cerebellum and nothing comes out of the cerebellum via this middle peduncle. The cerebral cortex and cerebellum have no direct communication with one another; their communicating fibers are relayed to one another through other nuclei. The cerebellar cortex projects specific corticobulbar fibers that are earmarked for pontine nuclei, the corticopontine fibers. These pontine nuclei then project into the cerebellum through the middle cerebellar peduncle as pontocerebellar fibers. Similarly, the cerebellum communicates indirectly with the cerebral cortex by projecting fibers, through the superior cerebellar peduncle, to the thalamus, where they can be relayed to the cerebral cortex.

The superior cerebellar peduncle is unique among the three cerebellar peduncles in that it is the only one that transmits cerebellar fibers out of the cerebellum. Specifically, it transmits cerebellar efferents to the thalamus, red nuclei, vestibular nuclei, and reticular nuclei. To add a twist, however, the superior cerebellar peduncle transmits one type of afferent fiber into the cerebellum. It transmits fibers of the anterior spinocerebellar tract, which carries complicated proprioceptive and other related sensory information.

LIMBIC SYSTEM

The limbic system consists of the cerebral limbic lobe and the limbic structures contained therein. It is the oldest region, phylogenetically, of the human brain. Limbic structures include the amygdala, hippocampus, fornix, and stria terminalis, as well as others (Figure B-18). As described previously, the amygdala, a nuclear mass, is located in the anterior aspect of the temporal lobe. Immediately posterior to it, located within the inferior horn of the lateral ventricle, is the hippocampus, a three-layered, ancient cortical structure. The hippocampus elaborates the fornix, which makes an arcing, C-shaped run around the thalamus to terminate largely in the mammillary nuclei of the ventral hypothalamus. From here, the mammillothalamic tract projects to the anterior thalamic nucleus, which, in turn, projects to the cingulate gyrus. The cingulate gyrus then projects into its associated deep white matter tract, the cingulum, which makes an arcing, C-shaped run around the periphery of the corpus callosum to eventually project back to the hippocampus. This neural loop is known as *Papez's circuit*. Another neural loop connects the amygdala to the hypothalamus and septal areas via the stria terminalis, a narrow tract of white matter that travels very closely to the C-shaped caudate nucleus.

Degenerative dementias that cause entorhinal cortical atrophy disrupt the normal functioning of the hippocampal formation, which can result in long-term memory loss and emotional and mood problems. Abnormalities of the limbic system have been implicated in thought disorders such as schizophrenia.

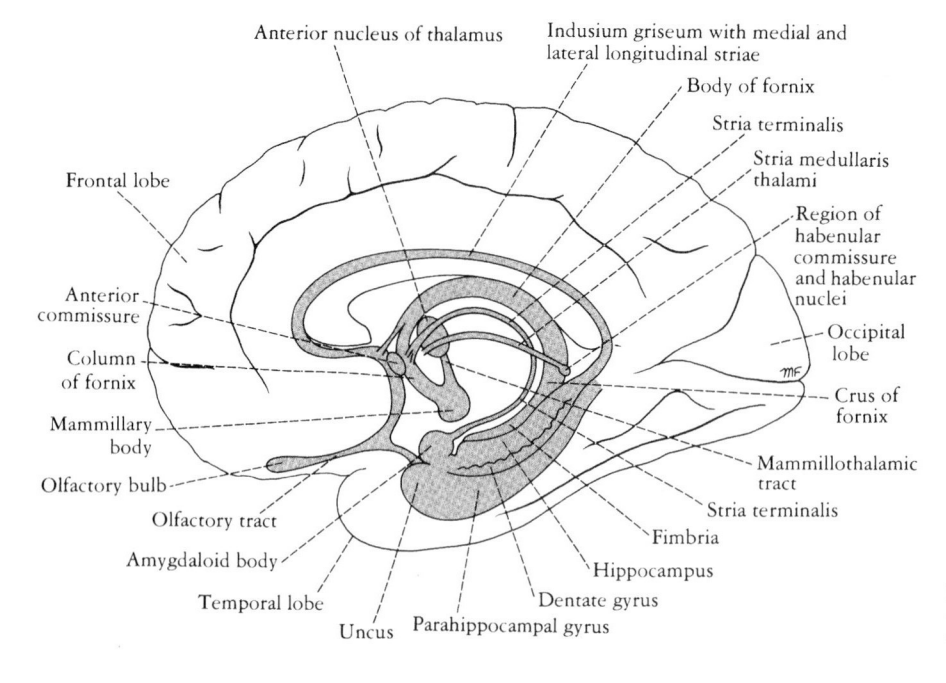

Figure B-18 The medial surface of the right cerebral hemisphere showing the parts of the limbic system.

CEREBRAL CORTEX

The cerebral cortex comprises a thin sheet of neuronal cell bodies and their local processes that covers essentially the entire (99%) surface of the telencephalon, from the frontal pole to the occipital pole to the temporal pole and everything in between, except for a very small area located on its ventromedial surface (Figure B-19). Tasks assigned to this thin sheet of gray matter include conscious sensory perception, the planning and execution of motor tasks, memory and cognition, language and musical skills, personality and imagination, and many others. Many of these tasks are assigned to specific regions of cerebral cortex; nearly all require integration between different cortical areas.

Four functional divisions of the cerebral cortex are conventionally identified:

1. Sensory
2. Motor
3. Limbic
4. Integrative or Associative

As described previously, there are five cerebral lobes. The frontal lobe is located anterior to the central sulcus and superior to the lateral sulcus, and is home to the primary motor cortex (Brodmann area 4) and premotor areas (Brodmann area 6), the language-related region, Broca's area (Brodmann areas 44 and 45, or pars opercularis and pars triangularis, respectively, of the inferior frontal gyrus), and the expansive prefrontal association area. Thus, a cerebrovascular accident (CVA) involving the frontal lobe can result in loss of motor function, Broca's aphasia, and personality and behavioral changes.

The parietal lobe is located posterior to the central sulcus and superior to the posterior extent of the lateral sulcus and is home to the primary (Brodmann areas 3, 1, 2) and secondary somatosensory cortices (Brodmann area 5), the language-related angular and supramarginal gyri, and the massive posterior parietal association area. Thus, a CVA involving the parietal lobe can result in loss of normal somatosensory function, various agnosias, and even visual changes.

The temporal lobe is found inferior to the lateral sulcus and is home to the auditory cortices (Brodmann areas 41, 42, and 22) and Wernicke's (receptive) speech area. The temporal lobe also likely plays an associative or integrative role for the neighboring visual cortices. Thus, a CVA involving the temporal lobe can result in loss of normal auditory function, Wernicke's aphasia, and even changes in normal visual function.

The occipital lobe occupies the posterior reaches of the cerebral hemispheres. Much of the occipital lobe is dedicated

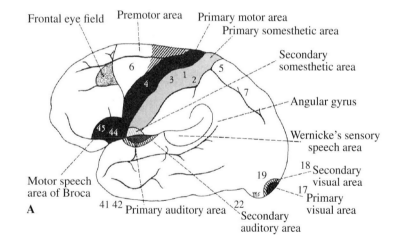

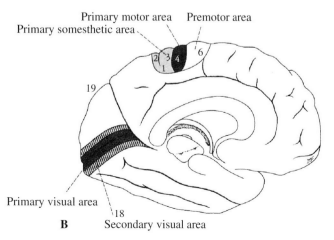

Figure B-19 Functional localization of the cerebral cortex. **A.** Lateral view of left cerebral hemisphere. **B.** Medial view of left cerebral hemisphere.

to the visual system, harboring the visual cortices. Thus, a CVA involving the occipital lobe nearly always results in loss of normal visual function.

The fifth cerebral lobe is the limbic lobe, which is found only on the medial aspect of the cerebral hemisphere and comprises the cingulate and parahippocampal gyri and the intervening isthmus. The C-shaped limbic lobe contains elements of the limbic system (e.g., the cingulum, hippocampal formation, fornix, and stria terminalis), as previously described.

Once considered a distinct lobe, the insula is an island of cortical tissue found tucked within the deepest reaches of the lateral sulcus. Composed of five or six small gyri, the insula is involved in gustatory sensation. It may also be related to limbic structures as well as other functions that have not yet been adequately described.

Cortex covers some 99% of the surface of the cerebrum. Approximately 90% of this coverage is composed of homotypical, six-layered neocortex. The remaining coverage is divided among phylogenetically older cortex types or allocortex (archicortex, paleocortex, and mesocortex) that have fewer than six layers.

Brodmann Areas

In the mid-19th century, Brodmann characterized the cytoarchitectural structure of the human cerebral cortex with tremendous precision. In fact, he described 52 different anatomic regions and posited that each distinct area, assigned a unique Brodmann area number, may have a distinct function. Research over the last 100 plus years has borne this out to a certain extent, but not absolutely. Thus, Brodmann area 4, found along much of the precentral gyrus, accounts very neatly for the primary motor cortex. This has also been found to hold true for the primary visual cortex (Brodmann area 17), Broca's area (Brodmann areas 44 and 45), and many others. In these cases, it is convenient and appropriate to refer to certain anatomic regions of the cerebral cortex by their Brodmann numbers, as is done in clinical practice.

Cortical processing of sensory information can be described as following series and parallel hierarchies. For series processing, subcortical afferents—largely thalamic—project to primary sensory areas, which project to local unimodal association cortices, which in turn project to the polymodal (or multimodal) association cortices, especially the posterior parietal association area (PPAA). In most cases, the PPAA ultimately sends projections to the prefrontal association area.

Cortical association areas serve to integrate different, and sometimes disparate, pieces of information into a more complex, cohesive, ordered unit. Sensory unimodal association areas integrate information from a single, primary sensory cortex. For example, consider the visual sense when an object is seen moving across a visual field. Different, specific aspects of the visual system are specialized to respond

maximally to very specific visual stimuli. Different visual system neurons encode for specific information regarding the object such as shape, size, color, motion, etc. Thus, the primary visual cortex (as well as the other primary sensory cortices) receives an enormous amount of sensory input that must be integrated in order to be fully comprehensible and useful. This function is carried out by an adjacent unimodal association cortex. For the visual system, this is Brodmann areas 18 and 19, located immediately adjacent to CN VI in the anterior aspect of the superior parietal lobule. Ultimately, many projections from these two areas are directed to the polymodal (or multimodal) PPAA located in Brodmann area 7, where they are integrated with other sensory information received from the other sensory cortices. The PPAA is the master sensory cortex; it functions to integrate all received sensory information into a cohesive, organized sensory picture. Ultimately, this integrated information is passed along to the prefrontal association area where motor responses are considered and planned.

It is important to note that the cortical sensory processing structure begins with simple, relatively unprocessed sensory information (although it is thought that thalamic nuclei undertake some level of processing of afferent stimuli, and are not simply relaying this information to cortical areas) and passes it along to successively higher cortical areas with successively higher degrees of processing. Thus, these systems move from the simple to the highly complex.

Although it is generally thought that most cortical sensory processing is performed in series, parallel processing also occurs. In parallel processing, shortcuts are made, skipping one or more cortical sensory processing steps. For example, thalamic efferents may be sent directly to a unimodal association area, bypassing the relevant primary sensory cortex. In the case of the visual system, for example, areas 18 and 19 will receive some direct thalamic projections, as well as (series) projections from its primary visual cortex (area 17). The massive PPAA will also receive its share of direct thalamic projections that skirt areas 17, 18, and 19. It is thought that this combination of series and parallel methods of cortical sensory processing enables a higher degree of cortical integration of sensory information.

Furthermore, as has been seen in the posterior column–medial lemniscus pathway and spinothalamic tracts, in the descending corticospinal tracts, and in the thalamic sensory nuclei, sensory projections maintain a topographic organization within the sensory cortices. For example, somatotopically organized thalamic projections synapse on the primary somatosensory cortex (S1) neocortical cells in a similar somatotopic pattern, such that an oddly shaped map of the human body is represented. This distorted *homunculus* is draped across the length of S1, located within the postcentral gyrus, with the grossly enlarged hand and face occupying much of its lateral and dorsolateral aspect, and the more understated lower limb found largely on its medial aspect. Those body areas that receive more innervation, such as the skin of the fingers and hands, and the skin and oral mucosa of the face, mouth, and tongue, have a greater amount of cerebral cortex dedicated to them. Conversely, the skin of the elbow or of the shin is represented by much smaller cortical areas.

Somatosensory Cortex

The posterior column–medial lemniscus pathway ultimately projects, by way of the VPL and VPM thalamic nuclei, to the primary somatosensory cortex (Brodmann areas 3, 1, 2) located largely within the postcentral gyrus of the parietal lobe. The anterolateral system, which includes the spinothalamic tract, also projects to this same gyrus via these same thalamic nuclei. And these somatotopically organized thalamic projections synapse on S1 neocortical cells in a similar somatotopic pattern, such that the aforementioned homunculus is represented.

As described earlier, S1 communicates directly with its adjacent unimodal association cortex. For the somatosensory system, this is Brodmann area 5 located immediately posterior to S1 in the posterior wall of the postcentral sulcus and the anterior aspect of the superior parietal lobule. Ultimately, many projections from area 5 are directed to the PPAA, located in Brodmann area 7, where they are integrated with other sensory information received from the other sensory cortices.

Visual Cortex

Thalamic efferent projections from the lateral geniculate nuclei via the optic radiations (or geniculocalcarine tract) are transmitted through the retrolenticular limb of the internal capsule to the primary visual cortex (V1), located within the cortex lining the calcarine sulcus in Brodmann area 17, as well as by its unimodal association cortex, Brodmann areas 18 and 19. It is also thought that parts of the temporal lobe serve to integrate visual information. Each of these three areas is retinotopically organized with specific cortical regions responsible for very specific qualities of the incoming visual information. The line of Gennari is believed to represent a broad and highly innervated internal granular layer (or layer IV) of the striate cortex. This line is often visible in gross sections to the unaided eye. The visual cortex also embodies both series and parallel elements. Finally, the PPAA receives a great deal of input from areas 18 and 19 as well as from the primary visual cortex.

Auditory Cortex

Thalamic afferent projections from the medial geniculate nuclei (i.e., the auditory radiations that are transmitted through the sublenticular limb of the internal capsule) are received by the primary auditory cortex, found within the cortex lining the transverse temporal gyri (Heschl's gyri) along the superior surface of the superior temporal gyrus, in Brodmann areas 41 and 42, and by the auditory associa-

tion cortex that inhabits most of the superior temporal gyrus in Brodmann area 22. Each of these three areas is tonotopically organized with specific cortical regions responsible for very specific qualities of the incoming auditory information. A specialized perisylvian language area, Wernicke's area, is located within the posterior aspect of area 22.

Vestibular Cortex

The vestibular cortex is thought to occupy the posterior aspect of the insula and adjacent parts of the inferior parietal lobule and superior temporal gyrus. Because this information is carried by CN VIII, the vestibulocochlear nerve, it is not surprising to find its cortex neighboring that of the auditory system (carried by the cochlear division of CN VIII). Ultimately, these cortical areas project to the nearby PPAA for further integration.

Olfactory and Gustatory Cortices

The olfactory cortex receives its afferent projections directly from fibers composing the olfactory tract; it is the only sense that is not first processed by the thalamus before reaching the cortex. Just as the optic nerve is a direct outgrowth of the diencephalon, the olfactory tract and bulb are a direct outgrowth of the telencephalon. The gustatory cortex is located within the medial surface of the frontal operculum and anterior insula.

Motor Cortices

First, just as the cortical sensory processing systems are organized (especially in their series mode) in a simple-to-complex manner, the cortical motor system is organized in the opposite fashion—complex to simple. Beginning with highly complex information originating in the prefrontal cortex, information is passed along to successively simpler cortical areas, the premotor area and primary motor cortex, ultimately ending in simple commands carried by corticospinal, corticobulbar, corticostriatal, and other descending fibers. In an oversimplified model, the sensory systems begin with very simple sensory data and end with highly integrated information, ultimately formulated within the prefrontal association area (PFAA). According to this model, this highly processed information then serves the motor system by determining the motor action or response that needs to be made next. This information (decision) is then passed along to the premotor area, where the exact strategy and supporting tactics are assembled in order to carry out the prefrontal strategic plan. The final step is for the premotor area to instruct the primary motor cortex to simply execute or implement its orders. As with the cortical sensory systems, the cortical motor system performs its function in both series and parallel fashions.

Prefrontal Association Area

As discussed previously, the PFAA, located anterior to the motor cortices, receives highly integrated sensory information from the PPAA. The PFAA also receives direct projections from the various primary cortices as well as from the unimodal sensory association areas. Furthermore, the PFAA also receives afferents from numerous subcortical structures, including the thalamus, basal ganglia, brainstem, cerebellum (by way of bulbar and thalamic projections), and ascending spinal cord projections. After receiving and processing a massive amount of cortical and subcortical input, the PFAA determines a motor action to be performed and passes this information along to the premotor area for further processing (series). In addition, the PFAA also contributes a number of descending fibers, such as those found in the corticospinal tracts and corticobulbar pathways (parallel). The PFAA also contains the frontal eye fields (Brodmann area 8) that help direct eye movements, as well as Broca's area (Brodmann areas 44 and 45), a key perisylvian language center for the production of (especially) oral language.

Premotor Area

Located in Brodmann area 6 immediately anterior to the primary motor cortex (Brodmann area 4), the premotor area is composed of the posterior reaches of the superior and middle frontal gyri as well as part of the inferior aspect of the precentral gyrus, located immediately superior to the lateral sulcus. As described earlier, the premotor cortex receives direct projections from its neighbor, the PFAA (in series). It also receives afferent projections from other cortical areas as well as from subcortical structures (in parallel) such as the basal ganglia, which aid in the selection and initiation of consciously willed movements; and the cerebellum, which helps provide instructions for the direction, timing, and force of voluntary, multijoint movements. The purpose (or at least one of the purposes) of the premotor area is to devises a specific strategy and plan for its consequential motor response, or the specific *What, When,* and *Where?* of the ultimate set of motor commands, and then to assemble the actual tactics, or the specific mechanisms of *How?* used to further process the devised strategic plans. In turn, in the series model, the premotor cortex next instructs the primary motor cortex to execute the ultimate motor command(s) originally devised by the PFAA. Some of these projections bypass the primary motor cortex and contribute directly to descending the corticospinal tracts and corticobulbar pathways, another example of parallel processing.

The premotor area comprises two functionally, although much less anatomically, distinct areas: the premotor cortex and the supplementary motor cortex, with the former located laterally, and the latter more dorsal and medial. The premotor cortex is generally activated when movements are planned in response to external sensory stimuli, whereas the supplementary motor cortex is involved with movements that are initiated internally, such as those requiring preparatory movement sequences from memory in the absence of visual clues.

Primary Motor Cortex

The primary motor cortex is located in Brodmann area 4, which covers much of the precentral gyrus. It is here that the execution or implementation of motor commands is carried out. In the series model, the primary motor cortex receives its commands directly from the premotor cortex, which receives it commands directly from the PFAA. And, in parallel fashion, the primary motor cortex also receives direct projections from other cortical areas and subcortical structures.

The primary motor cortex has its own specific homunculus that appears very similar to its neighboring primary somatosensory cortex homunculus. As with the somatosensory homunculus, motor areas contributing to the innervation of muscles of the face and hands and fingers occupy a disproportionately large area of cortex compared to anatomical regions that receive much less innervation, such as the elbow and shin. This enables greater motor control of the mouth, tongue, and neighboring areas, areas that play important roles in eating and speech. The expanded motor cortex dedicated to the fingers and hands affords the great dexterity required for their finely controlled movements.

Much of the output of the primary motor cortex is, ultimately, directed to the spinal cord; this is accomplished both directly and indirectly. Its direct projections comprise the corticospinal tract (CST) and the elements of the corticobulbar tract that synapse on the CN motor nuclei. The CST is also called the pyramidal tract, named not for the giant pyramidal cells (Betz cells) found, especially, in neocortical layer V or the internal granular layer, but for the pyramid-shaped elevations present on the ventral surface of the medulla. These bilateral collections of approximately 1,000,000 axons descend, in turn, through the anterior limb of the internal capsule, the cerebral peduncle, the basis pontis, pyramids of the medulla, and, ultimately, the spinal cord. Approximately 85% of these upper motor neurons decussate in the caudal medulla and descend as the contralateral lateral CST, located in the lateral funiculus. These neurons synapse largely on lower motor neurons located in the lateral aspect of the anterior horn, the axons of which innervate mostly distal limb musculature. The remaining 15% of corticospinal neurons pass through the medulla uncrossed into the anterior CST found in the ipsilateral anterior funiculus of the spinal cord, ultimately crossing to synapse with contralateral anterior horn cells that provide relatively minor innervation to proximal limb and axial muscles.

Interestingly, approximately only one-third of the lateral CST is composed of fibers that originate from the primary motor cortex; another third originates from the premotor area, and still another third from the primary somatosensory cortex. There are also small numbers of fibers that originate from other cortical areas. The anterior CST receives most of its fibers from the premotor area and a large number from the primary motor cortex.

Alzheimer's disease, the most common cause of degenerative dementia, eventually results in generalized cortical atrophy with accompanying neuritic plaques and neurofibrillary tangles. Other more focal degenerative dementias affect only specific cortical areas. Nevertheless, signs and symptoms vary according to the cortical areas being most affected. Thus, motor cortex atrophy can lead to apraxias, parietal lobe atrophy can lead to agnosias, frontal lobe atrophy can lead to short-term memory loss and Broca's aphasia, and temporal lobe atrophy can lead to Wernicke's aphasia.

THE AUTONOMIC NERVOUS SYSTEM

As described previously, the human nervous system comprises three major components: the CNS, the PNS, and the ANS. Each of these entities has sensory (afferent) and motor (efferent) components. The ANS has both central and peripheral components and comprises three major divisions: sympathetic, parasympathetic, and enteric. The ANS is responsible for the monitoring of, and providing normal routine adjustments to, vital physiological functions such as cardiovascular, pulmonary, GI, genitourinary, and blood pressure homeostasis. The ANS also innervates endocrine and exocrine glands, blood vessels, and smooth and cardiac muscle. Most of these adjustments are made below the level of consciousness, and are thus automatic (autonomic).

The sympathetic and parasympathetic divisions of the ANS share several similarities with the somatic portion of the central and peripheral nervous systems. They both have sensory and motor components, with their attendant ascending and descending pathways, and they also have simple reflex arcs. However, a fundamental difference exists between the two systems. The efferent component of the somatic component of the CNS and PNS requires a single neuron, whereas the efferent component of the ANS is always composed of two neurons. The cell body of the first neuron, the preganglionic neuron, in this short chain of motor command, is located within the CNS. The soma (cell body) of the second neuron, the postganglionic neuron, is located within specific ganglia located outside the CNS. The two divisions assemble their two-neuron efferent chain differently. In both cases, the preganglionic fibers are (thinly) myelinated, whereas the postganglionic fibers are unmyelinated.

Peripheral motor processes of the PNS all elaborate acetylcholine as a neurotransmitter. Similarly, both preganglionic and postganglionic parasympathetic neurons use acetylcholine as their neurotransmitter. Acetylcholine is also the neurotransmitter of choice for preganglionic sympathetic fibers; however, the postganglionic sympathetic elaborates a different neurotransmitter, norepinephrine.

Parasympathetic Division

The parasympathetic division of the ANS, as opposed to the *fight-or-flight* responses initiated by the sympathetic division, maintains many of the body's physiologic homeostatic functions in a state of *rest-and-digest*. In general, these two polar divisions elicit opposing effects (Table B-2).

The efferent or motor aspect of the parasympathetic division of the ANS is described as craniosacral outflow, because its preganglionic cell bodies are found within the brainstem cranial nuclei as well as in the sacral spinal cord. The four cranial nuclei that transmit preganglionic parasympathetic fibers are described below.

CN III (oculomotor nerve), in addition to conveying general somatic efferent (motor) fibers to four of the six extraocular muscles that move the ocular globe, also conveys preganglionic parasympathetic fibers. These fibers synapse in the ciliary ganglion (located posterior to the ocular globe in the bony orbit). The postganglionic fibers then innervate the pupillary sphincter muscle, which acts to decrease the size of the pupil, and the ciliary muscle, which affects the size and shape of the ocular lens.

CN VII (facial nerve) transmits preganglionic parasympathetic fibers to two ganglia: the submandibular ganglion (located near the submandibular gland), which provides postganglionic fibers to two salivary glands (sublingual and submandibular), and the pterygopalatine ganglion, which provides postganglionic fibers to the lacrimal (tear) gland.

CN IX (glossopharyngeal nerve) carries preganglionic parasympathetic fibers to the otic ganglion (so-named because of its proximity to the ear), which elaborates postganglionic fibers destined to innervate the parotid (salivary) gland.

Thus, there are four parasympathetic ganglia located in the head: ciliary, submandibular, otic, and pterygopalatine.

Finally, the fourth CN that conveys preganglionic parasympathetic fibers, CN X (vagus nerve), transmits these fibers to a wide array of structures outside the head. Even though it is indeed a CN (since its constituent nuclei are located within the brainstem), the parasympathetic division of the vagus does not innervate any structures within the head; however, its other four fiber types do supply such structures. Thus, the vagus (Latin for *wandering*) nerve, through its peripatetic course throughout the thoracic, abdominal, and pelvic cavities, provides parasympathetic innervation for all of the viscera contained therein except for the descending and sigmoid colon, the rectum, and the pelvic genitourinary organs. These organs are provided by preganglionic parasympathetic fibers present in the pelvic splanchnic nerves (S2–S4).

The cell bodies of the preganglionic parasympathetic neurons present in sacral spinal cord segments 2–4 are

TABLE B-2
THE AUTONOMIC NERVOUS SYSTEM

Structure or System	Sympathetic Effect	Parasympathetic Effect
Head		
Pupillary sphincter muscle	*no innervation*	Contracts (miosis)
Pupillary dilator muscle	Contracts (mydriasis)	*no innervation*
Superior tarsal muscle	Contracts (upper eyelid elevation)	*no innervation*
Ciliary muscle	*no innervation*	Contracts (accommodation)
Lacrimal gland	⇓ Secretion	⇑ Secretion
(3) Salivary glands	⇓ Secretion	⇑ Secretion
Pineal gland	⇑ Melatonin synthesis	*no innervation*
Cardiovascular System		
Heart rate and output	⇑	⇓
Arteries (skeletal muscle)	Constrict	*no innervation*
Arteries (skin)	Constrict	*no innervation*
Arteries (viscera)	Constrict	Dilate
Gastrointestinal System		
Motility	⇓	⇑
Sphincters	Contract	Relax
Secretion	⇓	⇑
Gallbladder	Relax	Contract
Urogenital System		
Bladder detrusor	Relax	Contract
Bladder sphincter	Contract	Relax
Seminal vesicles/vas deferens	Contract (during ejaculation)	*no innervation*
Penile/clitoral arteries	Constrict	Dilate
Skin		
Sweat glands	⇑ Secretion	*no innervation*
Piloerector muscles	Contract	*no innervation*
Others		
Bronchial muscles	Relax	Contract
Adrenal medulla	⇑ Secretion	*no innervation*

Adapted from Nolte, J. *The Human Brain: An Introduction to Its Functional Anatomy.* 5th Ed. St. Louis: Mosby; 2002.

found in the lateral aspect of the intermediate gray area, in a similar position as that of the preganglionic sympathetic neuronal cell bodies that are found in the lateral horn of intermediate gray matter of spinal cord levels T1–L2. The lightly myelinated axons of these preganglionic parasympathetic neurons are then carried within spinal nerves S2–S4, from which they quickly directly exit as pelvic

splanchnic nerves that are distributed to pelvic viscera, as described earlier.

Preganglionic parasympathetic fibers transmitted via the vagus and pelvic splanchnic nerves synapse with postganglionic neurons in ganglia located close to, or within the walls of, their target viscera. These ganglia are much less discrete than the ganglia of the somatic and sympathetic nervous systems. In the head, preganglionic parasympathetic neurons synapse with postganglionic parasympathetic neurons in four discrete ganglia, as noted above.

Sympathetic Division

In general, the sympathetic division of the ANS enables target cells and tissues, as well as the entire individual, to prepare for situations that require sudden, intense physical activity, traditionally known as the fight-or-flight response.

The cell bodies of sympathetic preganglionic neurons are located in the thoracic and upper lumbar spinal cord; thus, the sympathetic division of the ANS has a thoracolumbar distribution. There are two types of target ganglia of these sympathetic preganglionic neurons. The

TABLE B-3
PATTERNS OF DERMATOME-REFERRED PAIN

Organ Injured	Dermatomes
Diaphragm	C3–C4
Heart	T1–T4 (mainly left)
Stomach	T6–T9 (mainly left)
Gallbladder	T7–T8 (right)
Duodenum	T9–T10
Appendix	T–10 (right)
Reproductive organs	T10–T12
Kidney, ureter	L1–L2

paravertebral sympathetic chain is a collection of discrete ganglia that are interconnected by collections of preganglionic sympathetic fibers running along the posterior body wall just lateral to the vertebral bodies of the vertebral column. The chain extends from the base of the skull to the tip of the sacrum. There are also four individual preaortic (or prevertebral) ganglia—celiac, aorticorenal, superior mesenteric, and inferior mesenteric—that are located near the arterial branches of the abdominal aorta that their names describe.

Referred Pain

Along with general somatic afferents, sympathetic afferent fibers enter the spinal cord at levels T1–L2 via the dorsal root and dorsal horn, with their cell bodies stored for safekeeping in the dorsal root ganglion along with those of all afferent neurons that enter the spinal cord. Most of this sympathetic afferent traffic concerns information regarding visceral pain. Cardiac pain, such as angina pectoris, is conveyed through afferent sympathetic fibers that enter the spinal cord at levels T1–T4, and mainly only on the left side. General somatic afferent neurons that represent dermatomes T1–T4 also enter the spinal cord at these levels. It is presumed that there is some cross talk between pain-transmitting sympathetic afferents and pain-conducting somatic afferents, such that the latter may be stimulated by the former. Thus, cardiac pain may be felt (or referred) to one or more of dermatomes T1–T4 on the left side, which encompass the upper trunk and part of the upper limb, as pain in the upper left chest or back and pain radiating down the left upper limb. Table B-3 describes classic patterns of dermatome-referred pain.

Parasympathetic afferents that join the spinal cord at levels S2–S4, as well as those transmitted by CNs VII, IX, and X, concern information regarding physiologic visceral reflexes and do not normally reach the level of consciousness. Thus,

pain referred to dermatomes does not appear to exist with the parasympathetic division of the ANS.

Enteric Division

The enteric division of the ANS is unique in that it is a largely autonomous network of neurons that is associated solely with the GI tract. It consists of two interconnected plexuses of neurons—the myenteric plexus (of Auerbach) and the submucous plexus (of Meissner)—that are composed of visceral sensory neurons, interneurons, and visceral motor neurons, and is contained completely within the walls of the alimentary canal. The CNS, by way of the sympathetic and parasympathetic divisions of the ANS, helps to monitor and regulate GI functions but is not required for the normal functioning of the GI tract. In fact, the GI tract can function quite normally even when all connections with the CNS are broken.

RECOMMENDED TEXT AND ATLASES

Agur AMR, Dalley AF. *Grant's Atlas of Anatomy*. 11th Ed. Philadelphia: Lippincott Williams & Wilkins; 2005.

Carpenter MB. *Core Text of Neuroanatomy*. 4th Ed. Philadelphia: Lippincott Williams & Wilkins; 1991.

Haines DE. *Fundamental Neuroscience*. 2nd Ed. Philadelphia: Churchill Livingston; 2002.

Haines DE. *Neuroanatomy: An Atlas of Structures, Sections, and Systems*. 6th Ed. Philadelphia: Lippincott Williams & Wilkins; 2004.

Moore KL, Dalley AF. *Clinically Oriented Anatomy*. 4th Ed. Philadelphia: Lippincott Williams & Wilkins; 1999.

Netter FH. *Atlas of Human Anatomy*. 3rd Ed. New Jersey: Novartis; 2003.

Nolte J. *The Human Brain: An Introduction to Its Functional Anatomy*. 5th Ed. St. Louis: Mosby; 2002.

Putz R, Pabst R, eds. *Sobotta: Atlas of Human Anatomy*. 13th Ed. [CD-ROM]. Munich: Urban & Fischer; 2002.

Rohen JW, Yokochi C, Lutjen-Drecoll E. *Color Atlas of Anatomy: A Photographic Study of the Human Body*. 5th Ed. Philadelphia: Lippincott Williams & Wilkins; 2002.

Young PA, Young PH. *Basic Clinical Neuroanatomy*. Philadelphia: Lippincott Williams & Wilkins; 1997.

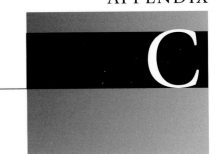

Resources for Geriatric Psychiatry

Maria I. Lapid

There is a wealth of resources available to assist clinicians and providers in caring for the elderly. While resources are readily accessible on the World Wide Web, the amount of information is staggering and navigation through the maze can be a challenge. This appendix contains a comprehensive list of helpful and practical resources relevant to the field of geriatric psychiatry that will better assist practitioners and caregivers in serving the needs of the elderly. The list provides current information, and is designed to help organize and guide a search for information. Every effort was done to ensure the accuracy of the references; however, an independent review by the reader is encouraged.

ADVANCE DIRECTIVES

Bazelon Center for Mental Health Law
   Provides templates for psychiatric advance directives.

Website: www.bazelon.org/advdir.html
Address: 1101 15th Street, NW, Suite 1212, Washington, DC 20005
Telephone: (202) 467-5730

National Academy of Elder Law Attorneys (NAELA)
   A nonprofit association that assists lawyers, bar organizations, and others who work with the elderly and their families, and promotes legal advocacy, education, and services with respect to elder law.

Website: www.naela.com
Address: 1604 N Country Club Road, Tucson, AZ 85716-3102
Telephone: (520) 881-4005

ADVOCACY

American Association of Retired Persons (AARP)
   A nonprofit organization that advocates for health, legal, and other issues on behalf of older Americans. Local chapters serve as clearinghouses for aging information, including many lifestyle issues, and provide various publications, including *Modern Maturity*.

Website: www.aarp.org
Toll-free: (800) 424-3410

American Society on Aging (ASA)
   A nonprofit organization committed to enhancing the knowledge and skills of those working with older adults and their families through educational programs and diversity initiatives, and sharing knowledge with professionals in the field of aging.

Website: www.asaging.org
Address: 833 Market Street, Suite 511, San Francisco, CA 94103 USA
Telephone: (415) 974-9600
Toll-free: (800) 537-9728

National Council of Senior Citizens
   An organization that operates as a research and issues advocacy group for seniors.

Website: www.seniorcoalition.com

National Council on the Aging (NCOA)
   A national network of organizations and individuals dedicated to improving the health and independence of older persons; increasing their continuing contributions to communities, society, and future generations; and building caring communities; also includes a voluntary network of

leaders from academia, business, and labor who support their mission and work.

Website: www.ncoa.org/
Address: 300 D Street, SW, Suite 801, Washington, DC 20024
Telephone: (202) 479-1200; (202) 479-6674 (TDD)

National Alliance for the Mentally Ill (NAMI)

A nonprofit, grassroots, self-help, support, and advocacy organization of consumers, families, and friends of people with severe mental illnesses. The site includes advocacy, education, and research resources.

Website: www.nami.org
Address: Colonial Place Three, 2107 Wilson Boulevard, Suite 300, Arlington, VA 22201-3042
Telephone: (703) 524-7600
Toll-free: (800) 950-6264

National Coalition of Mental Health and Aging

A mental health and aging coalition of agencies, organizations, and individuals working together to improve and increase mental health and substance abuse services to older adults.

Website: www.ncmha.org
Address: 3003 W. Touhy, Chicago, IL 60645
Telephone: (773)508-4745

National Conference of State Legislatures—Health Policy Tracking Service

Provides and tracks information on important developments in state legislation, policies, and programs affecting health.

Website: www.hpts.org
Address: 444 N Capitol Street, NW, Suite 515, Washington, DC 20001
Telephone: (202) 624-3567

National Mental Health Association (NMHA)

The country's oldest and largest nonprofit organization that addresses all aspects of mental health and mental illness. The site includes mental health information, advocacy materials, and links to local affiliates.

Website: www.nmha.org
Address: 2001 N Beauregard Street, 12th Floor, Alexandria, VA 22311
Toll-free: (800) 969-6642

National Organization for Rare Disorders (NORD)

A nonprofit, voluntary health agency dedicated to helping patients with rare diseases and their families, and assisting the organizations that serve them through programs of education, advocacy, research, and service.

Website: www.raredisease.org
Address: 55 Kenosia Avenue, PO Box 1968, Danbury, CT 06813-1968

Telephone: (203) 744-0100; (203) 797-9590 (TDD)
Toll-free: (800) 999-6673 (voicemail only)

ALZHEIMER'S DISEASE RESOURCES

Alzheimer's Association

The most helpful resource for individuals and families affected by Alzheimer's disease (AD) and related dementias; it promotes disease awareness and research, and offers information and advice, support services, referrals to community services. Local chapter phone numbers can be obtained from a 24-hour toll-free number.

Website: www.alz.org (USA)
             www.alzheimer.ca (Canada)
             www.alz.co.uk (International)
Address: 919 N Michigan Avenue, Suite 1100, Chicago, IL 60611
Telephone: (312) 335-8700; (312) 335-8882 (TTY)
Toll-free: (800) 272-3900

Alzheimer's Disease Education and Referral (ADEAR) Center

Provides information and publications on AD to individuals, families, caregivers, and health professionals. The Website includes several search engines, including one to find out about ongoing research trials.

Website: www.alzheimers.org
Address: PO Box 8250, Silver Spring, MD 20907-8250
Toll-free: (800) 438-4380 (English and Spanish)

Alzheimer Research Forum

An online scientific community of both health care professionals and nonprofessionals dedicated to developing treatments and preventions for AD. The Web site contains information on current theories, research, conferences, and resources.

Website: www.alzforum.org

Alzheimer's Association Safe Return Program

The Alzheimer's Association sponsors a program called Safe Return to assist in the event that an individual with dementia gets lost outside of the home. To get an application to register a person, call (800) 232-0851. There is a one-time $40 fee. One can also write to: Alzheimer's Association Safe Return Program, PO Box 3687, Chicago, IL 60690-3687.

CAREGIVER RESOURCES

Children of Aging Parents (CAPS)

A nonprofit, charitable organization with a mission to assist caregivers of the elderly or chronically ill with reliable information, referrals, and support. Its goal is to heighten public awareness that the health of the family caregivers is essential to ensure quality care of the nation's growing elderly population.

Website: www.caps4caregivers.org
Address: PO Box 7250, Penndel, PA 19047
Telephone: (800)227-7294

National Alliance for Caregiving (NAC)

A nonprofit coalition of more than 30 national organizations, with founding partners including the American Society on Aging, Department of Veterans Affairs, and National Association of Area Agencies on Aging, to support family caregivers and the professionals who serve them.

Website: www.caregiving.org
Address: 4720 Montgomery Lane, 5th Floor, Bethesda, MD 20814
Email: info@caregiving.org

Family Caregivers Alliance (FCA)

A nonprofit organization to address the needs of families and friends providing long-term care at home, with programs at national, state, and local levels to support and sustain caregivers.

Website: www.caregiver.org
Address: 690 Market Street, Suite 600, San Francisco, CA 94104
Telephone: (415) 434-3388
Toll-free: (800) 445-8106

CLINICAL GUIDELINES

National Guideline Clearinghouse

A resource for evidence-based clinical practice guidelines sponsored by the Agency for Health Care Research and Quality, US Department of Health and Human Services, in partnership with the American Medical Association and the American Association of Health Plans.

Website: www.guideline.gov

Expert Consensus Guidelines

Contains a wealth of detailed, state-of-the-art information on relevant topics in geriatrics, written specifically for professionals to assist with clinical decision-making.

Website: www.psychguides.com

GOVERNMENT AGENCIES

US Administration on Aging (AoA)

An agency in the US Department of Health and Human Services (DHHS) with the mission to promote the dignity and independence of older people and help society prepare for an aging population by providing home-based and community-based care for older persons and their caregivers.

Website: www.aoa.gov
Address: Administration on Aging, Washington, DC 20201
Telephone: (202) 619-0724

Centers for Medicare and Medicaid Services (CMS; formerly HCFA)

A federal agency within DHHS that runs the Medicare and Medicaid programs, two national health care programs that benefit about 75 million Americans. It works to improve quality of care to beneficiaries and better serve health care providers.

Website: www.cms.gov
Address: 7500 Security Boulevard, Baltimore, MD 21244-1850
Telephone: (410) 786-3000; (410) 786-0727 (TTY)
Toll-free: (877) 267-2323; (866) 226-1819 (TTY)

Medicare

The official United States government site for people with Medicare, which provides comprehensive information about benefits and services, comparisons of nursing homes and home health agencies, and various publications related to Medicare.

Website: www.medicare.gov
Helpline: 1-800-MEDICARE

National Institute on Aging (NIA)

One of the 25 institutes and centers of the National Institutes of Health (NIH) that provides leadership in aging research, training, health information dissemination, and other programs relevant to aging and older people. A very useful publication is the *Resource Directory for Older People*, available online (www.nia.nih.gov/health information/resourcedirectory.htm) or by calling 301-496-1752. The table of contents may be viewed at www.nia.nih.gov/rd/index.html.

Website: www.nih.gov/nia
Address: Building 31, Room 5C27, 31 Center Drive, MSC 2292, Bethesda, MD 20892
Telephone: (301) 496-1752;
             NIA Information Center: (800) 438-4380
Toll-free: (800) 222-2225; (800) 222-4225 (TTY)

National Institute on Alcohol Abuse and Alcoholism (NIAAA)

A federal agency that leads a national effort to reduce alcohol-related problems through research and education.

Website: www.niaaa.nih.gov
Address: 5635 Fishers Lane, MSC 9304, Bethesda, MD 20892-9304
Telephone: (301)443-3860

NIHSeniorHealth.gov

A Website of aging-related health information developed by the NIA and National Library of Medicine, both part of NIH; it is designed with senior-friendly features (large print, easy-to-read segments of information, simple navigation, talking function).

Website: nihseniorhealth.gov
Toll-free: (888) FIND-NLM (346-3656)

National Institute of Mental Health (NIMH)

A component of NIH with the mission to reduce the burden of mental illness and behavioral disorders through research on mind, brain, and behavior. The site provides information on research funding and clinical trials, as well as resources for practitioners, researchers, and the public.

Website: www.nimh.nih.gov
Address: 6001 Executive Boulevard, Room 8184, MSC 9663, Bethesda, MD 20892-9663
Telephone: (301) 443-4513; (301) 443-8431 (TTY)
Toll-free: (866) 615-NIMH (6464)

National Institute of Neurological Disorders and Stroke (NINDS)

A component of NIH that conducts, fosters, coordinates, and guides research on the causes, prevention, diagnosis, and treatment of neurological disorders and stroke, and supports basic research in related scientific areas.

Website: www.ninds.nih.gov/index.htm
Address: NIH Neurological Institute, PO Box 5801, Bethesda, MD 20824
Telephone: (301) 496-5751; (301) 468-5981 (TTY)
Toll-free: (800) 352-9424

Substance Abuse and Mental Health Services Administration (SAMHSA)

An agency of DHHS that works to improve care for those with substance abuse and mental illnesses. The Web site provides information on substance use by older adults and estimates of future impact on the treatment system.

Website: www.samhsa.gov/oas/aging/toc.htm
Address: Rm 12-105, Parklawn Building, 5600 Fishers Lane, Rockville, MD 20857
Telephone: (301) 443-4795

HOSPICE AND PALLIATIVE CARE

National Hospice and Palliative Care Organization (NHPCO)

Formerly the National Hospice Organization, it is the largest nonprofit membership organization representing hospice and palliative care programs and professionals in the United States. It works to improve end-of-life care and expand access to hospice care through advocacy, educational programs, materials, meetings and symposia, research, and monitoring Congressional and regulatory activities.

Website: www.nhpco.org
Address: 1700 Diagonal Road, Suite 625, Alexandria, Virginia 22314
Telephone: (703) 837-1500
Toll-free: (800) 646-6460
Fax: (703) 837-1233

PROFESSIONAL ORGANIZATIONS

American Academy of Neurology (AAN)

The central professional organization for neurologists and neuroscience professionals, dedicated to the care of patients with neurological disorders. The site assists in locating a referral for a neurologist who specializes in treating dementia and neurologic conditions associated with dementia.

Website: www.aan.com
Address: 1080 Montreal Avenue, St. Paul, MN 55116
Telephone: (651) 695-1940

American Association for Geriatric Psychiatry (AAGP)

The central, national professional organization for geriatric psychiatrists, dedicated to promoting the mental health and well-being of older people and improving care of those with late-life mental disorders.

Website: www.aagponline.org
Address: 7910 Woodmont Ave, Suite 1050, Bethesda, MD 20814-3004
Telephone: (301) 654-7850
Fax: (301) 654-4137

American Geriatrics Society (AGS)

A nonprofit organization for physicians and health care professionals, dedicated to improving the health and well-being of all older adults. The site provides information and resources for geriatrics health care professionals, the public, and other concerned individuals.

Website: www.americangeriatrics.org
Address: Empire State Building, 350 Fifth Avenue, Suite 801, New York, NY 10118
Telephone: (212) 308-1414
Fax: (212) 832-8646

American Psychiatric Association (APA)

The largest and most-recognized specialty society of United States and international member physicians that work to ensure accessible quality psychiatric diagnosis and treatment for all persons with mental disorders.

Website: www.psych.org
Address: 1000 Wilson Boulevard, Suite 1825, Arlington, VA 22209-3901
Telephone: (703) 907-7300

American Psychological Association (APA)

A professional organization of psychologists that coordinates activities related to aging through their Office on Aging, which serves as an information and referral source on aging issues. It develops and disseminates information pertaining to older adults to psychologists, other professionals, policymakers, and the public.

Website: www.apa.org
Address: 750 First Street, NE, Washington, DC 20002-4242
Telephone: (202) 336-5510; (202) 336-6123 (TDD/TTY)
Toll-free: (800) 374-2721

Gerontological Society of America (GSA)

A nonprofit professional organization in the field of aging that provides researchers, educators, practitioners, and policy makers with opportunities to understand, advance, integrate, and use basic and applied research on aging to improve the quality of life as one ages.

Website: www.geron.org
Address: 1030 15th Street, NW, Suite 250, Washington, DC 20005
Telephone: (202) 842-1275

International Psychogeriatric Association (IPA)

An international organization of professionals and scientists interested in psychogeriatrics with a mission to improve the mental health of older people everywhere through education, research, professional development, advocacy, health promotion, and service development.

Website: www.ipa-online.org
Address: 5215 Old Orchard Road, Suite 340, Skokie, IL 60077
Telephone: (847) 663-0574
Fax: (847) 663-0591

PROVIDER RESOURCES

American Association of Homes and Services for the Aging

An association representing not-for-profit nursing homes, continuing care retirement communities, assisted living and senior housing facilities, and home-based and community-based service providers committed to advancing the vision of healthy, affordable, and ethical aging services for America.

Website: www.aahsa.org
Address: 901 E Street, NW, Suite 500, Washington, DC 20004-2011
Telephone: (202) 783-2242

National Association of Area Agencies on Aging (N4A)

A nonprofit, government-funded organization that administers public funds, private grants, and donations for senior services, and provides services to enable older individuals to remain in their homes.

Website: www.n4a.org
Address: 1730 Rhode Island Avenue, NW, Suite 1200, Washington, DC 20036
Telephone: (202) 872-0888

National Association for Rural Mental Health (NARMH)

Provides rural providers, consumers, and advocates a forum to share problems, find solutions, and work cooperatively to improve rural mental health services. Membership is diverse, representing direct care, policy, academic, hospital, and community-based organizations, as well as those involved in professional mental health practice in rural areas.

Website: www.narmh.org
Address: 3700 W Division Street, Suite 105, St. Cloud, MN 56301
Telephone: (320) 202-1820

National Association of State Medicaid Directors (NASMD)

A bipartisan, professional, nonprofit organization of representatives of state Medicaid agencies that works to serve as a focal point of communication between the states and the federal government, and provides an information network among the states on issues pertinent to the Medicaid program.

Website: www.nasmd.org
Address: 810 First Street, NE, Suite 500, Washington, DC 20002-4267
Telephone: (202) 682-0100

National Association of State Mental Health Program Directors (NASMHPD)

An organization that advocates for the collective interests of state mental health authorities and their directors at the national level. It analyzes trends in the delivery and financing of mental health services, and builds and disseminates knowledge and experience reflecting the integration of public mental health programming in evolving healthcare environments.

Website: www.nasmhpd.org
Address: 66 Canal Center Plaza, Suite 302, Alexandria, VA 22314
Telephone: (703) 739-9333

RESEARCH

Alliance for Aging Research

A private, nonprofit advocacy organization dedicated to improving the health and independence of aging Americans. It works through the development, implementation, and advocacy of programs in medical and behavioral research into the aging process, professional and consumer health education, and public policy.

Website: www.agingresearch.org
Address: 2021 K Street, NW, Suite 305, Washington, DC 20006
Telephone: (202) 293-2856

American Federation for Aging Research (AFAR)

A research-funding organization that promotes healthier aging through biomedical research and supports the careers of scientists in aging research and geriatric medicine.

Website: www.afar.org
Address: 70 West 40th Street, 11th Floor, New York, NY 10018
Telephone: (212) 703-9977
Toll-free: (888) 582-2327

National Archive of Computerized Data on Aging (NACDA)

This organization has a mission to advance research on aging by helping researchers to utilize a broad range of datasets. By preserving and making available electronic data on aging in the United States, opportunities are provided for secondary analysis on major issues of scientific and policy relevance.

Website: www.icpsr.umich.edu/NACDA
Address: PO Box 1248, Ann Arbor, MI 48106-1248
Telephone: (734) 647-5000

SUICIDE PREVENTION

American Association of Suicidology (AAS)

A nonprofit organization that promotes suicide education and prevention through research, public awareness programs, public education, and training for professionals and volunteers. Membership includes mental health and public health professionals, researchers, suicide prevention and crisis intervention centers, school districts, crisis center volunteers, survivors of suicide, and persons with an interest in suicide.

Website: www.suicidology.org
Address: 4201 Connecticut Avenue, NW, Suite 408, Washington, DC 20008
Telephone: (202) 237-2280

American Foundation for Suicide Prevention (AFSP)

A foundation dedicated to advancing knowledge and prevention of suicide through education and support of research projects and suicide survivor programs.

Website: www.afsp.org
Address: 120 Wall Street, 22nd Floor, New York, NY 10005
Telephone: (212) 363-3500
Toll-free: (888) 333-2377

Suicide Awareness/Voices of Education (SAVE)

An organization with a mission to educate about suicide prevention, eliminate stigma, and support those touched by suicide.

Website: www.save.org
Address: PO Box 24507, Minneapolis, MN 55424-0507
Telephone: (612) 947-7998
Toll-free: 800-SUICIDE (800-784-2433) (hotline)

Suicide Prevention Action Network USA (SPAN USA)

A nonprofit organization with the goal of reducing the national rate of suicide by the year 2010.

Website: www.spanusa.org
Address: 5034 Odins Way, Marietta, GA 30068
Telephone: (770) 998-8819
Toll-free: (888) 649-1366

FINDING LOCAL RESOURCES

Drug and alcohol treatment providers
    findtreatment.samhsa.gov
Eldercare Locator
    www.eldercare.gov (or call 1-800-677-1116)
Geriatric psychiatrists
    www.aagponline.org/about/referrals.asp
Home health agencies
    www.medicare.gov/HHCompare/Home.asp
Hospice organizations
    www.nhpco.org/custom/directory/index.cfm
Nursing homes
    www.medicare.gov/NHCompare/home.asp
    www.nursinghomeinfo.com/search.html
Physicians (by medical specialty)
    http://dbapps.ama-assn.org/aps/amahg.htm

PUBLICATIONS—SCIENTIFIC PEER-REVIEWED JOURNALS

Obtained from the 2002 JCR Science Edition (http://isi10.isiknowledge.com/portal.cgi/jcr) using subject category "Geriatrics and Gerontology." This list is sorted by journal impact factor.

Neurobiology of Aging
Experimental Gerontology
Journals of Gerontology Series A-Biological Sciences and Medical Sciences
American Journal of Geriatric Psychiatry[a]
Journal of the American Geriatrics Society
Mechanisms of Ageing and Development
Dementia and Geriatric Cognitive Disorders[a]
Biogerontology
Drugs and Aging
Maturitas
International Journal of Geriatric Psychiatry[a]
Journals of Gerontology Series B-Psychological Sciences and Social Sciences
Age and Ageing
Aging Clinical and Experimental Research
Journal of the American Aging Association
Gerontology
Clinics in Geriatric Medicine
Journal of Geriatric Psychiatry and Neurology[a]

International Psychogeriatrics[a]
Geriatrics
Journal of Anti-Aging Medicine
Journal of Aging and Physical Activity
Archives of Gerontology and Geriatrics
Experimental Aging Research
Growth Development and Aging
Zeitschrift fur Gerontologie und Geriatrie
Ageing Research Reviews

[a]Psychiatric journals

PUBLICATIONS FOR CARE GIVERS— SELECTED BOOKS ON DEMENTIA AND CAREGIVING

Bell V, Troxel D. *The Best Friend's Approach to Alzheimer's Care.* Baltimore, MD: Health Professions Press; 1997.

Bridges BJ, Temairik. *Therapeutic Caregiving: A Practical Guide for Caregivers of Persons with Alzheimer's and Other Dementia-Causing Diseases.* Mill Creek, WA: BJB Publishing; 1998.

Fitzray BJ. *Alzheimer's Activities: Hundreds of Activities for Men and Women with Alzheimer's Disease and Related Disorders.* Windsor, CA: Rayve Productions; 2001.

Kuhn D, Bennett DA. *Alzheimer's Early Stages: First Steps in Caring and Treatment.* Alameda, CA. Hunter House; 1999.

Martin L. *The Nursing Home Decision: Easing the Transition for Everyone.* New York, NY; John Wiley & Sons; 1999.

Petersen RC. *Mayo Clinic on Alzheimer's Disease.* New York, NY: Kensington Publishing Corporation; 2002.

Powell L. *Alzheimer's Disease: A Guide for Families and Caregivers.* 3rd Ed. Cambridge, MA: Perseus Publishing; 2002.

Rabins PV, Mace NL. *The 36-Hour Day: A Family Guide to Caring for Persons with Alzheimer's Disease, Related Dementing Illness, and Memory Loss in Later Life.* Baltimore, MD: John Hopkins University Press; 1999.

Shenk D. The Forgetting. *Alzheimer's: Portrait of an Epidemic.* New York, NY: Doubleday; 2001.

Snowdon D. *Aging with Grace. What the Nun Study Teaches Us About Leading Longer, Healthier, and More Meaningful Lives.* New York, NY: Bantam Books; 2001.

Snyder L. *Speaking Our Minds: Personal Reflections from Individuals with Alzheimer's.* New York, NY: WH Freeman & Co.; 2000.

Strauss CJ. *Talking to Alzheimer's: Simple Ways to Connect When You Visit a Family Member or Friend.* Oakland, CA: New Harbinger Publications; 2002.

Warner ML, Warner M. *The Complete Guide to Alzheimer's-Proofing Your Home.* Revised Ed. West Lafayette, IN: Purdue University Press; 2000.

Zgola JM, Mace NL. *Doing Things: A Guide to Programming Activities for Persons with Alzheimer's Disease and Related Disorders.* Baltimore, MD: Johns Hopkins University Press; 1987.

PUBLICATIONS FOR PROFESSIONALS— TEXTBOOKS

Agronin ME. *Dementia: A Practical Guide.* Baltimore, MD: Lippincott Williams & Wilkins; 2003.

American Psychiatric Association. *Diagnostic and Statistical Manual of Mental Disorders.* 4th Ed. Text Revision. Washington, DC: American Psychiatric Publishing; 2000.

Blazer DG, Steffens DC, Busse EW, eds. *Textbook of Geriatric Psychiatry.* 3rd Ed. Washington, DC; American Psychiatric Publishing; 2004.

Coffey CE, Cummings JL, eds. *Textbook of Geriatric Neuropsychiatry.* 2nd Ed. Washington, DC; American Psychiatric Publishing, 2000.

Copeland JR, Abou-Saleh MT, Blazer DG, eds. *Principles and Practice of Geriatric Psychiatry.* 2nd Ed. New York: John Wiley & Sons; 2002.

Hazzard WR, Blass JP, Halter JB, Ouslander JG, Tinetti ME, eds. *Principle of Geriatric Medicine and Gerontology.* 5th Ed. New York, NY: McGraw-Hill Professional; 2003.

Jacobson SA, Pies RW, Greenblatt D. *Handbook of Geriatric Psychopharmacology.* 1st Ed. Washington, DC; American Psychiatric Publishing; 2002.

Kertesz A, Munoz DG. *Pick's Disease and Pick Complex.* New York, NY; Wiley-Liss; 1998.

Morrison MF, ed. *Hormones, Gender and the Aging Brain: The Endocrine Basis of Geriatric Psychiatry.* New York, NY; Cambridge University Press; 2000.

Nelson JC, ed. *Geriatric Psychopharmacology.* 1st Ed. New York, NY: Marcel Dekker; 1998.

Perry R, McKeith I, Perry E. *Dementia with Lewy Bodies: Clinical, Pathological, and Treatment Issues.* New York, NY; Cambridge University Press; 1996.

Post SG. *The Moral Challenge of Alzheimer Disease: Ethical Issues from Diagnosis to Dying.* Baltimore, MD: Johns Hopkins University Press; 2000.

Sadavoy J, Jarvik LF, Grossberg GT, Meyers BS, eds. *Comprehensive Textbook of Geriatric Psychiatry.* 3rd Ed. New York, NY: W.W. Norton & Company; 2004.

Salzman C, ed. *Clinical Geriatric Psychopharmacology.* 4th Ed. Baltimore, MD: Lippincott Williams & Wilkins; 2004.

MISCELLANEOUS LINKS

Accreditation Committee for Graduate Medical Education (ACGME) list of geriatric psychiatry training programs
www.acgme.org/adspublic
The 2003 US News & World Report ranking of hospitals with geriatric programs
www.usnews.com/usnews/health/hosptl/rankings/speci hqgeri.htm
Resource directory for older people
www.nia.nih.gov/rd/toc.html
(print a copy: www.nia.nih.gov/healthinformation/ resourcedirectory.htm)

Index

Pages followed by *f* indicate figures; pages followed by *t* indicate tables